PRIMARY CARDIOLOGY

PRIMARY
CARDIOLOGY

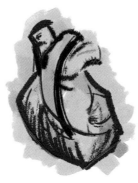

LEE GOLDMAN, M.D.
Julius R. Krevans Professor and
Chairman, Department of Medicine,
University of California, San Francisco
Associate Dean for Clinical Affairs,
University of California, San Francisco,
School of Medicine
San Francisco, California

EUGENE BRAUNWALD, M.D.
Vice President for Academic Programs,
Partners HealthCare System
Distinguished Hersey Professor of Medicine
Faculty Dean for Academic Programs at
Brigham and Women's Hospital and
Massachusetts General Hospital
Harvard Medical School
Boston, Massachusetts

W.B. SAUNDERS COMPANY
A Division of Harcourt Brace & Company
Philadelphia   London   Toronto   Montreal   Sydney   Tokyo

W.B. Saunders Company
A Division of Harcourt Brace & Company

The Curtis Center
Independence Square West
Philadelphia, Pennsylvania 19106

Library of Congress Cataloging-in-Publication Data

Primary cardiology / [edited by] Lee Goldman, Eugene Braunwald. — 1st ed.

   p.   cm.

  ISBN 0-7216-6402-4

  1. Heart—Diseases. 2. Cardiology.   I. Goldman, Lee, MD.
II. Braunwald, Eugene

   [DNLM: 1. Cardiovascular Diseases—diagnosis. 2. Cardiovascular
Diseases—therapy.   WG 120 P952 1998]

RC681.P72   1998   616.1′2—dc21

DNLM/DLC   97−50317

PRIMARY CARDIOLOGY   ISBN 0-7216-6402-4

Printed in the United States of America.

Last digit is the print number: 9 8 7 6 5 4 3 2 1

Dedicated to
Jill, Jeff, Daniel, and Robyn
and to
Elaine, Karen, Allison, Jill, Dana, Alex, Mara, Elise,
Cari, and Benjamin

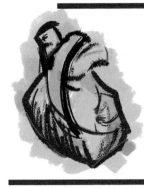

Contributors

JOSHUA S. ADLER, M.D.
Assistant Clinical Professor of Medicine,
   University of California, San Francisco;
   Assistant Chief of Staff, San Francisco
   Veterans Administration Medical Center,
   San Francisco, California
*Approach to the Patient Undergoing
Noncardiac Surgery*

MICHAEL H. ALDERMAN, M.D.
Professor and Chairman, Department of
   Epidemiology and Social Medicine,
   Albert Einstein College of Medicine,
   Bronx, New York
*Recognition and Management of Patients
with Hypertension*

ROBERT A. BARISH, M.D., M.B.A.
Professor of Surgery and Medicine,
   University of Maryland School of
   Medicine; Chief Executive Officer,
   UniversityCARE, University of
   Maryland Medicine, Baltimore,
   Maryland
Approach to Cardiovascular Emergencies

HENRY R. BLACK, M.D.
Charles J. and Margaret Roberts Professor
   of Preventive Medicine and Professor of
   Internal Medicine, Rush-Presbyterian-
   St. Luke's Medical Center; Chairman,
   Department of Preventive Medicine,
   Rush Medical College, Chicago, Illinois
Approach to the Patient with Hypertension

EUGENE BRAUNWALD, M.D.
Vice President for Academic Programs,
   Partners HealthCare System;
   Distinguished Hersey Professor of
   Medicine, Faculty Dean for Academic
   Programs at Brigham and Women's
   Hospital and Massachusetts General
   Hospital, Harvard Medical School,
   Boston, Massachusetts
The Clinical Examination; Recognition and

*Management of Patients with Acute
Myocardial Infarction; Recognition and
Management of Patients with Unstable
Angina; Recognition and Management of
Patients with Heart Failure*

BLASE A. CARABELLO, M.D.
Professor of Medicine, Charles Ezra Daniel
   Professor of Cardiology, Medical
   University of South Carolina; Ralph H.
   Johnson Veterans Administration
   Medical Center, Charleston, South
   Carolina
*Recognition and Management of Patients
with Valvular Heart Disease*

**KANU CHATTERJEE, M.B., F.R.C.P.(Lond.),
F.R.C.P.(Edin.), F.A.C.C., F.C.C.P.,
M.A.C.P.**
Professor of Medicine and Lucie Stern
   Professor of Cardiology, University of
   California, San Francisco, Medical
   School and Division of Cardiology,
   Moffitt-Long Hospital, San Francisco,
   California
*Recognition and Management of Patients
with Stable Angina Pectoris*

MELVIN D. CHEITLIN, M.D.
Emeritus Professor of Medicine, University
   of California, San Francisco; Staff,
   Cardiology Service and Former Chief of
   Cardiology, San Francisco General
   Hospital, San Francisco, California
*Recognition and Management of Adults with
Congenital Heart Disease*

GLENN M. CHERTOW, M.D., M.P.H.
Assistant Professor of Medicine, Harvard
   Medical School; Assistant Director of
   Dialysis Services, Brigham and
   Women's Hospital, Boston,
   Massachusetts
Approach to the Patient with Edema

G. WILLIAM DEC, M.D.
Associate Professor of Medicine, Harvard
Medical School; Medical Director,
Cardiac Transplantation Unit,
Massachusetts General Hospital, Boston,
Massachusetts
*Recognition and Management of Patients
with Cardiomyopathies*

ELYSE FOSTER, M.D., F.A.C.C.
Associate Professor of Clinical Medicine
and Anesthesia, University of California,
San Francisco; Director,
Echocardiography Laboratory, Moffitt-
Long Hospital, San Francisco, California
*Recognition and Management of Adults with
Congenital Heart Disease*

SAMUEL Z. GOLDHABER, M.D.
Associate Professor of Medicine, Harvard
Medical School; Staff Cardiologist and
Director, Anticoagulation Service,
Brigham and Women's Hospital, Boston,
Massachusetts
*Recognition and Management of Patients
with Pulmonary Embolism, Deep Venous
Thrombosis, and Cor Pulmonale*

LEE GOLDMAN, M.D.
Julius R. Krevans Professor and Chairman,
Department of Medicine, University of
California, San Francisco; Associate
Dean for Clinical Affairs, University of
California, San Francisco, School of
Medicine, San Francisco, California
*Evidence-Based Medicine; Clinical Decision-
Making; Approach to the Patient with Chest
Pain; Approach to the Patient Undergoing
Noncardiac Surgery*

NORA GOLDSCHLAGER, M.D.
Professor of Clinical Medicine, University
of California, San Francisco, School of
Medicine; Director, Coronary Care Unit
and ECG Laboratory, San Francisco
General Hospital, San Francisco,
California
*Recognition and Management of Patients
with Bradyarrhythmias*

MARK A. HLATKY, M.D.
Professor of Medicine and Professor and
Chair, Department of Health Research
and Policy and of Medicine
(Cardiovascular Medicine), Stanford
University School of Medicine, Stanford,
California
Approach to the Patient with Palpitations

WISHWA N. KAPOOR, M.D., M.P.H.
Falk Professor of Medicine, University of
Pittsburgh School of Medicine; Chief,
Division of General Internal Medicine,
and Vice-Chairman, Department of
Medicine, University of Pittsburgh
Medical Center, Pittsburgh, Pennsylvania
Approach to the Patient with Syncope

ADOLF W. KARCHMER, M.D.
Professor of Medicine, Harvard Medical
School; Chief, Division of Infectious
Diseases, Beth Israel Deaconess Medical
Center, Boston, Massachusetts
*Approach to the Patient with Infective
Endocarditis*

THOMAS H. LEE, M.D., S.M.
Associate Professor of Medicine, Harvard
Medical School; Medical Director,
Partners Community HealthCare, Inc.,
Boston, Massachusetts
Cardiac Noninvasive Testing

BEVERLY H. LORELL, M.D.
Associate Professor of Medicine, Harvard
Medical School; Director, Hemodynamic
Research Laboratory, Beth Israel
Deaconess Medical Center, Boston,
Massachusetts
*Recognition and Management of Patients
with Pericardial Disease*

JEROME F. X. NARADZAY, M.D.
Clinical Faculty, Division of Emergency
Medicine, University of Maryland,
Baltimore, Maryland; Attending
Physician, Department of Emergency
Medicine, Samaritan Medical Center,
Watertown; Course Medical Director,
Emergency Medical System, Jefferson
County, New York
Approach to Cardiovascular Emergencies

PATRICK T. O'GARA, M.D.
Assistant Professor of Medicine, Harvard
Medical School; Director, Clinical
Cardiology, Brigham and Women's
Hospital, Boston, Massachusetts
*Approach to the Patient with Cardiac
Enlargement; Recognition and Management
of Patients with Diseases of the Aorta:
Aneurysms and Dissection*

ROBERT A. O'ROURKE, M.D.
Charles Conrad Brown Distinguished
Professor in Cardiovascular Disease, The
University of Texas Health Science
Center, San Antonio; Director of
Coronary Care Unit, South Texas
Veterans Health Care System, Audie L.
Murphy Memorial Veterans Hospital;
Attending Cardiology Physician,
University Health System, Bexar County,
Texas
*Approach to the Patient with a Heart
Murmur*

ERNST J. SCHAEFER, M.D.
Professor of Medicine and Nutrition and
  Chief, Lipid Research Laboratory, Jean
  Mayer United States Department of
  Agriculture Human Nutrition Research
  Center on Aging at Tufts University;
  Director, Lipid and Heart Disease
  Prevention Clinic, New England Medical
  Center, Boston, Massachusetts
  *Recognition and Management of Patients
  with Lipoprotein Disorders*

MELVIN M. SCHEINMAN, M.D.
Professor of Medicine, University of
  California, San Francisco, San Francisco,
  California
  *Recognition and Management of Patients
  with Tachyarrhythmias*

RICHARD M. SCHWARTZSTEIN, M.D.
Assistant Professor of Medicine, Harvard
  Medical School; Divisions of Pulmonary
  and Critical Care Medicine and
  Emergency Medicine, Beth Israel
  Deaconess Medical Center, Boston,
  Massachusetts
  Approach to the Patient with Dyspnea

HAROLD C. SOX, M.D.
Joseph M. Huber Professor and Chair,
  Department of Medicine, Dartmouth
  Medical School; Dartmouth-Hitchcock
  Medical Center, Hanover, New
  Hampshire
  *Screening for Coronary Artery Disease and
  Its Risk Factors*

LYNNE WARNER STEVENSON, M.D.
Associate Professor of Medicine, Harvard
  Medical School; Clinical Director, Heart
  Failure Program, Brigham and Women's
  Hospital, Boston, Massachusetts
  *Recognition and Management of Patients
  with Heart Failure*

GEORGE E. THIBAULT, M.D.
Professor of Medicine, Harvard Medical
  School; Chief Medical Officer, Brigham
  and Women's Hospital, Boston,
  Massachusetts
  *Approach to the Patient with Dyspnea;
  Approach to the Patient with Edema*

NANETTE K. WENGER, M.D.
Professor of Medicine, Division of
  Cardiology, Department of Medicine;
  Consultant, Emory Heart Center, Emory
  University School of Medicine; Director,
  Cardiac Clinics, Grady Memorial
  Hospital, Atlanta, Georgia
  *Cardiovascular Disease in the Elderly and in
  Women*

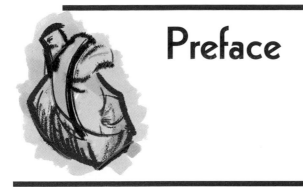

Preface

Despite a 40% decline in age-adjusted coronary heart disease death rates since the early 1960s, heart disease remains the leading cause of death in the United States. Cardiovascular symptoms, signs, and diseases continue to be a major determinant of office visits and hospital admissions. In the current era of managed care, the primary care physician is assuming increasing responsibility for the care of the patient with known or suspected cardiovascular disease, as well as for the prevention of such disease.

Although numerous texts address issues related to heart disease, *Primary Cardiology* has been conceived and designed to fill what we believe to be a critical gap—an authoritative, yet user-friendly text for primary care physicians, internists and family physicians—and other physicians who have not specialized in cardiovascular diseases. We believe that primary care physicians need and deserve a text that is far more sophisticated than a manual, yet more succinct and focused than an encyclopedic text written for the cardiovascular specialist. *Primary Cardiology* is designed to provide more clinically applicable information than is available in standard medical textbooks and to go beyond the texts in primary care and ambulatory care, which usually focus on conditions seen in outpatients.

Primary Cardiology is divided into three parts. Part 1 (Chapters 1 through 6) covers fundamental principles that underlie evidence-based medicine and the translation of advances in science to the practice of medicine. Part 2 (Chapters 7 through 16) emphasizes rational approaches to common presenting cardiovascular symptoms, signs, and situations frequently faced by the primary care physician. Part 3 (Chapters 17 through 31) focuses on the evaluation and management of a variety of cardiovascular disorders that the primary care physician commonly faces.

It is our hope that *Primary Cardiology,* which has been written by nationally recognized experts, all of whom serve as cardiovascular consultants, will capture the essence of the ideal consultative interaction, which quickly summarizes the most important evidence-based literature and provides a targeted approach to solving the problem at hand. The algorithms, flow diagrams, and practice guidelines in this book, whether based on consensus conferences or expert opinion, are the natural extension of the background and evidence on which they are based. Furthermore, each of these flow diagrams has been carefully color-coded to emphasize diagnostic approaches (in blue) and therapeutic recommendations (in green). We are grateful to our authors who worked so well with us in creating a new and different type of textbook. In our offices, Kathryn Saxon (Boston) and DeAnne Hill (San Francisco) were critical to the preparation of this book. At W.B. Saunders, we are grateful to our editor, Richard Zorab, and his Editorial Assistant, Jennifer Shreiner, Copy Editor Supervisor Mimi McGinnis, and Senior Production Manager Frank Polizzano.

No book with a new mission, especially a first edition, ever meets all of its goals. However, we hope that the readers, especially primary care physicians and internists who now render most cardiac care as well as trainees who aspire to these responsibilities, will find that *Primary Cardiology* fills an important niche, helps them to be better informed, and most importantly, aids them in the care of their patients on a daily basis.

LEE GOLDMAN, M.D.
EUGENE BRAUNWALD, M.D.

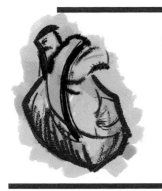

Contents

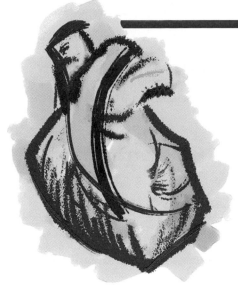

Part 1

CARDIOLOGIC PRINCIPLES FOR THE PRIMARY CARE PHYSICIAN

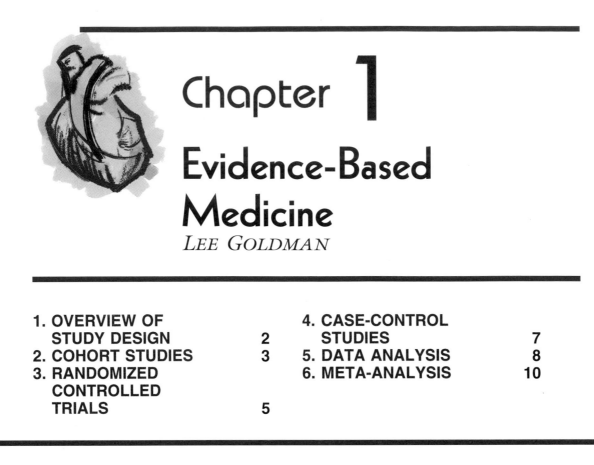

Chapter 1

Evidence-Based Medicine

LEE GOLDMAN

Decisions in cardiology, and for that matter, all of medicine, are increasingly being driven by objective evidence from well-designed clinical studies rather than by the experiential teachings of senior professors.[1-3] This evidence-based approach has led to the re-examination of virtually all of the accepted cardiologic practices of the past several decades. Some practices, such as the use of beta blockers for patients with ischemic heart disease, have been reinforced by such evidence, whereas others, such as the use of antiarrhythmic medications to treat asymptomatic ventricular arrhythmias, have not.

To understand evidence-based medicine, it is critical to appreciate key issues related to study design and the analysis of clinical data. These methods can be applied to questions of diagnosis, prognosis, cause, and therapy.

OVERVIEW OF STUDY DESIGN (Table 1–1)

Prospective cohort studies identify subjects *before* they have developed the outcome of interest—whether it is a diagnosis such as coronary artery disease in the Framingham Heart Study or whether an *endpoint such as death* occurs in a cohort of patients with known congestive heart failure—and then systematically observe those patients to determine who *develops the outcome.* Traditional *cohort* studies follow subjects without imposing any specific management interventions, so that their *natural his-*

tory can be determined and, if possible, explained in part by whatever baseline characteristics influence prognosis.

Prospective cohort studies are sometimes subdivided into *prolective* studies, which specifically gather baseline data as part of a planned clinical research study, and *retrolective* studies, which rely on clinical data that are routinely gathered for baseline description. Prospective studies that specifically assess therapeutic decisions are best designed as *randomized controlled trials,* which use the randomization process to distribute both known and unknown confounding factors (which might influence outcome) evenly among the patients receiving different randomized therapies. Although sophisticated, multivariate analytic techniques can theoretically adjust for measurable differences between patients who receive different nonrandomized treatments, the major benefit of randomization is that it should result in an unbiased distribution of the full range of unmeasured or poorly measured factors that may influence both treatment decisions and outcome.

Retrospective studies begin by selecting subjects in whom the outcome has already occurred and then look backward to assess potential predisposing risk factors. These studies are subject to a wide variety of biases related to the recall or recording of exposures and risk factors in the past and, hence, are weaker in study design than prospective cohort studies or randomized clinical trials. The most common type of retrospective study in the medical literature is the case-control study in which *cases* with the disease or outcome of interest are compared with *controls* who do not have the outcome in terms of their *relative exposures* to potential risk factors. This approach

Table 1-1	Overview of Study Design

I. Cohort study (prospective)
  A. To determine causes of a disease

Population free of disease ⟶ Sample followed ⟶ Incident cases of new disease

  B. To determine natural history in patients with a disease

Population of patients with a known disease ⟶ Sample followed ⟶ Cases with pre-specified outcomes (e.g., death or decline in functional status)

II. Case-control study (retrospective)
Patients with the disease or already with a pre-specified outcome ⟶ Look back to determine exposure to possible risk factors or causes

III. Cross-sectional study
Patients with characteristic of interest ⟷ Look at same time to see other characteristics

has also been used more recently to raise questions about the potential hazards of antihypertensive medications as risk factors for sudden death.

Cross-sectional studies compare characteristics and outcomes at the same point in time. For example, a study might report on the percentage of patients with congestive heart failure who have normal left ventricular systolic function.

COHORT STUDIES

Incidence

Cohort studies are ideal for determining the *incidence* of disease, which is the number of subjects who develop the new onset of disease divided by all of those who are at risk (Table 1–2). For example, the incidence of major bleeding in patients treated with oral anticoagulants may be 5% at 1 year and 3% in each subsequent year, for a cumulative incidence of 11% at 3 years. By comparison, *prevalence* refers to the total number of individuals with the disease at any given time. For example, there may be 6 million prevalent cases of coronary heart disease in the United States. By simple arithmetic, the prevalence of a given permanent disease is approximately equal to the annual incidence multiplied by the average life expectancy of patients with the disease.

In the incidence rate, the individuals who develop an endpoint are the numerator and the population or group

Table 1-2	Incidence and Prevalence

$$\text{Incidence (any given time period)} = \frac{\text{New cases}}{\text{Population at risk}} \bigg/ \text{Time period}$$

$$\text{Prevalence} = \frac{\text{Total cases}}{\text{Population at risk}}$$

$$\text{Prevalence} = \text{Incidence} \times \text{Average life expectancy}$$

of patients at risk is the denominator. The generalizability of a study will depend on whether the denominator is clinically relevant and represents the types of patients that a physician may see. For example, early studies of the natural history of mitral valve prolapse were based on patients referred to tertiary centers, presumably because of their higher risk characteristics. It is not surprising that this denominator was associated with many more outcome events (a higher incidence) than when subsequent studies evaluated the natural history of unselected consecutive patients with mitral valve prolapse in the general population.

Outcomes/Endpoints

In cohort studies, the outcome of interest may be death, a morbid event such as a myocardial infarction, functional status, quality of life, satisfaction, cost, or any other clinically cogent endpoint. For a study to be relevant for clinical practice, the endpoints must be clinically important and reproducible. To minimize bias, the investigators who determine whether an endpoint has occurred should be blinded as to the presence or absence of the putative risk factors for that endpoint.

Risk Factors

Although some texts distinguish risk factors for the development of a disease from prognostic factors that influence the subsequent course after the onset of the disease, this definition is somewhat artificial and should not obscure the fact that both types of studies use similar designs. Risk factors or prognostic factors may include the full spectrum of clinical data gathered by physicians, ranging from historical factors to the physical examination and laboratory data. The ability of these various clinical characteristics to predict risk or prognosis can be measured by their univariate association with the endpoint of interest or by their independent *multivariate* association. The impact of such factors may be measured in terms of their *absolute risk, relative risk,* and *attributable risk* (Table 1–3). Relative risk is calculated by dividing the incidence in subjects with the risk factor by the incidence in subjects without the risk factor. Many of the strongest risk factors for the development of coronary artery disease, such as smoking and hypercholesterolemia, have relative risks of about three or less. Another approach is to assess the attributable risk, which is the incidence of the endpoint in patients with the risk factor minus the incidence in those without the risk factor. When multiplied by the potential population at risk, the attributable risk provides an assessment of the magnitude of disease or disability that may be attributed to the risk factor in the entire population of interest.

Studies of Prognosis

In studies of prognosis, it is important that an *inception cohort* be assembled, so that patients are enrolled at a well-defined point along the course of their disease. For example, an inception cohort of patients with acute myo-

Table 1–3	Calculating Absolute Risk, Relative Risk, and Attributable Risk

Example 1:

Absolute incidence (risk) of death (death rate) per year in patients with a risk factor	15/1000 = 1.5%
Absolute incidence (risk) of death (death rate) per year in patients without a risk factor	5/1000 = 0.5%
Relative risk in patients with a risk factor compared with those without it	3.0
Risks attributable to risk factor	10/1000 = 1.0%

Example 2: Effect of a relative risk of 2.0 in a population of 1 million depending on the baseline absolute risk.

	Subjects without a Risk Factor	*Subjects with a Risk Factor*
Absolute risk	0.5%	1%
Relative risk		2.0
Attributable risk		0.5%
Population attributable risk		5000
Absolute risk	5%	10%
Relative risk		2.0
Attributable risk		5%
Population attributable risk		50,000

cardial infarction would enroll patients either at the time of the infarction or at some pre-specified later time, such as those who have survived hospital discharge or who have survived for 30 days. The construction of an inception cohort is especially important to avoid *lead-time bias,* by which patients who are diagnosed sooner will live longer and may be mistakenly thought to do better simply because their follow-up began at an earlier stage of their disease.

Case Fatality and Survival Curves

The *case fatality* rate is defined as the number of patients who die from an event or a disease divided by the total number with it. For some diseases, such as acute myocardial infarction, the case fatality rate has a relatively short time horizon, such as during the initial hospitalization. However, one might also determine that among patients with unoperated critical aortic stenosis, nearly all patients ultimately die from the aortic stenosis or its complications, thus yielding a disease-specific case fatality rate of nearly 100% over the lifetime of the patient.

The survival of a cohort is commonly measured by calculating a *survival curve,* in which the probability of survival is plotted against the time of follow-up. Alternatively, sometimes the Y-axis will instead plot the number of events, or the mortality rate. In either situation, *survival analysis* considers not only the number of events that occur but also their timing, and it recognizes that individual subjects in a study may be followed for various periods of time, either because they were enrolled at different times or because some are lost to follow-up. Thus, a survival curve will calculate a time-specific *hazard rate* and use the hazard rate to draw each subsequent

portion of the curve (Fig. 1–1). It is critical to recognize that the decline in the survival curve during any time interval is reflected by the percentage of endpoints among those patients who are at risk during the interval. Patients who are censored, either because their eligible follow-up time has not extended into this time period or because they were lost to follow-up, do not appear in either the numerator or the denominator. The comparison of prognosis between two groups requires that their entire survival curves be compared; comparison at just one point in time somewhere along the curve is subject to substantial bias by those who might pick that time because of what the data show.

Bias in Cohort Studies

One major potential bias in cohort studies relates to the ways in which the cohorts are selected. Theoretically, a cohort study *samples* a larger population of patients for whom the study subjects are supposed to be representative. If the cohort specifically selects sicker patients, those who have been referred to a certain medical center, those who have survived some particular stress or event, or those who just happen to be available, the cohort will not be *generalizable* to the broader sample from which it was theoretically drawn.

A second major bias in cohort studies relates to loss to follow-up. It can never be assumed that those who are lost to follow-up are completely represented by those for whom follow-up information is available. Although there is no magic rate of loss to follow-up that must be achieved in every study, the acceptable lost-to-follow-up rate depends on the rate of the endpoint of interest. For example, if 50% of patients with congestive heart failure die by the end of 2 years, a 3% or 4% lost-to-follow-up

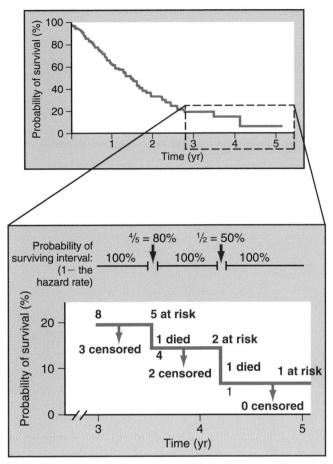

Figure 1–1

A typical Kaplan-Meier survival curve, with detail for one part of the curve. The curve considers the hazard rate (the deaths among the patients at risk) in each time period. (Adapted from Fletcher, R.H., Fletcher, S.W., and Wagner, E.H.: Clinical Epidemiology: The Essentials. 2nd ed. Baltimore, Williams & Wilkins, 1988.)

rate will have little effect on the assessment of risk factors or prognostic factors. By comparison, if an event is very uncommon, occurring in only 2% or so of patients, the same 3% or 4% lost-to-follow-up rate may introduce major biases if it is assumed that even 25% or 30% of those patients who are lost to follow-up had truly died.

A third major source of bias in cohort studies is the unblinding of investigators, so that those who are familiar with the potential risk factors are also identifying the outcome. In such circumstances, the risk factors may become self-fulfilling prophecies when potentially biased investigators are assessing them. This bias can be minimized by having different individuals assess risk factors and outcomes and by having strict definitions for both risk factors and outcomes.

The advantages of cohort studies include their ability to measure incidence, their ability to assess risk factors and prognostic factors before the outcome is known, and their potential ability to study multiple outcomes in the same patients. The disadvantages are the need to enroll many subjects if the outcome is uncommon or delayed, the need to follow patients for a protracted period of time,

and their inability to control for differences in medical treatments or to assess the true impact of various therapeutic interventions.

RANDOMIZED CONTROLLED TRIALS

Randomized trials represent a subgroup of cohort studies in which a treatment option is randomly allocated. Most studies randomly distribute half of the patients into two groups—one that receives the new, experimental treatment and the other that receives placebo or standard treatment. Placebo controls are always preferable because it is via the placebo that the patient is blinded as to treatment group. By blinding the patient, it is possible to include outcomes—such as functional status and quality of life—that might be biased by the patient's knowing which treatment he or she is receiving and also to encompass outcomes such as the use of medical resources. Ideally, the physicians who are caring for the patients are also blinded, and when both the patient and the caring physician have been blinded, the study is called *double-blind*. In many situations in cardiology, especially when comparing interventions such as angioplasty or coronary artery bypass grafting, it is impossible to blind either the patient or the caring physician. In such circumstances, the assessment of "hard" endpoints such as death and myocardial infarction is unlikely to be biased, but the measurement of "soft" endpoints such as quality of life may be influenced by the fact that both the patient and the physician know which treatment the patient received. For intermediate endpoints, such as hospitalization and functional status, it is important to be sure that the definitions were sufficiently stringent and reproducible to reduce bias. The core laboratories that interpret test results and the data and safety monitoring boards that decide whether to continue or terminate the trial should also be blinded as to group assignment so their judgments will not be biased.

Study Design

Although most clinical trials randomize patients evenly between two alternative strategies, some trials may randomize patients to more than two groups, especially if there is a low-dose and high-dose intervention to be compared with standard care.[3] Articles should explicitly detail the randomization process, which is usually via sealed envelopes or telephone relay of a centralized process generated by a random number sequence.[4]

Compliance

In randomized trials, one of the key issues is whether patients comply with the intervention. For a one-time intervention such as angioplasty or coronary artery bypass grafting, the issue of compliance seems straightforward. However, it is critical to remember that patients are enrolled in a randomized trial at the time that they are

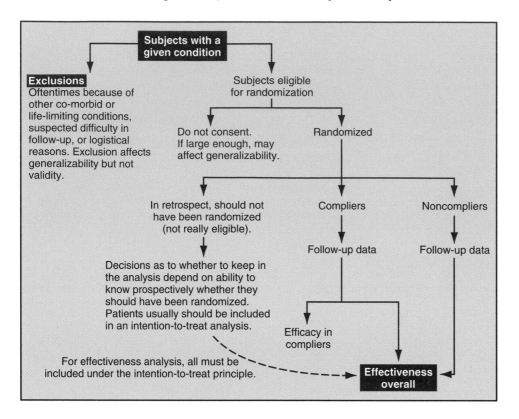

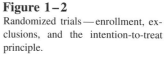

Figure 1–2

Randomized trials — enrollment, exclusions, and the intention-to-treat principle.

randomized, and there is always some interval between randomization and receipt of the assigned treatment. Even if patients do not receive the assigned treatment, be it a medication or a surgical intervention, they must remain in the group to which they were randomized under the *intention-to-treat principle* (Fig. 1–2). Patients who do not receive the assigned treatment are, by definition, fundamentally different from those who do, and it is critical that *all* patients be included in the final results of the study regardless of whether they received the assigned treatment or complied with it. It is only by such an intention-to-treat analysis that investigators can determine whether the treatment is *effective,* that is, it does more good than harm in those who are assigned to receive it at the time when a physician must make a clinical decision. For example, in the original Veterans Administration study of coronary artery bypass graft surgery compared with medical treatment for patients with stable angina, some argued that patients who were randomized to bypass graft surgery but died before receiving it should not be counted as "surgical deaths." At that time, however, it was common for patients awaiting elective surgery to wait many weeks, and therefore the *strategy* of choosing coronary artery bypass grafting compared with medical therapy had to include the waiting period for the invasive alternative. Otherwise, the sickest patients randomized to surgery, who of course were those most likely to die while awaiting it, would have been excluded from the surgical arm, thereby including only the less sick surgical patients and, hence, making surgery look better than it should have. Of course, if delay or noncompliance leads to a marked diminution in the effectiveness of the therapeutic alternative, one should try to find a new strategy

that will improve compliance. Sometimes the term *efficacious* is used to assess whether an intervention improves outcome in those who actually receive it and comply with it. Studies of *efficacy* normally serve as preludes to improved strategies that ultimately show whether the intervention is more *effective* as well.

Generalizability

A randomized trial will be *generalizable* to the types of patients who were included in it. Commonly, however, only a small subsample of patients with a given diagnosis is included in randomized trials. For example, patients with *co-morbid* conditions, which are conditions that are unrelated to the disease of interest but that may limit life expectancy, may be excluded because such conditions may compete with the disease of interest in terms of causing hospitalizations, morbidity, or mortality. By comparison, a randomized trial's *validity* is dependent only on the extent to which it followed the basic principles of study design in the patients who were included in it.

Analytic Issues

When evaluating the effect of an intervention, it is critical to be sure that the intervention and control groups were treated identically except for intervention itself. If, for example, a new medication is also combined with more aggressive follow-up or other concomitant care, it may be impossible to distinguish the benefits of the medication itself from the benefits of the other accompanying treatments.

Although randomization should create groups with equal baseline risk at the beginning of a trial, the randomization process itself is imperfect. One of the key tables in a randomized trial must compare the baseline characteristics of the intervention and control groups. Even if none of the factors differs significantly between the two groups, it is common to adjust for any baseline differences when reporting the effects of the study to be sure that the impact of the intervention is distinguished from any potential differences in baseline prognosis.

Magnitude of Effect

In assessing whether the results of a randomized trial may be useful for an individual physician, it is critical to understand the magnitude of the treatment effect.[4] Although randomized trials often report the percent reduction in the occurrence of an endpoint (similar to a decline in relative risk), for the individual patient and physician the absolute magnitude of the treatment effect (the change in absolute risk) may be critical in weighing the value of the intervention compared with other options. Another way to quantify the impact of an intervention is to estimate the number of patients who must be treated to achieve a particular benefit, such as the number of patients who must be treated to save a life or a year of life. For example, if an intervention reduces mortality from 6% to 4% in 1 year, there is an absolute 2% risk reduction, a relative 50% risk reduction, and 50 patients need to be treated for 1 year to save a life.

Subgroup Analyses

It is often tempting to perform *subgroup analyses* as part of randomized trials to determine whether certain types of patients are more likely to benefit or suffer from the intervention. Such subgroups should be specified before any data analysis to avoid biases inherent in multiple looks at the data. Within a randomized trial, any subgroup that is not pre-specified is subject to a wide variety of selection biases that may make the patients unrepresentative of others in the trial or even of nonrandomized patients who may have some similar characteristics. A reader must be especially wary of trials that compare *responders* to *nonresponders,* since responders may be intrinsically different in terms of their underlying prognosis.

Subgroup analyses are generally more likely to be valid when they are performed as part of a study in which the overall difference is large. When a study fails to show an overall difference, it is virtually always possible to identify by retrospective analysis some subgroups in whom the intervention was beneficial and others in which it appeared to be harmful; such findings may generate hypotheses for future testing but should not be considered definitive.

Other Biases

The *Hawthorne effect* describes the fact that decisions and care may improve simply because people realize they are being observed while participating in a trial, rather than because of the specific intervention itself. *Regression to the mean* describes the tendency for measurements that are the most extreme initially to move more toward the mean on remeasurement, even if there is no intervention. For example, if subjects are chosen based on their elevated blood pressures on one measurement, many will be selected based on a reading that is, for them, unusually high. On repeat measurement, the apparent improvement in blood pressure in many individuals will be a function of their fluctuation back toward their own mean blood pressure.

The major advantage of randomized trials is that they provide the least biased way to assess the benefit or harm of interventions. However, by definition, *randomized trials* are undertaken only to test something that is thought to be better than no treatment or the current standard of care. Hence, randomized trials are not performed with the intent of identifying interventions such as smoking, which are thought to be harmful. Randomized trials are also disadvantaged by their expense and logistical difficulties.

Quasi-Experimental Studies

In some situations, *quasi-experimental* approaches may be required because randomization is impractical or unreasonably expensive. Quasi-experimental designs are most appropriate in situations in which a program is being evaluated rather than when a treatment of individual patients is being studied. For example, if care at an institution is re-engineered in such a way that standard care can no longer be delivered or its delivery would be hopelessly *contaminated,* or influenced, by the intervention, it may be appropriate to have a control group from another institution or time period. Quasi-experimental designs are subject to a variety of biases, including the inability to be sure that patients seen in the intervention group are similar to those in a control group. In addition, temporal or secular changes unrelated to the intervention itself may be more important than the intervention. In interpreting quasi-experimental studies, it is critical to be sure there are adequate concurrent controls and that secular influences have been excluded or that adjustments have been made for them. One approach is to perform a *time series* study in which the program is implemented in some time periods and not in others, with these time periods alternated to provide an adequate control for secular and other influences.

CASE-CONTROL STUDIES

Since it is not ethical to randomize patients to receive interventions that are thought to be harmful, other study designs must be found to assess the cause of many diseases. In situations in which the risk factor is common and the outcome of interest occurs with a reasonably high frequency and in a reasonably short time frame, cohort studies can assess causative factors. However, in circumstances in which the outcome is unusual, an alternative design is the case-control study. In this approach, *cases* are patients with the disease and *controls* are subjects without it. These two groups are compared in terms of their *exposures* to various potential risk factors.[5]

Commonly, a case-control study will be *retrospective*, such that patients are identified after they already have the outcome (i.e., they are a *case*) and are then asked or surveyed to determine prior exposures. Alternatively, the cases may be the relatively few individuals who developed an endpoint as part of a cohort study, and to maximize both efficiency and power, they may be compared with randomly selected or matched control patients from that same cohort. In general, case-control studies become more powerful as the ratio of controls to cases increases to about 3 to 4 : 1, but there is little incremental power from further increasing the number of nondiseased controls in either a case-control or a cohort study. For example, in a large cohort study of 10,000 people, only 100 may develop intracranial bleeding, and it might be interesting to gather additional data on aspirin exposure or a family history of polycystic kidney disease. Rather than gathering the data on 9900 controls, the study might select 3 or 4 nonbleeding controls per case of bleeding and gather the additional data on this smaller sample. This *nested case-control* study within a larger cohort study is more efficient than including all of the cohort patients who did not develop the endpoint—especially if additional measurements must be made on patients who are included in the case-control study.

Case-control studies are subject to a number of biases, including how the cases and controls are defined and how the exposure is measured. Since the cases and controls may differ on a variety of factors other than the exposure being studied, it is common to adjust for these factors by using multivariate methods or by *matching* patients based on such attributes as age and sex.

In choosing cases and controls, it is important that the two groups be as similar as possible other than that the case has the outcome of interest. Potential exposures must be measured in similar ways in both groups, and it is critical to be sure that the exposure truly preceded the outcome. Furthermore, the conclusions of case-control studies are more likely to be valid if a clear dose-response gradient can be established, such that greater degrees of exposure result in a higher likelihood of disease or in more severe disease. Fox example, if smoking is associated with coronary disease, then more smoking should carry an even larger risk. When a case-control study identifies a potentially harmful exposure, consideration should be given to trying to confirm the harmful effect in a cohort study.

Since case-control studies arbitrarily select the numbers of patients with and without the disease, they cannot measure incidence or relative risk. Instead, they calculate an odds ratio (Table 1–4). Case-control studies are usually able to identify risk factors that have odds ratios of 2 or more, but they usually are not very useful for identifying exposures that increase the odds of an endpoint by less than that ratio.

Case-control studies suffer from the fact that the population at risk is generally undefined, the cases are selected based on their availability rather than by being sampled from a defined population, and the controls are selected by the investigator in hopes that they will somehow be appropriate for comparison with the cases. Exposure commonly must be recalled rather than being observed, and incidence rates and relative risk cannot be calculated. Nevertheless, case-control studies represent an efficient way to assess possible risk factors and were, for example, the method by which the increased cardiovascular risks associated with homocysteine were first noted.

DATA ANALYSIS

Statistics provide a mechanism for analyzing observations and determining whether clinically important differences exist.[3] Some clinical variables can be measured on a continuous scale, such as systolic blood pressure, so that a mean and standard deviation can be assessed. Others, such as the intensity of a systolic murmur, may be graded on an ordinal scale on which most individuals

Table 1–4	Calculation of the Odds Ratio in Case-Control Studies and Comparison with a Relative Risk Calculation from a Cohort Study		
	Cases with the Outcome	Controls without the Outcome	Total
Exposure present	A	B	A + B
Exposure absent	C	D	C + D
Total	A + C	B + D	
Odds ratio in a case-control study	$= \dfrac{\dfrac{A/(A + C)}{C/(A + C)}}{\dfrac{B/(B + D)}{D/(B + D)}}$	$= \dfrac{A/C}{B/D}$	$= \dfrac{AD}{BC}$
Relative risk in a cohort study	$= \dfrac{A/(A + B)}{C/(C + D)}$		

have a normal value (no murmur) and the number of patients with an abnormality declines as its severity increases.

Reproducibility or *reliability* refers to whether the same result would be obtained if the measurement were repeated. This should be contrasted with *validity,* which determines whether the measurement is an accurate reflection of reality. Ordinal measurements are oftentimes "soft" data that require clinical judgment rather than an automated machine. Nevertheless, assessment of functional status, quality of life, satisfaction, and the like can be "hardened" by standardized techniques that make them more reproducible. For example, standardized, validated questionnaires have been developed to measure functional capacity, health status, and quality of life with reproducibilities and validities that compare favorably with a typical radiographic test.

Since humans vary from time to time, it is not surprising that any measurement, be it blood pressure or functional status, may also vary. By statistical convention, measurements may be considered abnormal if there is less than 1 chance in 20 that they would be observed in a normal individual. However, for many laboratory tests, this statistical criterion is far too lenient, since just by chance each person would be abnormal on something if enough factors were measured. This principle of *multiple testing* demonstrates that statistical definitions of normal must be tempered by clinical judgment.

Specific types of statistical approaches are most appropriate for specific types of data (Table 1–5). Most of these tests can be performed easily by a variety of statistical packages on a personal computer.

Multivariate analyses can consider many potential factors and assess their importance independent of other factors. These various methods (Table 1–6) generally proceed by selecting the most important factor associated with the endpoint and then sequentially selecting the second most important factor, the third most important factor, and so on. Multivariate analyses can be used to assess the independent importance of risk factors or to adjust for a variety of known risk factors in determining whether an additional factor adds incremental importance.[2, 6]

When multiple factors are being tested, it may be more appropriate to define statistical significance as a less than 1 chance in 100 ($P < .01$) rather than as less than 1 chance in 20 ($P < .05$). Regardless of the definition of statistical significance, the question of clinical importance must also be addressed. In these situations, relative risk and attributable risk (Fig. 1–3) may be as important as the P value. For randomized trials, it may be appropriate to calculate the *number needed to treat,* that is, the number of patients who must receive an intervention to save one life or to avoid one endpoint.[3, 7, 8]

Table 1–6 Statistical Approaches

Parametric Multivariate Analyses

Create an equation that weights the various predictive factors and adds them up to give a score
$$ax_1 + bx_2 + cx_3 \ldots + \text{constant}$$ where a, b, and c are the respective weights for variables x_1, x_2, x_3.
Linear regression analysis: Preferred when the predictive variables are continuous (e.g., blood pressure) and the outcome is also continuous (e.g., left ventricular mass).
Logistic regression analysis: Preferred when the predictive variables are both continuous and dichotomous (e.g., blood pressure, family history of stroke) and the outcome is continuous (e.g., risk of stroke).
Discriminant analysis: Preferred when the outcome variable is in more than two ordered categories (e.g., no complications, major complications without death, death).

Recursive Partitioning Analysis

Sequentially splits subjects into subgroups based on factors that discriminate those with and those without the outcome of interest. Most useful when predictive factors are dichotomous and the outcome is dichotomous (e.g., live or die), especially if predictive factors have strong interrelationships.

Table 1–5 Overview of How to Choose Statistical Tests

Type of Measure	Comparison of Two Groups of Different Individuals to Each Other	Comparison of Same Individuals to Themselves—Two Measurements on Each	Comparison of Three or More Groups of Different Individuals	Comparison of Same Individuals to Themselves—Three or More Measurements on Each	Association of Two Different Variables with Each Other—Each Measured in the Same Individual
Continuous and either normally distributed or measured in many subjects (e.g., blood pressure)	Unpaired t test	Paired t test	Analysis of variance	Repeated measures analysis of variance	Pearson correlation coefficient or linear regression
Ordered but in few subjects or not normally distributed	Mann-Whitney rank sum test	Wilcoxon signed-rank test	Kruskal-Wallis statistic	Friedman statistic	Spearman rank correlation coefficient
Categorical—often dichotomous (two categories) and usually five or fewer categories	Chi-square test or Fisher exact test	McNemar's test	Chi-square test	Cochrane Q	Contingency coefficient

Adapted from Glantz, S.A. Primer of Biostatistics. 3rd ed. New York, McGraw-Hill, 1992. With permission of The McGraw-Hill Companies.

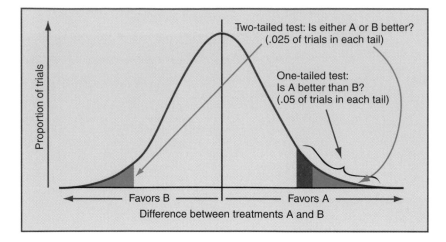

Figure 1–3
One-tailed and two-tailed tests of statistical significance, where $P_x = .05$. A larger observed difference in favor of treatment is required for statistical significance if the analysis is done assuming that either A or B might be better. (From Fletcher, R.H., Fletcher, S.W., and Wagner, E.H.: Clinical Epidemiology: The Essentials. 2nd ed. Baltimore, Williams & Wilkins, 1988.)

By convention, statistical tests may be considered *one-tailed* or *two-tailed*. A two-tailed test considers whether either of two options being compared may be better or worse than the other (see Fig. 1–3). A one-tailed test estimates the probability of whether option A is better than option B, but not the converse (the possibility that B may be better than A). Although clinical investigators are often tempted to use one-tailed tests, with the assumption that a new option may be better than a prior option but that it could not possibly be worse, statistical convention and most journals require that two-tailed tests be used. Simply put, the *P* value reported for a two-tailed test will be twice as large as the *P* value reported for a one-tailed test and, hence, is less likely to demonstrate conventional statistical significance.

It is common in medical literature to calculate *confidence intervals* around a point estimate. The 95% confidence interval indicates the range in which 95% of individuals are estimated to fall or the range in which the results are estimated to occur 95% of the time if the experiment were repeated multiple times.

Whereas the *P* value estimates the likelihood that an observed difference may be due to chance, the *power* of a study estimates the likelihood that it will be able to find a true difference if one exists (Table 1–7). Commonly, randomized trials are designed to have a power of at least 80% for finding a relevant difference if one, indeed, exists, but sometimes the power might be increased if it is extremely important to be sure that such a difference does not exist. A study's power is calculated before the study is conducted; when the final data are presented, they should be reported in terms of the confidence intervals around any observed differences.

META-ANALYSIS

Because even the largest studies oftentimes do not have a power sufficient to exclude a small difference, *meta-analysis* is a method for combining the results of randomized trials to increase aggregate sample size and see whether differences truly exist. Meta-analyses are more likely to be useful if the studies being combined are similar, if the studies represent current medical treatments, and if there is unlikely to be any *publication bias* such that only positive studies have been reported whereas negative studies have not.[9]

In formal meta-analyses, standardized methods are used to be sure that all potentially relevant studies have been identified, that they meet criteria for methodologic rigor, and that the results are combined in statistically appropri-

Table 1–7	Alpha and Beta Error: *P* Values and the Definition of Power		
		Truth in the Population from Which the Study Sample Was Chosen	
		Association	*No Association*
Findings in the study	Significant association (e.g., $P < .05$)	Correct	Type I (alpha) error* (association found by 1 in 20 chance even though it does not truly exist)
	Not a significant association (e.g., $P > .05$)	Type II (beta) error† (association not found, often because the study was too small to have a sufficient power to detect a statistically significant relationship)	Correct

*Usually the acceptable alpha error is .05 (1 in 20), but it may be .01 or lower.
†Usually the acceptable beta error is about .20 (1 in 5; power of 80%), but it may be .10 (power 90%) or even .05 (power 95%) if it is very important not to miss an association.

Odds Ratio (Log scale)

ALL CAUSE MORTALITY		T	C	Favors treatment						Favors control
STUDY				0.1	0.2	0.5	1	2	5	10
HDFP	1979	153/1202	178/1172							
ANBP	1981	7/293	9/289							
Sprackling	1981	48/60	44/60							
EWPHE	1985	135/416	149/424							
PPC	1986	50/419	69/465							
SHEP	1991	213/2365	242/2371							
STOP	1991	36/812	63/815							
MRC	1992	301/2183	315/2213							
Total		953/7750	1069/7809							
Odds ratio				0.88 (0.80 – 0.97)					P = .0092	

STROKE MORTALITY		T	C							
STUDY				0.1	0.2	0.5	1	2	5	10
HDFP	1979	17/1202	31/1172							
ANBP	1981	1/293	1/289							
EWPHE	1985	21/416	31/424							
PPC	1986	4/419	15/465							
SHEP	1991	10/2365	14/2371							
STOP	1991	4/812	15/815							
MRC	1992	37/2183	42/2213							
Total		94/7690	149/7749							
Odds ratio				0.64 (0.49 – 0.82)					P = .0005	

CHD MORTALITY		T	C							
STUDY				0.1	0.2	0.5	1	2	5	10
HDFP	1979	54/1202	58/1172							
ANBP	1981	1/293	4/289							
EWPHE	1985	29/416	47/424							
PPC	1986	25/419	28/465							
SHEP	1991	59/2365	73/2371							
STOP	1991	10/812	20/815							
MRC	1992	85/2183	110/2213							
Total		263/7690	350/7749							
Odds ratio				0.75 (0.64 – 0.88)					P = .00055	

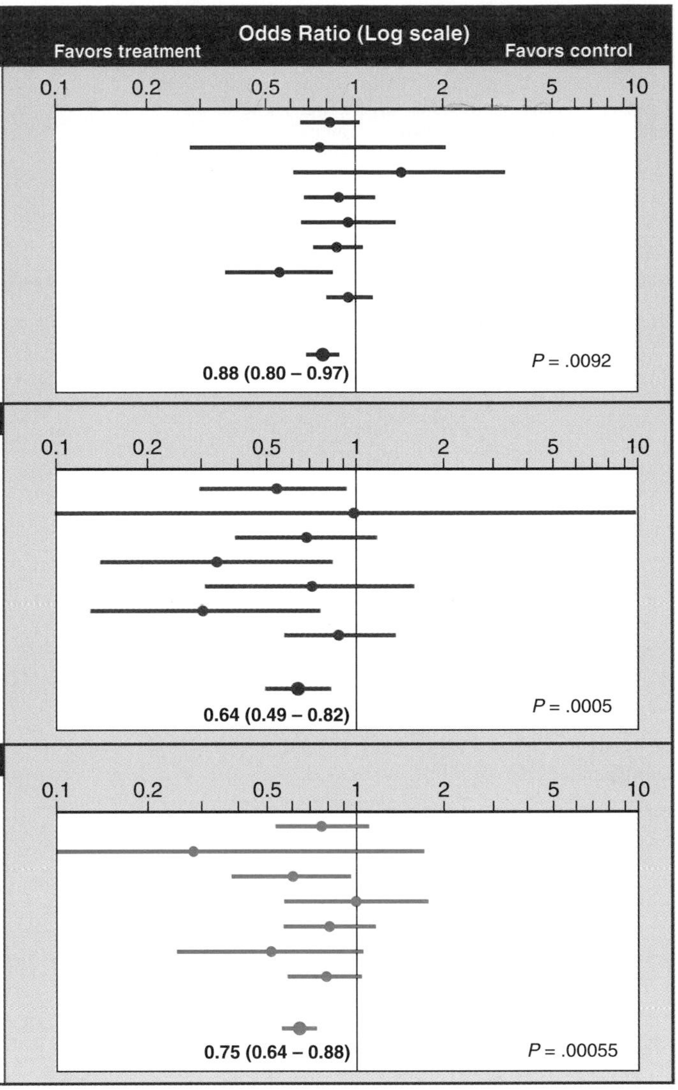

Figure 1–4

Results of meta-analysis of the effect on mortality of the treatment of hypertension in the elderly. The inclusion of more studies allows for a better point estimate of the true benefit and also a narrowing of the confidence intervals around this point estimate. *Left,* Absolute numbers. *Right,* Odds ratios and 95% confidence intervals. ANBP, Australian National Blood Pressure Study; EWPHE, European Working Party on High Blood Pressure in the Elderly; HDFP, Hypertension Detection and Follow-Up Program; MRC, Medical Research Council; PPC, Practice Primary Care; SHEP, Systolic Hypertension in the Elderly; STOP, Swedish Trial in Old Patients with Hypertension; VA, Veterans Administration Cooperative Study on Antihypertensive Agents. (Adapted from Insua, J.T., Sacks, H.S., Lau, T.-S., et al.: Drug treatment of hypertension in the elderly: A meta-analysis. Ann. Intern. Med. 121:355–362, 1994.)

ate ways. The results of meta-analyses are commonly demonstrated in a summary figure, which demonstrates the relative harm or benefit found in individual studies (with their 95% confidence intervals) as well as the pooled estimate of the effect of the intervention overall (Fig. 1–4).

In general, meta-analyses are more useful for summarizing the results of multiple large trials than those of very small studies that may be more subject to bias. Thus, meta-analyses appear to supplement rather than substitute for large clinical trials, and they are more useful when there is general consistency among the preceding trials than when they are used to resolve major differences among studies. For example, meta-analyses of thrombolysis predicted the results eventually found in large megatrials, but meta-analyses of the effects of magnesium and nitroglycerin in acute myocardial infarction have been discrepant with the results of the subsequent megatrials.

References

1. Oxman, A.D., Sackett, D.L., and Guyatt, G.H., for the Evidence-Based Medicine Working Group: Users' guides to the medical literature. I. How to get started. JAMA 270:2093–2095, 1993.
2. Fletcher R.H., Fletcher, S.W., and Wagner, E.H.: Clinical Epidemiology: The Essentials. 2nd ed. Baltimore, Williams & Wilkins, 1988.
3. Glantz, S.A.: Primer of Biostatistics. 3rd ed. New York, McGraw-Hill, 1992.
4. Guyatt, G.H., Sackett, D.L., and Cook, D.J., for the Evidence-Based Medicine Working Group: Users' guides to the medical literature. II.

How to use an article about therapy or prevention. A. Are the results of the study valid? JAMA 270:2598–2601, 1993.

5. Hulley, S.B., and Cummings, S.R.: Designing Clinical Research. Baltimore, Williams & Wilkins, 1988.

6. Laupacis, A., Wells, G., Richardson, W.S., and Tugwell, P., for the Evidence-Based Medicine Working Group: Users' guides to the medical literature. V. How to use an article about prognosis. JAMA 272:234–237, 1994.

7. Levine, M., Walter, S., Lee, H., et al., for the Evidence-Based Medicine Working Group: Users' guides to the medical literature. IV. How to use an article about harm. JAMA 271:1615–1619, 1994.

8. McQuay, H.J., and Moore, R.A.: Using numerical results from systematic reviews in clinical practice. Ann Intern Med 126:712–720, 1997.

9. Oxman, A.D., Cook, D., and Guyatt, G.H., for the Evidence-Based Medicine Working Group: Users' guides to the medical literature. VI. How to use an overview. JAMA 272:1367–1371, 1993.

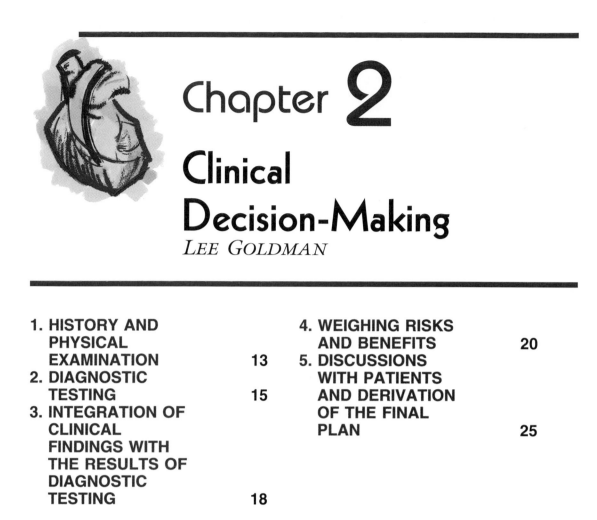

Chapter 2

Clinical Decision-Making

LEE GOLDMAN

Clinical decision-making is a complicated process based on experience, judgment, and reasoning that should simultaneously integrate information from the medical literature and a variety of other sources. Although *decision-making* should not be confused with *decision analysis,*[1] which is a quantitative method for analyzing medical information, it should incorporate the quantitative results of randomized clinical trials and other studies that form the substance of what is often called *evidence-based medicine* (see Chap. 1).

Medical decision-making generally proceeds through a five-step process that begins, *first,* with the physician's elicitation of pertinent historical information related to the chief complaint and history of present illness.[1] The past medical history and physical examination may be specially targeted to pursue possibilities uncovered by the original questioning in addition to providing a standard body of background information. *Second,* the physician may choose from a variety of diagnostic tests, which in cardiology oftentimes includes different options for obtaining the same type of information. For example, the left ventricular ejection fraction may be measured by echocardiography (transthoracic or transesophageal), by a radionuclide ventriculogram, or by a contrast ventriculogram. In the *third* step, the results of diagnostic tests are used to modify or adjust probabilities or hypotheses that were generated from the original history and physical examination. In the *fourth* phase, the potential risks and benefits of additional diagnostic tests and therapeutic interventions are compared so that the physician may develop a set of recommendations for the patient. *Fifth,* a plan or alternative plans are discussed with the patient, the patient's comparative preferences for various options are considered, and a plan is implemented.

HISTORY AND PHYSICAL EXAMINATION (See Chap. 3)

During the initial medical history, the physician should pursue complaints that may be cardiac in origin with the understanding that the importance of the cardiac abnormality may be far greater than the severity of the patient's presenting complaint.[2] For example, even very mild anginal pain may be the first key symptom for coronary artery disease. The same complaint would be far less important if it could be proved to be related to a musculoskeletal abnormality. Since even minor complaints that may be consistent with cardiac disease could be the first symptom of severe pathoanatomic abnormalities with dire and sudden clinical consequences, it is critical that complaints of chest discomfort, shortness of breath, dizziness, or edema be investigated in sufficient detail to determine whether or not they are early warning signs for important cardiac disease.

When investigating complaints potentially consistent with cardiac disease, an experienced physician will generate a list of important diseases that could cause the complaint and then ask additional questions in an order that helps determine whether the more serious potential causes of the symptom are present. In a process termed *iterative hypothesis* testing, the clinician will investigate sequentially the likelihood of various causes of the symptom or sign rather than asking all imaginable questions in a standardized order. For example, in a patient who complains of chest discomfort, the physician should focus on the location and quality of the discomfort and how it may be provoked or relieved. The physician should determine whether the pain is precipitated by exercise, emotion, eating, deep breathing, or changes in position (see Chap. 7). Depending on the responses, a series of questions would be used to try to reinforce or discard the diagnostic suspicion. For example, if the pain is pleuritic in nature, the physician would ask about prior viral symptoms and risk factors for venous thromboembolic disease. It must be emphasized that this focused approach does not obviate the need for a complete history and physical examination, and the history and physical examination should reinforce and influence each other.

Both the history and the physical examination will be more helpful if the physician is precise in the way questions are asked and in the way the physical examination is performed. Patients' responses to questions may vary from time to time, and it is often helpful to ask the same question in different ways to be sure that the responses are consistent. On physical examination, many of the key findings that are used for diagnostic decision-making, such as the presence and intensity of a murmur, may be poorly reproducible from time to time and from observer to observer.

Because of the poor reproducibility of many physical findings, it is important for the clinician to listen or observe carefully and also to look for corroborating information. For example, if the jugular veins appear to be distended, the finding of hepatomegaly, hepatojugular reflux, or peripheral edema would tend to confirm the abnormality. A precordial systolic murmur suspicious for aortic outflow obstruction may be confirmed by auscultation over the carotid arteries. In addition, by utilizing a variety of bedside maneuvers (see Chap. 13), careful cardiac auscultation often can accurately predict the cause of a systolic murmur.[3]

Diagnostic tests may be especially important to confirm suspicions raised by the history or physical examination. For example, the findings of bibasilar rales and a clearly enlarged heart on physical examination in a patient with dyspnea on exertion may be readily ascribed to congestive heart failure. However, the same apparent physical findings in the absence of symptoms of congestive heart failure would not be nearly so definitive and should prompt additional evaluation, such as with a chest radiograph, to assess whether congestive heart failure is present. Even when all the data support the diagnosis of congestive heart failure, a chest radiograph may be useful to assess the severity of the heart failure, and an echocardiogram may be critical for evaluating the cause and severity of any underlying left ventricular dysfunction or valvular abnormalities (see Chap. 4).

In weighing clinical information, physicians tend to have great difficulty in estimating accurate probabilities. Part of the problem is related to reliance on vague and ill-defined terms such as *often* or *unlikely*. Physicians also tend systematically to overestimate the probability that unusual conditions are present. For example, when a systolic murmur is heard in a patient with angina, congestive

---

Table 2–1   Definitions of Commonly Used Terms in Epidemiology and Decision-Making

Test Result	Disease State	
	Present	*Absent*
Positive	*a* (true positive)	*b* (false positive)
Negative	*c* (false negative)	*d* (true negative)

Prevalence (prior probability)	$= (a + c)/(a + b + c + d)$	= all patients with the disease/all patients tested
Sensitivity (true-positive rate)	$= a/(a + c)$	= true-positive test results/all patients with the disease
Specificity (true-negative rate)	$= d/(b + d)$	= true-negative test results/all patients without the disease
False-negative rate	$= c/(a + c)$	= false-negative test results/all patients with the disease
False-positive rate	$= b/(b + d)$	= false-positive test results/all patients without the disease
Positive predictive value	$= a/(a + b)$	= true-positive test results/all positive test results
Negative predictive value	$= d/(c + d)$	= true-negative test results/all patients with negative results
Overall accuracy	$= (a + d)/(a + b + c + d)$	= true-positive + true-negative test results/all tests
Likelihood ratio for a positive test	$= \dfrac{a/(a + c)}{b/(b + d)}$	= true-positive rate/false-positive rate
Likelihood ratio for a negative test	$= \dfrac{d/(b + d)}{c/(a + c)}$	= true-negative rate/false-negative rate

Adapted from Fauci A.S., Braunwald, E., Isselbacher, K.J., et al. (eds.): Harrison's Principles of Internal Medicine. 14th ed. New York, McGraw-Hill, 1998, p. 10.

heart failure, or syncope, it is vital to know whether critical aortic stenosis could be the cause. Even if the probability is very small that the murmur is related to aortic stenosis, a cardiac consultation or echocardiogram may still be important to be sure that this potentially fatal but curable cause is not present.

DIAGNOSTIC TESTING

No diagnostic test is perfect. Even a test such as coronary arteriography, which may be considered the gold standard for the diagnosis of coronary disease, has an imperfect correlation with autopsy findings. Similarly, a pulmonary angiogram, which is generally considered the gold standard for the diagnosis of pulmonary embolism, is also imperfect.

Since diagnostic tests provide useful but not perfect information, it is critical that their results be integrated with findings from the history and physical examination.[4] The history and physical examination provide a *prior probability* that a condition in question, such as critical aortic stenosis, is present. This probability can then be modified by the results of a diagnostic test, such as an echocardiogram. Although an echocardiogram should be an accurate way to determine the gradient across an aortic valve (see Chap. 25), this gradient may decline as a patient develops severe left ventricular dysfunction. Hence, a gradient of 50 or 60 mm Hg may represent only moderate stenosis in a patient with normal left ventricular function, whereas a gradient of 30 mm Hg may represent severe stenosis in a patient with markedly compromised left ventricular function. Therefore, cardiac catheterization with simultaneous measurement of both the aortic valve gradient and the cardiac output may be required to achieve the best possible in vivo estimate of the severity of aortic valve stenosis, with the recognition that even this estimate may not be perfect.

Since diagnostic tests do not provide perfect information, it is critical to understand the terminology that is commonly used to assess the accuracy of a diagnostic test (Table 2–1). Whereas the clinician tends to think about the patient in terms of the probability of a disease, such as critical aortic stenosis, after a test such as an echocardiogram, the postechocardiogram probability is dependent not only on the result of the echocardiogram but also on the pretest likelihood of aortic stenosis. This pretest likelihood in an individual patient is the equivalent of the *prevalence* of the disease in a population of patients with the same characteristics. Using this general approach, a single test, with known sensitivity and specificity, will yield different probabilities of disease depending on the pretest probability of the condition in question (Fig. 2–1).

The same phenomenon can be understood by looking from the population perspective. For example, the likelihood of different exercise test results among patients with differing severities of coronary artery disease is reasonably known from the medical literature. The prevalence of these varying severities of coronary disease in the population can also be estimated. Based on these two estimates, the expected results of exercise testing can be projected, and the likelihood of varying severities of disease, given a particular exercise test result, can be calculated (Fig. 2–2).

Sensitivity and Specificity

The sensitivity and specificity of a test do not depend on the prevalence of the disease in the population being studied or the probability of disease in the individual. However, both sensitivity and specificity are dependent on the *spectrum* of patients being studied. For example, if a new enzyme assay for the diagnosis of acute myocardial infarction is evaluated in 50 patients with obvious acute myocardial infarctions based on electrocardiographic criteria and 50 normal college students, it will appear to have a near-perfect sensitivity and specificity. If, however, the same test is applied to 100 patients with suspicious symptoms who are being evaluated as part of a rule-out myocardial infarction protocol, both the sensitivity and the specificity will be far lower; in fact, given the absence of a true gold standard, the precise sensitivity and specificity may be difficult if not impossible to determine.

For many diagnostic tests, the result is not dichotomous (i.e., normal vs. abnormal) but rather may be interpreted on a continuum.[4] Whether this continuum is the level of a cardiac enzyme, the number of millimeters of ST segment depression on exercise testing, or the measured gradient across a valve during Doppler echocardiography, judgment must be used to determine what value or values should guide medical decision-making. One way to assess this inherent tradeoff between defining normal so as to provide a high sensitivity (such as diagnosing a postangioplasty myocardial infarction as occurring in a patient with a minimal cardiac enzyme elevation) compared with emphasizing a high specificity (such as requiring a threefold or fourfold increase in cardiac enzyme values as a criterion for a postprocedure infarction) is to evaluate various definitions of an abnormal test result. This principle can be depicted by a *receiver operating characteristic curve,* which graphically displays the sensitivity and specificity associated with various test results (Fig. 2–3).

In many situations, tests may be valued because of their high sensitivity or high specificity but not both. For example, when an electrocardiogram shows 1 mm or more of ST segment elevation in two or more contiguous leads in a patient with acute chest pain, the likelihood of acute myocardial infarction is very high. In the absence of evidence for conditions such as acute pericarditis or aortic dissection, where the risks of thrombolysis are very high, these patients are considered appropriate for immediate thrombolysis or for catheterization with probable primary angioplasty, because the electrocardiogram result is unlikely to be a false positive (i.e., it is highly specific), and even if it is, the risks of aggressive therapy in the few false-positive cases are far outweighed by the benefits for the vast majority of true-positive cases. In other settings, a test may be valued because of its very high sensitivity. For example, cardiac enzyme abnormali-

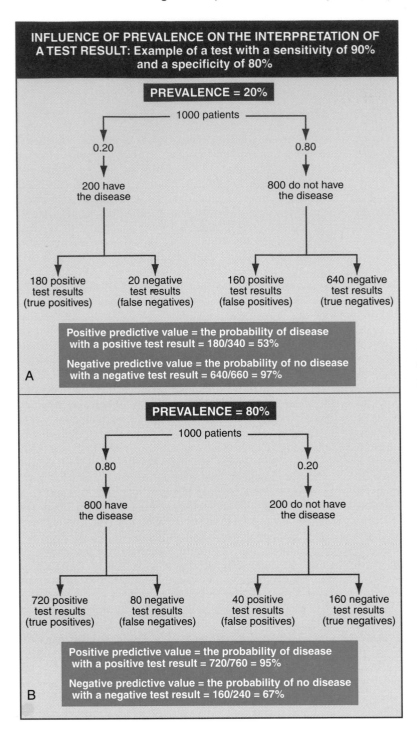

Figure 2–1
The influence of prevalence on the interpretation of a test result.

ties may represent false-positive elevations in patients with skeletal muscle trauma, alcohol ingestion, or a variety of other conditions but, unlike the electrocardiographic criteria of ST segment elevation, are virtually always found in patients with acute myocardial infarction. By combining a sensitive test with a specific test, such as the combination of cardiac enzymes with the electrocardiogram, a physician may be able to integrate information and avoid both false-positive and false-negative diagnoses. Alternatively, sometimes a single test, such as the pulmonary angiogram for the diagnosis of pulmo-

nary embolism, has a sufficiently high sensitivity and specificity to serve as the ultimate arbiter of clinical diagnosis, even though it is not a perfect predictor of pathoanatomy.

A set of principles for evaluating and applying the results of studies of diagnostic tests can be used as a general approach to interpreting the medical literature (Table 2–2). It is critical that a test be compared with the results of an independent gold standard performed and interpreted by people who do not know the results of the new test and that the sample of patients on

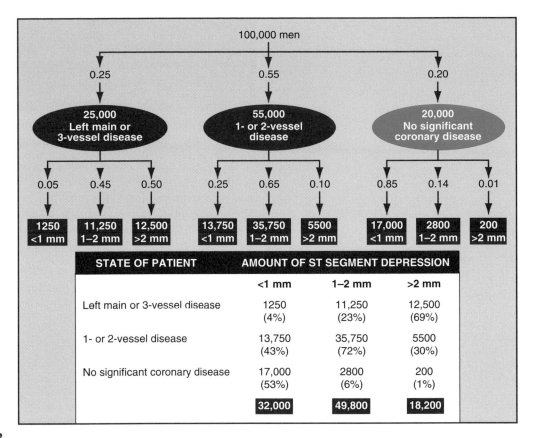

Figure 2–2

Cohort flow model of Bayes' rule used to interpret an exercise tolerance test in a 50-year-old man with typical angina. Consider a cohort of 100,000 such men: 25% have left main or three-vessel disease, 55% have one- or two-vessel disease, and 20% are free of significant coronary disease. If the conditional probabilities of less than 1 mm, 1 to 2 mm, and greater than 2 mm of ST segment depression are as shown and determine how many men from each diagnostic subgroup will have each finding, then of the 1250 + 13,750 + 17,000 (or 32,000) men with less than 1 mm of ST segment depression, 17,000, or 53%, will have no significant coronary disease, 43% will have one- or two-vessel disease, and 4% will have left main or three-vessel disease. (Redrawn from Bennett, J.C., and Plum, F. [eds.]: Cecil Textbook of Medicine. 20th ed. Philadelphia, W.B. Saunders, 1996, p. 79; based on data in Diamond, G.A., and Forrester, J.S.: Analysis of probability as an aid in the clinical diagnosis of coronary artery disease. N. Engl. J. Med. 300:1350, 1979. Copyright 1979, the Massachusetts Medical Society.)

Table 2–2   Evaluating and Applying the Results of Studies of Diagnostic Tests

Are the Results of the Study Valid?

Primary guides

   Was there an independent, blind comparison with a reference standard?
   Did the patient sample include an appropriate spectrum of patients to whom the diagnostic test will be applied in clinical
      practice?

Secondary guides

   Did the results of the test being evaluated influence the decision to perform the reference standard?
   Were the methods for performing the test described in sufficient detail to permit replication?

What Are the Results?

Are likelihood ratios for the test results presented or data necessary for their calculation provided?

Will the Results Help Me in Caring for My Patients?

Will the reproducibility of the test result and its interpretation be satisfactory in my setting?
Are the results applicable to my patient?
Will the results change my management?
Will patients be better off as a result of the test?

From Jaeschke, R., Guyatt, G.H., and Sackett, D.L., for the Evidence-Based Medicine Working Group. Users' guides to the medical literature. III. How to use an article about a diagnostic test. B. What are the results and will they help me in caring for my patients? JAMA 271:703–707, 1994. Copyright 1994, American Medical Association.

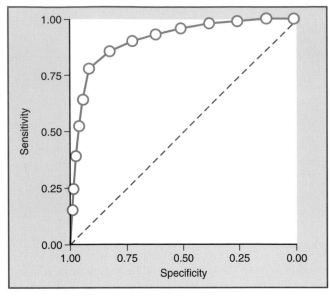

Figure 2–3

For any diagnostic test, an increase in sensitivity will be associated with an inherent tradeoff that lowers specificity. Better tests are associated with curves closer to the upper left hand corner, whereas tests near the 45-degree angle are of little value. The curve can be used to help decide the definition of a normal as compared with an abnormal test result.

whom the test is evaluated be similar to those in whom it would be used in clinical practice. Studies must also avoid biases inherent in situations in which the result of the new test being evaluated influences the decision to perform the gold standard test—for example, if the results of thallium scintigraphy influence the decision to perform coronary angiography, then the accuracy of the scintigram in the patients who do not undergo angiography is unknown. The information from the test must be provided in the form of sensitivity and specificity, so that the likelihood ratio can be calculated and used in subsequent Bayesian estimates.

INTEGRATION OF CLINICAL FINDINGS WITH THE RESULTS OF DIAGNOSTIC TESTING

The pretest probability of a disease, such as coronary artery disease, can be integrated with a test result, such as an exercise test, to determine a revised, posttest probability. In its quantitative form as defined by *Bayesian* analysis, these data can be combined mathematically to arrive at a precise probability (Fig. 2–4). In this example, the pretest probabilities are converted to the odds as in a gambling wager, then multiplied by the likelihood ratio (the sensitivity of the test divided by 1 minus the specificity of the test) to calculate aftertest odds, which are then converted back into a probability. This formal calculation may be possible in selected circumstances in which pretest diagnostic probabilities can be quantified accurately based on data from the literature and the sensitivity and specificity of a test are known. For example, by knowing the likelihood ratio associated with different results on a ventilation-perfusion scan (Table 2–3), the probability of acute pulmonary embolism in different types of patients with these scan findings can be estimated (Table 2–4). A similar, simple approach can help estimate the probability of coronary disease given varying results on exercise testing and thallium scintigraphy in patients with typical anginal pain, patients with atypical pain potentially consistent with coronary disease, or asymptomatic patients in the age range in which coronary disease is often found (Figs. 2–5 through 2–7). Similar information can also be generated via graphs that help integrate prior probabilities with diagnostic test results (Fig. 2–8). In other circumstances, such formal calculations may be impossible or inappropriate because of inadequate information on pretest probability or on the sensitivity or specificity of the diagnostic test, but the general Bayesian approach may still be helpful.

A key assumption in Bayesian analysis is that a test adds new, incremental information above and beyond

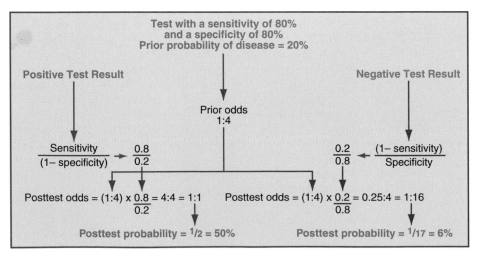

Figure 2–4

Bayesian analysis. Using odds and likelihood ratios to calculate a posttest probability.

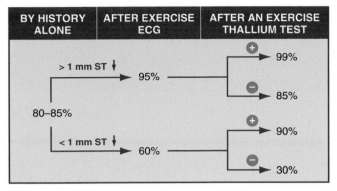

Figure 2–5

Approximate probability of coronary artery disease before and after noninvasive testing in a patient with typical angina pectoris. These percentages demonstrate how the sequential use of an electrocardiogram and an exercise thallium test may affect the probability of coronary artery disease in a patient with typical angina pectoris. (Redrawn from Branch, W.B., Jr. [ed.]: Office Practice of Medicine, 3rd ed. Philadelphia, W.B. Saunders, 1994, p. 45.)

what is already previously known. If a test simply duplicates prior information, it is not helpful. For example, an estimation of ejection fraction by a radionuclide ventriculogram does not add new, independent information to a similar estimation by echocardiography. In contrast, the information obtained by thallium or sestamibi scintigraphy appears to add incrementally to information obtainable from the history, physical examination, and standard exercise electrocardiogram.

The Threshold Approach

Diagnostic tests are most helpful when they change a probability across a decision-making threshold. Often-

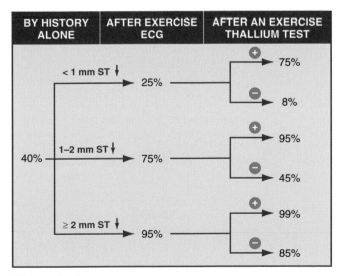

Figure 2–6

Approximate probability of coronary artery disease before and after noninvasive testing in a patient with atypical anginal symptoms. (Redrawn from Branch, W.B., Jr. [ed.]: Office Practice of Medicine, 3rd ed. Philadelphia, W.B. Saunders, 1994, p. 45.)

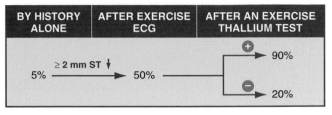

Figure 2–7

Approximate probability of coronary artery disease before and after noninvasive testing in an asymptomatic subject in the coronary artery disease age range. (Redrawn from Branch, W.B., Jr. [ed.]: Office Practice of Medicine, 3rd ed. Philadelphia, W.B. Saunders, 1994, p. 45.)

times, this threshold is not 50% but may well be far lower. For example, a test that lowers the probability of aortic dissection to 49% would not be considered reassuring, since the decision-making threshold for proceeding in the evaluation and potential treatment of this life-threatening condition should be lower. In such a situation, a test must be sensitive enough for detecting aortic dissection so that a negative test result reduces the probchability to a sufficiently low level. In other situations, it may be useful to divide patients into three different probability groups: one appropriate for immediate treatment, one appropriate for further testing, and one in which no further evaluation is indicated. Unfortunately, for many conditions the precise threshold that should guide clinical decision-making has not been determined.

Diagnostic tests may be useful for confirming a finding on physical examination, reassuring a patient, or reassuring the physician. However, they are most likely to be useful when they may lead to a sufficient change in diagnostic probabilities that the management of a patient will be altered.

In deciding whether or not to order a test, the physician must decide not only whether the test is sufficiently accurate (high sensitivity and specificity) for the condition in question but also how likely it is that the patient has the condition under consideration, what the adverse consequences would be if the condition were missed or the patient were inappropriately treated for a condition that is not present, and how likely it is that the test will have a sufficient impact on the probability of disease to then influence diagnosis or treatment.[4] In making these decisions, the physician must consider the benefits, risks, and costs of the test as well as other alternatives, such as continued observation or proceeding immediately to another test or empirical treatment.

Various studies of the ordering patterns and impact of cardiac nuclear medicine procedures and echocardiograms have found that such tests lead to an appropriate change in diagnosis in about 20% to 25% of cases and to an appropriate change in therapy in about 10% of cases in which they are ordered. These findings do not imply that all tests that do not lead to a change in diagnosis or management were inappropriate to order, unless they did not meet the criteria enumerated previously.

Table 2–3	Test Properties of Ventilation-Perfusion ($\dot{V}/\dot{Q}$) Scanning				
	Pulmonary Embolism				
	Present		*Absent*		
$\dot{V}/\dot{Q}$ Scan Result	*No.*	*Proportion*	*No.*	*Proportion*	Likelihood Ratio
High probability	102	102/251 = 0.406	14	14/630 = 0.022	18.3
Intermediate probability	105	105/251 = 0.418	217	217/630 = 0.344	1.2
Low probability	39	39/251 = 0.155	273	273/630 = 0.433	0.36
Normal/near normal	5	5/251 = 0.020	126	126/630 = 0.200	0.10
Total	251	—	630	—	—

From Jaeschke, R., Guyatt, G.H., and Sackett, D.L., for the Evidence-Based Medicine Working Group. Users' guides to the medical literature. III. How to use an article about a diagnostic test. B. What are the results and will they help me in caring for my patients? JAMA 271:703–707, 1994. Copyright 1994, American Medical Association.

Prediction Rules

Aggregated information from large numbers of patients in data banks or prospective cohort studies can be used to assess pretest probabilities for various diagnoses or outcomes. When appropriately validated in prospective testing, these probabilities can be used to guide clinical decision-making. For example, data on about 15,000 patients with chest pain have been used to derive and validate estimates of the likelihood that such patients will develop complications that require intensive care (Fig. 2–9). These initial probabilities can then be updated based on whether patients have developed evidence of an acute myocardial infarction, a life-threatening cardiac complica-

tion, or an intermediate cardiac complication to determine the subsequent likelihood of life-threatening complications (Table 2–5).

When probabilities are used to derive recommended decisions, they may be used to create a *prediction rule*. For prediction rules to be useful, they must be derived and tested in populations of patients that are relevant to the clinician and use clinical findings or diagnostic tests that are both readily available and reproducible.

WEIGHING RISKS AND BENEFITS

All clinicians intuitively compare the risks of tests and treatments with their likely benefits. In some situations, definitive data from large randomized trials may be available so that this process is simple and straightforward, such as the value of reperfusion therapy for acute myocardial infarction. In other situations, however, the individual patient may not be similar to those who have been included in randomized trials, or the precise question may not have been subjected to an appropriate trial. In these circumstances, decision analysis provides a quantitative method for comparing risks with benefits. It should be emphasized that formal decision analysis is oftentimes much too cumbersome to be utilized by the individual physician, but published decision analyses may help guide decisions in the absence of definitive data from randomized trials. However, decision analyses can be no more accurate than the data on which they are based, and sometimes the uncertainties are sufficiently large that the analyses cannot be considered conclusive.

Decision Analysis

A typical decision analysis (Fig. 2–10) considers the choices (decisions) the physician must make (the square box or node labeled *A*) as well as the probabilities of the various events that may depend on each decision (circular nodes *B–S*). For each of these probabilities, an estimate is commonly derived from the literature or based on the

Table 2–4	Pretest Probabilities, Likelihood Ratios (LRs) of Ventilation-Perfusion Scan Results, and Posttest Probabilities in Two Patients with Pulmonary Embolus	
Pretest Probability, % (Range)*	Scan Result (LR)	Posttest Probability, % (Range)*
78-Year-Old Woman with Sudden Onset of Dyspnea following Abdominal Surgery		
70 (60–80)	High probability (18.3)	97 (96–99)
70 (60–80)	Intermediate probability (1.2)	74 (64–83)
70 (60–80)	Low probability (0.36)	46 (35–59)
70 (60–80)	Normal/near normal (0.1)	19 (13–29)
28-Year-Old Man with Dyspnea and Atypical Chest Pain		
20 (10–30)	High probability (18.3)	82 (67–89)
20 (10–30)	Intermediate probability (1.2)	23 (12–34)
20 (10–30)	Low probability (0.36)	8 (4–16)
20 (10–30)	Normal/near normal (0.1)	2 (1–4)

From Jaeschke, R., Guyatt, G.H., and Sackett, D.L., for the Evidence-Based Medicine Working Group. Users' guides to the medical literature. III. How to use an article about a diagnostic test. B. What are the results and will they help me in caring for my patients? JAMA 271:703–707, 1994. Copyright 1994, American Medical Association.

*The values in parentheses represent a plausible range of pretest probabilities. That is, while the best guess as to the pretest probability is 70%, values of 60% to 80% would also be reasonable estimates.

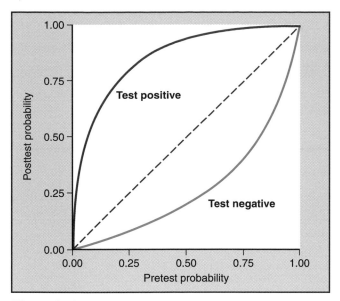

Figure 2-8

How the pretest probability affects the posttest probability of disease. The same test result has far different implications depending on the pretest probability.

best possible expert opinion. Each of the possible ultimate outcomes is then assigned a *utility* or relative value. An outcome of perfect health may be assigned a utility of 1.0, whereas death may be assigned an outcome of zero. Outcomes that are associated with survival in less than perfect health may be assigned utilities based on the cumulative quality of life associated with the outcome, such as life with angina, congestive heart failure, or after a cerebrovascular accident. After a utility corresponding with the outcome has been assigned to each terminal branch of the decision tree, all of the terminal branches related to a choice (decision) node can be summed and averaged to determine the *expected value* of the choices emanating from that node. The preferred decision would be the one that yields the highest average expected value after all of its potential outcomes have been considered.

Decision analyses often require estimates and sometimes even guesswork to assign the necessary probabilities and utilities. For example, although it is critical to adjust future years of life for their quality, especially in patients who may develop a complication such as intracranial hemorrhage or derive an advantage such as a smaller infarction with less congestive heart failure, these adjustments often cannot be determined accurately.

Since decision analysis is so inherently dependent on a variety of estimates, it is critical that *sensitivity analyses* be performed to demonstrate how conceivable differences in each of these estimates or assumptions will alter the ultimate conclusions. Many decision analyses consciously

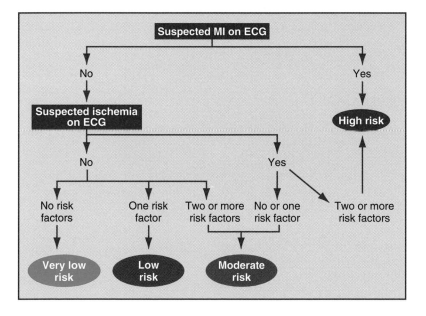

Figure 2-9

Derivation of four initial groups of patients with acute chest pain who are at varying risks of major complications on the basis of data available at the time of presentation in the emergency department. Myocardial infarction (MI) was suspected if the electrocardiogram (ECG) showed ST segment elevation of 1 mm or more or pathologic Q waves in two or more leads, and these findings were not known to be old. Ischemia was suspected if the ECG showed ST segment depression of 1 mm or more or T-wave inversion in two or more leads, and these findings were not known to be old. Risk factors included systolic blood pressure below 110 mm Hg, rales heard above the bases bilaterally on physical examination, and known unstable ischemic heart disease, defined as a worsening of previously stable angina, the new onset of postinfarction angina or angina after a coronary revascularization procedure, or pain that was the same as that associated with a prior myocardial infarction. The difference between each adjacent pair of risk groups was significant ($P < .001$) (see Table 2-5). (Redrawn with permission from Goldman, L., Cook, E.F., Johnson, P.A., et al. Prediction of the need for intensive care in patients who come to emergency departments with acute chest pain. N. Engl. J. Med. 334:1498-1504, 1996. Copyright © 1996 Massachusetts Medical Society. All rights reserved.)

Table 2–5	Rate of New Major Events, According to the Original Risk Group and as Updated on the Basis of the Occurrence of a Myocardial Infarction or Intermediate or Major Event after Admission.*							
	New Major Event							
	≤12 hr		>12–24 hr		>24–48 hr		>48–72 hr	
	Percentage of Patients (Number/Total Number)							
Risk Group	*Derivation Set*	*Validation Set*	*Derivation Set*	*Validation Set*	*Derivation Set*	*Validation Set*	*Derivation Set*	*Validation Set*
Very low risk	0.1 (5/6188)	0.2 (4/2596)	0.2 (14/7065)	0.2 (7/3394)	0.1 (4/6957)	0.1 (2/3333)	0.1 (9/6888)	0.2 (6/3288)
Low risk	0.7 (11/1511)	0.5 (5/918)	1.1 (16/1475)	1.0 (9/872)	0.5 (7/1377)	1.3 (11/816)	0.7 (9/1309)	0.7 (5/768)
Moderate risk	2.8 (55/1949)	1.1 (9/845)	3.5 (63/1790)	7.6 (28/367)	4.4 (88/1980)	7.5 (33/439)	3.5 (71/2035)	5.2 (25/483)
High risk	12.1 (125/1034)	7.6 (24/317)	24.9 (45/181)	12.8 (5/39)	12.7 (30/237)	18.1 (13/72)	12.0 (37/309)	18.0 (18/100)

From Goldman, L., Cook, E.F., Johnson, P.A., et al.: Prediction of the need for intensive care in patients who come to emergency departments with acute chest pain. N. Engl. J. Med. 334:1498–1504, 1996.

*For the first 12 hr, the risk groups correspond to those shown in Figure 2–9. For the other three intervals, the risk groups have been updated as follows: Patients at very low risk were those originally at very low or low risk who did not have a myocardial infarction or intermediate or major event before the period in question; patients at low risk were those originally at moderate or high risk who did not have a myocardial infarction or intermediate or major event before the period in question; patients at moderate risk were those who had a myocardial infarction or intermediate event but not a major event before the period in question, regardless of the original risk group; and patients at high risk were those who had a major event before the period in question, regardless of the original risk group. For both the derivation and the validation sets, all comparisons between risk groups for all periods were statistically significant (P < .05), except for the comparison between the low- and moderate-risk groups in the first 12 hr and the comparison between the moderate- and high-risk groups at >12–24 hr in the validation set.

use conservative estimates to demonstrate that an intervention is still valuable despite such conservatism, or may include more radical assumptions to prove that intervention is safe despite the most hazardous of assumptions.

Sometimes, decision analyses will demonstrate a dramatic difference between two options and definitively influence decision-making even in the absence of a randomized trial. In other situations, the analysis may reveal that the decision is a close call so that either alternative is reasonable, or suggest that unmeasured or unmeasurable

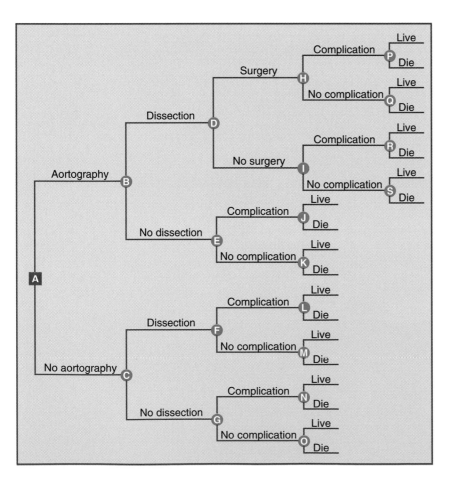

Figure 2–10

Simplified decision tree for the decision of whether or not to perform aortography in a patient who has a suspected aortic dissection, assuming surgery is performed only if the aortography is positive. The *square node* represents the decision point, and the *round nodes* denote the chance events for which probabilities can be estimated.

factors, such as a patient's preferences or local experience or expertise, should be the ultimate arbiter of decision-making. Even when the analysis seems to be definitive, care must be taken to be sure that other, unconsidered factors would not alter the conclusion.

In evaluating decision analyses, several general guidelines can help the reader determine whether the results are likely to be valid, what the results really mean, and whether the results are likely to help in the care of patients (Table 2–6). Decision analyses that follow these general principles are likely to be useful and may serve as the basis for decision-making in the absence of randomized trials; analyses that fail to meet these criteria propose a mathematical conclusion that is not justified by the evidence on which it is based.

Cost-Effectiveness Analysis

When decision analysis indicates that one alternative may be preferable to another, the physician must be aware of the potential incremental cost associated with any incremental benefit. A common approach to consider this question is *cost-effectiveness analysis*. In cost-effectiveness analysis, the incremental costs associated with a particular course of action are quantitatively compared with the incremental benefit. Commonly, costs are assessed in dollars, whereas effectiveness is measured in years of life saved or quality-adjusted years of life saved.[5]

In the estimate of cost, analyses commonly include the cost of the intervention (e.g., tests, medications, operations, hospitalizations), the cost of any adverse effects of the intervention, and the cost of treating diseases or problems that would not have occurred if the patient had not survived because of the intervention. Then, any savings from medications, tests, procedures, and hospitalizations that are avoided are deducted to determine the net costs.

For simplicity, most analyses include only disease-specific subsequent costs, so that the subsequent cost of cardiovascular disease (e.g., heart disease, stroke) is considered in a patient who is saved by thrombolysis, but the potential eventual cost of care for cancer or Alzheimer's disease among survivors is not.[6]

For example, consider a comparison of medication as compared with no medication in patients with hypercholesterolemia.[7] The costs would include the cost of the medication, tests needed to monitor the medication, and side effects of the medication, as well as costs associated with the potential treatment of coronary disease that may develop in the additional days of life gained by the intervention. The savings associated with the treatment program would include those related to the avoidance of subsequent myocardial infarctions, coronary procedures, or other medications.

The effectiveness of an intervention is estimated based on how it changes life expectancy or the quality of life. An intervention may be worthwhile because it prolongs life, improves quality, or does both.

In assessing both costs and benefits, it is important to determine when each will be realized. For many health care programs, costs must be incurred immediately in the form of medications or procedures, whereas the benefit may be delayed until well into the future. Since other events or unexpected developments may occur in the interim, the expectation or even promise of future benefit is

Table 2–6	Users' Guides for Clinical Decision Analysis

Are the Results Valid?

Were all of the important strategies and outcomes included?

Was an explicit and sensible process used to identify, select, and combine the evidence into probabilities?

Were the utilities obtained in an explicit and sensible way from credible sources?

Was the potential impact of any uncertainty in the evidence determined?

What Are the Results?

In the baseline analysis, does one strategy result in a clinically important gain for patients? If not, is the result a toss-up?

How strong is the evidence used in the analysis?

Could the uncertainty in the evidence change the result?

Will the Results Help Me in Caring for My Patients?

Do the probability estimates fit my patients' clinical features?

Do the utilities reflect how my patients would value the outcomes of the decision?

From Richardson, W.S., and Detsky, A.S., for the Evidence-Based Medicine Working Group: Users' guides to the medical literature. VII. How to use a clinical decision analysis? A. Are the results of the study valid? JAMA 273:1292–1295, 1995.

Table 2–7	Example of Costs, Effectiveness, and Cost-Effectiveness for a Hypothetical Intervention in 10,000 Patients for 5 Yr* (High-Risk Patients Versus Low-Risk Patients)

	High Risk		Low Risk	
	Untreated	*Treated*	*Untreated*	*Treated*
Annual death rate	10%	5%	1%	0.5%
Years of life saved†	0	5,209	0	614
Cost of treatment ($ millions) at $2,000/yr	0	90.5	0	99.0
Annual CABG rate	6%	3%	0.6%	0.3%
Cost/CABG	$20,000	$20,000	$20,000	$20,000
Annual MI rate	4%	2%	0.4%	0.2%
Cost/MI	$10,000	$10,000	$10,000	$10,000
Annual rate of other events	4%	2%	0.4%	0.2%
Cost/other event	$5,000	$5,000	$5,000	$5,000
Medical costs ($ millions)	70.0	39.7	8.8	4.4
Total cost ($ millions)	70.0	130.2	8.8	103.4
Total cost difference ($ millions)		60.2		94.8
Approximate cost/yr of life saved		$11,500		$155,000

Reprinted from *Journal of the American College of Cardiology*, Vol. 27, Goldman, L., Garber, A.M., Grover, S.A., and Hlatky, M.A.: Task Force 6. Cost effectiveness of assessment and management of risk factors, pp. 1020–1030, Copyright 1996, with permission from the American College of Cardiology.

Abbreviations: CABG, coronary artery bypass graft surgery; MI, myocardial infarction.

*Simplified so that the intervention reduces all risks by 50%, neither costs nor health effects discounted, all patients are assumed to die at midyear, and the analysis considers only the first 5 yr.

†By life-table analysis.

commonly not valued as highly as the realization of immediate benefit. This principle, which is commonly called *discounting,* is independent of monetary inflation and recognizes the common aphorism that a bird in the hand is worth two in the bush. In simple terms, if one had $10 to spend, one would rather see an immediate benefit than a promise of a similar benefit 5 years from now.

The Cost-Effectiveness Ratio

Very few health interventions both reduce costs and increase quality-adjusted life expectancy. In the calculation of a *cost-effectiveness ratio,* the relative benefit to be gained from an investment in different health programs can be assessed and compared. In such an approach, it is critical that the *incremental cost* and *incremental benefit* of the program be assessed.[8] For example, since streptokinase is already known to be beneficial at a reasonable cost compared with conservative treatment of patients with acute myocardial infarctions and ST segment eleva-

tion, any assessment of tissue plasminogen activator or primary angioplasty should be compared with streptokinase, unless the patient has a contraindication to it, rather than with conservative treatment.

Just as the interpretation of a diagnostic test depends not only on its own intrinsic sensitivity and specificity but also on the prior probability or prevalence in patients on whom it is being used, cost-effectiveness analysis depends not only on the cost and effectiveness of the intervention but also on the risk status of patients in whom the intervention is being considered. The same intervention may be associated with a very favorable cost-effectiveness ratio in high-risk patients but a much less favorable ratio in low-risk patients (Table 2–7). A common metric for a favorable cost-effectiveness ratio is the $35,000 to 45,000 per year of life saved by chronic renal dialysis, a cost that American society has indicated it is willing to pay.

It is oftentimes difficult to compare cost-effectiveness ratios from one study with those of another because of

Table 2–8 **Heart Disease Cost-Effectiveness Overview**

Strategy	Condition	Patient Targeting	Year	$/YLS or $/QALY*
Highly Cost-Effective (<$20,000/YLS or QALY)				
Lovastatin (20 mg/d)	Hyperlipidemia	2°, chol ≥250 mg/dl, men 45–54 yr old	1991	Saves $ and lives
Enalapril	CHF	EF ≤0.35	1994	Saves $ and lives
Nurse counseling manual	Smoking	Post-MI	1993	250
Physician counseling	Smoking	Men 50–54 yr old	1989	1,300
Beta blocker	Post-MI	High risk	1987	3,600
Lovastatin (20 mg/d)	Hyperlipidemia	2°, chol ≥250 mg/dl, women 45–54 yr old	1991	4,700
PTCA	Chronic CAD	Severe angina, 1 VD†	1990	8,700–10,200*
CABG	Chronic CAD	Severe angina, left main disease‡	1982	9,200*
Advice and nicotine gum	Smoking	Women 50–54 yr old	1989	13,000
Propranolol	Hypertension		1990	16,900
Usual care	Hypertension	Women 60 yr old	1990	18,000*
CABG	Chronic CAD	Mild angina, 3 VD§	1982	18,200*
Relatively Cost-Effective ($20,000–$40,000/YLS or QALY)				
Beta blocker	MI	Low risk	1987	20,200
Lovastatin (20 mg/d)	Hyperlipidemia	1°, chol ≥300 mg/dl, 3 RF, men 55–64 yr old	1991	20,200
Exercise	Prophylaxis	Men 35 yr old	1988	22,400*
Lovastatin (20 mg/d)	Hyperlipidemia	2°, chol <250 mg/dl, men 55–64 yr old	1991	22,900
Usual care	Hypertension	Men 40 yr old	1990	23,700*
Hydrochlorothiazide	Hypertension		1990	25,400
Captopril	Post-MI	EF ≤0.40	1995	28,400*
Community-wide screening	Hypertension	DBP ≥105 mm Hg	1976	29,700
ECG Ex testing	CAD	CAD (P = .60), men 55 yr old	1985	30,200* **
Oat bran	Hyperlipidemia	¶	1988	31,600
CCU	Possible MI	MI (P = .50)	1984	35,000
Angiography	CAD	CAD (P = .90), men 55 yr old	1985	37,000* **
ECG Ex testing	Asymptomatic	Men 60 yr old, ≥1 RF	1989	37,700
Borderline (>$40,000–$60,000)				
Lovastatin (20 mg/d)	Hyperlipidemia	1°, chol ≥300 mg/dl, 2 RF, men 55–64 yr old	1991	41,800
Usual care	Hypertension	DBP 95–104 mm Hg	1976	41,900
CABG	Chronic CAD	Severe angina, 2 VD§	1982	42,500*
Usual care	Hypertension	Men 20 yr old	1990	42,600*

Table 2–8   Heart Disease Cost-Effectiveness Overview *Continued*

Strategy	Condition	Patient Targeting	Year	$/YLS or $/QALY*
Borderline (>$40,000–$60,000) *Continued*				
Lovastatin (20 mg/d)	Hyperlipidemia	2°, chol <250 mg/dl, women 55–64 yr old	1991	48,600
Nifedipine	Hypertension		1990	48,900
Expensive (>$60,000–$100,000/YLS or QALY)				
Usual care	Hypertension	Women 20 yr old	1990	64,500*
Angiography	CAD	CAD (P = .60), men 55 yr old	1985	71,300* **
CABG	Chronic CAD	Severe angina, 1 VD§	1982	72,900*
CABG	Chronic CAD	Mild angina, 2 VD§	1982	72,900*
Lovastatin (20 mg/d)	Hyperlipidemia	1°, chol ≥300 mg/dl, 0 RF, men 55–64 yr old	1991	78,300
CCU	Possible MI	MI (P = .20)	1984	88,700
PTCA	Chronic CAD	Mild angina, 1 VD	1990	91,500*
Expensive (>$100,000/YLS or QALY)				
PTCA	Chronic CAD	Mild angina, 2 VD	1990	109,000*
Captopril	Hypertension		1990	111,600
Cholestyramine bulk drug	Hyperlipidemia	¶	1988	115,500
Cholestyramine	Hyperlipidemia	Chol 315 mg/dl, 45–49 yr old	1987	122,100
ECG Ex testing	Asymptomatic	Men 40 yr old	1989	124,400
Lovastatin (20 mg/d)	Hyperlipidemia	1°, chol ≥300 mg/dl, 0 RF, men 45–54 yr old	1991	148,500
CCU	Possible MI	MI (P = .10)	1984	177,400
CCU	Possible MI	MI (P = .05)	1984	373,800
Cholestyramine	Hyperlipidemia	Chol 315 mg/dl, 60–65 yr old	1987	1,055,000
CABG	Chronic CAD	Mild angina, 1 VD§	1982	1,142,000*
Lovastatin (20 mg/d)	Hyperlipidemia	1°, chol ≥300 mg/dl, 0 RF, women 35–44 yr old	1991	2,024,800

Reprinted from *Journal of the American College of Cardiology,* Vol. 27, Goldman, L., Garber, A.M., Grover, S.A., and Hlatky, M.A.: Task Force 6. Cost effectiveness of assessment and management of risk factors, pp. 1020–1030, Copyright 1996, with permission from the American College of Cardiology; adapted with permission from Kupersmith J, Holmes-Rovner M, Hogan A, et al.: Cost-effectiveness analyses in heart disease: ischemia, congestive heart failure, and arrhythmias. Prog. Cardiovasc. Dis. 37:307–348, 1995. References to each of the individual studies are included in this original publication.

Abbreviations: CAD, coronary artery disease; CCU, coronary care unit; CHF, congestive heart failure; chol, pretreatment cholesterol; d, day; DBP, diastolic blood pressure; ECG, electrocardiographic; Ex, exercise; MI, myocardial infarction; Pt, patient; RF, other risk factors; VD, vessel disease; 1°, primary prevention; 2°, secondary prevention.

* All values have been updated to 1993 $; values with an asterisk are shown in dollars per quality-adjusted life years ($/QALY); those without an asterisk are in dollars per year of life saved ($/YLS).

† Fifty-five-yr-old men with type A lesions and normal ventricular function.

‡ Saves both money and lives or quality-adjusted life years.

§ Analysis was of 55-yr-old man; ejection fraction (EF) ≥0.40.

¶ Patients were men (average age 48 yr), 38% smokers, cholesterol ≥265 mg/dl, low-density lipoprotein ≥190 mg/dl.

** Minimal willingness to pay; interventional strategy was coronary artery bypass graft surgery (CABG); percutaneous transluminal coronary angioplasty (PTCA) was not considered.

their varying assumptions. As noted previously, some analyses may have used particularly conservative or generous assumptions to prove a point, and it is difficult to update both the clinical and the cost assumptions of the studies that were performed in the past. Nevertheless, a recent compilation of the approximate cost-effectiveness ratios associated with a variety of cardiologic interventions can help put each into perspective (Table 2–8).

DISCUSSIONS WITH PATIENTS AND DERIVATION OF THE FINAL PLAN

In conjunction with quantitative estimates based on the medical literature and on the physician's experience, the patient's preferences must be taken into account. Although quantitative assessments of quality of life may be included in many decision analyses and cost-effectiveness analyses, these quantitative approaches are not ideally suited to the full consideration of the preferences, attitudes, and individuality of a single patient.

The physician must be cognizant of the benefits, risks, and costs of various options and be an advocate rather than a gatekeeper in advising the individual patient. In conjunction with the patient and the family, it is the physician's responsibility to help set priorities and make recommendations. Although physicians also have a responsibility to recognize the limits and restrictions of society and have a collective duty to try to influence societal priorities, the physician's responsibility to the individual patient is paramount. In an era of capitation and financial incentives to reduce unnecessary testing and treatments, physicians must be careful not to underutilize effective and worthwhile tests and treatments. It is also the physician's responsibility to be sure that the patient and family are fully informed about the various options so that the ultimate course of action is a collective decision based on the best available quantitative and qualitative information.

References

1. Richardson, W.S., and Detsky, A.S., for the Evidence-Based Medicine Working Group: Users' guides to the medical literature. VII. How to use a clinical decision analysis? A. Are the results of the study valid? JAMA 273:1292–1295, 1995.
2. Goldman, L.: Quantitative aspects of clinical reasoning. *In* Fauci, A.S., Braunwald, E., Isselbacher, K.J., et al. (eds.): Harrison's Principles of Internal Medicine. 14th ed. New York, McGraw-Hill, 1998, pp. 9–14.
3. Etchells, E., Bell, C., and Robb, K.: Does this patient have an abnormal systolic murmur? JAMA 277:564–571, 1997.
4. Jaeschke, R., Guyatt, G.H., and Sackett, D.L., for the Evidence-Based Medicine Working Group: Users' guides to the medical literature. III. How to use an article about a diagnostic test. B. What are the results and will they help me in caring for my patients? JAMA 271:703–707, 1994.
5. Goldman, L.: Cost awareness in medicine. *In* Fauci, A.S., Braunwald, E., Isselbacher, K.J., et al. (eds.): Harrison's Principles of Internal Medicine. 14th ed. New York, McGraw-Hill, 1998, pp. 49–52.
6. Detsky, A.S., and Naglie, I.G.: A clinician's guide to cost-effectiveness analysis. Ann. Intern. Med. 113:147–154, 1990.
7. Goldman, L., Garber, A.M., Grover, S.A., and Hlatky, M.A.: Task Force 6. Cost effectiveness of assessment and management of risk factors. J. Am. Coll. Cardiol. 27:1020–1030, 1996.
8. Kupersmith, J., Holmes-Rovner, M., Hogan, A., et al.: Cost-effectiveness analysis in heart disease. Part I: General principles. Prog. Cardiovasc. Dis. 37:161–184, 1994.

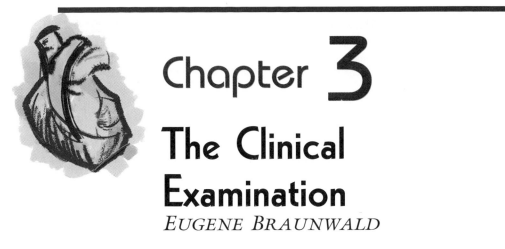

Chapter 3

The Clinical Examination

Eugene Braunwald

Since the development of the electrocardiograph by Einthoven and the x-ray by Roentgen a century ago, a series of ever more accurate noninvasive and invasive tests have been developed to characterize the structure and function of the cardiovascular system. However valuable these tests may be, they are not inexpensive, are sometimes uncomfortable or hazardous, and can provide conflicting information. The decision to undertake any specialized test of the cardiovascular system must be made in the light of the findings of the clinical examination, that is, the history and physical examination.[1] The primary care physician's findings on clinical examination are of the utmost importance in deciding whether specialized testing is to be performed, whether continued observation is advisable, whether the advice of a consultant should be sought, or whether the patient can be reassured that serious cardiovascular disease is not present.

Many cardiovascular conditions are part of systemic illnesses, and in conducting the clinical examination, the primary care physician must be aware of three major pitfalls: (1) failure to recognize cardiovascular manifestations in patients with recognized systemic illnesses frequently associated with heart disease, such as congenital heart disease in patients with the Down syndrome; (2) failure to recognize the presence of the underlying systemic disorder in a patient with recognized cardiovascular disease, such as thyrotoxicosis in a patient with unexplained atrial fibrillation; and (3) failure to recognize the cardiac cause of extracardiac manifestations of cardiac disease, such as severe jaundice in a patient with acute right ventricular failure. Table 3–1 lists a number of abnormalities found in the examination of the extremities, skin, eyes, and abdomen that may be observed in patients with cardiovascular disorders.

SYSTEMIC DISORDERS WITH CARDIOVASCULAR MANIFESTATIONS

The noncardiac history and physical examination are of critical importance because of the high frequency of cardiovascular manifestations in many systemic disorders. For example, endocrine abnormalities commonly have important cardiac manifestations; thyrotoxicosis can intensify angina and cause high-output heart failure; myxedema can be responsible for dilated cardiomyopathy and pericardial effusion; acromegaly often causes a dilated and hypertrophic cardiomyopathy. A number of endocrine disorders—Cushing's syndrome, primary hyperaldosteronism, pheochromocytoma, and hyperparathyroidism—may cause hypertension, whereas diabetes may be associated with premature and especially severe atherosclerotic coronary disease. Rheumatoid arthritis may be responsible for constrictive pericarditis, cardiac tamponade, and valvular heart disease, most commonly aortic regurgitation; systemic lupus erythematosus may be associated with mitral regurgitation and pericarditis; and systemic sclerosis may occur with pericarditis, systemic hypertension, pulmonary hypertension, and restrictive cardiomyopathy. Among hematologic disorders, chronic anemia may cause high-output heart failure; polycythemia is associated with an increased risk of clotting, including coronary thrombosis; and hemochromatosis can result in a restrictive cardiomyopathy.

A variety of tumors may metastasize to the pericardium and cause cardiac constriction or tamponade; myocardial metastases can cause a variety of arrhythmias. A number of cardiovascular disorders may occur during pregnancy, including pre-eclampsia manifested by hyper-

Table 3–1	Noncardiac Physical Findings in Cardiac Disorders	
Physical Finding	**Cause**	**Cardiac Condition**
General Appearance		
Shaking of body with each heartbeat	⇑ stroke volume	Severe aortic regurgitation, third degree AV block
Weight loss, malnutrition, cachexia	Reduced cardiac output, hypermetabolism	Advanced chronic heart failure
Marked obesity, somnolence, cyanosis	Impaired ventilation, pickwickian syndrome	Cor pulmonale
Long extremities, arm span > height, pubis-foot > head-pubis, arachnodactyly (spider fingers)	Marfan's syndrome	Thoracic aortic aneurysm, mitral valve prolapse
Bones and Skeleton		
Short stature, cubitus valgus, medial deviation of forearm	Turner's syndrome	Coarctation of the aorta, bicuspid aortic valve
Deformities of radius, thumb with extra phalanx	Holt-Oram syndrome	Familial atrial septal defect
Clubbing of the digits	Cyanosis	Congenital heart disease, cor pulmonale, pulmonary arteriovenous fistula, infective endocarditis
Severe kyphoscoliosis	Congenital	Cor pulmonale, Marfan's syndrome
Skin		
Bronze pigmentation of skin, loss of axillary and pubic hair	Hemochromatosis	Restrictive cardiomyopathy
Jaundice	Cardiac cirrhosis, hemochromatosis	Congestive heart failure, tricuspid valve disease, chronic constrictive pericarditis
Small, brown, macular lesions on head and trunk	Lentigines	Hypertrophic cardiomyopathy, pulmonary stenosis
Xanthoma, tuboeruptive (extensive surface of extremities), striatum pulmare (palmar and digital creases)	Subcutaneous deposits of cholesterol	Premature atherosclerosis
Small, tender, purplish, erythematous skin lesions in pads of fingers or toes	Osler's nodes	Infective endocarditis
Petechiae, especially under nail beds	Splinter hemorrhage	Infective endocarditis
Raised, nontender hemorrhagic lesions in palms or soles	Janeway's lesions	Infective endocarditis
Capillary hemangiomas in skin, lips, nasal mucosa, gastrointestinal tract	Hereditary telangiectasis (Osler-Weber-Rendu disease)	Pulmonary arteriovenous fistula with cyanosis
Eyes		
Exopthalmus and stare	Hyperthyroidism, ⇑ adrenergic tone	High output heart failure
Ptosis, dull, expressionless face	Myotonic dystrophy	AV block, arrhythmias
Ptosis with external ophthalmoplegia	Kearns-Sayre syndrome	Third-degree AV block
Blue sclerae	Osteogenesis imperfecta	Aortic dilatation, regurgitation, and dissection, mitral valve prolapse
Retinal changes	Arteriolar narrowing	Hypertension
Beading of retinal artery	Hypercholesterolemia	Atherosclerosis
White-centered retinal hemorrhage near optic disc	Roth spot	Embolization secondary to infective endocarditis
Retinal artery occlusion	Embolus	Atrial fibrillation, mitral stenosis, left atrial myxoma, atherosclerosis of ascending aorta or arch vessels
Cyanosis involving conjunctivae and mucous membranes (central cyanosis)	Arterial desaturation	Intracardiac or intrapulmonary right-to-left shunting
Cyanosis of cool, exposed extremities (peripheral cyanosis)	Impaired perfusion	Heart failure, shock, Raynaud's phenomenon
Abdomen		
Splenomegaly, hepatomegaly, ascites	Severe hepatic congestion	Constrictive pericarditis, tricuspid valve disease
Palpable, enlarged kidney	Polycystic renal disease	Hypertension
Systolic bruit over abdomen	Renal artery stenosis	Hypertension

Abbreviation: AV, atrioventricular.

tension, aggravation of symptoms in patients with congenital or valvular heart disease, and primary pulmonary hypertension. The skeletal muscular dystrophies can be associated with a variety of cardiac manifestations, including arrhythmias and dilated and restrictive cardiomyopathies. Chronic renal failure may be associated with pericarditis, systemic hypertension, and accelerated atherosclerosis.

THE HISTORY

Questionnaires and screening histories by nurses or assistants are often quite useful in focusing the physician's questioning, and directed interval histories can frequently be obtained by others, but the first definitive clinical examination is the responsibility of the physician and should not be delegated. There are important nuances that the physician can appreciate, and it is through taking a careful history that she or he can gain the patient's confidence, which is often necessary when agreement must be obtained to undergo complex, uncomfortable, and sometimes risky diagnostic maneuvers and therapeutic interventions. The history also often allows identification of the relationship between cardiovascular and noncardiovascular disease.

Initially, in obtaining the history, the patient should be encouraged to describe any complaints in his or her own way. This should be followed by directed interrogation regarding the onset, progression, and timing of symptoms as well as a description of their aggravating and alleviating conditions. A detailed general medical history, including occupational, family, and nutritional history, is of critical importance in the patient with known or suspected cardiovascular disease. For example, a history of recent infection, dental extraction, urogenital manipulation, or intravenous drug abuse is vital in the evaluation of patients with known or suspected congenital heart disease or acquired valvular abnormalities because the history may suggest the presence of infective endocarditis. A history of cigarette smoking, hypertension, hypercholesterolemia, or diabetes mellitus in the patient and a history of premature vascular disease in first-degree relatives are risk factors for coronary artery disease. Atherosclerosis is usually a diffuse vascular disease, and a history or clinical manifestations of extracoronary arterial disease — cerebral, renal, aortic, peripheral, or mesenteric vascular disease — raise the likelihood of the presence of coronary artery disease.

When symptoms suggestive of cardiac disease, such as dyspnea or chest pain, are present, their aggravation by activity and relief by rest support their cardiovascular origin. Symptoms at rest, of course, do not exclude serious cardiovascular disease, since most cardiac arrhythmias, Prinzmetal's angina, and paroxysmal nocturnal dyspnea characteristically occur at rest. The response to therapy is also a critical part of the history. Patients in whom hypertension is first diagnosed whose blood pressure fails to respond to adequate doses of two different classes of antihypertensive agents may have secondary rather than essential hypertension (see Chap. 11), whereas the failure of the initial administration of appropriate doses of loop diuretics to cause diuresis and improvement in patients with dyspnea and edema should throw some doubt on the diagnosis of congestive heart failure. On the other hand, the diagnosis of angina pectoris is supported when the threshold for exertional chest pain rises in patients receiving beta blockers or nitrates.

Dyspnea

This symptom, an abnormally uncomfortable awareness of breathing, may be caused by a wide variety of cardiac and pulmonary diseases, as well as by anxiety and severe obesity.[2] The mechanisms of dyspnea and the distinction among the various causes of this important symptom are described in Chapter 8.

It is useful to separate dyspnea into acute and chronic forms. *Acute dyspnea* occurs in pulmonary edema, pulmonary embolism, pneumonia, asthma, and other forms of airway obstruction. Tachyarrhythmias, acute myocardial infarction, and ruptured chordae tendineae can also cause acute dyspnea in persons who were previously well. *Chronic dyspnea* secondary to cardiac disease is often accompanied by orthopnea, third or fourth heart sounds, and cardiomegaly and usually responds to diuretic therapy. Dyspnea that awakens the patient from sleep and is relieved by sitting upright is characteristic of left ventricular failure (paroxysmal nocturnal dyspnea). In patients with chronic pulmonary disease, nocturnal dyspnea occurs earlier in the night than does cardiac dyspnea, usually immediately on assuming the recumbent position, and it rarely awakens the patient from sleep.[3] It is accompanied and relieved by cough and expectoration. Dyspnea occurring at rest, but not on exertion, and accompanied by sighing respiration is often due to an anxiety state.[4]

Chest Pain or Discomfort

This is one of the most common complaints faced by primary care physicians and is discussed in detail in Chapter 7. Despite the availability of a number of sophisticated and accurate noninvasive laboratory tests for the evaluation of chest pain, the history remains the cornerstone of diagnosis.[5] It is of critical importance for the primary care physician to recognize the discomfort associated with myocardial ischemia. Ischemic discomfort is characteristically described as a constricting, squeezing, or burning feeling or as a "heaviness" in the chest. Nonischemic discomfort is more likely to be described as "knifelike"—sharp, stabbing pain that may be aggravated by cough or respiration. Ischemic discomfort is most commonly retrosternal, in the anterior midthorax, in the arms, shoulders, neck, cheeks, teeth, forearms, and fingers, whereas pain localized to the left submammary area or that radiates to above the mandible or to below the umbilicus is usually not ischemic. Ischemic chest discomfort is usually provoked by exercise, excitement, cold weather, a heavy meal, or smoking a cigarette, and especially by a combination of these activities. Discomfort that occurs after cessation of exercise or is provoked by a particular body motion is usually not ischemic.

Effort angina (see Chaps. 7 and 18) usually lasts between 3 and 20 minutes. Exertion and emotion are frequent precipitants of stable angina, and relief by rest or administration of nitroglycerin is helpful in the diagnosis. Anginal discomfort may be accompanied by exertional dyspnea, which sometimes occurs without chest discomfort as an anginal equivalent. Angina at rest, which is characteristic of unstable angina (see Chap. 20), is often more severe than exertional angina, is usually described as frank pain, may awaken the patient from sleep (nocturnal angina), and may not be relieved by nitrates. When rest angina persists for more than 20 minutes, an electrocardiogram and serum markers are required to differentiate unstable angina from acute myocardial infarction. The chest pain of acute myocardial infarction is usually severe and generally persists for more than 30 minutes (see Chap. 19).

The primary care physician should be alert to the combination of chest pain and profuse diaphoresis, since this often signals a serious disorder, such as acute myocardial infarction or pulmonary embolism. The chest pain of acute myocardial infarction is often accompanied by nausea and vomiting, whereas the combination of chest pain and acute dyspnea occurs in myocardial infarction, pulmonary embolism, pneumothorax, and mediastinal emphysema. The pain of an expanding or rupturing thoracic aortic aneurysm is often severe and persistent and is localized to the interscapular region with radiation laterally and anteriorly (see Chap. 27).

Syncope (see Chap. 12)

The medical history is of critical importance in determining the cause of syncope. Vasovagal syncope, the most common cause of syncope, may occur in response to prolonged standing, emotional stress and physical exhaustion, pain, venipuncture, the sight of blood, or another emotion. Orthostatic hypotension may be precipitated by hypovolemia, dehydration, or the excessive administration of antihypertensive drugs. Syncope secondary to a cardiac arrhythmia (transient ventricular fibrillation or third-degree atrioventricular block) is usually virtually instantaneous in onset. Syncope accompanied by chest pain may occur in massive myocardial infarction. Exertional syncope is characteristic of aortic stenosis and hypertrophic obstructive cardiomyopathy. Syncope of cardiovascular origin is usually not associated with convulsive movements or a postsyncopal confusional state, and consciousness is usually regained promptly.

Edema (see Chap. 9)

Bilateral ankle edema, most prominent at the end of the day, is characteristic of congestive heart failure. This diagnosis is strongly supported when edema is accompanied by exertional dyspnea. Cardiac edema is usually preceded by a gain in weight of 5 to 10 lb, is symmetric, and progresses upward from the ankles to the shins, thighs, and genitalia. Cardiac edema that is *not* associated with orthopnea or severe dyspnea may be caused by chronic constrictive pericarditis or tricuspid stenosis. Bilateral ankle edema also occurs in patients with chronic bilateral thrombophlebitis. The presence of periorbital edema favors a renal origin, hypoproteinemia, myxedema, or angioneurotic edema. When the patient reports that edema has been limited to the upper extremities, neck, and face, obstruction of the superior vena cava should be considered. Unilateral edema of an extremity is most commonly caused by thrombophlebitis or lymphatic obstruction, and a history of ulceration and pigmentation of the legs may accompany edema due to venous disease. When jaundice accompanies edema, or when ascites precedes edema, the edema is often of hepatic origin.

Cyanosis

Cyanosis, like edema, is both a symptom, since it is frequently reported by the patient, and a physical finding, because it may be noted by the physician. It is a bluish coloration of the skin and mucous membranes and is

Table 3–2	Causes of Cyanosis

Central Cyanosis

Decreased arterial oxygen saturation
   Decreased atmospheric pressure—high altitude
   Impaired pulmonary function
      Alveolar hypoventilation
      Uneven relationships between pulmonary ventilation and perfusion
         (perfusion of hypoventilated alveoli)
      Impaired oxygen diffusion
   Anatomic shunts
      Certain types of congenital heart disease
      Pulmonary arteriovenous fistulas
      Multiple small intrapulmonary shunts
      Hemoglobin with low affinity for oxygen
Hemoglobin abnormalities
   Methemoglobinemia—hereditary, acquired
   Sulfhemoglobinemia—acquired
   Carboxyhemoglobinemia (not true cyanosis)

Peripheral Cyanosis

Reduced cardiac output
Cold exposure
Redistribution of blood flow from extremities
Arterial obstruction
Venous obstruction

From Braunwald, E.: Hypoxia, Polycythemia, and Cyanosis. *In* Fauci, A., Braunwald, E., Isselbacher, K.J., et al., (eds.): Harrison's Principles of Internal Medicine. 14th ed. New York, McGraw-Hill, 1998, pp. 205–210. Reproduced with permission of The McGraw-Hill Companies.

caused by an increased absolute quantity of reduced hemoglobin (>5 gm/dl) in the capillary bed just beneath the surface. It is recognized most readily in the nail beds, lips, and oral mucosa. There are two principal causes of cyanosis—central and peripheral (Table 3–2).

CENTRAL CYANOSIS. In this form of cyanosis, the arterial blood is unsaturated as a consequence of reduced inspired oxygen concentration—as occurs at a high altitude (usually above 10,000 ft)—or of impaired pulmonary function. It may occur transiently (as in acute extensive pneumonia) or chronically (as in advanced emphysema). Pulmonary edema can reduce oxygen diffusion from the alveoli to the pulmonary capillaries and thereby result in arterial unsaturation and cyanosis. Anatomic shunt, in which desaturated venous blood bypasses the pulmonary capillary bed, is an important cause of cyanosis. In adults, pulmonary arteriovenous fistulas and congenital cardiac malformation, such as Eisenmenger's syndrome and tetralogy of Fallot (see Chap. 26), are most commonly responsible for right-to-left shunting. Abnormalities of hemoglobin (see Table 3–2), including those with an abnormally low affinity for oxygen, are uncommon causes of central cyanosis.

Prolonged central cyanosis is usually accompanied by clubbing of the digits, that is, selective enlargement of the terminal phalanges of the fingers and toes (Fig. 3–1). Clubbing is *not* usually observed with cyanosis due to abnormalities of hemoglobin nor with peripheral cyanosis. In addition to chronic central cyanosis, clubbing is also frequent in patients with infective endocarditis, lung cancer, cystic fibrosis, bronchiectasis, and ulcerative colitis.

PERIPHERAL CYANOSIS. This form of cyanosis is more common than central cyanosis and is caused by

*assoc. c̄ central cyanosis
also c̄ lung ca, infective endo carditis
CF, UC, bronchiectasis*

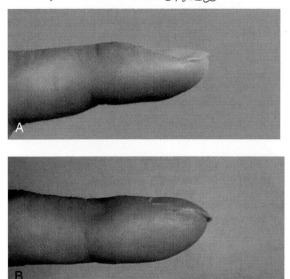

Figure 3–1

A, Profile of a normal finger. *B*, Profile of a clubbed finger, with bulbous enlargement of the terminal phalanx and convexity of the nail bed. (*A* and *B*, From Mir, M.A.: Atlas of Clinical Diagnosis. London, W.B. Saunders, 1995, pp. 199, 207.)

reduced blood flow to the extremities, particularly to distal portions, resulting in greater than normal extraction of oxygen from the hemoglobin in red cells traversing the capillary bed. Cutaneous vasoconstriction, as occurs with cold exposure, especially with cold immersion, can cause peripheral cyanosis. Blood flow to the periphery is also reduced in heart failure, both acute and chronic, shock, and with arterial obstruction. Venous obstruction, most commonly caused by thrombophlebitis, can cause cyanosis by dilating the subpapillary venous plexus.

Cough

Although it can be caused by a variety of inflammatory, allergic, or neoplastic disorders of the tracheobronchial tree, cough may be an important manifestation of left ventricular failure and frequently accompanies dyspnea, orthopnea, and paroxysmal nocturnal dyspnea. Cough secondary to left ventricular failure or mitral valve disease is usually dry and often nocturnal. In addition to pulmonary venous hypertension, cough may be caused by other cardiovascular conditions that compress the tracheobronchial tree,[6] including marked enlargement of the left atrium or pulmonary artery (which may also cause hoarseness by compressing the recurrent laryngeal nerve) and thoracic aortic aneurysm. Cough accompanied by frothy, pink sputum occurs in pulmonary edema, whereas yellowish mucoid sputum suggests an infection of the tracheobronchial tree. Hemoptysis most commonly reflects tracheobronchial disease, but it may be seen in four important cardiac conditions—mitral stenosis, pulmonary embolism, pulmonary edema, and pulmonary arteriovenous fistula.

Fatigue

This nonspecific symptom is present in many cardiovascular and noncardiovascular disorders. Fatigue is an important manifestation of low cardiac output and impaired systemic perfusion in heart failure. It may also be seen in heart failure after excessive diuresis. Profound fatigue is observed in patients with large myocardial infarcts as well as in patients with hypertension receiving antihypertensive therapy, in whom the blood pressure has been lowered too rapidly.

Palpitations

A variety of changes (see Chap. 10) in cardiac rhythm or rate can cause palpitations, an unpleasant awareness of rapid or forceful beating of the heart. A careful history is often helpful in identifying the cause of palpitations. An elevation of the stroke volume, valvular regurgitation, thyrotoxicosis, and marked bradycardia can all cause palpitations. When the patient takes his or her pulse, the rate, when regular, provides a clue to the mechanism underlying the palpitations. In many persons, the cause of palpitations cannot be uncovered despite careful workup, including a 48-hour ambulatory electrocardiogram. Anxiety is often responsible.

Drug-Induced Heart Disease

Cardiovascular manifestations of adverse reaction to drugs are shown in Table 3–3. The use of legal and illegal drugs is emerging as an increasingly important cause of heart disease. For this reason, it is critical for the primary care physician to obtain a careful drug history in evaluating patients with known or suspected cardiovascular disease. For example, quinidine, flecainide, and other class I antiarrhythmic agents may cause Q-T prolongation, torsades de pointes, and recurrent syncope (see Chap. 23). Lithium and tricyclic antidepressants may also be responsible for cardiac arrhythmias. Digitalis intoxication can cause atrial and ventricular tachyarrhythmias and atrioventricular block. Disopyramide, beta receptor blockers, verapamil, and diltiazem are cardiac depressants and may exacerbate (or rarely, induce) congestive heart failure. The excessive ingestion of alcohol can cause a chronic—often fatal—form of heart failure (alcoholic cardiomyopathy), and binge drinking can be responsible for acute decompensation, a variety of cardiac tachyarrhythmias and sudden death. Cocaine can cause myocarditis, coronary spasm, myocardial ischemia, myocardial infarction, and sudden death. Doxorubicin and cyclophosphamide can be responsible for both acute and chronic left ventricular failure as well as a variety of arrhythmias, whereas 5-fluorouracil can cause angina secondary to coronary spasm.

Assessing Cardiovascular Disability

The history is critical in evaluating cardiovascular disability. The New York Heart Association has proposed four classes ranging from no symptoms on "ordinary"

Table 3-3   Cardiovascular Manifestations of Adverse Reactions to Drugs

Acute Chest Pain (Nonischemic)

Bleomycin

Angina Exacerbation

Alpha blockers
Beta blocker withdrawal
Ergotamine
Excessive thyroxine
Hydralazine
Methysergide
Minoxidil
Nifedipine
Oxytocin
Vasopressin

Arrhythmias

Adriamycin
Antiarrhythmic drugs
Astemizole
Atropine
Anticholinesterases
Beta blockers
Daunorubicin
Digitalis
Emetine
Erythromycin
Guanethidine
Lithium
Papaverine
Phenothiazines, particularly thioridazine
Sympathomimetics
Terfenadine
Theophylline
Thyroid hormone
Tricyclic antidepressants
Verapamil

AV Block

Clonidine
Methyldopa
Verapamil

Cardiomyopathy

Adriamycin
Daunorubicin
Emetine
Lithium
Phenothiazines
Sulfonamides
Sympathomimetics

Fluid Retention/Congestive Heart Failure/Edema

Beta blockers
Calcium blockers
Carbenoxolone
Diazoxide
Estrogens
Indomethacin
Mannitol
Minoxidil
Phenylbutazone
Steroids
Verapamil

Hypotension (*see also* **Arrhythmias**)

Amiodarone (perioperative)
Calcium channel blockers, e.g., nifedipine
Citrated blood
Diuretics
Interleukin-2
Levodopa
Morphine
Nitroglycerin
Phenothiazines
Protamine
Quinidine

Hypertension

Clonidine withdrawal
Corticotropin
Cyclosporine
Glucocorticoids
Monoamine oxidase inhibitors with sympathomimetics
NSAIDs (some)
Oral contraceptives
Sympathomimetics
Tricyclic antidepressants with sympathomimetics

Pericarditis

Emetine
Hydralazine
Methysergide
Procainamide

Pericardial Effusion

Minoxidil

Thomboembolism

Oral contraceptives

From Wood, A.J.: Adverse reactions to drugs. *In* Fauci, A., Braunwald, E., Isselbacher, K.J., et al. (eds.): Harrison's Principles of Internal Medicine. 14th ed. New York, McGraw-Hill, 1998. Reproduced with permission of The McGraw-Hill Companies.
Abbreviations: AV, atrioventricular; NSAIDs, nonsteroidal anti-inflammatory drugs.

activity to symptoms at rest[7] (Table 3–4). The Canadian Cardiovascular Society Functional Classification provides a similar approach to the assessment of the severity of angina.[8] Goldman and associates have developed the so-called Specific Activity Scale based on the estimated metabolic cost of various activities. This scale is a more reproducible and better predictor of exercise tolerance than either of the other two scales.[9] Regardless of which scale is used, it is critical to determine whether the patient's disability is stable, increasing, or diminishing over time. This can be ascertained by comparing the symptoms elicited by any specific task, such as climbing two flights of stairs, currently and at some previous time (e.g., 6 months).

PHYSICAL EXAMINATION

Arterial Pressure

The indirect measurement of arterial pressure is described in Chapter 11.

Arterial Pulse

Palpation of the carotid pulse is most useful in assessing the central aortic pulse (Table 3–5). In examining this pulse, the right thumb should be applied to the left carotid artery in the lower third of the neck (see Fig. 3–8C). The volume, contour, frequency, and regularity of the pulse should be noted.[10, 11] Reduced carotid pulsations occur in shock and other conditions with markedly reduced stroke volume as well as in carotid atherosclerosis. The carotid pulse is diminished in amplitude and rises more slowly than normal (*pulsus parvus et tardus*) Fig. 3–2B) in patients with fixed, severe obstruction to left ventricular outflow (aortic valvular stenosis, congenital subaortic stenosis). In contrast, the arterial pulse is exaggerated in volume with a sharp rise in conditions in which the stroke volume is augmented, such as aortic regurgitation, arteriovenous fistula, and other causes of high cardiac output. The pulse rises more rapidly than normal when the arterial tree is inelastic, as occurs in patients with diffuse atherosclerosis as well as in the elderly.

An arterial pulse with two systolic peaks (*pulsus bisfer-*

Table 3–4 **A Comparison of Three Methods of Assessing Cardiovascular Disability**

Class	New York Heart Association Functional Classification	Canadian Cardiovascular Society Functional Classification	Specific Activity Scale
I	Patients with cardiac disease but without resulting limitations of physical activity. Ordinary physical activity does not cause undue fatigue, palpitation, dyspnea, or anginal pain.	Ordinary physical activity, such as walking and climbing stairs, does not cause angina. Angina with strenuous or rapid or prolonged exertion at work or recreation.	Patients can perform to completion any activity requiring ≤ 7 metabolic equivalents, e.g., can carry 24 lb up eight steps; carry objects that weigh 80 lb; do outdoor work (shovel snow, spade soil); do recreational activities (skiing, basketball, squash, handball, jog/walk 5 mph).
II	Patients with cardiac disease resulting in slight limitation of physical activity. They are comfortable at rest. Ordinary physical activity results in fatigue, palpitation, dyspnea, or anginal pain.	Slight limitation of ordinary activity. Walking or climbing stairs rapidly, walking uphill, walking or stair climbing after meals, in cold, in wind, or when under emotional stress, or only during the few hours after awakening. Walking more than two blocks on the level and climbing more than one flight of ordinary stairs at a normal pace and in normal conditions.	Patients can perform to completion any activity requiring ≤ 5 metabolic equivalents, e.g., have sexual intercourse without stopping, garden, rake, weed, roller skate, dance fox trot, walk at 4 mph on level ground, but cannot and do not perform to completion activities requiring ≥ 7 metabolic equivalents.
III	Patients with cardiac disease resulting in marked limitation of physical activity. They are comfortable at rest. Less than ordinary physical activity causes fatigue, palpitation, dyspnea, or anginal pain.	Marked limitation of ordinary physical activity. Walking one to two blocks on the level and climbing more than one flight in normal conditions.	Patients can perform to completion any activity requiring ≤ 2 metabolic equivalents, e.g., shower without stopping, strip and make bed, clean windows, walk 2.5 mph, bowl, play golf, dress without stopping, but cannot and do not perform to completion any activities requiring ≥ 5 metabolic equivalents.
IV	Patient with cardiac disease resulting in inability to carry on any physical activity without discomfort. Symptoms of cardiac insufficiency or of the anginal syndrome may be present even at rest. If any physical activity is undertaken, discomfort is increased.	Inability to carry on any physical activity without discomfort—anginal syndrome *may be* present at rest.	Patients cannot or do not perform to completion activities requiring ≥ 2 metabolic equivalents. *Cannot* carry out activities listed above (Specific Activity Scale, Class III).

From Goldman, L., Hashimoto, B., Cook, E.F., and Loscalzo, A.: Comparative reproducibility and validity of systems for assessing cardiovascular functional class: Advantages of a new specific activity scale. Circulation 64:1227, 1981. Copyright 1981 American Heart Association.

iens) occurs in patients with isolated aortic regurgitation (see Fig. 3–2C), with the combination of aortic regurgitation and stenosis, and with hypertrophic obstructive cardiomyopathy (see Fig. 3–2D). A double pulse in which the second peak occurs in diastole *(dicrotic pulse)* (see Fig. 3–2E) may occur in normal subjects with reduced peripheral resistance and hypotension (as in high fever) as well as in conditions in which a low stroke volume is ejected into an elastic aorta (heart failure, hypovolemic shock, cardiac tamponade).[12]

Table 3–5 **Diagnostic Significance of Visible and Palpable Carotid Arterial Pulse Waves**

Diagnosis	Carotid Arterial Pulse
Aortic stenosis	Early anacrotic notch, shudder, tardus and parvus rise, prolonged duration
Aortic insufficiency	Rapid rise, bifid peak, prolonged duration, reduced dicrotic notch, rapid runoff
Aortic stenosis and insufficiency	Bifid or bisferiens pulse
Hypertrophic cardiomyopathy	Rapid rise, early abrupt peak, plateau or gentle second hump (pulsus bisferiens)
Mitral stenosis	Smooth contour, normal or reduced amplitude and duration
Mitral insufficiency	Smooth contour, normal or reduced amplitude and duration
Left ventricular ischemia	Low amplitude
Left ventricular failure	Low amplitude, pulsus alternans
Constrictive pericarditis	Reduced amplitude, pulsus paradoxus
Pericardial tamponade	Reduced amplitude, pulsus paradoxus
Coarctation of aorta	Increased force, femoral delay or damping
Atherosclerosis	Reduced amplitude, thrill
Peripheral arteriovenous fistula	Rapid rise and runoff
Anemia, fever, sepsis thyrotoxicosis	Increased pulse amplitude and rate

From Evans, T.C., Giuliani, E.R., Tancredi, R.G., and Brandenburg, R.O.: Physical Examination. *In* Giuliani, E.R., Fuster, V., Gersh, B., et al. (eds.): Cardiology: Fundamentals and Practice. 2nd ed. Rochester, MN, Mayo Foundation, 1991, pp. 204–272. By permission of Mayo Foundation.

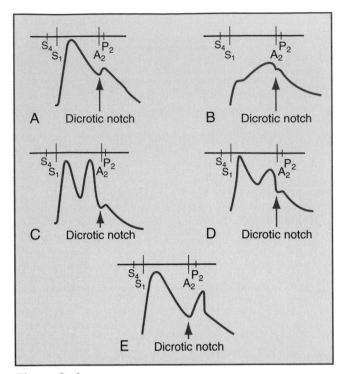

Figure 3–2

Schematic diagrams of the configurational changes in the carotid pulse and their differential diagnoses. Heart sounds are also illustrated. *A,* Normal. S_4, atrial sound; S_1, first heart sound; A_2, aortic component of the second heart sound; P_2, pulmonic component of the second heart sound. *B,* Anacrotic pulse with slow initial upstroke. The peak is close to the S_2. These features suggest fixed left ventricular outflow obstruction, such as occurs with valvular aortic stenosis. *C,* Pulsus bisferiens with both percussion and tidal waves occurring during systole. This type of carotid pulse contour is most frequently observed in patients with hemodynamically significant aortic regurgitation or combined aortic stenosis and regurgitation with dominant regurgitation. It is rarely observed in mitral valve prolapse or in normal individuals. *D,* Pulsus bisferiens in hypertrophic obstructive cardiomyopathy. It is rarely appreciated at the bedside by palpation. *E,* Dicrotic pulse results from an accentuated dicrotic wave and tends to occur in sepsis, in severe heart failure, in hypovolemic shock, in cardiac tamponade, and after aortic valve replacement. (*A–E,* From Chatterjee, K.: Bedside evaluation of the heart: The physical examination. *In* Chatterjee, K., and Parmley, W. [eds.]: Cardiology: An Illustrated Text/Reference. Philadelphia, J.B. Lippincott, 1991, pp. 3.11–3.51.)

Pulsus alternans is the condition in which strong and weak pulses alternate, although they occur with absolute regularity. It is detected best in a more peripheral vessel, such as the radial artery, and is accompanied by alternation in the intensity of Korotkoff's sounds during indirect sphygmomanometry. Pulsus alternans is often initiated by a premature ventricular contraction and is usually a sign of advanced myocardial failure. Not to be confused with pulsus alternans is *pulsus bigeminus,* in which a premature contraction follows every sinus beat and in which the weak beat follows a shorter interval.

Normally, the arterial pressure declines slightly (<10 mm Hg) during inspiration. An exaggerated decline *(pulsus paradoxus)* may be palpable as a diminished arterial pulse during inspiration, but as is the case for pulsus alternans, pulsus paradoxus is more readily detected by sphygmomanometry. It is a key finding in cardiac tamponade but may also be present in chronic constrictive pericarditis, hypovolemic shock, pulmonary embolism, and asthma or other conditions causing unusually wide respiratory swings in intrapleural pressure.

Peripheral Arterial Pulse

In patients suspected of having ischemic heart disease or peripheral arteriosclerosis, bilateral palpation of the common carotid, brachial, radial, femoral, dorsalis pedis, and posterior tibial arteries should be carried out. Diminished or absent pulses suggest obstruction. Systolic bruits are frequently audible at the site of obstruction. The abdominal aorta should be palpated, both above and below the umbilicus.

Jugular Venous Pulse

The pressure pulse in the right atrium is reflected in the pulsations of the internal jugular veins.[13] Their examination is best carried out on the right side of the neck, with the patient's head resting on a pillow at an angle at which the skin overlying the jugular vein is just visible at the angle of the mandible. The height of the jugular venous pressure is estimated as the top of the visible proximal vein. It is normally less than 4 cm above the sternal angle, corresponding to a right atrial pressure of 9 cm (the right atrium being 5 cm below the sternal angle) (Fig. 3–3). When the jugular veins are distended with the patient in the sitting position, the venous pressure is markedly elevated (Fig. 3–4). The jugular venous pressure is elevated in right heart failure irrespective of cause, tricuspid valve disease, pericardial constriction, pericardial tamponade, and obstruction of the superior

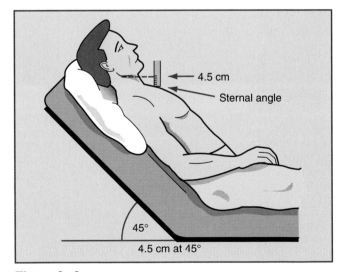

Figure 3–3

Venous pressure can be estimated by observing the upper level of internal jugular pulsations above the sternal angle. If it is over 4.5 cm at 45 degrees, it indicates an elevated right atrial pressure. (From Constant, J.: Bedside Cardiology. 4th ed. Boston, Little, Brown, 1993, p. 71. Reprinted by permission of Lippincott-Raven, Publishers.)

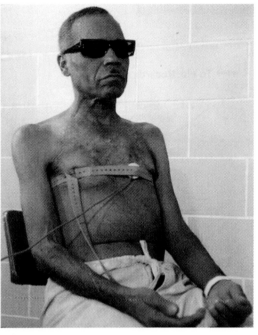

Figure 3–4

Visible external jugular venous distention extends to the mandibular level in a seated patient with effusive-constrictive pericarditis. Right atrial mean pressure was 20 mm Hg. (From Fowler, N.O.: Pericardial disease. *In* Abelmann, W.H. [vol. ed.]: Cardiomyopathies, Myocarditis, and Pericardial Disease. Braunwald, E. [ser. ed.]: Atlas of Heart Diseases. Vol. 2. Philadelphia, Current Medicine, 1995, pp. 13.1–13.16.)

vena cava. In Kussmaul's sign, which occurs typically in constrictive pericarditis and tricuspid stenosis, there is a paradoxical rise in jugular venous pressure during inspiration because the increased venous return from the reduction in intrapericardial pressure during inspiration cannot be accommodated in the right side of the heart.

The normal jugular venous pattern, reflecting the right atrial pressure pulse, consists of a presystolic expansion, the A-wave, caused by atrial contraction, followed in order by the X descent during atrial relaxation, the X^1 descent during early systole, the V-wave during late systole, and the Y descent in early diastole (Fig. 3–5). The A-wave is prominent in conditions in which right atrial emptying is impeded, such as tricuspid stenosis (Fig. 3–6), and in the presence of right ventricular hypertrophy of any cause, including pulmonary hypertension, pulmonic stenosis, and hypertrophy of the interventricular septum in patients with left ventricular hypertrophy. The A-wave disappears in atrial fibrillation (Fig. 3–7). In tricuspid regurgitation, the X′ descent is diminished, and the V-wave and Y descent are unusually prominent (Fig. 3–7). In tricuspid stenosis, the Y descent is attenuated. In constrictive pericarditis, both the X′ and the Y descents are prominent, causing a W-shaped jugular venous pulse. In cardiac tamponade, the X descent is most striking.

Cardiac Examination

Inspection and Palpation

The cardiac examination should begin with inspection and palpation of the thorax (Fig. 3–8). Both the fingers and the palm of the hand should be used (Fig. 3–9). The patient should be examined in both the supine and the left lateral positions. The timing of precordial movement is aided by simultaneous cardiac auscultation or palpation of the carotid arterial pulse.

Precordial prominence occurs in patients in whom cardiomegaly had developed before puberty. Left ventricular enlargement is suggested by displacement of the apex beat lateral to the midclavicular line and a hyperkinetic or sustained, forceful impulse (Fig. 3–10). Left ventricular

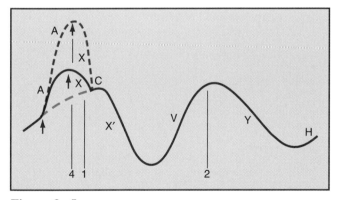

Figure 3–5

Jugular venous pulse. The normal contour is shown by the *solid line.* The A-wave *(a)* is absent in atrial fibrillation *(dashed green line).* The A-wave becomes large or giant when the right atrium contracts against a greater than normal volume of blood, a noncompliant or hypertrophied right ventricle, or a closing or closed tricuspid valve *(dashed blue line).* *Arrows* indicate the beginning and the end of the A-wave. The *numbers* represent the heart sounds. The fourth heart sound coincides with the peak of the large or giant A-wave. (From Evans, T.C., Giuliani, E.R., Tancredi, R.G., and Brandenburg, R.O.: Physical examination. *In* Giuliani, E.R., et al. [eds.]: Cardiology: Fundamentals and Practice. 2nd ed. St. Louis, Mosby–Year Book, 1991, pp. 204–272. By permission of Mayo Foundation.)

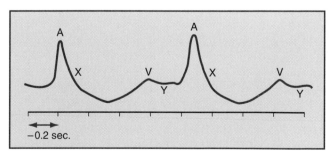

Figure 3–6

Jugular venous pulse in tricuspid stenosis, showing a large A-wave and a slow Y descent, the latter caused by difficulty in passive filling of the right ventricle. (From Fowler, N.O.: Cardiac Diagnosis and Treatment. 3rd ed. Hagerstown, MD, Harper & Row, 1980, p. 52.)

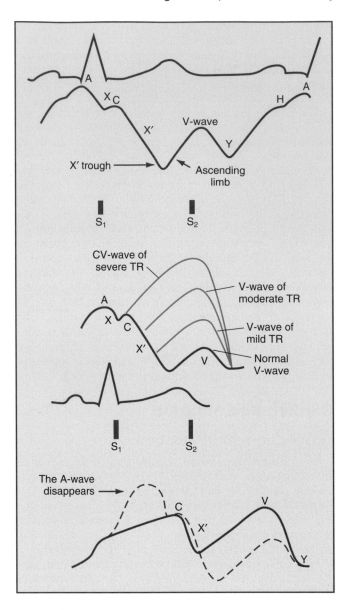

Figure 3–7

Top, Normal jugular venous pulse. The jugular V-wave is built up during systole, and its height reflects the rate of filling and the elasticity of the right atrium. Between the bottom of the Y descent (Y trough) and the beginning of the A-wave is the period of relatively slow filling of the "atrioventricle," or diastasis period. The wave built up during diastasis is the H-wave. The H-wave height also reflects the stiffness of the right atrium. S_1 and S_2 refer to the first and second heart sounds, respectively. *Center,* As the degree of tricuspid regurgitation (TR) increases, the X′ descent is increasingly encroached on. With severe TR, no X′ descent is seen, and the jugular pulse wave is said to be *ventricularized. Bottom,* The *red broken line* shows the normal jugular venous pulse and sinus rhythm. The *red solid line* indicates what occurs after the development of atrial fibrillation. The dominant descent in atrial fibrillation is almost always the Y descent; that is, it has the superficial appearance of the pulse wave of TR. (From Constant, J.: Bedside Cardiology. 4th ed. Boston, Little, Brown, 1993, pp. 81, 89, 93. Reprinted by permission of Lippincott-Raven, Publishers.)

Figure 3–8

A, Palpation of the anterior wall of the right ventricle by applying the tips of three fingers in the third, fourth, and fifth interspaces, left sternal edge *(arrows),* during full held exhalation. The patient is supine with the trunk elevated 30 degrees. *B,* Subxiphoid palpation of the inferior wall of the right ventricle (RV) with the relative position of the abdominal aorta (Ao) shown by the *arrow. C,* The bell of the stethoscope is applied to the cardiac apex while the patient lies in a partial left lateral decubitus position. The thumb of the examiner's free left hand is used to palpate the carotid artery for timing purposes. *D,* The soft, high-frequency early-diastolic murmur of aortic regurgitation or pulmonary hypertensive regurgitation is best elicited by applying the stethoscope's diaphragm very firmly to the mid-left sternal edge. The patient leans forward with breath held in full exhalation. *E,* Palpation of the left ventricular impulse with a fingertip *(arrow).* The patient's trunk is 30 degrees above the horizontal. The examiner's right thumb palpates the carotid pulse for timing purposes. *F,* Palpation of the liver. The patient is supine with knees flexed to relax the abdomen. The flat of the examiner's right hand is placed on the right upper quadrant just below the expected inferior margin of the liver; the left hand is applied diametrically opposite. *(A–F,* From Perloff, J.K.: Physical Examination of the Heart and Circulation. 2nd ed. Philadelphia, W.B. Saunders, 1990.)

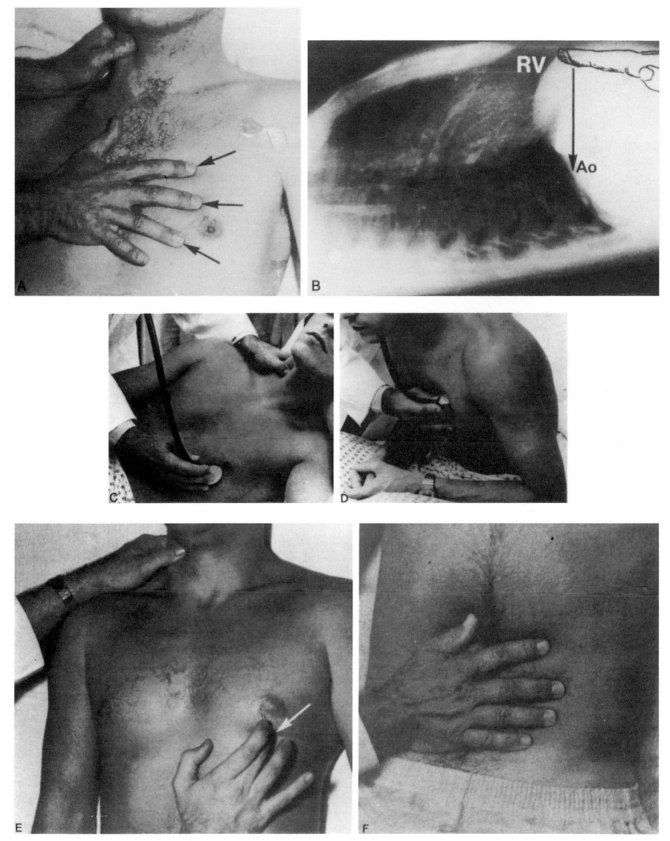

Figure 3–8
See legend on opposite page

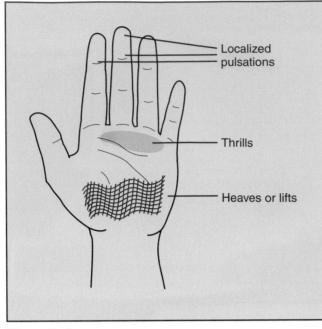

Figure 3–9
Although small localized movements are best perceived by the distal finger pads, thrills are best felt with the distal palm, whereas heaves or lifts are best felt with the proximal palm. (From Constant, J.: Bedside Cardiology. 4th ed. Boston, Little, Brown, 1993, p. 128. Reprinted by permission of Lippincott-Raven, Publishers.)

aneurysm produces a larger than normal area of systolic pulsation of the apex, whereas hypertrophic obstructive cardiomyopathy may cause a double outward thrust during systole. A presystolic apical thrust is palpable, usually with the patient in the left lateral decubitus condition, when the left atrial contribution to ventricular filling is augmented. This occurs in patients with sinus rhythm and left ventricular hypertrophy of any cause, myocardial ischemia, and myocardial fibrosis.[14] A systolic inward movement is characteristic of constrictive pericarditis.

Right ventricular enlargement or hypertrophy may be detected by a palpable anterior movement in the third or fourth intercostal space in the left parasternal region during systole. When pulmonary hypertension is present, the pulsation extends into the second intercostal space just left of the sternum. A palpable impulse simultaneous with the second heart sound reflects the presence of pulmonary hypertension.

Cardiac thrills are vibratory sensations best appreciated with the flat of the hand (see Fig. 3–9) and are palpable manifestations of loud (≥ grade IV/VI) murmurs with medium- or low-frequency components.

Auscultation

This should be carried out in a quiet room with the chest fully exposed and with the patient in the supine, sitting, and left lateral decubitus positions. The entire region between and including the cardiac apex and second intercostal space at the right sternal margin should be examined. Both the diaphragm (sensitive to high-pitched sounds) and the bell (sensitive to low-pitched sounds) of the stethoscope should be employed. Systematic and sequential attention should be directed to the heart sounds and the systolic and diastolic intervals.

Heart Sounds (Figs. 3–11 and 3–12)

The *first heart sound* is produced primarily by closure of the mitral valve; rarely, a second, softer component produced by tricuspid valve closure is audible.[15] The first heart sound is loudest when the mitral valve leaflets are widely apart at the onset of ventricular contraction, as occurs in mitral stenosis or with a short P-R interval. *Early-systolic sounds* (ejection sounds) are high-frequency events produced by the opening snap of stenotic, albeit mobile, aortic or pulmonic valves or by the ejection of blood into a dilated aorta or pulmonary trunk. Mid- to late-systolic sounds (often termed *clicks*) are caused most commonly by prolapse of the mitral valve, a condition in which the timing and intensity of the sounds are altered by respiration and other maneuvers (see Chap. 13).

The *second heart sound* is caused by closure of the semilunar valves and is heard best in the second left intercostal space along the sternal border. Splitting of the second heart sound is caused by the asynchronous closure of the valves (Table 3–6 and Fig. 3–13). Normally, the first component is caused by aortic closure, the second by pulmonic closure, and the time interval between the two components is increased by inspiration as right ventricular stroke rises and right ventricular systole lengthens in duration. A loud first (aortic) component of the second heart sound is present in systemic hypertension, and a loud second (pulmonic) component is heard in pulmonary hypertension. A decision tree for interpreting the second heart sound is shown in Figure 3–14. In *fixed splitting* of the second heart sound, the interval between the two components is unchanged and usually prolonged during the respiratory cycle. This auscultatory finding is a hallmark of atrial septal defect (see Chap. 26). In *paradoxical splitting* of the second heart sound, splitting is audible during exhalation and narrows or fuses during inspiration. It is caused by delayed aortic valve closure, most commonly complete left bundle branch block, but occasionally by chronic ischemic heart disease, severe systemic hypertension, left ventricular failure, pacing from the right ventricle, and left ventricular outflow tract obstruction.

Third and fourth heart sounds may originate from either ventricle[16] and are heard best with the bell of the stethoscope. Sounds from the left ventricle are best heard at the apex with the patient in the left decubitus position, whereas those from the right ventricle are most readily audible along the lower left sternal border in the supine position. The *third heart sound* (see Figs. 3–11 and 3–16) is often heard in normal children and young adults. When present after the age of 40 years, the third heart sound is abnormal and is caused by altered physical properties of the ventricle or an increase in the rate of ventricular filling in early diastole (Table 3–7). *Fourth heart sounds* may be audible in normal persons after the age of 50 years. Abnormal fourth heart sounds reflect increased

Type of movement and associated clinical condition		Location and accompanying features
NORMAL ADULT APEX IMPULSE	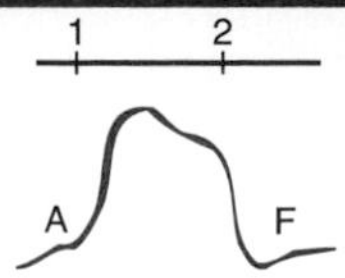	Cardiac apex; moderate systolic thrust; A- and F-waves usually imperceptible
HYPERKINETIC APEX IMPULSE Normal child Hyperdynamic states Ventricular septal defect Patent ductus arteriosus Mitral regurgitation Aortic regurgitation	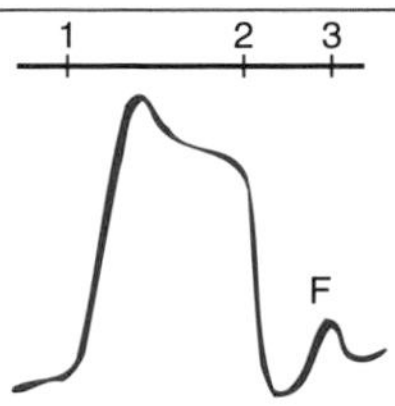	Exaggerated thrust at cardiac apex; F-wave may be palpable, coincident with S_3
HYPERKINETIC RIGHT VENTRICULAR IMPULSE Atrial septal defect Pulmonary regurgitation	**Same as above**	Maximal at left sternal edge in third and fourth intercostal spaces
SUSTAINED APEX IMPULSE Left ventricular hypertrophy, as in: Aortic stenosis Hypertension A variation that may occur in hypertrophic cardiomyopathy	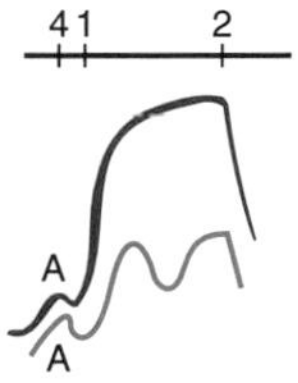	Maximal at cardiac apex; A-wave may be visible and palpable coincident with S_4
SUSTAINED RIGHT VENTRICULAR IMPULSE Right ventricular hypertrophy, as in: Pulmonary hypertension Pulmonary stenosis	**Same impulse as in "Sustained" above**	Maximal at left sternal edge in third and fourth intercostal spaces
ECTOPIC LEFT VENTRICULAR IMPULSE Ventricular aneurysm	**Same impulse as in "Sustained" above**	Maximal over mid-precordium rather than at apex
LEFT ATRIAL EXPANSION Severe mitral regurgitation	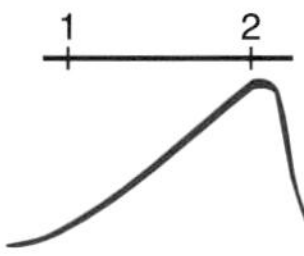	Left sternal edge or entire precordium; hyperkinetic apex impulse due to left ventricular volume overload
PULMONARY ARTERY PULSATION Pulmonary hypertension	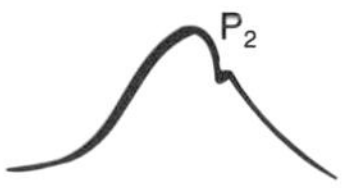	Second left intercostal space; palpable P_2
INWARD MOVEMENT DURING SYSTOLE Constrictive pericarditis Tricuspid regurgitation; primary	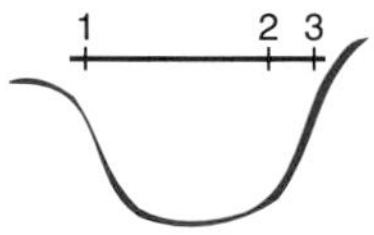	Cardiac apex or entire precordium; reversal of direction during systole as compared with preceding examples
DIASTOLIC MOVEMENTS Cardiomyopathy	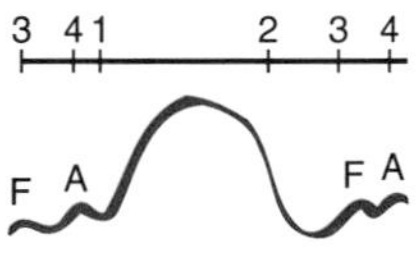	Cardiac apex; systolic movement may be inconspicuous; diastolic movements F and A correspond to S_3 and S_4, which may merge in tachycardia to form a summation gallop

Figure 3–10

Graphic representation of apical movements in health and disease. *Heavy line* indicates palpable features. P_2, pulmonic component of the S_2; A, atrial wave, corresponding to the fourth heart sound (S_4), or atrial gallop; F, filling wave, corresponding to the third heart sound (S_3), or ventricular gallop. (From Willis, P., IV: Inspection and palpation of the precordium. *In* Hurst, J.W. [ed.]: The Heart. 7th ed. New York, McGraw-Hill, 1990, p. 164.)

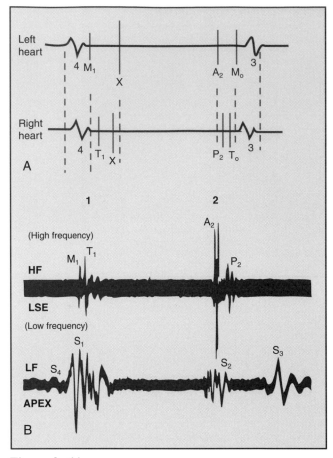

Figure 3–11

A, Diagrammatic representation of heart sounds originating from the left and right sides of the heart. Fourth (4) and third (3) heart sounds may originate from both sides, as may ejection sounds (X). Mitral valve closure (M_1), tricuspid valve closure (T_1), aortic valve closure (A_2), pulmonic valve closure (P_2), tricuspid valve opening (To), and mitral valve opening (Mo) are shown in relation to one another with respect to normal timing. *B,* Phonocardiograms recorded at the left sternal edge (LSE) using high-frequency filters (HF) and at the apex using low-frequency filters (LF) in a normal young individual. The components of the first heart sound (S_1) are seen to contain an initial low frequency (S_4) and two high frequencies—mitral (M_1) and tricuspid (T_1) valve closure. The second heart sound (S_2) contains two high-frequency components—aortic (A_2) and pulmonic (P_2) valve closure. The low-frequency third heart sound (S_3) is also seen. (*A* and *B,* From Sutton, G.C.: Examination of the cardiovascular system. *In* Julian, D.G., Camm, J.A., Fox, K.M., et al. [eds.]: Diseases of the Heart. London, Balliere-Tindall, 1989, p. 116.)

ventricular filling during atrial systole and occur in patients with sinus rhythm and ventricular hypertrophy, myocardial infarction, or ischemia (Table 3–8).

Other diastolic sounds include the opening snap of the mitral (rarely the tricuspid) valve. Valves producing this sound are usually stenotic but mobile. The time interval between the second heart sound and the opening snap of the mitral valve varies inversely with the height of the left atrial pressures (see Chap. 25). Opening snaps may be confused with widely split second heart sounds, but the second sound–opening snap interval narrows during inspiration (Fig. 3–15). Early-diastolic sounds also occur

in patients with chronic constrictive pericarditis, in whom they are known as pericardial *knocks* (Fig. 3–16*C*).

Heart murmurs are discussed in Chapter 13.

Examination of the Chest

Examination of the chest commences with inspection. Severe kyphoscoliosis and a markedly increased anteroposterior diameter may be a cause of cor pulmonale. Patients with chronic bronchitis or emphysema, an important cause of cor pulmonale, may have expiratory wheezes or poor transmission of breath sounds. Rales at the lung bases that do not clear with coughing as well as signs of pleural effusion are characteristic of heart failure.

Table 3–6 Abnormal Splitting of the Second Heart Sound

Persistent splitting
  Electrical delay of pulmonary component
    Right bundle branch block
    Left ventricular ectopic beats
    Preexcitation (left ventricular tract)
    Left ventricular pacemaker
  Mechanical delay of pulmonary component
    Pulmonary valve stenosis
    Subvalvular pulmonary obstruction
    Large pulmonary embolus
    Right ventricular dysfunction
  Decrease in pulmonary vascular impedance
    Dilatation of pulmonary artery
    Atrial septal defect
    After surgical repair of atrial septal defect
  Early aortic component
    Mitral regurgitation
    Ventricular septal defect
    Preexcitation (left ventricular tract)
Paradoxical splitting
  Electrical delay of aortic component
    Left bundle branch block
    Right ventricular ectopic beats
    Right ventricular pacemaker
    Coronary heart disease
  Mechanical delay of aortic component
    Aortic valve stenosis
    Hypertrophic cardiomyopathy
    Coronary heart disease
    Patent ductus arteriosus
    Aortic regurgitation
  Early closure of pulmonary valve
    Tricuspid regurgitation

From Evans, T.C., Giuliani, E.R., Tancredi, R.G., and Brandenburg, R.O.: Physical Examination. *In* Giuliani, E.R., Fuster, V., Gersh, B., et al. (eds.): Cardiology: Fundamentals and Practice. 2nd ed. Rochester, MN, Mayo Foundation, 1991, pp. 204–272. By permission of Mayo Foundation.

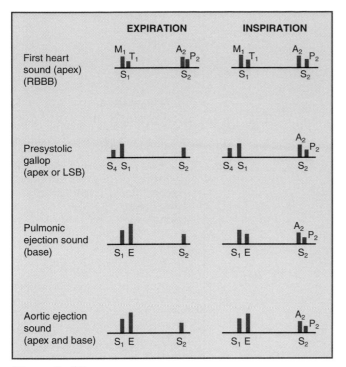

Figure 3–12

Splitting of the first heart sound (S_1), presystolic gallop sound (S_4), pulmonary ejection sound, and aortic ejection sound (E). Note that the pulmonary ejection sound is usually heard only at the base of the heart and may become louder during expiration. The aortic ejection sound is heard at both the base and the apex of the heart and may be audible in the carotid area. M_1, mitral valve closure; T_1, tricuspid valve closure; A_2, aortic valve closure; P_2, pulmonic valve closure; S_2, second heart sound; RBBB, right bundle branch block; LSB, left sternal border. (From Fowler, N.O.: Diagnosis of Heart Disease. New York, Springer-Verlag, 1991, p. 27.)

Table 3–7	Third Heart Sound (S_3), Ventricular Diastolic Gallop, Protodiastolic Gallop, and Pericardial Knock

Physiologic S_3—children and young adults
  Decreased prevalence with increasing age
Pathologic S_3
  Ventricular dysfunction—poor systolic function, increased end-diastolic and end-systolic volume, decreased ejection fraction, and high filling pressures
    Idiopathic dilated cardiomyopathy
    Ischemic heart disease
    Valvular heart disease
    Congenital heart disease
    Systemic and pulmonary hypertension
  Excessively rapid early-diastolic ventricular filling
    Hyperkinetic states
      Anemia
      Thyrotoxicosis
      Arteriovenous fistula
    Atrioventricular valve incompetence
    Left-to-right shunts
  Restrictive myocardial or pericardial disease
    Constrictive pericarditis (pericardial knock)
    Restrictive cardiomyopathy
    Hypertrophic cardiomyopathy?

From Shaver, J.A., and Salerni, R.: Auscultation of the heart. *In* Hurst, J.W. (ed.): The Heart. 7th ed. New York, McGraw-Hill, 1990. pp. 278, 281. Reproduced with permission of The McGraw-Hill Companies.

Examination of the Abdomen

The liver is usually enlarged in right ventricular failure. When the latter occurs acutely, rapid expansion of the hepatic capsule causes tenderness to palpation in the right upper quadrant. The liver may pulsate in tricuspid valve disease; pulsations are systolic in tricuspid regurgitation and presystolic in tricuspid stenosis. Timing of pulsations is aided by simultaneous auscultation. Firm pressure to the periumbilical region for about 20 seconds causes jugular vein expansion (the abdominojugular reflux) in the presence of right heart failure.[17] Palpation of the abdomen may reveal systolic expansion in the presence of an abdominal aortic aneurysm. Splenomegaly is sometimes seen in prolonged, severe right ventricular failure.

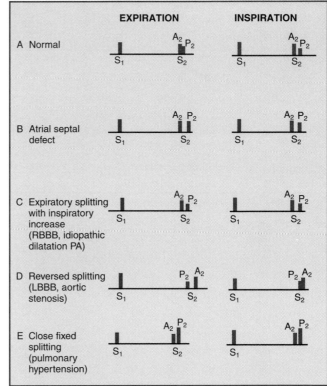

Figure 3–13

Demonstration of the relation of splitting of the S_2 to respiration in normal subjects *(A);* the fixed splitting of the S_2 heard in atrial septal defect *(B);* expiratory splitting of the S_2 with inspiratory increment as seen in right bundle branch block (RBBB) *(C);* reversed splitting of the S_2 associated with delayed aortic closure—most commonly caused by left bundle branch block (LBBB) *(D);* the close but audible and rather fixed splitting of S_2 characteristic of severe pulmonary hypertension associated with idiopathic or thromboembolic pulmonary hypertensive disease *(E).* S_1, first heart sound; A_2, aortic valve closure; P_2, pulmonic valve closure; PA, pulmonic artery. *(A–E,* From Fowler, N.O.: Diagnosis of Heart Disease. New York, Springer-Verlag, 1991, p. 31.)

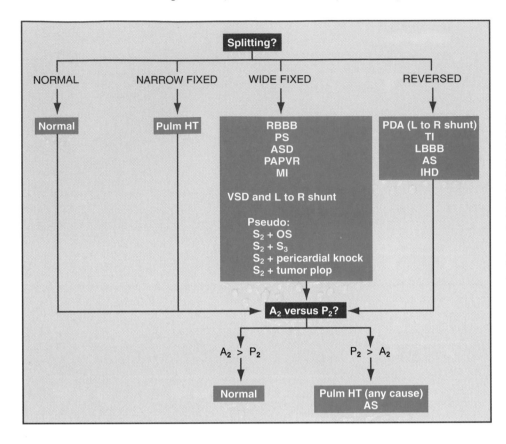

Figure 3–14

Decision tree for splitting of the S_2. Pulm HT, pulmonary hypertension; RBBB, right bundle branch block; PS, pulmonic stenosis; ASD, atrial septal defect; PAPVR, partial anomalous pulmonary venous return; MI, mitral insufficiency; VSD, ventricular septal defect; L to R shunt, left-to-right shunt; OS, opening snap; S_3, third heart sound; A_2, aortic valve closure; P_2, pulmonic valve closure; PDA, patent ductus arteriosus; TI, tricuspid insufficiency; LBBB, left bundle branch block; AS, aortic stenosis; IHD, ischemic heart disease. (From Sapira, J.D.: The Art and Science of Bedside Diagnosis. Munich, Baltimore, Urban & Schwartzenberg, 1990.)

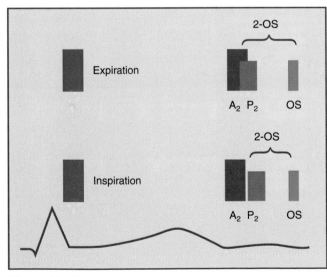

Figure 3–15

Respiration may give the false impression of a paradoxical split in a patient with an opening snap (OS) of the mitral valve because the P_2 moves away from the OS on expiration and toward the OS on inspiration. A_2, aortic valve closure. (From Constant, J.: Bedside Cardiology. 4th ed. Boston, Little, Brown, 1993, p. 182. Reprinted by permission of Lippincott-Raven, Publishers.)

Table 3–8	Fourth Heart Sound (S_4), Atrial Diastolic Gallop, and Presystolic Gallop

Physiologic—recordable, rarely audible
Pathologic
   Decreased ventricular compliance
      Ventricular hypertrophy
         Left or right ventricular outflow obstruction
         Systemic or pulmonary hypertension
         Hypertrophic cardiomyopathy
      Ischemic heart disease
         Angina pectoris
         Acute myocardial infarction
         Old myocardial infarction
         Ventricular aneurysm
      Idiopathic dilated cardiomyopathy
Excessively rapid late-diastolic filling secondary to vigorous atrial systole
   Hyperkinetic states
      Anemia
      Thyrotoxicosis
      Arteriovenous fistula
   Acute atrioventricular valve incompetence
Arrhythmias
   Heart block

From Shaver, J.A., and Salerni, R.: Auscultation of the heart. *In* Hurst, J.W. (ed.): The Heart. 7th ed. New York, McGraw-Hill, 1990. pp. 278, 281. Reproduced with permission of The McGraw-Hill Companies.

Figure 3–16

Diagnostic filling sounds. *A,* The fourth heart sound (S_4) occurs in presystole and is frequently called an atrial or presystolic gallop. S_1, first heart sound; S_2, second heart sound; *B,* The third heart sound (S_3) occurs during the rapid phase of ventricular filling. It is a normal finding and is commonly heard in children and young adults, disappearing with increasing age. When it is heard in the patient with cardiac disease, it is called a pathologic S_3 or ventricular gallop and usually indicates ventricular dysfunction or AV valvular incompetence. *C,* In constrictive pericarditis, a sound in early diastole, the pericardial knock (K) is heard earlier and is louder and higher pitched than the usual pathologic S_3. *D,* A quadruple rhythm results if both S_4 and S_3 are present. *E,* At faster heart rates, the S_3 and S_4 occur in rapid succession and may give the illusion of a middiastolic rumble. *F,* When the heart rate is sufficiently fast, the two rapid phases of ventricular filling reinforce each other, and a loud summation gallop (SG) may appear; this sound may be louder than either the S_3 or S_4 alone. (*A–F,* Reproduced with permission. *Examination of the Heart, Part 4: Auscultation,* 1990. Copyright © American Heart Association.)

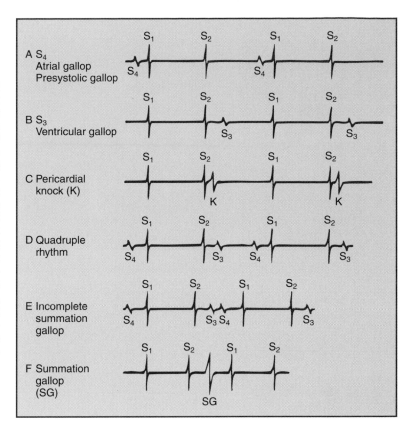

References

1. Braunwald, E.: The history. *In* Braunwald, E. (ed.): Heart Disease. 5th ed. Philadelphia, W.B. Saunders, 1997, pp. 1–14.
2. Mahler, D.A.: Dyspnea: Diagnosis and management. Clin. Chest Med. 8:215, 1987.
3. Wasserman, K.: Dyspnea on exertion. Is it the heart or the lungs? JAMA 248:2039, 1982.
4. Schmitt, B.P., Kushner, M.S., and Weiner, S.L.: The diagnostic usefulness of the history of the patient with dyspnea. J. Gen. Intern. Med. 1:386, 1986.
5. Christie, L.G., and Conti, C.R.: Sytematic approach to the evaluation of angina-like chest pain. Am. Heart J. 102:897, 1981.
6. Irwin, R.S., Curley, F.J., and French, C.L.: Chronic cough: The spectrum and frequency of causes, key components of the diagnostic evaluation, and outcome of specific therapy. Am. Rev. Respir. Dis. 141:640, 1990.
7. The Criteria Committee of the New York Heart Association: Nomenclature and Criteria for Diagnosis. 9th ed. Boston, Little, Brown, 1994.
8. Campeau, L.: Grading of angina pectoris. Circulation 54:422, 1975.
9. Goldman, L., Hashimoto, B., Cook, E.F., and Loscalzo, A.: Comparative reproducibility and validity of systems for assesssing cardiovascular functional class: Advantage of a new specific activity scale. Circulation 64:1227, 1981.
10. Perloff, J.K.: Physical Examination of the Heart and Circulation. 2nd ed. Philadelphia, W.B. Saunders, 1990.
11. O'Rourke, R.A., and Braunwald, E.: Physical examination of the cardiovascular system, in Fauci, A.S., Braunwald, E., et al. (eds.): Harrison's Principles of Internal Medicine, 14th ed. New York, McGraw-Hill, 1998, pp. 1231–1237.
12. Perloff, J.K., and Braunwald, E.: Physical examination of the heart and circulation. *In* Braunwald, E. (ed.): Heart Disease. 5th ed. Philadelphia, W.B. Saunders, 1997, pp. 15–52.
13. Constant, J.: Bedside Cardiology. 4th ed. Boston, Little, Brown, 1993.
14. Abrams, J.: Precordial palpation. *In* Horowitz, L.D., and Groves, B.M. (eds.): Signs and Symptoms in Cardiology. Philadelphia, J.B. Lippincott, 1985, pp. 156–177.
15. Waider, W., and Craige, E.: The first heart sound and ejection sounds. Echophonocardiographic correlation with valvular events. Am. J. Cardiol. 35:346, 1975.
16. Ishimitsu, T., Smith, D., Berko, B., and Craige, E.: Origin of the third heart sound: Comparison of ventricular wall dynamics in hyperdynamic and hypodynamic types. J. Am. Coll. Cardiol. 5:268, 1985.
17. Ducas, J., Magder, S., and McGregor, M.: Validity of the hepatojugular reflux as a clinical test for congestive heart failure. Am. J. Cardiol. 52:1299, 1983.

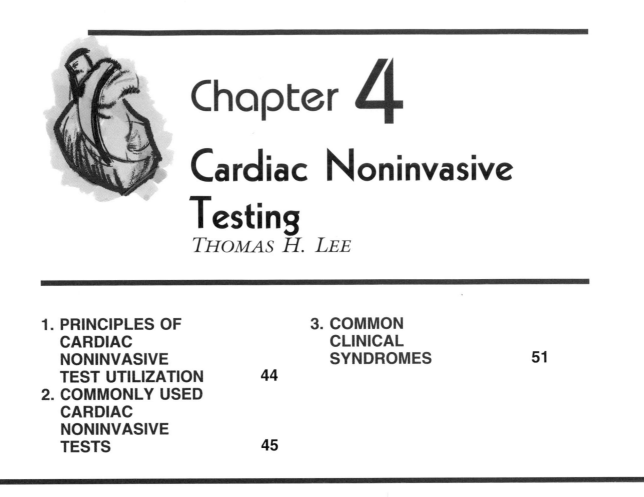

Chapter 4

Cardiac Noninvasive Testing

Thomas H. Lee

Noninvasive cardiac tests, including exercise electrocardiography, echocardiography, and radionuclide tests, can provide data to address several common questions that confront primary care physicians, including:

- Does the patient have coronary artery disease?
- Does the patient have severe coronary artery disease that might have a better prognosis if managed with percutaneous coronary angioplasty or coronary artery bypass graft surgery?
- Does the patient have abnormal left ventricular function?
- Does the patient have significant valvular heart disease?

In addition to helping physicians reach a diagnosis, cardiac noninvasive tests can also help monitor the impact of therapy and provide reassurance to the patient.

Although cardiac noninvasive tests generally yield accurate data, there is increasing pressure on primary care physicians to use these tests with discretion. The reasons include not only the costs and anxiety associated with the tests themselves but also the procedures that frequently result from the noninvasive tests. For example, treadmill exercise testing in a very low risk patient population (e.g., "executive-screening" programs) inevitably leads to suspicious results in some asymptomatic patients, which may subsequently lead to coronary angiography to resolve the question of whether the patient indeed has coronary disease. This "Pandora's box" phenomenon is supported by data demonstrating that regions in which there are high rates of use of noninvasive testing also tend to have high rates of use of coronary angiography and revascularization procedures.[1]

To improve the use of these tests, some managed care organizations are trying new strategies that actually restrict ordering of cardiac noninvasive tests to cardiologists in the belief that specialists have more insight into which patients are most likely to benefit from these tests. The impact of such strategies on patient outcomes, costs, and physician satisfaction is unclear, but primary care and other physicians clearly will need to use these tests appropriately in the years ahead. This chapter therefore includes three sections that describe:

1. General principles of test utilization as applied to noninvasive cardiac tests
2. The most frequently used cardiac noninvasive tests
3. Strategies for utilization of these tests for common clinical issues

PRINCIPLES OF CARDIAC NONINVASIVE TEST UTILIZATION

Like all tests, cardiac noninvasive tests are imperfect, and an understanding of their "performance characteristics" is an important skill for clinicians.[2] Key terms for descriptors of test performance, including sensitivity, specificity, positive and negative predictive value, and receiver operating characteristic curves, are discussed in Chapter 2. In cardiac noninvasive tests, it must be emphasized that these definitions provide a simplistic perspective on the interpretation of test results, since these tests rarely provide data in the form of a "yes" or "no" response. "Abnormal" and "normal" test results usually reflect an arbitrary threshold that is applied to quantitative information, such as the amount of ST segment depression seen on an electrocardiogram (ECG) during exercise testing. Even when an abnormality is apparently dichotomous, such as the presence or absence of defect on thallium scintigraphy, the classification of that abnormality is often based on a subjective interpretation of data.

The tradeoff between the true-positive and the false-positive rates associated with various definitions of "abnormal" is readily apparent in data on exercise ECGs. If the presence of 1 mm of ST segment depression is used to call an exercise test "positive," the test will have a high sensitivity for detection of coronary artery disease (Table 4–1), but it will also yield abnormal results in about 15% of patients without coronary artery disease. If the threshold is increased to 2 mm of ST segment depression, that false-positive rate will decrease, but at the expense of decreased sensitivity.

Exercise ECGs also demonstrate that the diagnostic performance of tests is complicated by variability in the definition of the outcome of interest. Exercise electrocardiography has a much higher sensitivity (80% or more) for detecting three-vessel or left main coronary disease than for detecting milder abnormalities (see Table 4–1). Therefore, even though a test may have an apparently poor sensitivity for detection of one outcome (e.g., the presence or absence of coronary disease), it may have a desirable sensitivity for detection of a more severe disease state that is actually of greater interest.

The principles for use of tests discussed in Chapter 2

are especially critical in cardiac noninvasive tests not only because these tests are expensive but also because of the consequences of false-positive or false-negative results. Unfortunately, controlled trials of the impact of cardiac noninvasive tests are likely never to be influential in guiding their use for several reasons. First, the "outcome" of such trials depends on what clinicians do with the information from a test, and standardization of management strategies that follow from various test results would be logistically and ethically difficult. Second, physicians usually have alternative methods for getting the information that they seek from noninvasive tests, including the use of invasive tests. Finally, the testing technologies themselves change so rapidly that by the time the outcomes from use or nonuse of the test could be measured, the findings would be irrelevant to current practice.

Therefore, guidelines for the use of noninvasive tests reflect analysis of data, opinion, and philosophy more than proven benefit of specific strategies. Improvement in the appropriateness of the use of these tests may be most likely to result from an increase in sophistication about their diagnostic performance among the clinicians who order these tests.

COMMONLY USED CARDIAC NONINVASIVE TESTS

Evaluation of Suspected Coronary Artery Disease

The least expensive—and often the most valuable—major test for evaluation of the patient with suspected coronary artery disease is *exercise electrocardiography,* also known as the exercise tolerance test. In addition to providing electrocardiographic data on the presence or absence of ischemia during exercise, this test addresses other key issues, including:
* What is the patient's functional capacity?
* At what level of exercise does ischemia develop?
* Does the patient develop symptoms such as chest pain with ischemia?

These data on functional capacity and patient symptoms are critical for assessment of prognosis and influence choices among therapeutic strategies.

The exercise tolerance test is associated with a surprisingly low complication rate, considering that it is based on pushing patients with suspected coronary disease to the limits of their physical capacity. Under proper supervision, the mortality can be expected to be less than 1 per 10,000 tests. Contraindications to exercise testing[3] are listed in Table 4–2.

Protocols

One protocol for exercise testing is the original Bruce protocol, which increases the grade of elevation and the speed of the treadmill at 3-minute intervals. The protocol begins with the treadmill moving at just 1.7 miles per

| Table 4–1 | Estimated Test Characteristics of the Exercise Tolerance Test and Exercise Thallium-201 |

ST Depression	Sensitivity	Specificity
Diagnosis of Coronary Disease		
≥1 mm	0.66	0.85
≥2 mm	0.33	0.97
≥3 mm	0.20	0.99
Thallium-201 scintigraphy		
Planar	0.83	0.88
SPECT	0.89	0.76
Positron emission tomography	0.87–0.97	0.78–1.00
Diagnosis of Left Main or Three-Vessel Coronary Disease		
≥1 mm	0.83	0.85
≥2 mm	0.67	0.76
≥3 mm	0.37	0.91
Thallium-201 scintigraphy	0.92	0.55

Adapted from Goldman, L., and Lee, T.H.: Noninvasive tests for diagnosing the presence and extent of coronary artery disease. J. Gen. Intern. Med. 1:258–265, 1986.
Abbreviation: SPECT, single-photon emission computed tomography.

Table 4–2	Contraindications to Exercise Testing

Unstable angina with recent rest pain
Untreated life-threatening cardiac arrhythmias
Uncompensated congestive heart failure
Advanced atrioventricular block
Acute myocarditis or pericarditis
Critical aortic stenosis
Severe hypertrophic obstructive cardiomyopathy
Uncontrolled hypertension
Acute systemic illness

From Chaitman, B.: Exercise stress testing. *In* Braunwald, E. (ed.): Heart Disease. 5th ed. Philadelphia, W.B. Saunders, 1997, p. 173.

hour with a 10% incline (stage 1), and only well-conditioned athletes can complete stage 7 (6.0 miles per hour at a 22% incline). The correlation is only approximate between exercise tolerance during treadmill testing and functional classification systems such as the New York Heart Association criteria, the Canadian Cardiovascular Society criteria, and the Specific Activity Scale, but patients are usually considered to be a functional class II if they can complete stage 1 of the Bruce protocol and class I if they can complete stage 2.

In most patients, the test is "symptom-limited"—that is, stopped when the patient develops fatigue, dyspnea, lightheadedness, chest pain, or pain elsewhere in the body (e.g., the legs) or when clear evidence of ischemia or arrhythmia is apparent on the ECG. In some settings, however, such as in the first days after acute myocardial infarction, the test may be stopped after some prespecified, low level of exertion has been reached.

A variety of other exercise test protocols are now used as or more often than the original Bruce protocol by many physicians (Table 18–2). For some protocols, the purpose of the test is not to push patients to their physical limits, but to determine whether it is safe for the patient to be discharged to home. Typically, the first stage of a modified Bruce protocol will be performed at 1.7 miles per hour at a 0% incline and the second stage will be performed at 1.7 miles per hour at a 10% incline. In many laboratories, tests for patients who are a few days post–acute myocardial infarction are even less strenuous, using the Naughton protocol. In the absence of symptoms or ECG observations that lead to cessation of the test, the Naughton protocol may be stopped at a level of exertion that is only the beginning of a conventional or even a modified Bruce protocol.

However, the modified Bruce protocol can also be used as a cautious way of assessing patients whose stability is uncertain. Examples include emergency department patients with acute chest pain without ECG changes,[4] those with potentially unstable arrhythmias or left ventricular dysfunction, and those with significant valvular disease—in short, patients in whom the safety of a standard exercise test is uncertain, but in whom the results of a test may be useful for management. In such cases, if the patient does not have evidence of ischemia during the first stage, the exercise test may continue as per a standard exercise test until limited by symptoms or ECG abnormalities.

Alternatives to walking on a treadmill must be considered for patients who cannot do so because of orthopedic or other problems. Bicycle protocols progressively increase workload from no or little resistance, usually stopping when the patient cannot pedal at least 40 cycles per minute. In subjects unfamiliar with bicycle exercise, the muscles required for such protocols are often not well developed, and tests are stopped at a lower cardiac workload than with treadmill exercise. Advantages of bicycle ergometry include less space requirements and the ability to get ECG tracings with less motion artifact.

Arm crank ergometry protocols—in which patients "pedal" with their arms—increase workloads incrementally at 2- or 3-minute stages. Because the arms of most people have less stamina than their legs, the peak heart rate achieved through such tests is usually only about 70% of that achieved with leg testing.

Interpretation

During and after exercise, the patient's ECG is monitored to detect evidence of ST segment changes or arrhythmia. Moderate ST segment depression is not necessarily diagnostic of ischemia, particularly if it occurs in the absence of chest pain or if the contour of the ST segment is upsloping (Fig. 4–1).[5] For this reason, tests are often not stopped at the first instant that ST segment depression becomes apparent.

Because so many types of information are collected during an exercise test, clinicians should specifically note several types of data when reviewing the results of this test:

- *How far did the patient go?* Ability to go 6 minutes or more of a standard Bruce protocol or 9 minutes on a modified protocol (see Table 18–2) indicates a normal work capacity.
- *What was the peak rate-pressure product?* Tests may be inconclusive if patients are unable to perform enough cardiac work to provoke ischemia. Multiplication of the peak systolic blood pressure and the peak heart rate provides a rough but easily calculated index of the heart's work—and tests with a double product that exceeds 18,000 (e.g., peak heart rate 100 beats/min, peak systolic blood pressure 180 mm Hg) are generally considered to be adequate. Beta-adrenergic blocking agents may compromise the ability of a patient to raise his or her heart rate to a level sufficient to precipitate an ischemic response.
- *Did the patient have symptoms and ECG changes?* The combination of these types of abnormalities is much more likely to be diagnostic of ischemia than either alone.
- *What did the ST segment depression look like?* ST segment depression should persist for at least 0.08 second (two of the little boxes) after the QRS complex for it to be considered significant, and it is much more likely to reflect ischemia if it is horizontal or downsloping in contour (see Fig. 4–1).[5] The greater the degree of ST segment depression, the more likely is coronary disease.
- *Does the patient have any characteristics that might affect the ECG response to exercise testing?* Digitalis

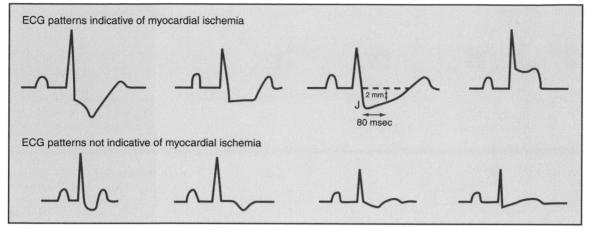

Figure 4–1

Electrocardiographic criteria suggestive of myocardial ischemia consist of at least 1 mm of J point depression with downsloping or horizontal ST segments; slowly upsloping ST segment depression, defined as 2 mm of ST depression measured 80 msec from the J point; and ST segment elevation. Patterns less suggestive of ischemia are included in the second row. (Redrawn from Goldschlager, N.: Use of the treadmill test in the diagnosis of coronary artery disease in patients with chest pain. Ann. Intern. Med. 97:383–388, 1982.)

and left ventricular hypertrophy can cause resting abnormalities of the ST segment that can be exacerbated by ischemia even in the absence of coronary disease. Conduction abnormalities, such as left bundle branch block or bypass tracts, may also lead to ST segment abnormalities.

- *Did the patient have any abnormal non-ECG responses to exercise?* The normal response to exercise is an increase in heart rate and in systolic blood pressure. Declines in blood pressure or failure to increase the rate-pressure product often reflect underlying cardiomyopathy or severe ischemia.

Alternatives to Exercise Electrocardiography

Many patients cannot perform sufficient physical exertion to unmask coronary artery disease or have ECGs that are difficult to interpret. For these patients, alternative technologies to exercise electrocardiography are now available. Virtually all of these alternatives are considerably more expensive and inconvenient to the patient than exercise electrocardiography. Furthermore, treadmill exercise is more typical physiologically of the type of cardiovascular work that provokes ischemia than are pharmacologic stressors. Therefore, for most patients, all of these alternatives should be considered second choices to exercise electrocardiography.

Most medical centers now perform pharmacologic stress tests using dobutamine, dipyridamole, or adenosine. Qualitative differences in the diagnostic performance of these agents are not considered to be sufficient at this time to choose among them.[6] Dipyridamole and adenosine cause coronary vasodilatation and thereby enhance coronary blood flow. The flow increase with these drugs is of less magnitude through stenotic arteries, leading to relative hypoperfusion that can be detected with radionuclide scanning. These relative perfusion defects may or may not be accompanied by myocardial ischemia; hence, echo-

cardiography is not as sensitive for detecting coronary artery disease as radionuclide scanning after administration of these agents.

Dobutamine in high doses can be used to induce myocardial ischemia by a different mechanism. Dobutamine raises heart rate, systolic blood pressure, and myocardial contractility, thereby causing a secondary increase in cardiac blood flow. This flow increase is less than that seen with dipyridamole or adenosine, but it still leads to perfusion defects suggestive of coronary disease.

The methods used to detect ischemia after such agents are given include radionuclide scintigraphy with thallium- or technetium-based agents or echocardiography. Thallium-201 is efficiently extracted from the circulation by viable myocardial cells, so that it distributes in proportion to regional blood flow. Therefore, images of the heart obtained shortly after thallium administration show reduced tracer concentrations in regions with relative hypoperfusion or nonviable myocardium (Figs. 4–2 and 4–3). Over several hours, these "defects" fill in owing to redistribution of the isotope if the myocardium is viable; where myocardium is dead, the defects persist. Lung activity of thallium-201 also provides prognostic information, since increased lung activity suggests elevated pulmonary venous pressures.

When thallium-201 is given to a patient undergoing treadmill exercise, it is injected through an intravenous line at peak exercise. The patient is asked to continue exercising for another 30 to 60 seconds, and images are obtained immediately and again 3 to 4 hours later. Thallium can also be used for patients who are believed to have rest ischemia. In such cases, serial imaging can demonstrate viable ischemic and nonviable myocardium.

Technetium-99m–based agents such as sestamibi have a shorter half-life (6 hours) than thallium-201 (73 hours), which allows injection of a larger dose, leading to improved count statistics during scanning. Technetium-99m is also characterized by higher emission energy levels and less scattered radiation than thallium-201, and it under-

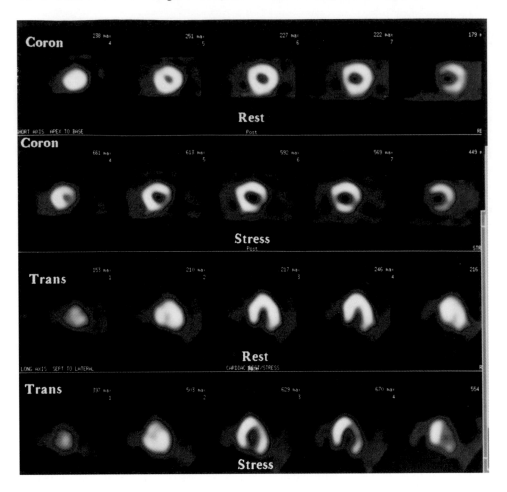

Figure 4–2
Myocardial perfusion scan shows moderate ischemia of the inferolateral wall of the left ventricle from base to apex with stress *(bottom right image)*. With rest, the region that was not perfused during pharmacologic stress receives normal blood flow, and the perfusion defect resolves *(third row, last image)*. Coron, coronal view; Trans, transverse view. (Courtesy of Finn Manting, M.D., Ph.D., Director, Nuclear Medicine, Brigham and Women's Hospital.)

goes only a small amount of washout after initial myocardial uptake. Therefore, the distinction between viable and nonviable myocardium requires two injections of the tracer—one during stress, and the other during rest. Research indicates that the diagnostic performance of technetium-99m perfusion tracers is similar to that of thallium-201 scintigraphy.

Echocardiography is becoming an increasingly popular technology for detection of ischemia for several reasons. First, this test is available with little or no advance notice at many institutions, so that it can be used to assess patients with chest pain syndromes on weekends and evenings, when nuclear testing may be difficult to arrange. Second, it detects ischemia through the imaging of new regional wall motion abnormalities or by demonstrating increased contractility when a patient is treated with an agent such as dobutamine. The "abnormal" results obtained with stress echocardiography have been shown to have adverse prognostic significance. For example, data from one study indicated that the presence of viable or ischemic myocardium helped in predicting risk for subsequent major cardiac complications.[7] Finally, this test also provides information on left ventricular function. The principal disadvantage is that echocardiography has a lower sensitivity for detecting mild coronary disease than other technologies.

For patients who undergo imaging with radionuclide agents, the basic instrument used in most laboratories is a "gamma camera" that encodes information on the distribution of the radioisotope onto a two-dimensional image. In recent years, rotating gamma cameras have been used to perform single-photon emission computed tomography (SPECT), which, in theory, improves sensitivity and specificity of diagnosis of coronary disease and delineation of the size of ischemic or infarcted myocardium. However, studies to date have not demonstrated higher specificity (see Table 4–1).

The use of positron emission tomography (PET) relies on tracers that emit two high-energy photons in opposite directions, allowing PET scanners to identify and localize true events and screen out the "noise" from random, scattered photons. This technology provides superior images compared with SPECT, but it requires considerably greater expense in the preparation of its tracers and the acquisition of scanning equipment. PET scanning can provide information for noninvasive detection of coronary disease and estimation of the severity of disease and can be used to assess myocardial viability. Experience to date indicates that PET using dipyridamole and either rubidium-92 or ^{13}N ammonia shows abnormal perfusion patterns in almost all patients with coronary disease, and specificity rates have ranged from 78% to 100%.[6] However, whether PET is superior to SPECT for routine diagnostic purposes is not clear. Therefore, whether the high costs of this technology will prevent its widespread dissemination remains uncertain.

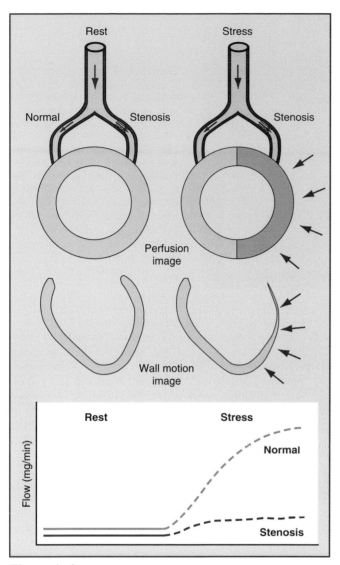

Figure 4–3

Principle of stress radionuclide imaging for the detection of coronary artery disease. Shown are (1) a normal coronary artery and an artery with significant stenosis *(top)*, (2) the myocardial territory (perfusion image), and (3) the ventricular wall (wall motion image) supplied by each artery. The graph *(bottom)* depicts coronary blood flow both at rest and during stress. (Redrawn from Beller, G.A.: Chronic ischemic heart disease. *In* Braunwald, E. [ed.-in-chief]: Essential Atlas of Heart Diseases. Philadelphia, Current Medicine, 1997, p. 3.6.)

A qualitatively different test is ambulatory electrocardiography, which uses ST segment data obtained over a period of up to 24 hours to diagnose ischemia. This test has been most widely used for patients with asymptomatic ischemia, and it has been shown to identify patients at high risk for major cardiac complications after noncardiac vascular surgery.

Choice of Tests

From the perspective of a primary care physician, the distinction among most of these tests may be less critical than is apparent at first. All of these tests have an excel-

lent sensitivity for detection of severe coronary artery disease and very good sensitivity for detection of any coronary disease. The best test at a given institution is likely to be the test that is performed most frequently because the specialists who perform the test are likely to be experienced in its interpretation.

The choice of tests may be influenced in some cases by patient-specific factors. Medications, including beta-adrenergic and calcium channel blocking agents and nitrates, may decrease the sensitivity of treadmill exercise tests; thus, if possible, discontinuation of these medications before a test intended to evaluate whether a patient has coronary disease is desirable. Pharmacologic perfusion imaging with dipyridamole or adenosine appears to be less influenced by antianginal drugs and can be considered as an alternative to exercise when medications cannot be stopped. However, for patients with known or probable coronary disease, the purpose of the test is often to assess the extent of myocardium in jeopardy at usual workloads. In these cases, it may be desirable to maximize medications before testing.

The treadmill ECG is less accurate in women, in part because of their lower pretest likelihood of coronary disease than men. Unfortunately, the sensitivity and specificity of thallium perfusion scans also appear to be lower in women than in men. Artifacts owing to breast attenuation also complicate interpretation of women's scans. In theory, technetium-99m scans should be less susceptible to artifacts introduced by breast tissue or breast implants.

Very obese patients can introduce a technical problem because the imaging tables used for SPECT scanning have weight limits that are often as low as 300 lb. Photon attenuation by soft tissue can render thallium-201 scans difficult to interpret in obese patients; in such patients, technetium-99m scans may provide better results.

In the absence of contraindications, exercise electrocardiography should be considered the initial test of choice because of the information it provides and its relatively low costs. Charges and costs for tests and procedures vary widely, but exercise electrocardiography is only about one-quarter as expensive as radionuclide alternatives. One study estimated the fee for exercise electrocardiography to be $330, versus $1200 for SPECT myocardial perfusion imaging and $1800 for PET myocardial perfusion imaging.[8]

Evaluation of Left Ventricular Function and Cardiac Anatomy

Echocardiography is potentially useful in almost all cardiac disorders and, with the addition of Doppler technology, has emerged as the principal ultrasonic technique for obtaining hemodynamic information. Echocardiography uses high-frequency sound waves to image cardiac anatomy and to assess the movement of cardiac structures.

Doppler analysis uses sound waves to evaluate blood flow, thus permitting detection of valvular regurgitation, stenosis, and intracardiac shunts. The principle of Doppler ultrasound is that red blood cells can reflect ultrasound

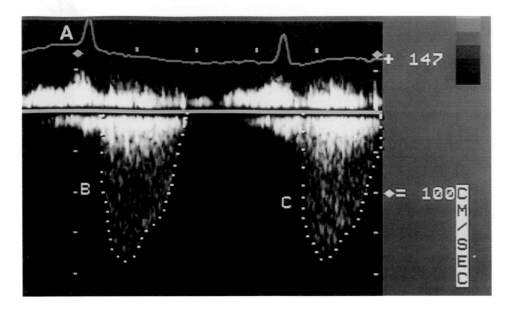

Figure 4-4

Doppler recording of blood flow through a stenotic aortic valve. The peak velocity is approximately 3700 cm/sec, which corresponds to a peak instantaneous gradient of 55 mm Hg. The accuracy of this method approaches cardiac catheterization. A, Electrocardiographic tracing. B and C, Recordings of blood flow during two consecutive heart beats. (Courtesy of Richard T. Lee, M.D., Brigham and Women's Hospital.)

signals generated by a crystal within a transducer and that the frequency of the reflected ultrasound waves is altered according to the relative motion of the red blood cells. The difference between the emitted and the reflected frequency is the *Doppler shift*. If the reflective surface is stationary, the emitted and reflected signals will have identical frequencies. If the reflective surface is moving away from the ultrasound source, the reflected signal will be shifted to a lower frequency. For accurate estimates of the red cell velocity, the ultrasound beam should be directed as parallel as possible to the column of blood being evaluated. Color flow Doppler assigns a red or blue color to blood flow moving toward or away from the transducer, respectively. Higher velocities are represented by brighter hues.

Doppler data can be used to estimate gradients across the aortic valve and thereby contribute to the assessment of the severity of aortic valvular stenosis. Significant valvular obstruction leads to turbulence, and the pressure drop across the valve during systole leads to increased flow velocity for the red blood cells that do cross the valve. From color-wave Doppler images, the peak flow velocities of the red blood cells can be calculated; these data can used to estimate the peak gradient across the valve (Fig. 4-4). Note that this "peak" gradient will be higher than the "mean" gradient, which is the figure usually provided in catheterization laboratory reports.

Doppler ultrasound is also highly useful for diagnosis of aortic insufficiency, since the regurgitant stream causes turbulence. The extent of the regurgitant jet is used to estimate the "grade" of aortic regurgitation on a I to IV scale. However, the most critical information in the noninvasive assessment of patients with aortic regurgitation is the patient's left ventricular size and function, which are evaluated via two-dimensional echocardiography.

Complications of ultrasound technology have not been demonstrated in human beings, but studies may be technically limited in patients with chronic obstructive lung disease or very obese patients.

Transesophageal echocardiography uses ultrasound technology in a manner that blurs the distinction between invasive and noninvasive tests. In this approach, an echocardiographic transducer at the end of a flexible endoscope is inserted into the esophagus and, for some views, the stomach, thereby providing views of the heart from the back and below, without the obstruction of lung tissue and the chest wall. Transesophageal echocardiography is particularly effective for the evaluation of prosthetic valves, abnormalities in the atria, vegetations, and aortic dissections (Fig. 4-5).

Among a number of new echocardiographic technologies, three-dimensional (3-D) echocardiography is emerging as a potential major clinical tool.[9] Current two-dimen-

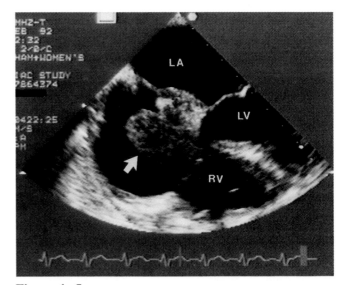

Figure 4-5

Transesophageal echocardiogram of a tumor in the heart. This patient had atrial fibrillation that led to the discovery of a possible mass by standard two-dimensional echocardiography. To better define the mass, an imaging probe was inserted into the esophagus. The large tumor occupying much of the right atrium and infiltrating the atrial septum *(arrow)* is a lymphoma. LA, left atrium; LV, left ventricle; RV, right ventricle. (Courtesy of Richard T. Lee, M.D.)

sional imaging methods are limited in their ability to evaluate some problems that are inherently 3-D. For example, the right ventricle is a complex asymmetric structure, and evaluating right ventricular size and systolic function reliably has plagued cardiologists for decades. In addition, the left ventricle, normally a symmetric ellipsoidal structure, becomes distorted and asymmetric after a myocardial infarction. Many other common cardiology diagnostic problems, including valvular regurgitation, aneurysms, congenital heart defects, and tumors, may be better approached with 3-D technology. Magnetic resonance imaging and ultrafast computed tomography are two technologies that can provide 3-D images of moving cardiac structures. However, these devices are over ten times more expensive than ultrasound devices, and the incremental benefit of using magnetic resonance imaging and ultrafast computed tomography is unclear for many cardiac diagnostic questions.

3-D echocardiography may be a widely available and inexpensive method in the near future. Existing clinical ultrasound machines can be coupled to a 3-D acquisition system, and the two-dimensional images are reconstructed by a computer to form moving 3-D pictures. The currently available 3-D systems are too slow for routine clinical use, and 3-D imaging is primarily a research tool. With faster computers and declining costs of digital storage, 3-D echocardiography may replace standard two-dimensional echocardiography.

Radionuclide ventriculography, an alternative to the echocardiogram, provides quantitative estimates of left ventricular function by calculating how much of a radionuclide tracer has been ejected from the left ventricle with each contraction. The radiation exposure is not clinically significant. Whether the more precise estimate of left ventricular function compared with echocardiography contributes to patient management is unclear, and this test does not provide an evaluation of valvular function. Furthermore, this test is more expensive than echocardiography. Therefore, radionuclide ventriculography should usually be considered a second choice to echocardiography.

Assessment of Cardiac Rhythm Disturbances

Although exercise electrocardiography is sometimes used to evaluate whether exercise-induced symptoms are due to arrhythmias, the procedure of choice for patients with known or suspected arrhythmias is long-term ECG monitoring, also known as Holter monitoring. Usually, a recorder the size of a small cassette player records two ECG channels for 24 hours. Newer variations on this technology allow patients to press a button after the occurrence of symptoms, causing the recorder to save the last several minutes of ECG activity. Patients with rare symptoms can wear such a "loop recorder" for periods as long as several months.

Assessment of Vasomotor Function

A test that is becoming more widely used outside of research settings is upright tilt testing, which can identify patients who have a vasodepressor or neurocardiogenic cause of syncope (see Chap. 12). Patients are strapped to a table in a horizontal position and then tilted upright for 20 to 45 minutes in an attempt to reproduce symptoms or cause syncope. Isoproterenol may be infused to provoke syncope in patients who are asymptomatic after initial testing. Although this test has a high false-positive rate for detection of neurocardiogenic syncope, some data indicate that it can be used to guide therapy in patients with a history of episodes of loss of consciousness.[10]

COMMON CLINICAL SYNDROMES

Evaluation of the Patient with Suspected Angina Pectoris

Chest pain and other symptoms consistent with angina pectoris suggest the possibility of coronary artery disease, but the differential diagnosis of chest pain also includes noncardiac conditions such as musculoskeletal chest pain, pulmonary disease, esophageal discomfort, and gastrointestinal abnormalities. The clinical assessment based on the history, physical examination, and review of the ECG usually allows clinicians to classify patients into one of three categories: (1) typical for angina pectoris, (2) atypical for angina pectoris but consistent with this diagnosis, and (3) clearly noncardiac chest pain. This categorization is critical to both the decision to order a noninvasive test for ischemia and the interpretation of the result. In patients with typical angina, the prevalence of coronary disease is high ($\geq 80\%$), and even a normal test result might not change the overall assessment of whether the patient is at high risk for coronary disease. In a patient at low risk for coronary disease because of atypical symptoms, an abnormal test result might not raise the possibility of coronary disease to a level at which coronary angiography or treatment with anti-ischemic medications seems warranted.

It is extremely important that the primary care physician have a clear idea of the purpose of noninvasive testing when it is ordered for patients with suspected coronary disease. The two most common principal reasons are:

• Estimation of the probability of any coronary disease
• Estimation of the probability of severe coronary disease that is associated with a poor prognosis with medical therapy, and therefore might warrant revascularization with angioplasty or bypass graft surgery

In this context, noninvasive tests for ischemia can be seen as most useful for *diagnosis* of coronary disease in patients who have an intermediate risk for this diagnosis, since in this population, a markedly positive result can essentially establish the diagnosis of coronary disease, whereas a clearly negative result can reduce that possibility to a low level.

These tests are also often useful for evaluation of overall *prognosis* in patients with typical angina, since certain subsets of patients with a worse prognosis with medical management have been found to have improved survival if they undergo coronary artery bypass graft surgery. These subsets include patients with left main coronary artery disease and three-vessel coronary disease in combination with mild to moderate left ventricular dysfunction.[11] One analysis concluded that exercise testing of patients with stable angina had a cost-effectiveness comparable with that of many accepted medical interventions if coronary angiography was performed for patients who were found to have 2 mm or more of ST segment depression.[12] Other signs during exercise testing that suggest that the patient may have a poor prognosis with medical therapy owing to high-risk coronary disease include short exercise duration and exercise-induced hypotension. On the other hand, even among patients with angina, good exercise tolerance predicts a benign short-term prognosis even in the presence of 2 mm or more of ST segment depression.[13]

These general recommendations can be used to identify patients for whom coronary angiography may be the most appropriate first strategy, without prior noninvasive testing. Such patients include those in whom the diagnosis of coronary disease must be excluded with essentially complete certainty, such as those with chest pain who have occupations with direct impact on the safety of others (e.g., airline pilots) or who have frequent need for sudden bursts of activity (e.g., police officers). Coronary angiography is also a reasonable test without prior noninvasive workup when the patient has a high probability of coronary disease that is likely to be treated with revascularization, such as those with angina at rest despite medical therapy or those with evidence of ischemia after acute myocardial infarction.

Guidelines for Use of Exercise Electrocardiography

An American College of Cardiology/American Heart Association (ACC/AHA) task force published guidelines for the use of exercise testing in 1997.[14] These guidelines rated the appropriateness of this test in various patient subsets according to three levels of appropriateness, including conditions for which or patients for whom there is general agreement that exercise testing is useful and effective (class I); conditions for which or patients for whom there is divergence of opinion with respect to its usefulness but the weight of evidence is either in favor of testing (class IIa) or less well established (class IIb); and conditions for which or patients for whom there is general agreement that exercise testing is not useful or effective and may even be harmful (class III).

The recommendations in these guidelines (Table 4–3) for use of exercise testing in patients with suspected or known coronary disease reflect the pretest probability of coronary disease (Table 4–4) as well as the situations in which exercise testing is most accurate. Exercise testing is most helpful in patients with an intermediate pretest probability who have normal baseline ECGs.

The ACC/AHA guidelines regarded exercise testing as valuable for the assessment of prognosis for patients with

coronary disease, but considered repetition at approximately 1-year intervals a reasonable if unproven (class II) strategy. The use of exercise tests to evaluate the response to therapy with cardiovascular drugs was also called a class II indication. However, the ACC/AHA Task Force discouraged the use of serial exercise tests to assess functional capacity in the course of an exercise rehabilitation program.

The ACC/AHA guidelines did not support the use of exercise testing in any setting to screen apparently healthy individuals or those with chest discomfort not thought to be of cardiac origin. However, the guidelines offered equivocal support (class IIb) for exercise testing of asymptomatic patients with special occupations or under certain specific circumstances (Table 4–5).

The difficult issue of when radionuclide tests should be used instead of exercise electrocardiography was addressed in a separate set of guidelines published in 1990 by a subcommittee of the American College of Physicians.[15] These guidelines, which antedated widespread use of technetium-based agents for detection of ischemic myocardium, concluded that thallium scintigraphy is clearly preferable to exercise electrocardiography alone when the resting ECG shows abnormalities impairing interpretation of changes or when information on the reversibility of ischemia in specific myocardial segments might influence the use of revascularization therapy.

High-risk features of noninvasive tests for ischemia that

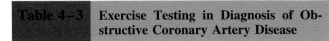

Table 4–3 Exercise Testing in Diagnosis of Obstructive Coronary Artery Disease

Class I

1. Adult patients (including those with complete right bundle branch block or less than 1 mm of resting ST depression) with an intermediate pretest probability of CAD (see Table 4–4), based on gender, age, and symptoms (specific exceptions are noted under Classes II and III below)

Class IIa

1. Patients with vasospastic angina

Class IIb

1. Patients with a high pretest probability of CAD by age, symptoms, and gender
2. Patients with a low pretest probability of CAD by age, symptoms, and gender
3. Patients with less than 1 mm of baseline ST depression and taking digoxin
4. Patients with electrocardiographic criteria for left ventricular hypertrophy and less than 1 mm of baseline ST depression

Class III

1. Patients with the following baseline ECG abnormalities:
   - Preexcitation (Wolff-Parkinson-White) syndrome
   - Electronically paced ventricular rhythm
   - Greater than 1 mm of resting ST depression
   - Complete left bundle branch block
2. Patients with a documented myocardial infarction or prior coronary angiography demonstrating significant disease have an established diagnosis of CAD; however, ischemia and risk can be determined by testing

From Gibbons, R.J., Balady, G.J., Beasley, J.W., et al.: ACC/AHA guidelines for exercise testing: Executive summary. A report of the American College of Cardiology/American Heart Association Task Force on Practice Guidelines (Committee on Exercise Testing). Circulation 96:345–354, 1997.
Abbreviations: CAD, coronary artery disease; ECG, electrocardiogram.

Table 4–4	Pretest Probability of Coronary Artery Disease by Age, Gender, and Symptoms*				
Age (yr)	Gender	Typical/Definite Angina Pectoris†	Atypical/Probable Angina Pectoris†	Nonanginal Chest Pain†	Asymptomatic†
30–39	Men	Intermediate	Intermediate	Low	Very low
	Women	Intermediate	Very low	Very low	Very low
40–49	Men	High	Intermediate	Intermediate	Low
	Women	Intermediate	Low	Very low	Very low
50–59	Men	High	Intermediate	Intermediate	Low
	Women	Intermediate	Intermediate	Low	Very low
60–69	Men	High	Intermediate	Intermediate	Low
	Women	High	Intermediate	Intermediate	Low

From Gibbons, R.J., Balady, G.J., Beasley, J.W., et al.: ACC/AHA guidelines for exercise testing: Executive summary. A report of the American College of Cardiology/American Heart Association Task Force on Practice Guidelines (Committee on Exercise Testing). Circulation 96:345–354, 1997.

*No data exist for patients <30 or >69 yr, but it can be assumed that prevalence of coronary artery disease increases with age. In a few cases, patients with ages at the extremes of the decades listed may have probabilities slightly outside the high or low range.

†High indicates >90%; intermediate 10%–90%; low, <10%; and very low, <5%.

make consideration of coronary angiography appropriate are summarized in Table 4–6.[14, 16]

Evaluation of the Patient with a Systolic Murmur

The potential causes and evaluation of systolic murmurs are reviewed in Chapter 13. In brief, several tests can provide information on the cause of systolic murmurs, including the chest x-ray, fluoroscopy, and radionuclide ventriculography. The most useful test, however, is echocardiography. In addition to visualization of valvular and septal abnormalities via echocardiographic images, Doppler analysis can be used to assess the severity of

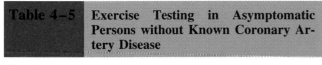

Table 4–5	Exercise Testing in Asymptomatic Persons without Known Coronary Artery Disease

Class I

1. None

Class IIb

1. Evaluation of persons with multiple risk factors*
2. Evaluation of asymptomatic men older than 40 yr and women older than 50 yr:
   - Who plan to start vigorous exercise (especially if sedentary)
   or
   - Who are involved in occupations in which impairment might impact public safety
   or
   - Who are at high risk for coronary artery disease due to other diseases (e.g., chronic renal failure)

Class III

1. Routine screening of asymptomatic men or women

From Gibbons, R.J., Balady, G.J., Beasley, J.W., et al.: ACC/AHA guidelines for exercise testing: Executive summary. A report of the American College of Cardiology/American Heart Association Task Force on Practice Guidelines (Committee on Exercise Testing). Circulation 96:345–354, 1997.

*Multiple risk factors are defined as hypercholesterolemia (cholesterol greater than 240 mg/dl), hypertension (systolic blood pressure greater than 140 mm Hg or diastolic blood pressure greater than 90 mm Hg), smoking, diabetes, and family history of heart attack or sudden cardiac death in a first-degree relative younger than 60 yr. An alternative approach might be to select patients with a Framingham risk score consistent with at least a moderate risk of serious cardiac events within 5 yr.

hemodynamic derangements caused by valvular disease, and the speed of red blood cell flow can be used to estimate the pressure gradient across the aortic valve in patients with aortic stenosis. Doppler analysis can also provide a qualitative (1+, 2+, and so on) description of the severity of mitral regurgitation.

In many patients, the nature of the valvular abnormality is not in question, but echocardiography is nevertheless useful for assessment of left ventricular function. For patients with mitral regurgitation, progressive dilatation of the left ventricular despite medical therapy with vasodilators should lead to consideration of valvular surgery to prevent irreversible ventricular dysfunction.

Guidelines

An ACC/AHA task force that developed guidelines for the use of echocardiography considered this test to be potentially useful in patients with systolic murmurs unless the physical examination made it extremely unlikely that the murmur was of organic origin (Table 4–7).[17] If a patient is felt to have a benign flow murmur, the clinician should exclude pathologic causes of increased cardiac output such as those described previously.

For patients with suspected mitral valve prolapse, confirmation of the diagnosis by echocardiography usually does not contribute to management, unless there is evidence on physical examination or chest x-ray that the patient has an enlarged left ventricle. Although the echocardiogram was used to define the entity of mitral valve prolapse, this test has a substantial false-positive rate for this diagnosis, and a slight alteration of the orientation of the transducer can lead to the appearance of mitral prolapse.

Syncope

Syncope is often benign, usually easily evaluated without expensive diagnostic testing, but occasionally the first evidence of a life-threatening disorder. The evaluation of patients with this condition is summarized in Chapter 12, but the use of noninvasive tests may well be in evolution for this syndrome. The most commonly used cardiac tests remain the ECG, which should be performed for all pa-

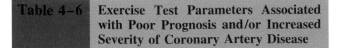

Table 4-6	Exercise Test Parameters Associated with Poor Prognosis and/or Increased Severity of Coronary Artery Disease

Exercise Electrocardiogram

1. Failure to complete stage II of Bruce protocol or equivalent workload (≤ 6.5 METS) with other protocols.
2. Failure to attain heart rate ≥ 120 beats/min (off beta blockers).
3. Time of onset, magnitude, morphology, and postexercise duration of abnormal horizontal or downsloping ST segment depression.
   Onset at heart rate < 120 beats/min or ≤ 6.5 METS.
   Magnitude ≥ 2.0 mm.
   Postexercise duration ≥ 6 min.
   Depression in multiple leads.
4. Systolic blood pressure response during or after progressive exercise.
   Sustained decrease of > 10 mm Hg or flat blood pressure response (≤ 130 mm Hg) during progressive exercise.
5. Other potentially important determinants.
   Exercise-induced ST segment elevation in leads other than aVR.
   Angina pectoris during exercise.
   Exercise-induced U-wave inversion.
   Exercise-induced ventricular tachycardia.

Thallium Scintigraphy

Abnormal thallium distribution in more than one vascular region at rest or with exercise that redistributes at another time:
   Abnormal distribution associated with increased lung uptake produced by exercise in the absence of severely depressed left ventricular function at rest.
   Enlargement of the cardiac pool of thallium with exercise.

Radionuclide Ventriculography

A fall in left ventricular ejection fraction of ≥ 0.10 during exercise.
A rest or exercise left ventricular ejection fraction of < 0.50, when suspected to be due to coronary artery disease.

Reprinted from *Journal of the American College of Cardiology*, Vol. 8, Schlant, R.C., Blomqvist, C.G., Brandenburg, R.O., et al.: Guidelines for exercise testing. A report of the American College of Cardiology/American Heart Association Task Force on Assessment of Cardiovascular Procedures (Subcommittee on Exercise Testing). pp. 725–738, Copyright 1986, with permission from the American College of Cardiology; and Pepine, C.J., Allen, H.D., Bashore, T.M., et al.: ACC/AHA guidelines for cardiac catheterization and cardiac catheterization laboratories. American College of Cardiology/American Heart Association Ad Hoc Task Force on Cardiac Catheterization. J. Am. Coll. Cardiol. 18:1149–1182, 1991.
Abbreviation: METS, metabolic equivalents.

tients over age 40 years or young patients with possible cardiac disease, and ambulatory electrocardiographic monitoring, which should be considered for patients with suspected cardiac syncope or those with no cause on history or physical examination.

A test that may become more routinely used in the future is head-up tilt-table testing, which some data indicate can be used to diagnose neurocardiogenic syncope and even to guide therapy. However, in the absence of a gold standard for diagnosis of neurocardiogenic syncope, the diagnostic performance of tilt-table testing is uncertain. Research in the next several years is likely to clarify the extent to which this test should be routinely considered and the actions that should follow from its results.

Rule Out Cardiac Source of Embolus

Emboli originating in the heart are believed to account for 15% of cerebrovascular ischemic strokes, and echocardiography is therefore an appropriate test for patients

with cerebral embolism and clinical evidence of heart disease. Because of a lower likelihood of cerebrovascular atherosclerosis as a cause of ischemic stroke in younger patients, echocardiography is also considered an appropriate test for patients with a cerebrovascular event who are younger than 45 years.[18] In such patients, potential sources of cardiac emboli include mitral valve prolapse and an intra-atrial communication.

Transesophageal echocardiography may be preferable to transthoracic echocardiography. The transesophageal procedure is more costly and uncomfortable for the patient, but this approach provides better views of the left atrium, left atrial appendage, and mitral valve, and it can also be used to assess possible atheroembolic sources in the ascending aorta. One algorithm has been proposed by DeRook and colleagues, although it has not been formally tested[19] (Fig. 4–6).

Assessment of Congestive Heart Failure

In the evaluation of the patient with an enlarged heart or clinical signs of congestive heart failure (see Chaps. 14 and 22), the goals of the clinician include detection or exclusion of valvular heart disease, congenital anomalies, pericardial effusion, and ischemic heart disease. The noninvasive test of choice is echocardiography, which provides data that address several issues:

- Does the patient have systolic or diastolic dysfunction?
- Is there structural heart disease such as valvular or congenital abnormalities?
- If the left ventricle is dilated, is there evidence of regional wall motion abnormalities, which would suggest damage due to coronary artery disease?

Echocardiography can be particularly useful in patients with clinical symptoms and signs of congestive heart failure, but who have a normal cardiac silhouette on chest x-

Table 4-7	Indications for Echocardiography in the Evaluation of Heart Murmurs

Indication	Class
1. A murmur in a patient with cardiorespiratory symptoms	I
2. A murmur in an asymptomatic patient if the clinical features indicate at least a moderate probability that the murmur is reflective of structural heart disease	I
3. A murmur in an asymptomatic patient in whom there is a low probability of heart disease but in whom the diagnosis of heart disease cannot be reasonably excluded by the standard cardiovascular clinical evaluation	IIa
4. In an adult, an asymptomatic heart murmur that has been identified by an experienced observer as functional or innocent	III

Reprinted from *Journal of the American College of Cardiology*, Vol. 29, Cheitlin, M.D., Alpert, J.S., Armstrong, W.F., et al.: ACC/AHA guidelines for the clinical application of echocardiography: Executive summary. A report of the American College of Cardiology/American Heart Association Task Force on Practice Guidelines (Committee on Clinical Application of Echocardiography), pp. 862–879, Copyright 1997, with permission from the American College of Cardiology.

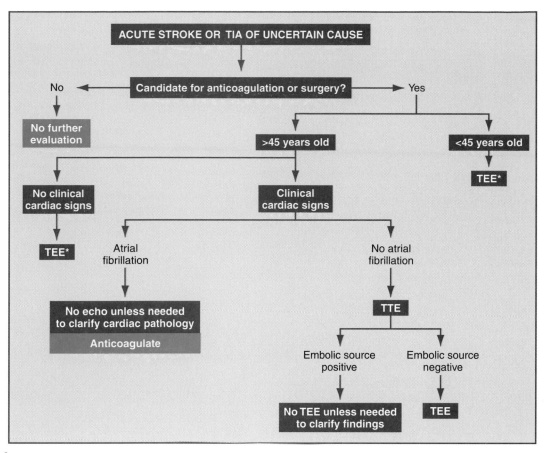

Figure 4–6

Algorithm for the use of transthoracic and transesophageal echocardiography for patients with suspected cardiac sources of emboli. *Because TTE and TEE are complementary, some clinicians may wish to do both. TIA, transient ischemic attack; TEE, transesophageal echocardiography; TTE, transthoracic echocardiography. (Redrawn from DeRook, F.A., Komess, K.A., Albers, G.W., and Popp, R.L.: Transesophageal echocardiography in the evaluation of stroke. Ann. Intern. Med. 117:922–932, 1992.)

ray. In such cases, the echocardiogram may reveal left ventricular diastolic dysfunction, restrictive cardiomyopathy, or evidence of pulmonary disease.

Serial echocardiograms are not necessary for patients with dilated cardiomyopathies unless there is the potential for an intervention such as valve replacement. For example, progressive dilatation of the left ventricle despite medical therapy warrants consideration of valvular surgery even if the patient is asymptomatic. However, if no such intervention is possible, and pharmacologic interventions are being adjusted according to the patient's symptoms and signs, then serial echocardiograms are unlikely to influence management.

References

1. Wennberg, D.E., Kellett, M.A., Dickens, J.D., Jr., et al.: The association between local diagnostic testing intensity and invasive cardiac procedures. JAMA 275:1161–1164, 1996.
2. Goldman, L., and Lee, T.H.: Noninvasive tests for diagnosing the presence and extent of coronary artery disease. J. Gen. Intern. Med. 1:258–265, 1986.
3. Chaitman, B.: Exercise stress testing. In Braunwald, E.: Heart Disease. 5th ed. Philadelphia, W.B. Saunders, 1997, p. 173.
4. Lewis, W.R., and Amsterdam, E.A.: Utility and safety of immediate exercise testing of low-risk patients admitted to the hospital for suspected acute myocardial infarction. Am. J. Cardiol. 74:987–990, 1994.
5. Goldschlager, N.: Use of the treadmill test in the diagnosis of coronary artery disease in patients with chest pain. Ann. Intern. Med. 97:383–388, 1982.
6. Ritchie, J.L., Bateman, T.M., Bonow, R.D., et al.: Guidelines for clinical use of cardiac radionuclide imaging. Report of the American College of Cardiology/American Heart Association Task Force on Assessment of Diagnostic and Therapeutic Cardiovascular Procedures (Committee on Radionuclide Imaging) developed in association with the American Society of Nuclear Cardiology. J. Am. Coll. Cardiol. 25:521–547, 1995.
7. Williams, M.J., Odabashian, J., Lauer, M.S., et al.: Prognostic value of dobutamine echocardiography in patients with left ventricular dysfunction. J. Am. Coll. Cardiol. 27:132–139, 1996.
8. Patterson, R.E., Eisner, R.L., and Horowitz, S.F.: Comparison of cost-effectiveness and utility of exercise ECG, single photon emission computed tomography, positron emission tomography, and coronary angiography for diagnosis of coronary artery disease. Circulation 91:54–65, 1995.
9. Gopal, A.S., Shen, Z., Sapin, P.M., et al.: Assessment of cardiac function by three-dimensional echocardiography compared with conventional noninvasive methods. Circulation 92:842–853, 1995.
10. Lippman, N., Stein, K.M., and Lerman, B.B.: Differential therapeutic responses of patients with isoproterenol-dependent and isoproterenol-independent vasodepressor syncope. Am. Heart J. 128:1110–1116, 1994.
11. Passamani, E., Davis, K.B., Gillespie, M.J., et al.: A randomized trial of coronary artery bypass surgery: Survival of patients with low ejection fraction. N. Engl. J. Med. 312:1665–1671, 1985.

12. Lee, T.H., Fukui, T., Weinstein, M., et al.: Cost-effectiveness of screening strategies for left main disease in patients with stable angina. Med. Decis. Making 8:268–278, 1989.

13. Podrid, P.J., Graboys, T.B., and Lown, B.: Prognosis of medically treated patients with coronary artery disease with profound ST segment depression during exercise testing. N. Engl. J. Med. 305: 1111–1116, 1981.

14. Gibbons, R.J., Balady, G.J., Beasley, J.W., et al.: ACC/AHA guidelines for exercise testing: Executive Summary. A report of the American College of Cardiology/American Heart Association Task Force on Practice Guidelines (Committee on Exercise Testing). Circulation 96:345–354, 1997..

15. American College of Physicians: Efficacy of exercise thallium-201 scintigraphy in the diagnosis and prognosis of coronary artery disease. Ann. Intern. Med. 113:703–704, 1990.

16. Pepine, C.J., Allen, H.D., Bashore, T.M., et al.: ACC/AHA guidelines for cardiac catheterization and cardiac catheterization laboratories. American College of Cardiology/American Heart Association Ad Hoc Task Force on Cardiac Catheterization. J. Am. Coll. Cardiol. 18:1149–1182, 1991.

17. Cheitlin, M.D., Alpert, J.S., Armstrong, W.F., et al.: ACC/AHA guidelines for the clinical application of echocardiography: Executive Summary. A report of the American College of Cardiology/American Heart Association Task Force on Practice Guidelines (Committee on Clinical Application of Echocardiography). J. Am. Coll. Cardiol. 29:862–879, 1997.

18. Cardiogenic brain embolism. Cerebral Embolism Task Force. Arch. Neurol. 43:71–84, 1986.

19. DeRook, F.A., Komess, K.A., Albers, G.W., and Popp, R.L.: Transesophageal echocardiography in the evaluation of stroke. Ann. Intern. Med. 117:922–932, 1992.

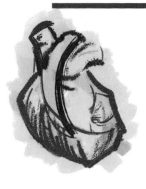

Chapter 5

Screening for Coronary Artery Disease and Its Risk Factors

HAROLD C. SOX

Screening means trying to detect a disease or its risk factors before they become clinically evident. Screening can improve the efficiency of *primary prevention,* which seeks to prevent a disease in people without evidence of the disease, by identifying high-risk individuals who are the most likely to benefit. Screening can also apply to *secondary prevention,* where the goal is to prevent subsequent manifestations of disease in those patients who have it. For example, screening for hyperlipidemia in persons with established coronary artery disease may lead to detection and modification of the risk factor and a consequent reduction in risk of angina, myocardial infarction, or sudden death.

This chapter focuses on the detection of asymptomatic coronary artery disease with tests commonly used by the primary physician, such as the resting electrocardiogram (ECG) and the stress ECG. It also addresses the detection of hypertension and hypercholesterolemia, two important modifiable risk factors for coronary artery disease.

ANALYTIC APPROACH

Probabilistic Reasoning

For the topic of screening, probabilistic reasoning is useful in understanding how new information, such as the results of a test, modifies the likelihood that a patient has a disease. The revision of a probability after obtaining new information is an application of Bayes' theorem, which allows the physician to calculate the posttest odds as the product of the pretest odds and the likelihood ratio (see Chap. 2). The likelihood ratio is another useful way to express the performance of a diagnostic test. Physicians often express test results as positive or negative, and so there is a likelihood ratio for a positive test result and one for a negative test result. Tests that have a very large likelihood ratio after a positive test or a very small (nearly zero) likelihood ratio after a negative test are the most useful. Tests with likelihood ratios close to 1.0 have little effect on the probability of disease.

Measurement of Test Performance Characteristics

The accurate measurement of a test's sensitivity, specificity, or likelihood ratio requires that all patients who meet defined inclusion criteria (e.g., healthy adults) undergo the index test (e.g., an exercise stress test) and immediately thereafter, regardless of the results of the index test, undergo the gold standard test (e.g., a perfect measure of myocardial ischemia). Few studies meet this criterion. The most common problem is "referral bias" or "workup bias," which occurs when the physician selects patients to undergo the gold standard test in part because the index test is abnormal. For example, a positive exercise test result influences a physician toward performing coronary arteriography. Arteriography is much less likely to be performed after a negative exercise test result. If the study population is patients who undergo arteriography, this practice pattern will deplete the study of patients with negative exercise tests, some of whom would have had positive arteriograms. A reduction in false-negative results leads to overestimating the true sensitivity relative to the results of the ideal study. By an analogous line of reasoning, a reduction in true-negative results underestimates specificity. Workup bias is endemic among studies of tests for coronary artery disease because the gold standard test, the coronary arteriogram, is costly and uncomfortable and has some risk.

One way to avoid workup bias is to use the subsequent development of coronary artery disease as the gold standard test to measure test performance. This approach is particularly useful in asymptomatic persons, in whom it is not realistic to perform a coronary arteriogram routinely. The problem with this approach is that it is not possible to be sure that coronary artery disease that occurs several years after a negative test was actually present when the test was performed nor that a person who remains asymptomatic is not about to have a major coronary event. This approach tends to underestimate sensitivity and specificity.

Epidemiologic Principles

The most important epidemiologic principle for understanding the rationale for applying a screening test is the relationship between *relative risk* and *absolute risk* (see Chap. 2). Absolute risk reduction is a better measure of the impact of an intervention than relative risk reduction. This principle is useful when interpreting the results of

clinical trials of screening or trials of treatment for disease detected by screening.

A test's ability to detect a presymptomatic abnormality is influenced not only by the technical characteristics of the test but also by the severity of the disease at the time of the screening. For example, a screening exercise test may detect inducible ischemia in a patient with a 60% stenosis in the left anterior descending coronary artery but not in a patient with a 10% stenosis. As individuals proceed along the continuum from normal to symptomatic (Fig. 5–1), screening tests become progressively more sensitive. In addition, early detection of disease may appear to increase life expectancy with the disease, not because of any improvements in treatment or outcome but simply because the patient is aware of the disease earlier in its natural history.

Chain of Evidence

The clinical trial with randomly assigned control subjects is the best way to measure the impact of screening and decide whether the evidence warrants a policy of screening.[1] There have been no randomized trials of screening for coronary artery disease or its risk factors, although there have been some important trials of treatment for hypertension and hypercholesterolemia in asymptomatic persons. When there have been no randomized trials of screening, the *chain of evidence* is a useful concept for deciding whether an intervention alters the important outcomes of the disease. In the case of screening, the following line of reasoning must be intact:

1. The test must detect presymptomatic, early-stage disease accurately, inexpensively, and safely.
2. Treatment in an early stage of disease must improve clinical outcomes.
3. The improved outcomes from screening must justify the overall cost of the screening test, subsequently indicated tests, and treatments (see Chap. 2).

Reference to Existing Guidelines

A number of leading professional societies and expert panels have recommended approaches to screening and prevention. The guidelines produced by these organizations usually have the following features: thorough review of the literature; a background article that summarizes the evidence and its quality; explanation of the rationale of the recommendation; and review by outside experts.

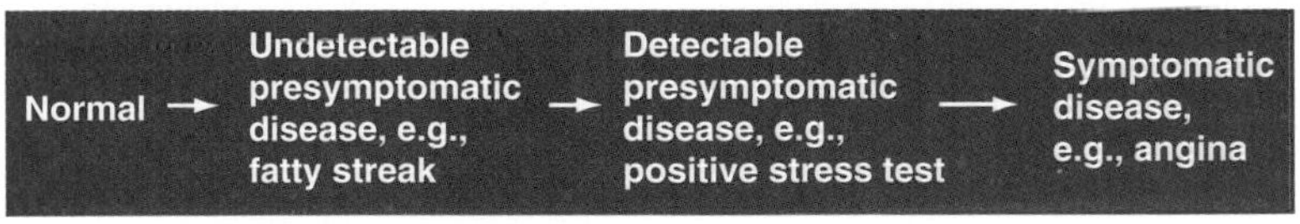

| Normal → | Undetectable presymptomatic disease, e.g., fatty streak | → | Detectable presymptomatic disease, e.g., positive stress test | → | Symptomatic disease, e.g., angina |

Figure 5–1

Progression of coronary artery disease. "Lead-time bias" is a hazard in interpreting the effect of screening on disease outcomes. Earlier detection may prolong life expectancy with the disease without prolonging the actual length of life, simply because the diagnosis occurs earlier in the patient's life. Screening tests usually become more sensitive as patients move toward the onset of symptomatic disease, which reflects more advanced disease.

These guidelines are important because they represent a serious effort to make an unbiased, evidence-based recommendation. Insurers usually base their decisions on the recommendations of independent expert panels such as the U.S. Preventive Services Task Force.

SCREENING FOR CORONARY ARTERY DISEASE

Resting ECGs and stress ECGs are the most popular screening tests for coronary artery disease in healthy adults. Since there have been no clinical trials of screening for coronary artery disease, the chain of evidence is the best approach for evaluating screening.

Incidence and Prevalence of Disease

About 500,000 people die of coronary artery disease in the United States each year, making it the leading cause of death. Its principal manifestations are angina pectoris, myocardial infarction, and sudden cardiac death. Sudden death is the first and only manifestation of coronary artery disease in approximately 18% of all coronary artery disease patients and occurs at the rate of 0.8 per 10,000 every 2 years in healthy men aged 45 years and younger and 6.0 per 10,000 in men aged 65 to 74 years according to data from the Framingham Heart Study.

Autopsies on apparently healthy people who died accidentally provide the best estimates of the prevalence of coronary artery disease in asymptomatic patients. In asymptomatic men, the prevalence of coronary artery disease was 4% in men aged 40 years or less and 11% in those 50 years or older. The corresponding prevalences in younger and older women were 0.7% and 5%, respectively. Risk factors for coronary artery disease increased the prevalence. In 60-year-old men, the prevalence of coronary artery disease was 5% with no risk factors and 16% with at least one risk factor; only 40% of men have no risk factors.[2]

The average 10-year incidence of coronary artery disease according to estimates from the Framingham Heart Study ranges from less than 1% in 30- to 34-year-old women to 24% in 70- to 74-year-old men.[3] Given the average life expectancy of persons with coronary artery disease, this approach is also useful for estimating coronary artery disease prevalence (Fig. 5–2). The Framingham Heart Study has developed a very useful clinical prediction rule for using age, gender, high-density lipoprotein (HDL) cholesterol, total cholesterol, systolic blood pressure, diabetes, cigarette smoking, and left ventricular hypertrophy on ECG to predict 5-year and 10-year incidence of coronary artery disease (Table 5–1).[3] Many internists use this table when counseling patients about their coronary risk.

Testing for Coronary Artery Disease in Asymptomatic Persons: A General Comment

Tests for myocardial ischemia often fail to identify healthy people who subsequently suffer unstable angina,

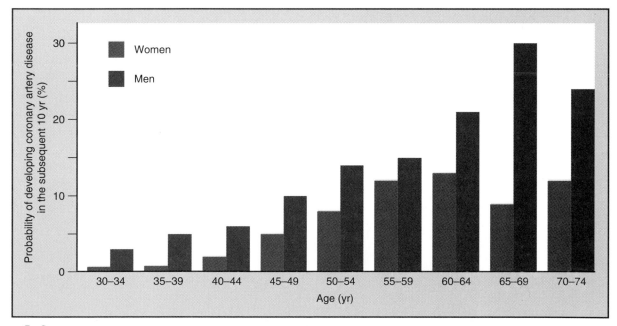

Figure 5–2

Probability of developing coronary artery disease in the subsequent 10 years, as estimated from the Framingham Study. If average life expectancy with new-onset coronary artery disease, including sudden death, is about 10 years, the 10-year incidence of coronary artery disease in a given age range would correspond approximately to the estimated prevalence in a population about 10 years older. (Data from Anderson, K.M., Wilson, P.W.F., Odell, P.M., and Kannel, W.B.: An updated coronary risk profile: A statement for health professionals. Circulation 83:356–362, 1991.)

Table 6-1   Framingham Cardiac Risk Predictor

1. Find points for each risk factor

Age (If Female) (yr)				Age (If Male) (yr)				HDL Cholesterol			
Age	Points	Age	Points	Age	Points	Age	Points	HDL	Points	HDL	Points
30	−12	41	1	30	−2	48–49	9	25–26	7	67–73	−4
31	−11	42–43	2	31	−1	50–51	10	27–29	6	74–80	−5
32	−9	44	3	32–33	0	52–54	11	30–32	5	81–87	−6
33	−8	45–46	4	34	1	55–56	12	33–35	4	88–96	−7
34	−6	47–48	5	35–36	2	57–59	13	36–38	3		
35	−5	49–50	6	37–38	3	60–61	14	39–42	2		
36	−4	51–52	7	39	4	62–64	15	43–46	1		
37	−3	53–55	8	40–41	5	65–67	16	47–50	0		
38	−2	56–60	9	42–43	6	68–70	17	51–55	−1		
39	−1	61–67	10	44–45	7	71–73	18	56–60	−2		
40	0	68–74	11	46–47	8	74	19	61–66	−3		

Total Cholesterol (mg/dl)				SBP (mm Hg)					Points	
Chol	Points	Chol	Points	SBP	Points	SBP	Points	Other factors	Yes	No
139–151	−3	220–239	2	98–104	−2	150–160	4	Cigarette smoking	4	0
152–166	−2	240–262	3	105–112	−1	161–172	5	Diabetes		
167–182	−1	263–288	4	113–120	0	173–185	6	Male	3	0
183–199	0	289–315	5	121–129	1			Female	6	0
200–219	1	316–330	6	130–139	2			ECG-LVH	9	0
				140–149	3					

2. Add points for all risk factors

‾‾‾‾‾ + ‾‾‾‾‾‾ + ‾‾‾‾‾ + ‾‾‾‾‾ + ‾‾‾‾‾‾‾ + ‾‾‾‾‾‾‾ + ‾‾‾‾‾‾‾ + ‾‾‾‾‾
(Age)   (Total chol)   (HDL)   (SPB)   (Smoking)   (Diabetes)   (ECG-LVH)   (Total)

Note: *Minus points subtract from total.*

3. Look up risk corresponding to point total

Points	Probability (%) 5 yr	Probability (%) 10 yr	Points	Probability (%) 5 yr	Probability (%) 10 yr	Points	Probability (%) 5 yr	Probability (%) 10 yr	Points	Probability (%) 5 yr	Probability (%) 10 yr
≤1	<1	<2	9	2	5	17	6	13	25	14	27
2	1	2	10	2	6	18	7	14	26	16	29
3	1	2	11	3	6	19	8	16	27	17	31
4	1	2	12	3	7	20	8	18	28	19	33
5	1	3	13	3	8	21	9	19	29	20	36
6	1	3	14	4	9	22	11	21	30	22	38
7	1	4	15	5	10	23	12	23	31	24	40
8	2	4	16	5	12	24	13	25	32	25	42

4. Compare with average 10-year risk

Age (yr)	Probability (%) Women	Probability (%) Men	Age (yr)	Probability (%) Women	Probability (%) Men	Age (yr)	Probability (%) Women	Probability (%) Men
30–34	<1	3	45–49	5	10	60–45	13	21
35–39	1	5	50–54	8	14	65–69	9	30
40–44	2	6	55–59	12	16	70–74	12	24

From Anderson, K.M., Wilson, P.W.F., Odell, P.M., and Kannel, W.B.: An updated coronary risk profile: A statement for health professionals. Circulation 83:356–362, 1991.

Abbreviations: HDL, high-density lipoprotein; Chol, cholesterol; SBP, systolic blood pressure; ECG-LVH, left ventricular hypertrophy by electrocardiography.

Table 5–2 Accuracy of Resting ECG Findings in Predicting the Diagnosis of Clinical CAD in Healthy Men in the Honolulu Heart Program over a Follow-Up Period of 12 Years*

Finding	Frequency	Sensitivity	Specificity	Likelihood Ratio (+)	Likelihood Ratio (−)	Probability of CAD if Finding Present	Probability of CAD if Finding Absent
ST segment depression	.013	.042	.989	3.8	.97	.24	.078
T-wave inversion	.023	.059	.980	3.0	.96	.20	.078

Adapted from Journal of Clinical Epidemiology, Vol. 41, Knutsen, R., Knutsen, S.E., Curb, J.D., et al.: The predictive value of resting electrocardiograms for 12-year incidence of coronary heart disease in the Honolulu Heart Program, pp. 293–302, Copyright 1988, with permission from Elsevier Science.

Abbreviations: ECG, electrocardiogram; CAD, coronary artery disease.

* The overall frequency of CAD events in the 12 years of observation was 80.8/1000, which corresponds to a .0808 probability of developing CAD.

acute myocardial infarction, and sudden cardiac death. The trigger event for these acute coronary syndromes is often the rupture of an atherosclerotic plaque, followed by thrombus formation and either infarction or rapidly progressive ischemia. Because these plaques may be relatively small and do not limit blood flow, some do not cause ischemia until they rupture, and therefore, they are very hard to detect by testing for myocardial ischemia. McHenry and coworkers showed that most apparently healthy men who developed symptomatic coronary artery disease after a negative stress test had unstable angina, acute myocardial infarction, or sudden cardiac death as their first manifestation.[4] By contrast, exertional angina was usually the first manifestation of coronary artery disease in apparently healthy men who had a prior positive stress ECG. A positive test for myocardial ischemia often reflects a coronary plaque that does obstruct blood flow and that may serve as the trigger for a superimposed thrombosis or as a "marker" for other, smaller plaques that rupture and actually cause the clinical event.

Diagnostic Testing: The Resting ECG

Accuracy of ECG Findings. The resting ECG is an imperfect indicator of existing coronary artery disease. In the Coronary Artery Surgery Study of men with stable angina pectoris, 29% with proven coronary artery disease had a normal ECG, implying a sensitivity of 71% for an abnormal ECG in predicting an abnormal coronary arteriogram. Q-waves, ST segment depression, and T-wave inversion had sensitivities of 29%, 34%, and 10%, respectively.[5] These findings may represent an overestimate of the true sensitivities because of workup bias (see earlier). In addition, the subjects had chest pain, and the results may not apply to healthy people.

There have been no studies of the sensitivity and specificity of the resting ECG in predicting the results of an immediate coronary arteriogram in asymptomatic persons. The Honolulu Heart Program used the subsequent development of coronary artery disease as the gold standard test to measure test performance in asymptomatic persons.[6] Table 5–2 shows the accuracy of a resting ECG in asymptomatic men in predicting coronary artery disease in a period of 12 years. Major abnormalities occurred infrequently in healthy men, and few men who later de-

veloped coronary artery disease had major abnormalities on the screening ECG. ECG abnormalities increased the odds of developing coronary artery disease, but the probability of being diagnosed with CAD increased to only about 20%. Absence of these ECG findings reduced the 12-year probability of a diagnosis of coronary artery disease only slightly.

In the Framingham Heart Study, routine ECGs performed at 2-year intervals detected a substantial number of myocardial infarctions that had not been diagnosed clinically. The proportion of myocardial infarctions that were "silent" was 20% in younger men but rose to over 50% in men aged 75 to 84 years (Table 5–3). These "silent" infarctions may be clinically significant if they are the rationale for secondary prevention of further coronary artery disease events (see Chap. 19) and because the death rate from surgery is relatively high during the 6 months following a known myocardial infarction. Still, the semiannual rate of previously unrecognized myocardial infarction is only 0.5 in 1000 in men aged 40 to 45 years.

Prognostic Value of ECG Findings. A variety of abnormalities on a resting ECG connote a higher risk of coronary artery disease death in apparently healthy middle-aged men (Table 5–4).[7] However, the ECG findings

Table 5–3 Detecting Previously Unrecognized MI on Routine ECG*

Age (years)	Men Unrecognized MIs (n/1000)	Men All MIs	Women Unrecognized MIs (n/1000)	Women All MIs
30–34	0.13	0.64	0.0	0.11
35–44	0.32	1.91	0.13	0.26
45–54	0.83	3.61	0.14	0.65
55–64	1.41	5.40	0.90	2.35
65–74	2.69	7.05	1.06	2.78
75–84	3.01	5.64	1.70	6.42

From Goldberger, A.L., and O'Konski, M.: Utility of the routine electrocardiogram before surgery and on general hospital admissions. Ann. Intern. Med. 105: 552–557, 1986.

Abbreviations: MI, myocardial infarction; ECG, electrocardiogram.

* These estimates assume a constant 10-year incidence. Data derived from 2282 men and 2845 women in the Framingham Study.

	Prognostic Value of Resting ECG Findings		
Finding	**Prevalence of Finding (% of ECGs)**	**Annual Deaths/1000 without Finding**	**Relative Risk of Cardiac Death if Finding Present**
Ventricular premature beats	1.6	1.1	3.6
Left axis deviation	2.7	0.5–2.0	2.0
Q-waves	1.4	1.9–4.7	4.6
T-wave inversion	4.3	1.9–3.8	2.6
ST segment depression	1.8	2.0–4.0	3.4
Any of several major findings	4.9	1.9–8.9	3.6

From Sox, H.C., Garber, A.M., and Littenberg, B.: The resting electrocardiogram as a screening test: A clinical analysis. Ann. Intern. Med. 111:489–502, 1990.

Abbreviation: ECG, electrocardiogram.

are infrequent, occurring in 1% to 5% of healthy men. Because the annual rate of coronary artery disease mortality is only 1 to 5 per 1000 per year, the attributable risk is small. Although these ECG findings do imply a worse mortality from coronary artery disease, the findings are infrequent, the baseline coronary artery disease death rate is very low, the prognosis is not much worse when the findings are present, and the attributable risk is small. As a result, these ECG findings alone should not cause undue alarm nor should they be the cause of interventions in otherwise healthy people.

In summary, a healthy person's resting ECG usually does not have the findings that increase the risk of coronary artery disease. These findings seldom presage major coronary artery disease events in apparently healthy people. The baseline risk of coronary artery disease is higher in persons with coronary artery disease risk factors, and these ECG findings will have greater significance. A routine ECG can detect a previously unsuspected myocardial infarction, but these events are infrequent even in older men.

Diagnostic Testing: The Stress ECG

Accuracy of Stress ECG Findings. In the ideal study of the accuracy of the stress ECG in asymptomatic persons, all subjects would undergo the index test (the stress ECG) and a gold standard test. The closest approximation to this ideal is three studies in which, following a maximal stress ECG, a total of 4333 apparently healthy men were monitored for 5 to 6 years for development of coronary artery disease (Table 5–5). An abnormal test (at least 1 mm ST segment depression) occurred in 10.4%. A total of 125 men (1.9%) developed coronary artery disease; the exercise ECG had been abnormal in 55. The sensitivity of the test was therefore 44%, with a false-positive rate (1-specificity) of 9%, a likelihood ratio after a positive test of 4.9, and a likelihood ratio after a negative test of 0.62.

Prognosis of Stress ECG Findings. An abnormal stress ECG increases the chance of dying of coronary artery disease, whereas a normal screening exercise ECG implies a lower subsequent death rate from coronary artery disease (Table 5–6). However, the principal question is whether these prognostic characteristics lead to a better outcome than expected without screening or treatment before development of symptoms. No clinical trials have addressed this question. A follow-up study of 50 initially asymptomatic men with positive stress tests and abnormal coronary arteriograms suggests that the onset of symptoms often precedes lethal events.[8] After 13.5 years of observation, 8 of the 9 men who died of coronary artery disease had developed angina pectoris before they died. The overall mortality was 1.5% per year.

The Resting ECG and Stress ECG as Screening Tests. In summary, the resting ECG and stress ECG are poor screening tests. They do not lower the probability of coronary artery disease very much because they have a low sensitivity. Furthermore, their low specificity and the low prevalence of coronary artery disease in asymptomatic people means that most positive tests will be false-positive results.

Effect of Early Detection and Treatment on Clinical Outcomes

To make a convincing case for doing a screening test, detection of disease when the patient is asymptomatic should improve clinical outcomes compared with waiting until the patient develops symptoms. As yet, there is no evidence that a positive test for coronary artery disease leads to behavior changes, medication, or surgery that improves quality of life or length of life in an apparently healthy person.

Asymptomatic persons with exercise ECG abnormalities are at increased risk of coronary artery disease, and antianginal drugs such as nitroglycerin, beta-adrenergic blockers, and calcium antagonists reduce the frequency and the duration of silent ischemic episodes detected with ambulatory ECG monitoring. As yet, however, there have been no completed studies of the effect of these agents on the incidence of major cardiac events or death in totally asymptomatic populations with silent ischemia detected by stress testing or by resting ECG abnormalities.

In patients with angina pectoris, coronary artery bypass grafting leads to longer survival than medical therapy if left main coronary artery, left anterior descending artery, or three-vessel disease is present[9] (see Chap. 18). The prevalence of these high-risk forms of coronary artery disease is probably quite low in healthy people, since they are very infrequent in people with atypical chest pain who have arteriography-proven coronary artery disease.[2]

There have been no studies of the efficacy of coronary artery bypass graft surgery in asymptomatic persons with coronary artery disease. Although patients with asymptomatic three-vessel coronary artery disease often experi-

Table 5-5	Accuracy of Stress ECG in Predicting Cardiac Events in Asymptomatic Men					
Frequency of Abnormal ECG Result	Sensitivity	Specificity	Likelihood Ratio (+)	Likelihood Ratio (−)	Probability of Developing CAD in 6 Years if Test Positive	Probability of Developing CAD in 6 Years if Test Negative
10.4%	.35	.91	4.9	.62	.127	.018

From Sox, H.C., Littenberg, B., and Garber, A.M.: The role of exercise testing in screening for coronary artery disease. Ann. Intern. Med. 110:456–469, 1989.
Abbreviations: ECG, electrocardiogram; CAD, coronary artery disease.
The overall 6-year incidence of CAD in healthy people in the studies used for this table was 28.8/1000, which corresponds to a 0.0288 probability of developing CAD in six years.

ence myocardial infarction or cardiac death, asymptomatic men with a positive exercise ECG and angiographically proven coronary artery disease commonly experience angina as a "warning sign" before one of these events.

The current lack of evidence that early detection of coronary artery disease alters its prognosis is a serious limitation in any argument for performing a resting ECG or exercise ECG as a screening test for coronary artery disease. The *possibility* that early detection of severe coronary artery disease might prolong life does not justify routine screening of large populations of asymptomatic persons.

Cost-Effectiveness

Because there have been no studies of the effectiveness of early treatment of asymptomatic coronary artery disease, there is no direct evidence that such treatment increases life expectancy. As a result, it is not possible to calculate the cost-effectiveness of screening by direct means. One cost-effectiveness decision model assumed that coronary artery bypass surgery is as effective in asymptomatic persons with high-risk coronary artery disease as it is in symptomatic persons.[2] Using this assumption, the cost of screening with an exercise test and the subsequent treatment including coronary angiography and coronary artery bypass surgery in men who were 40 years

Table 5-6	Prognostic Value of Stress ECG Findings		
Finding	Prevalence of Finding (% of Stress ECGs)	Annual Deaths/1000 with Finding	Relative Risk of Cardiac Death if Finding Present
Strongly positive result	2.2	12.7	5.0
All positive results	5.8	8.1	4.6
Normal result	94.2	.95	1.0

Adapted from Gordon, D.J., Ekelund, L.-G., Karon, J.M., et al.: Predictive value of the exercise tolerance test for mortality in North American men: The Lipid Research Clinics Mortality Follow-Up Study. Circulation 74:252–261, 1986.
Abbreviation: ECG, electrocardiogram.
The authors defined a "strongly positive" result as when the ST response was at least 2 mm depression (or elevation) or occurred within the first six minutes of exercise or occurred at a heart rate at or below 163 minus 0.66 times age.

of age was about $80,000 per extra year of life; and in women aged 40 and 60 years, it was about $215,000 and $48,000, respectively. In asymptomatic men aged 60 years, a policy of routine screening exercise ECG and subsequently indicated tests and treatments would prolong life by at most 12 days with a cost of about $25,000 per extra year of life. If the effect of bypass surgery on life expectancy in asymptomatic individuals is 50% of its effect in persons with angina pectoris, the cost rose to about $60,000 per extra year of life in 60-year-old men.

Recommendations of Expert Panels

The American College of Physicians[2, 7] and the U.S. Preventive Services Task Force[10] do not recommend routine exercise stress testing or a resting ECG in individuals with no cardiac risk factors, and the American College of Cardiology/American Heart Association[11] states that there is general agreement that the resting ECG is useful in persons aged 40 years or older and of little or no usefulness in persons under age 40 years (Table 5–7). The American College of Cardiology/American Heart Association states that there is general agreement that a routine exercise ECG is of little or no usefulness in average-risk individuals.[12] The organizations seem to agree that there is neither consensus nor any direct evidence about the effectiveness of doing an exercise test in certain groups: people whose job may place others at high risk (bus drivers and airline pilots), sedentary men about to undertake an exercise program, and people with cardiovascular risk factors (Table 4–5).

Table 5–8 shows an approach to using the resting ECG and the stress ECG to screen for coronary artery disease. These recommendations are conservative, as befits the dearth of good-quality evidence that screening for coronary artery disease accomplishes anything.

SCREENING FOR HYPERTENSION

Hypertension is common in America. The 1976 to 1980 National Health and Nutrition Examination Survey (NHANES) showed that 22% of adults had blood pressures exceeding 160/95 mm Hg. There has been remark-

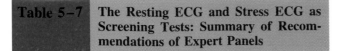

Table 5–7 The Resting ECG and Stress ECG as Screening Tests: Summary of Recommendations of Expert Panels

Resting ECG

American College of Physicians (1990; reaffirmed 1996)[7]

No CAD risk factors: Recommend against performing a resting ECG in men without evidence of cardiovascular disease or risk factors for CAD. Did not study the resting ECG in women but recommendations should apply to them.

CAD risk factors or other circumstances: Did not study the resting ECG in men with CAD risk factors.

U.S. Preventive Services Task Force (1995)[10]

No CAD risk factors: Insufficient evidence to recommend for or against screening middle-aged and older men and women with a screening resting ECG. Recommend against resting ECG in people without CAD risk factors, based on poor accuracy of test and cost of follow-up testing.

CAD risk factors or other circumstances: Reasonable to screen high-risk individuals if the results would alter management or if the individual is an airline pilot or bus driver.

American College of Cardiology/American Heart Association (1992)[11]

No CAD risk factors: Do a resting ECG in anyone who is undergoing a physical examination and is 40 years old or greater. Resting ECG is of little or no benefit before age 40 years if the person has no CAD risk factors or special job requirements.

CAD risk factors or other circumstances: Do an ECG in anyone, regardless of age, whose job requires cardiovascular fitness or is linked to public safety.

Stress ECG

American College of Physicians (1989; reaffirmed 1996)[2]

No CAD risk factors: Recommend against performing a stress ECG in adults without evidence of CAD.

CAD risk factors or other circumstances: Insufficient evidence to make a strong recommendation for or against doing a stress ECG in sedentary people who are about to undertake an exercise program, in persons whose occupations put others at risk, or in older men with one or more CAD risk factors.

U.S. Preventive Services Task Force (1995)[10]

Same recommendation as for resting ECG.

American College of Cardiology/American Heart Association (1997)[12]

No CAD risk factors: In apparently healthy individuals, there are no conditions for which there is general agreement that stress testing is justified.

CAD risk factors or other circumstances: There is divergence of opinion with respect to value and appropriateness of stress testing in persons with multiple CAD risk factors, in men over age 40 years or women over age 50 years who plan to start vigorous exercise, who have occupations in which impairment might impact public safety, or who are at high risk for CAD due to other diseases (e.g., chronic renal failure).

Abbreviations: ECG, electrocardiogram; CAD, coronary artery disease.

able progress in detection and treatment of hypertension in the United States. Since the 1971 to 1972 NHANES, the proportion of hypertensives who knew their diagnosis has risen from 51% to 84%, the proportion under treatment has risen from 36% to 73%, and the proportion under treatment whose blood pressure was less than 160/90 has risen from 16% to 55%.

Hypertension is an important risk factor for stroke and coronary artery disease. The risk rises continuously throughout the so-called normal range of blood pressure and on up to severe hypertension. Although cuff sphyg-

momanometry tends to overestimate blood pressure compared with intra-arterial measurement, all studies of the prognostic significance of hypertension and the effects of treatment are based on blood pressures taken under conditions similar to those in the physician's office (see Chap. 11).

Effect of Early Detection and Treatment on Clinical Outcomes

The case favoring screening for hypertension rests on the well-documented benefits of discovering hypertension in asymptomatic people. Many randomized, placebo-controlled clinical trials of treatment for hypertension form the body of evidence. In patients with severe diastolic hypertension (>114 mm Hg) and moderate diastolic hypertension (104 to 114 mm Hg), the Veterans Administration Cooperative Study provided definitive evidence that early treatment reduces cardiovascular events.[13, 14] The absolute risk reduction due to treatment was 21% over 3.3 years in men with moderate hypertension and 36% over 2.2 years in men with severe hypertension. These figures, which correspond to treating five moderately hypertensive patients for 3.3 years or three severely hypertensive patients for 2.2 years to prevent one cardiovascular complication, make a very strong case for screening.

People with newly discovered mild hypertension far outnumber those found to have moderate or severe hypertension, and the effects of treatment are harder to prove in this group. The largest placebo-controlled clinical trial was the Medical Research Council study, which randomized 8700 subjects to the treatment arm and 8654 to the placebo arm.[15] There was no effect on all-cause mortality or myocardial infarction. The stroke rate was 13 per 1000 in 5.5 years for the placebo group and 7 per 1000 for the treatment group. The risk reduction attributable to treatment was 6 strokes per 1000 in 5.5 years, which corresponds to treating 166 people for 5.5 years to prevent 1 stroke.

Screening should extend into the later years, since isolated systolic hypertension in the elderly is a risk factor for heart disease and stroke. The Systolic Hypertension in the Elderly Program was a placebo-controlled randomized trial involving 4736 people aged 60 years and above.[16] The mean systolic blood pressure during 5 years of follow-up was 155 mm Hg in the placebo group and 143 mm Hg in the treatment group. The baseline risk of stroke in the placebo group was 82 per 1000 persons in 5 years. The absolute reduction in 5-year risk of stroke was 30 strokes per 1000 persons, which corresponds to treating 33 people for 5 years to avoid 1 stroke, an almost fivefold higher impact compared with the effect of treating mild hypertension in the Medical Research Council trial. Treatment also reduced coronary heart disease. One hundred and four treatment group patients suffered the combined endpoint of nonfatal myocardial infarction or death from coronary artery disease compared with 141 placebo group patients (relative risk, 0.73; 95% confidence limits, 0.57 to 0.94). The absolute risk reduction due to treatment was 16 events per 1000, which corre-

Table 5–8	Summary Recommendations for Screening Resting ECG and Stress ECG	
	Resting ECG	**Stress ECG**
No CAD risk factors	Do not do (possible exception—older people)	Do not do
Relatively high risk for CAD (see Table 5–1)	Reasonable to do on individualized basis but not routinely No evidence for effect on outcomes Expert panel recommendations are discordant	Reasonable to do on individualized basis but not routinely No evidence for effect on outcomes Expert panel recommendations are discordant
Sedentary person about to start exercise program	Reasonable to do No evidence for effect on outcomes	Reasonable to do No evidence for effect on outcomes
Airline pilot/bus driver	Employer should set policy	Employer should set policy

Abbreviations: ECG, electrocardiogram; CAD, coronary artery disease.

sponds to treating 61 persons for 5 years to avoid 1 major coronary event.

Cost-Effectiveness

Several cost-effectiveness analyses have shown that screening for hypertension is an efficient way to use health care resources. Based on efficacy and current costs of therapy, it costs about $16,000 per quality-adjusted life year gained to screen men aged 40 years and about $23,000 for women of the same age.[17] Costs per quality-adjusted life year gained are higher for younger people and lower for older people (Table 5–9).

When to Start Screening and How Often to Screen: Recommendations of Expert Panels

Cost-effectiveness analysis suggests that it is appropriate to begin screening even at age 20 years, with costs that are reasonable in comparison with other health interventions.[17] The appropriate interval for rescreening is not known, but the incremental cost of measuring the blood pressure is very low, especially in the context of a visit to a physician. In general, one should screen more frequently (preferably yearly) in people whose blood pressure is close to a treatment threshold. Conversely, one can screen people with lower blood pressures at less frequent intervals, perhaps every several years.

The Joint National Committee on Detection, Evalua-

tion, and Treatment of Hypertension and the American Heart Association recommend taking the blood pressure at least once every 2 years if the systolic blood pressure is below 130 mm Hg and the diastolic blood pressure is below 85 mm Hg.[18] They recommend blood pressure measurement at least annually if the systolic blood pressure is 130 to 139 mm Hg or the diastolic blood pressure is below 85 to 89 mm Hg and more often if the blood pressure exceeds these levels. They recommend confirming an elevated reading (greater than 140 mm Hg systolic or 90 mm Hg diastolic) with two additional readings and basing the diagnosis on the average of the three readings. The American College of Physicians,[17] the Canadian Task Force on the Periodic Health Examination,[19] and the U.S. Preventive Services Task Force[10] all recommend taking the blood pressure at every medical visit or at least every 2 years (Table 5–10).

SCREENING FOR HYPERCHOLESTEROLEMIA

Hypercholesterolemia is an important risk factor for coronary artery disease. The relationship between serum cholesterol level and disease risk is approximately exponential. In the Hypertension Detection and Follow-up Program, the risk of coronary heart disease mortality rose from 1.0 to 1.7 from the first quintile (less than 181 mg/dl) to the third quintile (203 to 221 mg/dl) and then from 1.7 to 3.4 from the third to the fifth quintile (greater than 246 mg/dl).[20]

Table 5–9	Cost-Effectiveness of Screening for and Treating Hypertension in Various Age-Sex Groups					
	Men			**Women**		
	Age 20 years	*Age 40 years*	*Age 60 years*	*Age 20 years*	*Age 40 years*	*Age 60 years*
Marginal cost per patient ($)	281	491	456	76	255	363
Marginal increase in life expectancy (days)	4	11	20	1	4	11
Cost-effectiveness ($/quality-adjusted year)	29,291	16,280	8,374	44,412	23,216	12,404

Adapted from Littenberg, B., Garber, A.M., and Sox, H.C.: Screening for hypertension. Ann. Intern. Med. 112:192–202, 1990.

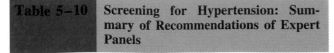

Table 5–10	Screening for Hypertension: Summary of Recommendations of Expert Panels

Canadian Task Force (1994)[19]

Fair evidence to measure blood pressure in all person aged 21 to 64 years by office sphygmomanometry. No recommendation about frequency of screening.

American College of Physicians (1990; reaffirmed 1996)[17]

Measure blood pressure on adults every time they seek care.

U.S. Preventive Services Task Force (1995)[10]

Excellent evidence to recommend periodic screening for all persons ≥21 years of age. The interval between blood pressure measurements is matter of preference, since the optimal interval is unknown.

Joint National Committee on Detection, Evaluation, and Treatment of High Blood Pressure (1993)[18]

Measure the blood pressure every 2 years if the diastolic pressure has been below 85 mm Hg and the systolic blood pressure has been below 130 mm Hg. Measure the blood pressure annually if the diastolic pressure has been between 85 and 90 mm Hg or the systolic blood pressure has been between 130 and 139 mm Hg. People with higher blood pressures require more frequent measurements.

The effect of serum cholesterol on coronary heart disease mortality in older persons is complex. Serum cholesterol rises gradually with age until 50 to 60 years and then remains constant. The effect of high cholesterol on the absolute risk of dying of coronary artery disease depends on the baseline risk of coronary artery disease mortality and the relative risk of dying of coronary artery disease if high cholesterol is present. With aging, the baseline risk of coronary artery disease mortality increases. The relative risk of an increased total cholesterol for coronary artery disease mortality decreases toward 1.0 with aging.[21] This effect is more pronounced in men, in whom the relative risk of increased total cholesterol for coronary artery disease mortality is 1.0 by age 80 years. Women aged 71 years and older with a total cholesterol greater than 240 mg/dl had a significant 1.8-fold increase in coronary heart disease mortality compared with women whose cholesterol was 161 to 199 mg/dl. Low HDL cholesterol is probably a significant predictor of coronary artery disease mortality in older persons, although less so than in younger people.[22]

Although the effect of cholesterol in the elderly is still subject to dispute, the evidence has consistently shown that the relative risk of an elevated cholesterol level for coronary heart disease mortality is much weaker in the elderly than in younger people. However, since the elderly have a much higher prevalence of coronary artery disease, the risk attributable to an elevated cholesterol level may be at least as high in the elderly.[23]

Testing for Hypercholesterolemia

A single measurement of serum cholesterol may mislead the physician. The concepts of sensitivity and specificity, so appropriate to a test for a disease, do not apply to a measure that places a person on a continuum of risk for developing a disease. One issue with serum cholesterol measurements, as with the measurement of blood pressure, is the degree to which the measured value reflects the true value. Standardization of method and performance in clinical laboratories is not as good as in the reference laboratories, and thus a single measurement may reflect substantial between-laboratory variation. Variability from test to test is an important factor, and there is both long-term and transient variability in a person's serum cholesterol. Nonetheless, a single determination predicts future levels and has been a strong predictor of the risk of coronary heart disease in the major long-term cohort follow-up studies, such as the Framingham Study. These studies used a standardized reference laboratory to measure serum cholesterol, thus minimizing variation due to technologic factors.

Effect of Early Detection and Treatment on Clinical Outcomes

Detection of hypercholesterolemia makes a difference. Many controlled clinical trials have shown that reduction of elevated serum cholesterol reduces coronary heart disease risk in asymptomatic middle-aged men. Pooled data from six placebo-controlled clinical trials of drug therapy involving approximately 37,000 asymptomatic men with high cholesterol have shown a 20% to 30% reduction in the incidence of coronary heart disease for a 10% reduction in serum cholesterol.[24]

Dietary changes are not nearly as effective as medications for reducing serum cholesterol.[25] A type I diet, in which saturated fat and total fat make up about 10% and 30% of total calories, respectively, reduces the serum cholesterol an average of 2%. A type II diet, which is considerably more restrictive, reduces total cholesterol by about 5% and also reduces HDL cholesterol.

The best tolerated, most effective, safest, most costly drugs are the statins. In the West of Scotland Study, a primary prevention trial in middle-aged men, pravastatin reduced total cholesterol by 20% and low-density lipoprotein (LDL) cholesterol by 26%, while increasing HDL cholesterol by 5%.[26] In that randomized, placebo-controlled trial, pravastatin reduced the primary endpoint, nonfatal myocardial infarction or death from coronary heart disease, by 31% (95% confidence interval, 17% to 43%). The absolute risk of this endpoint over 5 years was 79 patients per 1000 in the placebo group and 55 patients per 1000 in the pravastatin group. The absolute risk reduction was 24 patients per 1000, which corresponds to treating 40 persons for 5 years to prevent 1 endpoint. The West of Scotland Study was the first to show a statistically significant reduction in mortality from all causes, 4.1% to 3.2%. There were no excess deaths due to cancer.

Animal studies and trials using earlier medications such as clofibrate have raised the possibility that lipid-lowering agents can increase noncardiac mortality. However, multiple clinical trials of 3-hydroxy-3-methylglutaryl coenzyme

(HMG-CoA) reductase inhibitors, there was no increase in noncardiac mortality.[26–29]

Cost-Effectiveness

The cost-effectiveness of cholesterol screening and cholesterol treatment are very similar because the cost of testing is very small compared with the cost of lifetime treatment. Cost-effectiveness varies markedly depending on age, sex, and other risk factors. In 35- to 44-year-old men with a serum cholesterol of 300 mg/dl, taking 20 mg of lovastatin per day would cost $500,000 per extra year of life gained by preventing coronary artery disease.[30] The cost is much higher in women. Screening and treatment are progressively more cost-effective as the risk of a coronary artery disease event rises (see Table 5–1), especially in middle-aged men and in women ages 65 to 74 years. Screening men and women who have known coronary artery disease is highly cost-effective and may even reduce total costs in some subgroups.[30, 31]

When to Start Screening and How Often to Screen: Recommendations of Expert Panels

The most intense controversy about cholesterol screening concerns the age at which to begin screening. The National Cholesterol Education Program recommends commencing screening at age 20 years and continuing at 5-year intervals indefinitely[32] (Table 5–11). The essence of the argument is that a high serum cholesterol (greater than 160 mg/dl) is necessary for the endothelial cholesterol accumulation that leads to atherosclerotic plaque. Reducing a high serum cholesterol at the earliest time should minimize the development of arteriosclerotic plaque. The line of reasoning builds on pathophysiologic knowledge and the results of clinical trials of cholesterol lowering in middle-aged men, but it extrapolates this reasoning to young, low-risk adults, in whom there is no direct knowledge of the effects of treatment.

The American College of Physicians and the U.S. Preventive Services Task Force recommend starting at age 35 years in men and 45 years in women.[24] The Canadian Task Force on the Periodic Health Examination recommends measuring serum cholesterol in men aged 30 to 59 years who present to the doctor's office for any reason.[19] These organizations all recommend measuring serum cholesterol even in young people if they have risk factors for coronary heart disease or have known coronary heart disease. These groups underscore the importance of screening and treating only when the benefits exceed the harms. The benefits increase as people age and their baseline risk of coronary heart disease increases.[24] Coronary heart disease is very uncommon in young people (e.g., the death rate from coronary heart disease in men aged 35 years with a cholesterol of 280 mg/dl but no other risk factors is 27 per 100,000 per year). In the clinical trials in middle-aged men, treatment for only 5 years lowered the rate of coronary artery disease to the rate that would have

Table 5–11	Screening for Hypercholesterolemia: Summary of Recommendations of Expert Panels

Canadian Task Force (1994)[19]

No CAD risk factors: Perform a total cholesterol on all men aged 30–59 years. Repeat within 1–8 weeks if elevated. Repeat screening cholesterol every 5 years. No comment on screening women.

CAD risk factors or other circumstances: Consider testing when other CAD risk factors are present.

American College of Physicians (1996)[24]

No CAD risk factors: Performing a total cholesterol on all men aged 35–64 years and women aged 45–64 years is appropriate but not mandatory. Repeat within 1–8 weeks if elevated. Frequency of repeat testing depends on initial level: Every 5 years if initial level is close to a treatment threshold; less frequent testing if initial level is far from a treatment threshold (e.g., ≤160 mg/dl).

CAD risk factors or other circumstances: Perform a total cholesterol at any age if there are two or more CAD risk factors or a known familial lipid disorder, or if the patient has known arteriosclerotic vascular disease in any site.

U.S. Preventive Services Task Force (1995)[10]

No CAD risk factors: Perform a total cholesterol on all men aged 35–64 years and women aged 45–65 years. Appropriate interval for repeat testing is not known. Screen more frequently in people whose cholesterol is rising (middle-aged men, perimenopausal women, after weight gain). Screen less often in low-risk individuals (including a previous low cholesterol).

CAD risk factors or other circumstances: Screen adolescents and young adults with family history of lipid disorder, premature CAD in a first-degree relative, or major CAD risk factors.

National Cholesterol Education Program (1994)[32]

Measure nonfasting total cholesterol and HDL cholesterol at least every 5 years in all adults starting at age 20 years.

Abbreviations: CAD, coronary artery disease; HDL, high-density lipoprotein.

been expected if the person had always had the serum cholesterol achieved by the treatment. These results suggest that it is not necessary to maintain a low cholesterol for decades to achieve the benefits of treating high cholesterol. Therefore, it is logical to begin screening 5 to 10 years before the risk of coronary heart disease rises to an appreciable level. The American College of Physicians states that the evidence is insufficient to decide about cholesterol screening in symptomatic persons between ages 65 and 75 years and recommends against screening after age 75 years.[24]

Most expert groups recommend measuring serum cholesterol every 5 years. There is no empirical evidence pointing to this frequency or any other. Testing should be more frequent if a person's cholesterol is close to a threshold for beginning treatment and less frequent if the cholesterol is far from a treatment threshold.

Screening Tests for Other Risk Factors

Lipoprotein (a). Lipoprotein (a) (Lp[a]) is a macromolecular complex of apolipoprotein (a), which has a high degree of homology with plasminogen, and LDL. The function of Lp(a) is unknown. Although it does not have a defined role in atherogenesis, Lp(a) does compete with plasminogen for binding to the plasminogen receptor. A high serum level of Lp(a) is a risk factor for coronary artery disease, at least in persons with elevated serum LDL. Neither the statins nor anion-exchange resins reduce serum levels of Lp(a). Treatment with neomycin and niacin will reduce Lp(a) levels by 50%. The effect of reducing Lp(a) on the incidence of coronary artery disease is unknown. Therefore, even if there were an inexpensive, accurate assay for plasma Lp(a), the rationale for screening for Lp(a) is not convincing (see Chap. 29).

High-Density Lipoprotein. A low HDL level is an independent risk factor for coronary artery disease. A low-cholesterol, low–saturated fat diet reduces HDL levels, whereas niacin and the statins increase HDL cholesterol. Since an HDL level less than 35 mg/dl is a risk factor even in individuals with a normal total cholesterol, some experts recommend routine HDL screening in addition to total cholesterol. However, the effect of early detection and treatment of low HDL cholesterol in people with normal total cholesterol is unknown. Primary prevention trials in these patients should clarify the role of screening for isolated low HDL cholesterol.

Hyperhomocysteinemia. Elevated plasma levels of homocysteine increase the risk of myocardial infarction. In the Physicians Health Study, men initially free of myocardial infarction but in the top 5% of the cohort with respect to plasma homocysteine had a higher incidence of myocardial infarction in the ensuing 5 years than men whose levels placed them in the bottom 90% (relative risk of 3.4 after adjusting for other coronary artery disease risk factors).[33] In other studies, the magnitude of risk increased with increasing plasma levels of homocysteine. Still to be established is the mechanism by which elevated homocysteine levels increase the incidence of myocardial infarction, although there are hints that elevated levels alter thrombogenesis on vascular endothelium. Low levels of vitamins B_6 and B_{12} and folate increase plasma homocysteine. Modest doses of folic acid lower plasma homocysteine to normal.

Although as many as 20% of adults have homocysteine levels that are associated with a threefold increase in myocardial infarction, it is premature to screen for hyperhomocysteinemia except perhaps in patients with a strong family history of premature coronary heart disease or with known coronary heart disease themselves.[34] The measurement of plasma homocysteine requires gas-liquid chromatography and electrochemical procedures. More important to the decision to screen for this risk factor, there have been no clinical trials to document an effect of reducing elevated plasma homocysteine on the incidence of myocardial infarction.

RECOMMENDATIONS

Screening for risk factors for coronary artery disease in apparently healthy adults is worthwhile. Blood pressure can be measured every time an adult seeks care. It is very reasonable to begin screening for elevated serum cholesterol at age 35 years in men and at age 45 years in women. The physician should inquire about cigarette smoking. There is solid evidence that reducing these risk factors can reduce the incidence of coronary artery disease. The patient should be weighed and asked about diabetes because the presence of these risk factors should lower the threshold for screening for cholesterol and lowers the treatment threshold for hypertension and hypercholesterolemia. Dietary recommendations should stress a diet that keeps total fat less than 30% of total calories, saturated fat less than 10% of total calories, and cholesterol less than 300 mg per day. Exercise should be a part of the daily routine.

The value of screening for presymptomatic coronary artery disease is unknown. Certainly there is no direct evidence that screening resting or stress ECG testing reduces morbidity or mortality from coronary heart disease; if this is the standard of evidence, it would argue against such screening. When a patient asks for these screening tests, the physician should discuss the evidence. If the patient is intent on getting the test, it is reasonable to accede to her or his wishes, in part because the patient's preferences should carry particular weight when there is no solid, direct evidence pointing in one direction or the other.

References

1. Welch, H.G., and Black, W.C.: Evaluating randomized trials of screening. J. Gen. Intern. Med. 12:118–124, 1997.
2. Sox, H.C., Littenberg, B., and Garber, A.M.: The role of exercise testing in screening for coronary artery disease. Ann. Intern. Med. 110:456–469, 1989.
3. Anderson, K.M., Wilson, P.W.F., Odell, P.M., and Kannel, W.B.: An updated coronary risk profile: A statement for health professionals. Circulation 83:356–362, 1991.
4. McHenry, P.L., O'Donnell, J., Morris, S.N., and Jordan, J.J.: The abnormal exercise electrocardiogram in apparently healthy men: A predictor of angina pectoris as an initial coronary event during long-term follow-up. Circulation 70:547–551, 1984.
5. Coronary Artery Surgery Study (CASS): A randomized trial of coronary artery bypass surgery. Survival data. Circulation 68:939–950, 1983.
6. Knutsen, R., Knutsen, S.F., Curb, J.D., et al.: The predictive value of resting electrocardiograms for 12-year incidence of coronary heart disease in the Honolulu Heart Program. J. Clin. Epidemiol. 41:293–302, 1988.
7. Sox, H.C., Garber, A.M., and Littenberg, B.: The resting electrocardiogram as a screening test: A clinical analysis. Ann. Intern. Med. 111:489–502, 1990.
8. Erikssen, J. Silent ischemia. Herz 359–364, 1987.
9. Yusuf S., Zucker, D., Peduzzi, P., et al.: Effect of coronary artery bypass graft surgery on survival: Overview of 10-year results from randomised trials by the Coronary Artery Bypass Graft Surgery Trialists Collaboration. Lancet 344:563–570, 1994.
10. U.S. Preventive Services Task Force: Guide to Clinical Preventive Services. 2nd ed. Baltimore, Williams & Wilkins, 1995.
11. ACC/AHA Task Force Report. Guidelines for electrocardiography: A report of the American College of Cardiology/American Heart Association Task Force on assessment of diagnostic and therapeutic cardiovascular procedures (Committee on Electrocardiography). J. Am. Coll. Cardiol. 19:473–481, 1992.
12. Gibbons, R.J., Balady, G.J., Beasley, J.W., et al.: ACC/AHA guidelines for exercise testing. Executive Summary. A report of the American College of Cardiology/American Heart Association Task Force on Practice Guidelines (Committee on Exercise Testing). Circulation 96:345–354, 1997.
13. Veterans Administration Cooperative Study Group on Antihypertensive Agents: Effects of treatment on morbidity in hypertension.

Results in patients with diastolic blood pressures averaging 115 through 129 mm Hg. JAMA 202:1028–1034, 1967.

14. Veterans Administration Cooperative Study Group on Antihypertensive Agents: Effects of treatment on morbidity in hypertension. 3. Influence of age, diastolic blood pressure, and prior cardiovascular disease: Further analysis of side effects. Circulation 45:991–1004, 1972.

15. Medical Research Council Working Party: MRC trial of treatment of mild hypertension: Principal results. BMJ 291:97–104, 1985.

16. SHEP Cooperative Research Group: Prevention of stroke by antihypertensive drug treatment in older persons with isolated systolic hypertension: Final results of the Systolic Hypertension in the Elderly Program (SHEP). JAMA 265:3255–3264, 1991.

17. Littenberg, B., Garber, A.M., and Sox, H.C.: Screening for hypertension. Ann. Intern. Med. 112:192–202, 1990.

18. Joint National Committee on Detection, Evaluation, and Treatment of High Blood Pressure. The fifth report of the Joint National Committee on Detection, Evaluation, and Treatment of High Blood Pressure. (NIH Publication no. 93–1088.) Bethesda, MD, National Institutes of Health, 1993.

19. The Canadian Task Force on the Periodic Health Examination: Clinical Preventive Health Care. Health Canada, 1994.

20. Martin, M.J., Hulley, S.B., Browner, W.S., et al.: Serum cholesterol, blood pressure, and mortality: Implications from a cohort of 361,662 men. Lancet 2:933–936, 1986.

21. Kronmal, R.A., Cain, K.C., and Ye, Z.: Total serum cholesterol levels and mortality risk as a function of age: A report based on the Framingham data. Arch. Intern. Med. 153:1065–1073, 1993.

22. Corti, M.-C., Guralnik, J.M., Salive, M.E., et al.: HDL cholesterol predicts coronary heart disease mortality in older persons. JAMA 274:539–544, 1995.

23. Corti, M.C., Guralnik, J.M., Salive, M.E., et al.: Clarifying the direct relationship between total cholesterol levels and death from coronary heart disease in older persons. Ann. Intern. Med. 126:753–760, 1997.

24. Garber, A.M., Browner, W.S., and Hulley, S.B.: Cholesterol screening in asymptomatic adults, revisited. Ann. Intern. Med. 124:518–531, 1996.

25. Hunninghake, D.B., Stein, E.A., Dujovne, C.A., et al.: The efficacy of intensive dietary therapy alone or combined with lovastatin in outpatients with hypercholesterolemia. N. Engl. J. Med. 269:505–510, 1993.

26. Shepherd, M., Cobbe, S.M., Ford, I., et al.: Prevention of coronary heart disease with pravastatin in men with hypercholesterolemia. N. Engl. J. Med. 333:1301–1307, 1995.

27. Scandinavian Simvastatin Survival Study Group: Randomized trial of cholesterol lowering in 4444 patients with coronary heart disease: The Scandinavian Simvastatin Survival Study (4S). Lancet 344:1383–1389, 1994.

28. Byington, R.P., Jukema, J.W., Salonen, J.T., et al.: Reduction in cardiovascular events during pravastatin therapy: Pooled analysis of clinical events of the Pravastatin Atherosclerosis Intervention Program. Circulation 92:2419–2425, 1995.

29. Sacks, F.M., Pfeffer, M.A., Moye, L.A., et al., for the Cholesterol and Recurrent Events (CARE) Trial Investigators: The effect of pravastatin on coronary events after myocardial infarction in patients with average cholesterol levels. N. Engl. J. Med. 335:1001–1009, 1996.

30. Goldman, L., Weinstein, M.C., Goldman, P., et al.: Cost-effectiveness of HMG-CoA reductase inhibition for primary and secondary prevention of coronary heart disease. JAMA 265: 1145–1151, 1991.

31. Johannesson, M., Jönsson, B., Kjckshus, J., et al.: Cost-effectiveness of simvastatin treatment to lower cholesterol levels in patients with coronary heart disease. N. Engl. J. Med. 336:332–336, 1997.

32. Expert Panel on Detection, Evaluation, and Treatment of High Blood Cholesterol in Adults (Adult Treatment Panel II): Second report of the Expert Panel on Detection, Evaluation, and Treatment of High Blood Cholesterol in Adults. Circulation 89:1329–1445, 1994.

33. Stampfer, M.J., Malinow, R., Willett, W.C., et al.: A prospective study of plasma homocysteine and risk of myocardial infarction in US physicians. JAMA 268:877–881, 1992.

34. Nygård, O., Nordrehaug, J.E., Refsum H., et al.: Plasma homocysteine levels and mortality in patients with coronary artery disease. N. Engl. J. Med 337:230–236, 1997.

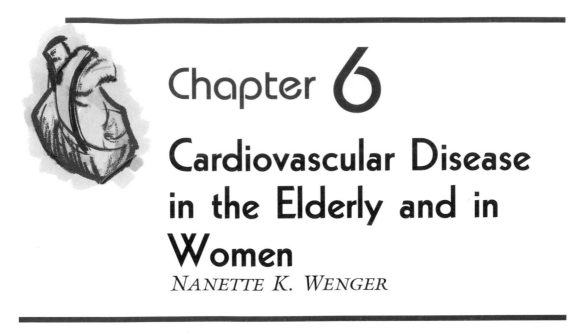

Chapter 6

Cardiovascular Disease in the Elderly and in Women

NANETTE K. WENGER

CARDIOVASCULAR DISEASE IN THE ELDERLY

Cardiovascular disease—especially coronary heart disease, hypertension, calcific aortic stenosis, and heart failure—increases dramatically with age,[1] and 83% of all cardiovascular deaths occur in elderly patients, defined here as those over 65 years. The percentage of all deaths due to cardiovascular diseases rises sharply with age (Fig. 6–1). The presentation of cardiovascular disease in elderly patients reflects both its superimposition on the physiologic and structural cardiovascular changes of normal aging, such as stiffening of the ventricle and arterial wall, and the progressively more frequent occurrence of atherosclerosis with longer exposure to coronary risk factors. The higher prevalence of co-morbid illnesses also adversely affects the response of elderly patients both to cardiac diseases and to the therapies for these conditions.

In elderly patients, it is the *physiologic* rather than the *chronologic* age that is of greater importance. The mental status, cognitive ability, emotional state, general physical well-being, family and social support systems, presence of co-morbid diseases, and the risks of and expectations for care must all be considered in clinical decision-making in elderly patients. Recent data suggest that in most patients between 65 and 75 years of age, other than directing attention to co-morbid conditions, which occur more frequently in this age group than in younger patients, diagnostic and management strategies can be similar. Data are limited for those patients between 75 and 84 years. In patients older than 85 years (the "oldest old"), decisions about cardiovascular diagnosis and therapy must be highly individualized.[2]

Coronary Heart Disease

It is estimated that more than 3.6 million elderly patients have coronary heart disease and approximately 60% of patients hospitalized for acute myocardial infarction (MI) in the United States are more than 65 years of age. By the eighth decade, coronary heart disease is present in about 20% of both men and women.

Angina Pectoris (see Chap. 18)

In elderly patients with asymptomatic coronary atherosclerosis, many of whom are not physically active, angina pectoris is often precipitated by the development of co-morbid conditions such as infection, blood loss, anemia, hypertension, hypotension, thyrotoxicosis, or arrhythmia rather than by physical activity, as occurs in younger adults. Exertional dyspnea and fatigue, instead of chest discomfort, may be the most prominent clinical manifestations of myocardial ischemia in elderly patients. Medical therapy is comparable for older and younger patients with angina pectoris, but particular attention must be directed to the identification and remediation of precipitating or exacerbating factors in the elderly. Also, because elderly patients often exhibit impaired baroreflex control of arterial pressure,[2] antianginal drugs—nitrates, beta blockers, and calcium antagonists—all of which lower arterial pressure, should be introduced more cautiously and at lower doses than in younger patients. In patients

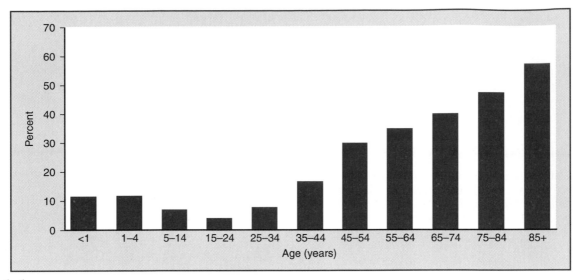

Figure 6–1

Percentage of all deaths due to cardiovascular disease by age in the United States, 1993. (From Morbidity and Mortality: 1996 Chartbook on Cardiovascular, Lung, and Blood Diseases. National Heart, Lung, and Blood Institute, National Institutes of Health, May 1996, p. 21.)

older than 80 years, it is advisable to commence treatment with one-half to two-thirds of the dosage used in younger adults and then to increase the dosage gradually as needed and as tolerated.

Advanced age is an important risk factor for mortality and nonlethal outcomes in both chronic stable angina and unstable angina.[3] Pharmacologic management is less intensive and coronary revascularization is utilized less frequently in patients over 75 years of age than in younger patients, potentially contributing to this less favorable outcome.

Coronary Revascularization

An 80% to 90% angiographic success rate, without excessive procedural complications, has been reported for percutaneous transluminal coronary angioplasty (PTCA) and other catheter-based interventions in patients up to the age of 75 years, even when multivessel angioplasty is undertaken. Coronary patency rates and functional improvements are comparable with those observed in younger patients; 5 years after successful PTCA, almost 75% of elderly patients are free of MI or the need for coronary artery bypass grafting (CABG). However, in octogenarians and even older patients, PTCA success rates are lower and procedural complication rates and mortality are higher than in younger patients.

Approximately one-half of all CABG operations are carried out in patients more than 65 years of age. Despite steady improvement in the outcome of surgery in all age groups, age is still an important relative risk factor for both morbidity and mortality.[4] In octogenarians undergoing elective CABG, hospital mortality is approximately 10% and serious complications occur in as many as one-third to one-half. Atherosclerotic emboli are an important complication in this group. However, the survivors of CABG are typically free of angina and have improved functional capacity, and their 5-year survival is similar to

that of age-matched individuals without symptomatic coronary artery disease. Both survival and freedom from angina were better with surgical than medical management in high-risk elderly patients in the Coronary Artery Surgery Study (CASS).[5] These favorable outcomes suggest that coronary revascularization may be undertaken in octogenarians who have disabling symptoms or who are at high risk, who do not have serious, life-threatening, or co-morbid illnesses, and who are otherwise suitable for the procedure. However, because catheter-based interventions are better tolerated than surgery, they may be the revascularization procedure of choice in patients over the age of 80 years if the coronary anatomy is suitable. Because *emergency* CABG is associated with a markedly increased risk of death in patients in this age group, early evaluation of severely symptomatic patients and referral for elective revascularization may be most appropriate.

Acute MI (see Chap. 19)

The clinical presentation of acute MI differs substantially in elderly compared with younger patients. Chest pain is less frequently the presenting manifestation; indeed, chest pain typical of acute MI is described by only one-third of patients older than 85 years. In the Cardiovascular Health Study,[1] 23% and 38% of community dwelling elderly men and women, respectively, with electrocardiographic evidence of MI did *not* report a history of infarction. The diagnosis of acute MI may be further obscured in this age group in that diagnostic CK-MB isoenzyme (isoenzyme of creatine kinase with muscle and brain subunits) elevations may occur in the presence of a normal or minimally elevated total creatine kinase level, probably reflecting the decrease in lean body mass with aging.

Because elderly patients are more likely to be asymptomatic or to have an atypical presentation of MI that does not include severe chest pain, on average they arrive in the hospital later than do younger patients. Also, these patients present with ST segment depression more frequently, and they often have co-morbid conditions (such as serious hypertension or a previous stroke) that serve as contraindications to thrombolytic therapy. Therefore, they are less likely than younger patients to receive thrombolytic therapy.

Data from large, randomized trials of thrombolytic therapy for acute MI have documented nearly comparable efficacy and *relative* benefits for patients under 65 years and those between 65 and 75 years, although the incidence of intracranial hemorrhage rises with advancing age.[6] Since patients between 65 and 75 years have a higher *absolute* risk of death with acute MI, the absolute benefit that they derive from thrombolysis is greater than it is in younger patients (see Fig. 19–6). Primary coronary angioplasty, if it can be accomplished within 4 to 6 hours of the onset of symptoms and by an experienced operator and team, is an attractive option for elderly patients with acute MI, especially those with an absolute or relative contraindication to coronary thrombolysis; a success rate of more than 90% for this procedure has been reported. However, data regarding both thrombolysis and primary angioplasty are limited for patients above the age of 75 years.

The diastolic dysfunction characteristic of aging myocardium (see Chap. 22) is accentuated by MI. Complications of acute MI, including pulmonary edema, heart failure, cardiogenic shock, conduction defects, arrhythmias, and cardiac rupture, all occur with increased frequency at elderly age. Nonetheless, hospital mortality from acute MI, although greater in elderly than in younger patients (Fig. 6–2), has improved in recent years, particularly among those under 85 years.

Predischarge exercise testing appears to be safe in appropriately selected elderly patients and offers prognostic information comparable with that in younger patients. Evidence of residual ischemia during exercise or pharmacologic testing (see Chap. 4) is associated with an increased risk of death or recurrent MI and warrants consideration for invasive intervention in elderly patients.

A number of studies have shown a lower use of thrombolytic therapy, PTCA, and CABG surgery in elderly patients with acute MI.[2, 3] Although it is unclear whether these lower rates are appropriate or inappropriate, even "low-technology" therapies such as aspirin, beta blocking drugs, and angiotensin-converting enzyme inhibitors appear to be underutilized in older patients, despite the documentation that such therapies provide long-term survival benefit in this group. Elderly patients, particularly elderly women, are also less likely to be referred to exercise cardiac rehabilitation,[7] despite the improvement in physical work capacity documented in such patients.

Modifiable coronary risk factors are highly prevalent in the elderly and also continue to influence the occurrence and recurrence of coronary events in this population (Table 6–1). Preventive approaches include the control of hypertension and weight, as well as dietary sodium and fat restriction, and emphasis on the discontinuation of cigarette smoking. Since hypercholesterolemia continues to confer increased risk in the elderly, at least to the age of 80 years, recommendations for the recognition and management of hyperlipidemia are similar to those for younger coronary patients. Older patients with coronary artery disease, both with elevated (Table 6–2) and with average (Table 6–3) cholesterol levels, benefit from cholesterol reduction.

Arterial Hypertension

(see Chaps. 11 and 21)

Hypertension occurs in more than half of the U.S. population above the age of 65 years. Systolic blood pressure continues to increase in most populations into the eighth and ninth decades, whereas diastolic pressure peaks in the sixth and seventh decades, so that there is a high prevalence of isolated systolic hypertension at elderly age. Using the definition of a systolic blood pressure exceeding 150 mm Hg and a diastolic pressure below 90 mm Hg for isolated systolic hypertension, one-third of elderly U.S. women and one-fifth of elderly men have isolated systolic hypertension.

The elderly patients in the Hypertension Detection and

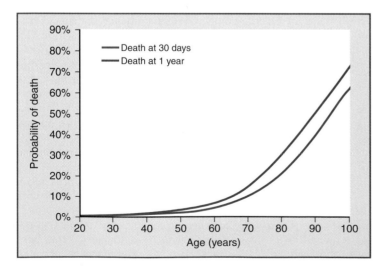

Figure 6–2

Probability of mortality in acute myocardial infarction at 30 days and 1 year as a function of age. (From White, H.D., Barbash, G.I., Califf, R.M., et al.: Age and outcome with contemporary thrombolytic therapy: Results from the GUSTO-I trial. Circulation 94:1826–1833, 1996.)

Table 6-1	Percentage Prevalence of Cardiovascular Risk Factors in the Elderly from the Framingham Study									
	Definite Hypertension		Hypercholesterolemia		Glucose Intolerance		Obesity		Cigarette Smoking	
Age	Men	Women	Men	Women	Men	Women	Men	Women	Men	Women
65–74	42.1	48.9	16.6	39.7	29.5	17.5	52.2	47.8	21.9	23.0
75–84	45.5	61.1	9.7	36.3	30.9	26.0	35.4	39.3	13.9	8.5
85–94	20.7	64.8	9.4	18.4	33.3	29.0	7.7	30.0	9.4	3.2

From Kannel, W.B.: Nutrition and the occurrence and prevention of cardiovascular disease in the elderly. Nutr. Rev. 46:68–78, 1988.

Follow-Up Program (HDFP), most of whom had mild diastolic hypertension, exhibited a greater than 60% reduction in mortality at 5 years with "stepped care," which focused on precise blood pressure control, compared with usual care.[8] In the Systolic Hypertension in the Elderly Program (SHEP), initial therapy with low-dose chlorthalidone and beta blockade added as needed was extremely effective and reduced the risk of stroke by 36% and of nonfatal and fatal cardiovascular events by 32%.[9] Elderly patients tolerated antihypertensive medication well and were adherent to therapy. A meta-analysis of trials in more than 15,000 patients 60 years or older showed a relative reduction in the risk of stroke and of cardiac morbidity and mortality similar to that observed in younger hypertensive patients.[10]

The impaired baroreflex control of arterial pressure in older patients may make them unusually sensitive to hypotensive drugs.[2] Accordingly, antihypertensive drug therapy in these patients should usually begin with half of the usual adult dose and should be increased slowly. The blood pressure goals should be similar to those in younger patients, with systolic pressure reduced to below 160 mm Hg and diastolic pressure below 90 mm Hg.

However, it may be desirable to attain these goals more gradually than in younger patients, with special attention to the avoidance of postural and postprandial hypotension and the maintenance of renal function.

Elderly patients appear to respond well to thiazide diuretics. Beta-adrenergic blockers should be used with care in patients with systolic dysfunction, atrioventricular conduction defects, obstructive pulmonary disease, or peripheral vascular disease, all of which are more common at elderly age. Alpha-adrenergic blockers are useful antihypertensives in older men with prostatic hypertrophy.

Valvular Heart Disease
(see Chap. 25)

Aortic stenosis secondary to degenerative calcification is the most frequent valvular lesion that requires surgical correction in elderly patients. Angina, syncope, presyncope, dizziness, and heart failure, the cardinal symptoms of hemodynamically significant calcific aortic stenosis at any age, appear later in the course in patients who are inactive physically. Additionally, at elderly age, these symptoms may be incorrectly attributed to ischemic heart disease or noncardiac disorders.

In patients of any age, the most important feature in the recognition of aortic stenosis on physical examination is the late-peaking, harsh systolic murmur at the base of the heart that radiates along the carotid arteries (see Chap. 13). The diagnosis of aortic stenosis may be more difficult in the elderly because their stiffer arterial vessels may mask the classic slow-rising carotid pulse and low pulse pressure and lead to persistence of systolic hypertension even with critical aortic stenosis. In the elderly, the transmission of the aortic systolic murmur along the carotid arteries may be erroneously attributed to a primary carotid bruit caused by cerebrovascular disease. Hyperexpansion of the lungs and dorsal kyphosis, both of which occur more commonly in the elderly, may obscure the forceful apical impulse of left ventricular hypertrophy and mask even the systolic murmur and thrill at the base of the heart.

Aortic valve replacement is generally indicated in elderly patients who remain symptomatic despite medical therapy and in the absence of life-limiting co-morbid illness. This procedure can be performed at an acceptable risk even in octogenarians who are in New York Heart Association class III or class IV. In one series, periopera-

Table 6-2	Influence of Gender and Age on the Effects of Simvastatin		
	No. (%) of Patients		
	Placebo	Simvastatin	Relative Risk* (95% CI)
Death			
Women	25 (6.0)	27 (6.6)	1.12 (0.65–1.93)
Men	231 (12.8)	155 (8.5)	0.66 (0.53–0.80)
Age <60 yr	89 (8.1)	55 (5.2)	0.63 (0.45–0.88)
Age ≥60 yr	167 (14.8)	127 (11.0)	0.73 (0.58–0.92)
Major Coronary Event			
Women	91 (21.7)	59 (14.5)	0.65 (0.47–0.91)
Men	531 (29.4)	372 (20.5)	0.66 (0.58–0.76)
Age <60 yr	303 (27.6)	188 (17.6)	0.61 (0.51–0.73)
Age ≥60 yr	319 (28.3)	243 (21.0)	0.71 (0.60–0.86)

From Scandinavian Simvastatin Survival Study Group: Randomised trial of cholesterol lowering in 4444 patients with coronary heart disease: The Scandinavian Simvastatin Survival Study (4S). Lancet 344 (8934):1383–1389, © by The Lancet Ltd, 1994.
Abbreviation: CI, confidence interval.
*Calculated by Cox regression analysis.

Table 6–3	Expected Number of Cardiovascular Events Preventable by Treating 1000 Patients with Pravastatin for 5 Years*		
Event	Unselected Patients	Patients ≥60 Yr of Age (n)	Women
Fatal coronary heart disease	11	27	10
Clinical nonfatal myocardial infarction	26	46	83
Coronary artery bypass grafting	25	32	34
Percutaneous transluminal coronary angioplasty	37	20	66
Stroke or transient ischemic attack	13	25	28
Other cardiovascular event	38	57	7
All cardiovascular events	150	207	228
Patient with ≥1 event prevented	51	71	97

From Sacks, F.M., Pfeffer, M.A., Moye, L.A., et al., for the Cholesterol and Recurrent Events Trial Investigators: The effect of pravastatin on coronary events after myocardial infarction in patients with average cholesterol levels. N. Engl. J. Med. 335:1001–1009, 1996.

*It is assumed that pravastatin was given to three hypothetical groups of patients with a history of myocardial infarction and a total cholesterol level of less than 240 mg/dl: 1000 otherwise unselected patients, 1000 patients 60 years or older, and 1000 female patients.

tive mortality was 2.5% in patients below the age of 70 years, 7.3% over age 70 years, and 12.5% in those over 80 years.[11] A 5-year survival of approximately 75% may be anticipated among patients older than 80 years, with maintenance of improved cardiac functional status in a large majority of the survivors.

Mitral stenosis in elderly, as in younger, patients is usually due to rheumatic fever. However, calcification of the valve apparatus, a common finding in the elderly, makes their stenotic mitral valve less suitable for balloon valvuloplasty. *Mitral regurgitation* in this age group is most commonly caused by mitral annular calcification, ischemic dysfunction of a papillary muscle, or mitral valve prolapse. These conditions are often amenable to operative repair and may not require valve replacement.

Heart Failure (see Chap. 22)

In the United States, heart failure is the most common hospital discharge diagnosis in patients more than 65 years of age, and a large majority of patients with heart failure are elderly. Heart failure is an increasingly frequent cause of death, having risen by more than 45% in patients 75 to 89 years in the past two decades.

Heart failure is both underdiagnosed and overdiagnosed in elderly patients, who may fail to report dyspnea, cough, ankle edema, or easy fatigability because they inappropriately attribute these manifestations to aging. Heart failure in the elderly may present as diminished cognitive function and behavioral disturbance resulting from a reduction in cerebral blood flow. Sometimes, the presenting complaint is profound fatigue rather than exertional dyspnea. Conversely, physicians may mistakenly attribute to congestive heart failure the ankle edema of venous stasis, the reduced exercise tolerance secondary to increased lung stiffness, and the breathlessness of the physical deconditioning common at elderly age.

Heart failure in the elderly is often precipitated by uncontrolled hypertension, unrecognized acute MI, or the development of atrial fibrillation and other arrhythmias. However, co-morbid conditions such as intercurrent infections, fever, fluid overload, acute blood loss, anemia, renal insufficiency, dietary indiscretion, or poor compliance with a medical regimen, all of which are more common in elderly patients, must also be considered, and the management of these conditions is of critical importance in the treatment of heart failure. Nonsteroidal anti-inflammatory drugs, which are frequently used by elderly patients to treat musculoskeletal disorders, can precipitate heart failure by causing sodium and water retention or by inducing renal dysfunction.

The evaluation of heart failure and the search for its cause are similar in older and younger adults. The assessment of ventricular function can be accomplished most readily by echocardiography or radionuclide angiography. The major challenge is to differentiate systolic from diastolic dysfunction. Diastolic dysfunction secondary to interstitial fibrosis and ventricular scarring is characteristic of the aging heart, and as many as 40% of elderly patients hospitalized for heart failure have preserved systolic function. The prevalence of cardiac amyloidosis increases with aging and causes predominantly diastolic dysfunction, often accompanied by arrhythmias, conduction disturbances, and abnormalities of peripheral vascular tone (see Chap. 31).

Because of reduced glomerular filtration rates in the elderly,[2] digoxin clearance is reduced and the dose of this drug should, in general, be lowered to 0.125 mg/day in patients 70 years or older.

CARDIOVASCULAR DISEASE IN WOMEN

Coronary Heart Disease

Although coronary heart disease has traditionally been considered to be a disease of men, it is, in fact, responsible for almost 250,000 deaths annually and is the leading cause of death among adult women in the United States.[12–14] Coronary heart disease in women who undergo natural menopause occurs on average 10 years later than in men (Table 6–4), whereas women who undergo early natural menopause or bilateral oophorectomy develop coronary heart disease at a younger age. At whatever age it occurs, a decline in ovarian function increases the risk for developing coronary heart disease, in part related to raised low-density lipoprotein (LDL) and lowered high-density lipoprotein (HDL) levels.

Coronary heart disease is associated with substantial morbidity in women as well; over one-third of women aged 45 to 64 years of age with coronary heart disease are disabled by symptoms of their illness, and this per-

Table 6–4	Incidence of CHD, by Age and Sex: 30-Year Follow-Up, Framingham Study			
	Annual Rate*			
	CHD		*MI*	
Age (yr)	*Men*	*Women*	*Men*	*Women*
35–44	5	1	3	—
45–54	11	4	5	1
55–64	19	10	9	3
65–74	23	14	12	6
75–84	30	22	18	8
85+	—	41	—	24
35–64	13	6	6	2
65–94	25	16	13	7

From Kannel, W.B., and Abbott, R.D.: Incidence and prognosis of myocardial infarction in women: The Framingham Study. *In* Eaker, E.D., Packard, B., Wenger, N.K., et al. (eds.): Coronary Heart Disease in Women. New York, Haymarket Doyma 1987, pp. 208–214.

Abbreviations: CHD, coronary heart disease; MI, myocardial infarction.

*Per 1000.

centage increases to more than 55% in those 75 years or older. After clinical manifestations of coronary heart disease appear, the outcomes in women are less favorable than those in men. This mandates careful attention to coronary risk reduction and aggressive evaluation of chest pain syndromes in women of all ages. The initial clinical presentation of coronary heart disease in women most frequently is angina, both stable and unstable, whereas MI or sudden death is a more common presentation in men.

Coronary Risk Factors and Their Reduction

Risk factors such as hypertension, hypercholesterolemia, cigarette smoking, obesity, diabetes mellitus, and a sedentary lifestyle are each present in more than 25% of U.S. women aged 20 to 74 years. Each of these appears to increase the relative risk of coronary heart disease by a similar magnitude in women as in men, although diabetes is a more powerful risk attribute for women (Table 6–5) and treatment appears to confer a similar relative benefit. For example, in the SHEP study, control of isolated systolic hypertension reduced the occurrence of stroke and of fatal and nonfatal cardiovascular events in both genders.[8] In the Scandinavian Simvastatin Survival Study (4S), pharmacologic cholesterol lowering reduced major coronary events as much in women as in men (see Table 6–2).[15] In the Cholesterol and Recurrent Events (CARE) trial of cholesterol lowering in post-MI patients with average cholesterol levels for the population (e.g., 209 mg/dl), pravastatin caused a 46% reduction in death or recurrent infarction in women, compared with a 20% reduction in men, a difference that was statistically significant (see Table 6–3).[16] Non–insulin-dependent diabetes, insulin resistance, and upper body obesity often occur in combination and may be accompanied by low HDL cho-

lesterol and elevated triglycerides. This combination of coronary risk factors, sometimes referred to as *syndrome X,* is common in women.

There has been a smaller reduction in coronary risk factors in women than in men in the United States during the past two decades, probably because less attention has been directed toward risk reduction in women despite benefit that is equivalent to that in men. Cigarette smoking has not decreased in women (as it has in men) and remains an important risk factor for coronary artery disease (see Table 6–5). The prevalence of coronary risk factors is higher among women with less favorable socio-economic circumstances and education, and intensive risk reduction is especially warranted in these groups.

HORMONE REPLACEMENT. The Postmenopausal Estrogen/Progestin Intervention (PEPI) trial addressed a risk intervention unique to women.[17] An increase in HDL cholesterol and decreases in LDL cholesterol and fibrinogen levels occurred with oral estrogen alone and with several combinations of estrogen and progestin (Fig. 6–3). Importantly, none of the hormone regimens increased blood pressure or weight, although all were associated with modest increases in triglycerides. Because one-third of the women with a uterus, who were randomized to unopposed estrogen therapy, developed adenomatous or atypical endometrial hyperplasia, a premalignant lesion, a regimen including a progestin appears indicated in such women. Unopposed estrogen may be used in women who have undergone hysterectomy.

Data from the Cardiovascular Health Study showed that postmenopausal estrogen use was associated with a lower cardiovascular risk well into the eighth decade of life.[18] Both the Nurses' Health Study and meta-analyses suggest a reduction of approximately 40% in death from coronary heart disease in women using postmenopausal hormone therapy.[12, 13] However, these are observational studies; a reduction of coronary events and deaths with hormone replacement therapy has not been demonstrated in a prospective, randomized clinical trial. Hormone therapy also causes a marked reduction in osteoporosis and osteoporotic fractures, a reduction in menopausal symptoms, but a modest increase in venous thromboembolism and in the risk of breast cancer.

While awaiting the results of ongoing clinical trials and

Table 6–5	Relative Risk of Coronary Heart Disease by Sex: Follow-Up of NHANES I	
Risk Factor	**Men RR (95% CI)**	**Women RR (95% CI)**
Hypertension	1.5 (1.3, 1.7)	1.5 (1.3, 1.8)
Cholesterol	1.4 (1.2, 1.6)	1.1 (0.9, 1.2)
Diabetes	1.9 (1.5, 2.5)	2.4 (1.9, 3.0)
Overweight	1.3 (1.1, 1.5)	1.4 (1.2, 1.6)
Smoking	1.6 (1.4, 1.8)	1.8 (1.5, 2.1)

Source: *MMWR* 1992:41:528.

From Wenger, N.K.: Coronary heart disease in women: Risk factors, prevention and treatment. Cardiology Special Edition 3:1–5, 1997.

Abbreviations: NHANES, National Health and Nutrition Examination Survey; RR, relative risk, CI, confidence interval.

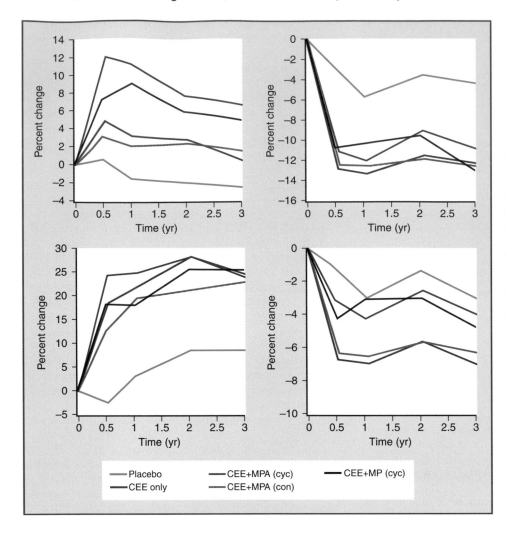

Figure 6–3
Effects of hormone replacement on lipid levels in postmenopausal women. Mean percent change from baseline by treatment arm for high-density lipoprotein cholesterol *(top left)*, low-density lipoprotein cholesterol *(top right)*, triglycerides *(bottom left)*, and total cholesterol *(bottom right)*. CEE, conjugated equine estrogen; MPA, medroxyprogesterone acetate; cyc, cyclical administration; con, administered daily continuously; MP, micronized progesterone. (From The Writing Group for the PEPI Trial: Effects of estrogen or estrogen/progestin regimens on heart disease risk factors in postmenopausal women. The Postmenopausal Estrogen/Progestin Interventions [PEPI] Trial. JAMA 273: 199–208, 1995. Copyright 1995, American Medical Association.)

based on the totality of the available evidence, hormone replacement therapy appears to exert health benefits that outweigh risks in many postmenopausal women. It is most likely to provide benefit for women with established coronary heart disease and in those with risk factors for coronary heart disease. However, it is not recommended for women with a personal history of breast cancer, and caution is advisable in women with a history of breast cancer in a first-degree relative, as well as in those at risk for venous thromboembolism.

Angina Pectoris

Based on data from the Framingham Heart Study, angina pectoris was initially considered to be the major initial manifestation of coronary heart disease in women, in whom it was thought to have a benign prognosis.[19] Subsequent observations, however, have shown that the chest pain in many of the women in the Framingham Study probably was not secondary to coronary heart disease. The CASS registry documented that 50% of women (compared with 17% of men) referred by their physicians for evaluation of chest pain considered to be of sufficient severity to merit evaluation for CABG surgery had minimal or no atherosclerotic obstruction in their epicardial

coronary arteries at coronary arteriography.[20] Women with angina are usually older than men and more often have vasospastic or microvascular angina and angina that is precipitated by mental stress. Thus, a critical task in the management of women with chest pain syndromes is to differentiate those with coronary heart disease (whose prognosis is at least as serious as it is in men) from those whose chest pain is due to noncoronary causes and who have a favorable prognosis. The history is less valuable in the diagnosis of angina pectoris in women than it is in men (Table 6–6), and objective confirmatory testing is required.

Diagnostic Testing and Risk Stratification (Table 6–7)

Although exercise electrocardiography is the cornerstone of the noninvasive evaluation of myocardial ischemia (see Chap. 4), it is less predictive in women than it is in men.[13] Exercise electrocardiography is associated with a higher false-positive rate in women than in men. In large part, this is related to the lower pretest probability of coronary heart disease in premenopausal women than in comparably aged men, rendering a false-positive test more likely (see Chap. 1). Conversely, older women,

Table 6–6	Gender Differences in Probability of CAD or W/M = (%)					
Age (yr)	Nonanginal Chest Discomfort (pCAD)		Atypical Chest Discomfort (pCAD)		Typical Angina (pCAD)	
	Women	Men	Women	Men	Women	Men
35	0.01 (14%)	0.07	0.03 (13%)	0.23	0.26 (37%)	0.70
45	0.05 (42%)	0.12	0.12 (27%)	0.44	0.52 (60%)	0.87
55	0.10 (50%)	0.20	0.30 (56%)	0.54	0.70 (76%)	0.92
65	0.17 (71%)	0.24	0.50 (76%)	0.67	0.85 (92%)	0.93

From Patterson, R.E., Cloninger, K., Churchwell, K.B. et al.: Special problems with cardiovascular imaging to assess coronary artery disease in women. *In* Julian, D.G., and Wenger, N.K. (eds.): Women and Heart Disease. London, Martin Dunitz, 1997, pp. 91–115.

Abbreviations: CAD, coronary artery disease; pCAD, probability of developing clinical manifestations of coronary artery disease in next 7 years in Framingham Study; W/M, (%) ratio of probability (p) of CAD for women as a percentage of pCAD for men with same age and chest discomfort (likelihood ratio).

in whom the pretest probability of coronary heart disease is higher, are more often unable to perform adequate exercise than are men and therefore more often have an inconclusive test result. The negative predictive value of a normal exercise electrocardiogram for excluding the diagnosis of coronary heart disease is comparable in women and men.

Exercise thallium scintigraphy and technetium-99m-sestamibi imaging have approximately equivalent sensitivities and specificities in women and men and both appear to be more accurate than exercise electrocardiography. Myocardial perfusion scintigraphy following pharmacologic stress with adenosine or dipyridamole is particularly useful in older women who are unable to exercise. Exer-

Table 6–7	Difficulties Diagnosing CAD in Women	
Diagnostic Tool	**R or R/S**	**Compared with Men, Women Show:**
History of chest discomfort	R/S	More false (+)
ECG-ST	R/S	More false (+) owing to unknown factors (estrogens?)
SPECT MPI ± LV function	R/S	More false (+) owing to soft tissue attenuation
		Radiation risk if pregnant
LV function (RNA)	R/S	More false (+) owing to different hemodynamic responses in women: less increase in LVEF and more increase in LVED volume, less increase in systolic BP
		Radiation risk if pregnant
		Gender-related differences in attenuation make little difference
LV function (Echo)	R/S	Same as above (but no radiation), and
		Often difficult to acquire images of all walls of left ventricle owing to more limited "window" in women
PET MPI ± LV function	R/S	Best current test because gender-related differences in attenuation are corrected
		Radiation risk if pregnant but less radiation with ^{82}Rb versus with other radionuclide methods
MRI: LV function and MPI	R/S	Promising, but more validation is needed
MRA	R	Gender differences in attenuation will not alter cardiovascular images
UFCT: LV function and MPI	R/S	Promising, but more validation is needed
Angiography (contrast)	R	Radiation risk if pregnant
		Gender differences in attenuation will have little effect on cardiovascular images
UFCT: Coronary calcification in arterial walls	R	Preliminary data showing less Ca^{2+} in women
		Radiation risk if pregnant
		Gender differences in attenuation will have little effect on cardiovascular images
Cardiac catheterization with contrast coronary angiography	R	More arterial access complications owing to smaller size of arteries in women
		Radiation risk if pregnant
		Gender differences in attenuation will have little effect on cardiovascular images

From Patterson, R.E., Cloninger, K., Churchwell, K.B., et al.: Special problems with cardiovascular imaging to assess coronary artery disease in women. *In* Julian, D.G., and Wenger, N.K. (eds.): Women and Heart Disease. London, Martin Dunitz, 1997, pp. 91–115.

Abbreviations: CAD, coronary artery disease; R, rest only; R/S, rest and stress; (+), positive; ECG-ST, electrocardiographic ST segments; SPECT, single-photon emission computed tomography with thallium-201 or technetium-99m-sestamibi; MPI, myocardial perfusion imaging; LV, left ventricular; RNA, radionuclide angiocardiography; LVEF, left ventricular ejection fraction; LVED, left ventricular and end-diastolic; BP, blood pressure; Echo, echocardiography; PET, positron emission tomography; MRI, magnetic resonance imaging; MRA, magnetic resonance angiography; UFCT, ultrafast computed tomography.

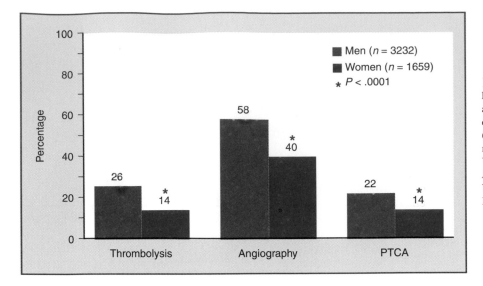

Figure 6–4

Frequencies of utilization of thrombolytics, angiography, and angioplasty in the Myocardial Infarction Triage and Intervention (MITI) registry. PTCA, percutaneous transluminal coronary angioplasty. (From Roger, V.L., and Gersh B.J.: Myocardial infarction. *In* Julian, D.G., and Wenger, N.K. [eds.]: Women and Heart Disease. London, Martin Dunitz, 1997, p. 144.)

cise and pharmacologic stress echocardiography appear to have similar sensitivity and specificity in women and in men.

Acute MI (see Chap. 19)

Although acute MI was less often the initial presentation of coronary heart disease in women than in men in the Framingham Heart Study, women who incurred MI had more morbidity and a higher mortality than did men. Even with the contemporary reduction in mortality from acute MI, the hospital mortality in women in the Myocardial Infarction Triage and Intervention (MITI) Registry was 16% compared with 11% in men, and the use of thrombolytic therapy, angiography, and angioplasty was lower (Fig. 6–4).[21] Women are twice as likely as men to die in the early weeks of convalescence after MI, and they experience reinfarction more frequently. They also have higher rates of stroke, shock, heart failure, recurrent chest pain, and cardiac rupture than do men, and their risk of intracranial hemorrhage with thrombolytic therapy is higher.

Thrombolytic therapy confers equal benefit for survival in women and in men, despite an excess of bleeding complications among women. It is uncertain whether the typical fixed-dosage regimen for thrombolytic therapy results in higher plasma levels of thrombolytic drugs in women (owing to their lower body mass) and thereby engenders increased bleeding. Although thrombolytic therapy reduces acute MI mortality rates in both genders, it has not altered the gender differentials (Fig. 6–5).[22] In the Global Use of Strategies to Open Occluded Coronary Arteries (GUSTO) trial, unadjusted 30-day mortality rates for women were more than twice those for men (13.1% vs. 4.8%).[23]

The explanation for these gender differences is not clear, although the older average age of women who sustain MI appears to be an important contributor. Despite higher left ventricular ejection fractions in women than in men both at hospital admission and at hospital discharge, the prognosis for women experiencing MI remains unfavorable in that they have an increased incidence of post-MI angina and heart failure. Importantly, women appear less eligible for reperfusion therapy than men, in great part because of their later arrival at the hospital after the onset of chest pain. The challenge is to recognize the importance of coronary heart disease as a clinical problem in women, particularly older women, and to target educational programs and family and social support systems to accelerate their access to emergency care.

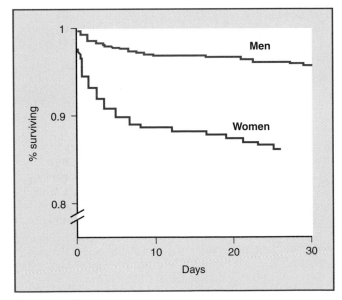

Figure 6–5

Kaplan-Meier analysis of the effect of gender on the unadjusted 30-day mortality rate in women (13.1%) versus men (4.8%) (*P* < .0001). (Reprinted from *Journal of the American College of Cardiology,* Vol. 29, Woodfield, S.L., Lundergan, C.F., Reiner, J.S., et al.: Gender and acute myocardial infarction: Is there a different response to thrombolysis?, pp. 35–42, Copyright 1997, with permission from the American College of Cardiology.)

The role of lower rates of post-MI risk stratification and referral for myocardial revascularization in women remains to be ascertained.

Unrecognized MI is more common among women than among men. Atypical presentations with neck, shoulder, and abdominal pain, as well as dyspnea without pain, occur more frequently in women. A higher incidence of older age and diabetes mellitus in women with MI increases the likelihood of both silent and unrecognized MI.

Clinicians should be attuned to the morbidity related to the psychosocial complications of acute MI, which are more common in women. These include anxiety, depression, sexual dysfunction, and guilt about illness. Despite their early resumption of high-intensity household tasks, return to remunerative work is less frequent and more delayed in women than in men.

Myocardial Revascularization

During the decade from the mid-1980s to the mid-1990s, there has been an almost threefold increase in the rates of myocardial revascularization procedures in women, both CABG surgery and PTCA or other transcatheter revascularization procedures. Although the rate at which coronary arteriography is performed may be somewhat lower in women than in men, it is now clear that *after* coronary arteriography, a comparable approach to myocardial revascularization is employed in both genders. However, even today, women hospitalized for MI are less likely than men to have risk stratification procedures performed before hospital discharge or in the early posthospital period,[3] although the frequency of use of these procedures has increased in recent years. It is uncertain whether this is appropriate or inappropriate, since many women, because of older age or co-morbidity, may not be candidates for myocardial revascularization. Also, it is unclear whether more women than men refuse these procedures when they are recommended.

Women who undergo PTCA tend to be older and are less likely to have had prior MI, but they are more likely to have heart failure, unstable angina, hypertension, hypercholesterolemia, and diabetes mellitus than their male counterparts and therefore are at higher procedural risk. Hospital mortality after angioplasty remains higher for women, probably because of older age and a higher prevalence of co-morbid illnesses. Women also have a higher incidence of complications, including acute coronary occlusion and groin bleeding. Women have less subsequent surgical revascularization after PTCA; whether this is a favorable or unfavorable feature remains to be ascertained. Women with unstable angina are less likely than men to receive intensive anti-ischemic therapy or to undergo coronary angiography or coronary revascularization.[3]

In the CASS trial, the risk of perioperative mortality after CABG surgery was 4.5% for women compared with 1.9% for men. More recent data from the MITI Registry, in which the overall surgical mortality was higher because CABG was carried out in higher-risk patients, the hospital mortality was 13% in women compared with 6%

in men.[24] Women also have a higher incidence of graft occlusion, are less likely to receive an internal mammary artery graft, report less symptomatic relief, and more frequently experience perioperative infarction and heart failure. This reduced efficacy may well influence the referral of sicker women for operation. Nonetheless, women who survive the perioperative period have 15-year survival rates comparable with those for men. However, women are more likely to experience adverse psychosocial outcomes after surgical revascularization, with more frequent depression and lesser and later resumption of preoperative activities, including employment.

In all reports of coronary revascularization, female gender has been associated with both an excessive mortality rate and an excess of surgical complications among survivors.[13] However, in most reported series of both CABG surgery and PTCA, women were older than men and had greater functional impairment and more severe and unstable angina pectoris and were therefore more likely to require urgent or emergent procedures. Furthermore, women have smaller coronary arteries than men, presumably related to their smaller body size, and as a consequence, more technical problems that may limit the completeness of myocardial revascularization in women.

Arterial Hypertension

(see Chaps. 11 and 21)

There is an equal prevalence by gender among the 50 million adults with hypertension in the United States. However, hypertension is somewhat more frequent among men than women before the age of 60 years, with the age-associated increase in systolic blood pressure more pronounced in women, so that after this age, more women than men have hypertension. Isolated systolic hypertension is particularly prominent among elderly women. Clinical trials suggest comparable benefit from the control of hypertension in women and in men.

Congenital Heart Disease

(see Chap. 26)

Contraception poses a problem for women with congenital heart disease in whom pregnancy is contraindicated. Oral contraceptives are inadvisable for women with cyanotic heart disease because of the increased risk of thromboembolism, and intrauterine devices should not be used in the majority of patients with congenital heart disease because of the risk of infective endocarditis. Barrier methods and controlled-release progestin (Norplant) are recommended in such patients. Tubal ligation should be considered for women with primary pulmonary hypertension or the Eisenmenger syndrome, for whom pregnancy poses especially high risks (Table 6–8).

Valvular Heart Disease

(see Chap. 25)

Mitral stenosis occurs more commonly in women than in men, whereas aortic valve disease is more common in

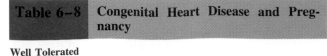

Table 6–8 Congenital Heart Disease and Pregnancy

Well Tolerated

Uncomplicated septal defects
Mild or moderate pulmonary or aortic stenosis
Corrected tetralogy of Fallot
Hypertrophic cardiomyopathy (usually)
Acyanotic Ebstein's anomaly
Corrected transposition without signficant other defects

Moderate Risk

Coarctation of the aorta
Cyanosed mother with pulmonary stenosis

High Maternal and Fetal Risk

Pulmonary hypertension
    In the Eisenmenger syndrome (with reversed central shunt)
    Residual after closure of nonrestrictive ventricular septal defect
Univentricular circulation after the Fontan operation

High Fetal Risk

Cyanotic mother with pulmonary stenosis

From Oakley, C.M.: Heart disease and heart surgery during pregnancy. *In* Julian, D.G., and Wenger, N.K. (eds.): Women and Heart Disease. London, Martin Dunitz, 1997, pp. 195–213.

men. Mitral stenosis is, occasionally, diagnosed for the first time during pregnancy, when the increased cardiac output or the development of atrial fibrillation results in pulmonary edema. If hemodynamic stabilization with medical therapy, which usually involves the administration of diuretics and beta blocking drugs, is unsuccessful, balloon valvotomy may be the treatment of choice.

Mechanical Prosthetic Heart Valves

The hypercoagulable state of pregnancy increases the risks of thromboembolism, and therefore careful attention to anticoagulation in pregnant women with prosthetic cardiac valves is mandatory. There is risk of embryopathy when warfarin is administered during the first trimester of pregnancy, and the use of subcutaneous heparin during this period is only in part protective. Before delivery, the patient may be switched from warfarin to subcutaneous heparin; this drug can be discontinued at the onset of labor and reinstated, along with warfarin, shortly after delivery. Because of these problems with anticoagulants, it is usually advised that women with prosthetic valves avoid pregnancy or that valve replacement be deferred until the completion of pregnancy. Balloon valvuloplasty for mitral stenosis or aortic stenosis or mitral valve repair for mitral regurgitation should be employed whenever possible in women who are, or plan to become, pregnant. Bioprosthetic valves, which do not pose a risk of thromboembolic complications, exhibit limited durability in women of childbearing age and are not satisfactory alternatives.

Antibiotic prophylaxis against infective endocarditis at delivery is recommended for women with prosthetic heart valves (see Chap. 16).

Peripartum Cardiomyopathy (see Chap. 31)

Unexplained heart failure within 1 or 2 months before or 6 months after delivery is termed *peripartum cardiomyopathy*. The cause is unknown, but it occurs more commonly with multiple pregnancies. The age, parity, and race of the mother appear to have little effect on the incidence of this condition. The severity ranges from mild heart failure to severe pulmonary edema, and the degree of cardiac enlargement varies comparably. The diagnosis of peripartum cardiomyopathy requires exclusion of other causes of cardiac failure. The management is that of heart failure due to systolic dysfunction (see Chap. 22).

The prognosis of peripartum cardiomyopathy varies markedly in that some patients recover promptly and others partially, whereas a minority may progress to the need for cardiac transplantation. However, rejection rates with cardiac transplantation are higher in women with prior pregnancies than in men. Even in patients who recover from peripartum cardiomyopathy with apparently normal ventricular function, subsequent pregnancy may be associated with recurrent cardiomyopathy and should therefore be discouraged.

References

1. Mittelmark, M.B., Psaty, B.M., Rautaharju, P.M., et al.: Prevalence of cardiovascular diseases among older adults. The Cardiovascular Health Study. Am. J. Epidemiol. 137:311–317, 1993.
2. Lakatta, E.G., Gerstenblith, G., and Weisfeldt, M.L.: The aging heart: Structure, function and disease. *In* Braunwald, E. (ed.): Heart Disease. 5th ed. Philadelphia, W.B. Saunders, 1997, pp. 1687–1703.
3. Stone, P.H., Thompson, B., Anderson, H.V., et al.: Influence of race, sex, and age on management of unstable angina and non–Q-wave myocardial infarction. The TIMI III Registry. JAMA 275:1104–1112, 1996.
4. Tsai, T.P., Chaux, A., Matloff, J.M. et al.: Ten-year experience of cardiac surgery in patients aged 80 years and over. Ann. Thorac. Surg. 58:445–451, 1994.
5. Gersh, B.J., Kronmal, R.A., Schaff, H.V., et al., and the Participants in the Coronary Artery Surgery Study: Comparison of coronary artery bypass surgery and medical therapy in patients 65 years of age or older. A nonrandomized study from the Coronary Artery Surgery Study (CASS) Registry. N. Engl. J. Med. 313:217–224, 1985.
6. White, H.D., Barbash, G.I., Califf, R.M., et al.: Age and outcome with contemporary thrombolytic therapy: Results from the GUSTO-I Trial. Circulation 94:1826–1833, 1996.
7. Wenger, N.K., Froelicher, E.S., Smith, L.K., et al: Cardiac rehabilitation. Clinical Practice Guideline no. 17. AHCPR Publication no. 96–0672. Rockville, MD, U.S. Department of Health and Human Services, Public Health Service, Agency for Health Care Policy and Research, and the National Heart, Lung, and Blood Institute, October 1995.
8. Hypertension Detection and Follow-Up Program Cooperative Group: Five-year findings of the Hypertension Detection and Follow-Up Program: II. Mortality by race, sex and age. JAMA 242:2572–2577, 1979.
9. SHEP Cooperative Research Group: Prevention of stroke by antihypertensive drug treatment in older persons with isolated systolic hypertension. Final results of the Systolic Hypertension in the Elderly Program (SHEP). JAMA 265:3255–3264, 1991.
10. MacMahon, S., and Rodgers, A.: The effects of blood pressure reduction in older patients: An overview of five randomized controlled trials in elderly hypertensives. Clin. Exp. Hypertens. 15:967–978, 1993.

11. Craver, J.M., Weintraub, W.S., Jones, E.L., et al.: Predictors of mortality, complications, and length of stay in aortic valve replacement for aortic stenosis. Circulation 78(Suppl I):I-85–I-90, 1988.

12. Julian, D.G., and Wenger, N.K. (eds.): Women and Heart Disease. London, Martin Dunitz, 1997.

13. Douglas, P.S.: Coronary artery disease in women. *In* Braunwald, E. (ed.): Heart Disease. 5th ed. Philadelphia, W.B. Saunders, 1997, pp. 1704–1714.

14. Wenger, N.K., Speroff, L., and Packard, B.: Cardiovascular health and disease in women. N. Engl. J. Med. 329:247–256, 1993.

15. Scandinavian Simvastatin Survival Study Group. Randomised trial of cholesterol lowering in 4444 patients with coronary heart disease: The Scandinavian Simvastatin Survival Study (4S). Lancet 344: 1383–1389, 1994.

16. Sacks, F.M., Pfeffer, M.A., Moye, L.A., et al., for the Cholesterol and Recurrent Events Trial Investigators: The effect of pravastatin on coronary events after myocardial infarction in patients with average cholesterol levels. N. Engl. J. Med. 335:1001–1009, 1996.

17. The Writing Group for the PEPI Trial: Effects of estrogen or estrogen/progestin regimens on heart disease risk factors in postmenopausal women. The Postmenopausal Estrogen/Progestin Interventions (PEPI) Trial. JAMA 273:199–208, 1995.

18. Manolio, T.A., Furberg, C.D., Shemanski, L., et al., for the CHS Collaborative Research Group: Associations of postmenopausal estrogen use with cardiovascular disease and its risk factors in older women. Circulation 88:2163–2171, 1993.

19. Kannel, W.B., and Feinleib, M.: Natural history of angina pectoris in the Framingham Study. Prognosis and survival. Am. J. Cardiol. 29:154–163, 1972.

20. Kennedy, J.W., Killip, T., Fisher, L.D., et al.: The clinical spectrum of coronary artery disease and its surgical and medical management, 1974–1979. The Coronary Artery Surgery Study. Circulation 66(Suppl III):III-16–III-23, 1982.

21. Maynard, C., Litwin, P.E., Martin, J.S., et al. Gender differences in the treatment and outcome of acute myocardial infarction. Results from the Myocardial Infarction Triage and Intervention Registry. Arch. Intern. Med. 152:972–976, 1992.

22. Woodfield, S.L., Lundergan, C.F., Reiner, J.S., et al.: Gender and acute myocardial infarction: Is there a different response to thrombolysis? J. Am. Coll. Cardiol. 29:35–42, 1997.

23. Lee, K.L., Woodlief, L.H., Topol, E.J., et al.: Predictors of 30-day mortality in the era of reperfusion for acute myocardial infarction. Circulation 91:1659–1668, 1995.

24. Maynard, C., and Weaver, W.D.: Treatment of women with acute MI. New findings from the MITI Registry. J. Myocard. Ischemia 4: 27–37, 1992.

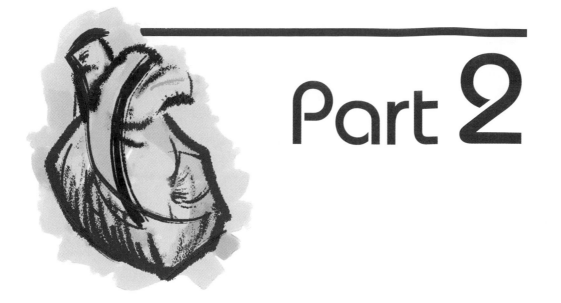

Part 2

APPROACH TO COMMON CARDIAC PROBLEMS

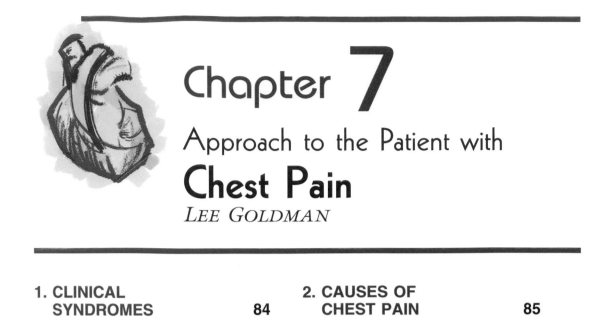

Chapter 7

Approach to the Patient with

Chest Pain

LEE GOLDMAN

Chest pain is a common symptom that may represent a condition as serious as an acute myocardial infarction (MI) or as benign as a strained thoracic chest muscle. A patient's concern about chest pain is often unrelated to the severity of the symptom but related rather to the possible underlying cause. Similarly, the physician must remember that the intensity of chest pain is often unrelated to the importance of the underlying condition.[1] Many patients with serious coronary artery disease may complain of a vague discomfort rather than severe pain, whereas inflammatory costochondritis may lead to severe pain.

The diagnosis of the cause of chest pain must take into account the chest pain syndrome itself, the associated symptoms and signs, and an appreciation for the patient's other general characteristics. For example, the likely cause of burning substernal chest pain will be different in a patient whose pain is associated with diaphoresis and shortness of breath than in a patient whose pain is precipitated by lying flat after a large meal. Furthermore, the same chest pain and associated symptoms would be much more likely to represent coronary artery disease if they were found in a 60-year-old man than in a 20-year-old woman.

Chest pain is one of the most frequent problems encountered in primary care and is one of the most frequent causes for hospital admission. Coronary artery disease, a leading cause of chest pain, remains the most common cause of death in the United States. Every complaint of chest pain must be taken seriously, but the physician must choose appropriately from among a wide range of diagnostic tests and possible therapeutic trials.

CLINICAL SYNDROMES

Patients who complain of chest pain can quickly be put into one of three general categories: acute chest pain of recent onset, which may be ongoing and persistent; episodic, recurrent chest pain, with each individual episode lasting for minutes rather than hours; or persistent pain, which may continue for hours or even days with variable fluctuation in intensity. By placing an individual patient in one of these three general categories, the physician may focus the evaluation on the various causes of chest pain (Table 7–1).

For some causes, such as coronary artery disease, chest pain may be of sudden, new onset, as with an acute MI, or recurrent and episodic, as with angina (Table 7–2). When the anginal pain occurs more frequently or at lower levels of stress or even at rest, the episodes suggest unstable rather than stable angina. Other causes of insufficient coronary arterial flow, such as are found with valvular aortic stenosis, hypertrophic cardiomyopathy, or microvascular angina, also tend to be recurrent and episodic. By comparison, the pain of acute pericarditis may be of sudden acute onset, may be recurrent and episodic during the acute phase of pericarditis or during periodic recurrences, or may persist for hours or days as a dull ache.

Among vascular causes, aortic dissection commonly presents as severe acute pain with a discrete onset. Much less commonly, patients with chronic aortic dissections may have intermittent episodes of pain associated with extension of the dissection. Acute pulmonary embolism may be associated with severe pain at the time of onset. If the pulmonary embolism leads to pulmonary infarction and irritation of the pleural surface, it may be associated with recurrent episodic pain, especially pain associated with deep breathing. The pain of pulmonary hypertension and right ventricular strain may be of sudden onset but is more commonly associated with exertion or other stress that leads to increased pulmonary blood flow and hence increased pulmonary blood pressure in the face of an elevated pulmonary vascular resistance.

Pain from pneumonia or pleuritis may be of acute on-

Table 7–1 Some Causes of Chest Discomfort

	New, Acute, Often Ongoing	Recurrent, Episodic	Persistent, Even for Days
Cardiac			
Coronary artery disease	+	+	
Aortic stenosis		+	
Hypertrophic cardiomyopathy		+	
Pericarditis	+	+	+
Vascular			
Aortic dissection	+		
Pulmonary embolism	+	+	
Pulmonary hypertension	+	+	
Right ventricular strain	+	+	
Pulmonary			
Pleuritis or pneumonia	+	+	+
Tracheobronchitis	+	+	+
Pneumothorax	+		+
Tumor			+
Mediastinitis or mediastinal emphysema	+		+
Gastrointestinal			
Esophageal reflux	+	+	+
Esophageal spasm	+	+	+
Mallory-Weiss tear	+		
Peptic ulcer disease	+	+	+
Biliary disease	+	+	
Pancreatitis		+	+
Musculoskeletal			
Cervical disk disease		+	+
Arthritis of the shoulder or spine		+	+
Costochondritis	+	+	+
Intercostal muscle cramps	+	+	+
Interscalene or hyperabduction syndromes		+	+
Subacromial bursitis	+	+	+
Other			
Disorders of the breast		+	+
Chest wall tumors			+
Herpes zoster	+		+
Emotional	+	+	+

From Fauci, A.S., Braunwald, E., Isselbacher, K.J., et al. (eds.): Harrison's Principles of Internal Medicine. 14th ed. New York, McGraw-Hill, 1998, p. 58. Reproduced with permission of The McGraw-Hill Companies.

set at the time of initial pleural irritation, may be recurrent at times of deep breathing or other maneuvers that stretch or irritate the pleura, or may be persistent because of pleural irritation (Table 7–3). Pain from a pneumothorax is usually sudden and acute and then persists until the pneumothorax resolves spontaneously or by treatment. Pain from lung tumors is commonly persistent for days or longer.

Most of the various gastrointestinal causes of chest discomfort are acute in onset, but many may also be recurrent and episodic. Most gastrointestinal causes of discomfort can be related to eating, vomiting, or other associated gastrointestinal signs or symptoms.

Musculoskeletal chest discomfort can be acute and of sudden onset, especially when related to costochondritis,

muscle cramps or injuries, or bursitis. Musculoskeletal complaints can also be recurrent and episodic, usually in association with movements that can be directly related to the involved structures. In differentiating recurrent episodic musculoskeletal chest pain from angina pectoris, the relationship to specific movements is vital. Many musculoskeletal complaints cause persistent chest discomfort, and this lack of relationship to activity may be an important way to discriminate musculoskeletal chest pain from coronary artery disease.

CAUSES OF CHEST PAIN

Myocardial Ischemia

Myocardial ischemia may be of acute and sudden onset, such as with acute MI, or recurrent and episodic, such as with angina pectoris from atherosclerosis or other causes of coronary stenosis. It may also be seen in patients with normal epicardial coronary arteries but with abnormalities of coronary vascular tone or of the coronary microvascular circulation. Patients with nonatherosclerotic causes of coronary stenosis, such as may be found with collagen vascular diseases, syphilis, or coronary artery dissection, also develop coronary ischemia. Myocardial ischemia may also be found in patients with congenital anomalies of the coronary arteries, including the congenital absence of one or more important coronary arteries, a coronary artery that originates from the pulmonary artery rather than the aorta, or even rarely from a coronary arteriovenous fistula. Myocardial ischemia can also occur with totally normal coronary arteries, both anatomically and functionally, if markedly increased oxygen demand is not matched by oxygen supply. For example, in patients with valvular aortic stenosis or hypertrophic cardiomyopathy, myocardial ischemia may develop, especially with exercise, because diastolic coronary flow is not adequate to supply the needs of the hypertrophic, stressed myocardium.

When chest pain is caused by an abnormality in the coronary artery, the abnormality may range from a total, anatomic occlusion to an endothelial or functional abnormality associated with a normal lumen at the time of coronary arteriography. A sudden, total occlusion of a coronary artery, usually by intrinsic thrombosis but occasionally by embolization, commonly causes an acute MI, although occasionally it may be asymptomatic in a patient with impaired pain response or with adequate, pre-existing collateral vessels. In patients with a chronic total occlusion, angina pectoris may then develop because circulation to the affected myocardium via collaterals may be adequate at rest but not during exercise or other stress.

FIXED CORONARY STENOSES. These generally do not impair resting coronary blood flow substantially until they occlude about 70% to 90% of the cross-sectional area of the coronary lumen. However, stenoses of 50% of luminal diameter, which corresponds to about 70% of cross-sectional area, are frequently associated with ischemia during exercise or other stress. Since myocardial oxygen extraction tends to be near maximal at all

Table 7–2   Cardiovascular Causes of Chest Pain

Condition	Location	Quality	Duration	Aggravating or Relieving Factors	Associated Symptoms or Signs
Angina	Retrosternal region; radiates to or occasionally isolated to neck, jaw, epigastrium, shoulder, or arms—left common	Pressure, burning, squeezing, heaviness, indigestion	<2–10 min	Precipitated by exercise, cold weather, or emotional stress; relieved by rest or nitroglycerin; atypical (Prinzmetal's) angina may be unrelated to activity, often early morning	S_4, or murmur of papillary muscle dysfunction during pain
Rest or unstable angina	Same as angina	Same as angina but may be more severe	Usually <20 min	Same as angina, with decreasing tolerance for exertion or at rest	Similar to stable angina, but may be pronounced. Transient cardiac failure can occur
Myocardial infarction	Substernal and may radiate like angina	Heaviness, pressure, burning, constriction	Sudden onset, 30 min or longer but variable	Unrelieved by rest or nitroglycerin	Shortness of breath, sweating, weakness, nausea, vomiting
Pericarditis	Usually begins over sternum or toward cardiac apex and may radiate to neck or left shoulder; often more localized than the pain of myocardial ischemia	Sharp, stabbing, knifelike	Lasts many hours to days; may wax and wane	Aggravated by deep breathing, rotating chest, or supine position; relieved by sitting up and leaning forward	Pericardial friction rub
Aortic dissection	Anterior chest; may radiate to back	Excruciating, tearing, knifelike	Sudden onset, unrelenting	Usually occurs in setting of hypertension or predisposition such as Marfan's syndrome	Murmur of aortic insufficiency, pulse or blood pressure asymmetry; neurologic deficit
Pulmonary embolism (chest pain often not present)	Substernal or over region of pulmonary infarction	Pleuritic (with pulmonary infarction) or angina-like	Sudden onset; minutes to <1 hr	May be aggravated by breathing	Dyspnea, tachypnea, tachycardia; hypotension, signs of acute right heart failure, and pulmonary hypertension with large emboli; rales, pleural rub, hemoptysis with pulmonary infarction
Pulmonary hypertension	Substernal	Pressure; oppressive		Aggravated by effort	Pain usually associated with dyspnea; signs of pulmonary hypertension

From Andreoli, T.E., Bennett, J.C., Carpenter, C.C.J., and Plum, F.: Evaluation of the patient with cardiovascular disease. *In* Cecil Essentials of Medicine. 4th ed. Philadelphia, W.B. Saunders, 1997, p. 11.
Abbreviations: S_4, fourth heart sound.

times, increased oxygen supply can be provided only by increased coronary flow. The major determinant of total coronary flow is coronary vascular resistance; in response to exercise, adrenergic stimuli, and most substances that dilate peripheral arteries, the coronary arteries also dilate. The resulting decrease in coronary resistance permits the increased blood flow that is required to meet the myocar-dial demands of exercise and stress. In patients with an abnormal coronary arterial endothelium, vasodilatation may not occur in response to typical vasodilatory stimuli; in some circumstances, paradoxical vasoconstriction may occur. Although impaired coronary vasodilatation may oc-cur in the absence of any evident pathoanatomic abnor-malities, it is more common in patients with hypercholes-

Table 7–3 **Noncardiac Causes of Chest Pain**

Condition	Location	Quality	Duration	Aggravating or Relieving Factors	Associated Symptoms or Signs
Pneumonia with pleurisy	Localized over involved area	Pleuritic localized		Painful breathing	Dyspnea, cough, fever, dull to percussion, bronchial breath sounds, rates, occasional pleural rub
Spontaneous pneumothorax	Unilateral	Sharp, well localized	Sudden onset, lasts many hours	Painful breathing	Dyspnea; hyperresonance and decreased breath and voice sounds over involved lung
Musculoskeletal disorders	Variable	Aching	Short or long duration	Aggravated by movement; history of muscle exertion or injury	Tender to pressure or movement
Herpes zoster	Dermatomal in distribution		Prolonged	None	Vesicular rash appears in area of discomfort
Esophageal reflux	Substernal, epigastric	Burning, visceral discomfort	10–60 min	Aggravated by large meal, postprandial recumbency; relief with antacid	Water brash
Peptic ulcer	Epigastric, substernal	Visceral burning, aching	Prolonged	Relief with food, antacid	
Gallbladder disease	Epigastric, right upper quadrant	Visceral	Prolonged	May be unprovoked or follows meal	Right upper quadrant tenderness may be present
Anxiety states	Often localized over precordium	Variable; often location moves from place to place	Varies; often fleeting	Situational	Sighing respirations, often chest wall tenderness

From Andreoli, T.E., Bennett, J.C., Carpenter, C.C.J., and Plum, F.: Evaluation of the patient with cardiovascular disease. *In* Cecil Essentials of Medicine. 4th ed. Philadelphia, W.B. Saunders, 1997, p. 12.

terolemia or those who smoke, and the abnormal reflex may disappear when cholesterol levels are reduced or smoking ceases. Patients with obstructive atherosclerotic coronary disease also commonly have impaired coronary vasodilatation or paradoxical vasoconstriction, sometimes at the sites of atherosclerotic stenoses and sometimes in locations in which coronary arteriography does not reveal any gross abnormalities.

Vasoactive substances, such as cocaine, may cause inappropriate coronary vasoconstriction and even spasm sufficient to obliterate the coronary lumen and cause severe ischemia or even MI. Patients with Prinzmetal's angina have spontaneous, severe vasoconstriction that may occur at rest, when typical coronary vasodilator stimuli are lacking, or paradoxically with exercise.

Coronary artery emboli may originate from infectious endocarditis, clot in the left atrium or left ventricle, marantic endocarditis in patients with metastatic malignancies, Libman-Sacks endocarditis, clot on prosthetic heart valves, or even paradoxical emboli originating in the venous system and shunting to the left side of the heart via a ventricular septal defect, atrial septal defect, or patent foramen ovale.

Acute MI can be caused by any sudden occlusion of a coronary artery, ranging from intrinsic thrombus to embolus to internal dissection or external compression of a coronary artery.

Acute MI (see Chap. 19)

Clinical Presentation

The pain of acute MI is classically described as constriction, tightness, pressure, or squeezing discomfort centered in the mid-substernal region and often radiating to the left shoulder, neck, or arm. It is classically associated with diaphoresis and may be accompanied by shortness of breath, nausea, or a feeling of impending doom. It classically builds in intensity over a period of 5 to 10 minutes before reaching peak intensity. The pain may begin with exercise or stress, but it most commonly occurs without warning or an obvious immediate precipitating cause. Although acute MI is statistically more likely to occur in the early morning hours, it may happen at any time of day.

Analyses of large numbers of patients evaluated for acute chest pain, however, reveal that many patients do not have this typical presentation, and many patients without acute MI or even acute myocardial ischemia may have many of the characteristics that are usually thought to be typical for acute ischemia. For example, pain that is described as aching, burning, indigestion, or gas is nearly as likely to represent acute MI as is pain that is described as pressure, squeezing, tightness, or constriction. Pain is much less likely to represent acute MI if it is described as stabbing or knifelike or as sharp when the term *sharp* is not being used as a synonym for severe but rather to describe the feeling of the pain.

When pain radiates from the chest to the left shoulder, neck, or left arm, the likelihood that it represents acute MI is about threefold higher than when chest pain does not radiate to these locations. It must be remembered, however, that innervation of the thoracic dermatomes is not sufficiently precise for the location or radiation of pain to be considered definitive from a diagnostic perspective. Furthermore, severe pain from any source may stimulate adjacent dermatomes. Therefore, esophageal spasm may cause pain radiation indistinguishable from that of an acute MI.

The pain of acute MI may also radiate to the jaw, teeth, right arm, back, or abdomen. Nevertheless, concomitant back pain should raise the possibility of aortic dissection or musculoskeletal causes, whereas radiation to the abdomen should increase suspicion for the various gastrointestinal causes of acute chest discomfort. The pain of acute myocardial ischemia rarely radiates to the lower abdomen or legs.

Diaphoresis may accompany any discomfort that evokes severe sympathetic stimulation or parasympathetic response. Diaphoresis tends to be more common in larger, more severe, more obvious MIs, in which diagnosis by other means is often easier.

Shortness of breath may accompany acute MI because of concomitant left heart failure related to left ventricular dysfunction caused by the myocardial ischemia. Subjective shortness of breath may also develop in patients who are in severe pain or who are anxious or hyperventilating because of the acute pain syndrome.

Physical Examination

Pain is much less likely to represent acute MI if it can be reproduced by localized chest palpation. However, since many patients will have discomfort on vigorous chest palpation, it is critical to determine whether the patient's complaints are truly reproduced by relatively modest chest palpation as compared with when vigorous chest manipulation produces a different pain syndrome.

The physical examination may be totally normal in patients with acute MI unless there is concomitant heart failure or other complications (see Chap. 19).

Diagnostic Testing

The single most important piece of laboratory information in the patient with possible acute MI is the electrocardiogram (ECG).[2, 3] The ECG will show ST segment elevation or Q-waves not known to be old in about 40% to 45% of patients with acute MI. An additional 30% to 40% of patients will have ST segment depression or T-wave inversion not known to be old on the initial ECG.

In patients with such electrocardiographic changes and a clinical presentation consistent with acute MI, rapid triage to an acute care setting and institution of emergent treatment is mandatory.

For patients with a clinical presentation that might be consistent with acute MI but that might also represent unstable angina pectoris (see Chap. 20), a combination of clinical factors can be used to estimate the approximate probability of acute MI (Fig. 7–1). The recent development of chest pain evaluation units (see later) provides a low-cost, efficient mechanism for a brief but focused evaluation in such patients.

Angina

Myocardial ischemia (without infarction) that occurs at rest, with less exertion than with prior angina, or for the first time is commonly called *unstable angina* (see Chap. 20). The typical pain of angina resembles that of an acute MI except it is commonly transient, lasting for minutes, and is relieved by cessation of the precipitating activity or by nitroglycerin.

Angina is commonly precipitated by any stimulus that increases myocardial oxygen demand, including exertion or emotion (see Chap. 18). It may also be precipitated by stimuli that increase peripheral vascular resistance, such as exposure to cold, or that cause selective vasodilatation, such as a heavy meal. Angina may also be precipitated by tachycardia from any cause.

In a substantial proportion of patients, symptomatic angina or asymptomatic myocardial ischemia may develop without any prior evidence of increased myocardial oxygen demand, peripheral vasoconstriction or dilatation, or tachycardia. In such situations, intrinsic changes in coronary arteries themselves, sometimes precipitated by paradoxical responses to stimuli that usually cause coronary arterial vasodilatation, precipitate ischemia.

Whereas most patients will complain of chest pain, others may relate an ill-described discomfort or note only shortness of breath or fatigue. The discomfort is usually sufficiently severe to cause the patient to slow down or cease activity. The pain usually persists for no more than 5 to 30 minutes; persistent discomfort may represent an acute MI or, in the absence of other evidence for myocardial ischemia, a noncoronary cause. The pain is typically relieved within 5 minutes by sublingual nitroglycerin, which may also delay the onset of pain during exertion. Pain that resolves in less than 1 minute or that is precipitated by deep breathing or changes in position is unlikely to be angina.

The chest pain syndrome of myocardial ischemia is similar regardless of whether the cause is intrinsic coronary atherosclerosis or the other coronary and noncoronary causes of myocardial ischemia. The underlying cause of the myocardial ischemia is often evident by careful history and physical examination, although it may occasionally require diagnostic coronary angiography.

Physical Examination

The physical examination is often totally normal in patients with acute myocardial ischemia. The ischemia

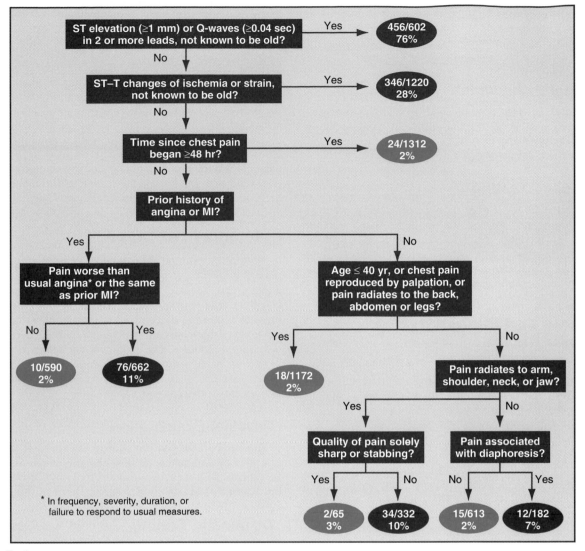

Figure 7–1

Flow diagram for estimating the risk of acute myocardial infarction (MI) in emergency departments in patients with acute chest pain. For each clinical subset, the numerator is the number of patients with the set of presenting characteristics who developed an MI, whereas the denominator represents the total number of patients presenting with that characteristic or set of characteristics. (Adapted from Pearson, S.D., Goldman, L., Garcia, T.B., et al.: Physician response to a prediction rule for the triage of emergency department patients with chest pain. J. Gen. Intern. Med. 9:241–247, 1994.)

and resulting left ventricular dysfunction may precipitate a third or fourth heart sound or evidence of pulmonary congestion. Papillary muscle ischemia may cause a late systolic mitral regurgitant murmur. Ischemia caused by aortic valvular stenosis or obstructive hypertrophic cardiomyopathy may be accompanied by the typical murmur.

Diagnostic Testing

An ECG during pain will commonly be abnormal in patients with acute myocardial ischemia. Between spontaneous episodes of discomfort, myocardial ischemia may be precipitated by exercise or pharmocologic maneuvers and be detected by electrocardiography, radionuclide scintigraphy, or echocardiography.

Pericarditis (see Chap. 29)

Pericarditis can cause pain that is acute, episodic and recurrent, or persistent.[1] Since the pericardium, except for the inferior parietal surface, is insensitive to pain, most of the discomfort associated with pericarditis is caused by inflammation of the adjacent parietal pleura. Although virtually all pericarditis is inflammatory, infectious causes are commonly associated with more severe pain, whereas noninfectious causes are associated with less pain. In patients with more acute inflammation, irritation of the relatively insensitive pericardium or surface of the heart may cause a persistent pain that can be confused with acute MI when it first begins or with noncardiac causes when it persists.

Depending on the site of pleural and diaphragmatic

irritation, the pain may be anterior or upper abdominal or felt in the back or tip of the shoulder. The pain is typically pleuritic and commonly exacerbated by having the patient in a sitting position and leaning forward.

Physical Examination

Pericarditis is often accompanied by a detectable pericardial friction rub. If there is sufficient fluid to cause pericardial tamponade, typical findings include jugular venous distention, pulsus paradoxus, and hypotension.

Diagnostic Testing

The chest radiograph may show cardiomegaly, whereas an echocardiogram will be the most sensitive test for detecting an increase in pericardial fluid. However, it must be remembered that acute pericarditis may cause pain and an associated pericardial friction rub in the absence of a detectable increase in pericardial fluid.

Systemic and Pulmonary Vascular Disease

An acute aortic dissection (see Chap. 27) usually causes the abrupt onset of severe discomfort that is commonly felt in the center of the chest with an ascending aortic dissection and in the back with a descending aortic dissection. The pain commonly persists for hours, requires substantial doses of analgesics, and is unrelated to exercise, breathing, or changes in position.

Pulmonary emboli (see Chap. 30) can cause acute chest discomfort, sometimes associated with acute hypoxia, hypotension, and even syncope. The pain of an acute pulmonary embolism may be substernal and may mimic an acute MI. With smaller emboli, there may be no acute pain at the time of embolization but rather pleuritic pain, which may be caused by focal pulmonary infarction and associated with a pleural friction rub. Pulmonary hypertension of any cause may produce right ventricular strain and pain similar to angina pectoris.

Physical Examination

The hallmark of an acute aortic dissection is asymmetry in blood pressure above as compared with below the site of dissection (see Chap. 27). An ascending aortic dissection, which may affect all of the great vessels and therefore not cause a blood pressure discrepancy, may be associated with retrograde dissection affecting the right coronary artery and hence causing ischemia or infarction in the distribution of that artery, or it may dissect back into the pericardium and cause acute pericardial tamponade with its associated signs and symptoms.

Pulmonary emboli may cause an acute rise in pulmonary vascular resistance and acute right-sided heart failure, often evidenced on physical examination by a loud pulmonic second sound. Similar findings are present chronically in patients with long-standing pulmonary hypertension. Focal pulmonary infarction is often associated with a detectable pleural rub at the site of infarction.

Many patients will have some evidence of pre-existing underlying venous thrombotic disease.

Diagnostic Testing

A routine chest radiograph may show evidence of aortic dissection. When the diagnosis is seriously suspected, transesophageal echocardiography is probably the best screening test. For suspected pulmonary embolism, the diagnostic evaluation may begin with a pulmonary ventilation-perfusion scan or proceed directly to pulmonary angiography. In some patients, documentation of peripheral venous disease may be sufficient for making acute diagnostic and therapeutic decisions (see Chap. 30).

Pulmonary Diseases

Most acute pulmonary causes of chest discomfort will present with pleural pain, which is typically described as a sharp and stabbing pain that is related to breathing or coughing. The pain of tracheobronchitis may be described more as a burning discomfort, whereas tumors commonly cause persistent discomfort that is often unrelated to breathing or activity. The pain of a pneumothorax is commonly of acute onset and is severe and disabling, although smaller pneumothoraces may be associated with less severe, persistent pain.

Physical Examination

The hallmark of the physical examination is the detection of a pleural rub at or near the site of the discomfort. In patients with a pneumothorax, focal hyperinflation and the absence of breath sounds are often diagnostic.

Diagnostic Testing

The chest radiograph will commonly detect pulmonary causes of chest discomfort. However, patients with postviral pleurisy may have a normal chest radiograph or minimal atelectasis that may be indistinguishable from the changes found in patients with pulmonary embolization and infarction. In such situations, diagnostic testing to exclude the possibility of pulmonary embolism is often required (see Chap. 30).

Gastrointestinal Conditions

Esophageal pain can be caused by direct irritation of the esophagus, usually by acid reflux from the stomach, or from esophageal obstruction, spasm, or injury.[4] Acid reflux commonly produces a burning discomfort that is exacerbated by alcohol, aspirin, and some foods. The pain is usually relieved promptly by antacids or dairy products, and sometimes by other food or water. Acid reflux is usually exacerbated by lying down or by anything that causes eructation, such as the swallowing of air. The pain is typically most noticed in the morning, when the acid is not neutralized by food, or about an hour after eating.

Esophageal spasm, which may be precipitated by acid

reflux, often causes a deep, visceral pain that may be difficult to distinguish from myocardial ischemia.[5] When severe, the pain of esophageal spasm may radiate to the left arm or shoulder, although such radiation is not typical. Esophageal obstruction from tumor or achalasia is commonly associated with dysphagia, the regurgitation of undigested food, or loss of weight. Esophageal injury, such as a Mallory-Weiss tear caused by especially strenuous vomiting, causes acute chest pain.

The pain of a duodenal or gastric ulcer or of gastritis typically occurs 60 to 90 minutes after meals, when postprandial acid production is no longer neutralized by food in the stomach. As with acid reflux into the esophagus, it is usually relieved within minutes by antacids or dairy products.

The pain of an ulcer or gastritis is commonly epigastric but often radiates to the substernal area. It rarely will radiate to the neck, shoulder, or arms.

Cholecystitis commonly presents as an aching pain, sometimes with colicky spasms, 60 to 90 minutes after a meal. It is more commonly felt predominantly in the right upper quadrant, but epigastric, chest, and even back pain are not uncommon.

The pain of pancreatitis is commonly described as a steady aching, which may be worsened by eating. The pain of pancreatitis, like that of a posterior penetrating ulcer that irritates the pancreas, commonly radiates to the back.

The presence of a gastrointestinal abnormality does not guarantee that the chest discomfort is related to it. Hiatal hernia, gallstones, and even ulcers may be asymptomatic. To make differential diagnosis even more difficult, acid reflux into the esophagus may occasionally precipitate coronary vasospasm, sometimes with resulting myocardial ischemia as well as esophageal spasm.[5]

Physical Examination

In patients with ulcer disease, gastritis, pancreatitis, and gallbladder disease, careful physical examination will usually reveal epigastric or right upper quadrant tenderness. In patients with esophageal conditions, however, the physical examination is commonly normal.

Diagnostic Testing

When gastrointestinal causes of chest discomfort are suspected, the evaluation should include specific tests to assess the possible causes: barium swallow or endoscopy for esophageal disease; upper gastrointestinal series or endoscopy for the stomach and duodenum; or ultrasonography commonly as the first test for the gallbladder or pancreas.

In some situations, the difficulty in diagnosing esophageal causes of chest discomfort may warrant a Bernstein test, in which acid is dripped into the esophagus in attempt to precipitate the patient's typical pain. Esophageal manometry may also be used to document the temporal coexistence of pain and detectable esophageal spasm. However, it is critical that the physician be confident that myocardial ischemia is not the cause of the chest discomfort before ascribing it to esophageal causes.

Musculoskeletal Abnormalities

Chest discomfort may be caused by costochondritis, bursitis, arthritis of the shoulder or spine, cervical disk disease, tendonitis, intercostal muscle cramps, and other abnormalities of the thoracic musculature, skeleton, and nerve roots. Only rare patients will have classic Tietze's syndrome with objective swelling, redness, and warmth over a costochondral joint.

Physical Examination

The pain of the various neuromuscular abnormalities may be of acute onset but is often repeatedly precipitated by particular movements, changes in position, or local palpation. Localized palpation of the cervical and thoracic spine, shoulder, pectoral area, and chondrosternal and costochondral junctions is critical for diagnosing or excluding these various syndromes.

Diagnostic Testing

Most neuromusculoskeletal causes of chest pain are diagnosed by the physical examination, with subsequent testing required only for potentially serious disk disease or shoulder or joint disease.

Emotional and Psychiatric Conditions

A sensation of tightness or aching in the chest may often accompany emotional and psychiatric conditions, including panic disorder. Commonly the pain from these emotional conditions persists for 30 minutes or more and is unrelated to exertion or movement. The patient may have other evidence of emotional disorders, and evaluation for possible panic disorder may be very helpful.

Physical Examination

In patients with emotional disorders, the physical examination is typically normal. Chest palpation may reveal various degrees of discomfort but not usually suggestive of any serious neuromuscular or skeletal abnormality.

Diagnostic Testing

Ascribing severe chest discomfort to an emotional disorder is a diagnosis of exclusion. Patients will often require some degree of diagnostic testing to be confident that acute myocardial ischemia is not the underlying cause of the discomfort, especially if the patient has other risk factors for coronary disease.

Approach to the Patient with New, Acute, Often Ongoing Pain

In the patient with new, acute, ongoing pain, emergent stabilization and treatment often cannot await definitive diagnosis. If there is evidence for circulatory collapse or respiratory insufficiency, this emergent treatment (see Chaps. 17 and 19) will be critical to maximize the likelihood of a favorable outcome.

Even when the assessment of vital signs indicates that emergency treatment is not required, the history and physical examination should be focused and goal-oriented, usually being performed simultaneously with an emergent ECG. If the history, physical examination, and ECG suggest possible aortic dissection, pulmonary embolism, or other acute, noncoronary conditions, diagnosis and treatment must proceed expeditiously (Figs. 7–2 and 7–3; see Chaps. 27 and 30). If the history, physical examination, or ECG, or any combination of these, suggests a potential coronary artery cause, the evaluation must quickly focus on whether urgent reperfusion therapy, with either intravenous agents or angioplasty, should be pursued (see Chap. 19).

If the ECG shows ST segment elevation or Q-waves in two or more leads that are not known to be old, the probability of acute MI in the setting of new, acute, often ongoing chest pain is about 75%. If the ECG does not have these changes but shows ST segment depression of 1 mm or more or T-wave inversion suggestive of ischemia in two or more leads and not known to be old, the probability of acute MI is in the 15% to 25% range. Although the probability is somewhat higher in a patient with a more typical history and somewhat lower in a patient with a decidedly atypical history, patients with these ST–T-wave changes and a history of new, acute, often ongoing pain should be considered as having unstable angina until proved otherwise. Treatment generally will include aspirin, intravenous heparin, and agents to reduce myocardial oxygen demand (see Chap. 19).

Patients without Major Electrocardiographic Changes

When the chest pain is potentially of coronary cause but the patient does not have electrocardiographic changes of ischemia or infarction, further evaluation and treatment may be indicated if the clinical presentation is otherwise

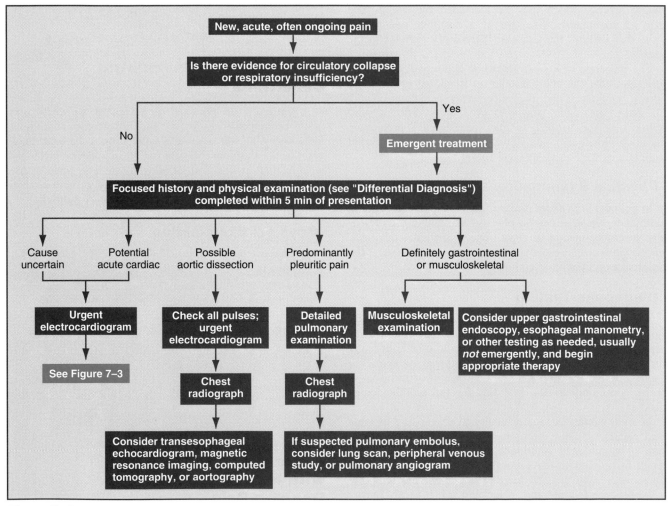

Figure 7–2

Diagnostic approach to the patient with new, acute, often ongoing chest pain. (From Goldman, L.: Chest discomfort and palpitation. *In* Fauci, A.S., Braunwald, E., Isselbacher, K.I., et al. [eds.]: Harrison's Principles of Internal Medicine. 14th ed. New York, McGraw-Hill, 1998, p 61. Reproduced with permission of The McGraw-Hill Companies.)

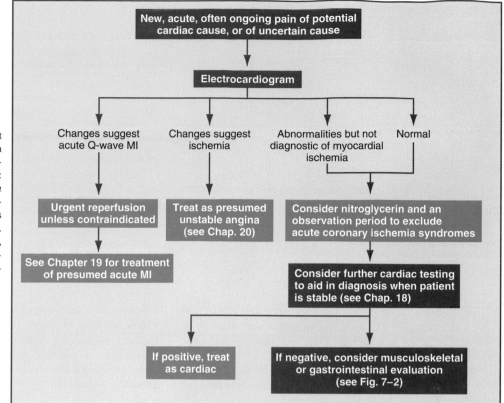

Figure 7–3

Diagnostic approach to the patient with new, acute, often ongoing pain of potential cardiac cause or of uncertain cause. (From Goldman, L.: Chest discomfort and palpitation. *In* Fauci, A.S., Braunwald, E., Isselbacher, K.I., et al. [eds.]: Harrison's Principles of Internal Medicine. 14th ed. New York, McGraw-Hill, 1998, p 62. Reproduced with permission of The McGraw-Hill Companies.)

consistent with acute ischemic heart disease. In addition to multivariate algorithms that have attempted to distinguish patients with sufficiently high likelihoods of acute ischemic heart disease as compared with those with very low probabilities (see Fig. 7–2), further observation will generally be indicated for patients with a clear worsening of a known anginal syndrome, whether the worsening is in terms of the pain's duration, frequency, intensity, or lack of response to rest, nitroglycerin, or interventions that have been successful in the past. For patients without electrocardiographic changes and no prior history of ischemic heart disease, the highest-risk patients are middle-aged men with typical angina radiating to the neck, shoulder, or arms. However, angina may present in atypical ways, and the physician must always consider the possible risks of inappropriate discharge of a patient with possible new onset of ischemic heart disease.[6–9]

Intensive Care Units Versus Stepdown/ Intermediate Care Units

Patients with electrocardiographic changes of infarction or ischemia are usually recommended for initial admission to an intensive care unit because of their increased risk of developing acute complications that will require this level of care (Table 7–4; see also Fig. 2–9). Similarly, patients with other high-risk characteristics should be admitted directly to intensive care, whereas patients at moderate risk are commonly appropriate for admission to

a stepdown or intermediate care unit.[10] Depending on clinical characteristics and the probability of acute MI or unstable angina, low-risk patients are appropriate for either stepdown/intermediate care or a chest pain evaluation unit (see later), and very low-risk patients are appropriate for either a chest pain evaluation unit or discharge.

Chest Pain Evaluation Units

Substantial data indicate that a 6- to 12-hour observation period in a chest pain evaluation unit or a coronary observation unit is an appropriate, cost-effective alternative for patients without electrocardiographic changes or evident complications in whom the possibility of new-onset ischemic heart disease is sufficiently high to make discharge inadvisable. These chest pain evaluation or coronary observation units are generally evaluation areas in the emergency department itself, existing short-stay units newly equipped with cardiac monitors, or otherwise empty beds newly converted to observation status.[11, 12] These units typically provide continuous electrocardiographic monitoring to detect life-threatening arrhythmias. However, the nursing services are usually provided at a typical ward level, with the expectation that patients will feed themselves, ambulate to the bathroom on their own, and so on. Patients are eligible for admission only if they have a low probability for acute MI, have no other complications or ongoing chest discomfort, have no ischemic electrocardiographic changes on admission, and require

Table 7–4 Rate of First Major Event According to the Level of Risk Identified in the Emergency Department

| | First Major Event [number of patients/total number (%)] | | | |
| | ≤12 hr | | >12–24 hr | |
Risk	Derivation Set	Validation Set	Derivation Set	Validation Set
High	125/1043 (12.1)	24/317 (7.6)	36/909 (4.0)	10/293 (3.4)
Moderate	55/1949 (2.8)	9/845 (1.1)	36/1894 (1.9)	18/836 (2.2)
Low	11/1511 (0.7)	5/918 (0.5)	14/1500 (0.9)	11/912 (1.2)
Very low	5/6188 (0.1)	4/2596 (0.2)	12/6182 (0.2)	5/2592 (0.2)
Area under the ROC curve†	0.89	0.84	0.79	0.77

From Goldman, L., Cook, E.F., Johnson, P.A., et al. Prediction of the need for intensive care in patients who come to emergency departments with acute chest pain. N. Engl. J. Med. 334:1498–1502, 1996. Copyright 1996 Massachusetts Medical Society. All rights reserved.

Abbreviation: ROC, receiver-operating characteristic.

* The derivation of the risk groups is shown in Figure 2–9.

† None of the differences between the derivation set and the validation set was significant.

no intravenous medications. Patients must be transferred if they develop any of these findings, recurrent angina, or evidence of acute MI. In essence, these units provide the availability of rapid treatment and resuscitation should a life-threatening arrhythmia develop, as well as the rapid institution of appropriate treatment for any evidence of unstable angina or acute MI.

In a number of studies, patients admitted to chest pain evaluation or observation units have rates of acute MI in the 1% to 3% range, with even lower rates of complications potentially requiring intensive care. By providing appropriate monitoring and nursing availability without the other aspects of intensive care, these units provide the same documented safety with costs that are about one-third those of a stepdown or intermediate unit. The advent of these units allows physicians to have a lower threshold for admitting more patients with complaints that are atypical of acute ischemic heart disease but that make the physician uncomfortable about discharge. The 6- to 12-hour length-of-stay and lower costs allow more patients to be admitted for observation than previously, while still reducing costs as well as the potential morbidity and mortality of inappropriate discharge.

The 6- to 12-hour length-of-stay in these units should be adequate for diagnostic purposes. In general, if a patient is initially admitted with a 5% or so probability of acute MI, this probability will be reduced to less than 1% by 6 to 12 hours of sequential ECGs and cardiac enzyme determinations. Newer enzyme assays including troponin T, troponin I, and creatine kinase (CK) MB isoforms appear to be more sensitive than traditional CK-MB isoenzymes for diagnosing acute MI, especially in the early hours after the onset of symptoms, while being equally or more specific in terms of identifying patients without acute MI.[13–16] Myoglobin is perhaps the most sensitive assay, but it achieves this sensitivity at the expense of a markedly diminished specificity. At the current time, these various enzyme assays all appear to be sufficiently insensitive to allow for a single determination to be used to exclude the possibility of acute MI. However, by about

6 hours after the beginning of observation, two negative values on any of these assays will make acute MI very unlikely in patients whose initial probabilities are in the 5% range. In patients with initially higher probabilities, more prolonged observation periods of 12 to 24 hours are generally indicated.

Recommended Triage Approach

By considering the ECG, a history of prior known coronary artery disease, and evidence of other complications, patients with known or suspected coronary disease as a cause of acute, new, often ongoing pain can be quickly recommended for one of three different in-hospital strategies: coronary intensive care, intermediate care/stepdown unit, or evaluation/observation unit (Table 7–5). These recommendations, which are based on both clinical and cost data, provide an efficient, high-quality strategy for this often-challenging group of patients.[17]

Approach to the Patient With Recurrent, Episodic Pain

Although the patient with recurrent, episodic pain may be having an acute MI superimposed on prior angina, recurrent pulmonary emboli, or even chronic aortic dissection, most patients with this syndrome have less acute conditions for which a complete history and physical examination will be necessary to make the diagnosis (Fig. 7–4). The physician should focus on the description of the pain, what precipitates and relieves it, its location and quality, the patient's age and gender, and other coronary risk factors.

In determining whether the pain is typical, atypical, or highly unlikely to represent coronary ischemia, precipitating factors such as rapid walking, exercise, or sexual activity suggest angina, as does pain that is relieved

Table 7–5	**Recommended Triage Strategies for Patients With Acute Chest Pain Who Do Not Otherwise Require Intensive Care Because of the Need to Treat Ongoing, Life-Threatening Conditions***

Intensive Care

1. Major ischemic electrocardiographic changes in two or more leads, not known to be old:
   a. ST elevation of 1 mm or more or Q-waves of 0.04 sec or more
   or
   b. ST depression of 1 mm or more or T-wave inversion consistent with ischemia
   or
2. Any two of the following, with or without major electrocardiographic changes:
   a. Unstable known coronary disease (in terms of frequency, duration, intensity, or failure to respond to usual measures)
   b. Systolic blood pressure below 110 mm Hg
   c. Major new arrhythmias (new-onset atrial fibrillation, atrial flutter, sustained supraventricular tachycardia, second-degree or complete heart block, or sustained or recurrent ventricular arrythmias)
   d. Rales above the bases

Intermediate Care/Stepdown Unit

Patients who do not meet criteria for intensive care but who either:
1. Have one unstable characteristic:
   a. Unstable known coronary disease
   b. Systolic blood pressure below 110 mm Hg
   c. Rales above the bases
   d. Major arrhythmias (new-onset atrial fibrillation, atrial flutter, sustained supraventricular tachycardia, second-degree or complete heart block, or sustained or recurrent ventricular arrhythmias)
2. A patient with new onset of very typical ischemic heart disease that meets the clinical criteria for unstable angina (see Chap. 20) and that is occurring now at rest or with minimal exertion

Evaluation/Observation unit

1. Other patients with new-onset symptoms that may be consistent with ischemic heart disease but that are not associated with electrocardiographic changes or a convincing diagnosis of unstable ischemic heart disease at rest or with minimal exertion
2. Some patients with known coronary disease whose presentation does not suggest a true worsening but for whom further observation is thought to be beneficial

Home With Office Follow-Up In 7–10 Days to Determine Whether Further Testing Is Needed

Other patients

---

*Except in patients in whom other serious noncoronary causes of chest pain are being considered, such as possible aortic dissection or pulmonary embolism, the triage will be dictated by the appropriate evaluation for these possible diagnoses.

within several minutes after rest or taking nitroglycerin. By comparison, pain that is precipitated by deep breathing or coughing suggests a pleural or pericardial cause, whereas pain exacerbated by other movements or by palpation is most typical for neuromuscular or skeletal causes.

Physical Examination

The physical examination should be comprehensive and not limited to the cardiopulmonary systems. For example, the skin examination should search for xanthelasma and cyanosis. Lymphadenopathy would raise the possibility of a malignancy. The chest wall must be inspected and palpated to search for neuromusculoskeletal causes of chest discomfort. A pulmonary examination should search for evidence of congestive heart failure, pleural rubs, or pneumonia. The cardiac examination should include a careful evaluation of possible third or fourth heart sounds, papillary muscle dysfunction, aortic valvular stenosis, or obstructive hypertrophic cardiomyopathy. A pericardial friction rub or increased pulmonic second sound would raise the possibilities of pericarditis and pulmonary embolism/pulmonary hypertension, respectively. The abdominal examination is critical for the diagnosis of cholecystitis or pancreatitis and may also be abnormal in peptic ulcer disease.

It is important to emphasize that the same clinical syndrome may have very different implications in individuals with different underlying risks of coronary artery disease based on age, gender, and pre-existing hypertension, hypercholesterolemia, smoking status, and other factors. Nevertheless, no single piece of evidence can either diagnose or exclude coronary artery disease, and the physician must be suspicious of a reasonably consistent history in an otherwise low-risk patient, just as an atypical presentation in a high-risk patient demands further evaluation.

Diagnostic Testing

Most patients with recurrent, episodic chest pain caused by myocardial ischemia will have normal ECGs in the intervals between painful episodes, although some may have resting abnormalities or evidence of prior MI. Based on the combination of data from the history, physical examination, and resting ECG, the physician should be able to categorize the pain as typical angina, atypical but possible angina, or very unlikely to represent angina. In general, these categories correspond to about an 80%, 40%, and 5% probability, respectively, for coronary artery disease if the patient undergoes diagnostic coronary arteriography.

For most patients with recurrent episodic pain, the evaluation can proceed on an ambulatory basis over a period of days or even weeks. However, if unstable angina is suspected, urgent evaluation, often with hospitalization as described for new, acute chest pain, is indicated. In patients with new-onset angina that is stable (see Chap. 18), an ambulatory evaluation is reasonable but should proceed expeditiously (see Chap. 19).

Myocardial ischemia may be detected by typical electrocardiographic changes, scintigraphic abnormalities, or wall motion abnormalities on echocardiography. Myocardial ischemia may be precipitated by exercise or by a pharmacologic stress (see Chap. 4). None of these tests is perfect, but they can be integrated with findings on the history and physical examination to evaluate patients with recurrent, episodic chest discomfort (see Figs. 2–5 through 2–7). Although negative test results cannot exclude the possibility of myocardial ischemia in patients with a typical history, a sequence of a negative exercise ECG and perfusion scintigram makes coronary disease very unlikely in a patient with atypical chest discomfort.

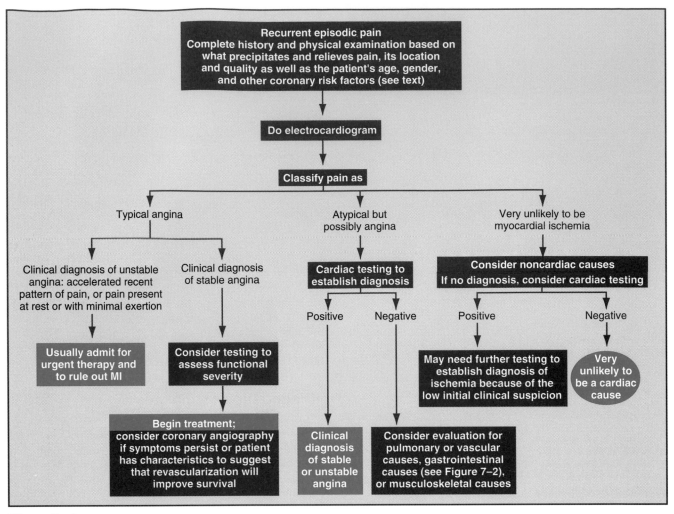

Figure 7–4

Diagnostic approach to the patient with recurrent, episodic chest pain. MI, myocardial infarction. (From Goldman, L.: Chest discomfort and palpitation. *In* Fauci, A.S., Braunwald, E., Isselbacher, K.I., et al. [eds.]: Harrison's Principles of Internal Medicine. 14th ed. New York, McGraw-Hill, 1998, p 62. Reproduced with permission of The McGraw-Hill Companies.)

These negative tests also generally imply a relatively favorable prognosis even if undiagnosed myocardial ischemia is present.

Evaluation of Patients with Persistent Pain

When pain persists for hours or even days, it is highly unlikely to be caused by myocardial ischemia in the absence of an acute MI. The clinician should suspect musculoskeletal abnormalities, gastrointestinal diseases, and less commonly, pulmonary disease or pericarditis. The history must be comprehensive, as emphasized under Approach to the Patient with Recurrent, Episodic Pain.

Physical Examination

A comprehensive physical examination is mandatory to assess possible musculoskeletal, gastrointestinal, and pulmonary abnormalities. Careful consideration should be given to any other focal or systemic diseases for which abnormalities in the neck, chest, or upper abdomen may coexist.

Diagnostic Testing

The diagnostic evaluation of persistent pain can be accomplished in the ambulatory setting and rarely requires hospitalization. As directed by the history and physical examination, further testing with a chest radiograph, upper gastrointestinal endoscopy, or abdominal ultrasonography should be considered. In some patients, further testing may be required to reassure the patient that coronary artery disease is not present even though the pain syndrome is highly atypical. In patients with a suggestive history, echocardiography may be useful to evaluate the possibility of pericarditis, although pericarditis and a pericardial friction rub may be present in the absence of increased pericardial fluid or other pericardial abnormalities detectable by echocardiography. Injection of a suspected musculoskeletal source of chest discomfort, such as costochondritis or bursitis, with local anesthetic may be critical to making the diagnosis.

Careful consideration should be given to the possibility that the patient with persistent pain is suffering from an emotional condition that has previously been undiagnosed or underappreciated. In such patients, this diagnosis of exclusion may require some degree of prior diagnostic testing to exclude other conditions of concern to the patient or physician.

References

1. Goldman, L.: Chest discomfort and palpitation. *In* Fauci, A.S., Braunwald, E., Isselbacher, K.J., et al. (eds.): Harrison's Principles of Internal Medicine. 14th ed. New York, McGraw-Hill, 1998, pp. 58–65.
2. Baxt, W.G., and Skora, J.: Prospective validation of artificial neural network trained to identify acute myocardial infarction. Lancet 347: 12–16, 1996.
3. Goldman, L., Cook, E.F., Brand, D.A., et al.: A computer protocol to predict myocardial infarction in emergency department patients with chest pain. N. Engl. J. Med. 318:797–803, 1988.
4. Singh, S., Richter, J.E., Hewson, E.G., et al.: The contribution of gastroesophageal reflux to chest pain in patients with coronary artery disease. Ann. Intern. Med. 117:824–830, 1992.
5. Chauhan, A., Mullins, P.A., Taylor, G., et al.: Cardioesophageal reflux: A mechanism for "linked angina" in patients with angiographically proven coronary artery disease. J. Am. Coll. Cardiol. 27:1621–1628, 1996.
6. Goldman, L., Cook, E.F., Johnson, P.A., et al.: Prediction of the need for intensive care in patients who come to emergency departments with chest pain. N. Engl. J. Med. 334:1498–1504, 1996.
7. Gomez, M.A., Anderson, L., Karagounis, L.A., et al.: An emergency department–based protocol for rapidly ruling out myocardial ischemia reduces hospital time and expense: Results of a randomized study (ROMIO). J. Am. Coll. Cardiol. 28:25–33, 1996.
8. Lee, T.H., Juarez, G., Cook, E.F., et al.: Ruling out acute myocardial infarction: A prospective multicenter validation of a 12-hour strategy for patients at low risk. N. Engl. J. Med. 324:1239–1246, 1991.
9. Pozen, M.W., D'Agostino, R.B., Selker, H.P., et al.: A predictive instrument to improve coronary-care-unit admission practices in acute ischemic heart disease: A prospective multicenter clinical trial. N. Engl. J. Med. 310:1273–1278, 1984.
10. Tosteson, A.N.A., Goldman, L., Udvarhelyi, S., and Lee, T.H.: Cost-effectiveness of a coronary care unit versus an intermediate care unit for emergency department patients with chest pain. Circulation 94:143–150, 1996.
11. Gaspoz, J., Lee, T.H., Weinstein, M.C., et al.: Cost-effectiveness of a new short-stay unit to "rule out" acute myocardial infarction in low-risk patients. J. Am. Coll. Cardiol. 24:1249–1259, 1994.
12. Roberts, R.R., Zalenski, R.J., Mensah, E.K., et al.: Costs of an emergency department–based accelerated diagnostic protocol vs. hospitalization in patients with chest pain: A randomized controlled trial. JAMA 278:1670–1676, 1997.
13. Gibler, W.B., Young, G.P., Hedges, J.R., et al.: Acute myocardial infarction in chest pain patients with nondiagnostic ECGs: Serial CK-MB sampling in the emergency department. The Emergency Medicine Cardiac Research Group. Ann. Emerg. Med. 331:504–512, 1992.
14. Newby, L.K., Califf, R.M., Guerci, A., et al.: Early discharge in the thrombolytic era: An analysis of criteria for uncomplicated infarction from the Global Utilization of Streptokinase and t-PA for Occluded Coronary Arteries (GUSTO) Trial. J. Am. Coll. Cardiol. 27:625–632, 1996.
15. Puleo, P.R., Meyer, D., Wathen, C., et al.: Use of a rapid assay of subforms of creatine kinase MB to diagnose or rule out acute myocardial infarction. N. Engl. J. Med. 331:561–566, 1994.
16. Hamm, C.W., Goldman, B.U., Heeschen, C., et al.: Emergency room triage of patients with acute chest pain by means of rapid testing for cardiac troponin T or troponin I. N. Engl. J. Med. 337: 1648–1653, 1997.
17. Roberts, R., and Kleinman, N.S.: Earlier diagnosis and treatment of acute myocardial infarction necessitates the need for a "new diagnostic mind-set." Circulation 89:872–881, 1994.

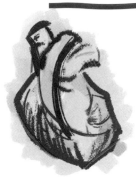

Chapter 8

Approach to the Patient with

Dyspnea

RICHARD M. SCHWARTZSTEIN AND
GEORGE E. THIBAULT

Shortness of breath or dyspnea afflicts patients both acutely and chronically; it is often associated with great discomfort, anxiety, and emotional distress; and it may be associated with serious disability. It may be a sign only of a sedentary lifestyle or of a potentially life-threatening illness. Everyone, if pushed to the limits of aerobic capacity, will experience shortness of breath. Two of the most central questions for the primary care physician faced with a patient with dyspnea are: Is it an indication of a pathologic finding or is it a manifestation of normal physiology? If the former, is it secondary to heart disease or lung disease?

There are no data on the prevalence of dyspnea in the general population, but certain epidemiologic facts suggest the problem is quite large. Coronary artery disease is the leading cause of mortality in the United States, and breathlessness may be a symptom of angina or myocardial infarction.[1] Congestive heart failure (CHF) is the most common reason for hospitalization among Medicare patients, and dyspnea is the most common symptom in patients with this condition. In addition, there are approximately 25 million people in the United States who suffer from asthma and chronic obstructive lung disease, resulting in 17 million physician office visits a year, usually for complaints of breathlessness, at a cost of over $10.4 billion.[2]

Given the magnitude of these clinical problems and the central role of dyspnea in the symptoms experienced by patients with heart and lung disease, it is imperative that the primary care physician have a solid understanding of the physiology and qualities of dyspnea and an organized and rational approach to the patient with this complaint.

PHYSIOLOGY OF DYSPNEA

Respiratory sensations that are commonly grouped under the term *dyspnea* appear to arise in one of several ways.[3] There are primary sensations associated with increased neural activity within the motor cortex as messages are sent to the ventilatory muscles, within the brain stem respiratory centers under conditions associated with increased "respiratory drive," and from stimulation of receptors in the lungs, chest wall, and upper airways (Fig. 8–1). In addition, the intensity of dyspnea appears to increase when there is a dissociation between the incoming information from peripheral receptors that tells the brain how much the lungs and chest moved and how much air flow was generated and the outgoing neural traffic from the brain.[4]

When there is a mechanical load on the respiratory system, for example, airways obstruction or restrictive lung disease, the motor cortex must increase the neural

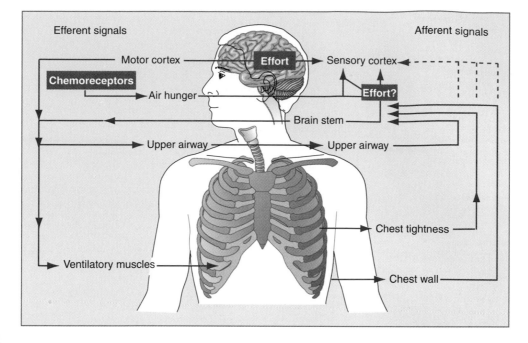

Figure 8–1
Afferent and efferent signals that contribute to dyspnea. The sensations that make up "dyspnea" arise from signals within the central nervous system, from chemoreceptors, and from receptors in the lungs, chest wall, and upper airway. Although afferent information from airway, lung, and chest wall receptors most likely passes through the brain stem before reaching the sensory cortex, the *dashed lines* indicate uncertainty about whether some afferents bypass the brain stem and project directly to the sensory cortex. (From Manning, H.L., and Schwartzstein, R.M.: Pathophysiology of dyspnea. N. Engl. J. Med. 333:1547–1553, 1995.)

discharge to the respiratory muscles to activate the muscles sufficiently to generate an appropriate ventilatory response. At the same time that these neural impulses are transmitted to the muscles, a corresponding impulse is transmitted to the sensory cortex. Thus, the individual is able to perceive the increased neural activity that is felt as an increased sense of "effort" or "work of breathing." This mechanism also appears to underlie the respiratory discomfort associated with neuromuscular weakness, for example, in association with myasthenia gravis.

Acute changes in blood gases, for example, acute hypoxia or hypercapnia, stimulate the respiratory centers in the brain stem and lead to an increase in ventilation. These conditions are also associated with respiratory distress, usually a sense of "air hunger" or an urge to breathe more. These sensations may arise directly from information emanating in the chemoreceptors or may be processed through the respiratory centers in the medulla. Stimulation of receptors in the lungs may also cause an increase in both ventilation and respiratory discomfort, for example, in patients with asthma or pulmonary embolism, although the exact neural pathways that account for these findings have not been fully elucidated.

Bronchoconstriction produces a sensation of chest tightness, even in patients with spinal cord injury who are deprived of sensory information from their chest wall. These findings suggest that the sensation arises from stimulation of mechanoreceptors in the lung. Inhaled lidocaine, which presumably blunts the activity of airway receptors, was shown in one study to reduce the intensity of dyspnea arising from bronchoconstriction.[5]

A mismatch between the efferent activity originating in the brain and the afferent information arising in the lungs, upper airways, ventilatory muscles, and chest wall appears to increase the intensity of dyspnea. This observation, which originally was thought to apply only to tension and corresponding length changes in respiratory muscles and was termed *length-tension inappropriateness*,[6] has been generalized to include information from the upper airways and lungs and is referred to as *efferent-reafferent dissociation*.[7] Several studies have demonstrated, for example, that the dyspnea associated with acute hypercapnia is better tolerated when subjects are able to breathe with larger tidal volumes[8] and that the application of mechanical vibrators to the chest wall may reduce the intensity of breathing discomfort associated with resistive loads.[9]

Clinical Pathophysiology

When confronted with a patient complaining of dyspnea, one can place the vast majority of individuals into one of two broad categories: cardiovascular dyspnea and respiratory dyspnea (Fig. 8–2).

Cardiovascular Dyspnea

Within the category of cardiovascular dyspnea, one should consider three subsets. Patients with *high cardiac outputs*—for example, secondary to anemia or shunts—frequently complain of dyspnea with exertion. The exact mechanism underlying this symptom has not been elucidated, but the symptom may reflect either reduced oxygen delivery to the tissues or increased pulmonary vascular pressures necessary to maintain the elevated cardiac out-

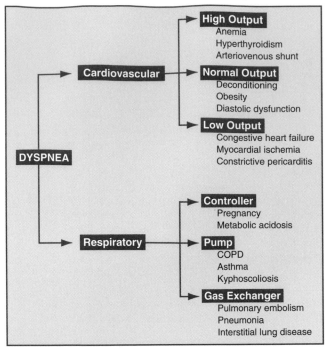

Figure 8–2

Clinical pathophysiology of dyspnea. When confronted with a patient with shortness of breath of unclear cause, it is useful to begin the analysis with a consideration of the broad pathophysiologic categories that explain the vast majority of cases. COPD, chronic obstructive pulmonary disease.

put. Individuals with *normal cardiac output,* particularly if they are obese or deconditioned, also develop breathlessness with exertion. Ultimately what separates the average person from the trained athlete is the level of cardiovascular fitness that is determined not only by the heart's ability to increase stroke volume and cardiac output during stress but also by the ability of the peripheral muscles to extract and utilize oxygen, thereby delaying the onset of anaerobic metabolism. An early shift from aerobic to anaerobic processes places added strain on the respiratory system to the extent that greater levels of ventilation are required to compensate for the evolving metabolic acidosis. In addition, the buildup of lactic acid in the muscles may also contribute to breathing discomfort.

Patients with obesity generally fall into this category unless their obesity is so great as to cause abnormalities in the pulmonary pump (see later). Individuals with no true physiologic cause for their breathing discomfort, for example, anxiety or psychogenic dyspnea, may be considered within the category of normal cardiac output.

A special group of patients with cardiovascular dyspnea and a normal cardiac output are those with diastolic dysfunction. These patients usually have a stiffened left ventricle and a normal cardiac output at rest. With exercise, the heart must increase its rate to a greater extent than stroke volume because of the inability of the left ventricle to dilate. Furthermore, to achieve the cardiac output needed to sustain the metabolic activity of exercise

in these patients, the left ventricular diastolic pressure must increase, leading to an elevation of the pulmonary capillary pressure and shortness of breath. A similar mechanism is probably responsible for ischemia-induced dyspnea in patients with normal left ventricular systolic function. It is important to note that some patients with myocardial ischemia will not experience chest pain and that dyspnea may be the only sign of acute coronary insufficiency. In these patients, shortness of breath is considered to be an "anginal equivalent."

The third subset of patients within the category of cardiovascular dyspnea includes those with a *low cardiac output.* Classically, these are the patients with compromised left ventricular systolic function or pericardial disease. Forward flow is reduced, and the system compensates by increasing the filling pressures within the chambers of the heart. As a result, there may be increased lung water as well as increased pressures within the pulmonary circulation, both of which may lead to dyspnea.

Respiratory Dyspnea

This category can also be divided into three subsets. Patients with disorders of the *respiratory controller,* that is, conditions that result in stimulation of the medullary center that determines the rate and depth of breathing, have a greater neural drive to breathe than would be expected on the basis of the metabolic needs for oxygen uptake or carbon dioxide elimination. Common examples of this type of derangement include the dyspnea associated with early pregnancy or with aspirin overdoses. In the former, the elevated levels of progesterone induce hyperventilation and dyspnea well before the uterus enlarges sufficiently to compromise motion of the diaphragm. In the latter, the direct effect of aspirin on the respiratory centers in the brain stem leads to hyperventilation and, in some cases, respiratory distress. Conditions in which the controller is stimulated are often associated with a sensation of "air hunger" or an "urge or need to breathe."

The second subset of patients with respiratory dyspnea has abnormalities of the *ventilatory pump.* Once the respiratory controller has determined how rapidly and deeply the individual must breathe, neural impulses from the brain must be translated into movement of air into and out of the alveoli. To accomplish this task, one must have a functioning ventilatory pump, which consists of the peripheral nerves connecting the controller to the ventilatory muscles, the muscles of ventilation, the supporting skeleton for these muscles, the pleura that transmits pressure changes generated by the muscles to the lungs, and the airways that serve as a conduit for airflow. Dysfunction of any of these components of the ventilatory pump—for example, spinal cord injury, myopathies, kyphoscoliosis, pleural fibrosis, and airways obstruction—may lead to breathing discomfort, most often associated with an increased sense of effort or work of breathing.

The third, and probably most common, subset of patients with respiratory dyspnea presenting to primary care physicians comprises those patients with abnormalities in the *gas exchanger,* that is, alveoli and pulmonary capillaries. Ultimately the goal of the respiratory system is to provide oxygen to the blood and to carry away carbon dioxide. To achieve this goal, one must have a functioning gas exchanger. Derangements of the gas exchanger generally result in hypoxia or hypercapnia or in an increased ventilation to compensate for the ventilation/perfusion abnormalities. A gas exchange problem exists in conditions such as pneumonia, pulmonary edema, pulmonary embolism, asthma, and chronic obstructive pulmonary disease (COPD).

Patients presenting with dyspnea can usually be characterized by placement within one or more of these subsets. It is helpful if one can determine that the problem is primarily cardiovascular versus respiratory, although the reality is that many individuals may manifest a mixed picture. Nevertheless, the practical approach to the patient with breathing discomfort ultimately makes better sense if the pathophysiology has been clarified.

WORKUP OF THE PATIENT WITH DYSPNEA

The History

Definitions of *dyspnea* have included "difficult, labored, uncomfortable breathing," "an awareness of respiratory distress," "the feeling of air hunger," and "an uncomfortable sensation of breathing."[10] It is important when considering dyspnea to avoid confusing the symptom, that is, what a patient describes about sensations he or she is experiencing, with a physical sign, that is, something the physician observes, such as a rapid respiratory rate or the use of accessory muscles of ventilation. Common to these definitions is the concept of "discomfort" in the act of breathing. In addition, it is apparent that there may be more than one sensation lumped together under the heading of dyspnea.

Physicians readily conceive of different qualities of pain and use the information about these qualities to aid them in the differential diagnosis. For example, a "burning" chest discomfort suggests a gastrointestinal cause, whereas a "pressure-like" discomfort raises the specter of myocardial ischemia (see Chap. 7). Formal studies of pain established that different pain syndromes are characterized by unique sets of phrases[11-13] and that these phrases can be utilized to distinguish various types of headache and facial pain.

Although physicians, even those in general good health, commonly experience a variety of pains during their lives—for example, headaches, stomach upset, bruises, and fractures—and thereby develop a vocabulary with which to communicate with their patients, they tend to have limited experience with dyspnea. In the absence of cardiopulmonary pathology, the only breathing discomfort a physician may experience is likely to be associated with exercise. Is that sensation the same as that experienced by the patient with asthma, COPD, pulmonary embolism, CHF, or angina? What information can the physi-

cian draw on to construct questions for her or his patient to elicit the qualities of dyspnea?

Descriptions of Dyspnea

It has now been shown that dyspnea, like pain, comprises multiple, qualitatively distinct sensations.[14-17] Normal subjects made breathless with a series of respiratory tasks easily distinguished the sensations associated with these experiences. Clusters of phrases emerged to characterize the various types of induced dyspnea.[14] Similarly, when presented with a list of phrases used by patients and subjects to describe breathing discomfort, patients with different cardiopulmonary diseases selected unique clusters of verbal descriptors as representative of their dyspnea. Each condition tends to be associated with more than one phrase; some phrases or expressions are used to characterize more than one condition; and each condition is associated with a unique set of phrases.[15-17] These features of the vocabulary chosen by patients suggest that more than one mechanism is probably responsible for dyspnea in a given pathologic state, that different disease states may share common mechanisms for producing respiratory discomfort, and that each condition has a unique set of physiologic factors that produces its particular discomfort.

Studies of the *language of dyspnea* have provided insight into the physiology of respiratory distress for categories of disease and into the specific pathologic conditions causing symptoms in individual patients. The sensitivity and specificity of these tools, however, remain to be determined. Nevertheless, although more work needs to be done in this area, there appear to be at least four sensations that can give the physician clues to the underlying diagnosis.

The sensation of "chest tightness or constriction" is commonly associated with bronchoconstriction, even when measurements of lung function fall within the normal range. Although these studies have focused on the bronchoconstriction of reactive airways disease, that is, classic asthma, it is possible that patients with cardiac asthma, for example, bronchial narrowing from acute changes in pulmonary capillary wedge pressure, may experience similar sensations.

Patients with severe degrees of airway obstruction describe a sense of increased "work or effort of breathing." This sensation also appears to be present in patients with interstitial lung disease and in most clinical situations in which there is a mechanical load on the respiratory system or the breathing muscles are weakened, that is, an abnormality of the ventilatory pump.

The sensation of "air hunger, urge to breathe, or need to breathe" characterizes conditions associated with an increased respiratory drive, for example, acute hypercapnia, early pregnancy, pulmonary vascular disease, and pulmonary edema.[10] These conditions are linked by the common pathophysiology of stimulation of the respiratory controller.

Finally, the sensation of "heavy breathing" or "rapid breathing" without an accompanying sense of difficulty moving air in and out of the lungs appears to characterize the dyspnea associated with deconditioning. This sensation may be present in otherwise healthy individuals as well as in patients who have gradually reduced their activity level owing to a cardiopulmonary disorder and now are limited primarily by their low level of fitness.[18, 19] The association between various qualitative descriptors of dyspnea and pathophysiologic mechanisms of shortness of breath is summarized in Table 8–1.

Questioning the Patient

When obtaining a history of dyspnea, it is important to question the patient about the quality of the breathing discomfort.[20, 21] One should start with an open-ended question designed to elicit the patient's spontaneous response. However, it is not uncommon for the patient to answer with a quizzical expression, since this may be the first time anyone has posed this particular question. Under these circumstances, the next step is to provide the patient with some alternative phrases (Table 8–2) and to ask whether one or more phrases describe the sensation he or she is experiencing. It is also important to ask the patient if he or she experiences different kinds of respiratory discomfort at different times or under different circumstances, since this may signify the coexistence of two conditions, with each more prominent at different times—for example, COPD and increased airways reactivity, COPD and CHF, or asthma and deconditioning. Although patients may at first have difficulty describing their sensations, they often are quite adamant that the dyspnea associated with a respiratory infection is different from that associated with walking up the stairs. As noted previously, deconditioning may be the factor that ultimately limits activity in patients with many forms of cardiopulmonary disease. An awareness of this fact is critical, since the level of deconditioning may be improved with an exercise program independently of the responsiveness of the patient's underlying cardiopulmonary disorder to specific therapy.

In addition to the quality of the dyspnea, the timing of

Table 8–1	The Language of Dyspnea — Association of Qualitative Descriptors and Pathophysiologic Mechanisms of Shortness of Breath
Descriptor	**Pathophysiologic Mechanism**
Chest tightness or constriction	Bronchoconstriction, interstitial edema (asthma, myocardial ischemia)
Increased work or effort of breathing	Airways obstruction, neuromuscular disease, chest wall disease (chronic obstructive pulmonary disease, moderate to severe asthma, myopathy, kyphoscoliosis)
Air hunger, need to breathe, urge to breathe	Increased drive to breathe (congestive heart failure, pulmonary embolism, moderate to severe airways obstruction)
Heavy breathing, rapid breathing, breathing more	Deconditioning

Table 8–2	Qualitative Descriptors of Dyspnea That May Be Incorporated into a Patient Interview When Eliciting a History of Shortness of Breath*

My chest feels tight.
My chest is constricted.

My breathing is heavy.
I am panting.
I feel that I am breathing more.

My breathing requires effort.
My breathing requires more work.

I feel that I am suffocating.
I feel that I am smothering.

I feel a hunger for more air.
I cannot get enough air.

My breathing is shallow.
I cannot take a deep breath.

Note: Phrases are grouped into clusters based on the studies of the language of dyspnea in normal subjects and patients.[9, 13]

dyspnea and the factors that precipitate episodes of respiratory discomfort are also important to identify. Does the discomfort occur at rest or only with exertion? Is it episodic or continuous? Dyspnea that occurs with exertion may be a manifestation of a variety of disease states that become evident because of the increased metabolic demands of the activity. For example, COPD or interstitial lung disease may indicate the development of an acute physiologic change, such as bronchospasm or myocardial ischemia, or may merely reflect the relative cardiovascular conditioning of the individual. Whereas chronic dyspnea at rest usually indicates severe structural lung or heart disease, episodic breathing discomfort at rest invariably indicates an acute derangement that is reversible. Asthma and myocardial ischemia are examples of the latter.

Identification of factors that precipitate the dyspnea and symptoms associated with the respiratory discomfort are also important clues to the cause of the patient's problem. Dyspnea resulting from exposure to fumes, scents, or cigarette smoke is usually the result of constriction of reactive airways in asthma and COPD. Inhalation of cold air may be a trigger for asthma. Hot, humid days with high levels of air pollution typically provoke dyspnea in patients with COPD. Associated symptoms such as pleuritic chest pain and fever may indicate the presence of a respiratory infection or pulmonary embolism, whereas chest pressure, diaphoresis, and nausea along with dyspnea are clues that the patient is suffering from myocardial ischemia.

Special Forms of Dyspnea

Orthopnea, the presence of dyspnea when lying flat, is most commonly a sign of CHF. The redistribution of blood volume from dependent portions of the body to the central circulation with an attendant increase in pulmonary capillary wedge pressure leads to interstitial edema and dyspnea. However, other conditions may also present in this fashion. For example, patients with a paralyzed diaphragm experience breathing discomfort in the supine position because of the cephalad displacement of the diaphragm secondary to the forces exerted by the abdominal contents. This places a greater burden on the remaining accessory muscles of ventilation, which are responsible for generating a negative intrapleural pressure.

Nocturnal dyspnea typically is a manifestation of CHF. Paroxysmal nocturnal dyspnea usually occurs in patients with peripheral edema whose interstitial fluid is reabsorbed into the circulation during the night, leading to increased intracardiac pressures. It is less well known that bronchial asthma may also present as nocturnal dyspnea. One cause of nocturnal asthma is thought to be the reflux of acid from the stomach into the esophagus, which triggers a reflex, mediated by the vagus nerve, and leads to bronchospasm. Intermittent aspiration of gastric contents, a lower level of endogenous steroid, or a trough in the serum level of medications may also play a role in triggering nocturnal asthma in some patients.

Physical Examination

The first part of any physical examination should be a general assessment of the patient's condition from a distance, what we call the "view from the door." Is the patient comfortable or does she or he appear to be in distress? What is the patient's color? Is he or she cyanotic? What position does the patient assume? Is she or he sitting back easily in the chair or is she or he leaning forward with hands braced on the knees or on a table, that is, the tripod position? The latter permits the patient to recruit additional chest wall muscles to aid in respiration and, along with large swings in pleural pressure, evidenced by intercostal or supraclavicular retractions, is a good indicator of moderate to severe obstructive lung disease. The use of breathing with pursed lips is also a fairly typical finding in patients with emphysema in whom it may decrease breathing discomfort by slowing the respiratory rate and reducing hyperinflation, by improving oxygenation, and by changing transmural pressures across the walls of the airways.

The patient's vital signs offer additional diagnostic clues. Acute dyspnea in association with an increase in the pulse–systolic pressure product, that is, an elevated heart rate and blood pressure, should always raise the possibility of acute myocardial ischemia. A very rapid respiratory rate, usually with a shallow breathing pattern, is most typical of patients with low pulmonary compliance or "stiff lungs," for example, CHF or interstitial fibrosis. *Pulsus paradoxus* refers to the normal fall in systolic pressure during inspiration. When this is exaggerated, that is, greater than 10 mm Hg, it is a clue either to very large negative intrathoracic pressures, as seen in patients with severe airways obstruction, or to cardiac tamponade.

The Chest

The examination of the chest provides additional helpful diagnostic clues. Careful *inspection of the chest* should precede auscultation. Intercostal retractions due to intrapleural pressure swings are associated with airways obstruction. The patient's chest wall should be evaluated for symmetry of movement, and this is best done by observing the patient from behind. Deformities of the chest wall, such as kyphoscoliosis, impose a mechanical load on the ventilatory pump. The movement of the lateral rib cage during inspiration should be noted. Under normal circumstances, the lateral chest wall moves outward as the diaphragm descends. However, in patients with COPD and marked hyperinflation, the diaphragm is in a flattened position and contraction of the muscle results in the inward motion of the lateral chest wall.

Auscultation of the chest may reveal focal findings suggestive of pneumonia or diffuse findings compatible with asthma, COPD, interstitial lung disease, or CHF. *Rales* are short, high-pitched inspiratory sounds produced by the sudden equalization of pressure in terminal bronchioles as collapsed alveoli pop open. When lungs are "stiff," that is, have a reduced compliance because of interstitial inflammation or edema, there is a tendency for alveoli to collapse at low lung volumes at the end of exhalation. With the next inspiration, alveoli are reopened and rales are heard. The rales associated with interstitial inflammation and fibrosis are very short, distinct sounds and are often described as "dry rales." In contrast, the rales heard in patients with CHF may have a thicker, slightly gurgling sound and are termed "wet rales." *Rhonchi,* coarse large airway sounds, are found in patients with increased mucus production. Wheezes, the product of turbulent flow through narrow airways, may be heard in asthma, COPD, and CHF, that is, "cardiac asthma."

Extremities

Finally, the examination of the patient with dyspnea should include careful inspection of the extremities. Cyanosis is found in patients with at least 5 gm/100 ml of desaturated hemoglobin (individuals with severe anemia will not appear cyanotic even with very marked degrees of hypoxia). The presence of peripheral edema may indicate right ventricular dysfunction or local venous insufficiency. If the edema is due to increased pressures in the right heart, one should also see elevation of the jugular venous pulse and, in some cases, an enlarged, congested liver. Peripheral edema secondary to local factors in the legs may be associated with deep venous thrombosis and pulmonary emboli. Calf pain with dorsiflexion of the foot is suggestive of deep venous thrombosis, as is a palpable cord. However, one must remember that 50% of patients with deep venous thrombosis have a normal physical examination. Finally, although clubbing of the digits is found in patients with congenital heart disease and right-to-left shunts, pulmonary arteriovenous fistula, lung cancer, interstitial fibrosis, and chronic inflammatory conditions of the lung, it is *not* associated with COPD alone.

Laboratory Evaluation

Patients being evaluated for dyspnea of unknown cause should have a *chest radiograph.* An enlarged heart and redistribution of blood flow to the apices of the lung may indicate mild CHF, and the shape of the cardiac silhouette will provide important clues regarding the cause of the heart failure. Patients with COPD may have large lung volumes secondary to gas trapping from early collapse of airways. Approximately 90% of patients with interstitial lung disease will have abnormal findings on chest radiograph at the time of clinical presentation. Radiographic findings of pneumonia, a common cause of dyspnea, may precede abnormal physical findings on examination. Pulmonary embolism may be suggested by the presence of atelectasis or a small pleural effusion, although most patients with pulmonary embolism will have a normal chest film. In patients with subacute or chronic dyspnea in whom there is a question about possible cardiac dysfunction, an *echocardiogram* can provide much useful information. The contractile status of the ventricles is easily determined, as is the competency of the cardiac valves. In addition, an estimate can be made of the pulmonary artery pressures that, if elevated, may be an indication of left ventricular failure, severe parenchymal lung disease, or occult pulmonary vascular disease. Finally, the pericardium can be viewed to evaluate the patient for pericardial effusion or infiltrative process.

The assessment of cardiovascular dyspnea should always include a *hematocrit* to eliminate anemia as the explanation for exertional shortness of breath. In general, a hematocrit above 30 is unlikely to explain moderate to severe dyspnea.

The *oxygen saturation,* that is, the measurement of the percentage of hemoglobin saturated with oxygen, has virtually become the "fifth vital sign." The ready availability of pulse oximeters and their ease of use have made them a mainstay of emergency departments and inpatient units, and they are now beginning to appear in the office setting as well. A low oxygen saturation, that is, below 90%, may immediately suggest to the primary care physician that the patient likely has a major problem with gas exchange. One must be cautious, however, in the setting of a relatively normal oxygen saturation, that one does not dismiss the patient's shortness of breath as an insignificant issue.

Because of the sigmoid shape of the hemoglobin-oxygen association/dissociation curve, the oxygen saturation is relatively insensitive to changes in the arterial partial pressure of oxygen (Pa_{O_2}) above 60 to 65 mm Hg. Consequently, a patient's Pa_{O_2} may drop by 10 to 15 mm Hg with relatively little change in the oxygen saturation. This problem is further complicated by the presence of hyperventilation. When a patient hyperventilates, as often occurs during an acute asthma attack or pulmonary embolism, the Pa_{CO_2} drops and the Pa_{O_2} rises. The gas exchange abnormality—reflected by the alveolar-arterial oxygen pressure difference ($P(A - a)O_2$), which is calculated with values for Pa_{O_2} and Pa_{CO_2} obtained from an arterial blood gas (Fig. 8 3)—remains abnormal while the oxygen saturation may be completely normal. Thus, one may be fooled by a patient who has a normal oxygen saturation yet a very abnormal $P(A - a)O_2$ and a very deranged gas exchanger. The $P(A - a)O_2$ should be calculated whenever underlying pulmonary disease or pulmonary vascular disease is suspected.

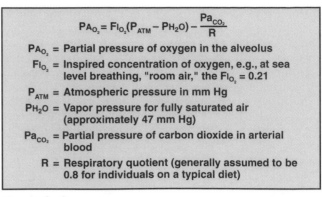

$$PA_{O_2} = FI_{O_2}(P_{ATM} - PH_2O) - \frac{Pa_{CO_2}}{R}$$

PA_{O_2} = Partial pressure of oxygen in the alveolus

FI_{O_2} = Inspired concentration of oxygen, e.g., at sea level breathing, "room air," the FI_{O_2} = 0.21

P_{ATM} = Atmospheric pressure in mm Hg

PH_2O = Vapor pressure for fully saturated air (approximately 47 mm Hg)

Pa_{CO_2} = Partial pressure of carbon dioxide in arterial blood

R = Respiratory quotient (generally assumed to be 0.8 for individuals on a typical diet)

Figure 8–3

Alveolar gas equation. Using the alveolar gas equation, one can calculate the partial pressure of oxygen in the alveolus. Then, knowing the arterial PO_2 obtained from a blood gas, the alveolar-arterial oxygen gradient ($P(A - a)O_2$) can be determined. An abnormal gradient indicates a problem with the gas exchanger, specifically, any cardiopulmonary process that worsens ventilation-perfusion inequalities or impairs diffusion of oxygen into the pulmonary capillary will result in an increase in the $P(A - a)O_2$.

Pulmonary Function Testing

Assessment of the ventilatory pump and gas exchanger is further enhanced by the information provided by pulmonary function testing. Spirometric testing provides data on airways obstruction. Simple spirometers are now available for use by primary care physicians in their offices, and these devices can be helpful in detecting mild bronchospasm or airways obstruction. The measurement of lung volumes must be performed in a formal pulmonary function laboratory, and is important in assessing the full extent of COPD or to determine whether restrictive lung disease is present, that is, to detect reductions in total lung capacity. Respiratory muscle strength is assessed with measurement of the maximal inspiratory and expiratory pressures and should be determined if there is a suspicion of neuromuscular disease.

The lungs' *diffusing capacity* measured with carbon monoxide (DL_{CO}) provides insight into the status of the membrane between the pulmonary capillaries and the alveoli. In diseases that result in destruction of lung tissue (e.g., emphysema or pulmonary fibrosis) or inflammation of the pulmonary interstitium, the DL_{CO} is reduced. In contrast, patients with mild CHF will have an increase in pulmonary vascular blood volume and a mild increase in the DL_{CO}. In general, patients who demonstrate a drop in oxygen saturation with exercise also have a reduced DL_{CO}.

In the vast majority of cases, the history, physical examination, and elements of the laboratory evaluation outlined previously will provide the answer to the question, "What is the cause of this patient's respiratory discomfort?" In some circumstances, a presumptive diagnosis can be made that leads to a therapeutic trial, for example, a diuretic for subtle volume overload or a bronchodilator for probable intermittent bronchoconstriction. In a small number of cases, however, the answer is still unclear. At this point, a cardiopulmonary exercise test can be extremely helpful.

Cardiopulmonary Exercise Testing

Cardiopulmonary exercise testing incorporates measurements of respiratory and cardiovascular system function under conditions of dynamic large muscle group activity. Utilizing either treadmill or bicycle exercise, the physician assesses a patient's functional capacity and aerobic performance and looks for patterns of physiologic abnormality at the point that the patient indicates she or he cannot continue to exercise (Table 8–3). The test is particularly useful for patients in whom it is uncertain after preliminary evaluation whether derangements in the cardiovascular system or in the respiratory system are the explanation for the dyspnea.[22, 23]

The major indications for cardiopulmonary exercise testing in patients with dyspnea include (1) to search for an explanation for symptoms the cause of which remain obscure after completing the evaluation outlined previously; (2) to determine the relative contributions of cardiac and pulmonary processes to a patient's functional limitation when multiple causes may be present; and (3) to determine a patient's functional capacity when there appears to be a discrepancy between the physiologic data and a patient's reported exercise tolerance, that is, when one suspects that the individual should be able to do more than he or she states.

Exercise testing is particularly helpful in ascertaining whether cardiovascular deconditioning is the major source of a patient's functional limitation and in assessing whether occult myocardial ischemia is the explanation for respiratory distress when the preliminary evaluation is unrevealing. It is not uncommon for an individual who begins to experience respiratory discomfort with activities to alter her or his lifestyle in ways that reduce the chance that she or he will become short of breath. Over time, the individual becomes deconditioned and the heart is not able to generate as high a cardiac output nor are the

skeletal muscles of the limbs able to extract and utilize oxygen as efficiently. Subsequently, the patient experiences dyspnea performing activities that had been easily accomplished in the past. The response may be to curtail lifestyle even further. A vicious circle is established with diminishing exercise capacity and increasing symptoms.

Not uncommonly, the patient attributes this decline in functional status to worsening of her or his underlying lung or heart disease. Patients with asthma, for example, who report that they are limited by their lung disease, have been found in many cases to be deconditioned rather than restricted by fixed airways obstruction or exercise-induced bronchoconstriction.[18] Exercise capacity correlates better with their general level of physical activity than the severity of their asthma. Patients with severe COPD have also been shown to develop lactic acidosis with minimal activity and to improve their aerobic capacity with an exercise program, that is, their level of conditioning was a major element in their functional limitation.[24] Physicians must be cautious in assuming that all of a patient's dyspnea is due to the underlying pulmonary process.

Most exercise testing for patients with a complaint of dyspnea is performed utilizing a treadmill or bicycle ergometer. Treadmill testing, to the extent that it more closely reproduces the predominant activity of the individual, that is, walking, is usually preferable. However, some patients, particularly the elderly, have difficulty coordinating their pace with the machine or have so much anxiety about "falling off" that reliable measurements cannot be made. In these circumstances, an exercise bicycle is used.

ENDPOINTS. The primary endpoints of the test are symptoms, cardiovascular changes, and gas exchange abnormalities. If the patient terminates the test because he or she is too uncomfortable, one must ask the patient what actually caused him or her to stop. Observation of the patient during the exercise often provides useful information as one assesses the patient's response. For example, the patient, while complaining of significant distress, may appear quite comfortable with little increase in ventilation or alteration in vital signs, suggesting the individual may be malingering or may have a very low threshold for discomfort after months or years of doing little activity. If the patient states that he or she stopped exercising because of "shortness of breath," one should pursue the question further by inquiring about the explicit sensations. As described previously in the discussion of the language of dyspnea, there are many sensations subsumed by the generally used term *shortness of breath,* and these descriptors can give one useful information about the cause of the symptom. It is useful to ascertain whether the sensation that caused the patient to stop exercising during the test was the same as that he or she feels at home under similar or different conditions. One should also be sure that the patient has stopped because of breathing discomfort rather than leg pain or general fatigue. The latter two symptoms commonly accompany peripheral vascular disease or the deconditioned state.[19]

If the patient does not complain of symptoms, the exercise test will be stopped if there is evidence that the

---

Table 8–3	**Cardiopulmonary Exercise Testing**

Indications

Evaluate a patient with dyspnea of unclear cause after history, physical examination, and standard laboratory evaluations fail to yield a diagnosis

Assess relative contributions of cardiovascular and respiratory system to a patient's functional limitation

Determine patient's functional capacity

Measurements

Electrocardiogram
Heart rate
Blood pressure
Oxygen consumption
Carbon dioxide production
Anaerobic threshold
Oxygen saturation
Forced vital capacity and forced expiratory volume in 1 sec before and after exercise

patient has reached the limits of cardiovascular performance or if there is evidence of myocardial ischemia (see Chap. 4) or significant hypoxemia. Cardiac output rises by increasing either stroke volume or heart rate. Achievement of greater than 85% of the predicted heart rate indicates one is nearing maximal cardiac output. A significant rise or fall in systemic blood pressure, usually with typical electrocardiogram (ECG) changes, is suggestive of myocardial ischemia and indicates that the test should be terminated. At a minimum, an oxygen saturation is monitored with a pulse oximeter to screen for hypoxemia.

During the test, multiple *physiologic measurements* are made. As noted previously, respiratory function is monitored with a pulse oximeter and, in many cases, with serial arterial blood gases and minute ventilation.

If the heart rate reaches greater than 85% of predicted at a low workload, one has evidence that cardiovascular function is contributing to the patient's exercise limitation. As discussed previously (under Clinical Pathophysiology), cardiovascular limitations may occur in the setting of both "normal" myocardial function (e.g., deconditioning) and abnormal function (e.g., heart failure). In a patient with a well-functioning myocardium, cardiac output is increased by a combination of stroke volume and heart rate, with a preference toward stroke volume. As the limits of stroke volume are reached, further increases in cardiac output require a rising heart rate. Thus, as the heart rate approaches the patient's predicted maximum, one has an indication that the maximal cardiac output is being reached. However, patients who develop acute myocardial ischemia may develop shortness of breath because of associated elevations in pulmonary capillary pressures before achieving this high a heart rate. Decreases in blood pressure, which may result from failure of the cardiac output to rise in the presence of exercise-induced peripheral vasodilatation, may be caused by myocardial ischemia and accompanied by typical ECG changes.

The *anaerobic threshold*, that is, the level of oxygen consumption above which the body begins to employ anaerobic metabolism to support its energy needs during exercise, can also be measured during the exercise test. The total body oxygen consumption is determined by the quantity of oxygen delivered to the tissues and the fraction of that oxygen that can be extracted by the tissues. Oxygen delivery is primarily dependent on the patient's hemoglobin, the percentage of hemoglobin saturated with oxygen, and the cardiac output. The ability to extract oxygen from the tissues is related to the density of capillaries in the tissue and the biochemical status of the cell, that is, whether the mitochondria and enzymes are primed to utilize oxygen. In a deconditioned person, the heart has a reduced ability to increase cardiac output, which limits oxygen delivery, and the muscles are not in an optimal biochemical state to extract and utilize oxygen. Consequently, the anaerobic threshold is reached at lower workloads than those in the well-conditioned athlete. If the anaerobic threshold is low, a metabolic acidosis develops as the body produces lactic acid, a byproduct of anaerobic metabolism. This acid load poses an additional stress to the respiratory system, since the anaerobic metabolism

Table 8–4	Patterns of Abnormality in Cardiopulmonary Exercise Testing*

Cardiovascular Limitation

Heart rate ≥85% of predicted maximum
Low anaerobic threshold
Reduced maximal oxygen consumption
Drop in blood pressure with exercise
Arrhythmias or ischemic changes on ECG
Does not achieve maximal predicted ventilation
Does not have significant desaturation

Respiratory Limitation

Achieves or exceeds maximal predicted ventilation
Significant desaturation (<90%)
Stable or increase dead space–to–tidal volume ratio
Development of bronchospasm with falling FEV_1
Does not achieve 85% of predicted maximal heart rate
No ischemic ECG changes

Abbreviations: ECG, electrocardiogram; FEV_1, forced expiratory volume in 1 sec.

* Note: All features will not be present in a particular case and there may be elements of both cardiovascular and respiratory causes of shortness of breath. One looks for the predominant pattern in assessing the etiology of the patient's exercise limitation.

must be compensated for by increasing ventilation. This may drive the patient to an early ventilatory limit.

PATTERNS OF ABNORMALITY. In assessing the patient's response to the exercise test, one looks for patterns of abnormality (Table 8–4). Patients with impaired cardiovascular function (other than acute ischemia) as the primary explanation for the exercise limitation demonstrate high heart rates at low workloads. Metabolic acidosis will occur early during exercise; that is, there is a low anaerobic threshold. In addition, they will have a maximal oxygen consumption well below what is predicted for their age and size. The ventilation achieved during exercise, on the other hand, does not reach the maximal level achievable by the respiratory system. As noted previously, patients with myocardial ischemia will demonstrate changes in the ECG, abnormal hemodynamic responses, or new rales on examination during exercise.

Patients with a respiratory cause of their exercise limitation will have a maximal ventilation that reaches or exceeds the predicted value, a significant decline in oxygen saturation (<90%), or a rise in the dead space–to–tidal volume ratio. The heart rate does not reach 85% of the predicted maximum, the anaerobic threshold is in the normal range, and the ECG does not show ischemic changes.

The interpretation of exercise tests must consider the patient's motivation to perform the test and her or his ability to tolerate uncomfortable sensations. The staff supervising the test should encourage the patient to provide a maximal effort and should note whether this is achieved.

DISTINGUISHING CARDIAC FROM PULMONARY DYSPNEA

Faced with a patient with subacute or chronic dyspnea, the primary care physician should first try to identify the broad pathophysiologic cause. Key elements in the history include the quality of the sensation and the timing and precipitating factors for the symptom. Patients with CHF will generally report a sense of air hunger, of not being able to get enough air, or having an increased urge to breathe. Patients with COPD and interstitial lung disease will complain primarily of increased work or effort of breathing, whereas patients with asthma will relate a sense of chest tightness and constriction or a sense of not being able to get a deep breath. Although patients with intermittent myocardial ischemia also may experience chest tightness or heaviness, there is more of a "painful" aspect to the chest discomfort.

Both cardiac and pulmonary causes of dyspnea are precipitated by exertion. However, the onset of dyspnea in association with cold air, inhalation of fumes, or respiratory infections generally points toward a pulmonary origin. Nocturnal dyspnea is a strong clue to the presence of CHF, especially if peripheral edema is present. Such patients usually achieve relief within several minutes with assumption of the upright position, redistribution of intravascular fluid, and a decrease in pulmonary capillary wedge pressure. However, nocturnal breathlessness may also be a manifestation of asthma, usually as a result of gastroesophageal reflux or a trough in levels of medications. Cough is often present with asthma, and the symptoms are not as quickly relieved in the upright posture.

After a comprehensive history and physical examination, an empirical trial of therapy is often an appropriate way to try to establish the diagnosis. For example, if dyspnea is relieved by diuretic therapy that induces a weight loss of 2 kg or more, the diagnosis of heart failure is supported. Alternatively, improvement in or elimination of respiratory distress after the institution of a beta-agonist inhaler is strong evidence for the presence of airways reactivity in asthma or COPD.

When additional testing is required, the chest radiograph, two-dimensional echocardiogram with Doppler imaging, and pulmonary function tests provide important data. The classic findings of a large heart (see Chap. 14), upper-zone vascular redistribution, increased vascular markings, and pleural effusions all point toward the diagnosis of CHF. A completely normal chest radiograph in a patient with intermittent dyspnea suggests the possibility of myocardial ischemia. Patients with COPD typically have evidence of hyperinflation and loss of normal pulmonary vascular markings, whereas those with interstitial lung disease have reduced lung volumes and increased interstitial lines. This last group can often be distinguished from those with CHF by the presence of a normal-sized heart and the absence of pleural effusions.

Pulmonary function tests in patients with CHF typically show low-normal or mildly reduced lung volumes (total lung capacity, functional residual capacity, and vital capacity) and may have concomitant mild airways obstruction (reduced forced expiratory volume in 1 sec [FEV_1] and maximal mid flows). The diffusing capacity in mild CHF is normal or slightly increased, reflecting the increased pulmonary vascular volume associated with elevated pulmonary capillary wedge pressure. In the presence of pulmonary edema, the diffusing capacity is reduced. This finding of a normal to elevated diffusing capacity in mild CHF may be helpful in distinguishing patients with this condition from those with interstitial fibrosis who also demonstrate low lung volumes and increased interstitial markings on chest radiograph but have a reduced pulmonary diffusing capacity. Patients with COPD and asthma typically have airways obstruction with normal to elevated lung volumes and often have evidence of air trapping, with an increased ratio of residual volume to total lung capacity.

If the diagnosis is still uncertain despite the considerations discussed previously, cardiopulmonary exercise testing may be indicated. Table 8–4 summarizes the patterns of abnormality on exercise testing that assist one in distinguishing cardiac from pulmonary dyspnea.

Dyspnea in the Presence of Normal Physical Examination and Physiologic Testing

It is not uncommon for patients with dyspnea to present with a normal physical examination, chest radiograph, ECG, echocardiogram, and pulmonary function tests. At this point, the possibilities of psychogenic dyspnea and malingering should be considered. Patients with psychogenic dyspnea include those with anxiety disorders, who tend to hyperventilate and experience the increased ventilation as distressing. Typically, these patients have evidence of a respiratory alkalosis with low arterial pressure of carbon dioxide (PCO_2) and a normal $P(A - a)O_2$. Psychogenic dyspnea also includes patients who have become hypersensitive to respiratory sensations after long periods of reduced physical activity. These individuals may experience the increased ventilation associated with even mild exercise as a distressing and, in their minds, abnormal sensation. Finally, there are persons who may complain of symptoms in an effort to gain worker's compensation or some other benefit. The cardiopulmonary exercise test and arterial blood gases are generally quite effective at eliminating the possibility of organic disease in these patients.

Case Examples

To illustrate the application of this approach to the patient with shortness of breath, the evaluation of three patients who presented with shortness of breath is documented. Figure 8–4 provides an overview of the algorithm for the evaluation.

CASE 1. A 53-year-old man complains of shortness of breath walking up hills and when carrying objects up stairs. He is comfortable at rest and walking on flat ground. When he experiences dyspnea, which he describes as a sensation of "chest tightness," he stops and rests and the sensation disappears after a few minutes. He has not had any shortness of breath at rest. He denies a chronic cough and does not think he has heard himself wheeze. The patient smokes one pack of cigarettes each day and has a history of hypertension treated with a diuretic. He has no other significant medical history.

On physical examination, the patient is a moderately

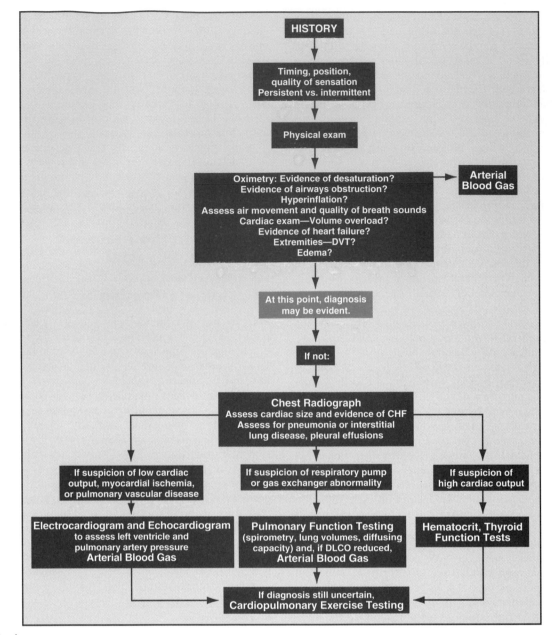

Figure 8–4

Algorithm for the evaluation of the patient with dyspnea. The pace and completeness with which one approaches this framework depend on the intensity and acuity of the patient's symptoms. In the patient with severe, acute dyspnea, an arterial blood gas may be one of the first laboratory evaluations, for example, whereas it might not be obtained until much later in the workup in a patient with chronic breathlessness of unclear cause. A therapeutic trial of a medication, for example, a bronchodilator, may be instituted at any point if one is fairly confident of the diagnosis based on the data available at that time. DVT, deep venous thrombosis; CHF, congestive heart failure; DLCO, diffusing capacity of the lung for carbon monoxide.

obese, middle-aged man who is comfortable sitting at 90 degrees. The blood pressure is 135/92 mm Hg with no pulsus paradoxus. The heart rate is 88 beats per minute and regular, and the respiratory rate is 16 breaths per minute. The examination otherwise reveals mild hyperinflation of the chest with a flattened diaphragm, a mild decrease in air movement throughout, but no wheezes or rales. Cardiac evaluation is notable for a jugular venous pulsation at 8 cm, a normal precordial impulse, and a fourth heart sound. Abdominal examination is normal and there is no clubbing or edema.

DISCUSSION. On the basis of the history and physical examination, it is apparent that the patient has at least mild COPD, but the quality of his dyspnea is more suggestive of CHF than the increased work of breathing or sense of effort typical of patients with emphysema. The intermittent nature of the symptoms and their quality are consistent with reactive airways disease or myocardial ischemia. The patient does not appear to have CHF at rest.

A chest radiograph shows a borderline enlarged heart and hyperinflated lung fields but no infiltrates or effusions. An ECG reveals evidence of left ventricular hypertrophy. Because it is still unclear whether the patient is suffering from COPD or ischemia, pulmonary function tests are obtained. The spirometry demonstrates mild to moderate obstructive lung disease.

A trial of albuterol inhaler is started, but the patient continues to experience exertional symptoms despite an increase in his FEV_1. He is then referred for a cardiopulmonary exercise test. Before the test, he is given a dyspnea questionnaire. Using the questionnaire, he indicates that his respiratory discomfort is characterized primarily as a sense of "not getting enough air, needing more air." There is also an element of "chest tightness." During the test, the patient experiences his symptoms at a moderate level of work. At the point that he stops, his heart rate is 80% of predicted and his blood pressure has risen to 200/110 mm Hg. The ECG demonstrates ischemic changes in the anterior precordial leads that resolve quickly after discontinuing the exercise. At peak exercise, he has not reached his ventilatory limit and oxygen saturation is 94%. There is no drop in FEV_1 with exercise. The test confirms the presence of significant coronary artery disease as the cause of the patient's symptoms.

CASE 2. A 76-year-old woman with a history of both COPD and CHF has been hospitalized frequently for respiratory distress, and it is difficult to determine which of her problems is primarily responsible for her symptoms. Her examination often demonstrates wheezes and scattered rales. The chest radiograph shows the hyperinflation and reduced lung markings of emphysema. The patient insists that she knows whether the problem is "too much fluid" or whether her "emphysema is acting up," despite the fact that she has difficulty explaining the differences in her sensations. Because of the patient's inability to characterize the quality of her dyspnea, a more directed history is obtained utilizing a number of phrases offered to her. She then indicates that she has increased work and effort of breathing when her COPD is worse, and she has a sense of air hunger and suffocating feeling when her CHF is the primary problem. Although there is clearly some overlap in the sensations, there are elements that distinguish the cause of her symptoms, lead to better communication between patient and physician, and serve as guidelines for therapy.

CASE 3. A 55-year-old woman has a history of tuberculosis treated with chemotherapy. One year ago, she had an episode of pleuropericarditis, which was felt to be an early manifestation of systemic lupus erythematosus. She has experienced shortness of breath with exertion over the past 3 months. Particular difficulties are encountered walking up stairs or inclines or when carrying bundles. She has no cough or fevers. Her weight has increased approximately 20 lb in the previous year. The patient denies orthopnea and nocturnal dyspnea, although her husband thinks he has heard her wheeze on occasion at night. The patient has a 20 pack-year history of smoking, which she discontinued 6 months before presentation. She has a sedentary lifestyle and has not participated in regular aerobic activity since her episode of pleuropericarditis.

The past medical history is notable for borderline hypertension. Her only medications are atenolol, conjugated estrogens (Premarin), and medroxyprogesterone acetate (Provera). On physical examination, the patient is a moderately obese woman who appears comfortable sitting at 90 degrees. The blood pressure is 140/85 mm Hg with no pulsus paradoxus, the heart rate is 92 beats per minute, and the respiratory rate is 16 breaths per minute. The examination is within normal limits except for a mild decrease in air movement bilaterally and the presence of a fourth heart sound on cardiac examination.

At this point, one is faced with a broad differential diagnosis. The possibilities may be organized utilizing the construct outlined in Figure 8–2. With respect to cardiovascular causes of dyspnea, the patient may have anemia related to systemic lupus and, as a result, a high output state. She is obese and sedentary and may be deconditioned, that is, normal output cardiac dyspnea. Alternatively, with her history of hypertension, she may be experiencing silent ischemia with activity leading to transient CHF. Given the history of pericarditis, a constrictive pericardial process with associated impact on cardiac output could also be contributing to her limitation.

From the standpoint of possible respiratory causes for her shortness of breath, the hormone therapy could be stimulating her drive to breathe and contributing to dyspnea if there are additional explanations for limited respiratory reserve. Her obesity may be placing some limits on her ability to move air in and out of her chest. If the history of possible wheezing is confirmed to represent airways obstruction, intermittent bronchospasm might be having the same effect. Respiratory muscles may be further compromised by diaphragmatic weakness, a complication of systemic lupus erythematosus. Interstitial pneumonitis associated with systemic lupus or recurrent pulmonary emboli in the setting of silent thromboembolic disease in a sedentary, obese individual could produce hypoxia and dyspnea.

How is the differential diagnosis narrowed? On further questioning, the patient indicates that when she exerts herself, she is "breathing heavily" and "huffing and puffing." She feels she needs to "get more air in." She denies chest tightness or difficulty in moving the air in and out of her chest and feels her lungs expand fully with each breath. These descriptions suggest that deconditioning or a process that resulted in increased respiratory drive, for example, pulmonary vascular disease or anemia, might be the underlying cause of the symptom.

The initial laboratory evaluation includes a chest radiograph to assess the pulmonary interstitium of the lung, the cardiac silhouette, and the presence of pleural effusions. There is evidence of upper-zone scarring consistent with the history of tuberculosis and some basilar atelectasis but no CHF, interstitial changes, or pleural effusions. The heart is borderline enlarged. Pulmonary function tests reveal borderline low lung volumes with very mild airway obstruction and a normal diffusing capacity. The maximal inspiratory and expiratory pressures are within normal limits, and the oxygen saturation is 96%.

Several options are now available. One could begin an empirical trial of bronchodilators, given a history suggesting some wheezing and mild obstruction on pulmonary function testing. The patient could be started on an exercise program to treat deconditioning on the basis of the qualitative descriptors of her dyspnea and the relatively unimpressive workup to this point. Additional studies could be performed in an effort to further define the nature of the problem. Because the patient is concerned about possible cardiac disease and is anxious to have a definitive diagnosis, a cardiopulmonary exercise test was recommended. Although a standard cardiac stress test would provide information about possible myocardial ischemia, a cardiopulmonary exercise test would yield additional data about exercise-induced bronchospasm and pulmonary vascular disease.

The patient terminated the exercise test because of a combination of fatigue and shortness of breath. Again, she described the quality of breathing discomfort primarily as "heavy breathing." At the point that she stopped, she had reached 88% of her maximal heart rate. She was at only 75% of her predicted maximal ventilation, did not drop her oxygen saturation, and had a normal response in her dead space–to–tidal volume ratio. There was no exercise-induced bronchoconstriction. The patient reached anaerobic threshold at a relatively low workload, without ECG changes to suggest ischemia, and the blood pressure response was normal. The patient's dyspnea was attributed to her obesity and deconditioning. She was started on an exercise program with improvement in functional capacity.

This case illustrates how one can approach even complicated patients with shortness of breath in a systematic way. With attention to the quality of dyspnea and a reasoned approach to laboratory testing, the physician can distinguish cardiac and respiratory causes of this symptom.

ACUTE DYSPNEA

The approach to the patient with acute respiratory distress still includes the basic physiologic principles, essentials of history taking and physical examination outlined previously. However, this group of patients, in addition to dyspnea, usually has symptoms such as chest pain, cough, or fever, and the differential diagnosis for the shortness of breath is somewhat different (Table 8–5).

Cardiac disease, especially acute ischemia, leads the list of conditions to be considered in a patient with acute

dyspnea and risk factors for coronary artery disease. Acute myocardial infarction or unstable angina is frequently associated with diaphoresis, nausea, and chest discomfort in addition to dyspnea. The physical examination may reveal an increase in pulse and blood pressure, bibasilar rales, an elevated jugular venous pulse, as well as third or fourth heart sound gallops. Ischemic changes on the ECG are diagnostic, as is the response to nitrate therapy. Cardiac tamponade is a much less common cause of acute dyspnea but may be seen in patients with pericarditis or malignant pericardial effusions and after chest injuries.

Respiratory system derangements associated with acute dyspnea include infections, airways obstruction, pulmonary emboli, and pneumothorax. Acute bronchitis and pneumonia are generally associated with cough, sputum, and fever and may impair gas exchange as well as increase airways resistance. Obstruction of the upper airway, as is seen with anaphylaxis and foreign body aspirations, is often accompanied by stridor, an inspiratory sound produced by turbulent flow through a narrowed trachea as the internal diameter of the upper airway is diminished during inhalation. Acute lower airway obstruction, for example, asthma, may be observed with acute respiratory infections or after exposure to cold air or allergens.

Acute pulmonary embolism should be considered in patients with risk factors for venous thrombosis — for example, long periods of immobilization or lower extremity trauma, the presence of adenocarcinoma and a hypercoagulable state, the use of oral contraceptives, the peripartum state, and the presence of CHF. Pleuritic chest pain is frequently present, and the ECG generally demonstrates a sinus tachycardia. Evidence of right ventricular hypertrophy on the ECG, right ventricular dilatation on the echocardiogram, and typical changes on pulmonary ventilation/perfusion scintigraphy (see Chap. 30) are also helpful in establishing the diagnosis. It should be recalled that a normal arterial blood gas determination does not exclude the presence of acute pulmonary embolism in a patient who otherwise has a good history for the condition.

The combination of acute dyspnea and pleuritic chest pain should also raise the possibility of a pneumothorax. Spontaneous pneumothoraces may occur in tall, thin persons who often have small blebs at the apices of the lung. Patients with asthma are at somewhat increased risk of spontaneous pneumothorax, as are individuals with *Pneumocystis carinii* pneumonia. One must also consider this diagnosis in those patients with chest trauma and acute shortness of breath.

Table 8–5	Causes of Acute Dyspnea

Cardiac

Myocardial ischemia
Congestive heart failure
Hypertensive urgency or emergency
Cardiac tamponade

Pulmonary

Drug overdose with hyperventilation (e.g., aspirin, ethylene glycol)
Acute bronchitis
Pneumothorax
Pulmonary embolism
Upper airway obstruction

IMPLICATIONS FOR THERAPY

If a specific disease process can be identified as the cause of a patient's shortness of breath, an attempt is made to reverse the pathologic state and alleviate the dyspnea. Bronchodilators are administered for airways obstruction; diuretics and vasodilators are prescribed for

CHF (see Chap. 22); nutritional supplementation is prescribed or blood is transfused in the patient with anemia; supplemental oxygen is given to the patient with significant oxygen desaturation. It is also important to consider whether the patient has more than one cause of dyspnea. Are there qualitatively different sensations under different circumstances? The physician must be sensitive to the role of deconditioning in the deterioration of persons who have become increasingly sedentary over months to years. It is possible that the patient may have COPD or CHF. But the presence of either of these conditions may not be the sole reason for the patient's disability. Is the COPD actually the reason the patient is no longer able to do his or her own shopping? If deconditioning is identified, exercise programs may be of benefit even in patients with marked airways obstruction.

SUMMARY

Dyspnea, or shortness of breath, is a complex symptom comprising multiple, qualitatively distinct sensations. It may result from a range of cardiac and pulmonary pathophysiologic derangements. Attention to the nuances of the history and physical examination will provide considerable insight into the cause of a patient's breathing discomfort. A focused laboratory evaluation provides the additional information needed to make a diagnosis in the majority of cases. For more complicated cases or when it is suspected that deconditioning or myocardial ischemia has been superimposed on chronic lung disease, cardiopulmonary exercise testing can be extremely useful.

References

1. Cook, D.G., and Shaper, A.G.: Breathlessness, lung function and risk of heart attack. Eur. Heart J. 9:1215–1222, 1988.
2. Higgins, M.: Epidemiology of obstructive pulmonary disease. In Casaburi, R., and Petty, T.L. (eds.): Principles and Practice of Pulmonary Rehabilitation. Philadelphia, W.B. Saunders, 1993, pp. 10–17.
3. Wasserman, K., and Casaburi, R.: Dyspnea: Physiological and pathophysiological mechanisms. Ann. Rev. Med. 140:1021–1027, 1989.
4. Manning, H.L., and Schwartzstein, R.M.: Pathophysiology of dyspnea. N. Engl. J. Med. 333:1547–1553, 1995.
5. Taguchi, O., Kikuchi, Y., Hida, W., et al.: Effects of bronchoconstriction and external resistive loading on the sensation of dyspnea. J. Appl. Physiol. 71:2183–2190, 1991.
6. Campbell, E.J.M., and Howell, J.B.L.: The sensation of breathlessness. Br. Med. Bull. 19:36–40, 1963.
7. Schwartzstein, R.M., Manning, H.L., Weiss, J.W., et al.: Dyspnea: A sensory experience. Lung 168:185–199, 1990.
8. Remmers, J.E., Brooks, J.G., and Tenney, S.M.: Effect of controlled ventilation on the tolerable limit of hypercapnia. Respir. Physiol. 4:78–90, 1968.
9. Manning, H.L., Basner, R., Ringler, J., et al.: Effect of chest wall vibration on breathlessness in normal subjects. J. Appl. Physiol. 71:175–181, 1991.
10. Schwartzstein, R.M., and Cristiano, L.M.: Qualities of respiratory sensation. In Adams, L., and Guz, A. (eds.): Respiratory Sensation. New York, Marcel Dekker, 1993, pp. 125–154.
11. Melzack, R.: The McGill pain questionnaire: Major properties and scoring methods. Pain 1:277–299, 1975.
12. Hunter, M., and Philips, C.: The experience of headache—An assessment of the qualities of tension headache pain. Pain 10:209–219, 1981.
13. Melzack, R., Terrence, C., Fromm, G., et al.: Trigeminal neuralgia and atypical facial pain: Use of the McGill pain questionnaire for discrimination and diagnosis. Pain 27:297–302, 1986.
14. Simon, P.M., Schwartzstein, R.M., Weiss, J.W., et al.: Distinguishable sensations of breathlessness induced in normal volunteers. Am. Rev. Respir. Dis. 140:1021–1027, 1989.
15. Simon, P.M., Schwartzstein, R.M., Weiss, J.W., et al.: Distinguishable types of dyspnea in patients with shortness of breath. Am. Rev. Respir. Dis. 142:1009–1014, 1990.
16. Elliott, M.W., Adams, L., Cockroft, A., et al.: The language of breathlessness: Use by patients of verbal descriptors. Am. Rev. Respir. Dis. 144:826–832, 1991.
17. Mahler, D.A., Harver, A., Lentine, T., et al.: Descriptors of breathlessness in cardiorespiratory diseases. Am. J. Respir. Crit. Care Med. 154:1357, 1996.
18. Garfinkel, S.K., Kesten, S., Chapman, K.R., et al.: Physiologic and nonphysiologic determinants of aerobic fitness in mild to moderate asthma. Am. Rev. Respir. Dis. 145:741–745, 1992.
19. Killian, K.J., Leblanc, P., Martin, D.H., et al.: Exercise capacity and ventilatory, circulatory, and symptom limitation in patients with chronic airflow limitation. Am. Rev. Respir. Dis. 146:935–940, 1992.
20. Schwartzstein, R.M.: Are you fluent in the language of dyspnea? J. Respir. Dis. 17:322–328, 1996.
21. Schwartzstein, R.M.: The language of dyspnea. In Mahler, D.A. (ed.): Dyspnea. London, Marcel Dekker, 1998, pp. 35–62.
22. Killian, K.J., and Jones, N.L.: The use of exercise testing and other methods in the investigation of dyspnea. Clin. Chest Med. 5:99–108, 1984.
23. Wasserman, K., Hansen, J.E., Sue, D.Y., et al.: Principles of Exercise Testing and Interpretation. Philadelphia, Lea & Febiger, 1994.
24. Sue, D.Y., Wasserman, K., Moricca, R.B., et al.: Metabolic acidosis during exercise in patients with chronic obstructive pulmonary disease. Chest 94:931–938, 1988.

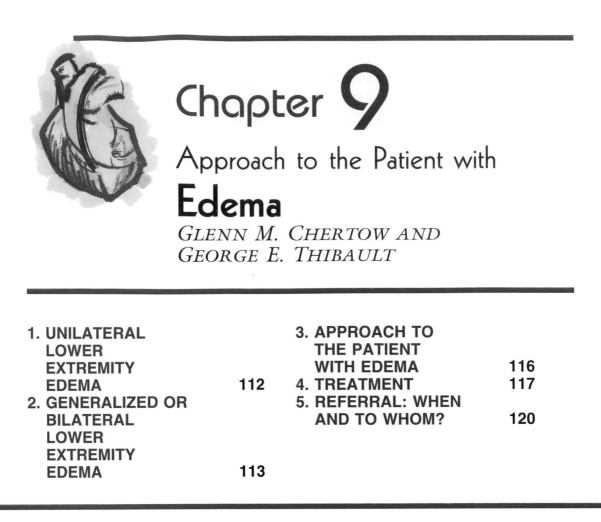

Chapter 9

Approach to the Patient with
Edema

GLENN M. CHERTOW AND
GEORGE E. THIBAULT

Edema of the lower extremities is commonly observed by the primary care physician, and it may reflect a broad spectrum of conditions. The common thread among all causes of edema is elevation of capillary pressure, due to either increased venous pressure or impaired lymphatic drainage. There are many differences, however, in the pathophysiology, diagnostic approach, and treatment of edema, depending on its cause.[1] In this chapter, the common causes of edema encountered in primary care practice are described, focusing on the differentiation between systemic edematous disorders (cardiac, hepatic, and renal diseases) and more localized disease. In addition, a practical approach to differential diagnosis and therapy is presented.

UNILATERAL LOWER EXTREMITY EDEMA

Edema is often considered to be a sign of advanced cardiac, hepatic, or renal disease. However, in primary care practice, *unilateral* lower extremity edema is at least as common as bilateral or generalized edema, and the diagnostic approach and management of these conditions are markedly different (Table 9–1).[2]

A key element in the clinical evaluation of unilateral lower extremity edema is the presence or absence of pain. Painful edema points strongly to the presence of deep venous thrombosis (DVT) or a musculoskeletal disorder. DVT may involve both lower extremities, but one leg usually predominates and manifests clinically with leg swelling, erythema, and pain (see Chap. 30). Occasionally, pain is alleviated with dorsiflexion of the foot, the so-called Homans sign. Often, a history of trauma or immobility can be elicited. A history of DVT or of neoplastic disease, particularly mucin-producing adenocarcinomata of the gastrointestinal tract (e.g., colorectal, pancreatic, cholangiocarcinoma), should further heighten suspicion for DVT.

The tape measure is the simplest diagnostic tool for the evaluation of unilateral edema. It should be placed circumferentially around the mid calf at the same distance below the patella on each leg; marking the site may assist in serial examinations. Although there may be some variability in calf muscle size among normal individuals, asymmetry in circumference in excess of 1 to 2 cm is probably of clinical significance. Doppler examination is a sensitive and specific method for evaluating DVT in the thigh;[3] it is less accurate for determining DVT in the calf. Impedance phlethysmography has also been widely used, but it is operator-dependent and less accurate than venous

Table 9–1	Causes of Unilateral Lower Extremity Edema

With Pain

Deep venous thrombosis
Postphlebitic syndrome
Popliteal cyst rupture
Gastrocnemius rupture
Cellulitis
Psoas or other abscess

Without Pain

Deep venous thrombosis
Postphlebitic syndrome
Other venous insufficiency
   After saphenous vein harvest
   Varicosities
Lymphatic obstruction/lymphedema
   Carcinoma, including cervical, colorectal, prostate
   Lymphoma
   Retroperitoneal fibrosis
   Sarcoidosis
   Filariasis

ultrasonography.[4] Although venography remains the gold standard, its disadvantages include its inconvenience, the need for radiocontrast, and the risk of inducing venous trauma. A strongly positive serum test for D-dimer (a fibrinogen breakdown product) can be used to support the diagnosis of DVT.

The *postphlebitic syndrome* is a relatively common complication following DVT.[5] It is often associated with mild to moderate discomfort and persistent leg swelling and sometimes with pitting edema. Asymmetric painless edema of a lower extremity is often due to chronic venous insufficiency. The latter is observed increasingly at the site of previous saphenous vein harvest as the number of patients who have undergone coronary bypass surgery grows; this form is of little clinical concern, unless it causes pain or functional limitations or leads to secondary infection.

Lymphatic obstruction should be considered as a cause of lower extremity edema when there is no history of trauma or venous system disease. Lymphatic obstruction is most commonly caused by malignant disease in the retroperitoneum. Other causes include retroperitoneal fibrosis, either idiopathic or drug-related (e.g., methysergide).[6] The diagnosis is usually made by computed tomography with oral and intravenous contrast enhancement.

A *ruptured popliteal (Baker's) cyst* is often confused with DVT.[7] It typically presents with the relatively rapid development of unilateral leg edema and pain. A subtle clinical clue is the presence of petechiae around and below the lateral malleolus. Gastrocnemius rupture with local hemorrhage may also be confused with DVT and other causes of lower extremity edema.[8] This process can result in significant pain and enlargement of the diameter of the leg. However, it rarely results in edema per se. Muscle rupture is best confirmed with magnetic resonance imaging. Skin and soft tissue infections may cause edema and can occasionally be confused with DVT. Cellulitis, usually caused by gram-positive cocci that colonize the skin (e.g., *Staphylococcus, Streptococcus*), can result in unilateral leg swelling with erythema that is often streaky in nature, pain, and systemic signs and symptoms, including fever and leukocytosis.

The *treatment* of unilateral lower extremity edema should be cause-directed. Most cases are best managed conservatively, with leg elevation and analgesics when required. Diuretics should not be employed. Anticoagulation is the cornerstone of treatment for DVT (see Chap. 30).

GENERALIZED OR BILATERAL LOWER EXTREMITY EDEMA

In ambulatory individuals, the lower extremities are the predominant site of edema accumulation owing to the effects of gravity on hydrostatic pressure. On the other hand, edema is more uniformly distributed, or more localized to the dependent presacral region, in patients who are predominantly supine throughout the day. Distinct sites of edema (e.g., facial, upper extremity) usually indicate local vascular or lymphatic complications. Generalized edema is the result of systemic sodium retention (Fig. 9–1); the three most common causes are congestive heart failure (CHF), cirrhosis, and the nephrotic syndrome. The mechanisms of generalized edema include (1) an increase in capillary pressure secondary to an elevation in central venous pressure, as occurs in heart failure; (2) primary renal retention of sodium and water, as occurs in primary renal disease; and (3) a reduction in cardiac output that triggers renal vasoconstriction and activation of the renin-angiotensin-aldosterone system, both of which cause retention of sodium and water.[1]

Congestive Heart Failure
(see Chap. 22)

CHF secondary to right heart failure caused by left ventricular systolic dysfunction or valvular heart disease is the most common and well-recognized cause of generalized edema. Generalized edema occurs less frequently in patients with diastolic dysfunction. High-output CHF may also present with sodium retention and edema.[9] The most common causes of the latter are anemia, thyrotoxicosis, beriberi, and large arteriovenous fistulas.

Right ventricular failure without preexisting left heart failure also frequently results in severe bilateral lower extremity edema (and occasionally ascites). Acute right ventricular failure occurs most frequently in the presence of a massive pulmonary embolism (see Chap. 30) or a large right ventricular infarction, which occurs most commonly with a large inferoposterior myocardial infarction (see Chap. 19). Chronic right ventricular failure (when not secondary to left ventricular failure) occurs in the presence of severe pulmonary hypertension. Frequent causes of the latter are chronic obstructive pulmonary disease, obstructive sleep apnea, chronic pulmonary embolization, and primary pulmonary hypertension. Severe edema is a common feature of chronic constrictive peri-

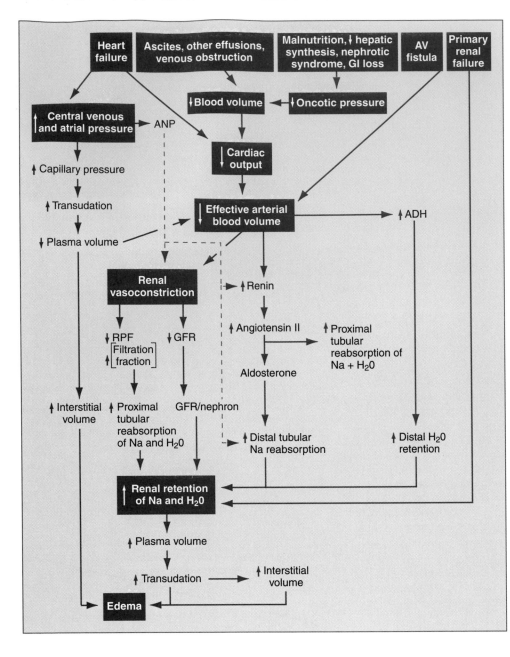

Figure 9–1

Sequence of events leading to the formation and retention of salt and water and the development of edema. Inhibitory influences are shown by *dashed lines.* GI, gastrointestinal; AV, atrioventricular; ANP, atrial natriuretic peptide; ADH, antidiuretic hormone; RPF, renal plasma flow; GFR, glomerular filtration rate. (Redrawn from Braunwald, E.: Edema. *In* Fauci, A.S., Braunwald, E., Isselbacher, K.J., et al. [eds.]: Harrison's Principles of Internal Medicine, 14th ed. New York, McGraw-Hill, 1998, p. 212. Reproduced with permission of The McGraw-Hill Companies.)

carditis (see Chap. 28). Edema of cardiac origin is generally accompanied by elevated jugular venous pressure, which is usually detectable on physical examination (see Chap. 3).

Hepatic Cirrhosis

Cirrhosis is the end-result of a variety of chronic liver diseases, of which Laënnec's cirrhosis (alcoholic liver disease) is the most common. Edema is a hallmark of decompensated cirrhosis, although the mechanisms of edema formation are still open to debate.[10] Edema of hepatic origin tends to be localized in the lower extremities and the abdominal cavity (ascites), depending on the severity of portal hypertension. Central venous pressure is rarely increased in the absence of concomitant cardiac disease. Other physical findings such as jaundice and pal-

mar erythema and abnormal liver function tests can be used to support the diagnosis of cirrhosis (Table 9–2).

Nephrotic Syndrome

Nephrotic syndrome is defined as the presence of urinary protein excretion rates in excess of 3.0 gm/day, complicated by generalized edema, severe hypoalbuminemia, hypercholesterolemia, and a hypercoagulable state. The hypercholesterolemia involves primarily low-density lipoprotein that increases the risk of accelerated atherosclerosis. The hypercoagulable state is attributable to renal losses of antithrombin III and other inhibitors of the coagulation cascade and can lead to renal vein thrombosis and pulmonary embolism.[11]

The most common causes of nephrotic syndrome in adults include membranous nephropathy, diabetic ne-

Table 9–2	Principal Causes of Generalized Edema: History, Physical Examination, and Laboratory Findings		
Organ System	**History**	**Physical Examination**	**Laboratory Findings**
Cardiac	Dyspnea with exertion prominent—often associated with orthopnea—or paroxysmal nocturnal dyspnea	Elevated jugular venous pressure, ventricular (S_3) gallop; occasionally with displaced or dyskinetic apical pulse; peripheral cyanosis, cool extremities, small pulse pressure when severe	Elevated urea nitrogen–to–creatinine ratio common; elevated uric acid; serum sodium often diminished; liver enzymes occasionally elevated with hepatic congestion
Hepatic	Dyspnea infrequent, except if associated with significant degree of ascites; most often a history of ethanol abuse	Frequently associated with ascites; jugular venous pressure usually normal or low; blood pressure typically lower than in renal or cardiac disease; one or more additional signs of chronic liver disease (jaundice, palmar erythema, Dupuytren's contracture, spider angiomata, male gynecomastia or testicular atrophy, caput medusa); asterixis and other signs of encephalopathy may be present	If severe, reductions in serum albumin, cholesterol, other hepatic proteins (transferrin, fibrinogen); liver enzymes may or may not be elevated, depending on the cause and acuity of liver injury; tendency toward hypokalemia, respiratory alkalosis; magnesium and phosphorus often markedly reduced if associated with ongoing ethanol intake; uric acid typically low; macrocytosis from folate deficiency
Renal	Usually chronic; associated with uremic signs and symptoms, including decreased appetite, altered (metallic or fishy) taste, altered sleep pattern, difficulty concentrating, restless legs or myoclonus; dyspnea can be present, but generally less prominent than in heart failure	Blood pressure often high; hypertensive or diabetic retinopathy in selected cases; nitrogenous fetor; periorbital edema may predominate; pericardial friction rub in advanced cases with uremia	Elevation of serum creatinine and urea nitrogen most prominent; also frequent hyperkalemia, metabolic acidosis, hyperphosphatemia, hypocalcemia, anemia (usually normocytic)

Abbreviation: S_3, third heart sound.

phropathy, focal segmental glomerulosclerosis, human immunodeficiency virus (HIV)–associated nephropathy, diabetic nephropathy, minimal change disease, and multiple myeloma (and other plasma cell dyscrasias, including primary amyloid). Patients with diabetic nephropathy are at increased risk of atherosclerotic vascular complications (e.g., myocardial infarction, stroke) compared with diabetics without nephropathy. It is advisable to attempt lipid-lowering therapy with 3-hydroxy-3-methylglutaryl coenzyme A (HMG-CoA) reductase inhibitors in these patients.[12]

Hypertension, another important risk factor for coronary atherosclerosis, is frequent in membranous nephropathy[13] and focal segmental glomerulosclerosis, both important causes of nephrotic syndrome and edema.

Drug-Induced Edema

(Table 9–3)

The nonsteroidal anti-inflammatory drugs (NSAIDs) are the most commonly used agents that promote edema formation. Salt and water retention are due primarily to constriction of the renal microvasculature. In addition to causing edema, the NSAIDs can counteract the effects of various antihypertensive agents, including diuretics, and thereby complicate the management of hypertension.[14]

Several commonly prescribed antihypertensive agents have been linked to the development of edema. The first-generation calcium channel antagonists verapamil, diltiazem, and nifedipine have been reported to cause edema

in up to 5% to 10% of patients. The incidence of edema with the newer, longer-acting preparations, such as amlodipine, appears to be lower. Although the exact mechanisms are unknown, the enhanced renal sodium and water reabsorption related to reflex sympathetic response appears likely. The direct-acting vasodilators, such as hydralazine, minoxidil, and nitroglycerin, used in the treatment of hypertension or CHF may cause edema and

Table 9–3	Drugs Associated with Edema Formation

Nonsteroidal anti-inflammatory drugs
Antihypertensive agents
    Direct arterial/arteriolar vasodilators
        Minoxidil
        Hydralazine
        Clonidine
        Methyldopa
        Guanethidine
    Calcium channel antagonists
    Alpha-adrenergic antagonists
Steroid hormones
    Corticosteroids
    Anabolic steroids
    Estrogens
    Progestins
Cyclosporine
Growth hormone
Immunotherapies
    Interleukin-2
    OKT3 monoclonal antibody

require the initiation or intensification of a diuretic regimen. Alpha-adrenergic antagonists, which are used occasionally in the treatment of hypertension and now are used frequently for urinary symptoms associated with prostatism, also cause edema. Usually, the edema associated with calcium antagonists and vasodilators can be managed with low to moderate doses of thiazide diuretics, which are also useful adjuncts in the management of hypertension. The principal mechanism involved in edema associated with all of these agents appears to be activation of the sympathetic nervous system, leading to sodium retention.

The adrenal corticosteroids and sex hormones are two other classes of drugs that promote salt and water retention and edema formation. Hydrocortisone and, to a lesser extent, prednisone and methylprednisolone promote sodium retention via their effects on the aldosterone-sensitive sodium channel in the cortical collecting duct of the nephron. Mild degrees of hypokalemia and metabolic alkalosis may also accompany their use.

APPROACH TO THE PATIENT WITH EDEMA

The edematous patient who presents to the primary care physician poses several important challenges. First, it is essential to ensure that the edema is not a sign of a life-threatening condition, such as acute CHF. A careful, directed clinical examination and electrocardiogram are most useful (Fig. 9–2).

The History

The history provides the majority of diagnostic clues. Queries should focus on the *five D*s of edema: *d*istribution (unilateral or bilateral), *d*uration (acute or chronic), *d*egree (severity), *d*olor (pain), and associated *d*iseases (heart disease, liver disease, renal disease, diabetes, cancer, arthritis, thromboembolism). It should first be determined whether the edema is unilateral or bilateral, and

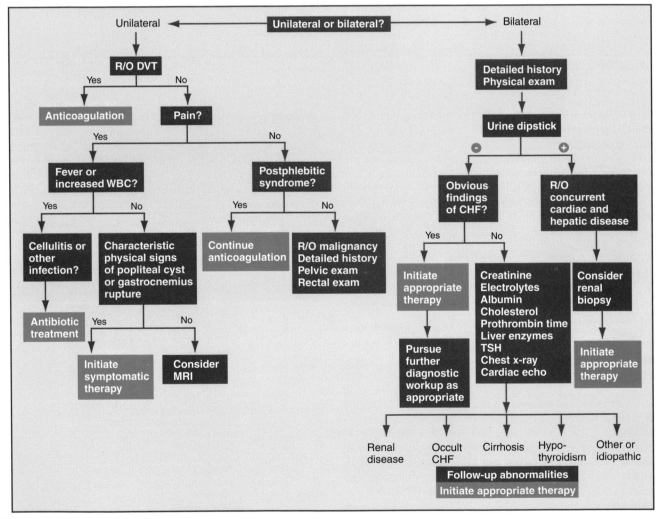

Figure 9–2

Diagnostic approach to the patient with edema. R/O, rule out; DVT, deep venous thrombosis; WBC, white blood cell count; MRI, magnetic resonance imaging; CHF, congestive heart failure; TSH, thyroid-stimulating hormone.

next, whether it is painful or pain-free. Most patients with *unilateral* leg edema should have lower extremity Doppler studies to rule out DVT, unless an alternative diagnosis can be easily established by the history and physical examination. More extensive workup may be required in a patient with a history of abdominal or pelvic malignancy. If the patient has not undergone routine health maintenance checks, a digital rectal examination and bimanual pelvic examination should be performed. If malignancy is suspected as the cause of lower extremity edema, pelvic ultrasonography or computed tomography may be indicated to investigate abnormalities in the retroperitoneal space.

In the presence of *bilateral* edema, a broader differential diagnosis should be entertained, and a detailed history is likely to help narrow the differential. Symptoms of CHF (e.g., exertional dyspnea, orthopnea, paroxysmal nocturnal dyspnea, nocturia) and a history of valvular heart disease or myocardial infarction should be carefully sought, since they point to cardiac disease as the likely cause of the edema.

A history of alcohol abuse or hepatitis or symptoms of active hepatitis (e.g., jaundice, nausea) suggest the possibility of liver disease as a cause. A history of renal disease or a change in the frequency or nature of urinary output (e.g., hematuria, "foamy" urine) suggests a renal cause for the edema. A history of symptoms of thyroid disease should also be elicited. Finally, a detailed drug and dietary history is important for diagnostic clues and also for designing a therapeutic regimen.

Physical Examination

An elevated jugular venous pressure is frequently found in edema associated with CHF or renal disease but is rare in cirrhosis. On cardiac examination, a third heart sound (S_3) gallop indicative of left ventricular systolic dysfunction, the presence of heart murmurs indicative of valvular lesions, or the signs of pulmonary hypertension and cor pulmonale (a loud second pulmonic sound [P_2] and right ventricular heave) all point to the presence of heart disease. Physical signs of chronic liver disease (see Table 9–2) should also be sought.

Laboratory Studies

In most instances, after careful clinical examination, the condition most likely responsible for the edema will be apparent. If there is still diagnostic uncertainty, the following screening laboratory studies are advisable (Table 9–4): serum sodium (low values may occur with CHF, cirrhosis, or hypothyroidism), serum albumin (extremely low values [< 2.0 gm/dl] are seen with nephrotic syndrome; moderate reductions [2.5–3.5 gm/dl] are often seen with cirrhosis), serum creatinine (elevated in renal failure), and urine dipstick (3+ protein is usually indicative of protein loss in excess of 500 mg/day). Thyroid-stimulating hormone should also be measured in the evaluation of edema of uncertain cause, given the high incidence of occult hypothyroidism, particularly among elderly women. Typically, mild to moderate degrees of

Table 9–4	Recommended Laboratory Screening for the Outpatient with Edema

Serum sodium
Serum albumin
Serum creatinine
Urine dipstick
Thyroid-stimulating hormone

hypothyroidism do not result in myxedema or sufficient cardiac disease to promote substantial edema formation. Other serum chemistries to assess liver function, such as alanine aminotransferase and lactate dehydrogenase, are not sufficiently sensitive nor specific to be useful on initial screening. Additional laboratory tests, such as prostate-specific antigen (to evaluate for metastatic prostate carcinoma), should be reserved for specific clinical settings, and after more common causes of edema have been excluded.

Imaging studies are helpful in a relatively small fraction of patients. Echocardiography may be useful for confirming findings on cardiac examination and for providing a quantitative estimate of left ventricular function and pulmonary artery pressure, as well as aortic, mitral, and tricuspid valve function. Abdominal ultrasound can confirm the diagnosis of cirrhosis by demonstrating hepatic nodularity and splenomegaly. Renal ultrasound can be used to assess kidney size and the chronicity of renal disease; longer duration of disease tends to be associated with smaller kidneys. Diabetic nephropathy and HIV-associated nephropathy are two exceptions to this rule, as affected kidneys tend to be large and to remain so through most of the clinical course.

Patients with chronic or bilateral edema can often be managed on an ambulatory basis with an intensification of oral diuretic therapy, or modification of other medications (e.g., vasodilators), without requiring hospitalization. However, an acute worsening of edema may represent progression of the underlying disease state (e.g., the development of myocardial ischemia in the presence of left ventricular dysfunction or the occurrence of spontaneous bacterial peritonitis in the presence of cirrhosis), which should be carefully investigated by clinical and laboratory examination during an outpatient evaluation and which might lead to the need for hospitalization.

TREATMENT

Dietary Modifications

Sodium restriction is the principal dietary intervention for generalized edema, irrespective of its cause. It may be effective by itself, but it is usually employed as an adjunct to diuretic therapy. The daily intake of sodium should be restricted to less than 3 gm. This can be accomplished by eliminating the salt shaker from the table. Restriction to below 1½ gm may be of additional benefit, and this requires the elimination of salt in cooking as well. Further reduction requires foods low in sodium content, but the poor palatability of such a diet makes adherence and maintenance far less likely. It is important to advise patients to avoid the use of canned or other prepared foods, particularly soups and canned vegetables.

Stringent water restriction (>1 L/day) is typically reserved for patients with dilutional hyponatremia associated with advanced CHF or hepatic cirrhosis. There may be some benefit to modest water restriction (1–2 L/day) in other cases.

Changes in Body Position

Like dietary sodium restriction, bed rest in the supine position is moderately effective in the treatment of CHF and other edematous states and enhances the more powerful action of diuretics.[15] Venous pressure in the lower extremities is reduced in the supine position. This promotes redistribution of interstitial fluid to the intravascular compartment, leading ultimately to diuresis. The latter is mediated in part by atrial distention, leading to the synthesis and secretion of atrial natriuretic peptide, which promotes generalized vasodilatation, increased renal blood flow, filtration fraction, and natriuresis.

Diuretics (Table 9–5)

These drugs remain the cornerstone of the treatment of edema. Three classes of diuretics are widely used.

Thiazides

The thiazide diuretics, alone or in combination with distal tubule or potassium-sparing diuretics, are among the most frequently prescribed drugs, both for the treatment of essential hypertension (see Chap. 21) and in the management of edema.

The thiazides are well absorbed, have a peak onset of action between 2 and 6 hours, and have a duration of action between 12 and 24 hours or more, thereby allowing once-daily administration. Like loop diuretics (see later), thiazides are less effective in patients with renal insufficiency.

The site of action of thiazides is the distal convoluted tubule. In contrast to the loop diuretics, thiazides exert no effect on the tonicity of the renal medulla and thereby do not impair the capacity to concentrate urine. Patients with renal hypoperfusion due to moderate or severe CHF or cirrhosis may have elevated levels of vasopressin, and the use of thiazide as the only diuretic can lead to hyponatremia.

Table 9–5	Some Commonly Used Diuretic Agents			
Drug	**Site**	**Half-Life**	**Potency**	**Comments***
Furosemide	THAL	1 hr	++++	Most commonly used loop diuretic agents, po dose 2–3 × equivalent IV dose, half-life prolonged with renal insufficiency and congestive heart failure
Bumetanide	THAL	1–1.5 hr	++++	Higher cost than furosemide, similar therapeutic profile, half-life not prolonged in patients with renal insufficiency
Ethacrynic acid	THAL	1–4 hr	++++	Highest risk is ototoxicity, occasionally used in patients with allergic reaction to other loop diuretics
Torsemide	THAL	3-hr, active metabolites 3 or more hr	++++	Longest-acting loop diuretic
HCTZ	DCT	10–12 hr	++	Prototype thiazide agent effective at doses as low as 6.25 mg, half-life prolonged with renal insufficiency and congestive heart failure
Chlorthalidone	DCT	~3 day	++	Commonly used, similar to HCTZ
Indapamide	DCT	12–24 hr, active metabolites	++	Reported to cause less hyperlipidemia than other thiazides
Metolazone	DCT ± PCT	8–14 hr	+++	Potent agent, distal and proximal tubular activity, effective even at very low GFR
Acetazolamide	PCT	4–8 hr	+	Weak diuretic, leads to hypokalemia and metabolic acidosis, occasionally used in glaucoma and refractory seizure disorders and to alkalinize urine
Spironolactone	CCD	1–1.5 hr, metabolites 9–60 or more hr	+	Long half-life owing to active metabolites, half-life prolonged with renal insufficiency, antiandrogen side effects, promotes hyperkalemia and mild metabolic acidosis
Amiloride	CCD	6–9 hr	+	Well-tolerated, promotes hyperkalemia and mild metabolic acidosis, half-life prolonged with renal insufficiency
Triamterene	CCD	1 6 hr	+	Extremely weak diuretic, rarely used alone
Aminophylline	VASC ± DCT	3–9 hr	+	Weak diuretic, adenosine antagonist, low therapeutic profile, half-life prolonged with congestive heart failure
Dopamine	PCT, VASC	<30 min	++	Promotes natriuresis, may increase renal blood flow, widely used in critically ill patients

Abbreviations: THAL, thick ascending limb of loop of Henle; po, by mouth; IV, intravenous; HCTZ, hydrochlorothiazide; DCT, distal convoluted tubule; PCT, proximal convoluted tubule; GFR, glomerular filtration rate; CCD, cortical collecting duct; VASC, vascular.
* Thiazide class effects: hypokalemia, hypomagnesemia, hyponatremia, hyperuricemia, hypochloremic metabolic alkalosis, hyperglycemia, hypercalcemia, hyperlipidemia. Loop diuretic class effects: hypokalemia, hypomagnesemia, hypochloremic metabolic alkalosis, hypocalcemia, hyperuricemia, hyperglycemia, hypercholesterolemia.

The dose of thiazide diuretics utilized has been reduced in recent years, from the 50 to 100 mg of hydrochlorothiazide per day (or its equivalent) typically used in the past to the doses of 6.25 to 25 mg/day that are currently employed. This reduction occurred because the higher doses exerted marginal natriuretic and antihypertensive effects while increasing the incidence and severity of a variety of metabolic complications, including hypokalemia, hypomagnesemia, hypochloremic metabolic alkalosis, hyperuricemia, and hyperglycemia.

Loop Diuretics

Loop diuretics (e.g., furosemide, bumetanide, ethacrynic acid, and torsemide) are so named because their action is localized to the Na-K-2Cl transporter in the thick ascending limb of the loop of Henle. This transporter is responsible, in part, for maintaining the osmotic gradient within the renal medulla, allowing the maximal concentration of urine.

The onset of action of loop diuretics is rapid, within 5 minutes when given intravenously and within 30 to 60 minutes when given by mouth. The duration of action is relatively short (6–8 hr, somewhat longer with torsemide), requiring twice-daily doses in many patients. Compared with the thiazide diuretics, loop diuretics are more potent (i.e., they promote a larger and more brisk natriuresis) and are better suited for the treatment of edematous disorders. As a result of Na-K-2Cl transporter inhibition, the medullary osmotic gradient is diminished in patients treated with loop diuretics, thereby reducing the risk of hyponatremia in states of vasopressin excess. Furthermore, these drugs exert a direct venodilatory effect, which provides additional relief in the acute management of pulmonary edema. However, owing to their rapid and powerful diuretic effects, loop diuretics may induce a number of electrolyte abnormalities, including hypokalemia, hypomagnesemia, hypochloremic metabolic alkalosis, and hypocalcemia. Hyperuricemia and hyperglycemia occur less frequently than with thiazides.

A low dose of furosemide (e.g., 20 mg/day) is appropriate in patients with edema secondary to CHF despite moderate dietary sodium restriction. Escalating doses (particularly if CHF is accompanied by renal insufficiency) to as high as 240 mg/day may be required. If symptoms persist despite such large doses, the causes of diuretic resistance should be considered (Table 9–6; see also later discussion). In refractory patients, thiazides (intravenous chlorothiazide or oral metolazone), potassium-sparing agents, or dopamine, or a combination of these may be added to loop diuretics.

Diuretics Acting on the Distal Tubule (Potassium-Sparing Diuretics)

Spironolactone, amiloride, and triamterene, the three major drugs in this class, are weak diuretics when administered alone but are valuable in treating edema when used in combination with thiazide or loop diuretics. These agents are effective in augmenting sodium excretion in cases of edema refractory to a single agent, and by their

Table 9–6	Potential Causes of (Loop) Diuretic Resistance

Excessive dietary sodium intake
Diminished intestinal absorption
Distal nephron hypertrophy with chronic use
Severe hypoalbuminemia
Profound hypoperfusion
Mineralocorticoid excess
Renal failure

potassium- and magnesium-retentive properties, they may abrogate the most serious electrolyte disturbances caused by thiazide or loop diuretic agents when the latter are prescribed alone.

Although the clinical effects of these diuretics on urinary electrolyte concentrations are similar, that is, natriuresis and potassium retention, their mechanisms of action differ. Spironolactone is a competitive inhibitor of aldosterone-sensitive sodium transport, whereas amiloride and triamterene act by direct inhibition of the sodium transport channels in the cortical collecting duct. The pharmacokinetics and side effects of this class of diuretic differ considerably; spironolactone may cause gynecomastia and other effects related to its steroid structure, and it has a longer duration of action (24–48 hr) than amiloride (12–24 hr); the latter is better tolerated. Triamterene is now rarely employed, given its low potency and risk of intraluminal crystallization and interstitial nephritis in patients with volume depletion or azotemia.[16]

The distal diuretic agents are useful in patients with edema secondary to advanced hepatic cirrhosis who are in a state of intense stimulation of the renin-angiotensin-aldosterone system. The prolonged half-life and active metabolites of spironolactone allow for once-daily dosing in most cases. In contrast to loop diuretics, the reduction in plasma volume induced by spironolactone is gradual and is less likely to provoke worsening renal function in patients with advanced hepatic disease. However, these agents may lead to hyperkalemia, particularly in the presence of renal dysfunction, diabetes, and the coadministration of angiotensin-converting enzyme inhibitors.

When prescribing potassium-sparing diuretics to patients with edematous disorders, the drugs should be started in low doses and gradually escalated so as to avoid hyperkalemia. Amiloride is the agent of choice in this class of drugs, owing to its excellent tolerability and relatively short half-life.

Diuretic Resistance

One or more of the factors listed in Table 9–6 are usually operative in patients with diuretic resistance whose generalized edema cannot be controlled. The most important of these factors is *excessive dietary sodium intake*. Although most patients with edematous disorders are instructed to limit their sodium intake, the prescription of diuretic agents and the brisk urine output that can ensue after their initiation often provide a false sense of security, leading to liberalization of the diet. This problem can be particularly troublesome with the once-daily use of a short-acting loop diuretic, such as furosemide. In this case, there may be 4 to 6 hours of negative fluid balance, whereas edema recurs during the remainder of the day. This problem is best dealt with by re-establishing appropriate dietary sodium restriction. Also, the use of twice-daily diuretics may be necessary.

A second common cause of diuretic resistance in the presence of chronic use of a loop diuretic is *hypertrophy of the distal nephron*.[17] The adaptation to a sustained reduction in plasma volume is upregulation of the sodium-retentive effects of the distal nephron. This phenomenon has been confirmed pathologically and serves as the physiologic basis for sequential nephron blockade (see later).[18]

Severe *renal hypoperfusion*, as occurs in advanced CHF or cirrhosis, is another cause of diuretic resistance. If the fraction of solute absorbed in the proximal nephron results in insufficient delivery of filtrate to the distal sites of action of diuretics, the latter will be ineffective. Renal failure also often results in diuretic resistance, as the reduction in glomerular filtration leads to reduced delivery of drug to the site of action within the tubular lumen. Therefore, progressively higher doses of diuretics are required in patients with renal insufficiency. Oral thiazides (with the exception of metolazone) are generally ineffective in patients with glomerular filtration rates less than 20 to 30 ml/min.

Decreased gastrointestinal absorption of diuretics, as occurs in the presence of bowel wall edema, may further limit active drug delivery. The use of NSAIDs, corticosteroids (see earlier) and states of relative mineralocorticoid excess (including Cushing's syndrome and the pharmacologic use of prednisone or hydrocortisone) may lead to diuretic resistance by increasing sodium reabsorption in the distal nephron. If withdrawal of these drugs is not possible, the addition of amiloride or spironolactone to furosemide may be helpful. Finally, moderate to severe degrees of hypoalbuminemia may impede the response to furosemide therapy through mechanisms described later.[19]

Management of Diuretic Resistance. Diuretic resistance can often be overcome by withdrawal of offending agents and strict adherence to a low-sodium diet or an increase in the dose or frequency of diuretic administered. If these measures are ineffective, sequential nephron blockade, produced by a combination of furosemide or bumetanide and metolazone (5–10 mg one to three times per week), may be the most effective means of overcoming diuretic resistance. This combination is particularly effective in patients with chronic exposure to loop diuretics, in whom sodium retention in the distal nephron is enhanced and who are therefore more sensitive to metolazone or another thiazide. Close monitoring of electrolyte and acid-base status in this setting is essential, since there is risk of hypokalemia and hypochloremic alkalosis.[20] The addition of amiloride or spironolactone to a loop diuretic may also be extremely effective. However, the concomitant use of angiotensin-converting enzyme inhibitors may preclude the use of the potassium-sparing diuretics because of the risk of hyperkalemia.

Patients most likely to benefit from a continuous intravenous infusion of a loop diuretic are those with chronic loop diuretic exposure (e.g., patients with New York Heart Association class III and IV CHF) or renal insufficiency. The use of a large-bolus dose of furosemide (120–240 mg) followed by a continuous infusion (5–30 mg/hr) appears to be well tolerated and effective in the treatment of refractory edema.

Albumin administration is useful in the treatment of edema associated with severe hypoalbuminemia (<2.5 gm/dl) and that associated with the nephrotic syndrome. The delivery of furosemide to the active luminal site of the nephron is reduced in this condition because furosemide is highly protein (albumin) bound. If albumin (12.5 to 25 gm) is administered along with furosemide, more of the latter can be delivered to the active site, resulting in an augmentation of the diuresis. In this case, parenteral albumin is effective, not because of its role in modifying Starling forces, but simply in its capacity as a transporter of the diuretic to its site of action.

REFERRAL: WHEN AND TO WHOM?

A large majority of patients with edema present initially to the primary care physician who can implement the strategy outlined previously in a cost-effective manner. Referral to a specialist is advisable in patients in whom the cause of the underlying condition remains obscure or in whom it is far advanced, such as severe CHF. Similarly, patients with chronic liver disease can usually be well managed by generalists, unless and until complications ensue. Patients with edema caused by the nephrotic syndrome or chronic renal failure should be referred to nephrologists.

Patients with edema secondary to DVT generally do not require referral to a specialist, unless the episodes are recurrent or there is a strongly positive family history, raising the possibility of an inherited hematologic disorder (e.g., antithrombin III, protein C or S, or Factor V Leiden deficiency). Patients suspected of having edema secondary to advanced malignancy (leading to either lymphatic obstruction or a hypercoagulable state) may benefit from chemotherapy, radiotherapy, or debulking procedures, depending on the type and extent of tumor, and generally warrant consultation with an oncologist.

References

1. Braunwald, E.: Edema. *In* Fauci, A.S., Braunwald, E., Isselbacher, K.J., et al. (eds.): Harrison's Principles of Internal Medicine. 14th ed. New York, McGraw-Hill, 1998, pp. 210–214.
2. Merli, G.J., and Spandorfer, J.: The outpatient with unilateral leg swelling. Med. Clin. North Am. 79:435–447, 1995.
3. Lensing, A.W., Pandoni, P., Brandjes, D., et al.: Detection of deep-vein thrombosis by real-time B-mode ultrasonography. N. Engl. J. Med. 320:342–345, 1989.
4. Heijboer, H., Buller, H.R., Lensing, A.W., et al.: A comparison of real-time compression ultrasonography with impedance plethysmography for the diagnosis of deep-vein thrombosis in symptomatic outpatients. N. Engl. J. Med. 329:1365–1369, 1993.
5. Johnson, B.F., Manzo, R.A., Bergelin, R.O., and Strandness, D.E., Jr.: Relationship between changes in the deep venous system and the development of the postthrombotic syndrome after an acute

episode of lower limb deep vein thrombosis: A one- to six-year follow-up study. J. Vasc. Surg. 21:307–313, 1995.

6. Farrell, W.J., Nolan, J.J., and Tessitore, A.: Unilateral leg edema, migraine, and methysergide. A clinical presentation of retroperitoneal fibrosis. JAMA 207:1909–1911, 1969.

7. Brady, H.R., Quigley, C., Stafford, F.J., et al.: Popliteal cyst rupture and the pseudothrombophlebitis syndrome. Ann. Emerg. Med. 16:1151–1154, 1987.

8. McClure, J.: Gastrocnemius musculotendinous rupture: A condition confused with thrombophlebitis. South. Med. J. 77:1143–1145, 1984.

9. Schrier, R.W.: Pathogenesis of sodium and water retention in high-output and low-output cardiac failure, nephrotic syndrome, cirrhosis, and pregnancy. N. Engl. J. Med. 319:1127–1134, 1989.

10. Martin, P.-Y., and Schrier, R.W.: Renal sodium excretion and edematous disorders. Endocrinol. Metab. Clin. North Am. 24:459–479, 1995.

11. Llach, F.: Hypercoagulability, renal vein thrombosis, and other thrombotic complications of nephrotic syndrome. Kidney Int. 28:429–439, 1985.

12. Rabelink, A.J., Hene, R.J., Erkelens, D.W., et al.: Effects of simvastatin and cholestyramine on lipoprotein profile in hyperlipidaemia of nephrotic syndrome. Lancet 2:1335–1338, 1988.

13. Cattran, D.C., Pei, Y., and Greenwood, C.: Predicting progression in membranous glomerulonephritis. Nephrol. Dial. Transplant. 7:48–52, 1992.

14. Pope, J.E., Anderson, J.J., and Felson, D.T.: A meta-analysis of the effects of nonsteroidal anti-inflammatory drugs on blood pressure. Arch. Intern. Med. 153:477–484, 1993.

15. On bedresting in heart failure. [Editorial.] Lancet 336:975–976, 1990.

16. Fairley, K.F., Woo, K.T., Birch, D.F., et al.: Triamterene-induced cystalluria and cylinduria: Clinical and experimental studies. Clin. Nephrol. 26:169–173, 1986.

17. Wilcox, C.S., Mitch, W.E., Kelly, R.A., et al.: Response of the kidney to furosemide. I. Effects of salt intake and renal compensation. J. Lab. Clin. Med. 102:450–458, 1983.

18. Channer, K.S., McLean, K.A., Lawson-Matthew, P., and Richardson, M.: Combination diuretic treatment in severe heart failure: A randomised controlled trial. Br. Heart J. 71:146–150, 1994.

19. Inoue, M., Okajima, K., Itoh, K., et al.: Mechanism of furosemide resistance in analbuminemic rats and hypoalbuminemic patients. Kidney Int. 32:198–203, 1987.

20. Black, W.D., Shiner, P.T., and Roman, J.: Severe electrolyte disturbances with metolazone and furosemide. South. Med. J. 71:380–381, 385, 1978.

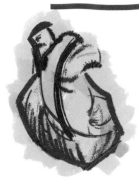

Chapter 10

Approach to the Patient with

Palpitations

MARK A. HLATKY

Palpitations are a common symptom,[1, 2] defined as an uncomfortable awareness of the heartbeat. It is important to recognize there is a distinction between the symptom of palpitations and the presence of cardiac arrhythmias. A patient can have an uncomfortable awareness of normal sinus rhythm or of sinus tachycardia owing to anxiety or to particularly forceful contraction of the heart. Conversely, cardiac arrhythmias may be asymptomatic, or they may cause other symptoms such as dizziness, syncope, shortness of breath, fatigue, or chest pain instead of palpitations. Palpitations and arrhythmia are closely related phenomena, but they are not synonymous.

Cardiac arrhythmias can arise from any form of heart disease or even from a structurally normal heart. Palpitations and arrhythmias can therefore represent anything from a benign but annoying condition to a foreshadowing of sudden cardiac death. The physician must have an organized approach to evaluation and management of the patient with palpitations in order to establish the diagnosis, prognosis, and therapy efficiently and effectively.

The physician evaluating a patient with palpitations should recall the interrelated but distinct concepts of (1) the symptom (palpitations), (2) the functional disturbance (arrhythmia), (3) the substrate (underlying heart disease), and (4) the precipitating factors. The goal of the physician's investigation should be to evaluate each of these dimensions of the patient's problem and thereby provide a sound basis for further management.

DETERMINING THE CAUSE OF PALPITATIONS

Clinical History

A complete history is the first step in the evaluation of palpitations and provides information about all dimensions of the patient's problem (Table 10–1). A complete description of the palpitations should be sought, first by having the patient describe the problem in his or her own words, then through specific questions. Timing is a key element characterizing palpitations. How long does each episode last? How often do the episodes occur? What was the patient doing at the time the episode began? Are episodes more common at certain times of the day or on certain days of week? When did the symptom begin? Responses to questions about timing provide information about the type of arrhythmia (if any) responsible and suggest precipitating factors. It is important to ask about the details of the episode, including whether the sensation is brief or prolonged ("skipped beat," "flip-flop"), whether the heartbeat is regular or irregular ("is it regular, like a clock?"), and whether the onset and termination of the episode are gradual or abrupt ("like a light switch?"). The physician should help the patient by tapping out examples of a regular or irregular rhythm or by having the patient tap out the rhythm he or she has experienced. The presence of coexisting symptoms such as dizziness, lightheadedness, chest pain, shortness of breath, and sweating may

Table 10-1 Clinical History in Evaluation of Palpitations

Symptoms of Palpitations

Duration of episode
Frequency of episodes
Associated chest pain, dyspnea, lightheadedness?
How does episode start? How does episode stop?

Underlying Heart Disease

Angina, prior myocardial infarction
Valvular heart disease
Congenital heart disease
Cardiomyopathy
Coronary risk factors
Congestive heart failure
Prior antiarrhythmic therapy

Precipitating Factors

Psychologic stress
Exercise
Caffeine, alcohol, cocaine, amphetamines
Thyroid disease
Anemia, hypoxemia

provide useful information about the likely effects of an arrhythmia on cardiac output and blood pressure.

The circumstances in which the palpitations occur provide information about the likelihood they are due to an arrhythmia as well as precipitating factors. In what activities was the patient engaged when struck by palpitations? Mental stress and anxiety may lead to an overawareness of sinus rhythm or may precipitate cardiac arrhythmia in a patient with an appropriate substrate. Exercise, caffeine, alcohol, and drugs such as cocaine or amphetamines may all precipitate episodes of arrhythmia. Noncardiac disorders such as anemia, hyperthyroidism, and hypoxemia may lead to tachycardia and symptomatic palpitations.

History-taking in patients with palpitations should also address the likelihood of underlying heart disease. Coronary heart disease may be suggested by symptoms of chest pain, a history of prior myocardial infarction, cardiac risk factors (age, gender, smoking, hypertension, hyperlipidemia, diabetes, family history), and atherosclerosis in other vascular beds. Valvular or congenital heart disease may be suggested by a history of cardiac murmurs, rheumatic fever, or cyanosis or by symptoms of congestive heart failure.

Physical Examination

Since palpitations are episodic, it is likely that the patient will be between spells at the time of the physical examination. In these circumstances, standard cardiac examination is aimed at detecting evidence of the presence of underlying heart disease. Cardiac murmurs may be a sign of valvular heart disease, congenital heart disease, or hypertrophic cardiomyopathy. Signs of congestive heart failure, such as a third heart sound (S_3) gallop, elevated jugular venous pressure, rales, or peripheral edema are important evidence of serious associated cardiac disease. Bruits over the carotid or femoral arteries or diminished peripheral pulses provide evidence of a tendency toward

atherosclerosis, raising the likelihood of underlying coronary artery disease.

Physical examination during a symptomatic attack provides information about the cardiac arrhythmia and its hemodynamic consequences. The rate and regularity of the heartbeat are key observations regarding the arrhythmia, and documentation by electrocardiography is crucial. The physical examination during an episode provides evidence of atrial activity through the jugular venous pulse and by the first heart sound (S_1): intermittent cannon A-waves or variations in the intensity of S_1 suggest atrioventricular (AV) dissociation. The consequences of the arrhythmia on perfusion should be evaluated as well. Adequacy of cardiac output and blood pressure can be assessed by level of consciousness, perfusion of the extremities, and urine output. It is important to recall that patients with ventricular tachycardia may have an adequate blood pressure and cardiac output, especially if they are supine.

The Electrocardiogram

The electrocardiogram (ECG) is the single most valuable laboratory study in a patient with palpitations, and it provides information about both the arrhythmia and the presence of underlying heart disease. A resting 12-lead ECG should be performed in every patient at the time of initial evaluation as well as during an episode of palpitations.

ECGs recorded between episodes of palpitations provide evidence regarding the arrhythmia substrate. Particular attention should be paid to the P-wave, PR interval, presence of delta waves or abnormal Q-waves, and the QT interval. Left or right atrial enlargement increases the likelihood of supraventricular arrhythmias. A short PR interval or delta wave provides evidence for accessory AV pathways that form the substrate for supraventricular tachycardia. Q-waves consistent with myocardial infarction suggest that a substrate for ventricular tachycardia may exist. Left or right ventricular hypertrophy suggests underlying structural heart disease. Prolongation of the QT interval may dispose the patient toward torsades de pointes or other forms of ventricular tachycardia.

An ECG recorded at the time of symptoms is the definitive diagnostic study to document the presence and type of arrhythmia. Tracings taken during an arrhythmia may be challenging to interpret and may need to be reviewed with a physician experienced in electrocardiography. Computerized ECG analysis of arrhythmias should be regarded with great suspicion, since subtle aspects of the tracing may be missed by the computer. The basic principles of arrhythmia evaluation on the 12-lead ECG are simple, and yet application of these principles to interpret tracings may be difficult. The key elements in interpreting an ECG with an arrhythmia are (1) evidence of atrial activity, (2) relationship between atrial and ventricular complexes, (3) regularity or irregularity, (4) ventricular rate, (5) width and morphology of the QRS complexes, and (6) duration of tachycardia.

Narrow-complex tachycardias (QRS duration < 0.10 sec) indicate that the ventricles are being activated in the usual fashion through the normal conduction system. With rare exceptions, a narrow-complex tachycardia is supraventricular in origin. An irregular narrow-complex tachycardia without defined P-waves suggests atrial fibrillation (see Fig. 23–3), whereas a regular narrow-complex tachycardia suggests atrial flutter (see Fig. 23–4) or other supraventricular tachycardia. Flutter waves are most visible in the inferior leads (II; III; aVF). AV node blockade by increasing vagal tone or by pharmacologic means (beta blockade, adenosine, verapamil, diltiazem) may either slow the ventricular response and bring out flutter waves or terminate supraventricular arrhythmias in which the AV node is part of a reentrant circuit (see Chap. 23).

Wide-complex tachycardia may be due to ventricular tachycardia or to supraventricular tachycardia with aberration. The most specific feature for ventricular tachycardia is evidence of AV dissociation. The presence of AV dissociation establishes the arrhythmia as ventricular tachycardia, whereas its absence is consistent with either a supraventricular or a ventricular origin. In the absence of AV dissociation, suggestive evidence is provided by the QRS morphology. Although many schemes have been proposed to distinguish ventricular tachycardia from supraventricular tachycardia with aberration (see Fig. 23–1), all are based on the fundamental principle that the QRS complex widens in supraventricular tachycardia as a result of rate-related conduction delay through the usual conducting system, whereas the QRS complex is wide in ventricular tachycardia because the ventricle is being activated from an abnormal site. Thus, aberrantly conducted supraventricular tachycardia tends to have fairly typical right or left bundle branch block configuration, whereas in ventricular tachycardia the QRS complex tends to have an unusual morphology. The wider the complex, the more likely it is that the arrhythmia is ventricular tachycardia, since conduction through the myocardium is particularly slow.

Initial Evaluation

After taking a careful clinical history, performing the physical examination, and reviewing the ECG, the physician will have to decide whether further evaluation is necessary and, if so, to select the appropriate diagnostic tests. The key issues are (1) establishing the diagnosis of which arrhythmia (if any) is causing the patient's symptoms and (2) evaluating the risk for death or serious complications. Empirical therapy of palpitations without establishing the underlying arrhythmia is unwise, as an inappropriate or ineffective drug may be chosen. Since antiarrhythmic agents may actually exacerbate arrhythmias and often have significant side effects, empirical therapy may worsen rather than alleviate the patient's problem. If symptoms are severe enough to warrant therapy, a diagnosis should be established first.

The differential diagnosis of palpitations includes heightened awareness of a normal heartbeat as well as supraventricular and ventricular arrhythmias. The probability of serious arrhythmias as a source of palpitations is increased in the presence of underlying structural heart disease, which is more likely in older patients because the prevalence of ischemic heart disease and congestive heart failure increases with age. The likelihood of life-threatening ventricular arrhythmia is increased by evidence of these and other disease processes that affect the ventricles. Conversely, in younger patients without structural heart disease, the probability of supraventricular arrhythmia is greater, as is the possibility of heightened awareness of isolated premature beats or of noncardiac causes of palpitations.

Several series of patients seen in primary care settings provide information on the clinical epidemiology of palpitations.[3, 4] Weber and Kapoor evaluated 190 patients who presented to the emergency department, medical clinics, or inpatient services at the University of Pittsburgh.[3] The population had an average age of 46 years, 61% were female, and 32% had a history of cardiac disease. Specific arrhythmias were found to be causative in 41% of the patients, most commonly atrial fibrillation, supraventricular tachycardia, or premature atrial or ventricular beats. Ventricular tachycardia was documented in only 4 (2%) patients. Psychiatric disorders were the cause of palpitations in 30% of the patients, with panic attacks accounting for almost all the diagnoses. Other specific diagnoses accounted for another 13% of the patients, and in 16% of patients the cause of the palpitations was unknown. Four factors were independently predictive of a cardiac cause for palpitations: male sex, a history of heart disease, a description of an irregular heartbeat, and a duration of palpitations of more than 5 minutes.[3]

Psychologic stress, palpitations, and arrhythmias are closely intertwined. Stress leads to increased levels of sympathetic drive and circulating catecholamines, which in turn increase heart rate and contractility. Patients who are particularly anxious, hyperventilating, or suffering from panic attacks may complain of palpitations owing to a heightened awareness of sinus tachycardia. The clinician should not, however, simply dismiss as benign symptoms of palpitations in the setting of psychologic stress. A wide variety of serious arrhythmias may also be precipitated by increased levels of circulating catecholamines in patients with an appropriate arrhythmia substrate.

Documentation of the Arrhythmia

Palpitations and arrhythmias are by nature transient phenomena. Spontaneous arrhythmias may be documented by continuous ambulatory electrocardiography (Holter monitoring) or by intermittent recordings of an ECG during symptoms (event monitors). Arrhythmias may also be provoked by exercise testing or programmed electrical stimulation.

Holter Monitoring

Continuous ambulatory electrocardiography (also known as *Holter monitoring* after its developer) is a valuable means of assessing frequent palpitations. The patient has several electrodes placed on the torso, and two or more electrocardiographic leads are recorded from 24 to 72 hours. Correlation between symptoms and the cardiac rhythm is a key feature of ambulatory monitoring, and patients should be carefully instructed to record their symptoms in a diary and to note the time indicated on the Holter monitor itself. The test provides much less information in patients who are unable to keep an accurate symptom diary.

Ambulatory monitoring is diagnostic only when a patient experiences her or his typical symptom of palpitations while wearing the monitor and records the type and time of the symptoms in a diary (Table 10–2). If an arrhythmia is recorded at the same time that the patient notes palpitations, a positive link between symptoms and a cardiac arrhythmia is established, and the precise arrhythmia responsible may be identified. Conversely, if typical symptoms occur when the ECG recording shows sinus rhythm, the documented dissociation between symptoms and arrhythmia provides the physician reassurance and a basis for symptomatic management. The ambulatory monitoring result is ambiguous when either no symptoms occur or the patient experiences atypical symptoms. No useful information is provided by the combination of no symptoms and no recorded arrhythmias (Table 10–2). The combination of no recorded symptoms with minor arrhythmias (e.g., premature supraventricular or ventricular beats) also provides little useful information because isolated premature beats are very common in the normal population.[2] Short runs of supraventricular tachycardia or ventricular tachycardia in the absence of symptoms provide suggestive, but not definitive, evidence that an arrhythmia may be the cause of the patient's symptoms. These equivocal results of ambulatory monitoring are usually not strong enough evidence to lead to treatment, but they do suggest the need for further evaluation. Most ominous in an asymptomatic patient is sustained ventricular tachycardia (i.e., 30 sec or more in duration). This finding warrants very careful evaluation, usually in consultation with an arrhythmia specialist.

Event Monitors

If episodes of palpitations are infrequent, it is unlikely that 24 hours or even 72 hours of ambulatory ECGs will provide diagnostic information. A convenient alternative is an event monitor, in which the patient wears or carries a small electrocardiographic recording device and activates it when experiencing symptoms, thus recording the ECG in the device for later playback and analysis. The smaller size and intermittent recording behavior of this device allow it to be worn or carried for prolonged periods of time. The information provided is similar to that of continuous ECG recorders (see Table 10–2). Event monitors require a conscious patient with the cognitive abilities to recognize an arrhythmia and activate the device. In patients unable to use the event recording system, several 24-hour recordings may be needed.

A recent study enrolled patients with palpitations to receive in random order a Holter monitor for 48 hours or an event monitor for up to 3 months.[5] A recording was made during symptoms in 67% of patients with the event monitor versus 35% of patients with a Holter monitor ($P < .001$). Half of the yield of the event recorder was in

Table 10–2 Ambulatory Electrocardiography in Evaluating Palpitations

Symptom	Concurrent Rhythm	Interpretation
Present	Sinus rhythm	Symptoms not due to arrhythmia
Present	Arrhythmia (sustained or not)	Establishes arrhythmia as cause of symptoms
None	Sinus rhythm	No diagnostic information
None	Premature atrial or ventricular beats	No diagnostic information
None	Runs of PVCs or PACs	Suggestive but not definitive
None	Supraventricular tachycardia >30 sec duration	Suggestive but not definitive
None	Ventricular tachycardia	Very suggestive of life-threatening arrhythmia

Abbreviations: PVCs, premature ventricular contractions; PACs, premature atrial contractions.

the first few days of use, and the remaining events were recorded within 30 days. The cost of evaluation in this study was actually lower with event monitors than with the Holter monitor.[5]

Clinical guidelines suggest that a 24-hour ambulatory ECG is the test of choice to document arrhythmias in patients with daily palpitations. For those with less frequent palpitations, the guideline suggests a single 24-hour ambulatory ECG to characterize baseline arrhythmia, followed by an event monitor if the patient did not experience any symptoms during the first 24 hours.[6]

Exercise Testing

Exercise testing is more useful for the evaluation of ischemic heart disease than of arrhythmia. For patients who describe palpitations as a direct result of physical exertion, however, exercise testing is a reasonable method of evaluation. In some young patients with catecholamine-induced ventricular tachycardia, the arrhythmia may be brought out only by exercise testing.

Electrophysiologic Study

Invasive electrophysiologic study (EPS) (see Chap. 23) has a very high diagnostic yield in patients with suspected arrhythmia, but it should be used only after evaluation by an ambulatory ECG or an event monitor, with virtually the only exception being patients resuscitated from a cardiac arrest or those with other life-threatening symptoms.

EPS attempts to provoke arrhythmias by the controlled introduction of premature atrial or ventricular beats. In patients with the appropriate substrate, a sustained reentry arrhythmia can be induced. Patients with an accessory AV connection may have AV reciprocating tachycardia induced, and those with a prior myocardial infarction may have sustained ventricular tachycardia induced. Other arrhythmias reliably induced and studied by EPS are supraventricular tachycardia and atrial flutter. Each of these arrhythmias occurs using a reentry mechanism in a fixed anatomic substrate and thus is ideal for evaluation by EPS.

EPS is not as useful in inducing arrhythmias that arise from transient substrates, such as ventricular fibrillation resulting from myocardial ischemia or electrolyte disorders. Arrhythmias due to mechanisms other than reentry —including torsades de pointes, multifocal atrial tachycardia, and ectopic atrial tachycardia—are also not induced reliably by EPS. Very aggressive stimulation protocols may induce nonclinical arrhythmias in some patients. Thus, although EPS is an extremely valuable laboratory test, it is neither 100% sensitive nor 100% specific in the evaluation of arrhythmias.

The main role for EPS is to guide therapy in patients with established arrhythmias. Radiofrequency ablation may be used in selected symptomatic patients with Wolff-Parkinson-White syndrome, supraventricular tachycardia, atrial flutter, and certain uncommon forms of ventricular tachycardia (see Chap. 23).[7] Antiarrhythmic therapy may be guided by findings at EPS in patients with established arrhythmias. The use of EPS as a purely diagnostic test in patients with palpitations is limited. Clinical guidelines based on expert opinion strongly endorse EPS only in patients in whom ECG recordings fail to establish a diagnosis (Table 10–3).

Table 10–3	AHA/ACC Guidelines for Use of Diagnostic Tests in Patients with Palpitations*

Ambulatory Electrocardiography[6]

Class I   Palpitation, syncope, dizziness
Class II   Shortness of breath, chest pain, or fatigue (not otherwise explained, episodic and strongly suggestive of an arrhythmia as the cause because of a relation of the symptom with palpitation)
Class III Symptoms not reasonably expected to be due to arrhythmia

Electrophysiologic Study[7]

Class I   1. Patients with palpitations who have a pulse rate documented by medical personnel as inappropriately rapid and in whom electrocardiographic recordings fail to document the cause of the palpitations.
          2. Patients with palpitations preceding a syncopal episode
Class II   Patients with clinically significant palpitations, suspected to be of cardiac origin, in whom symptoms are sporadic and cannot be documented; studies are performed to determine the mechanisms of arrhythmias, to direct or provide therapy, or to assess prognosis
Class III Patients with palpitations documented to be due to extracardiac causes (e.g., hyperthyroidism)

Echocardiography[11]

Class I   1. Arrhythmias with evidence of heart disease
          2. Family history of genetic disorder associated with arrhythmias
Class II   1. Arrhythmias commonly associated with, but without evidence of, heart disease
          2. Atrial fibrillation or flutter
Class III 1. Palpitation without evidence of arrhythmias
          2. Minor arrhythmias without evidence of heart disease

Abbreviations: AHA/ACC, American Heart Association/American College of Cardiology.

  * Class I, general agreement the test is useful and indicated; class II, frequently used, but there is a divergence of opinion with respect to its utility; class III, general agreement the test is not useful.

ASSESSING RISK DUE TO ARRHYTHMIA

Therapy in patients with palpitations due to cardiac arrhythmia is aimed at relief of symptoms and reduction of the risk due to the arrhythmia. The risk of the arrhythmia to the patient is jointly determined by (1) the type of arrhythmia responsible for the patient's symptoms and (2) the type and severity of the patient's underlying heart disease, if any.

Atrial Arrhythmias

Atrial arrhythmias do not generally pose a risk of death because transmission of atrial electrical activity to the ventricles is regulated by the AV node. Rapid atrial flutter or atrial fibrillation, for instance, can be conducted directly to the ventricles only when the protection of the AV node fails, as in some cases of Wolff-Parkinson-White syndrome, or in patients in whom drug therapy accelerates AV nodal conduction (e.g., quinidine or procainamide without an AV node suppressant). Patients with severe underlying heart disease such as hypertrophic cardiomyopathy, congestive heart failure, or critical coronary artery disease, however, may experience circulatory collapse as a result of rapid atrial rates, myocardial ischemia, or loss of effective atrial contraction.

Patients with atrial arrhythmias are also at risk for stroke due to emboli. The risk is highest in patients with chronic atrial fibrillation or flutter in whom ineffective atrial contraction leads to stasis and formation of intra-atrial thrombi. Patients with valvular heart disease, congestive heart failure, hypertension, or a history of thromboembolism are at highest risk of stroke,[8] but chronic anticoagulation is generally recommended in most patients with chronic atrial fibrillation and no contraindications (see Chap. 23).

Ventricular Arrhythmias

Patients with ventricular arrhythmias are at increased risk of sudden cardiac death because of the potential for deterioration of the arrhythmia to ventricular fibrillation. Epidemiologic studies in patients with recent myocardial infarction suggest a gradient of increasing risk with increasing complexity of the arrhythmia. The lowest-risk category is associated with isolated premature ventricular beats, with somewhat higher risk associated with couplets or triplets of ventricular premature beats—the next higher level of risk associated with nonsustained ventricular tachycardia (>3 beats but <30 sec)—and the highest level of risk is associated with sustained ventricular arrhythmia (≥ 30 sec or requiring countershock for termination). The frequency of the arrhythmia and the highest level of complexity together establish the risk of death. The greatest information is conveyed by the level of complexity; at any level of complexity, risk increases with more frequent arrhythmias.[9]

The risk posed by ventricular arrhythmias is also deter-

[handwritten note at top of page:] risk of sudden death in vent. arrhythmia ∝ to decreases in LV systolic fnx

mined by the presence and severity of underlying heart disease. Frequent premature ventricular beats are associated with low risk in a young patient with a structurally normal heart,[10] and yet these are associated with a considerably higher risk in an older patient with congestive heart failure due to prior myocardial infarction. Left ventricular systolic function is particularly important in assessing the risk of patients with ventricular arrhythmia.[11] Patients with normal left ventricular function are generally at low risk, perhaps because they are more able to maintain cardiac output and blood pressure in the face of ventricular tachycardia, and perhaps because of the greater difficulty in inducing ventricular fibrillation in a ventricle of normal size and function. Conversely, patients with poor ventricular function are at higher risk in the presence of ventricular arrhythmia because the poorer mechanical function of the ventricles may not support an adequate blood pressure or cardiac output during ventricular tachycardia (leading to secondary ventricular fibrillation), or because a dilated and scarred ventricle may be more susceptible to primary ventricular fibrillation. Regardless of the underlying mechanism, the risk of sudden death is inversely proportional to left ventricular function, and for any level of ventricular arrhythmia, patients with lower left ventricular ejection fraction have a worse prognosis. Evaluation of the state of left ventricular function is such a powerful predictor of outcome in patients with ventricular arrhythmias that it is reasonable and appropriate to evaluate left ventricular ejection fraction in virtually every patient with documented ventricular arrhythmia in whom a decision regarding therapy needs to be made.[11]

SUMMARY AND RECOMMENDATIONS

The goals of evaluation in a patient with palpitations are to (1) establish the arrhythmia, if any, responsible for the patient's symptoms and (2) evaluate the risk posed by the arrhythmia in light of the nature and severity of the patient's underlying heart disease, if any. All patients should receive a careful history and physical examination as well as a 12-lead ECG. Based on this information, the physician should first assess the likelihood of underlying structural heart disease and the potential risk to the patient (Fig. 10–1). In patients without evidence of structural heart disease, risk is low and decisions about further testing may be made solely on the basis of severity and frequency of symptoms. In patients with structurally normal hearts and either mild symptoms or symptoms consisting of only brief skipped beats, no further testing is necessary. Patients with structurally normal hearts with symptoms frequent enough to require medication for control, however, should have the arrhythmia documented first.

Patients with evidence of structural heart disease or with features suggesting increased risk (e.g., associated presyncope or syncope) should have a 24-hour ambulatory ECG recorded unless an ECG during an episode of palpitations is already available. Patients who have no symptoms during a 24-hour recording should receive an event monitor to record symptoms unless they would be unable to use the device. EPS should generally be reserved for patients with arrhythmias documented by non-

Figure 10–1

Diagnostic approach to the patient with palpitations.

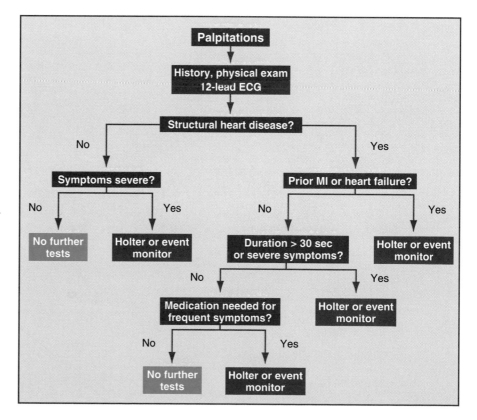

invasive methods in whom further therapy depends on an invasive evaluation. Patients with clinical evidence of underlying heart disease and documented ventricular arrhythmias should generally receive an echocardiogram to evaluate left ventricular function and hence the risk of serious adverse effects due to the arrhythmia. The therapy of specific arrhythmias based on this information is outlined in Chapter 23.

References

1. Kroenke, K., Arrington, M.E., and Mangelsdorff, A.D.: The prevalence of symptoms in medical outpatients and the adequacy of therapy. Arch. Intern. Med. 150:1685–1689, 1990.
2. Lochen, M.-L., Snaprud, T., Zhang, W., and Rasmussen, K.: Arrhythmias in subjects with and without a history of palpitations: The Tromso study. Eur. Heart J. 15:345–349, 1994.
3. Weber, B.E., and Kapoor, W.N. Evaluation and outcomes of patients with palpitations. Am. J. Med. 100:138–148, 1996.
4. Barsky, A.J., Cleary, P.D., Coeytaux, R.R., and Ruskin, J.N.: The clinical course of palpitations in medical outpatients. Arch. Intern. Med. 155:1782–1788, 1995.
5. Kinlay, S., Leitch, J.W., Neil, A., et al.: Cardiac event recorders yield more diagnoses and are more cost-effective than 48-hour Holter monitoring in patients with palpitations. A controlled clinical trial. Ann. Intern. Med. 124:16–20, 1996.
6. ACC/AHA Task Force Report: Guidelines for ambulatory electrocardiography. A report of the American College of Cardiology/American Heart Association Task Force on Assessment of Diagnostic and Therapeutic Cardiovascular Procedures (Subcommittee on Ambulatory Electrocardiography). J. Am. Coll. Cardiol. 13:249–258, 1989.
7. ACC/AHA Task Force Report: Guidelines for clinical intracardiac electrophysiological and catheter ablation procedures. A report of the American College of Cardiology/American Heart Association Task Force on Practice Guidelines (Committee on Clinical Intracardiac Electrophysiologic and Catheter Ablation Procedures), developed in collaboration with the North American Society of Pacing and Electrophysiology. J. Am. Coll. Cardiol. 26:555–573, 1995.
8. The Stroke Prevention in Atrial Fibrillation Investigators: Predictors of thromboembolism in atrial fibrillation: I. Clinical features of patients at risk. Ann. Intern. Med. 116:1–5, 1992.
9. Maggioni, A.P., Zuanetti, G., Franzosi, M.G., et al., GISSI-2 Investigators: Prevalence and prognostic significance of ventricular arrhythmias after acute myocardial infarction in the fibrinolytic era. GISSI-2 results. Circulation 87:312–322, 1993.
10. Kennedy, H.L., Whitlock, J.A., Sprague, M.K., et al.: Long-term follow-up of asymptomatic healthy subjects with frequent and complex ventricular ectopy. N. Engl. J. Med. 312:193–197, 1985.
11. ACC/AHA Task Force Report: ACC/AHA guidelines for the clinical application of echocardiography. A report of the American College of Cardiology/American Heart Association Task Force on Practice Guidelines (Committee on Clinical Application of Echocardiography). J. Am. Coll. Cardiol. 29:862–879, 1997.

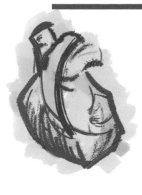

Chapter 11

Approach to the Patient with
Hypertension

HENRY R. BLACK

Although it was not possible to measure blood pressure accurately and noninvasively until early in the 20th century, *more Americans now visit health care providers because of hypertension than for any other reason.* Because of the frequency of hypertension in the general population (Fig. 11–1), every primary care physician needs to understand how to measure blood pressure, how to define hypertension, how to confirm the diagnosis, and finally, how to evaluate persons with hypertension in order to properly assess their risk and plan and implement a successful therapeutic program (see also Chap. 21).

DEFINITION OF HYPERTENSION

In the United States, hypertension has for many years been defined as a diastolic blood pressure of 90 mm Hg or more. Those persons with diastolic blood pressure between 90 and 104 mm Hg were said to have *mild* hypertension; those with diastolic blood pressure between 105 and 114 mm Hg, as having *moderate* hypertension; and those with diastolic blood pressure of 115 mm Hg or higher, as having *severe* hypertension. Those with systolic blood pressure of 160 mm Hg or higher and diastolic blood pressure less than 90 mm Hg were said to have *isolated systolic hypertension;* and those with diastolic blood pressure of less than 90 mm Hg and systolic blood pressure from 140 to 159 mm Hg had *borderline isolated systolic hypertension.*

Although these definitions have served us well, they were drastically revised in 1993 with the report of the Fifth Joint National Committee on the Detection, Evaluation, and Treatment of High Blood Pressure (JNC V; Table 11–1).[1] This system has eliminated the modifiers such as "mild" and "moderate" and has instead introduced the concept of *stages* of hypertension, much as is done in the classification of neoplastic diseases. This change reflects the growing understanding that "mild" hypertension was an inappropriate designation. The prognosis of hypertensive patients depends as much or more on whether end-organ damage or other risk factors are present or absent than it does on the level of blood pressure. "Mild" implies benign and suggests incorrectly to the clinician and the patient that they need not be too concerned. Seventy percent of diastolic hypertensive patients have blood pressures in this range (90 to 104 mm Hg), and more than half of the deaths and disability attributable to hypertension occur in individuals with this level of diastolic blood pressure.

This new system also recognizes the importance of systolic blood pressure in defining the prognosis of a hypertensive individual. Since the early 1970s, it has been known that systolic blood pressure is closely correlated with all of the complications attributable to hypertension (mortality, coronary heart disease, cerebrovascular disease, left ventricular hypertrophy, congestive heart failure, loss of renal size and function). Furthermore, the Systolic

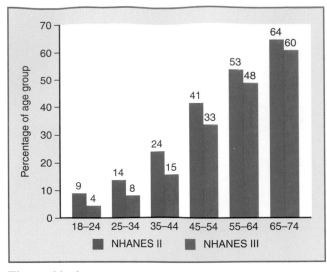

Figure 11–1

Prevalence of hypertension in U.S. adults according to data from the National Health and Nutrition Examination Surveys (NHANES) conducted during 1976 through 1980 (NHANES II) and 1988 through 1991 (NHANES III). Hypertension is defined as mean blood pressure of 140/90 mm Hg or higher based on three readings taken on a single occasion or the use of antihypertensive medications. (Redrawn from Centers for Disease Control and Prevention, National Center for Health Statistics: National High Blood Pressure Education Program Working Group report on primary prevention of hypertension. Arch. Intern. Med. 153:186–208, 1993.)

Hypertension in the Elderly Program (SHEP) showed that treating elderly patients with isolated systolic hypertension dramatically reduced hypertension-related cardiovascular disease and made it impossible to ignore systolic blood pressure.

The stages of hypertension in JNC V were selected because the levels of systolic and diastolic blood pressure impart approximately the same risk. When using this system, the clinician measures blood pressure and then classifies the patient based on the higher of the stages to which the measurement would assign the patient. For example, a person with a blood pressure of 160/94 mm Hg is considered to have stage 2 hypertension, as would another whose blood pressure is 142/106 mm Hg. Those patients with acute end-organ damage, regardless of stage,

are said to have *hypertensive crises*. When hypertensive encephalopathy or pulmonary edema supervenes, these are considered to be *hypertensive emergencies* and require parenteral treatment.

Although this new classification is a major improvement over earlier stratification systems, it still needs further modification. Only 1% of Americans have stage 3 or 4 hypertension, and therefore, these two separate categories may not be needed. Also, the new classification does not highlight the importance of co-morbid conditions on prognosis, although the JNC V authors did suggest that the clinician should specify whether the patient had co-morbidity, such as diabetes mellitus or an elevated serum cholesterol, or end-organ damage, such as left ventricular hypertrophy or renal failure.[1]

The JNC V classification also failed to appreciate the importance of a *wide pulse pressure* (the difference between systolic and diastolic blood pressure), which has been found to be associated with a highly significant independent increase in cardiovascular risk, especially in older persons.[2] Patients with a wide pulse pressure (≥60 to 70 mm Hg) often have an elevated systolic *and* a low or normal diastolic blood pressure. In the absence of aortic regurgitation (or an arteriovenous fistula), such a pattern suggests that the arterial system, particularly the large arteries, is noncompliant, as occurs in the presence of severe atherosclerosis and in elderly patients.

MEASUREMENT OF BLOOD PRESSURE

In 1896, Rivi-Rocci successfully measured blood pressure noninvasively in humans. He compressed the brachial artery with a cuff and used palpation to estimate systolic blood pressure. Janeway, in 1901, first appreciated that sounds emanated from these arteries when the cuff was deflated, whereas Korotkoff, a surgical resident from Russia, published his description of the auscultatory method of estimating blood pressure in 1905. He described the sounds made when arteries are compressed above systolic levels and then slowly released. These "Korotkoff sounds" still form the basis of most noninvasive measurements of blood pressure. It is conventional to deem the systolic blood pressure to be that number when clear and repetitive tapping sounds are first heard (Korotkoff phase 1). Diastolic blood pressure is taken to be the pressure at which sounds disappear (Korotkoff phase 5). Should sounds continue on to zero, then both Korotkoff phase 5 and Korotkoff phase 4 (muffling of the sounds) should be recorded. In general, phase 1 sounds correlate very well with intra-arterial measurements of systolic blood pressure, and true diastolic blood pressure is between phases 4 and 5.

Technique of Blood Pressure Measurement

Many expert groups have evaluated the techniques of blood pressure measurement and generally agree on the following basic principles:

	Systolic Blood Pressure (mm Hg)	Diastolic Blood Pressure (mm Hg)
Table 11–1 **Classification of High Blood Pressure**		
Category		
Optimal	<120	<80
Normal	<130	<85
High normal	130–139	85–89
Stage 1 hypertension	140–159	90–99
Stage 2 hypertension	160–179	100–110
Stage 3 hypertension	180–209	110–119
Stage 4 hypertension	≥210	≥120

Adapted from The Joint National Committee on Detection, Evaluation, and Treatment of High Blood Pressure: The fifth report of the Joint National Committee on Detection, Evaluation, and Treatment of High Blood Pressure (JNC V). Arch. Intern. Med. 153:154–182, 1993.

- Multiple measurements made in the health provider's office on several occasions at least a week apart are necessary to establish an individual's true "casual" blood pressure. Other techniques, such as home or ambulatory blood pressure monitoring, add important information but do not substitute for office measurements.
- The subject should sit or lie quietly for at least 5 minutes before the measurements are made and the pressure should be measured at least 30 minutes after eating, exercising, smoking a cigarette, or drinking a caffeine-containing beverage. In the elderly, who are prone to postprandial hypotension, an even longer wait may be appropriate. Since bladder or bowel distention may also raise blood pressure, the subject should not have a distended bladder or bowel when the reading is taken. The measurement should be made with the arm supported and at the level of the heart.
- An appropriate-sized cuff must be used to avoid overestimating blood pressure (if the cuff is too narrow) or underestimating it (if the cuff is too wide). The width of the inflatable bladder should be 40% of the mid-arm circumference. A variety of cuffs should be available in any office that measures blood pressure, including a "regular" cuff (12 × 23 cm) for those with a mid-arm circumference less than 33 cm, a "large" cuff (15 × 33 cm) for those with a mid-arm circumference of 33 to 41 cm, and a "thigh" cuff for those with even larger arms. The bladder of the cuff should nearly encircle the arm.
- Although mercury sphygmomanometers are generally considered to be the most accurate, concern about the toxicity of mercury has intensified and many states have prohibited their use. Aneroid manometers should be calibrated with a known standard at least every 6 months. Only a few commercially available electronic devices measure blood pressure accurately enough to be recommended.
- The cuff should be carefully placed on the *bare* arm, and the bell or diaphragm of a well-functioning stethoscope should be placed over the brachial artery in the antecubital fossa. The systolic blood pressure should be estimated first by palpation—the pressure at which the pulse disappears and reappears on deflation is used. The cuff should then be inflated to 20 to 30 mm Hg above this level and deflated slowly (2 to 3 mm Hg/sec). Once the systolic blood pressure is noted, the deflation should be continued until the sounds disappear (the diastolic blood pressure).
- The readings should be recorded to the nearest 2 mm Hg. Care must be taken to avoid rounding the numbers to the nearest zero. More than one measurement should be made (within 1 to 5 min), and these should be averaged and reported as the blood pressure for that visit.
- Blood pressure should be measured in both arms at the first visit, and the observers should record both and note which arm has the higher reading. If there is more than a 10-mm Hg difference between the measurements in both arms, the reading in the arm with the higher pressure should be used and the possibility of an atherosclerotic obstruction of an artery in an upper extremity or coarctation of the aorta should be considered. Measurement of blood pressure in the legs may also be helpful if a coarctation is a realistic clinical possibility. It is helpful to check for postural hypotension by measuring blood pressure in the standing position after 1 to 3 minutes. This is clearly necessary in the elderly and in any subject who complains of dizziness or who is being treated with an agent that may cause postural hypotension.

Although blood pressure measurement is one of the most commonly performed office procedures, the steps described previously are rarely followed and the inaccuracy of the measurement may be as high as 15 mm Hg. Since care providers other than physicians (nurses, medical assistants, paramedics) frequently record blood pressure, the responsible physician must be assured that these individuals are properly trained so that their measurements can be relied on. Properly functioning equipment must be provided if readings are to be accurate. All too frequently, sphygmomanometers are in poor repair, leading to incorrect diagnoses and the potential for improper management. In the past two decades, it has become possible to measure blood pressure in settings other than the physician's office or hospital clinic and the use of home blood pressure monitoring and ambulatory blood pressure monitoring has increased dramatically.

Home Blood Pressure Monitoring

Home monitoring is particularly appealing, since it is inexpensive and directly involves the hypertensive patient in his or her care. Some specialists in the care of patients with hypertension feel that most of those with hypertension should purchase or be given a sphygmomanometer and be trained in the technique of blood pressure measurement. Those with poor hearing or problems with manual dexterity can overcome these barriers by using automated devices or enlisting a spouse or friend to make the measurements. Hypertensive patients who use home monitoring must be made aware of the variations in blood pressure with time of day and that criteria for "normal" blood pressure are based on office measurements. It is well established that home readings are lower than office readings, especially in hypertensive subjects. However, home readings tend to correlate better with hypertensive end-organ damage than do physician measurements obtained in the office. The latter also are much more prone to be increased due to the "white-coat effect," an increase in blood pressure due to anxiety or the "alerting reaction" provoked by the presence of a doctor or other care provider. In addition to eliminating or greatly reducing white-coat hypertension, home monitoring is useful for detecting low blood pressure that corresponds to symptoms of weakness, dizziness, or near syncope and in the assessment of the efficacy of therapy.

Although home measurements can be valuable, they must be interpreted with caution. Many factors, including posture, time of day, alcohol intake, exercise, food, and stress, all contribute to the variability of blood pressure, especially in a setting other than the physician's office.

Hypertensive subjects who are monitoring their blood pressure should take readings at a predetermined time of day (e.g., an hour after awakening and when they return from work), and all readings should be recorded and reported to the physician for interpretation, regardless of how the patient "feels" that day. Although patients who can measure blood pressure themselves should be encouraged to obtain a measurement if they feel dizzy or lightheaded, in some hypertensive subjects measuring blood pressure at home can become an obsession and should be discouraged.

Although many instruments are available for home blood pressure monitoring, the accuracy of almost all electronic and automated devices has been questioned. It is often useful to ask patients to bring the device to the office and to calibrate it against the physician's reading. It is clear that home monitoring has a place in the management of hypertensive subjects, but until reliable instruments are widely available and both providers and patients are properly educated as to how and when to measure blood pressure at home, its role can be only adjunctive to office care.

Ambulatory Blood Pressure Monitoring

(Table 11–2)

Ambulatory blood pressure monitoring has a much better defined role in the diagnosis and management of hypertension than does home blood pressure recording. This technique allows for measurement of blood pressure throughout the day and night and provides as many as 80 to 100 separate blood pressure readings during a 24-hour period. This enables the clinician to evaluate blood pressure in settings other than the provider's office and does

Table 11–2	Advantages and Disadvantages of Ambulatory Blood Pressure Monitoring

Advantages

Can take many BP measurements during 24-hr period
Measures diurnal variation (BPs during sleep)
Measures BP during daily activities
Can identify "white-coat" hypertension
No "alerting response"
No placebo effect
Apparent better correlation with target organ damage than other methods of BP measurement

Disadvantages

Cost
Limited availability of equipment
Disruption of daily activities from noise or discomfort (e.g., sleep quality, flaccid arm during measurement)
Lack of "normal" data and treatment guidelines
Lack of long-term prospective studies demonstrating utility compared with traditional (and much less expensive) BP measurements

From Elliott, W.J., and Black, H.R.: Special situations in the management of hypertension. *In* Hollenberg, N.K. (vol. ed.): Hypertension: Mechanisms and Therapy. Braunwald, E. (ser. ed.): Atlas of Heart Diseases. Vol. 1. Philadelphia, Current Medicine, 1995, pp 12.1–12.17.
Abbreviation: BP, blood pressure.

so without the inherent bias of self-measurement, where patients may report only some of the readings. It also elucidates the circadian pattern of the subject's blood pressure.

Currently available devices are battery-driven, lightweight, and reasonably quiet, reducing discomfort and embarrassment for the subject. The instrument can be programmed to measure blood pressure as frequently as necessary. Most clinicians obtain readings three or four times per hour during the waking hours and once or twice per hour at night. Discomfort is minor and tolerable, and most subjects are able to sleep through the measurements.

The devices measure blood pressure in one of two ways. Either a microphone detects Korotkoff sounds (auscultatory method), which are then converted into blood pressure readings, or oscillations from the brachial artery are measured (oscillometric method), which are converted in a similar fashion. Some devices use both methods; some require that electrocardiogram (ECG) leads be placed on the chest so that measurements can be gated to the R-wave, optimizing the detection of the Korotkoff sounds. Both techniques report the individual readings and provide average readings for the day, the night, and the 24-hour period and are programmed to discard measurements considered to be artifactual. The percentage of systolic blood pressure measurements above 140 mm Hg or diastolic blood pressure above 90 mm Hg, the so-called systolic or diastolic loads, can be obtained. The American Society of Hypertension suggested the ranges for each of these parameters, shown in Table 11–3.[3]

Both techniques have problems. Auscultatory measurements are very sensitive to ambient noise and may produce considerable artifact. They often fail to make measurements if the environment is not quiet, as during automobile driving. The oscillometric method is also prone to artifact if the subject has a tremor. This method measures systolic and mean blood pressures and calculates diastolic blood pressure; these calculations are not always precise. Nevertheless, most of the available instruments do provide accurate and reproducible measurements and important insight into blood pressure patterns. Patients in whom ambulatory blood pressure measurements are recorded should keep a diary as to their condition or circumstances at the time the readings are taken. This enables the physician and the subject to understand the relationship between events of daily living and blood pressure, and can help ascertain whether low or high blood pressure readings are associated with symptoms.

The National High Blood Pressure Education Program has reported that average blood pressures vary by age.[4] The cost of performing ambulatory blood pressure monitoring on *all* hypertensive patients is clearly prohibitive and it is often not covered by health insurance. The measurements, however, are very helpful in a number of common clinical situations (Table 11–4).

Diagnosis and Prognosis

Perhaps as many as 20% of persons with stage 1 hypertension and 5% of those with stage 2 will have blood pressure in the normal or borderline range during ambula-

Table 11–3	American Society of Hypertension Values for Home and Ambulatory Blood Pressure Monitoring

BP Measure	Probably Normal	Borderline	Probably Abnormal
Systolic average (mm Hg)			
Awake	<135	135–140	>140
Asleep	<120	120–125	>125
24-hr	<130	130–135	>135
Diastolic average (mm Hg)			
Awake or asleep	<85	85–90	>90
24-hr	<80	80–85	>85
Systolic load (%)*			
Awake or asleep	<15	15–30	>30
Diastolic load (%)†			
Awake	<15	15–30	>30
Asleep	<15	15–30	>30

Reprinted by permission of Elsevier Science Inc. from Pickering, T.: Recommendations for the use of home (self) and ambulatory blood pressure monitoring, American Journal of Hypertension, Vol. 9, pp. 1–11. Copyright 1995 by American Journal of Hypertension, Inc.

Abbreviation: BP, blood pressure.

*Percentage of systolic blood pressure measurements above 140 mm Hg

†Percentage of diastolic blood pressure measurements above 90 mm Hg

tory blood pressure monitoring. These persons are referred to as "white-coat hypertensives." This condition is more common in women than in men and in the elderly than in young adults. In hypertensive subjects who report that readings outside of the office—taken by themselves or others—are always lower than the office measurements, ambulatory blood pressure monitoring can avoid unnecessary antihypertensive therapy. On the other hand, several studies suggest that white-coat hypertensives have larger hearts and more metabolic abnormalities than true normotensives, suggesting that this form of hypertension is merely an intermediate stage between normal blood pressure and sustained hypertension.[5] Whereas pharmacologic therapy may not be necessary in these individuals, lifestyle modification (weight loss, exercise, alcohol reduction, and salt restriction) is warranted in order to prevent the development of sustained hypertension. If demonstrable target organ damage (left ventricular hypertrophy, vascular bruits, hypertensive retinopathy, microalbuminuria, renal insufficiency) or significant co-morbidity (diabetes or glucose intolerance, dyslipidemias, cigarette smoking) is present, ambulatory blood pressure measurement is probably not necessary, since active therapy and

Table 11–4	Uses of Ambulatory Blood Pressure Monitoring

Diagnosis and Prognosis
Evaluation of suspected "white-coat" hypertension
Evaluation of refractory hypertension
Evaluation of circadian pattern of blood pressure
Symptoms
Evaluation of dizziness and syncope
Evaluation of relationship of blood pressure to clinical events
Evaluation of the Efficacy of Antihypertensive Agents

careful follow-up are indicated, regardless of the ambulatory blood pressure monitoring measurements.

The pattern of ambulatory blood pressure measurements can also contribute important diagnostic and prognostic information. Hypertensive subjects can be divided into "dippers" and "nondippers" based on their ambulatory recordings. Dippers show at least a 10% drop in average blood pressure when they are asleep than when awake and they tend to have less end-organ damage and a substantially better prognosis than nondippers.[6]

ASSESSING "REFRACTORY" HYPERTENSIVE PATIENTS. A number of hypertensive subjects appear not to respond to what should be adequate therapy. In some of these, an ambulatory blood pressure monitoring study is valuable in assessing the response to treatment outside the office. It may possibly save them a risky and expensive evaluation for secondary hypertension or the addition of potentially poorly tolerated and expensive drugs to their regimen.

ASSESSING SYMPTOMS. Ambulatory blood pressure monitoring also can be helpful in assessing symptoms suggestive of hypotension and determining whether nocturnal angina or left ventricular failure is triggered by increases in blood pressure.

EVALUATION OF THE HYPERTENSIVE PATIENT

The initial office evaluation of the hypertensive patient should be directed at:

- Confirming the diagnosis
- Assessing the patient's risk for cardiovascular disease
- Determining the cause of the patient's hypertension, that is, excluding the presence of secondary hypertension
- Screening for other important medical problems
- Obtaining information to guide therapy

Although it is clear that extensive and expensive laboratory studies are rarely necessary in the evaluation of the hypertensive patient, the primary care physician must be able to recognize when additional studies or consultation with a specialist is appropriate and warranted. Delaying the discovery of a potentially curable form of hypertension places the patient at unnecessary risk. Failing to properly assess whether end-organ damage or co-morbidity is present may lead to inappropriate therapeutic choices or delay proper treatment.

Confirming the Diagnosis

Blood pressure should be measured under relaxed and controlled conditions after appropriate rest (usually at least 5 minutes) and taken by someone whose ability to do the measurement has been certified. The American Heart Association has shown that 10% to 15% of adults cannot properly hear Korotkoff sounds, and it is wrong to assume that measurements reported by every observer are accurate. Excellent commercial training programs are available that can be used both to train and to validate the competence of observers. The technique for blood pressure measurement described previously (p. 131) should be meticulously followed, and individuals who measure blood pressure should be recertified on a regular basis.

In order to be considered "hypertensive," an individual's blood pressure should be shown to be elevated (the average of two or three readings taken a few minutes apart in the sitting position) at least twice or three times at visits separated by a week or more. Measurements should be made in the supine and the standing positions in subjects with a history suggesting postural hypotension. Patients who exhibit wide disparities in blood pressure and who are hypertensive on some measurements but normotensive on others may need additional measurement or may have ambulatory blood pressure monitoring performed to confirm that they are hypertensive. Treatment should *not* be initiated until the diagnosis is proved, although in rare circumstances—such as when stage 3 or 4 hypertension or active end-organ damage is present—treatment may need to be started after a single set of measurements.

Assessing Risk

Although the highest levels of blood pressure are clearly associated with the highest levels of risk, particularly for cerebrovascular disease, hypertension is just one of several important cardiovascular risk factors. Numerous epidemiologic assessments have shown that the impact of risk factors on outcomes are additive, perhaps even multiplicative. Thus, it is inappropriate to concentrate simply on the level of blood pressure without also knowing about whether other cardiovascular risk factors (lipid abnormalities, cigarette smoking, diabetes mellitus) are also present and, if so, for how long and how severe they are. Hypertensive subjects with other risk factors require earlier and more aggressive treatment. Patients with end-organ damage are also at substantially higher risk and need to be approached more aggressively than those hypertensive subjects free of clinical or subclinical disease.

The key to assessing risk is to ascertain whether the patient already has overt cardiovascular disease, such as a prior myocardial infarction, has experienced angina pectoris or heart failure, or has had any symptoms suggestive of cardiovascular disease. Hypertensive patients should be carefully queried about symptoms that suggest coronary artery disease, cerebrovascular disease, congestive heart failure, peripheral vascular disease, diabetes mellitus, and chronic renal disease.

The interpretation of chest pain in hypertensive subjects may be difficult. Hypertensive patients are at significant risk of aortic dissection, which most commonly presents as an emergency. They may also have small vessel coronary artery disease and develop chest pain that is atypical for angina pectoris. Very often this chest pain syndrome is associated with left ventricular hypertrophy and diastolic dysfunction. The latter is common in patients with a hypertensive cardiomyopathy, and exertional dyspnea is the most common symptom in these patients.

The clinician should determine whether there is a *family history* of premature cardiovascular disease, diabetes, sudden death, and especially hypertension. Information as to how severe the hypertension has been in affected family members, when it began, and what other conditions accompanied it should be noted. Details of the family history may bear large dividends as more inherited hypertension syndromes are identified. Some inherited conditions, such as glucocorticoid suppressible hyperaldosteronism and Liddle's syndrome, may respond to specific therapy.

It must then be determined whether other risk factors, such as an elevated cholesterol or glucose intolerance, have ever been diagnosed and whether the patient is a current or past cigarette smoker. Not only does a history of cigarette smoking substantially increase cardiovascular risk but smokers are much more likely to have peripheral vascular disease, cerebrovascular disease, and renovascular disease; the latter could be the cause of the patient's hypertension (see p. 139).

DETERMINING THE CAUSE OF HYPERTENSION. Whereas 95% of hypertensive patients have essential (or idiopathic or primary) hypertension, that is, the condition in which the specific cause cannot at present be determined, it is important to identify the 5% with secondary hypertension (Table 11–5). Although it is not always possible to cure secondary hypertension—other than when it is due to a drug or substance that can be eliminated—it is still extremely important not to miss the diagnosis, since conventional therapy is often ineffective (see under Secondary Hypertension).

SCREENING FOR OTHER IMPORTANT MEDICAL PROBLEMS. The clinician should not miss the opportunity to use the initial office visit for hypertension to screen for other important medical conditions, especially those that might be subclinical but could be discovered with simple measures. Thus, the initial evaluation of the hypertensive subject should also include those procedures judged to be of value in any routine general medical examination and that have not already been provided to the patient.

Guide to Therapy

With more than 70 antihypertensive agents available in 1998 and more planned to be introduced soon, therapy for hypertension should be individualized. The initial evaluation should be directed at discovering historical, clinical, or laboratory features that might influence the choice of treatment (see Chap. 21).

Much of the most important information needed in the initial evaluation can be gleaned from a carefully performed history, a "directed" physical examination, and a few inexpensive and safe laboratory tests.

Medical History

In addition to assessing risk, a careful drug, environmental, and nutritional history is important during the initial evaluation of a hypertensive patient and throughout subsequent management. It is particularly important to

Table 11–5	Types of Hypertension

I. Systolic and Diastolic Hypertension

A. Primary, essential, or idiopathic
B. Secondary
  1. Renal
    a. Renal parenchymal disease
      (1) Acute glomerulonephritis
      (2) Chronic nephritis
      (3) Polycystic disease
      (4) Diabetic nephropathy
      (5) Hydronephrosis
    b. Renovascular
      (1) Renal artery stenosis
      (2) Intrarenal vasculitis
    c. Renin-producing tumors
    d. Renoprival
    e. Primary sodium retention (Liddle's syndrome, Gordon's syndrome)
  2. Endocrine
    a. Acromegaly
    b. Hypothyroidism
    c. Hyperthyroidism
    d. Hypercalcemia (hyperparathyroidism)
    e. Adrenal
      (1) Cortical
        (a) Cushing's syndrome
        (b) Primary aldosteronism
        (c) Congenital adrenal hyperplasia
        (d) Apparent mineralocorticoid excess (licorice)
      (2) Medullary: Pheochromocytoma
    f. Extra-adrenal chromaffin tumors
    g. Carcinoid
    h. Exogenous hormones
      (1) Estrogen
      (2) Glucocorticoids
      (3) Mineralocorticoids
      (4) Sympathomimetics
      (5) Tyramine-containing foods and monoamine oxidase inhibitors
  3. Coarctation of the aorta
  4. Pregnancy-induced hypertension
  5. Neurologic disorders
    a. Increased intracranial pressure
      (1) Brain tumor
      (2) Encephalitis
      (3) Respiratory acidosis
    b. Sleep apnea
    c. Quadriplegia
    d. Acute porphyria
    e. Familial dysautonomia
    f. Lead poisoning
    g. Guillain-Barré syndrome
  6. Acute stress, including surgery
    a. Psychogenic hyperventilation
    b. Hypoglycemia
    c. Burns
    d. Pancreatitis
    e. Alcohol withdrawal
    f. Sickle cell crisis
    g. Postresuscitation
    h. Postoperative
  7. Increased intravascular volume
  8. Alcohol and drug use

II. Systolic Hypertension

A. Increased cardiac output
  1. Aortic valvular insufficiency
  2. Atrioventricular fistula, patent ductus
  3. Thyrotoxicosis
  4. Paget's disease of bone
  5. Beriberi
  6. Hyperkinetic circulation
B. Rigidity of aorta

From Kaplan, N.M: Systemic hypertension: Mechanisms and diagnosis. *In* Braunwald, E. (ed): Heart Disease. 5th ed. Philadelphia, W.B. Saunders, 1997, pp. 807–839.

ascertain whether the patient is taking any drug, prescription or over-the-counter, or both, or other substance that might elevate the blood pressure (Table 11–6). Of particular concern are nonsteroidal anti-inflammatory drugs and sympathomimetic amines (such as phenylpropanolamine and pseudoephedrine, which are common ingredients in cold and allergy preparations); both of these classes of drugs are now available over-the-counter. Hypertensive subjects should be cautioned to not use drugs in either of these classes on a chronic basis and to try to obtain relief of pain with acetaminophen and of the symptoms of nasal congestion with antihistamines, if possible. If these other modalities are ineffective, the patient may be permitted to use nonsteroidal anti-inflammatory drugs and sympathomimetic amines in acute situations but for only very brief periods of time.

Estrogen/progestin-containing drugs used for contraception will raise blood pressure in some women, although rarely with the low doses now used. If feasible, women who are taking oral contraceptives should discontinue them, perhaps for as long as 6 months, to be sure that they are not the cause of hypertension. Conjugated estrogens with or without progesterone when given for postmenopausal hormone replacement do not raise blood pressure. Hypertensive patients on hormone replacement therapy do *not* need to adjust their regimen.

Other prescription drugs are known to raise blood pressure or interfere with antihypertensive drugs. These include cyclosporine, erythropoietin, corticosteroids, methylxanthines such as theophylline, monoamine oxidase inhibitors, and tricyclic antidepressants. Cocaine and other

Table 11–6	Substances That Can Raise Blood Pressure

Nonsteroidal anti-inflammatory drugs
Sympathomimetic amines
Contraceptive hormones
Methylxanthines (theophylline)
Cyclosporine
Erythropoietin
Cocaine
Caffeine*
Nicotine*
PCP

Abbreviation: PCP, phenylcyclohexyl piperidine (angel dust).
*Short duration.

illicit drugs such as phenylcyclohexyl piperidine (PCP; angel dust) also elevate blood pressure. It is essential to ascertain whether a hypertensive patient has taken any of these agents. Some environmental agents, particularly chromium and lead, may contribute to raising blood pressure, and the individual's exposure to these and other toxins should be determined.

The diet should be evaluated at the initial examination. Salt and saturated (animal) fat intake should be estimated. If salt is not added to the food at the table or in the cooking, the diet is acceptable (<2.3 gm or 100 mEq of Na^+/day) and further salt reduction is not likely to reduce blood pressure substantially. Although not all hypertensive subjects will experience a reduction in blood pressure on a low-salt diet and an increase on a high-salt diet, those who are salt-sensitive will likely benefit from reducing dietary sodium. It is rarely necessary or worthwhile to formally test a patient's salt sensitivity. However, it should be appreciated that in general, blacks, the elderly, diabetic patients, and obese hypertensive subjects are more responsive than others to reducing salt intake.

In addition to keeping salt intake from being excessive, adequate quantities of potassium, magnesium, and calcium should be ingested. The nutritional history should include questions about dairy product intake and whether any mineral or vitamin supplements are being used. Since obesity is a major problem for hypertensive subjects, the initial nutritional history should focus on the caloric intake and the eating pattern. Of all lifestyle modifications, weight loss is the most successful and should be encouraged from the outset.[1]

Social History

Although *alcohol* in moderation (one to two usual-sized drinks per day [24 oz of beer, 8 oz of wine, or 3 oz of spirits]) protects against coronary artery disease, excessive alcohol intake (four drinks or more per day) raises blood pressure. In some patients, reducing or stopping alcohol intake can have very salutary effects on blood pressure. Although *cigarette smokers* tend to be less obese than nonsmokers and populations of smokers have, on the average, lower blood pressures than nonsmokers, it is important to determine whether hypertensive patients smoke and, if so, to induce them to discontinue. Smoking a single cigarette acutely raises blood pressure and heart rate, owing to the nicotine-induced stimulation of catecholamine secretion. This effect disappears in 15 minutes, and it is recommended that blood pressure be taken by at least this interval after smoking.

The history should also ascertain whether the hypertensive leads a *sedentary lifestyle* and whether she or he is interested or able to engage in regular recreational exercise. Even limited aerobic exercise, such as brisk walking 30 minutes three times a week, may reduce blood pressure and improve cardiovascular prognosis. Snoring, daytime sleepiness, and other clinical features of sleep apnea should be noted, since the latter is an underappreciated and underdiagnosed form of secondary hypertension. This information is particularly necessary in obese hypertensive patients. Although it has not yet been shown that reducing *stress* can reliably lower blood pressure, the

home and work environment should be assessed in order to discover any psychosocial issues—such as a lack of finances, transportation, or social supports—that might raise blood pressure or complicate the ultimate therapeutic plans.

In addition, the medical history should carefully ascertain the patient's prior experience with antihypertensive and other agents and be sensitive to any cultural factors or health beliefs that could hinder diagnostic or therapeutic plans.

Physical Examination

The "directed" physical examination in the hypertensive patient should pay special attention to weight and features consistent with secondary hypertension, especially those that were suggested by the medical history.

- The pattern of fat distribution should be noted. Android obesity (waist-to-hip ratio >0.95) is associated with increased cardiovascular risk, whereas gynecoid obesity (waist-to-hip ratio <0.85) is not. Android obesity is also a feature of syndrome of insulin resistance, sleep apnea, and glucocorticoid excess states.
- The patient's skin should be carefully examined looking for café-au-lait spots and axillary freckles, which are cutaneous signs of neurofibromatosis and possibly a pheochromocytoma. Cutaneous signs of hyperlipidemia, such as tendon xanthomata and xanthelasma, should be noted.
- The fundoscopic examination is important. The presence of hypertensive retinopathy (grade 1: arterial tortuosity, silver-wiring; grade 2: arteriovenous crossing changes [arteriovenous nicking]; grade 3: hemorrhages or exudates; grade 4: papilledema) provides definite evidence of end-organ damage.
- The neck should be examined to assess the status of the carotid circulation, and bruits should be listened for.
- The chest should be auscultated for evidence of heart failure and bronchospasm, the presence of which would alter the therapy.
- The examination of the heart should be meticulous. Special attention should be directed to detecting the presence of cardiomegaly, gallops, and murmurs.
- The abdominal examination is one of the most important parts of the "directed" physical examination in hypertensive patients. The examiner should carefully auscultate looking for abdominal bruits, a sign of renal artery stenosis. The search for bruits should include all four quadrants and the back. Diastolic or continuous bruits are common in renovascular hypertension. Systolic bruits in young and thin hypertensive subjects may not indicate arterial pathology.
- The legs and groin should be examined for evidence of peripheral vascular disease (bruits and decreased or absent pulses), since this indicates diffuse atherosclerosis that may also involve the renal artery. The presence of edema should be carefully evaluated.
- The neurologic examination need not be extensive in a hypertensive patient with no history suggesting prior cerebrovascular disease, but it should be com-

plete if a history of stroke or transient ischemic attacks has been elicited.

Laboratory Testing

In most hypertensive patients only a few inexpensive and simple laboratory tests are needed as part of the routine initial and subsequent evaluations. In selected patients, however, extensive testing is not only appropriate but also often necessary to avoid missing secondary hypertension and delaying proper treatment. The laboratory tests that are appropriate for all hypertensives are shown in Table 11–7 and can be divided into those that are done to assess risk, establish cause, screen for important common diseases, and finally, guide therapy.

For uncomplicated hypertensive patients whose history and physical examination offer nothing to suggest a secondary cause of hypertension, the simple battery of tests in Table 11–7 is all that is needed. A full lipid profile and measurement of fasting serum glucose are indicated in hypertensive patients because the prevalence of the syndrome of insulin resistance is high. It is very common to find hypertensive patients with both high serum triglyceride levels and low levels of high-density lipoprotein cholesterol and elevated serum glucose concentrations. The presence of these additional risk factors mandates more aggressive therapy and closer follow-up than would be needed in a hypertensive patient free of these or any other important cardiovascular risk factor.

Routine measurement of serum creatinine and a full urinalysis are recommended for three reasons. The first is to assess risk, since hypertensives with renal insufficiency and proteinuria have a worse prognosis than those free of these abnormalities. Second, these tests are useful in identifying secondary hypertension. Patients with hypertension secondary to chronic renal disease usually have an elevated serum creatinine and may have an abnormal urinalysis with proteinuria and formed elements in the sediment. Third, knowledge of the level of the serum creatinine will guide therapy, since hypertensives with reduced renal function (glomerular filtration rates <30 ml/min) usually do not respond to thiazide diuretics.

The ECG provides important but limited information in most hypertensive subjects. The finding of old myocardial infarction in a patient with no prior history of an event is useful information but is uncommon. The ECG is not a sensitive screening test for left ventricular hypertrophy. In a survey of the Framingham cohort, only 6.7% of those with left ventricular hypertrophy by ECG satisfied the ECG criteria for left ventricular hypertrophy.[7] However, ECG evidence of left ventricular hypertrophy is a potent risk factor for adverse outcome (Fig. 11–2). In blacks, the specificity of the ECG is low, indicating that there are a substantial number of false-positive ECGs for left ventricular hypertrophy in that population. In hypertensive patients who have no other evidence of end-organ damage and stage 1 or 2 hypertension, a two-dimensional directed M-mode or "limited echocardiogram" for measurement of left ventricular wall thickness *may* provide useful information about risk and *may* be worth the cost.

Since hypothyroidism is a cause of secondary hyperten-

Table 11–7	Laboratory Tests Appropriate for All Hypertensive Patients

Assessing Risk

Lipid profile including TC,* HDL-C,* TG*
Serum glucose*
Serum creatinine
Urinalysis including microscopic
12-lead electrocardiogram

Establishing Cause

Serum potassium
Serum creatinine
Urinalysis
?TSH or serum thyroxine level

Screening for Common Asymptomatic Diseases

Complete blood count
Serum calcium
?Stool sample for occult blood, PSA or mammogram in age-appropriate patients

Guiding Therapy

Lipid profile including TC,* HDL-C,* TG*
Serum glucose*
Serum creatinine

Abbreviations: TC, total serum cholesterol; HDL-C, high-density lipoprotein cholesterol; TG, serum triglycerides; TSH, thyroid-stimulating hormone; PSA, prostate-specific antigen.
*Preferably fasting.

sion and often missed, especially in the elderly, a thyroid-stimulating hormone or serum thyroxine measurement may be helpful. It is *not* necessary to measure plasma renin activity (PRA) routinely to screen for secondary causes of hypertension.

Very few screening tests are needed as part of the routine evaluation. These include a serum calcium to look for asymptomatic hyperparathyroidism. If the patient is on schedule to have routine laboratory screening for cancer such as a mammogram, stool for occult blood, or prostate-specific antigen, these could be ordered as part of the evaluation for hypertension.

Several of the laboratory tests ordered for other reasons also serve as a guide to therapy. Abnormalities in the lipid profile, serum glucose, serum uric acid, and serum creatinine, for example, might affect the choice of therapy.

SECONDARY HYPERTENSION

Clues to the presence of secondary hypertension are often provided by a "directed" medical history. Many patients with essential hypertension report an isolated elevated reading some time in their 20s or 30s that was not reproducible or sustained until their 40s or beyond. The level of their blood pressure gradually rises until it reaches a level that is considered to be hypertensive. In the majority of hypertensive subjects, a single drug, if correctly chosen, will effectively control blood pressure, at least at the outset.

Patients with secondary hypertension usually present

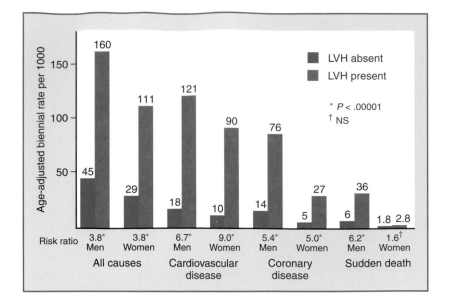

Figure 11-2

Mortality and morbidity associated with left ventricular hypertrophy (LVH) as evidenced by electrocardiogram. Subjects were men and women aged 35 to 94 years during a 36-year follow-up of the Framingham Study. (Redrawn from Kannel W.B.: Natural history of cardiovascular risk. *In* Hollenberg, N.K. [vol. ed.]: Hypertension: Mechanisms and Therapy. Braunwald, E. [ser. ed.]: Atlas of Heart Diseases. Vol. 1. Philadelphia, Current Medicine, 1995, pp. 5.1–5.22.)

with a very different history. Instead of the gradual onset of elevated blood pressure, they usually have a relatively abrupt onset of hypertension, often presenting at a higher stage and with considerable end-organ damage. For many years, it was believed that essential hypertension rarely, if ever, starts after the age of 50 years and that hypertensive patients whose problem began that late in life were likely to have a secondary cause. It is now realized that essential hypertension, especially when manifest as isolated systolic hypertension, can begin at any age; the *new* onset of elevated blood pressure below the age of 30 years or after 50 years should alert the clinician to the possibility of a secondary cause for the hypertension. Thus, the history of the patient's presentation of hypertension should be carefully documented. At what age did it start? How high has the pressure been? Were all prior readings in the normal range? Was it discovered on a routine visit or did the patient have clinical problems related to the elevation of blood pressure or related end-organ damage?

Since patients with secondary hypertension do not respond as well to antihypertensive drugs as do those with essential hypertension, the history of the patient's response to treatment must be ascertained. What drugs were used and at what doses? Did the patient respond initially and then fail? This is a common story in patients with essential hypertension who then develop secondary hypertension, especially atherosclerotic renovascular hypertension.[8]

The response to treatment may also offer important clues to the presence and type of secondary hypertension. Were angiotensin-converting enzyme (ACE) inhibitors or angiotensin II–receptor blockers particularly effective, as one might expect in a patient with renovascular hypertension? Did one of these agents result in a significant but reversible loss of renal function, as also might occur with renovascular hypertension? Was the response to an alpha-adrenoreceptor blocker extremely good, whereas a beta-adrenoreceptor blocker raised blood pressure, as might occur in a patient with a pheochromocytoma? Did even low doses of a thiazide or related diuretic lower potassium excessively and did the patient on a thiazide remain hypokalemic while on an ACE inhibitor or angiotensin II–receptor blocker and potassium supplementation, as is often seen in patients with hypertension caused by excess mineralocorticoid? Were ACE inhibitors or angiotensin II–receptor blockers totally ineffective, as might also occur in patients with mineralocorticoid-excess hypertension?

Laboratory Testing for Secondary Hypertension

All forms of secondary hypertension are unusual in the general hypertensive population. When interpreting tests in a population with a low prevalence of the disease in question, the *sensitivity* of a test (the percentage of those with the disease who have a positive test [see Chap. 2]) cannot be relied on, but rather the *positive predictive value* (the percentage of positive tests done that are true positives) of the test is critical. The predictive value of a test depends on the prevalence of the disease in the patient for whom the test was ordered. Therefore, the medical history, physical examination, and routine laboratory studies are used to select those hypertensive patients who have a higher likelihood of having a particular secondary cause of hypertension. The value of testing is substantively enhanced in this group of patients.

When the medical history, physical examination, or a routine laboratory finding suggests that a patient might have secondary hypertension, establishing or excluding that diagnosis with the proper selection of further laboratory testing is important, especially in patients whose blood pressure is difficult to control. The choice of tests and the order in which they are obtained should depend

Table 11–8	Testing for Renovascular Hypertension: Clinical Index of Suspicion as a Guide to Selecting Patients for Workup

Low (Should Not Be Tested)

Stage 1 or 2 hypertension, in the absence of clinical clues

Moderate (Noninvasive Tests Recommended)

Stage 4 hypertension
Hypertension refractory to standard therapy
Abrupt onset of sustained stages 2 to 4 hypertension at age <20 yr
Hypertension with a suggestive abdominal bruit (long, high-pitched, and localized to the region of the renal artery)
Stages 2 to 4 hypertension (diastolic blood pressure exceeding 105 mm Hg) in a smoker, in a patient with evidence of occlusive vascular disease (cerebrovascular, coronary, peripheral vascular), or in a patient with unexplained but stable elevation of serum creatinine

High (May Consider Proceeding Directly to Arteriography)

Stage 4 hypertension with either progressive renal insufficiency or refractoriness to aggressive treatment, particularly in a patient who has been a smoker or has other evidence of occlusive arterial disease
Accelerated or malignant hypertension (grade III or IV retinopathy)
Hypertension with recent elevation of serum creatinine, either unexplained or reversibly induced by an angiotensin-converting enzyme inhibitor
Moderate to severe hypertension with incidentally detected asymmetry of renal size

Modified from Mann, S.J., and Pickering, T.G.: Detection of renovascular hypertension: State of the art: 1992. Ann. Intern. Med. 117:845, 1992.

not only on the prior probability of finding the disease in question but also on considerations of safety, availability, and cost.

Renovascular Hypertension

Patients with this form of secondary hypertension often have stage 3 or 4 hypertension and considerable end-organ damage and are at risk of losing renal function. At least 80% of cases of renovascular hypertension are caused by atherosclerosis, with only 10% to 15% being due to fibromuscular dysplasia.[8] The remainder are due to unusual causes such as vasculitis, extrinsic bands that cross the renal arteries, and trauma.[9] *Fibromuscular dysplasia,* a distinctive form of arteriopathy, tends to affect young white women in whom blood pressure tends to rise abruptly to stage 3 or 4. *Atherosclerotic renal artery stenosis* is a disease of older individuals. Characteristically, these patients develop hypertension after age 55 or 60 years or have a history of hypertension that had been relatively easy to control and that now has become refractory. A large proportion of these patients have evidence of vascular disease elsewhere (carotids, coronaries, and peripheral circulation, in particular) and the majority are cigarette smokers, often heavy smokers. Although it is more common in whites, blacks can also develop renovascular hypertension.[10]

Laboratory Tests

The objective of laboratory testing in patients suspected of having renovascular hypertension is not only to verify that arterial lesions are present but also to determine that the lesion discovered is, in fact, the cause of the patient's hypertension. A guide to the selection of patients for testing for renovascular disease is given in Table 11–8 and suggested workup is shown in Figure 11–3. The types of testing used to confirm the clinical suspicion that a patient has renovascular hypertension are either biochemical or use a variety of imaging techniques (Table 11–9).

Measurement of serum potassium (which, if low, might indicate hyperaldosteronism) or of PRA (which, if high, might confirm activation of the renin-angiotensin-aldosterone system) has no role in the further case finding for renovascular hypertension. Even measuring the PRA after captopril (the so-called captopril test) has a sensitivity of only 60% to 70%, although better results have been obtained in some series.[11] Measuring the renal vein renin levels on each side and computing the renal vein renin ratio was a very popular approach until recently. The

Figure 11–3
The workup for renovascular hypertension depends on the index of clinical suspicion. (Modified from Siragy, H.M., and Carey, R.M.: Hypertension: Kidney, sodium and the renin-angiotensin system. *In* Hollenberg, N.K. [vol. ed.]: Hypertension: Mechanisms and Therapy. Braunwald, E. [ser. ed.]: Atlas of Heart Diseases. Vol. 1. Philadelphia, Current Medicine, 1995, pp. 3.1–3.16.)

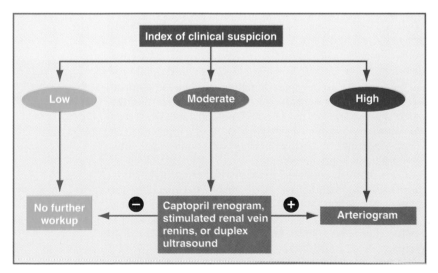

Table 11–9	Detection of Renovascular Hypertension

Biochemical

Serum potassium
Plasma renin activity
Renal vein renin activity
Split renal function tests

Imaging

Rapid sequence intravenous pyelography
Renography
Captopril (or enalaprilat) renography
Intra-arterial digital subtraction angiography
Standard angiography
Duplex renal ultrasound
Magnetic resonance angiography

sensitivity and specificity for detection of renovascular hypertension with this test are approximately 75%, unacceptably low for an invasive procedure that requires special expertise and sophisticated measurements.

Rapid-sequence intravenous pyelography and standard renal scanning were the earliest noninvasive imaging studies used for diagnosing renovascular hypertension. Even though in expert hands they have a sensitivity approaching 65% to 70% for scanning and 75% for pyelography, neither has a place any longer. Renal duplex ultrasound has the advantage of being totally noninvasive and widely available. In some laboratories, the sensitivity approaches 90% to 95%. The presence of gas or abdominal fat may make it difficult to visualize the renal artery. Magnetic resonance imaging (MRI) is a new approach to visualization of the renal arteries that appears to be promising. Dye is not needed, making it safer than angiography and less invasive. However, until the quality of the images improves and the cost becomes lower, this technique is not likely to be widely used.

The two imaging modalities currently favored are isotopic renography with labeled hippurate (a measure of renal blood flow) or diethylenetriaminepenta-acetic acid (DTPA, a measure of glomerular filtration) and intra-arterial digital subtraction angiography.[8,11] The overall sensitivity and specificity of the former, a minimally invasive test, which detects a discrepancy between perfusion of the two kidneys, are well over 90%, especially in patients whose prior probability of having renovascular hypertension is judged to be high. Only ACE inhibitors and angiotensin II–receptor blockers need to be stopped before performing the test, and adverse reactions from the single dose of captopril are rare. The captopril renal scan also provides functional information. If the time to peak activity is initially normal and becomes abnormal after captopril ("captopril-induced changes"), the likelihood of cure or improvement after revascularization is high. Intra-arterial digital subtraction angiography has become the invasive procedure of choice to definitively demonstrate the arterial lesion. Although an arterial puncture is required, the needle used is small and the dye load is modest.

When considering whether to proceed with these studies, the clinician must consider how the data will be used.

In a number of hypertensive patients with renovascular hypertension, the blood pressure is adequately controlled with medical therapy. If the risk of surgery or angioplasty is viewed as unacceptably high or if the patient would not consent to having a revascularization procedure should a remediable lesion be discovered, further evaluation may not be appropriate.

Pheochromocytoma

Patients with pheochromocytoma are almost always symptomatic on presentation. They usually have a characteristic cluster of complaints that occur in paroxysms or "spells." The description of the spell tends to be typical and the same in each patient and may occur several times a day or be separated by weeks or months. Often there is a characteristic trigger (postural change, foods, trauma, pain, drugs) that, if present, should greatly increase the index of suspicion for pheochromocytoma. However, the hypertension is *not* usually paroxysmal, as is often stated, with some blood pressure readings elevated and some normal. Instead, most measurements are in the hypertensive range, although wide variability is the rule. The three most common symptoms of pheochromocytoma are headache, diaphoresis, and palpitations.[12] Many other symptoms, particularly anxiety, weakness, and tremulousness, are also quite frequent. The pattern of symptoms can provide guidance as to the predominant hormone secreted by the tumor. When norepinephrine is the primary hormone, pallor is usually noted; flushing is more prominent if epinephrine is dominant.

Laboratory Tests

Whereas it is possible and sometimes desirable to manage hypertensive patients with renovascular hypertension or mineralocorticoid-excess states with medical therapy, it is almost always imperative to remove a pheochromocytoma. As with renovascular hypertension, once the clinical presentation suggests that a pheochromocytoma may be the cause of the patient's hypertension, a variety of the tests are available to confirm the diagnosis (Table 11–10).

Once pheochromocytoma is suspected, the next step is

Table 11–10	Diagnostic Tests for Pheochromocytoma

Biochemical

Urinary free catecholamines
Urinary vanillylmandelic acid
Urinary metanephrines
Plasma catecholamines (or metanephrines)
Clonidine suppression test

Imaging Studies

Computerized axial tomography
Magnetic resonance imaging
^{131}I-meta-iodobenzylguanidine
Abdominal ultrasound
Adrenal vein or vena caval drainage
Angiography

obtaining biochemical confirmation of an increase in cate-cholamine production. Measurements of 24-hour urinary excretion of total catecholamines (norepinephrine, epi-nephrine, or dopamine) or of their metabolites (vanillyl-mandelic acid or metanephrine) are equally sensitive and specific in the diagnosis (both approximately 85% and 90%).[12] When two or three of these compounds are mea-sured and several samples are sent, both sensitivity and specificity improve. Attention must be paid to the condi-tions under which the sample is collected. To reduce false-positive results, the patient should be in a nonstress-ful situation when the sample is obtained.

When the urinary assays are borderline, the measure-ment of plasma catecholamines may be useful. If plasma catecholamine (norepinephrine plus epinephrine) levels exceed 2000 pg/ml in the basal state, the presence of a pheochromocytoma is likely. If the levels are less than 1000 pg/ml, the diagnosis is highly unlikely, whereas in patients with plasma catecholamine levels between 1000 and 2000 pg/ml, the clonidine suppression test may be useful. If plasma catecholamine levels do not suppress after administration of 0.3 mg of oral clonidine in an appropriately prepared and monitored patient, a further aggressive search for a pheochromocytoma is warranted.

The choice of which initial imaging procedure to ob-tain is also controversial. Computerized axial tomography (CAT) scanning is a highly sensitive imaging modality that will locate nearly all pheochromocytomas, especially those located in the adrenal gland. MRI has the advantage of not requiring contrast material (which is sometimes necessary with CAT scanning) and is also helpful in dif-ferentiating pheochromocytomas from other adrenal or ab-dominal masses. MRI can also be very helpful in localiz-ing nonadrenal or nonabdominal pheochromocytomas.

The use of ^{131}I-meta-iodobenzylguanidine scanning has been particularly helpful when a pheochromocytoma is suspected but is not clearly located with CAT scanning or MRI. This radiopharmaceutical is a guanethidine analog that is concentrated in pheochromocytomas and other neural crest tumors. Using total-body scanning helps to localize the tumor if the initial CAT scan is negative or equivocal. The sensitivity of this test exceeds 90%, but it is still not uniformly available.

Mineralocorticoid-Excess States

Patients with this secondary form of hypertension present a history that is very similar to those with essen-tial hypertension, with the exception of symptoms related to hypokalemia. They may have muscle weakness and muscle cramps from the effects of potassium depletion on skeletal muscle and nocturia, polyuria, and polydipsia secondary to hypokalemic nephropathy. Glucose intoler-ance and hyperglycemia may be present. End-organ dam-age is typically less severe than would have been ex-pected from the level of blood pressure. Although benign aldosterone-producing adrenal adenomas (50% to 60%) and idiopathic bilateral adrenal hyperplasia (30% to 50%) are the most common forms of mineralocorticoid-excess hypertension, the ingestion of large quantities of licorice, which contains glycyrrhizic acid (which stimulates miner-alocorticoid receptors), or the use of chewing tobacco laced with licorice flavoring can cause the same clinical and metabolic features.

Laboratory Tests

A low serum potassium that is discovered as part of the routine evaluation of a hypertensive patient is the most important clue that a mineralocorticoid-excess state may be present. Hypokalemia, especially a serum level of 3.2 mEq/L or less, when not secondary to thiazide ther-apy, indicates that mineralocorticoid-excess hypertension is likely. Hypertensive patients who are hypokalemic on low-dose thiazide therapy (≤25 mg of hydrochlorothia-zide or chlorthalidone) and whose serum potassium stays below normal (3.5 mEq/L) despite potassium supplemen-tation or the concomitant use of drugs that interfere with the renin-angiotensin-aldosterone system (ACE inhibitors or angiotensin II–receptor blockers) may have mineralo-corticoid-excess hypertension.

As is the case for renovascular hypertension and pheo-chromocytoma, the further tests available to confirm the diagnosis of mineralocorticoid-excess hypertension in-clude biochemical and imaging studies (Table 11–11). In addition to confirming the diagnosis of mineralocorticoid-excess hypertension, the clinician must also attempt to distinguish aldosterone-producing adrenal adenomas from idiopathic bilateral adrenal hyperplasia and from unusual causes of mineralocorticoid-excess hypertension such as tumors producing other mineralocorticoids (e.g., deoxy-corticosterone), glucocorticoid-suppressible hyperaldoster-onism, adrenal carcinoma, and drug-induced hyperaldo-steronism (licorice).

In order to properly assess the renin-angiotensin-aldos-terone system, the hypertensive patient should not be tak-ing any drug that may perturb the system. Beta-adrenore-ceptor blockers suppress PRA; ACE inhibitors and angiotensin II–receptor blockers increase PRA, and thia-zide diuretics increase both PRA and plasma aldosterone. Calcium antagonists, especially nifedipine, may suppress aldosterone secretion. These drugs should be discontinued for at least 2 weeks before evaluation. Clonidine or al-

Table 11–11	Diagnostic Studies for Mineralocor-ticoid-Excess States

Biochemical

Serum potassium
Plasma renin activity
Plasma aldosterone
Plasma aldosterone/renin ratio
Urinary aldosterone
Plasma 18-hydroxycorticosterone
Plasma 18-oxocortisol
Plasma 18-hydroxycortisol
Adrenal vein sampling for aldosterone

Imaging Studies

Abdominal ultrasound
Computerized axial tomography
Iodocholesterol scanning
Adrenal venography

pha-adrenoreceptor blockers should be given to control blood pressure during this washout. The PRA and plasma aldosterone should be measured in a state in which aldosterone secretion would normally be suppressed, such as volume expansion or when an adequate sodium intake (>200 mEq/day) has been ingested. Plasma aldosterone levels may be appropriately elevated if the patient is volume depleted, and the PRA may be suppressed because of other conditions such as diabetes mellitus or advancing age. Owing to the normal diurnal variation in plasma levels of aldosterone, measurements should be carried out in the morning, when levels are highest.

Two 24-hour urine collections should be carried out on consecutive days, after a week on the high-salt diet. PRA and plasma aldosterone should be measured in the morning. Total aldosterone and sodium should be measured on each urine sample. This protocol will allow the clinician to confirm that plasma and primary aldosterone are elevated, that PRA is suppressed, and that the findings were not due to interfering drugs, volume depletion, or diurnal changes in plasma aldosterone.

Once the diagnosis of primary aldosteronism is confirmed, it should be determined whether the patient has an adenoma or bilateral adrenal hyperplasia. This distinction is of great importance because adenomas are generally removed surgically or through a laparoscope, whereas patients with bilateral adrenal hyperplasia should be treated with spironolactone and antihypertensive agents. CAT scanning is useful in identifying adrenal adenomas, but the diagnostic accuracy is not nearly as high as it is with pheochromocytomas because adenomas may be well below the 7-mm sensitivity range of CAT scanning. MRI does not appear to improve much on this accuracy. Adrenal venography or adrenal vein sampling may be employed in cases where the results of the noninvasive methods are not diagnostic.

Even if an adrenal mass is located, some feel that biochemical proof that the patient has a functioning adenoma is necessary. Nonfunctioning adrenal adenomas are at least as common as those that produce aldosterone. Adenomas can be distinguished from hyperplasia by measuring the postural effects on plasma aldosterone and 18-hydroxycorticosterone.[13] Patients with adenomas show a fall in plasma aldosterone and 18-hydroxycorticosterone levels from the supine to the upright position. The levels of these hormones in patients with bilateral adrenal hyperplasia, whose renin-angiotensin-aldosterone system is still responsive to normal stimuli, will rise under these conditions.

In selected patients, in whom the possibility of glucocorticoid-suppressible hyperaldosteronism has been raised, a dexamethasone suppression test or a genetic analysis may be appropriate.

Other Forms of Secondary Hypertension

The clinician should inquire into symptoms characteristic of sleep apnea, both hyperthyroidism and hypothyroidism, and Cushing's syndrome because these disorders may be associated with hypertension. Absent or diminished femoral pulses, particularly in children or young adults, suggest coarctation of the aorta.

PATIENT EDUCATION

The approach to the hypertensive patient is not complete until the clinician provides adequate education and advice about the problem. Patients should understand that

- Hypertension is not a disease, but rather a pathophysiologic condition that increases the likelihood of developing a cardiovascular or cerebrovascular complication,[14] but not one that will inevitably do so.
- Blood pressure measurements vary, and those taken in the health provider's office should be followed most closely. Self-measurement can be very useful in monitoring and understanding the day-to-day fluctuations in blood pressure but is not sufficient to direct therapy.
- Although hypertension is rarely cured, it can almost always be successfully treated.
- Systematic introduction of both lifestyle modification and drug therapy, if necessary, is the most effective approach to lowering blood pressure.
- If started on drugs to control hypertension, patients will probably require them indefinitely, unless they make substantive changes in their lifestyle.
- Patients should be strongly encouraged to stay on their regimen and keep their appointments for follow-up visits.

References

1. The Joint National Committee on Detection, Evaluation, and Treatment of High Blood Pressure: The Fifth Report of the Joint National Committee on Detection, Evaluation, and Treatment of High Blood Pressure (JNC V). Arch. Intern. Med. 153:154, 1993.
2. Madhavan, S., Ooi, W.L., Cohen, H., and Alderman, M.: Relation of pulse pressure and blood pressure reduction to the incidence of myocardial infarction. Hypertension 23:395–401, 1994.
3. Pickering T: Recommendations for the use of home (self) and ambulatory blood pressure monitoring. Am. J. Hypertension 9:1–11, 1995.
4. The National High Blood Pressure Education Program Coordinating Committee: National High Blood Pressure Education Program Working Group report on ambulatory blood pressure monitoring. Arch. Intern. Med. 150:2270–2280, 1990.
5. Weber, M.A., Neutel, J.M., Smith, D.H.G., and Graettinger, W.F.: Diagnosis of mild hypertension by ambulatory blood pressure monitoring. Circulation 90:2291–2298, 1994.
6. Verdecchia, P., Porcellati, C., Schillaci, G., et al.: Ambulatory blood pressure: An independent predictor of prognosis in essential hypertension. Hypertension 24:793–801, 1994.
7. Levy, D., Garrison, R.J., Savage, D.D., et al.: Prognostic implications of echocardiographically determined left ventricular mass in the Framingham Heart Study. N. Engl. J. Med. 322:1561–1566, 1990.
8. Setaro, J.F., Saddler, M.C., Chen, C.C., et al.: Simplified captopril renography in diagnosis and treatment of renal artery stenosis. Hypertension 18:289–298, 1991.
9. Stair, D.C., Rios, W.A., and Black, H.R.: Atypical causes of curable renovascular hypertension: A review. Prog. Cardiovasc. Dis. 33:185–210, 1990.
10. Svetkey, L.P., Kadir, S., Dunnick, N.R., et al.: Similar prevalence of renovascular hypertension in selected blacks and whites. Hypertension 17:678–683, 1991.

11. Mann, S.J., and Pickering, T.G.: Detection of renovascular hypertension: State of the art: 1992. Ann. Intern. Med. 117:845–853, 1992.
12. Stein, P.P., and Black, H.R.: A simplified diagnostic approach to pheochromocytoma: A review of the literature and report of one institution's experience. Medicine 70:46–66, 1991.
13. Melby, J.C.: Primary aldosteronism. Kidney Int. 26:769–778, 1984.
14. Williams, G.H.: Hypertensive vascular disease, *In* Fauci, A.S., Braunwald, E., Isselbacher, K.J., et al. (eds.): Harrison's Principles of Internal Medicine. 14th ed. New York: McGraw-Hill, 1998, pp. 1380–1394.

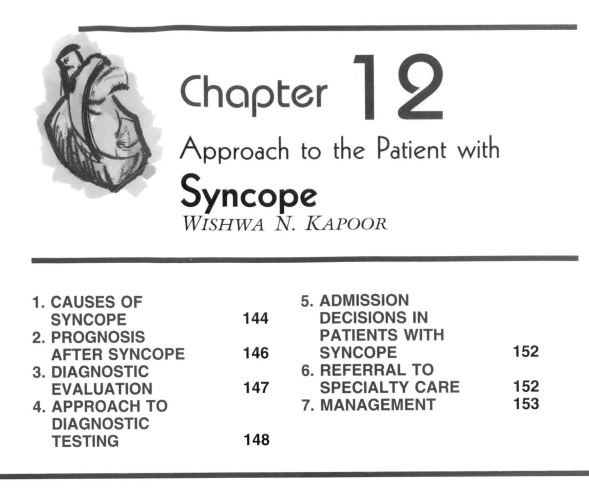

Chapter 12

Approach to the Patient with

Syncope

WISHWA N. KAPOOR

Syncope is defined as a sudden temporary loss of consciousness associated with a loss of postural tone with spontaneous recovery not requiring electrical or chemical cardioversion. Patients with syncope account for 1% to 6% of hospital admissions and up to 3% of emergency department visits. Loss of consciousness is very common in healthy young adults in the community (reported by 12% to 48%), although most do not seek medical attention. Syncope is also a frequent and recurrent symptom in the elderly; a 6% incidence and 23% prevalence of previous episodes were found in one long-term care institution.[1]

Studies have shown that patients with cardiac causes of syncope have a higher 1-year mortality than patients with noncardiac or unknown causes of syncope. The majority of deaths in patients with cardiac causes are sudden. Thus, identifying and treating cardiac causes of syncope are two of the most important issues in the management of patients with syncope.

Primary care physicians are the initial point of contact for the majority of patients with syncope. The questions that the primary care physician needs to address are (1) What is the cause of patient's symptoms? (2) How serious is the potential cause? (3) What tests should be ordered? (4) How rapidly does the workup need to be done? and (5) When should the patient be referred to subspecialists?

CAUSES OF SYNCOPE

Although syncope has a large differential diagnosis, the causes can be classified into four broad categories (Table 12–1). The first category is neurally mediated or neurocardiogenic syncope, which is loss of consciousness resulting from sudden reflex vasodilatation or bradycardia. The entities under this group include syndromes such as vasovagal, vasodepressor, situational, and carotid sinus syncope. A neurally mediated reflex mechanism is also implicated for syncope in association with exercise, especially immediately postexercise in individuals without structural heart disease. Neurally mediated syncope may also occur with the use of drugs, such as nitroglycerin, that decrease venous return to the heart in an upright position. Syncope with aortic stenosis, hypertrophic cardiomyopathy, supraventricular tachycardias, and paroxysmal atrial fibrillation and that related to pacemakers (i.e., pacemaker syndrome) also appear to result from neurally mediated mechanisms. These entities are grouped under cardiac causes for this review because of the potentially worse prognosis for some and specific treatment considerations in the others.

The second broad category is orthostatic hypotension, which may result from age-related physiologic changes, medications, volume depletion, and diseases affecting the autonomic nervous system[2] (Table 12–2 shows the

Table 12-1	Causes of Syncope

Reflex-Mediated Vasomotor Instability	Decreased Cardiac Output
Vasovagal	**Obstruction to Flow**
Situational	Obstruction to LV outflow or inflow
Micturition	Aortic stenosis, obstructive
Cough	hypertrophic cardiomyopathy
Swallow	Mitral stenosis, myxoma
Defecation	Obstruction to RV outflow or inflow
Carotid sinus syncope	Pulmonic stenosis
Neuralgias	PE, pulmonary hypertension
High altitude	Myxoma
Psychiatric disorders	**Other Heart Disease**
Others (exercise, selected drugs)	Pump failure
Orthostatic Hypotension	MI, CAD, coronary spasm
	Tamponade, aortic dissection
Neurologic Diseases	**Arrhythmias**
Migraines	Bradyarrhythmias
TIAs	Sinus node disease
Seizures	Second- and third-degree
	atrioventricular block
	Pacemaker malfunction
	Drug-induced bradyarrhythmias
	Tachyarrhythmias
	Ventricular tachycardia
	Torsades de pointes (e.g.,
	associated with congenital long
	QT syndromes or acquired QT
	prolongation)
	Supraventricular tachycardia

Abbreviations: TIAs, transient ischemic attacks; LV, left ventricular; RV, right ventricular; PE, pulmonary embolism; MI, myocardial infarction; CAD, coronary artery disease.

obstruction, resulting in syncope (see Table 12–1). The mechanism of exertional syncope in entities that cause left ventricular outflow obstruction is widely believed to be neurally mediated responses. In these situations, exercise leads to an increase in left ventricular systolic pressure without a corresponding increase in aortic pressure. This discrepancy may result in excessive stimulation of left ventricular mechanoreceptors, leading to inhibition of sympathetic and activation of parasympathetic tone through cardiac vagal afferent fibers.

Syncope occurs in up to 42% of patients with severe aortic stenosis, commonly with or just after exercise. Myocardial ischemia is also often present during syncope (even in patients without coexistent coronary artery disease), but the role of ischemia in causing syncope is not well understood. Syncope is prognostically important in aortic stenosis, with an average survival of 2 to 3 years after its onset in the absence of valve replacement.

In patients with hypertrophic cardiomyopathy, syncope has similar pathophysiology and is reported in up to 30% of patients. Left ventricular outflow obstruction is worsened by an increase in contractility, a decrease in chamber size, or a decrease in afterload and distending pressure. Thus, Valsalva's maneuver, a severe coughing paroxysm, or specific drugs (e.g., digitalis) may precipitate hypotension and syncope. Ventricular tachycardia is reported in approximately 25% of adult patients with hypertrophic cardiomyopathy and is an important cause of syncope. Predictors of syncope include age less than 30 years, left ventricular end-diastolic volume index under 60 ml/m², and nonsustained ventricular tachycardia. Ex-

causes of orthostatic hypotension). Postprandial syncope occurs especially in the elderly owing to hypotension after meals. A systolic blood pressure decline of 20 mm Hg or more after a meal has been reported in up to 36% of elderly nursing home residents, and this occurs at 45 to 60 minutes in most patients; however, this decline rarely leads to symptoms.

The third category is neurologic disorders, which are infrequent causes of syncope. These disorders include transient ischemic attacks (TIAs), migraines, and seizures. Syncope due to TIAs almost exclusively involves the vertebrobasilar territory. Migraines may be basilar artery–related, or syncope may be a response to severe pain. Seizures may be atonic, temporal lobe epilepsy, or unwitnessed grand mal seizures.

The fourth category includes a large group of cardiac causes that can be divided into diseases associated with severe obstruction to cardiac output, ischemia, and rhythm disturbances.

Obstruction to Flow

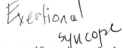

Exertional syncope is a common manifestation of obstruction to flow in which cardiac output is fixed and does not rise with exercise. Structural lesions of either the left or the right side of the heart may lead to outflow

Table 12-2	Causes of Orthostatic Hypotension

Primary

Autonomic failure with multiple system atrophy (Shy-Drager syndrome)

Secondary

General medical disorders (diabetes, amyloid, alcoholism)
Autoimmune disease (Guillain-Barré syndrome, mixed connective tissue disease, rheumatoid arthritis, Eaton-Lambert syndrome, systemic lupus erythematosus)
Metabolic disease (vitamin B_{12} deficiency, porphyria, Fabry's disease, Tangier disease)
Hereditary sensory neuropathies, dominant or recessive
Central brain lesions (vascular lesion or tumors involving the hypothalamus and midbrain, e.g., craniopharyngioma, multiple sclerosis, Wernicke's encephalopathy)
Spinal cord lesions
Familial dysautonomia
Aging

Drugs

Tranquillizers (phenothiazines, barbiturates)
Antidepressants (tricyclics; monoamine oxidase inhibitors)
Vasodilators (prazosin, hydralazine, calcium channel blockers)
Centrally acting hypotensive drugs (methyldopa, clonidine)
Adrenergic neuron-blocking drugs (guanethidine)
Alpha-adrenergic blocking drugs (phenoxybenzamine, labetalol)
Ganglion-blocking drugs (hexamethonium, mecamylamine)
Angiotensin-converting enzyme inhibitors (captopril, enalapril, lisinopril)

Adapted from Bannister, S.R. (ed): Autonomic Failure. 3rd ed. New York, Oxford University Press, 1992, pp. 1–20. Reprinted by permission of Oxford University Press.

tensive hypertrophy and ventricular tachycardia are associated with poorer prognosis.

Effort syncope commonly occurs in pulmonary hypertension (up to 30% in primary pulmonary hypertension) and severe pulmonic stenosis. Patients with congenital heart disease (e.g., tetralogy of Fallot, patent ductus arteriosus, and interventricular or interatrial septal defects) can experience syncope with effort or crying owing to sudden reversal of a left-to-right shunt and a fall in arterial oxygen saturation.

Approximately 10% to 15% of patients with pulmonary embolism have syncope, which is more common in patients with massive embolism (>50% obstruction of the pulmonary vascular bed). Pulmonary embolism may result in acute right ventricular failure and may lead to increased right ventricular filling pressure, decreased stroke volume, decreased cardiac output, hypotension, and subsequent loss of consciousness. Alternatively, activation of cardiopulmonary mechanoreceptors in the setting of increased force of ventricular contraction may be the cause of syncope.

Atrial myxomas may result in obstruction of the mitral or tricuspid valve, leading to symptoms of cardiac failure and, rarely, syncope. Mitral stenosis may cause severe obstruction to outflow, leading to exertional syncope, or loss of consciousness may be caused by atrial fibrillation with rapid ventricular response, pulmonary hypertension, or a cerebral embolic event.

Other Organic Heart Disease

Approximately 5% to 12% of elderly patients with acute myocardial infarction present with syncope. Loss of consciousness may be due to (1) sudden pump failure resulting in a decline in cardiac output and blood flow to the brain and (2) rhythm disturbance such as ventricular tachycardia or bradyarrhythmias. Neurocardiogenic reflexes may also be activated by acute inferior infarction or ischemia involving the right coronary artery. Unstable angina and coronary artery spasm have also been rarely associated with syncope. Syncope is a rare manifestation (in ≤5%) of patients with aortic dissection.

Arrhythmias

(see Chaps. 23 and 24)

Tachyarrhythmias reduce the time available for diastolic filling of the ventricles and cause such a marked reduction in stroke volume that cardiac output declines despite the increase in heart rate, especially with atrial fibrillation or ventricular tachycardia, in which effective atrial kick is lost. The diminished cardiac volume and vigorous ventricular contraction of supraventricular tachycardias and paroxysmal atrial fibrillation also may activate cardiac mechanoreceptors and cause neurally mediated syncope. Syncope in Wolff-Parkinson-White syndrome may be related to the rapid rate of reciprocating supraventricular tachycardia or to a rapid ventricular response over the accessory pathway during atrial fibrillation.

Sick sinus syndrome includes sinus bradycardia,

Table 12–3	Prevalence of Various Causes of Syncope	
Cause	Mean Prevalence (%)	Range of Prevalence (%)
Reflex-Mediated		
Vasovagal	18	8–37
Situational	5	1–8
Carotid sinus	1	0–4
Orthostatic hypotension	8	4–10
Medications	3	1–7
Psychiatric	2	1–7
Neurologic	10	3–32
Cardiac		
Organic heart disease	4	1–8
Arrhythmias	14	4–38
Unknown	34	13–41

pauses, arrest, or exit block. Supraventricular tachycardia or atrial fibrillation may also occur in association with bradycardia, or atrial fibrillation may occur with a slow ventricular response (tachycardia-bradycardia syndrome). Syncope is reported in 25% to 70% of patients with sick sinus syndrome.

Ventricular tachycardias generally occur in patients with structural heart disease. Polymorphic ventricular tachycardia (torsades de pointes) may lead to syncope in the setting of syndromes of congenital prolongation of Q-T interval (with or without deafness) as well as acquired long Q-T syndromes, which occur with drugs, electrolyte abnormalities, and central nervous system disorders. Antiarrhythmic drugs, including quinidine, procainamide, disopyramide, flecainide, encainide, amiodarone, and sotalol, are the most common cause of torsades de pointes.

How Often Are Causes of Syncope Assigned?

Studies of consecutive, generally unselected patients from the 1980s are available to estimate the comparative likelihood of the causes of syncope[3–6] (Table 12–3). The most common causes are vasovagal syncope, organic heart diseases, arrhythmias, orthostatic hypotension, and seizures. The cause of syncope was not diagnosed in 34%. However, the proportion of patients who are currently undiagnosed is probably substantially lower because many cardiovascular testing modalities were not available at the time of these studies. With wider use of event monitoring, tilt testing, electrophysiologic studies (EPS), attention to psychiatric illnesses, and recognition that syncope in the elderly may be multifactorial, a larger fraction are now diagnosable.

PROGNOSIS AFTER SYNCOPE

The 1-year mortality of patients with cardiac causes of syncope has been consistently high, ranging between 18%

Poor prognosis in syncope reflects underlying cardiac disease

and 33%. These rates have been higher than those in patients with a noncardiac cause (0% to 12%) or in patients with an unknown cause (6%). The incidence of sudden death in patients with cardiac causes was also markedly higher compared with the other two groups. Even after adjustments for differences in co-morbid conditions that may affect prognosis, cardiac syncope remains an independent predictor of mortality and sudden death.

Several studies have addressed the question of whether syncope predisposes to increased risk of mortality independent of underlying diseases. In the Framingham study, patients less than 60 years of age experiencing syncope who did not have cardiovascular or neurologic diseases had similar rates of mortality, sudden death, stroke, and myocardial infarction regardless of whether they had a history of syncope. In a study of patients with advanced heart failure, poor left ventricular function was associated with a high risk of sudden death, regardless of the cause of syncope. A recent comparative outcome study of unselected patients with and without syncope showed that underlying cardiac and noncardiac diseases are associated with increased mortality independent of syncope.[7] Thus, the presence of underlying cardiac disease in patients with syncope predicts a worse prognosis. Every attempt should be made to define the underlying structural heart disease in syncope patients and to treat the cardiac diseases to reduce the probability of mortality and sudden death.

There is an important difference in prognosis between cardiac syncope and neurally mediated or neurocardiogenic syncope. Neurocardiogenic syncope has excellent long-term prognosis, although recurrences are common and constitute a major reason for seeking medical care. Similarly, syncope associated with psychiatric disease has no increased mortality but has 1-year recurrence rates of 26% to 50%.

In patients presenting with syncope, the recurrence rate is 34% over 3 years of follow-up.[8] Although recurrences are associated with fractures and soft tissue injury in 12% of patients, they do not predict an increased risk of mortality or sudden death.

DIAGNOSTIC EVALUATION

The history, physical examination, and electrocardiogram (ECG) form the cornerstone of the initial evaluation of patients with syncope and can be used to risk-stratify patients and plan further diagnostic testing.

History, Physical Examination, and Baseline Laboratory Tests

The history and physical examination identify a potential cause of syncope in approximately 45% of patients.[9] Additionally, organic cardiac diseases causing syncope (e.g., pulmonary hypertension, aortic stenosis, pulmonary embolism) are usually suspected clinically and can then be confirmed by specific testing.

A detailed history surrounding the events leading to the episode, the description of symptoms during loss of consciousness, and symptoms after the event are useful in diagnosing specific entities. Table 12–4 shows symptoms that are often helpful in leading to consideration of specific diagnoses. For example, a history of precipitating factors and presence of autonomic symptoms may lead to diagnosis of vasovagal syncope. Similarly, loss of consciousness during or immediately after micturition, cough, defecation, or swallowing may be diagnosed as situational syncope. Neurologic symptoms of brain stem ischemia concurrent with a brief loss of consciousness suggest TIAs, basilar artery migraines, and subclavian steal syndrome. A detailed drug history may provide clues to possible drug-induced syncope.

Specific findings that are particularly helpful on physical examination include orthostatic hypotension, cardiovascular signs, and neurologic examination. Orthostatic hypotension is generally defined as a decline of 20 mm Hg or more in systolic pressure on assuming an upright position. However, this finding is reported in up

---

Table 12–4   Clinical Features Suggestive of Specific Causes

Symptom or Finding	Diagnostic Consideration
After sudden unexpected pain, unpleasant sight, sound, or smell	Vasovagal syncope
During or immediately after micturition, cough, swallow, or defecation	Situational syncope
With neuralgia (glossopharyngeal or trigeminal)	Bradycardia or vasodepressor reaction
On standing	Orthostatic hypotension
Prolonged standing at attention	Vasovagal
Well-trained athlete after exertion	Neurally mediated
Changing position (from sitting to lying, bending, turning over in bed)	Atrial myxoma, thrombus
Syncope with exertion	Aortic stenosis, pulmonary hypertension, pulmonary embolus, mitral stenosis, obstructive hypertrophic cardiomyopathy, coronary artery disease, neurally-mediated
With head rotation, pressure on carotid sinus (as in tumors, shaving, tight collars)	Carotid sinus syncope
Associated with vertigo, dysarthria, diplopia, and other motor and sensory symptoms of brain stem ischemia	TIA, subclavian steal, basilar artery migraine
With arm exercise	Subclavian steal
Confusion after episode	Seizure

Abbreviation: TIA, transient ischemic attack.

to 24% of the elderly and is frequently not associated with symptoms. Thus, the clinical diagnosis of orthostatic hypotension should incorporate the presence of symptoms (e.g., dizziness and syncope) in association with a decrease in systolic blood pressure.

Orthostatic hypotension is detected by measuring supine blood pressure and heart rate after the patient has been lying down for at least 5 minutes. Standing measurements should be obtained immediately and repeated for at least 2 minutes. These measurements should be continued for 10 minutes if there is a high suspicion of orthostatic hypotension but a drop in blood pressure is not found earlier. Sitting blood pressures are not reliable for detection of orthostatic hypotension and should not be used.

Cardiovascular findings may help diagnose specific entities. Differences in the pulse intensity and blood pressure (generally >20 mm Hg) in the two arms are suggestive of aortic dissection or subclavian steal syndrome. Attention to cardiovascular examination for aortic stenosis, hypertrophic obstructive cardiomyopathy, pulmonary hypertension, myxomas, and aortic dissection may uncover clues to these entities.

Initial laboratory blood tests are generally not abnormal, nor do they lead to a diagnosis. Hypoglycemia, hyponatremia, hypocalcemia, or renal failure is found in 2% to 3% of patients, but these are seen more often in patients who are eventually diagnosed as having seizures rather than syncope. These abnormalities are often suspected clinically.

APPROACH TO DIAGNOSTIC TESTING

The clinical assessment and ECG are the initial steps in the evaluation of patients with syncope. As noted in Figure 12–1, this assessment may lead to a diagnosis or provide suggestive evidence for specific entities (e.g., signs of aortic stenosis or idiopathic hypertrophic subaortic stenosis). These clues can be pursued with further testing to confirm or exclude these entities as the causes of syncope. In a large group of patients, however, the initial clinical evaluation does not lead to a specific diagnosis or point to a potential cause of syncope. These patients can be divided into two groups: those with structural heart disease or abnormal ECG and those without underlying heart disease. Patients with structural heart disease or abnormal ECG should undergo Holter monitoring (or monitoring in a telemetry unit), and if diagnostic arrhythmias are found, treatment can be initiated. Patients with nondiagnostic or negative Holter monitoring but with multiple syncopal episodes can be further evaluated using loop monitoring. Patients with nondiagnostic loop monitoring or those with one or rare episode of syncope should undergo EPS for the evaluation of possible arrhythmic syncope.

In patients without structural heart disease or abnormal ECG but with multiple episodes of syncope, tilt testing and psychiatric evaluation should be considered as the initial areas of investigation (see Fig. 12–1). Loop monitoring may be also be considered for detection of arrhythmias (especially bradyarrhythmias or supraventricular tachycardias) in patients with clinical suspicion of arrhythmic syncope but without known structural heart disease. Patients with one episode of syncope can be followed closely without further workup, if clinical evaluation is negative and psychiatric illnesses are not clinically suggested as a cause of syncope.

12-Lead ECG

An ECG is recommended in all patients with syncope,[9] since abnormalities found on ECG may guide further evaluation or make a specific diagnosis. In one study, approximately 50% of the patients had an abnormal ECG, including bundle branch block, old myocardial infarction, and left ventricular hypertrophy. However, causes of syncope are rarely assigned (in <5% of patients) on the basis of the ECG and rhythm strip because of the transient nature of arrhythmias.

Prolonged ECG Monitoring

Ambulatory monitoring is often difficult to interpret when it is used for the diagnostic evaluation of patients with syncope because of the rarity of symptoms during monitoring.[10] In studies using 12 or more hours of monitoring, approximately 4% of patients had symptoms concurrently with arrhythmias. In another 17% of patients, symptoms were reported but no arrhythmias were found, thus potentially excluding arrhythmias as a cause of symptoms. In approximately 79% of patients, there were no symptoms, but brief arrhythmias were found in 13%.[11] In the absence of symptoms during monitoring, finding brief or no arrhythmias does not exclude arrhythmic syncope. Brief arrhythmias are nonspecific and can be found in asymptomatic healthy individuals. Additionally, absence of arrhythmias on monitoring does not exclude arrhythmic syncope, since they are episodic and may not be captured during monitoring. In patients with a high pretest probability of arrhythmias, such as brief sudden loss of consciousness without prodrome, patients with abnormal ECG, or those with structural heart disease, further evaluation is needed to establish or exclude arrhythmias as a cause of syncope.

One study evaluated the yield of Holter monitoring for a duration longer than 24 hours.[12] Extending the duration of monitoring to 72 hours increased the yield of brief arrhythmias from 14% during the first day to an additional 11% during the second day and a further increase of 4% during the third day. However, none of the arrhythmias found during the second and third days of monitoring was associated with symptoms. Therefore, 24 hours of monitoring is sufficient in the initial evaluation of patients with syncope when arrhythmias are suspected clinically.

Long-Term Ambulatory Loop Event Monitoring

Loop ECG monitoring is a noninvasive test enabling patients to be monitored for prolonged periods of times

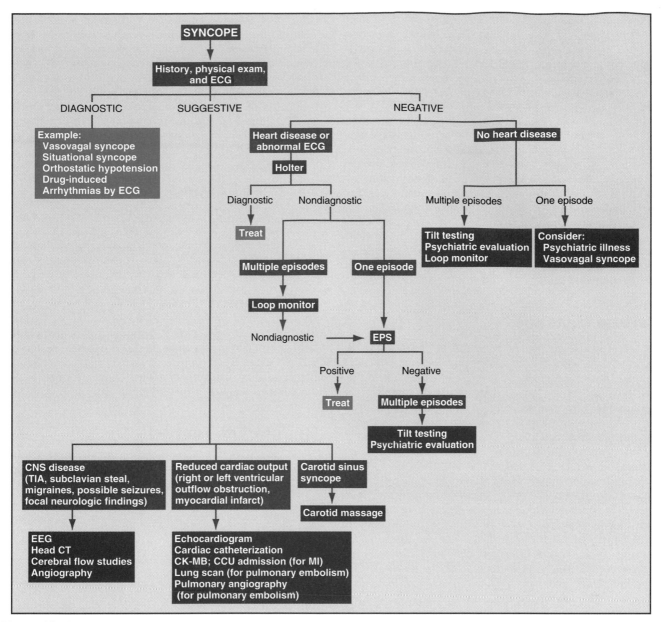

Figure 12–1

Diagnostic approach to the patient with syncope. ECG, electrocardiogram; EPS, electrophysiologic study; CNS, central nervous system; EEG, electroencephalogram; CT, computed tomography; CK-MB, CK-MB isoenzyme of creatine kinase; CCU, coronary care unit; MI, myocardial infarction.

(such as for a month or more).[10] Loop monitors generally use two chest ECG leads that are continuously worn and connected to a small recorder. Loop monitors can be activated after a syncopal episode and can record 2 to 5 minutes of rhythm strip before the activation and 30 to 60 seconds of the rhythm after the activation. Tracings can be transmitted via telephone. Loop monitoring is attractive because it provides the capability of ECG recording during a symptomatic period. Studies of loop monitoring show that arrhythmias with symptoms are found in 8% to 20% of patients.[13] In an additional 12% to 27%, there are symptoms without concurrent arrhythmias. This test is recommended in patients with recurrent syncope when there is a high probability of a recurrent event during the monitoring period.

Electrophysiologic Studies

EPS is an invasive modality often requiring hospital admission (see Chap. 23). EPS utilizes electrode catheters and electrical stimulation protocols to determine (1) cardiac conduction system abnormalities that may be associated with bradyarrhythmias and (2) evidence of tachyarrhythmias as a potential cause of syncope. There is a great deal of variation in protocols for EPS. Protocols for programmed ventricular stimulation generally include a minimum of three extra stimuli at one ventricular site. More aggressive protocols, such as ventricular stimulation at two sites and the use of isoproterenol, are associated with high rates of false-positive results. A large number of findings are nonspecific and difficult to utilize in management decisions. The findings most helpful diagnostically in patients with syncope include (1) induction of sustained monomorphic ventricular tachycardia, (2) prolonged corrected sinus node recovery time (> 1000 msec), (3) prolonged His-ventricle interval greater than 90 msec, and (4) spontaneous or induced infra-His block.[10]

In patients with structural heart disease or abnormal ECG, the diagnostic yield of EPS is approximately 50%. In patients without structural heart disease, the diagnostic yield is approximately 10%. The structural heart diseases in these studies include coronary artery disease, congenital or valvular heart disease, and cardiomyopathy. Particularly important ECG findings include bundle branch block, prior myocardial infarction, and evidence of bypass tract. Bradyarrhythmias are much more likely to be diagnosed in patients with conduction disease on the surface ECG, but the sensitivity and specificity of EPS for detection of bradyarrhythmias are low.[14]

Carotid Massage

Carotid sinus syncope is diagnosed in patients who are found to have carotid sinus hypersensitivity and who have reproduction of spontaneous symptoms during carotid sinus massage. In the absence of symptom reproduction, carotid sinus syncope is likely when carotid sinus hypersensitivity is found and (1) spontaneous episodes are related to activities that press or stretch the carotid sinus or (2) the patient has recurrent syncope with a negative evaluation.

Carotid sinus hypersensitivity is detected by carotid sinus massage. Carotid sinus massage is generally performed in the supine position and repeated in the sitting and standing positions if the vasodepressor variety of carotid hypersensitivity is suspected and the supine test is negative. Noninvasive ECG and blood pressure monitoring are needed for the interpretation of the results. Mixed cardioinhibitory and vasodepressor response is diagnosed when carotid sinus massage is performed after cardioinhibitory response is abolished with atropine or atrioventricular sequential pacing. The duration of massage has varied from 5 to 40 seconds, but recent studies have used 6 to 10 seconds. Simultaneous bilateral massage should never be done. At least 15 seconds should be allowed between massage from one side to the other. Complications of carotid sinus massage include prolonged asystole, ventricular fibrillation, transient or permanent neurologic deficit, and sudden death. Complication rates are considered extremely low (incidence of neurologic complications < 0.2%); however, in patients with cerebrovascular disease, the test should be done only if all other diagnostic modalities are exhausted and the pretest probability of carotid sinus syncope remains high.

Carotid sinus massage is recommended when symptoms are suggestive of carotid sinus syncope (see Table 12–4) and in elderly patients with unexplained syncope.

Echocardiogram

An echocardiogram is recommended when clinical assessment suggests organic cardiac disease as a possible cause of syncope (e.g., clinical findings of possible aortic stenosis, hypertrophic cardiomyopathy, pulmonary hypertension). Echocardiography in the absence of clinical evidence of organic heart diseases as causes of syncope rarely reveals unexpected findings that lead to a cause for syncope. Even in patients with known heart disease, the usefulness of the echocardiogram is low unless obstruction to inflow or outflow is suspected. This test is not recommended for screening purposes in patients with syncope.

Exercise Testing

An exercise ECG is recommended for the evaluation of symptoms with exercise and for the diagnosis of ischemia or exercise-induced tachyarrhythmias. This test is also recommended for the evaluation of postexertional syncope in patients without clinical structural heart disease. The yield of exercise testing in the diagnosis of the cause of syncope is very low (< 1%). Exercise testing is useful as an ancillary diagnostic tool for evaluation of ischemic heart disease in patients with arrhythmic syncope, particularly ventricular tachycardia. In these patients, in addition to the treatment of ventricular arrhythmias, exercise testing or cardiac catheterizations, or both, are often needed for the management of underlying cardiac disease.

Upright Tilt Testing

Maintaining the patient in an upright position for a brief duration on a tilt table has become a common means of testing for predisposition to vasovagal syncope. The pathophysiologic mechanism of syncope with upright tilt testing is not entirely understood. It is widely accepted that hypotension or bradycardia during upright tilt testing is equivalent to spontaneous vasovagal syncope. This is supported by the fact that the temporal sequence of blood pressure and heart rate changes during tilt testing is similar to that of spontaneous spells. Additionally, catecholamine release immediately before tilt-induced syncope is similar to that in spontaneous vasovagal faint.

Upright posture leads to pooling of blood in the lower limbs, resulting in decreased venous return. The normal compensatory response to upright posture is reflex tachycardia, more forceful contraction of the ventricles, and vasoconstriction. However, in individuals susceptible to vasovagal syncope, this forceful ventricular contraction, in the setting of a relatively empty ventricle, may activate the cardiac mechanoreceptors, triggering reflex hypotension or bradycardia. Catecholamine release is also important in precipitating syncope. Catecholamines increase ventricular contraction and thereby may also activate the nerve endings responsible for triggering this reflex. Thus, catecholamines have been used to facilitate positive responses during upright tilt testing.

Tilt testing is generally performed by cardiology services in electrophysiology laboratories. Table 12–5 shows general procedures for tilt testing.[15, 16] The testing is done using a motorized tilt table with a footboard support where position can be changed rapidly. Testing is often performed with the patient in a fasting state, and vasoactive drugs (e.g., calcium channel blockers, vasodilators,

Table 12–5	Tilt-Table Testing Technique
Laboratory	Quiet, dim lighting, comfortable temperature
	20–45-min supine equilibration period
Patient	Fasting overnight or for several hours before procedure
	Parenteral fluid replacement
	Follow-up studies at similar times of day
Recordings	Minimum of three ECG leads continuously recorded
	Beat-to-beat blood pressure recordings using the least intrusive means (may not be feasible in children)
Table	Footboard support
	Smooth, rapid transitions (up and down)
Tilt angle	60–80° acceptable
	70° becoming most common
Tilt duration	Initial drug-free tilt 30–45 min
Pharmacologic provocation	Isoproterenol (infusion preferred)
Supervision	Nurse or laboratory technician experienced in tilt-table technique and cardiovascular laboratory procedures
	Physician in attendance or in proximity and immediately available

Adapted from *Journal of the American College of Cardiology,* Vol. 28, Benditt, D.G., Ferguson, D.W., Grubb, B.P., et al., Tilt table testing for assessing syncope, pp. 263–275, Copyright 1996, with permission from the American College of Cardiology.
Abbreviation: ECG, electrocardiogram.

diuretics) are withheld before testing (for approximately 5 half-lives). It is preferable to measure blood pressure noninvasively during upright tilt testing (e.g., with a blood pressure cuff or digital plethysmography), since invasive intra-arterial catheterization may provoke vasovagal reactions (decrease specificity in older patients) and increase the cost and complexity of testing.

Two general types of testing procedures (Table 12–6) include upright tilt testing alone (passive testing) and tilt testing in conjunction with a chemical agent.[17] The vast majority of the reported studies employ passive testing or use isoproterenol after a brief period of passive tilt testing. Protocols using other agents (e.g., edrophonium, intravenous or sublingual nitroglycerin) are not recommended for general use because of limited data on their accuracy.

Widely used passive tilt testing protocols utilize a tilt angle of 60 degrees for a total duration of 30 to 45 minutes. Common protocols with isoproterenol use an initial passive phase for 10 to 15 minutes at 80 degrees. If an endpoint of the study is not reached, the patient is brought to a supine position and isoproterenol infusion is started at a rate of 1 μg/min and the patient is retilted for 10 to 15 minutes. If the patient does not develop an endpoint, he or she is again brought to a supine position and the isoproterenol infusion rate is increased. This tilting procedure is continued with increasing doses of isoproterenol until a positive response or another endpoint (e.g., maximal dose of 3 to 5 μg/min, adverse effects, or development of severe tachycardia) is reached. The positive response is syncope or presyncope in association with hypotension or bradycardia. There are many variations of this protocol, including titrating isoproterenol infusion rates to increase the baseline heart rate by 20%.

Approximately 50% of patients with unexplained syn-

Table 12–6	Commonly Used Tilt Protocols

Passive (Drug-Free) Protocols

30–45 min of drug-free tilt
Angle 60–80°

Protocols Using Isoproterenol

Use isoproterenol if drug-free tilt is negative (for 30–45 min)
Return patient to supine position
Begin infusion of isoproterenol at 1 μg/min
After 10 min of supine, retilt for 10 min
Repeat procedure until maximal infusion rates (3 μg/min)
Another common protocol—infuse isoproterenol to raise heart rate by 20% after returning patient to a supine position; retilt once heart rate is ≥20% of baseline

Endpoint of a Positive Test

Hypotension or bradycardia and reproduction of symptoms

cope have a positive response to passive tilt testing (Table 12–7). With isoproterenol, overall positive responses are approximately 66%, two-thirds of which occur during the isoproterenol phase. With either type of testing, approximately two-thirds of the responses appear to be cardioinhibitory (defined as bradycardia with or without associated hypotension) and the remaining are pure vasodepressor reactions (defined as hypotension without significant bradycardia). The higher proportion of positive responses with chemical stimulation is probably due to augmentation with isoproterenol, although the effect of angle and duration of testing and other variables is not entirely clear.

The sensitivity of tilt testing can be calculated by examining patients with a clinical diagnosis of vasovagal syncope, since there are no other gold standards. Using this approach, the sensitivity of tilt testing is 67% to 83%. Specificity has generally been evaluated by performing upright tilt testing in subjects without prior syncope. With passive tilt testing, specificity has been variable and has ranged between 0% and 100%, although an overall rate is approximately 90%. The overall specificity of upright tilt testing with isoproterenol is approximately 75%, with a range of 35% to 100%.

When repeat testing is performed on the same day or days later, a reproducibility of 65% to 85% is reported,

Table 12–7	Positive Responses in Patients With Unexplained Syncope*	
	% Positive	**Range†**
Passive tilt only	49	26–90
Isoproterenol tilt, passive phase	23	0–57
Isoproterenol phase	48	12–81
Overall	64	39–87

Adapted from American Journal of Medicine, Vol. 97, Kapoor, W.N., Smith, M., and Miller, N.L., Upright tilt testing in evaluating syncope: A comprehensive literature review, pp. 78–88, Copyright 1994, with permission from Excerpta Medica Inc.
* Summary of results from studies reported in the literature.
† Range refers to percentage of positive responses reported from the studies in the literature.

except for one study that has shown a lack of reproducibility.[18] An initial negative study is rarely positive on repeat testing.

INDICATIONS. Upright tilt testing is recommended in patients with recurrent unexplained syncope in whom cardiac causes have been excluded or are not likely. Initial testing is recommended using a passive protocol for 45 to 60 minutes.[16] In patients with a negative passive test and a high likelihood of neurally mediated syncope clinically (e.g., a young patient with concurrent autonomic symptoms), additional testing with isoproterenol is recommended. It is not possible to recommend any one protocol for this test. Women of childbearing age should undergo a pregnancy test before tilt testing, since the tilt testing should be avoided in pregnant women. Older patients (age >50 years) or patients with a history of ischemic heart disease should also undergo stress testing before tilt testing, since isoproterenol and precipitating hypotension are best avoided in patients with significant ischemic heart disease. Tilt testing is generally contraindicated in patients with cerebrovascular disease.

Neurologic Testing

Skull films, lumbar puncture, radionuclide brain scan, and cerebral angiography do not generally yield diagnostic information for a cause of syncope in the absence of clinical findings suggestive of a specific neurologic process. Studies of electroencephalograms in syncope have shown that in 1% of patients, an epileptiform abnormality was found; almost all of these were suspected clinically.[19] Treatment based on electroencephalography was initiated in 1% to 2% of patients. Head computed tomography scans are rarely useful to assign a cause, but these are needed if subdural bleed owing to head injury or seizure as a cause of syncope is suspected.

Rarely, specific tests of autonomic function may be useful to define the cause of diseases responsible for postural hypotension or when no clear reason for orthostasis is apparent. These tests are not recommended routinely, since clinical data with a focus on autonomic symptoms, diseases causing orthostatic hypotension, and drugs frequently provide clues to the cause of orthostatic hypotension, and there is often little need for additional diagnostic testing or for therapy selection.

Psychiatric Assessment

Psychiatric illnesses need to be considered as a cause of syncope, especially in young patients and those with multiple syncopal episodes who also have other nonspecific complaints. High clinical suspicion for these disorders is needed, since they are often not diagnosed in medical patients. The disorders that may cause syncope include generalized anxiety and panic disorders, major depression, somatization disorder, and alcohol and substance abuse. Screening instruments for these disorders are available and recommended. A high rate of recurrence of syncope in these patients makes detection of these illnesses especially important.[20]

ADMISSION DECISIONS IN PATIENTS WITH SYNCOPE

Most syncope patients presenting to primary care physicians can be evaluated and treated as outpatients. Patients should be admitted to the hospital if a rapid diagnostic evaluation is deemed necessary mainly because of concerns about serious arrhythmias, sudden death, newly diagnosed serious cardiac disease (e.g., aortic stenosis, myocardial infarction), and new onset of seizure or stroke (Table 12–8). Patients with evidence of possible acute ischemia or infarction on ECG, chest pain, congestive heart failure, and those taking medications capable of provoking malignant arrhythmias should be admitted. Occasionally, admission may also be needed for treatment when the cause is clear (e.g., management of dehydration or subarachnoid bleed). In the large group of patients with unexplained syncope after initial history, physical examination, and ECG, risk stratification for arrhythmias and sudden death should guide the admission decision. Factors related to these two outcomes include the presence of structural heart disease and an abnormal ECG.

Elderly patients are often hospitalized for rapid workup because of the concern about the asymptomatic presence of underlying heart disease (especially coronary disease). Additionally, there is often a concern that recurrence of syncope may result in severe injury, such as fractures or a subdural bleed.

REFERRAL TO SPECIALTY CARE

Since syncope has a large differential diagnosis, multiple consultations are frequently requested for diagnostic evaluation and management. The primary care physician can utilize the initial clinical assessment for judicious use of specialty services. Specialty consultation can be approached as follows:

HISTORY AND PHYSICAL EXAMINATION LEAD TO A DIAGNOSIS OF A SPECIFIC CAUSE. The entities found as causes of syncope can often be treated without the need for consultation. Examples in-

Table 12–8	Admission Decision

Admission Generally Indicated

History	CAD, CHF, ventricular arrhythmias, chest pain
Physical examination	AS, focal neurologic findings
ECG	Ischemia, arrhythmias, long Q-T, BBB

Admission Often Indicated

Sudden LOC with injury, frequent spells
Suspicion of CAD or arrhythmias
Age >70 yr, severe orthostatic hypotension

Abbreviations: CAD, coronary artery disease; CHF, congestive heart failure; AS, aortic stenosis; ECG, electrocardiogram; BBB, bundle branch block; LOC, loss of consciousness.

clude volume depletion, cough syncope, clinical vasovagal syncope, and neuralgia.

HISTORY AND PHYSICAL EXAMINATION SUGGEST SPECIFIC ENTITIES. In these instances, further testing is generally needed to confirm or exclude the entities under consideration. Obtaining the results of specific testing is recommended before consultations, since the results of testing may determine the need for consultation. For example, when aortic stenosis or hypertrophic cardiomyopathy is considered clinically, an echocardiogram may be useful to include or exclude the diagnosis. If the possibility of specific cardiac conditions is still a consideration after appropriate noninvasive testing, cardiology consultation for cardiac catheterization may be needed.

UNEXPLAINED SYNCOPE. In these situations, the following consultation may be needed:

1. If arrhythmias are under consideration clinically (such as in patients with structural heart disease) and Holter and loop monitoring have been nondiagnostic, EPS may be needed for diagnosis and therapy. Consultation by a cardiac electrophysiologist is recommended under these circumstances.
2. If neurally mediated syncope is a major consideration, tilt testing is often needed for diagnosis. Consultation with a cardiac electrophysiologist is recommended, although the primary care physician can effectively manage these patients after the results of testing are received.

MANAGEMENT ISSUES. Rarely, patients with syncope have multiple possible causes. This situation commonly arises in the elderly who may have cardiovascular diseases, may be taking multiple medications, and may have orthostatic hypotension. In these situations, the primary care physician should work closely with multiple specialists to coordinate the care of the patient.

MANAGEMENT

Treatment of neurally mediated syncope includes patient education, pharmacologic agents, and dual-chamber pacing. All patients should be instructed on ways of preventing episodes by avoiding provocative factors and by maneuvers that prevent loss of consciousness. Patient education includes avoiding triggers such as prolonged standing, heat, large meals, fasting, lack of sleep, alcohol, and dehydration. Patients should be instructed to assume a supine position when premonitory symptoms occur and to avoid activities that may lead to serious injury.

Drug therapy should be reserved for patients with recurrent syncope who have not responded to nonpharmacologic measures. Table 12–9 shows drugs often used for neurally mediated syncope. Most widely used treatments include beta blockers and salt in combination with fludrocortisone. The data on the effectiveness of treatments are primarily uncontrolled case series, although one randomized trial of atenolol showed improvement in symptoms in the treated group at 1 month.

Dual-chamber pacemakers have rarely been used to treat neurally mediated syncope that is associated with severe bradycardia or asystole. Studies using temporary pacing show improvement in cardiac index and blood pressure on repeat tilt testing as well as amelioration of symptoms. However, there are no long-term studies to show the effectiveness of pacemakers in the treatment of vasovagal syncope.

Table 12–9	Commonly Used Therapies for Recurrent Vasovagal Syncope
Therapies	**Dose**
Beta blockers	
Atenolol	25–200 mg/day
Metoprolol	50–200 mg/day
Propranolol	40–160 mg/day
Disopyramide	200–600 mg/day
Fludrocortisone	0.1–1 mg/day
Fluoxetine	20–40 mg/day
Scopolamine patch	1 patch every 3 days
Theophylline	6–12 mg/kg/day

References

1. Lipsitz, L.A., Wei, J.Y., and Rowe, J.W.: Syncope in an elderly, institutionalized population: Prevalence, incidence, and associated risk. Q. J. Med. 55:45–55, 1985.
2. Lipsitz, L.A.: Orthostatic hypotension in the elderly. N. Engl. J. Med. 321.952–956, 1989.
3. Day, S.C., Cook, E.F., Funkenstein, H., and Goldman, L.: Evaluation and outcome of emergency room patients with transient loss of consciousness. Am. J. Med. 73:15–23, 1982.
4. Kapoor, W.N.: Evaluation and outcome of patients with syncope. Medicine 69:160–175, 1990.
5. Martin, G.J., Adams, S.L., Martin, H.G., et al.: Prospective evaluation of syncope. Ann. Emerg. Med. 13:499–504, 1984.
6. Silverstein, M.D., Singer, D.E., Mulley, A., et al.: Patients with syncope admitted to medical intensive care units. JAMA 248: 1185–1189, 1982.
7. Kapoor, W.N., and Hanusa, B.H.: Is syncope a risk factor for poor outcomes? Comparison of patients with and without syncope. Am. J. Med. 100:646–655, 1996.
8. Kapoor, W.N., Peterson, J., Wieand, H.S., and Karpf, M.: Diagnostic and prognostic implications of recurrences in patients with syncope. Am. J. Med. 83:700–708, 1987.
9. Linzer, M., Yang, E.H., Estes, M., III, et al.: Diagnosing syncope: Part 1: Value of history, physical examination, and electrocardiography. Ann. Intern. Med. 126:989–996, 1997.
10. Linzer, M., Yang, E.H., Estes, M., III, et al.: Diagnosing syncope: Part 2: Unexplained syncope. Ann. Intern. Med. 127:76–86, 1997.
11. DiMarco, J.P., and Philbrick, J.T.: Use of ambulatory electrocardiographic (Holter) monitoring. Ann. Intern. Med. 113:53–68, 1990.
12. Bass, E.B., Curtiss, E.I., Arena, V.C., et al.: The duration of Holter monitoring in patients with syncope: Is 24 hours enough? Arch. Intern. Med. 150:1073–1078, 1990.
13. Linzer, M., Pritchett, E.L.C., Pontinen, M., et al.: Incremental diagnostic yield of loop electrocardiographic recorders in unexplained syncope. Am. J. Cardiol. 66:214–219, 1990.
14. Klein, G.J., Gersh, B.J., and Yee, R.: Electrophysiological testing: The final court of appeal for diagnosis of syncope? Circulation 92: 1332–1335, 1995.
15. Benditt, D.G., Remole, S., Bailin, S., et al.: Tilt table testing for evaluation of neurally-mediated (cardioneurogenic) syncope: Rationale and proposed protocols. Pacing Clin. Electrophysiol. 14:1528–1537, 1991.
16. Benditt, D.G., Ferguson, D.W., Grubb, B.P., et al.: ACC expert consensus document. Tilt table testing for assessing syncope. J. Am. Coll. Cardiol. 28:263–275, 1996.

17. Kapoor, W.N., Smith, M., and Miller, N.L.: Upright tilt testing in evaluating syncope: A comprehensive literature review. Am. J. Med. 97:78–88, 1994.

18. Brooks, R., Ruskin, J.N., Powell, A.C., et al.: Prospective evaluation of day-to-day reproducibility of upright tilt-table testing in unexplained syncope. Am. J. Cardiol. 71:1289–1292, 1993.

19. Davis, T.L., and Freemoon, F.R.: Electroencephalography should not be routine in the evaluation of syncope in adults. Arch. Intern. Med. 50:2027–2029, 1990.

20. Kapoor, W.N., Fortunato, M., Hanusa, B.H., and Schulberg, H.C.: Psychiatric illnesses in patients with syncope. Am. J. Med. 99:505–512, 1995.

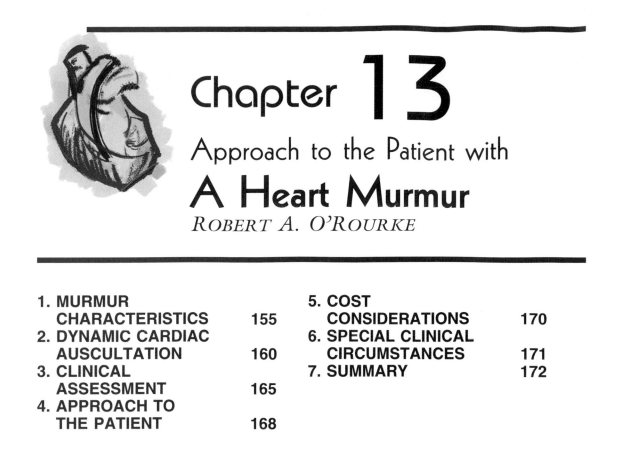

Chapter 13

Approach to the Patient with
A Heart Murmur

ROBERT A. O'ROURKE

Cardiac murmurs are present on physical examination in many individuals with and without cardiac disease. A murmur heard during cardiac auscultation may have no pathologic significance or may be an important clue to the presence of valvular, congenital, or other structural abnormalities of the heart. Most cardiac murmurs do not signify cardiac disease, and many are related to physiologic increases in blood-flow velocity. The common "innocent" mid-systolic vibratory murmur heard loudest at the pulmonic area and left sternal edge in children and young adults does not indicate cardiac disease. A soft, short mid-systolic murmur heard best in the aortic area in asymptomatic often hypertensive elderly patients is commonly due to aortic leaflet thickening (sclerosis) and no stenosis. In such circumstances, assessment of the cardiac murmur often requires little, if any, additional diagnostic testing.[1, 2]

In other instances, a heart murmur may be an important clue to the diagnosis of otherwise undetected cardiac disease (e.g., valvular aortic stenosis) that, even in the absence of cardiac symptoms, is clinically important or may define the reason for cardiac symptoms.[3] In these situations, various noninvasive or invasive cardiac tests may be necessary to establish a firm diagnosis and to form the basis for rational treatment of the underlying disorder. Echocardiography with Doppler color-flow imaging is particularly useful in this regard. It is the purpose of this chapter to define cardiac murmurs, their auscultatory characteristics, methods for improving the accuracy of their interpretation, and the circumstances in

which various degrees of further diagnostic workup are indicated with an emphasis on reducing unnecessary costs due to additional testing that is not needed.

The traditional auscultatory method of assessing cardiac murmurs has been based on their timing, configuration, location, pitch, intensity, and duration. It is necessary to use this information in making important decisions that are dependent on the correct interpretation of cardiac murmurs. As listed in Table 13–1, such decisions concern the need for antibiotic prophylaxis for endocarditis or the prevention of recurrent rheumatic fever, the necessity of restricting physical activity, and the need for further cardiac evaluation utilizing various noninvasive or invasive diagnostic techniques. Also, the precise interpretation of an isolated heart murmur is important in determining the risk of noncardiac surgery in a patient with no other evidence of cardiac disease.

MURMUR CHARACTERISTICS

Cardiac murmurs result from vibrations set up in the blood stream and the surrounding heart and great vessels as a result of turbulent blood flow that arises when blood velocity becomes critically high owing to high flow or flow through an irregular or narrow area, or a combination of both. The production of murmurs has been attributed to three main factors: (1) high blood-flow rate

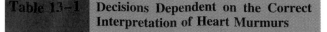

Table 13–1	Decisions Dependent on the Correct Interpretation of Heart Murmurs

Antibiotic prophylaxis for endocarditis
Antibiotic prophylaxis for rheumatic fever
Restriction of activity
Need for further cardiac evaluation
Risk assessment of noncardiac surgery

through normal or abnormal orifices, (2) forward flow through a narrowed or regular orifice into a dilated vessel or chamber, and (3) backward or regurgitant flow through an incompetent valve, septal defect, or patent ductus arteriosus. Often, more than one of these factors are operative.[4, 5]

Intensity

The intensity (loudness) of murmurs is usually graded from I to VI. A grade I murmur is so soft (faint) that it can be heard only with great effort, and a grade II murmur is faint but can be readily heard. A grade III murmur is moderately loud, and a grade IV murmur is very loud. A grade V murmur is extremely loud and can be heard when only the edge of the stethoscope is in contact with the chest; it is not heard if the stethoscope is removed from the skin. A grade VI murmur is exceptionally loud and can be heard with the stethoscope slightly removed from contact with the chest. Experience has shown that the systolic murmurs of grade III or higher intensity are more likely to be hemodynamically significant and due to cardiac disease. Systolic thrills are often palpable owing to murmurs of grade IV or louder intensity.

The loudness of the murmur relates directly to the velocity of blood flow across the site of murmur production, and the velocity is determined by the pressure difference that drives the blood across the murmur-producing site. For example, high velocity of flow through a small ventricular septal defect produces a loud systolic murmur, often accompanied by a thrill, whereas a large flow at low velocity through an atrial septal defect produces no murmur. The loudness of a murmur as auscultated at the chest wall is also determined by the transmission characteristics of the tissues interposed between the source of the murmur and the stethoscope. Obesity, obstructive lung disease, and the presence of moderate to large pericardial or pleural effusions diminish the intensity of a murmur, whereas a thin ectomorphic body habitus or severe weight loss augments it.

Frequency

The frequency (pitch) of a murmur is also directly related to the velocity of blood flow at the site of the murmur's origin.[6] The low velocity flow due to a small pressure gradient across a stenotic mitral valve causes a low-pitched, rumbling murmur, whereas the large diastolic pressure gradient across a regurgitant aortic valve results in a high-pitched murmur. Sometimes, the frequency components of the same systolic murmur will vary at different sites of auscultation. Often, the systolic murmur of aortic stenosis or sclerosis is higher pitched at the apex than at the base. Some murmurs may have an unusual musical quality. These include the diastolic murmur of a ruptured or retroverted aortic leaflet and the systolic "whoop" or "honk" of mitral valve prolapse.[3]

Timing and Configuration

The *timing* of the heart murmur relative to the cardiac cycle and its configuration are important considerations for defining its cause (Table 13–2). The separation of systole and diastole is usually easy because systole is considerably shorter at normal heart rates. However, with tachycardia, the relative duration of diastole shortens and the two intervals become similar. During tachycardia, the auscultator can usually time the murmur by simultaneous palpation of the carotid artery or can relate it to the second heart sound (S_2), which is usually the louder sound at the base. With S_2 defined, murmurs can be accurately identified as occurring in systole or diastole. When sinus tachycardia is present, carotid sinus pressure may temporarily slow the heart rate, enabling the differentiation of systole from diastole. When premature contractions are occurring, the first sound after the compensatory pause is the first heart sound (S_1).

The *configuration* of a murmur may be crescendo, decrescendo, crescendo-decrescendo (diamond-shaped), or plateau. The precise time of onset and time of cessation of a murmur due to cardiac pathology depend on the point in the cardiac cycle at which an adequate pressure difference between two chambers appears and disappears (Fig. 13–1). Systolic murmurs are generally classified as holosystolic (pansystolic) murmurs or mid-systolic (systolic ejection) murmurs. Certain other murmurs may not begin until mid or late systole, particularly those due to papillary muscle dysfunction. These are called *late-systolic* murmurs. The murmur of mitral valve prolapse also commonly occurs as a late-systolic murmur.

Diastolic murmurs are usually divided into early high-pitched diastolic murmurs such as those due to aortic or pulmonic regurgitation, mid-diastolic murmurs such as those due to blood flow across a stenotic mitral or tricuspid valve, and presystolic murmurs, which occur for the same reason in patients with a gradient between the atria and the ventricles and in sinus rhythm. A continuous murmur can usually be separated from a systolic plus a diastolic murmur because it begins in systole and continues through S_2, where it peaks into diastole.[2, 6]

Systolic Murmurs

Holosystolic (pansystolic) murmurs are generated when there is flow between chambers that have widely different pressures throughout systole, such as the left ventricle and either the left atrium or the right ventricle. The pressure gradient occurs early in contraction and lasts until relaxation is almost complete. Therefore, holosystolic murmurs begin with S_1 before aortic ejection and at the area of maximal intensity, and they end after S_2. Holosystolic murmurs are caused by mitral and tricuspid regurgitation, ventricular septal defects, and certain aortopulmonary

Table 13–2	Principal Causes of Heart Murmurs

A. Organic Systolic Murmurs
  1. Midsystolic (ejection)
    a. Aortic
      (1) Obstructive
        (a) Supravalvular—supra-aortic stenosis, coarctation of the aorta
        (b) Valvular—AS and sclerosis
        (c) Infravalvular—HOCM
      (2) Increased flow, hyperkinetic states, AR, complete heart block
      (3) Dilatation of ascending aorta, atheroma, aortitis, aneurysm of aorta
    b. Pulmonary
      Obstructive
        (a) Supravalvular—pulmonary arterial stenosis
        (b) Valvular—pulmonic valve stenosis
        (c) Infravalvular—infundibular stenosis
      (2) Increased flow, hyperkinetic states, left-to-right shunt (e.g., ASD, VSD)
      (3) Dilatation of pulmonary artery
  2. Pansystolic (regurgitant)
    a. Atrioventricular valve regurgitation (MR, TR)
    b. Left-to-right shunt to ventricular level
B. Early-Diastolic Murmurs
  1. AR
    a. Valvular: rheumatic deformity; perforation postendocarditis, posttraumatic, postvalvulotomy
    b. Dilatation of valve ring: aorta dissection, annuloectasia, cystic medial necrosis, hypertension
    c. Widening of commissures: syphilis
    d. Congenital: bicuspid valve, with VSD
  2. Pulmonic regurgitation
    a. Valvular: postvalvulotomy, endocarditis, rheumatic fever, carcinoid
    b. Dilatation of valve ring: pulmonary hypertension; Marfan's syndrome
    c. Congenital: isolated or associated with tetralogy of Fallot, VSD, pulmonic stenosis
C. Mid-Diastolic Murmurs
  1. MS
  2. Carey-Coombs murmur (mid-diastolic apical murmur in acute rheumatic fever)
  3. Increased flow across nonstenotic mitral valve (e.g., MR, VSD, PDA, high-output states, and complete heart block)
  4. Tricuspid stenosis
  5. Increased flow across nonstenotic tricuspid valve (e.g., TR, ASD, and anomalous pulmonary venous return)
  6. Left and right atrial tumors
D. Continuous Murmurs
  1. PDA
  2. Coronary AV fistula
  3. Ruptured aneurysm of sinus of Valsalva
  4. Aortic septal defect
  5. Cervical venous hum
  6. Anomalous left coronary artery
  7. Proximal coronary artery stenosis
  8. Mammary soufflé
  9. Pulmonary artery branch stenosis
  10. Bronchial collateral circulation
  11. Small (restrictive) ASD with MS
  12. Intercostal AV fistula

A and *C*, Modified from Oram, S. (ed.): Clinical Heart Disease. London, Heinemann, 1981. *D*, Modified from Fowler, N.O. (ed.): Cardiac Diagnosis and Treatment. Hagerstown, MD, Harper & Row, 1980.

Abbreviations: AS, aortic stenosis; HOCM, hypertrophic obstructive cardiomyopathy; AR, aortic regurgitation; ASD, atrial septal defect; VSD, ventricular septal defect; MR, mitral regurgitation; TR, tricuspid regurgitation; MS, mitral stenosis; PDA, patent ductus arteriosus; AV, arteriovenous.

shunts. Although the typical high-pitched murmur of mitral regurgitation usually continues throughout systole, the murmur may vary in configuration. The murmur of tricuspid regurgitation associated with pulmonary hypertension is holosystolic and frequently increases during inspiration. Not all patients with mitral or tricuspid regurgitation or ventricular septal defect have holosystolic murmurs, and changes in murmur intensity with various maneuvers described later in this chapter are often useful for their correct interpretation.[2, 6]

Mid-systolic (systolic ejection) murmurs, often crescendo-decrescendo or diamond-shaped, occur when blood is ejected across the aortic or pulmonic outflow tracts. The murmur starts shortly after S_1, when the ventricular pressure rises sufficiently to open the semilunar valve. As ejection increases the murmur is augmented, and as ejection declines it diminishes. The murmur ends before the ventricular pressure falls enough to permit closure of the aortic or pulmonic leaflets. In the presence of normal semilunar valves, an increased flow rate—as occurs in states of elevated cardiac output (e.g., fever, thyrotoxicosis, anemia, and pregnancy), ejection of blood into a dilated vessel beyond the valve, or increased transmission of sound through a thin chest wall—may cause this murmur. Most benign "innocent" murmurs that present in children and young adults are mid-systolic, due to high velocity, and originate from either the aortic or the pulmonic outflow tracts. Valvular or subvalvular obstruction to either ventricle may also cause such a mid-systolic murmur with the intensity being related to the velocity of blood flow across the obstructed area.

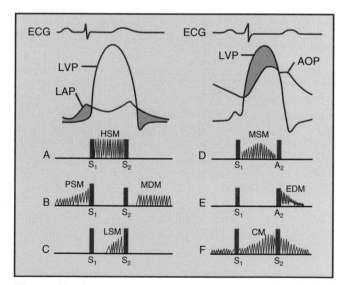

Figure 13–1

Schematic representation of the major types of abnormal murmurs and the associated pressure recordings. ECG, electrocardiogram; LVP, left ventricular pressure; LAP, left atrial pressure; AOP, aortic pressure; S_1, first heart sound; S_2, second heart sound; A_2, aortic second sound; HSM, holosystolic murmur; PSM, presystolic murmur; MDM, mid-diastolic murmur; LSM, late-systolic murmur; MSM, mid-systolic murmur; EDM, early-diastolic murmur; CM, continuous murmur. (Redrawn from Crawford, M.H., and O'Rourke, R.A.: A systematic approach to the bedside differentiation of cardiac murmurs and abnormal sounds. Curr. Probl. Cardiol. 1:1–42, 1977.)

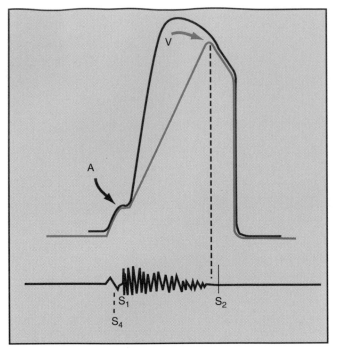

Figure 13–2

Ventricular and atrial pressure pulses with phonocardiogram illustrating the mechanism of the *early*-systolic murmur of acute severe mitral regurgitation or low-pressure tricuspid regurgitation. The V-wave reaches ventricular pressure at end systole *(upper curved arrow),* so regurgitant flow diminishes or ceases. The murmur is therefore early systolic and decrescendo, paralleling the hemodynamic pattern of regurgitation. S_1, first heart sound; S_2, second heart sound; S_4, fourth heart sound. The A-wave *(lower curved arrow)* is due to left or right atrial contraction. (From Perloff, J.K.: Heart sounds and murmurs: Physiological mechanisms. *In* Braunwald, E. [ed.]: Heart Disease. 4th ed. Philadelphia, W.B. Saunders, 1992, pp. 43–63.)

The murmur of *aortic stenosis* is the typical left-sided mid-systolic murmur due to heart disease. Sclerosis of the aortic leaflets without a left ventricular–aortic systolic pressure gradient often causes a similar murmur. If the aortic valve is heavily calcified, the aortic closure sound (A_2) may be soft or inaudible; as a result, the length and configuration of the murmur are more difficult to determine. Mid-systolic murmurs also occur in patients with mitral regurgitation or, less frequently, tricuspid regurgitation resulting from papillary muscle dysfunction. Such murmurs due to mitral regurgitation are commonly misinterpreted as aortic stenosis or sclerosis, particularly in elderly patients.

The patient's age and the site of maximal murmur intensity are useful in determining the significance of mid-systolic murmurs.[7] Thus, in the young adult with a thin chest and a high velocity of blood flow, a faint or moderate mid-systolic murmur heard only in the pulmonic area usually has no clinical significance, whereas a louder murmur in the aortic area may indicate congenital aortic stenosis. In elderly patients, pulmonic flow murmurs are rare but aortic systolic murmurs are common and may be due to aortic valve sclerosis, valvular aortic stenosis, or aortic dilatation. Mid-systolic aortic and pul-

monic murmurs are intensified by various maneuvers, as indicated later. Echocardiography is often necessary to separate a prominent and exaggerated benign mid-systolic murmur from one due to congenital or acquired aortic valve stenosis.[4–6]

Early-systolic murmurs are less common; they begin with S_1 and end in mid systole. In large ventricular septal defects with pulmonary hypertension and small muscular ventricular septal defects, the shunting at the end of systole may be insignificant, with the murmur limited to early systole. An early-systolic murmur is often due to tricuspid regurgitation occurring in the absence of pulmonary hypertension. This murmur is common in drug addicts with active or prior infective endocarditis, in whom a tall regurgitant right atrial V-wave reaches the level of the normal right ventricular pressure in late systole; thus, there is no pressure difference or murmur in late systole. In patients with acute mitral regurgitation and a large V-wave in a nondilated left atrium, a loud early-systolic murmur is often heard; this murmur decreases in late systole as the pressure difference between left ventricle and left atrium diminishes (Fig. 13–2).

Late-systolic murmurs are soft or moderately loud, high-pitched murmurs at the left ventricular apex that start well after ejection and end before or at S_2. They are likely caused by ischemia, by infarction or dysfunction of the mitral papillary muscles, or by left ventricular dilatation. These murmurs may be heard in patients with chronic ischemic heart disease only during angina, but they are also commonly present in patients with myocardial infarction or dilated cardiomyopathy. Late-systolic murmurs in patients with mid-systolic clicks are the result of late-systolic mitral regurgitation due to prolapse of the mitral leaflet(s) into the left atrium.[2, 3]

Diastolic Murmurs

Early-diastolic murmurs begin with or shortly after S_2 when the associated ventricular pressure drops sufficiently below that in the aorta or pulmonary artery. High-pitched murmurs of aortic regurgitation or pulmonic regurgitation due to pulmonary hypertension are generally decrescendo, consistent with the rapid decline in the volume or rate of regurgitation during diastole. Faint, high-pitched murmurs of aortic regurgitation are often heard only when the diaphragm of the stethoscope is held firmly over the left mid-sternal border while the patient sits, leans forward, and holds a breath in full expiration.[2, 5, 6] The diastolic murmur of aortic regurgitation is enhanced by an acute elevation of the arterial pressure such as occurs with multiple maneuvers, discussed later.

The diastolic murmur of pulmonic regurgitation *without* pulmonary hypertension such as may occur with congenital heart disease, endocarditis, or other diseases directly affecting the pulmonic valve (e.g., carcinoid syndrome) is low to medium pitched. The onset of this murmur is slightly delayed because the regurgitant flow is minimal at pulmonic valve closure, when the reverse pressure gradient responsible for the regurgitation is minimal.[6]

Mid-diastolic murmurs usually originate from the mitral and tricuspid valves, occur during early ventricular filling, and are due to a relative disproportion between valve orifice size and diastolic blood-flow velocity. Such murmurs may be quite loud despite only slight atrioventricular valve stenosis when there is normal or increased blood flow. Conversely, these murmurs may be faint or inaudible at rest despite severe stenosis if the cardiac output is very low. When the obstruction is marked, the diastolic murmur is longer; its duration is more reliable than its intensity for indicating the severity of valve stenosis.[2, 5, 6]

The low-pitched, mid-diastolic murmur of mitral stenosis usually follows an opening snap. It is best detected with the bell of the stethoscope placed over the site of the left ventricular impulse with the patient turned to the left side. The murmur of mitral stenosis is often localized to the left ventricular apex. In tricuspid stenosis, the mid-diastolic murmur is usually confined to a relatively small area along the left sternal edge and is generally louder during inspiration.

Mid-diastolic murmurs may be due to turbulent blood flow across the mitral valve in patients with ventricular septal defect, patent ductus arteriosus, or mitral regurgitation and across the tricuspid valve in patients with atrial septal defect or tricuspid regurgitation. These murmurs usually occur after a third heart sound (S_3) and only with large left-to-right shunts or severe atrioventricular valve regurgitation. A soft mid-diastolic murmur may be heard in patients with acute rheumatic fever owing to inflammation of the mitral valve leaflets or severe mitral regurgitation.[1-3]

In severe, chronic aortic regurgitation, a low-pitched diastolic murmur (Austin Flint murmur) is often present at the left ventricular apex; it may be either mid-diastolic or presystolic. This murmur originates at the anterior mitral valve leaflet when blood flow simultaneously enters the left ventricle from both the aortic root and the left atrium.[2, 5, 6]

Presystolic murmurs begin during the period of ventricular filling that follows atrial contraction and therefore occur in sinus rhythm. They are usually due to mitral or tricuspid stenosis. These are low pitched and usually crescendo in configuration, reaching peak intensity at the time of a loud S_1. The presystolic murmur is related to the atrioventricular valve gradient, which may be augmented by right or left atrial contraction. It is often present in patients with tricuspid stenosis and sinus rhythm. A right or left atrial myxoma may occasionally cause either mid-diastolic or presystolic murmurs similar to those of tricuspid or mitral stenosis.[2]

Continuous Murmurs

These arise from high- to low-pressure shunts that persist through the end of systole and the beginning of diastole (see Table 13-2). Thus, they begin in systole, peak near S_2, and continue into part or all of diastole. A patent ductus arteriosus causes a continuous murmur when the pressure in the pulmonary artery is much below that in the aorta. The murmur is louder when the systemic arterial pressure is raised and softer when it is lowered. When pulmonary hypertension is present, the diastolic portion may disappear. Surgically produced connections such as the subclavian–pulmonary artery anastomosis result in murmurs similar to that of a patent ductus arteriosus. Continuous murmurs may result from congenital or acquired systemic arteriovenous fistula, coronary arteriovenous fistula, anomalous origin of the left coronary artery from the pulmonary artery, and communications between an aortic sinus of Valsalva and the right side of the heart. Continuous murmurs may also occur in patients with a small atrial septal defect with a high left atrial pressure. Continuous murmurs may also be due to abnormal blood-flow patterns in constricted systemic or pulmonary arteries. For example, a continuous murmur in the back may occur with coarctation of the aorta, and pulmonary embolism may cause continuous murmurs in partially occluded vessels.[2, 5, 6]

Continuous murmurs may be caused by rapid blood flow through a tortuous bed in nonconstricted arteries, as occurs within the bronchial arterial collateral circulation in patients with severe pulmonary outflow obstruction and cyanosis. The "mammary soufflé," a physiologic murmur heard over the breasts during late pregnancy and early postpartum, may be systolic or continuous.[8] The innocent cervical venous hum is a continuous murmur that is usually heard over the medial aspect of the right supraclavicular fossa with the patient upright. It is usually louder during diastole and can be immediately abolished by digital compression of the ipsilateral internal jugular vein. Transmission of a loud venous hum to the left infraclavicular area may result in an incorrect clinical diagnosis of patent ductus arteriosus.[3]

Location and Radiation of Murmurs

The location on the chest wall where the murmur is best heard and the areas to which it radiates can be helpful in identifying the cardiac structure from which it originates. The location and radiation of a murmur of aortic stenosis are influenced by the direction of the high-velocity jet within the aortic root. In valvular aortic stenosis, the murmur is usually maximal in the second right intercostal space, with radiation into the neck. In supravalvular aortic stenosis, the murmur is usually loudest, even higher, with greater radiation to the right carotid artery. In hypertrophic cardiomyopathy, the mid-systolic murmur is generated within the left ventricular cavity, is usually loudest at the lower left sternal edge and apex, and radiates little, if at all, to the neck. By contrast, the murmur of mitral regurgitation is most often loudest at the cardiac apex. It may radiate to the left sternal border and base of the heart when the posterior mitral leaflet is involved, or to the axilla or back when the anterior leaflet is more seriously affected. In the latter case, the regurgitant blood is directed toward the posterior left atrial wall. However, the location and radiation of a murmur are multifactorial and are determined by its site of origin, its intensity, and duration of blood flow as well as by the physical characteristics of the chest. For example, in elderly patients, the murmur of aortic stenosis is often loudest at the left ventricular apex.

DYNAMIC CARDIAC AUSCULTATION

Attentive cardiac auscultation during dynamic changes in cardiac hemodynamics (Table 13–3) often enables the careful observer to deduce the correct origin and significance of a cardiac murmur. The maneuvers discussed in this chapter for evaluating heart murmurs during dynamic cardiac auscultation include respiratory variation, the Valsalva maneuver, exercise, postural changes, use of pharmacologic agents, postpremature beat, and transient arterial occlusion.[7, 9, 10]

Respiratory Variation

Normal inspiration decreases intrathoracic pressure, thus increasing venous return to the right side of the heart and dilatation of the pulmonary circulation. As the right ventricular volume increases, so does the stroke volume, due partly to the Frank-Starling mechanism and also to lessened impedance to right ventricular ejection. Respiratory changes in systemic flow are most prominent in the sitting or standing position when venous return is normally lower. In the supine position, venous return is higher and the changes with inspiration are less marked. Therefore, it is useful to observe auscultatory changes during inspiration with the patient in both the supine and the seated positions. If normal respiration does not produce the expected changes in the intensity of murmurs or sounds, the patient should be directed to take slightly deeper breaths. However, maximal inspiration should be avoided because this can result in a partial Valsalva maneuver with possible opposing hemodynamic results.

Respiration is the best maneuver for differentiating between cardiac murmurs originating in the right and the left sides of the heart. Inspiration will accentuate most auscultatory events originating in the right heart, including the murmurs of tricuspid and pulmonic valve regurgitation or stenosis, each of which will become louder during inspiration. Insignificant mid-systolic murmurs across the pulmonic outflow tract will also increase in intensity. Conversely, expiration causes a decrease in lung volume, placing the heart closer to the anterior chest wall, and pulmonary venous flow is augmented as well. Therefore, left-sided murmurs originating at the mitral or aortic valve are usually loudest during expiration and diminish or are unchanged with inspiration.

Variations in the normal splitting of S_2 during inspiration often provide an important clue to the presence of heart disease, particularly in patients with a mid-systolic murmur. Normal splitting of A_2 and the second pulmonic sound (P_2) may be widened by the late activation of the right ventricle, such as occurs with prolonged ventricular contraction because of a right ventricular pressure load (e.g., pulmonic stenosis), or by delayed pulmonic valve closure because of reduced impedance of the pulmonary vasculature (e.g., idiopathic dilatation of the pulmonary artery). In patients with left-to-right shunting through an atrial septal defect, pulmonary vascular impedance may be decreased to a point where augmented venous return during inspiration will not affect right heart flow or stroke

Table 13–3	Maneuvers Used to Change the Intensity of Cardiac Murmurs

Respiratory variation
Valsalva maneuver
Exercise
Postural changes
After a premature contraction
Pharmacologic interventions
Transient arterial occlusion

volume. In this case, inspiration produces little, if any, additional separation between the two components of S_2, and it remains widely split, resulting in the so-called fixed splitting of S_2 that occurs in patients with atrial septal defect in addition to the mid-systolic pulmonic murmur that is present.[4, 5]

Careful evaluation of the timing of the two components of S_2 during respiration can be quite helpful in assessing the significance of a murmur. The aortic component of S_2 may occur early when there is decreased resistance to left ventricular ejection, as occurs with mitral regurgitation and ventricular septal defect. By contrast, late aortic valve closure may cause the aortic component of S_2 to occur after the pulmonic component during expiration. Thus, maximal splitting occurs during expiration and results in reversed (paradoxical) splitting of S_2. Prolonged left ventricular ejection, such as occurs with severe aortic stenosis, may produce reversed splitting of S_2. Reversed splitting of S_2 in a patient with a loud, late-peaking mid-systolic murmur at the base usually indicates very severe aortic stenosis.

The Valsalva Maneuver

The Valsalva maneuver is a useful method for determining the likely cause of various cardiac murmurs. The maneuver is a two-part process with a straining period followed by a relaxation period, each of which has importance in characterization of heart murmurs (Fig. 13–3).[7, 10]

The Valsalva maneuver is performed by having the patient forcefully attempt to exhale against a closed glottis after taking a normal breath. The examiner should place a hand on the patient's abdomen to be sure that the muscles are tightening. An alternative method is to have the patient exhale into a manometer to maintain a level of 40 mm Hg or greater for the duration of the maneuver. When the Valsalva maneuver is performed, the intrathoracic pressure will be elevated considerably, thus increasing both end-systolic and end-diastolic ventricular pressures. The pulmonary vasculature is emptied into the left atrium and left ventricle, resulting in a small initial rise in systemic arterial pressure. Subsequently, venous return to the right heart is inhibited by the higher intrathoracic pressure, the right and then the left ventricular outputs decline, and systemic arterial pressure falls.

The Valsalva maneuver usually is performed for about 10 seconds while the examiner listens to intensity changes in heart murmurs. The maneuver should be dis-

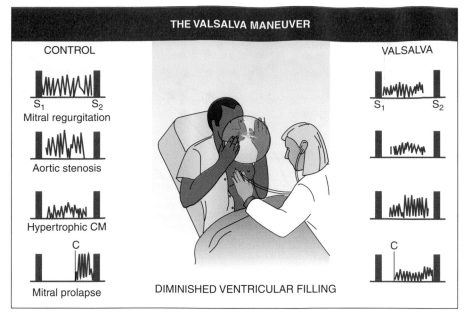

Figure 13–3

Changes in four left-sided systolic murmurs during the strain phase of the Valsalva maneuver. S_1, first heart sound; S_2, second heart sound; CM, cardiomyopathy; C, systolic click. (From Grewe, K., Crawford, M.H., and O'Rourke, R.A.: Differentiation of cardiac murmurs by auscultation. Curr. Prob. Cardiol. 13:669–721, 1988.)

continued after 10 seconds to prevent symptoms (e.g., syncope) due to the reduced cardiac output and blood pressure. The maneuver briefly decreases myocardial blood flow and should not be used in patients with known myocardial ischemia or recent infarction. Most cardiac murmurs and sounds diminish in intensity during the Valsalva maneuver because of the decreased ventricular filling and cardiac output.

The murmur of mitral valve prolapse is one of only two murmurs that will increase in intensity or duration with the Valsalva maneuver. The decrease in left ventricular volume during straining causes earlier mitral leaflet(s) prolapse in systole, usually increasing the length and often the intensity of the systolic murmur. Occasionally, a musical "whoop" will be induced by the Valsalva maneuver.[3]

The murmur of hypertrophic cardiomyopathy is the only other murmur that will increase in intensity with the Valsalva maneuver. The degree of left ventricular outflow tract narrowing due to abnormal motion of the anterior mitral leaflet toward the hypertrophic interventricular septum varies depending on left ventricular volume. When the volume is diminished, as during the strain phase of the Valsalva maneuver, the outflow tract pressure gradient increases and the murmur is louder. Although highly specific, not all patients with hypertrophic cardiomyopathy will exhibit an increase in mid-systolic murmur intensity with the Valsalva maneuver.

During release of straining, the second phase of the Valsalva maneuver, the intrathoracic pressure returns to normal and there is sudden augmentation of right and then left ventricular filling and cardiac output. The delay in filling between right and left heart chambers often aids in the differentiation of murmurs of right and left heart origin. Murmurs generated in the right heart usually return to baseline intensity within 1 to 4 heartbeats after release of straining. Left-sided murmurs often require 5 to 10 cardiac cycles to return to baseline intensity. Thus, in patients with aortic or mitral valve stenosis or regurgita-

tion, a ventricular septal defect, or other left-sided lesions, there is a decrease in intensity of the murmur during straining and a gradual return to baseline during relaxation. In patients with tricuspid stenosis or regurgitation, or pulmonic stenosis or regurgitation, the murmur will also soften during straining, but its intensity will return to baseline almost immediately on release of the Valsalva maneuver. This is the response observed in most young patients with innocent mid-systolic heart murmurs.

Exercise

All forms of exercise increase the heart rate and cardiac output and may be clinically useful in differentiating various heart murmurs. However, it is impractical for hospitalized, uncooperative, or deconditioned patients to perform many types of dynamic exercise. Thus, isometric exercise in the form of sustained handgrip is often used during cardiac auscultation in the office or at the bedside. Usually, the patient is instructed to squeeze the examiner's finger or another object, such as a rolled towel, as tightly as possible with one or both hands while auscultatory changes are assessed. In more precise studies, the use of a calibrated dynamometer can measure the amount of force applied to the handle. The patient should be instructed to breathe normally and to squeeze with only the forearm so that the chest remains relaxed and a simultaneous Valsalva maneuver does not confuse the results. A minimum of 60 to 90 seconds usually elapses before a significant heart rate and blood pressure response are noted. Sustained handgrip rapidly increases the heart rate, cardiac output, and both systolic and diastolic arterial pressure. There is a quick return to baseline values after cessation of the maneuver. Although isometric exercise causes a lesser increase in heart rate and cardiac output than does isotonic exercise, blood pressure increases are usually greater. When the effort expended exceeds 50% of the subject's maximal voluntary contraction, there is a substantial increase in systemic vascular resistance as well as an increase in heart rate, cardiac output, and arterial pressure.[7, 10]

The rise in systemic arterial pressure during isometric exercise augments the systolic pressure gradient between the left ventricle and the left atrium or right ventricle, and the murmurs of mitral regurgitation and ventricular septal defect increase in intensity. The late-systolic murmur of a mitral valve prolapse is usually louder during handgrip. The increased aortic diastolic blood pressure increases the murmur of aortic regurgitation. Murmurs of aortic stenosis and hypertrophic cardiomyopathy usually soften or are unchanged during handgrip because of the higher aortic pressure.

Since myocardial oxygen demand is increased with isometric exercise, ischemia of the papillary muscles may result in patients with coronary artery disease. New murmurs of mitral regurgitation may be heard during a handgrip but are rarely associated with chest pain. However, patients with acute or recent myocardial infarction should not undergo isometric exercise.

Handgrip exercise is an excellent maneuver for assessing patients with rheumatic mitral valve disease. Systolic murmurs of mitral regurgitation and the diastolic rumbling murmur of mitral stenosis are accentuated by the elevated blood pressure and tachycardia during handgrip.

Postural Changes

Cardiac auscultation of the patient in only the supine position fails to provide important information that can be obtained about heart murmurs from changes in position. Postural changes are particularly useful for separating the mid-systolic murmur of valvular aortic stenosis or aortic sclerosis from those associated with hypertrophic cardiomyopathy or mitral valve prolapse (Fig. 13–4).

When the patient assumes the upright position, venous return diminishes owing to gravitational pooling, thereby decreasing ventricular filling pressures. The stroke volume declines, causing a reflex rise in the heart rate and systemic vascular resistance. Most heart murmurs soften with these hemodynamic changes, a response similar to that observed with the Valsalva maneuver that also decreases ventricular filling pressures. Exceptions are the systolic murmurs of hypertrophic cardiomyopathy and mitral valve prolapse; they often become louder and longer when the patient is sitting or stands owing to the smaller left ventricular volume. Pulmonic mid-systolic flow murmurs are usually softer when the patient stands but will still get louder during inspiration in the upright position, similar to most right-sided heart murmurs.[7, 10]

Cardiac auscultation while the patient squats rapidly from the upright position is a useful diagnostic maneuver. Squatting is an effective way to assess the physiologic changes of increased ventricular filling volumes. During squatting, the patients should rest on their heels with the hips laterally flexed. With the physician sitting throughout the examination, the patient can be auscultated immediately on reaching the standing and squatting positions with a minimum of effort.

During squatting, compression of the femoral arteries causes the mean aortic pressure to rise abruptly and remain at a level higher than that at rest. Also, reflex bradycardia is observed. Venous return to the heart is augmented because of increased pressure in the legs and abdominal cavity. For patients unable to perform the squatting maneuver owing to age or musculoskeletal disease, the examiner can passively bend the patient's knees toward the abdomen ("jackknifing") while the patient is in the supine position and produce similar physiologic and auscultatory changes as those that occur during squatting.

Right heart volume and flow are augmented by the increase in venous return during squatting. As the left-sided pressures increase, so do the murmurs of mitral regurgitation, ventricular septal defect, and aortic regurgi-

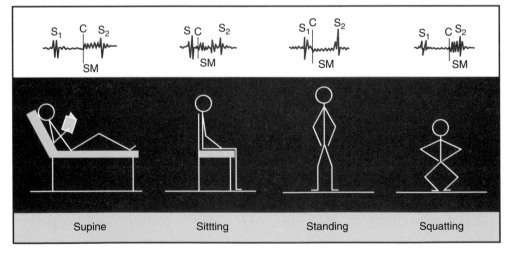

Figure 13–4

Postural maneuvers that affect the click(s) (C) and late-systolic murmur (SM) of mitral valve prolapse. A change from supine to sitting or standing causes the click to become earlier and the murmur longer, although softer. Conversely, squatting delays the timing of the click, and the murmur gets shorter but louder. S_1, first heart sound; S_2, second heart sound. (From Devereux, R., Perloff, J.K., Reichek, N., and Josephson, M.: Mitral valve prolapse. Circulation 54:3, 1976.)

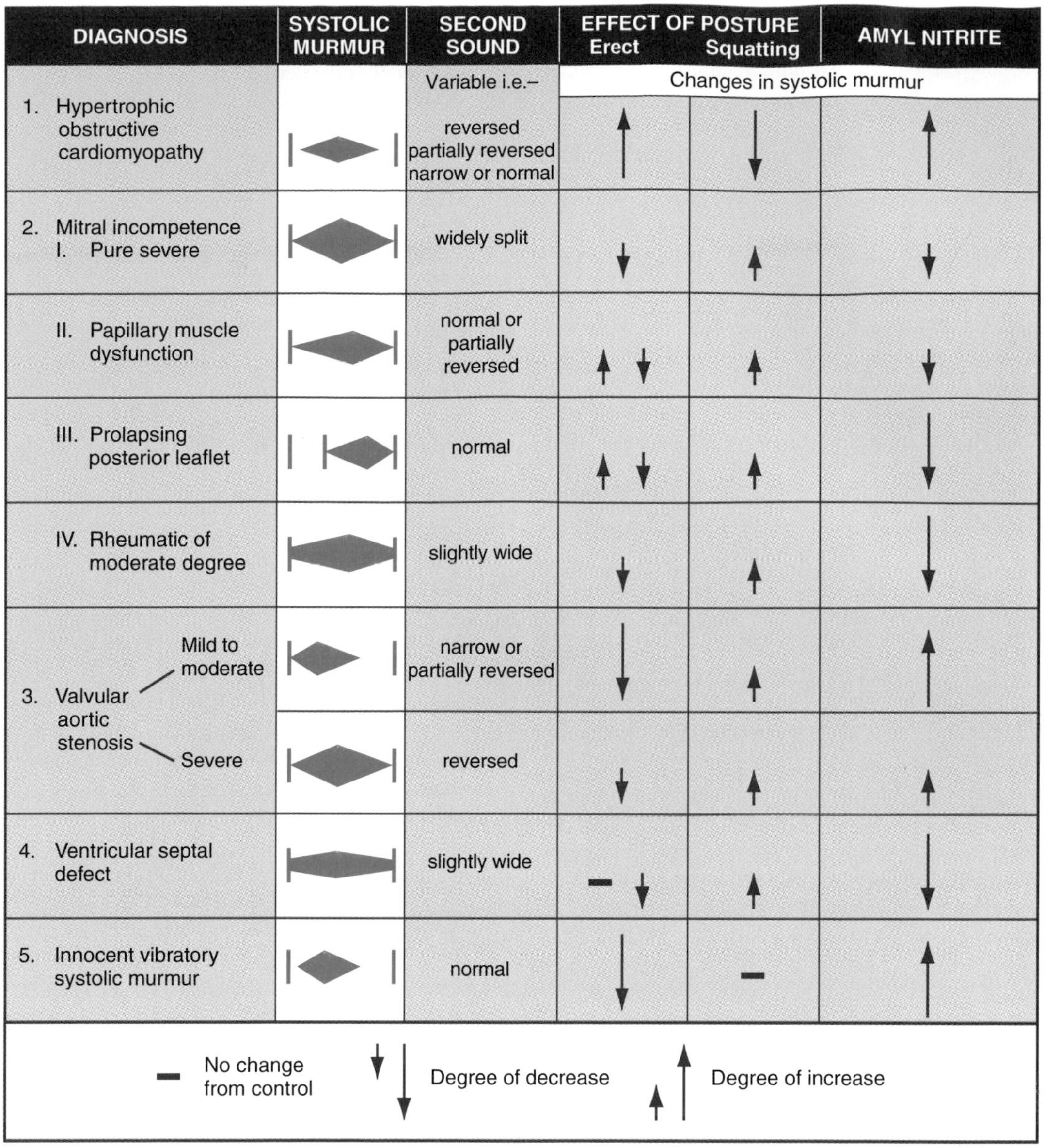

DIAGNOSIS	SYSTOLIC MURMUR	SECOND SOUND	EFFECT OF POSTURE Erect	Squatting	AMYL NITRITE
			Changes in systolic murmur		
1. Hypertrophic obstructive cardiomyopathy	◆	Variable i.e.– reversed partially reversed narrow or normal	↑	↓	↑
2. Mitral incompetence I. Pure severe	◆	widely split	↓	↑	↓
II. Papillary muscle dysfunction	◆	normal or partially reversed	↑ ↓	↑	↓
III. Prolapsing posterior leaflet	◆	normal	↑ ↓	↑	↓
IV. Rheumatic of moderate degree	◆	slightly wide	↓	↑	↓
3. Valvular aortic stenosis — Mild to moderate	◆	narrow or partially reversed	↓	↑	↑
3. Valvular aortic stenosis — Severe	◆	reversed	↓	↑	↑
4. Ventricular septal defect	◆	slightly wide	— ↓	↑	↓
5. Innocent vibratory systolic murmur	◆	normal	↓	—	↑

— No change from control ↓ Degree of decrease ↑ Degree of increase

Figure 13–5
Diagram of the character of the systolic murmur and of the second heart sound in five conditions demonstrates the effects of posture and amyl nitrite inhalation on the intensity of the murmurs. (Modified from Barlow, J.B.: Perspectives on the Mitral Valve. Philadelphia, F.A. Davis, 1987, p. 138.)

tation. The larger left ventricular volume and higher arterial pressure reduce any aortic outflow pressure gradient in hypertrophic cardiomyopathy, thus diminishing the mid-systolic murmur. Also, owing to the same mechanism, the late-systolic murmur of mitral valve prolapse will be softer and the systolic click-murmur complex will often begin later in systole, closer to S_2.

Changes in murmur intensity during standing may become more evident when the patient stands abruptly from the squatting position. Thus, auscultation during standing, squatting, and then standing again may produce diagnostic changes in murmur intensity. An example is the mid-systolic murmur of hypertrophic cardiomyopathy, which usually becomes louder during standing, much softer during squatting, and still louder when the patient stands again (Fig. 13–5).

All four of the previously described methods for altering the intensity of cardiac murmurs depend on normal function of the autonomic nervous system, required for inducing the changes in hemodynamics responsible for the auscultatory results. Therefore, in patients with heart failure and other conditions that affect autonomic nervous system function, the usefulness of these maneuvers for determining the cause of heart murmurs is diminished.

Changes after a Premature Contraction

Variations in murmur intensity in the first beat after a premature beat can provide important information concerning the cause of the murmur. During the compensatory pause, right and left ventricular filling is increased and the aortic and pulmonic diastolic pressures decline, thus enhancing stroke volume and promoting forward blood flow. Also, ventricular function is augmented after a premature beat because of the increase in end-diastolic ventricular volume (Frank-Starling effect). Similar hemodynamic responses usually occur in patients with atrial fibrillation and are due to changing R-R intervals and varying cardiac cycle length.[7, 10]

Mitral regurgitation murmurs usually do not change in intensity after a long cardiac cycle. Although left ventricular end-diastolic and forward flow are each greater after a premature beat and the regurgitant flow across the mitral valve early in systole is also enhanced, the increase in mitral regurgitant flow after a premature beat is confined primarily to the period of isovolumic contraction when the aortic valve is still closed.[11] During the latter half of systole after the aortic valve opens, the regurgitant volume is actually lessened, whereas the forward stroke volume is greater. The net result is little change in mitral regurgitant flow in the beat after a long cardiac cycle and thus no apparent change in murmur intensity.

The increased ventricular filling and decreased aortic impedance accentuate turbulent flow across a stenotic or sclerotic aortic valve. Systolic murmurs of aortic stenosis or sclerosis are louder in the first beat after the premature beat. In aortic stenosis at the valvular, supravalvular, and discrete subvalvular levels, the systolic pressure gradient across the left ventricular outflow tract increases after the extra-systolic beat and the systolic murmur intensifies. The systolic murmur of hypertrophic cardiomyopathy is more variable, although it usually gets louder. Insignificant pulmonic and mid-systolic murmurs and the murmur of pulmonic stenosis are also louder in postpremature beats.

In examining a patient with atrial fibrillation or premature beats, the effect of changing cycle length on murmur intensity can be useful for differentiating between the systolic murmurs of mitral regurgitation and left ventricular outflow tract turbulence. Also, no active patient participation is required and the results are not dependent on normal function of the autonomic nervous system.

Pharmacologic Maneuvers Used to Change the Intensity of Cardiac Murmurs

In the past, many drugs were used to aid in the correct identification of heart murmurs by modifying cardiovascular hemodynamics. They have been employed less commonly in recent years owing to the advent of other maneuvers and the emergence of two-dimensional (2-D) and Doppler echocardiography. The most common drug still used for this purpose is amyl nitrite, the volatile ester of nitrous acid. It is administered by inhalation and works very rapidly; its important hemodynamic effect occurs in the first 10 to 30 seconds after inhalation for two to three rapid, deep breaths.[7, 10]

Amyl nitrite is a potent vasodilator that causes an immediate decline in the systemic arterial pressure within 15 seconds after drug inhalation but lasts only about 30 sec-onds. The left ventricular size decreases, and left ventricular ejection is enhanced. Reflex tachycardia develops within 30 to 60 seconds after inhalation, thus increasing the cardiac output.

The most common clinical use of amyl nitrite is in separating systolic murmurs of aortic from mitral origin (see Fig. 13–5). In the first 15 seconds after inhalation, the rapid decline in arterial pressure increases the forward flow. The mid-systolic murmurs of aortic stenosis or sclerosis increase in intensity owing to the increased turbulence in the left ventricular outflow tract. The murmur of hypertrophic cardiomyopathy becomes louder as well. Left-sided regurgitant systolic murmurs, such as mitral regurgitation, become shorter and softer, particularly in the last half of systole. Owing to the decrease in aortic diastolic pressure, amyl nitrite diminishes the murmur of aortic regurgitation.

Blood flow to the right heart is increased with the use of amyl nitrite, which augments right-sided murmurs. Thus, systolic murmurs owing to tricuspid regurgitation will be louder. The diastolic murmur of tricuspid stenosis is augmented by the tachycardia and enhanced cardiac output. The murmur of pulmonic stenosis and insignificant pulmonic flow murmurs are increased as well.

Inhalation of amyl nitrite is useful in differentiating between the low-pitched diastolic murmur of mitral stenosis and the Austin Flint mitral diastolic murmur heard in severe aortic regurgitation. Amyl nitrite reduces the regurgitant flow across the aortic valve (owing to the decline in blood pressure and systemic vascular resistance), thereby lessening the intensity of the Austin Flint murmur. In contrast, the murmur owing to mitral stenosis is louder with amyl nitrite, particularly during the tachycardia response.

Although relatively safe, amyl nitrite should be given to a patient only in the supine position and is contraindicated for use in patients with severe aortic stenosis or unstable angina pectoris.

Transient Arterial Occlusion

The maneuvers described previously are traditional additions to the routine cardiac examination that can be used to help delineate various auscultatory findings. However, the usefulness of these maneuvers may be limited in some instances. Active patient participation may be difficult to obtain owing to musculoskeletal disease or altered mental status. Some patients unintentionally perform two maneuvers with opposing hemodynamic effects at the same time. For example, patients frequently perform the Valsalva maneuver during sustained handgrip exercise or when squatting.

Thus, in 1985, a new maneuver was developed that does not require drug administration or patient participation.[9] Transient arterial occlusion is performed by placing sphygmomanometers around the upper portions of both arms and inflating the cuffs simultaneously to 20 to 40 mm Hg above the patient's systolic blood pressure for 20 seconds. Aortic pressure is not increased by this maneuver, but aortic impedance is. Transient arterial occlusion reliably augments the left-sided regurgitant murmurs caused by aortic regurgitation, mitral regurgitation, and ventricular septal defect. When compared with squatting, transient arterial occlusion was a better method for increasing the intensity of left-sided regurgitant lesions and resulted in fewer false-positive diagnoses (Table 13–4). Also, this maneuver has a sensitivity equal to that of sustained handgrip exercise or inhalation of amyl nitrite for detection of left-sided regurgitant murmurs. Importantly, this maneuver can be applied to almost all patients and is a reproducible technique that is easy to perform.

Systematic Dynamic Auscultation

When performing the cardiac examination, the observer should systematically use various maneuvers to test possible murmur causes. Some maneuvers are more sensitive and specific than others (see Table 13–4).[10] A logical, efficient approach to the patient with a cardiac murmur often enables the physician to reach a reasonable conclusion about the importance of the murmur in question.

Initial auscultation will reveal whether a murmur occurs during systole or diastole. The next step should always be to listen carefully during respiration, since this is a very specific method of identifying right-sided or left-sided murmurs.

The right-sided systolic murmurs of tricuspid regurgitation and pulmonic stenosis both increase in intensity during inspiration with the patient in the upright position. Classically, the tricuspid regurgitant murmur is holosystolic and heard at the lower left sternal edge, whereas the murmur of pulmonic stenosis and the insignificant pulmonic flow murmur are mid-systolic, crescendo-decrescendo, and loudest at the left upper sternal edge.

Systolic murmurs that are not augmented or decrease with inspiration are left-sided in origin. The application of dynamic auscultation for distinguishing murmurs owing to mitral regurgitation, ventricular septal defect, valvular aortic stenosis or sclerosis, hypertrophic cardiomyopathy, or mitral valve prolapse is often useful. Murmurs of hypertrophic cardiomyopathy and mitral valve prolapse become louder or longer during the Valsalva maneuver, and the murmurs of both diminish or become shorter during squatting.

Several useful maneuvers can be used to differentiate murmurs of mitral regurgitation and ventricular septal defects from aortic valvular disease.[7, 10] The presence of occasional premature beats or atrial fibrillation may lead to a relatively easy differentiation of valvular aortic stenosis from mitral regurgitation. Murmurs owing to flow across a normal or obstructed semilunar valve become louder with inhalation of amyl nitrite, whereas those of mitral regurgitation and ventricular septal defects become softer. Transient arterial occlusion and sustained handgrip exercise will augment murmurs of mitral regurgitation and ventricular septal defects; the systolic murmur of valvular aortic stenosis changes little, if at all. The presence of an aortic ejection sound, a soft or absent A_2, reversed splitting of S_2, and a fourth heart sound (S_4) are additional clues to the diagnosis of aortic valve stenosis.[2, 5, 6]

If initial auscultation reveals a diastolic murmur, it usually indicates cardiovascular pathology. Thus, the physi-

Table 13–4	Sensitivity and Specificity Value of Maneuvers in the Identification of Systolic Murmurs			
Maneuver	Response	Murmur	Sensitivity (%)	Specificity (%)
Inspiration	↑	RS	100	88
Expiration	↓	RS	100	88
Valsalva maneuver	↑	HC	65	96
Squat to stand	↑	HC	95	84
Stand to squat	↓	HC	95	85
Leg elevation	↓	HC	85	91
Handgrip	↓	HC	85	75
Handgrip	↑	MR & VSD	68	92
Transient arterial occlusion	↑	MR & VSD	78	100
Amyl nitrite	↓	MR & VSD	80	90

Modified with permission from Lembo, N.J., Dell'Italia, L.J., Crawford, M.H., et al.: Bedside diagnosis of systolic murmurs. N. Engl. J. Med. 318:1572–1578, 1988. Copyright 1988 Massachusetts Medical Society. All rights reserved.
Abbreviations: RS, right-sided; HC, hypertrophic cardiomyopathy; MR, mitral regurgitation; VSD, ventricular septal defect.

cian should be certain that the auscultatory finding is definitely present because there are important implications for further diagnostic evaluation, antibiotic prophylaxis, and possible restriction of activity. As with systolic murmurs, the initial evaluation should be careful auscultation during respiration, since augmentation of a diastolic murmur during inspiration indicates a right-sided origin and either tricuspid stenosis or pulmonic regurgitation. Diastolic murmurs that soften during inspiration and are louder during expiration are due to either mitral stenosis or aortic regurgitation or are Austin Flint murmurs. Diastolic murmurs that return to baseline intensity in the first few cardiac cycles after release of a Valsalva maneuver are usually of right-sided cause; later return to baseline intensity implies a left-sided origin. Discrimination between the murmurs of mitral stenosis and those of aortic regurgitation can be difficult at times, despite the fact that the murmurs are usually of different pitch, different diastolic timing, and maximal at different auscultatory sites. Both diastolic murmurs are increased with handgrip and squatting, and both are attenuated in the upright position. Although inhalation of amyl nitrite enhances the diastolic murmur of mitral stenosis and will soften the diastolic murmur of aortic regurgitation, the correct interpretation of diastolic and continuous murmurs is usually established by Doppler echocardiography.

CLINICAL ASSESSMENT

Symptoms or No Symptoms

An important consideration in a patient with a cardiac murmur is the presence or absence of symptoms that may be related to the cause of the heart murmur that is present on cardiac auscultation. For example, symptoms of syncope, anginal chest pain, or congestive heart failure in a patient with a mid-systolic murmur will usually result in a more aggressive approach than that for a patient with a similar mid-systolic murmur who has none of these symptoms. Symptomatic patients should have at least a 2-D echocardiographic assessment with Doppler flow velocity recordings to rule in or rule out the presence of significant aortic valve stenosis. A history of thromboembolism or possible infective endocarditis should also result in a more extensive workup. The presence of systemic embolism in a patient with a cardiac murmur is an indication for 2-D echocardiographic assessment of cardiac chambers and valves for evidence of thrombosis or vegetations and for Doppler echocardiographic flow velocity measurements for the detection of valvular stenosis or regurgitation. In the presence of mitral valve disease, particularly when atrial fibrillation is present, transesophageal echocardiography may be necessary to demonstrate the presence of left atrial thrombus or vegetations.

In patients with cardiac murmurs and clinical findings suggestive of endocarditis, (e.g., fever, petechiae, positive blood cultures, hematuria), 2-D echocardiography with Doppler flow velocity imaging is again indicated. In some cases where the infection involves the mitral valve, or an infected valve prosthesis is suspected, transesophageal echocardiography may be necessary to determine the presence or absence of vegetations and abscesses.

Conversely, many asymptomatic children and young adults with grade II/VI midsystolic murmurs without a history suggestive of cardiac disease and no other cardiac physical findings need no further cardiac workup after the initial history and physical examination. A particularly important group are the large number of *asymptomatic* elderly patients, many with systemic hypertension, who have mid-systolic murmurs due to sclerotic aortic valve leaflets or flow into tortuous, noncompliant great vessels, or a combination of these. Such murmurs must be distinguished from murmurs due to valvular aortic *stenosis,* which is prevalent in this age group. The absence of left ventricular hypertrophy on electrocardiogram (ECG) and a normal chest x-ray are reassuring and less costly than routine echocardiography.

Physical Findings

The presence of other physical findings, either cardiac or noncardiac, may provide important clues to the significance of a cardiac murmur. For example, in a heroin addict who presents with fever, petechiae, Osler's nodes, and Janeway lesions, a right-sided mid-systolic murmur likely represents tricuspid regurgitation without pulmonary hypertension. Also, the diastolic murmur of aortic regurgitation and the mid- to late-systolic murmur of mitral valve prolapse are common in patients with the Marfan syndrome. A soft systolic murmur at the apex is more likely to indicate mitral regurgitation due to coronary artery disease in a patient with uncontrolled systemic hypertension and tuberous xanthomas.[2]

Associated cardiac findings frequently provide important information concerning cardiac murmurs. Fixed splitting of S_2 during inspiration and expiration in a patient with a grade II/VI mid-systolic murmur in the pulmonic area and left sternal border likely indicates an atrial septal defect. Left ventricular dilatation on precordial palpitation, an elevated jugular venous pressure, and bibasilar pulmonary rales favor the diagnosis of mitral regurgitation in a patient with a grade II/VI holosystolic murmur at the cardiac apex. A slow-rising, diminished arterial pulse suggests severe aortic stenosis in a patient with a grade II/VI mid-systolic murmur at the upper intercostal spaces.

ECG and Chest X-Ray

Whereas echocardiography usually provides more specific and often quantitative information concerning the significance of a heart murmur and may be the only test needed, the ECG and chest x-ray are often already obtained and readily available. The absence of ventricular hypertrophy, atrial dilatation, arrhythmias, conduction abnormalities, prior infarction, and evidence of active ischemia on ECG interpretation provides useful negative information at a relatively low cost when the murmur is likely insignificant. The presence of abnormal findings on the ECG, such as ventricular hypertrophy or a prior myocardial infarction, will usually lead to more extensive evaluation, including 2-D and Doppler echocardiography.

Posteroanterior and lateral chest x-rays often yield qualitative information concerning cardiac chamber size, pulmonary arterial blood flow, pulmonary venous blood flow, and cardiac calcifications in patients being assessed with cardiac murmurs. When abnormal findings are present on chest x-ray, 2-D and Doppler echocardiography are commonly performed. The presence of normal posteroanterior and lateral chest x-rays as well as a normal ECG is likely in patients with insignificant mid-systolic cardiac murmurs, particularly in younger age groups, in females, and when the murmur is less than grade III in intensity. Many of these asymptomatic patients may need neither an ECG nor a chest x-ray when a careful cardiac examination indicates an insignificant vibratory mid-systolic heart murmur and no abnormal cardiac or noncardiac findings.

Echocardiography

Echocardiography is an important noninvasive method for assessing the significance of various cardiac murmurs in certain patients by the accurate imaging of cardiac structures and function and the flow-direction of velocities within cardiac chambers and vessels.[4–6] 2-D echocardiography may indicate the presence of abnormal valvular motion and morphology, but it usually does not indicate the severity. Using the Doppler effect, direction of shift in ultrasound frequency is used to determine the direction of flow of the red cells in relation to transducers. The direction of flow is displayed as a spectral velocity profile with the profile oriented toward the transducer for blood coming toward it and away from the transducer for blood flowing away from it.

The direction of flow can also be depicted by using color coding of velocity shapes within the cardiac chambers, with red depicting blood flow toward the transducer and blue indicating blood flow moving away from the

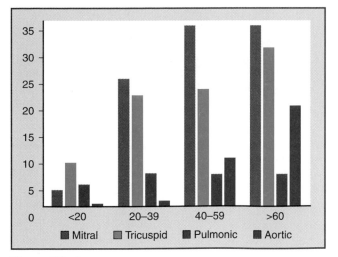

Figure 13–6

Percent incidence of mitral, tricuspid, pulmonic, and aortic regurgitation by Doppler echocardiography in clinically normal subjects at various ages. (Modified from Choong, C.Y., Abascal, V.M., and Weyman, J.: Prevalence of valvular regurgitation by Doppler echocardiography in patients with structurally normal hearts by 2-dimensional echocardiography. Am. Heart J. 117:636–642, 1989.)

transducer. Not only can the direction of flow of the red cells be assessed, but also the red blood cell velocity can be measured. This velocity information can be used to quantify flow and measure pressure within cardiac chambers. Using the modified Bernoulli equation ($P = 4V^2$), the peak instantaneous velocity (V) across the region can be converted to the peak instantaneous pressure gradient (P) across it. The area of a valve can be calculated to assess the severity of stenosis by using the rate of velocity decrease (pressure half-time) or incorporating the flow through the valve (continuity equation). Thus, by measuring the increase in Doppler velocity across the valve, the extent of valvular stenosis can be quantitated accurately. Using the Doppler principle, valvular regurgitation and intracardiac shunts can be estimated by showing the extent of abnormal velocity jet into the receiving chamber.

Although 2-D echocardiography and Doppler color-flow imaging can provide important information concerning patients with cardiac murmurs, they are not necessary tests for all patients with cardiac murmurs and usually add little but expense in the evaluation of asymptomatic patients with short grade I to II mid-systolic murmurs, otherwise normal physical findings, and no history suggestive of cardiac disease.

It is important to consider that many recent studies indicate that with improved sensitivity of Doppler ultrasound devices, valvular regurgitation may be detected through the tricuspid and pulmonic valves in a very high percentage of young healthy subjects and through left-sided valves in a variable but lower percentage.[12–15] In a recent study of 200 healthy Japanese subjects, mitral regurgitation could be detected by Doppler in up to 45% of individuals; tricuspid regurgitation in up to 70%; and pulmonic regurgitation in up to 88%, even though these patients were healthy, had no cardiac auscultation evidence of heart disease, and had normal ECGs.[14] "Normal"

aortic regurgitation is encountered much less frequently and its incidence increases with advancing age (Fig. 13–6). Thus, echocardiographic interpretations of mild or trivial (physiologic) valvular regurgitation may lead to the echocardiographic diagnosis of cardiac disease in patients without clinical heart disease.

The valvular regurgitation signal in healthy subjects is usually localized in the immediate proximity of the coaptation site of the valve leaflets and is much less widely distributed in the receiving chamber than in patients studied with pathologic valve regurgitation. Various criteria have been developed for the diagnosis of "physiologic" valvular regurgitation of the tricuspid, mitral, or pulmonic valves that may be considered to be normal findings when detected at the level of the leaflets.[13] There is, unfortunately, a gray zone where normal meets abnormal as well as variations in the prevalence of observed valvular regurgitation in specific patient populations. An incorrect diagnosis of abnormal regurgitation ("echocardiographic heart disease") may be less frequent if such tests are not ordered routinely in asymptomatic patients with insignificant short mid-systolic murmurs who have no other evidence of cardiac disease by physical examination. General recommendations for performing 2-D and Doppler echocardiography in patients with heart murmurs are listed in Table 13–5. Of course, individual exceptions to these indications may exist. For example, an asymptomatic 60-year-old with a short grade II mid-systolic murmur and ECG evidence of left ventricular hypertrophy may require echocardiography to determine the presence of valvular aortic stenosis.

Cardiac Catheterization

Cardiac catheterization and angiography can provide important information concerning the presence and severity of valvular obstruction, valvular regurgitation, and intracardiac shunting. These are not necessary in most patients with cardiac murmurs and normal echocardiograms, but they provide added information in some patients in whom the echocardiogram has established the presence of significant heart disease as the cause of the cardiac murmur. Cardiac catheterization with coronary arteriography to assess the presence of coronary disease is performed routinely in most adult patients aged 35 years and older who are being considered for cardiac surgery to correct either valvular heart disease or congenital heart disease.

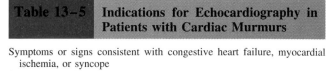

Table 13–5	Indications for Echocardiography in Patients with Cardiac Murmurs

Symptoms or signs consistent with congestive heart failure, myocardial ischemia, or syncope
Symptoms or signs consistent with infective endocarditis or thromboembolism
Any diastolic or continuous murmur
All holosystolic and late-systolic murmurs
Any mid-systolic murmur of grade III or more intensity
Additional abnormal physical findings on cardiac palpation or auscultation

APPROACH TO THE PATIENT

The evaluation of the patient with a heart murmur may vary greatly depending on many of the considerations discussed previously. These include the intensity of the cardiac murmur, its timing in the cardiac cycle, its location and radiation, and its response to various physiologic maneuvers. Also of importance are the presence or absence of cardiac and noncardiac symptoms and whether other cardiac or noncardiac physical findings suggest that the cardiac murmur is clinically significant. The skill and confidence of the cardiac auscultator, the relative costs of various diagnostic approaches, and the accuracy and reliability of additional tests in the laboratory where they are performed are also important factors. One systematic approach to the patient with a heart murmur is depicted in Figure 13–7. This algorithm is particularly applicable to children and adults under age 40 years.

Patients with definite diastolic heart murmurs or continuous murmurs not due to a cervical venous hum or a mammary soufflé during pregnancy are candidates for 2-D and Doppler echocardiography. If the results of echocardiography indicate significant heart disease, a cardiac consultation is generally obtained. An echocardiographic examination is also recommended for patients with apical or left sternal edge pansystolic or late-systolic murmurs, for those with mid-systolic murmurs of grade III or more in intensity, and for those with softer mid-systolic murmurs in whom dynamic cardiac auscultation suggests a definite cardiac diagnosis (e.g., hypertrophic cardiomyopathy). The suggested approach is to proceed with 2-D and Doppler echocardiography, with cardiac consultation if abnormal results are obtained.

More specifically, further cardiac evaluation including echocardiography or cardiac consultation, or both, is recommended for patients in whom the intensity of a systolic murmur increases during the Valsalva maneuver, becomes louder when the patient assumes the upright position, and decreases in intensity when the patient squats. These responses during dynamic auscultation suggest the diagnosis of either hypertrophic cardiomyopathy or mitral valve prolapse. Additionally, further cardiac assessment is indicated when a systolic murmur increases in intensity during transient arterial occlusion, becomes louder during sustained handgrip exercise, or does not increase its intensity either in the cardiac cycle following a premature ventricular contraction or after a long R-R interval in patients with atrial fibrillation. The diagnosis of mitral regurgitation or ventricular septal defect is likely.

In many patients with grade I/II mid-systolic murmurs, an extensive workup is not necessary. This applies particularly to children and young adults who are asymptomatic, have an otherwise normal cardiac examination, and have no other physical findings associated with cardiac disease. In these patients, there is no need for routine echocardiography or other tests that increase the cost of health care delivery. However, echocardiography is indicated in certain patients with grade I/II mid-systolic murmurs. These include patients with symptoms or signs consistent with infective endocarditis or thromboembolism and those with symptoms or signs consistent with congestive heart failure, myocardial ischemia, or syncope. Echocardiography also usually provides an accurate diagnosis in patients with other abnormal physical findings on cardiac palpitation or auscultation, the latter including specific changes in the intensity of the systolic murmur during certain physiologic maneuvers as described previously. When the diagnosis is in doubt in asymptomatic patients after auscultation, the presence of an abnormal ECG or chest x-ray usually leads to echocardiography (Fig. 13–8). In elderly asymptomatic patients with limited functional activity, echocardiography will separate patients with soft mid-systolic aortic murmurs owing to aortic sclerosis from those with valvular aortic stenosis.

Whereas 2-D and Doppler echocardiography are important tests for those patients with a moderate to high likelihood that a cardiac murmur is clinically important, it must be re-emphasized that trivial, minimal, or physiologic valvular regurgitation—especially affecting the mitral, tricuspid, or pulmonic valves—is detected by color-flow imaging techniques in many otherwise normal pa-

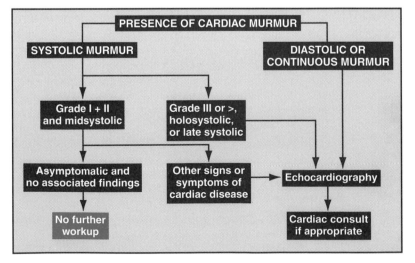

Figure 13–7

An approach to the workup of a patient with a cardiac murmur, depending on whether the murmur is likely innocent or due to cardiac pathology. This algorithm is particularly relevant to children and adults under age 40 years and utilizes echocardiography before cardiac consultation.

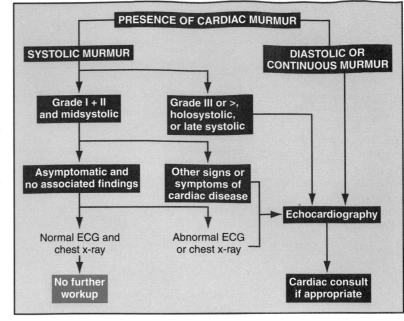

Figure 13–8

An alternative "echocardiography-first" approach to the evaluation of a heart murmur that also uses the results of the electrocardiogram (ECG) and chest x-ray in asymptomatic patients with soft mid-systolic murmurs and no other physical findings. This algorithm is useful in patients over age 40 years in whom the prevalence of coronary artery disease and aortic stenosis increases as the cause of systolic murmurs.

tients and including many patients who have no heart murmur at all. This must be considered when using echocardiogram results to guide decisions concerning asymptomatic patients in whom echocardiography was used to assess the clinical significance of an isolated heart murmur.

A cardiac consultation *without additional cardiac testing* costs considerably less than routine echocardiography and is an alternative method for assessing the significance of a cardiac murmur when the primary physician believes that further evaluation is necessary (Fig. 13–9). The relative cost depends on whether the cardiac consultation includes the ordering of a large number of additional tests for many patients who have no underlying cardiac disease. This alternative approach may be most useful in the evaluation of children with loud innocent vibratory systolic murmurs and in adults with insignificant but loud

mid-systolic murmurs during high blood-flow states, such as pregnancy or severe anemia. It may also be the better approach for asymptomatic patients who are elderly and have short faint mid-systolic murmurs due to flow across thickened aortic leaflets, such as commonly occur in patients with hypertension; such murmurs often differ from those due to valvular aortic stenosis or significant mitral regurgitation. If the cardiac consultant orders echocardiography for all patients referred for evaluation with heart murmurs, this is clearly not cost-effective. The absence of left ventricular hypertrophy on an ECG and the presence of a normal cardiac size without pulmonary venous congestion on chest x-ray may aid in the evaluation of the asymptomatic elderly patient with an insignificant short soft mid-systolic murmur without the need for more costly cardiac consultation and echocardiography (Fig. 13–10).

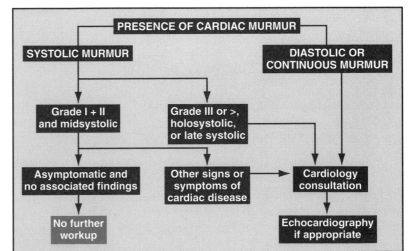

Figure 13–9

This approach for assessing patients with heart murmurs uses cardiac consultation rather than the echocardiogram as the initial step for those patients with increased likelihood of having cardiac disease. This approach is particularly useful in situations where the cardiac consultant does not order routine echocardiography in all patients referred for evaluation of heart murmurs.

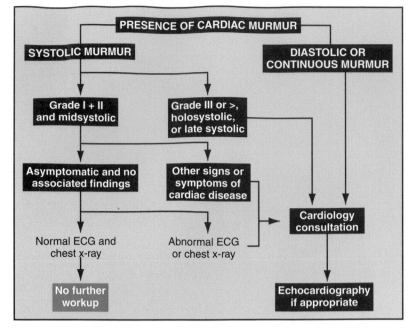

Figure 13–10

This modification of the "cardiac consultation—first" approach for the evaluation of heart murmurs uses the results of the electrocardiogram (ECG) and chest x-ray in asymptomatic patients with soft mid-systolic murmurs and no other physical findings. Cardiac consultation is usually obtained for asymptomatic patients who have left ventricular hypertrophy by electrocardiography or have cardiomegaly or pulmonary venous congestion by chest x-ray.

COST CONSIDERATIONS

Very little data consider the cost-effectiveness of various approaches to the patient undergoing medical evaluation because of the presence of a cardiac murmur. Optimal auscultation by well-trained examiners who can recognize an insignificant mid-systolic murmur with confidence using dynamic cardiac auscultation as indicated results in the less frequent use of expensive additional testing to define murmurs that do not indicate cardiac pathology. Unfortunately, cardiac auscultation is less emphasized in medical and postgraduate medical training than in previous years owing to the more popular high-technology tests that are available for assessing patients with suspected or definite cardiac disease.

The relative costs of a cardiac consultation, posteroanterior and lateral chest x-rays, an ECG, Doppler and 2-D echocardiography, and cardiac catheterization without coronary arteriography are indicated in Figure 13–11. When needed, cardiac consultation alone is relatively inexpensive but many patients with heart murmurs being referred for cardiac consultation have chest x-rays, ECGs, and 2-D and Doppler echocardiograms recorded routinely before or after the consultation visit. Thus, if a cardiac consultation routinely results in the ordering of echocardiography and other noninvasive tests, the accumulated cost is greater than if cardiac consultation is obtained only in patients with echocardiographic evidence of heart disease as the cause of a cardiac murmur.

Since echocardiography available directly to primary care physicians represents an alternative strategy to cardiac consultation for heart murmur evaluation, Danford and associates[16] used a decision-analysis model to compare the costs of two diagnostic strategies: (1) perform echocardiography first, refer to a cardiologist, if appropriate; and (2) cardiologist evaluates murmur, echocardiography if appropriate. Of the 236 pediatric patients with innocent systolic murmurs in the referral-first strategy group, the pediatric cardiologists ordered an echocardiogram in only 25%. Of those patients with trivial and significant heart disease, the cardiologists ordered an echocardiogram in 53% and 88%, respectively. In the echocardiography-first group, 77% had innocent murmurs, 15% had trivial heart disease, and 8% had potentially significant disease. Echocardiography-first strategy costs

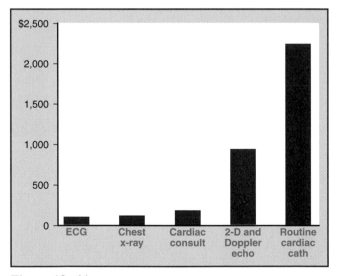

Figure 13–11

The relative costs of the cardiac evaluation using laboratory plus interpretation fees for an electrocardiogram (ECG), posteroanterior and lateral chest x-rays, two-dimensional (2-D) and Doppler echocardiography, and cardiac catheterization without coronary arteriography are compared with the cost of an initial cardiac consultation alone. If the cardiac consultation routinely includes an ECG, chest x-ray, and echocardiogram, it will be less cost-effective than the initial use of 2-D and Doppler echocardiography with further cardiac consultation only if the results are abnormal.

averaged $257 more than referral-first strategy costs. Thus, pediatric cardiac consultation appeared to be the preferred approach provided that cardiac consultation costs are moderate, echocardiographic costs are moderate to high, and the rate at which the cardiologist orders echocardiography for patients with innocent murmurs is low. In the author's experience, the percentage of patients undergoing routine echocardiography if referred to adult cardiologists because of a heart murmur is much higher. There are no prospective data concerning the cost-effectiveness of the approaches indicated in Figures 13–7 through 13–10, but the echocardiography-first approach in patients with clinical indications for further evaluation appears logical at this time.

SPECIAL CLINICAL CIRCUMSTANCES

Innocent Murmur

The so-called innocent murmur is heard at rest in patients with normal cardiovascular systems and normal hemodynamics. Innocent murmurs are usually soft, are of short duration, and are heard in early to mid systole at the left sternal edge and the pulmonic area. In children, they are vibratory in quality and available evidence suggests that they are caused by aortic turbulence. Innocent murmurs can also originate at vessel branch points owing to increased flow velocity or turbulence as the vessel becomes tortuous or smaller. These extra-cardiac murmurs are typically heard in the neck (e.g., brachiocephalic) or abdomen.[2, 3, 7]

Insignificant murmurs due to pulmonic turbulence will increase with inspiration and decrease with expiration and are softer when the patient is upright. Insignificant murmurs of left-sided or right-sided origin will increase with any maneuver that augments blood flow, such as squatting, exertion, or anxiety. The murmur will be intensified in the cardiac cycle after a premature beat. The straining phase of the Valsalva maneuver will decrease the intensity of the insignificant murmur, whereas isometric handgrip exercise has no effect on the auscultatory findings.

Physiologic maneuvers will help distinguish the murmurs of mitral regurgitation or tricuspid regurgitation from insignificant outflow murmurs, which can sound quite similar. However, differentiating between insignificant and pathologic aortic or pulmonic murmurs is more difficult and is best done by exclusion. Subjects with benign murmurs will usually be asymptomatic and have no other physical findings of cardiac disease. The most useful negative auscultatory finding is the absence of an ejection sound, since mild to moderate aortic or pulmonic valvular stenosis is usually associated with this finding.

Pregnancy

It is important to identify women with cardiovascular abnormalities before or during pregnancy so that proper endocarditis antibiotic prophylaxis can be considered during a complicated labor and delivery. This task is more difficult if the initial cardiac examination is done after early pregnancy because the intensity of some murmurs changes greatly during the altered hemodynamics of pregnancy. Cardiac output begins to increase during the first trimester, possibly as early as the 10th week, and remains elevated through the third trimester. Simultaneously, systemic vascular resistance falls during the first and second trimesters and is maintained at a lower level, often with a decrease in mean arterial pressure. The circulating blood volume is increased, and an insignificant mid-systolic murmur and a physiologic S_3 are present in the majority of pregnant women.[7, 8]

In the nonpregnant state, murmurs of mitral or aortic regurgitation vary in intensity and duration with changes in arterial blood pressure. During pregnancy, these murmurs will often be softer than in the nonpregnant state owing to the reduced systemic vascular resistance. When no reduction in intensity of aortic and mitral regurgitant murmurs occurs during pregnancy, it is often due to the onset or exacerbation of maternal systemic hypertension. Bilateral maximal handgrip exercise and transient arterial occlusion are useful methods for increasing left-sided regurgitant murmurs in pregnant patients. Patients with either mitral regurgitation or aortic regurgitation usually do well during pregnancy because the physiologic hemodynamic changes minimize the volume of regurgitant flow. However, antibiotic endocarditis prophylaxis is indicated. The murmurs of mitral stenosis and tricuspid regurgitation usually become louder during pregnancy owing to the changes in cardiac output and systemic vascular resistance that occur.

Mammary soufflé is a continuous murmur heard at the left sternal edge in many pregnant or lactating women when the patient is supine. It results from blood flow through the superficial mammary arteries of the breast. When present, this continuous murmur can be heard as early as the second or third trimester and can persist during lactation. The Valsalva maneuver has no effect on the mammary soufflé, differentiating it from the continuous murmur due a venous hum, which disappears during the Valsalva maneuver. Assuming an upright posture will cause the mammary soufflé to fade or disappear. The schematic approaches to the assessment of cardiac murmurs depicted in Figures 13–7 through 13–10 pertain during pregnancy as well.

Heart of the Athlete

Physicians caring for athletes need to be aware of the physiologic effects of training because some of the cardiovascular changes can mimic pathologic heart disease. An erroneous diagnosis of heart disease in a normal athlete may have major unfortunate consequences, including the limitation of physical activity.

The physical examination of athletes can elicit many findings that would be considered abnormal in less well conditioned individuals. Accurate history-taking will help place abnormal physical findings in proper perspective. Cervical venous hums may be heard over the neck owing to the large stroke volume and increased cardiac output.

Cardiac enlargement is manifested as a displaced apical impulse or right ventricular lift. The presence of an S_3 is usual owing to rapid filling of the left ventricle in early diastole. Approximately half of all athletes will have an audible S_4 for unknown reasons.[7]

Murmurs are very common in this population. They are usually insignificant mid-systolic murmurs due to the increased stroke volume. Rarely, a mid-diastolic low-pitched murmur occurs owing to the augmented blood flow across atrioventricular valves. Having the patient assume an upright posture will cause a decrease or disappearance of both systolic and diastolic murmurs. The approaches to the assessment of the murmur indicated in Figures 13–7 through 13–10 also apply to this group.

Mitral Valve Prolapse
(See also Chap. 25)

Mitral valve prolapse is defined as the systolic posterior movement of one or both mitral valve leaflets into the left atrium, often resulting in mitral regurgitation. Mitral valve prolapse occurs when the left ventricular volume falls below a certain critical level during systole. The hallmark finding on physical examination is the mid-systolic click; it may or may not be followed by a late-systolic murmur. The timing of the auscultatory findings during systole can be altered by various maneuvers, with the response often indicating a definite diagnosis.[1, 3, 7]

Maneuvers that modify the left ventricular end-diastolic volume will affect the click-murmur timing during systole. Interventions such as the Valsalva maneuver or assuming an upright posture will decrease the left ventricular volume and cause the critical volume at which prolapse occurs to be achieved earlier in systole; as a result, the click-murmur complex moves closer to S_1. Submaximal isometric handgrip exercise also moves the click-murmur complex to an earlier point in systole because the associated tachycardia reduces the left ventricular volume and increases contractility.

Maneuvers that increase either the left ventricular volume or the afterload will move the click-murmur complex to a later point in systole. Therefore, bradycardia such as is induced with beta blocker therapy will increase the left ventricular volume and the systolic clicks or murmur moves toward S_2. Rapid squatting increases aortic pressure and afterload and enhances venous return. Thus, the left ventricular volume is enlarged, and the click-murmur complex begins later in systole. It is particularly useful to have the patient stand up rapidly from the squatting position because this markedly reduces the left ventricular volume and moves the click-murmur complex to a much earlier point in systole.

Systolic clicks are not necessarily specific for a mitral valve prolapse, and some patients with prolapse have a mid-systolic click without a late-systolic murmur. Systolic clicks can mimic a split S_1 or an early-systolic ejection sound. An important physical finding is movement of the click with maneuvers, because ejection sounds and a split S_1 never occur in mid or late systole. Changes in the systolic timing of the murmur during various maneuvers are important when a mitral valve prolapse occurs with only a systolic murmur and no click. This presentation is often seen in patients with a mitral valve prolapse.

The author recommends 2-D and Doppler echocardiography for all patients with definite or suspected mitral valve prolapse. This is not only to confirm the diagnosis, which the echocardiogram will fail to detect in up to 10% of clinically certain cases, but more importantly also to assess left atrial size, left ventricular size and function, the extent of mitral leaflet redundancy, and the presence and severity of mitral regurgitation. The risk of complications including infective endocarditis and thromboembolism, and subsequent need for mitral valve surgery, correlates with the severity of the echocardiographic findings.

The late-systolic murmur of hypertrophic cardiomyopathy (see Chap. 31) can be confused with the murmur of mitral valve prolapse, although patients with hypertrophic cardiomyopathy rarely have mid-systolic clicks. Both murmurs have a similar response to changes in posture, squatting, and standing. The Valsalva maneuver is a useful method to differentiate between the two conditions. In hypertrophic cardiomyopathy, the murmur is markedly louder during the straining phase of the Valsalva maneuver, whereas in mitral valve prolapse, the murmur is longer but usually not louder and sometimes softer. More reliable is the variance in the murmur after a premature beat; it is much louder in hypertrophic cardiomyopathy, but unchanged in mitral valve prolapse. Additionally, transient arterial occlusion will reliably increase the intensity of mitral regurgitant murmurs in mitral valve prolapse but has little effect on the murmur of hypertrophic cardiomyopathy. 2-D and Doppler echocardiography will confirm the correct diagnosis.

SUMMARY

The diagnostic evaluation of a patient with a cardiac murmur varies considerably, depending on many factors. Careful and accurate cardiac auscultation forms the cornerstone for the subsequent approach. Most patients who have associated abnormal cardiac findings and those with symptoms suggesting cardiovascular disease will undergo 2-D and Doppler echocardiography. Cardiac consultation is appropriate when the echocardiographic findings are abnormal or as an alternative first approach when the murmur is likely significant.

Conversely, many asymptomatic patients with grade I/II mid-systolic murmurs and no associated abnormal cardiac findings need no further diagnostic testing after the history and physical examination.

When the primary physician is uncertain as to the significance of a cardiac murmur after careful auscultation, including the use of physiologic maneuvers to alter its intensity, the two alternatives are initial cardiac consultation and echocardiography with subsequent cardiac consultation, if appropriate. If the consultant is likely to order echocardiography in the majority of patients sent for further evaluation, an echocardiogram requested by the primary physician, and referral only if the echocardiogram is abnormal, may be the most cost-effective approach.

References

1. Abrams, J.: Essentials of Cardiac Physical Diagnosis. Philadelphia, Lea & Febiger, 1987, pp. 145–183.
2. O'Rourke, R.A., and Braunwald, E.: Physical examination of the cardiovascular system. *In* Fauci A.S., Braunwald, E., Isselbacher, K.J., et al. (eds.): Principles in Internal Medicine. 14th ed. New York, McGraw-Hill, 1998, pp. 1230–1237.
3. Harvey, W.P.: Cardiac pearls. Dis. Mon. 20:45–116, 1994.
4. Shaver, J.A.: Cardiac auscultation: A cost-effective diagnostic skill. Curr. Probl. Cardiol. 20:441–530, 1995.
5. Shaver, J.A., and Salerni, R.: Auscultation of the heart. *In* Schlant, R.A., and Alexander, R.W. (eds.): The Heart. 8th ed. New York, McGraw-Hill, 1994, pp. 253–314.
6. Perloff, J.K.: Heart sounds and murmurs: Physiological mechanisms. *In* Braunwald, E. (ed.): Heart Disease. 5th ed. Philadelphia, W.B. Saunders, 1997, pp. 15–51.
7. Grewe, K., Crawford, M.H., and O'Rourke, R.A.: Differentiation of cardiac murmurs by auscultation. Curr. Probl. Cardiol. 13:699–721, 1988.
8. McAnulty, J.H., Morton, M.J., and Ueland, K.: The heart and pregnancy. Curr. Probl. Cardiol. 13:589–665, 1988.
9. Lembo, N.J., Dell'Italia, L.J., Crawford, M.H., et al.: Diagnosis of left-sided regurgitant murmurs by transient arterial occlusion: A new maneuver using blood pressure cuffs. Ann. Intern. Med. 105: 368–670, 1986.
10. Lembo, N.J., Dell'Italia, L.J., Crawford, M.H., et al.: Bedside diagnosis of systolic murmurs. N. Engl. J. Med. 318:1572, 1988.
11. Karliner, J.S., O'Rourke, R.A., Kearney, D.J., et al.: Haemodynamic explanation of why the murmur of mitral regurgitation is independent of cycle length. Br. Heart J. 35:397–401, 1973.
12. Choong, C.Y., Abascal, V.M., and Weyman, J.: Prevalence of valvular regurgitation by Doppler echocardiography in patients with structurally normal hearts by 2-dimensional echocardiography. Am. Heart J. 117:636–642, 1989.
13. Sahn, D.J., and Maciel, B.C.: Physiological valvular regurgitation. Doppler echocardiography and the potential for iatrogenic heart disease. Circulation 78:1075–1077, 1988.
14. Yoshida, K., Yoshikawa, J., and Shakudo, M.: Color Doppler evaluation of valvular regurgitation in normals. Circulation 78:840–847, 1988.
15. Kostucki, W., Vandenbossche, J.-L., Friart, A., et al.: Pulsed Doppler regurgitant flow patterns of normal valves. Am. J. Cardiol. 58: 309–313, 1986.
16. Danford, D.A., Nasir, A., and Gumbiner, C.: Cost assessment of the evaluation of heart murmurs in children. Pediatrics 91:365–368, 1993.

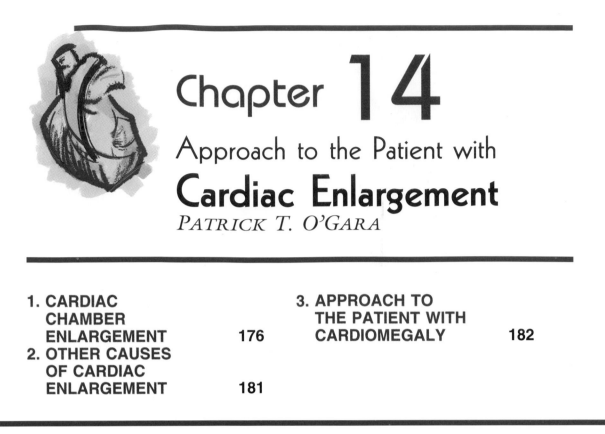

Chapter 14

Approach to the Patient with
Cardiac Enlargement

PATRICK T. O'GARA

At autopsy, the weight of the heart ranges from 280 to 340 gm in adult men and from 230 to 280 gm in adult women. The heart increases in size and weight with age, a process that is more pronounced in men. In clinical practice, the first clue to the presence of cardiomegaly is usually provided by the radiologic examination, but it may also be derived from the physical findings. When the adult heart is viewed in the posteroanterior (PA) projection, it generally measures 12 cm from base to apex, 8 to 9 cm in the transverse direction, and on lateral films, 6 cm in the anteroposterior (AP) direction.

Cardiac enlargement is commonly detected by physical examination or by chest radiography. In some patients, cardiac enlargement may be the first sign of previously undiagnosed cardiac disease, so this finding should prompt a careful search for the cause of the enlargement, based on an integrated assessment of the key features of the history, physical examination, and other findings on laboratory examination.

Physical Examination

(see also Chap. 3)

Observation of the chest wall, palpation of the cardiac impulse, and percussion of the lateral border of cardiac dullness provide a first approximation of heart size, posi-tion, and shape.[1] The left ventricular apex beat should not fall outside the mid-clavicular line or more than 10 cm to the left of the mid-sternal line and should occupy an area not more than 3 cm in diameter or lower than the fifth intercostal space. Any further leftward or downward displacement or enlargement of the apical impulse usually signifies an increase in heart size. Although the characteristics of the apex beat are best appreciated by palpation with the patient in the left lateral decubitus position, the location of the apex should always be ascertained with the patient supine and the trunk elevated to approximately 30 degrees.

The location and character of the apex beat are also dependent on the configuration and thickness of the thoracic cage, which must be taken into account in estimating cardiomegaly. Tall, asthenic individuals with a thin chest wall tend to have a vertically oriented heart, the lateral border of which may extend only a few centimeters from the midline. However, the apical impulse is well transmitted through the chest wall and may appear unusually prominent. The opposite occurs in short, muscular, or obese persons. Patients with chronic obstructive lung disease and barrel chest deformity with flattened diaphragms tend to have displacement of the cardiac impulse—in this case, the right ventricle—into the subxiphoid area. In such patients, left-sided cardiac enlargement can be very difficult to appreciate, but when the signs of left ventricular enlargement are apparent on

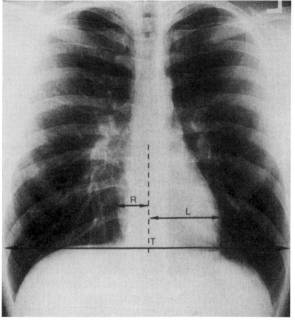

Figure 14–1
Measurement of heart size. Transverse cardiac diameter = R + L. Cardiothoracic ratio = (R + L)/T. (From Rubens, M.B.: Chest x-ray in adult heart disease. *In* Julian, D.G., Camm, A.J., Fox, K.M., et al. [eds.]: Diseases of the Heart. 2nd ed. London, W.B. Saunders, 1996, p. 258.)

physical examination, the true enlargement is usually quite severe. Conversely, in patients with pectus excavatum or a straight back deformity with loss of the normal dorsal spine kyphosis and a reduced AP chest diameter, the left ventricular apex beat can be displaced laterally in the absence of true cardiac enlargement. The presence of these two deformities can be confirmed on clinical examination.

Chest Radiography

Enlargement of the heart may first be detected as an incidental finding on a chest radiograph that is obtained for the evaluation of other processes.[2] Cardiomegaly on chest radiography is commonly defined by a cardiothoracic ratio of 0.50 as measured on the PA film. The widest transverse dimension of the cardiac silhouette is compared with the maximal width of the thoracic cage (Fig. 14–1). Assessment of relative cardiac size is less accurate on films obtained in the AP projection because of magnification artifact. Alterations in lung volume also detract from the reliability of this estimate. The cardiothoracic ratio is falsely elevated when lung volumes are low, as during exhalation, and may be misleadingly small with hyperinflation, as occurs in emphysema. Both pectus excavatum and straight back syndrome can exaggerate the size of the cardiac silhouette and increase the cardiothoracic ratio on the PA projection (Fig. 14–2). Relative cardiac volume can be estimated by measuring the long

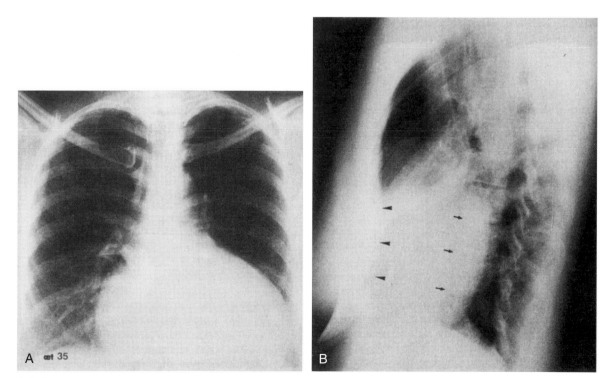

Figure 14–2
Straight back. *A,* On the frontal film, the heart appears markedly enlarged. *B,* The lateral film shows that the dorsal spine is straightened, the thoracic anteroposterior diameter is decreased, and the heart is compressed between sternum *(arrowheads)* and spine *(arrows).* (*A* and *B,* From Rubens, M.B.: Chest x-ray in adult heart disease. *In* Julian, D.G., Camm, A.J., Fox, K.M., et al. [eds.]: Diseases of the Heart. 2nd ed. London, W.B. Saunders, 1996, p. 260.)

axis (L) and short axis (S) on the frontal view and the AP diameter (D) on the lateral view (Fig. 14–3). The calculation is made as follows:

Relative cardiac volume (in ml/m² BSA)

$$= \frac{L \times S \times D \times K}{BSA \ (in \ ml/m^2)}$$

L, S, K, and D are expressed in centimeters and the constant K, the enlargement factor, is related to the distance between the x-ray tube and the film and is 0.42 for the usual 6-foot film. (BSA means body surface area.) Values exceeding 490 ml/m² in women and 540 ml/m² in men denote definite cardiac enlargement. Other imaging methods (echocardiography, computed tomography [CT], magnetic resonance imaging [MRI]) that are more accurate than the plain chest radiogram are available for the measurement of cardiac size and for following changes.

Differential Diagnosis

The list of disorders associated with cardiomegaly is long, but it can often be pared substantially by careful attention to the history and physical examination. In most patients, additional testing can be pursued thereafter in a focused, hierarchical, and cost-effective manner. A pathoanatomic approach to the differential diagnosis, based on the actual structures shown to be enlarged, is a useful starting point (Table 14–1).

CARDIAC CHAMBER ENLARGEMENT

The normal radiographic anatomy of the heart and the location of the four chambers and great vessel are shown in Figure 14–4.

Left Ventricle

On physical examination, dilatation of the left ventricle is evidenced by a leftward and downward displacement of the cardiac apex and enlargement of the latter. The PA radiogram also shows such displacement (Fig. 14–5A). The enlarged left ventricle may extend posterior to the esophagus on the lateral view (Fig. 14–5B). Enlargement of the left ventricle is especially well seen on the left anterior oblique view (Fig. 14–6A).

Left ventricular dilatation occurs in response to the chronic volume overload that accompanies significant mitral or aortic regurgitation, conditions readily identified by their characteristic murmurs (see Chaps. 13 and 25); their severity can be estimated by the presence of associated symptoms or additional findings on physical examination, such as a thrill, third heart sound, or pulmonary rales. Unusual causes of left ventricular volume overload in the adult include a previously unrecognized patent ductus arteriosus, ventricular septal defect, and arteriovenous fistula, malformations that are usually recognizable by their auscultatory findings. Volume overload and left ventricular dilatation are also observed in high cardiac output

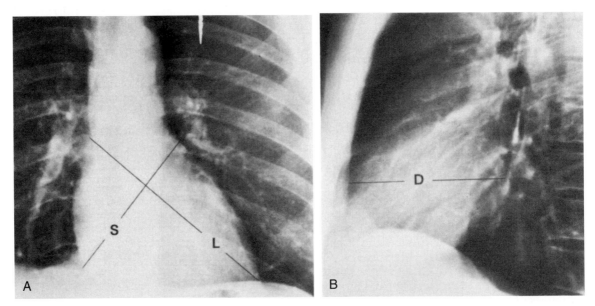

Figure 14–3
Measurement of relative cardiac volume. *A,* Frontal projection. The long axis of the heart (L) is measured from the break in the right cardiac contour, where the superior vena cava joins the right atrium, to the apex of the heart. The short diameter (S) extends from the right cardiophrenic angle to the junction of the left atrial and pulmonary artery segments. This line is roughly perpendicular to the long axis. *B,* Lateral view. The widest anteroposterior dimension of the cardiac silhouette constitutes the depth of the heart (D). If the posterior border of the heart cannot be clearly identified, the anterior margin of the barium-filled esophagus can be used as the boundary for this measurement. (*A* and *B,* From Baron, M.G.: Radiological and angiographic examination of the heart. *In* Braunwald, E. [ed.]: Heart Disease. 3rd ed. Philadelphia, W.B. Saunders, 1988, p. 151.)

Table 14–1	Cardiac Enlargement: Differential Diagnosis

Cardiac chamber enlargement
  Chronic volume overload
    Mitral or aortic regurgitation
    Left-to-right shunt (PDA, VSD, AV fistula)
  Cardiomyopathy
    Ischemic
    Nonischemic
  Decompensated pressure overload
    Aortic stenosis
    Hypertension
  High-output states
    Severe anemia
    Thyrotoxicosis
  Bradycardia
    Severe sinus bradycardia
    Complete heart block
Left atrium
  LV failure of any cause
  Mitral valve disease
  Myxoma
Right ventricle
  Chronic LV failure of any cause
  Chronic volume overload
    Tricuspid or pulmonic regurgitation
    Left-to-right shunt (ASD)
  Decompensated pressure overload
    Pulmonic stenosis
    Pulmonary artery hypertension
      Primary
      Secondary (PE, COPD)
    Pulmonary veno-occlusive disease
Right atrium
  RV failure of any cause
  Tricuspid valve disease
  Myxoma
  Ebstein's anomaly
Multichamber enlargement
  Hypertrophic cardiomyopathy
  Acromegaly
  Severe obesity
Pericardial disease
  Pericardial effusion with or without tamponade
  Effusive constrictive disease
  Pericardial cyst, loculated effusion
Pseudocardiomegaly
  Epicardial fat
  Chest wall deformity (pectus excavatum, straight back syndrome)
  Low lung volumes
  AP chest x-ray
  Mediastinal tumor, cyst

Abbreviations: PDA, patent ductus arteriosus; VSD, ventricular septal defect; AV, arteriovenous; LV, left ventricular; ASD, atrial septal defect; PE, pulmonary embolism; COPD, chronic obstructive pulmonary disease; RV, right ventricular; AP, anteroposterior.

states, such as those associated with anemia and thyrotoxicosis, and in conditions that cause a high stroke volume, such as chronic severe sinus bradycardia or complete heart block.

As it attempts to compensate for the reduction in cardiac output resulting from impairment of contractile performance in response to any injury or process, the left ventricle dilates. Ischemic damage (myocardial infarction) is the most common cause of contractile impairment. A previous history of myocardial infarction or the presence of pathologic Q-waves on the electrocardiogram (ECG) suggest an ischemic origin for the enlargement. An anterior or apical infarction, associated with Q-waves in the precordial leads, may also render the left ventricular impulse dyskinetic on palpation. Occasionally in such patients, the chest radiogram reveals an angulated distortion of the left heart border to suggest the presence of a left ventricular aneurysm (see Fig. 14–6B).

Dilated cardiomyopathy[3] (see Chap. 31) causes not only left ventricular but also generalized cardiac dilatation (Fig. 14–7A). Whereas the majority of patients with a nonischemic, dilated cardiomyopathy do not have an identifiable cause, the history and physical examination should focus on those processes that are most commonly responsible or that may be potentially reversible. Clues to toxic (alcohol, doxirubicin [Adriamycin]), infectious (myocarditis), metabolic (hypothyroidism, hemochromatosis, pheochromocytoma), and genetic (familial, Duchenne's) origins should be sought.

Left ventricular dilatation can also complicate the late stages of pressure overload from long-standing, uncorrected, and severe aortic stenosis or systemic hypertension. In their earlier stages, these conditions lead to concentric left ventricular hypertrophy that may not be associated with obvious enlargement of the heart. Thus, although the cardiac impulse in pressure overload hypertrophy may be vigorous, enlarged, and sustained on physical examination, it is usually not displaced and the cardiac silhouette on chest x-ray may be normal, despite the presence of ECG evidence of left ventricular hypertrophy. Over time, replacement fibrosis, wall thinning, and progressive systolic dysfunction occur and lead to cardiac dilatation, a low-output state, and clinical heart failure. Left ventricular enlargement may then become evident on radiography.

Left Atrium

Enlargement of the left atrium usually cannot be appreciated on physical examination. Rarely, the systolic expansion of the left atrium can be palpated as a mid-late-systolic lift in patients with severe mitral regurgitation. Radiologic enlargement of the left atrium is suggested by several signs: (1) a prominent, convex upper portion of the left heart border (see Figs. 14–7B and 14–9A); (2) posterior displacement of the barium-filled esophagus on the lateral projection (Fig. 14–8); (3) a "double density" near the right heart border (representing the left atrial wall) (Fig. 14–9A); (4) posterior and superior displacement of the left main stem bronchus (Fig. 14–9B); and (5) splaying of the carina beyond 75 degrees.

The left atrium commonly enlarges in the presence of conditions that elevate the left ventricular diastolic pressure. These include left ventricular pressure or volume overload, or both, or left ventricular systolic or diastolic dysfunction, as progressively higher left atrial pressures are required to fill the failing ventricle. In chronic mitral regurgitation, in which the volume load is directed into the left atrium, this chamber can attain massive propor-

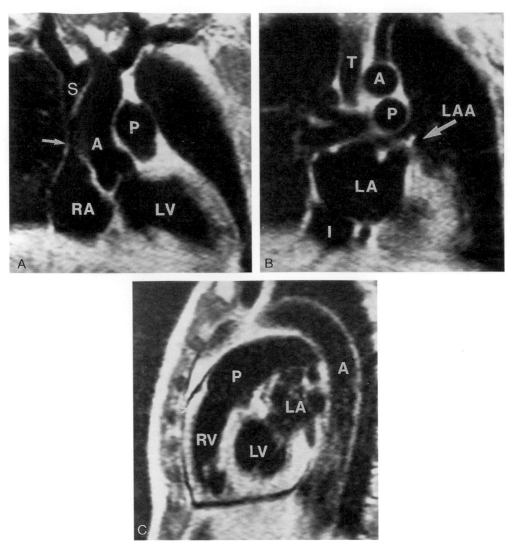

Figure 14-4

Normal radiographic anatomy. Magnetic resonance images. *A,* Coronal section at the level of the aortic valve. The right border of the cardiac silhouette is formed by the superior vena cava (S) and the right atrium (RA). The *arrow* indicates the caval-atrial junction. The lower portion of the left cardiac border is formed by the left ventricle (LV). A, ascending aorta; P, main pulmonary artery. *B,* Coronal section at the level of the left atrium (LA). The upper portion of the left cardiac border is formed by the ascending aorta, main pulmonary artery, and left atrial appendage (LAA, *arrow*). I, inferior vena cava; T, trachea. *C,* Sagittal section near midline. The right ventricle (RV) forms the anterior surface of the heart, abutting the sternum. The main pulmonary artery extends upward and posteriorly from the ventricle. The posterior border of the heart is formed by the left atrium and left ventricle. (*A–C,* From Baron, M.G.: Radiology of the heart. *In* Bennett, J.C., and Plum, F. [eds.]: Cecil Textbook of Medicine. 20th ed. Philadelphia, W.B. Saunders, 1996, p. 181.)

tions. A thin-walled, capacious left atrium can accommodate a large volume load without much increase in pressure.

The left atrium can enlarge independently of the left ventricle in the presence of obstruction to mitral inflow, as in mitral stenosis (see Fig. 14–7*B*) or, less commonly, left atrial myxoma. The former can usually be identified by the characteristic auscultatory findings, but is rarely "silent" and identifiable only by echocardiography. In general, the left atrium enlarges to a greater extent with significant mitral regurgitation than with mitral stenosis (see Fig. 14–9). Radiographic or echocardiographic calcification in the wall of an enlarged left atrium signifies a chronic process usually associated with organized mural/endocardial thrombi.

Right Ventricle

Enlargement of the right ventricle on physical examination is suggested by a prominent parasternal impulse that is medial to the left ventricular apex beat. Sometimes, the right ventricle enlarges so that it occupies the entire precordial area and the left ventricle cannot be palpated because it has been displaced posteriorly. Under this circumstance, tricuspid murmurs may be incorrectly identified as mitral in origin unless care is taken to examine

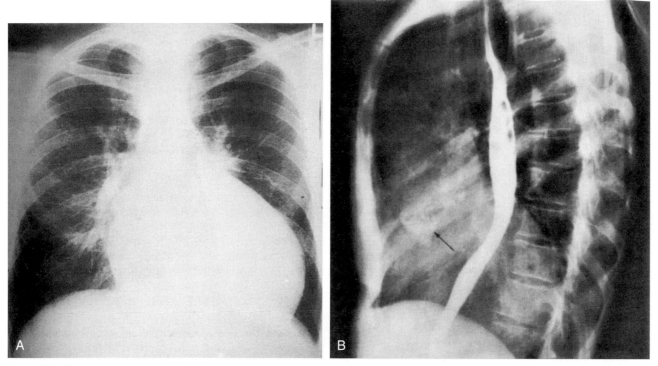

Figure 14–5

A, Left ventricular enlargement. Congestive cardiomyopathy. Gross cardiac enlargement. Frontal film shows a convex left heart border with a downwardly displaced apex. Note the redistribution of blood flow and bilateral basal interstitial lines. *B,* Dilatation of the left ventricle in aortic valve disease. Lateral view. The left ventricle is markedly enlarged and extends posterior to the esophagus. The aortic valve is densely calcified *(arrow).* The indentation on the anterior wall of the midesophagus is caused by the moderately dilated left atrium. There was no evidence of mitral valve disease. (*A,* From Rubens, M.B.: Chest x-ray in adult heart disease. *In* Julian, D.G., Camm, A.J., Fox, K.M., et al. [eds.]: Diseases of the Heart. 2nd ed. London, W.B. Saunders, 1996, p. 275. *B,* From Baron, M.G.: Radiological and angiographic examination of the heart. *In* Braunwald, E. [ed.]: Heart Disease. 3rd ed. Philadelphia, W.B. Saunders, 1988, p. 145.)

the neck veins and identify the changes characteristic of tricuspid valve disease (see Chaps. 3 and 25) and to listen for changes in the murmurs with inspiration. In patients with barrel chest deformity, an enlarged right ventricle may be directed inferiorly and the impulse will best be appreciated in the subxiphoid area. Other signs of right heart failure, such as ascites or edema, may be present.

Right ventricular enlargement can be difficult to detect on chest radiograms. An increase in the transverse dimension of the cardiac silhouette on the PA film, with a concave upward displacement of the lower left heart border (Fig. 14–10), may also signify right ventricular enlargement but is much less specific. The lateral view is especially helpful because the enlarged right ventricle encroaches on the upper retrosternal space (Fig. 14–11A).

The most common cause of right ventricular enlargement is left ventricular failure or mitral stenosis with chronic elevations of the pulmonary venous and arterial pressures leading to right ventricular systolic dysfunction. With left-sided cardiac abnormalities of sufficient severity to cause right ventricular enlargement, clinical and radiographic signs of pulmonary congestion are usually evident. When such signs are absent, primary lesions in the pulmonary parenchyma and pulmonary vascular bed should be sought.

The right ventricle can also enlarge as a result of the chronic volume overload associated with atrial septal de-

fect (see Fig. 26–1) or from tricuspid or pulmonic valve regurgitation. Tricuspid regurgitation is most commonly due to annular dilatation resulting from a gradual and progressive increase in the size of a failing right ventricle. Primary tricuspid regurgitation, however, is seen with endocarditis, carcinoid (fenfluramine-phentermine), myxomatous degeneration, trauma, and rheumatic involvement. Significant pulmonic regurgitation is unusual and typically results from dilatation of the pulmonic annulus in the presence of severe pulmonary hypertension.

Right ventricular pressure overload can also result in right ventricular enlargement. Pulmonary hypertension and uncorrected pulmonic valve stenosis (see Fig. 14–10A) are the two important causes. The former can be primary (idiopathic) or secondary to Eisenmenger's syndrome (see Chap. 26), pulmonary thromboembolic disease, or obstructive lung disease (see Chap. 30).

Right Atrium

Enlargement of the right atrium cannot be detected by physical examination. Determination of right atrial size is quite difficult on chest radiogram until there is marked enlargement, suggested by bowing of the right heart border with rightward displacement, well away (>6 cm)

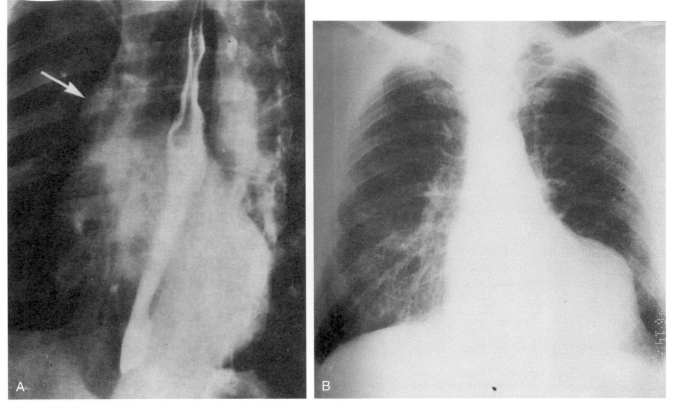

Figure 14–6

A, Left ventricular enlargement, left anterior oblique view. The cardiac silhouette is enlarged downward, to the left, and posteriorly, indicating dilatation of the left ventricle. The ascending aorta is widened *(arrow). B,* Left ventricular aneurysm. There is a localized bulge on the left heart border. (*A,* From Baron, M.G.: Radiological and angiographic examination of the heart. *In* Braunwald, E. [ed.]: Heart Disease. 3rd ed. Philadelphia, W.B. Saunders, 1988, p. 150. *B,* From Rubens, M.B.: Chest x-ray in adult heart disease. *In* Julian, D.G., Camm, A.J., Fox, K.M., et al. [eds.]: Diseases of the Heart. 2nd ed. London, W.B. Saunders, 1996, p. 275.)

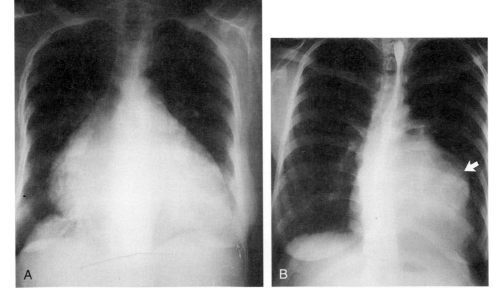

Figure 14–7

A, Dilated cardiomyopathy. There is diffuse dilatation of the heart in this woman with systemic lupus erythematosus. *B,* Mitral stenosis. The left atrial border is prominently convex *(arrow).* The aorta is small in this 19-year-old patient with mitral stenosis. (*A* and *B,* From Steiner, R.M., and Levin, D.C.: Radiology of the Heart. *In* Braunwald, E. [ed.]: Heart Disease. 5th ed. Philadelphia, W.B. Saunders, 1997, pp. 226, 227.)

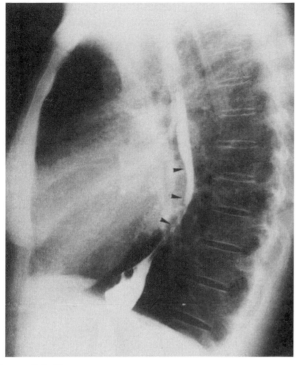

Figure 14–8

Left atrial enlargement. Mitral stenosis. The body of the left atrium is displacing the barium-filled esophagus posteriorly *(arrowheads)*. (From Rubens, M.B.: Chest x-ray in adult heart disease. *In* Julian, D.G., Camm, A.J., Fox, K.M., et al. [eds.]: Diseases of the Heart. 2nd ed. London, W.B. Saunders, 1996, p. 272.)

from the midline (see Fig. 14–11*B*). Care must be taken to exclude left atrial enlargement as the cause of this displacement. The right atrium enlarges chiefly in the presence of right ventricular failure of any cause, as well as in tricuspid stenosis or regurgitation (see Fig. 14–11*B*) (see Chap. 25). Ebstein's anomaly of the tricuspid valve (see Fig. 14–11*C*) (see Chap. 26) and right atrial myxoma are rare causes.

OTHER CAUSES OF CARDIAC ENLARGEMENT

Increased Myocardial Mass

The most frequent causes of cardiomegaly secondary to a marked increase in myocardial (predominantly left ventricular) wall thickness are hypertension, aortic stenosis, and hypertrophic cardiomyopathy. The last may be suspected on the basis of the family history, a characteristic heart murmur, and ECG evidence of left ventricular hypertrophy in the absence of aortic stenosis or systemic hypertension (see Chap. 31).

Patients with marked chronic obesity may also have an increased cardiac size that is greater than that predicted by gender and body surface area. Pathologic studies in these patients have demonstrated both cavity dilatation and eccentric hypertrophy that may occur in the absence of coronary artery disease or hypertension.

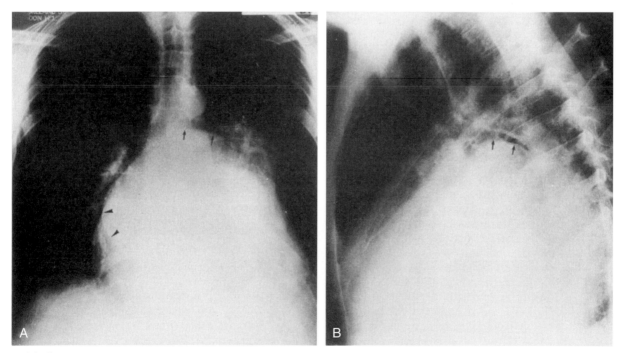

Figure 14–9

A and *B*, Left atrial enlargement in mitral regurgitation. The body of the left atrium is grossly enlarged, displacing the left bronchus *(arrows)* superiorly and posteriorly. A double density is visible over the right heart *(arrowheads)*. (*A* and *B*, From Rubens, M.B.: Chest x-ray in adult heart disease. *In* Julian, D.G., Camm, A.J., Fox, K.M., et al. [eds.]: Diseases of the Heart. 2nd ed. London, W.B. Saunders, 1996, p. 272.)

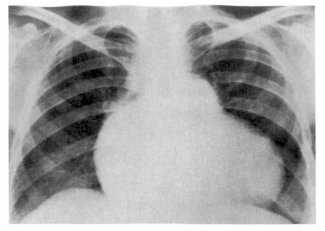

Figure 14–10

Pulmonic valvular stenosis with right heart failure. Congenital stenosis of the pulmonic valve in a 38-year-old woman. The shadow of the heart is widened to the left, and the cardiac apex is rounded and elevated because of dilatation of the right ventricle. The tricuspid valve was regurgitant, and the right atrium is markedly enlarged. The main pulmonary artery is dilated, and there is decreased vascularity of the lungs. (From Baron, M.G.: Radiological and angiographic examination of the heart. *In* Braunwald, E. [ed.]: Heart Disease. 3rd ed. Philadelphia, W.B. Saunders, 1988, p. 160.)

Pericardium

Pericardial effusions in excess of 200 ml usually result in cardiac enlargement that can be detected on physical examination or chest radiogram. Although signs of cardiac tamponade (hypotension, pulsus paradoxus, elevated jugular venous pressure) are powerful evidence that cardiac enlargement is secondary to pericardial disease (see Chap. 28), a leftward displacement of the lateral border of percussion dullness combined with a muffling of the heart sounds may be early signs of pericardial effusions without tamponade. The history can provide clues regarding a potential cause of pericardial disease (acute infection, neoplasm, radiation, tuberculosis, uremia, cardiac surgery).

The classic appearance of pericardial effusion on the chest radiogram is that of an enlarged "water-bottle" heart that sits on the diaphragm with effacement of the normal contours of the cardiomediastinal silhouette (Fig. 14–12*A*). On the lateral film, a distinct stripe separating the subepicardial fat from the subxiphoid fat (epicardial fat pad sign) is a highly specific sign for a pericardial effusion (Fig. 14–12*B–D*), but it is a relatively insensitive sign and is present in no more than one-quarter of patients with this condition. Calcification of the pericardium is present in as many as one-half of patients with constrictive pericarditis, but the overall size of the cardiac silhouette in these patients is usually normal, unless a significant pericardial effusion coexists, that is, effusive-constrictive disease is present.

Pericardial cysts or loculated effusions are unusual, asymmetric protrusions away from the cardiac border that are typically identified as incidental findings on chest x-ray. These do not equate with cardiomegaly and can be further characterized by echocardiography or CT scanning.

Epicardium

Patients with marked obesity, in whom it is difficult to appreciate heart size on physical examination, may display cardiac enlargement on the PA chest film in the absence of chamber dilatation, severe hypertrophy, or pericardial effusion. In these cases, the apparent enlargement is due to a generous epicardial fat pad that extends leftward and inferiorly from the left ventricular apex. Occasionally, the rounded contour of the left ventricular apex can be apparent through the triangular fat pad on the chest radiogram, thus exposing the latter as the cause of the increase in heart size. An analogous increase in epicardial fat also occurs in patients with Cushing's syndrome or those on large doses of adrenocorticoid hormone. Delineation of epicardial fat as the cause of cardiomegaly usually requires additional imaging with echocardiography or CT scanning.

Great Vessels; Mediastinal Structures

The great vessels can enlarge either with or independently from the cardiac chambers, but they are usually distinguishable on the basis of their location, contour, and projection. Expansion of the central pulmonary artery segments can be readily discerned on PA chest films (Fig. 14–13*A*) and is usually accompanied by right ventricular enlargement. Poststenotic or aneurysmal dilatation of the proximal ascending aorta can sometimes be appreciated on the PA chest film as a rounded bulge along the upper right heart border above the right atrium (Fig. 14–13*B*). Such enlargement may be accompanied by a palpable right upper parasternal pulsation on physical examination. However, enlargement of the great vessels does not result in cardiomegaly per se without an associated abnormality such as left ventricular enlargement secondary to significant aortic regurgitation in the presence of an aneurysm of the ascending aorta.

APPROACH TO THE PATIENT WITH CARDIOMEGALY

Because cardiac enlargement may accompany serious heart disease that may adversely affect long-term survival if it is not treated appropriately, it is imperative to delineate its cause and to understand the associated pathophysiologic derangements. Retaking a more directed history can be very useful, especially if the patient was referred for an apparently unrelated problem and the cardiomegaly was detected incidentally. A careful cardiovascular examination, with auscultation in several positions and after provocative maneuvers, may elicit additional clues. An

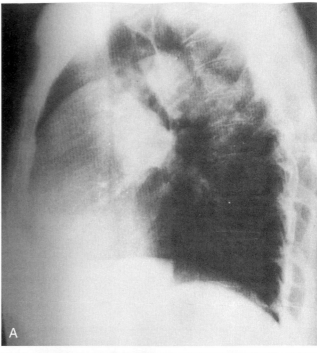

Figure 14–11

A, Right ventricular enlargement; lateral view. Primary pulmonary hypertension. There is increased contact of the anterior aspect of the heart with the sternum. The right ventricular outflow tract is prominent. *B,* Right atrial enlargement in congenital tricuspid stenosis. The right heart border is prominent; the superior vena cava is dilated *(arrowheads). C,* Ebstein's anomaly. There is globular cardiac enlargement due to severe tricuspid regurgitation and right heart enlargement. The pulmonary blood flow is reduced. (*A* and *B,* From Rubens, M.B.: Chest x-ray in adult heart disease. *In* Julian, D.G., Camm, A.J., Fox, K.M., et al. [eds.]: Diseases of the Heart. 2nd ed. London, W.B. Saunders, 1996, pp. 271, 270. *C,* From Steiner, R.M., and Levin, D.C.: Radiology of the heart. *In* Braunwald, E. [ed.]: Heart Disease. 5th ed. Philadelphia, W.B. Saunders, 1997, p. 234.)

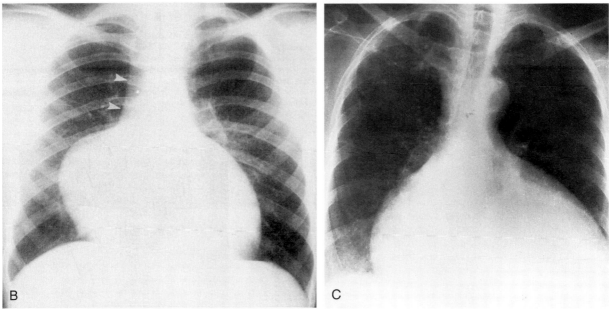

ECG should be obtained routinely. Further evaluations as outlined later can then be undertaken (Fig. 14–14).

Echocardiography/Doppler

Echocardiography is the single most useful initial imaging study and is generally the first test of choice in patients with evidence of cardiac enlargement on physical or radiographic examination. In patients in whom technically adequate studies can be performed, two-dimensional transthoracic echocardiography with Doppler flow imaging provides an accurate assessment of chamber dimensions, wall thickness, global and regional ventricular function, valvular morphology and function, great vessel size and orientation, and pericardial characteristics. The technique is safe and reproducible and can also be used to assess the response to any therapies initiated.

Some clinical examples of the utility of echocardiography in patients with cardiac enlargement include (1) the assessment of left ventricular size and systolic function, both global and regional, in patients with cardiomegaly and suspected coronary artery disease; (2) the change in left ventricular size, shape, and function in the weeks after myocardial infarction; (3) delineation of valvular pathology and estimation of its physiologic significance in patients with cardiac enlargement and heart murmurs; (4) serial evaluation of left ventricular size and function in

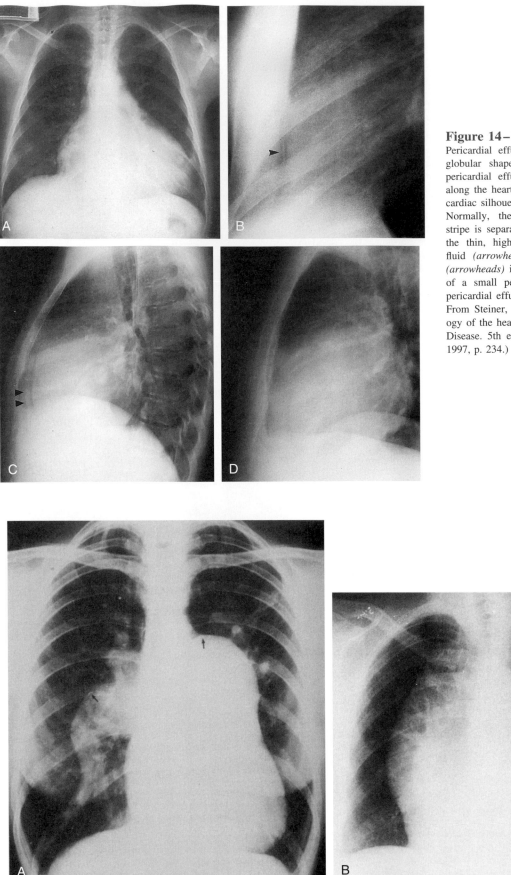

Figure 14–12

Pericardial effusion. *A,* The heart assumes a globular shape following development of a pericardial effusion. The normal indentations along the heart borders are effaced so that the cardiac silhouette is smooth and featureless. *B,* Normally, the subepicardial radiolucent fat stripe is separated from the subxiphoid fat by the thin, higher-density stripe of pericardial fluid *(arrowhead). C,* The pericardial stripe *(arrowheads)* is wider than it is in *B* because of a small pericardial effusion. *D,* A large pericardial effusion is present *(arrows). (A–D,* From Steiner, R.M., and Levin, D.C.: Radiology of the heart. *In* Braunwald, E. [ed.]: Heart Disease. 5th ed. Philadelphia, W.B. Saunders, 1997, p. 234.)

Figure 14–13

A, Atrial septal defect with Eisenmenger's syndrome. The central pulmonary arteries are enormously dilated, and there is dramatic peripheral pruning. Pulmonary arterial calcification *(arrows)* indicates severe chronic pulmonary arterial hypertension. *B,* Large aneurysm of the ascending aorta. The descending aorta is diffusely calcified and mildly dilated. *(A* and *B,* From Rubens, M.B.: Chest x-ray in adult heart disease. *In* Julian, D.G., Camm, A.J., Fox, K.M., et al. [eds.]: Diseases of the Heart. 2nd ed. London, W.B. Saunders, 1996, pp. 266, 276.)

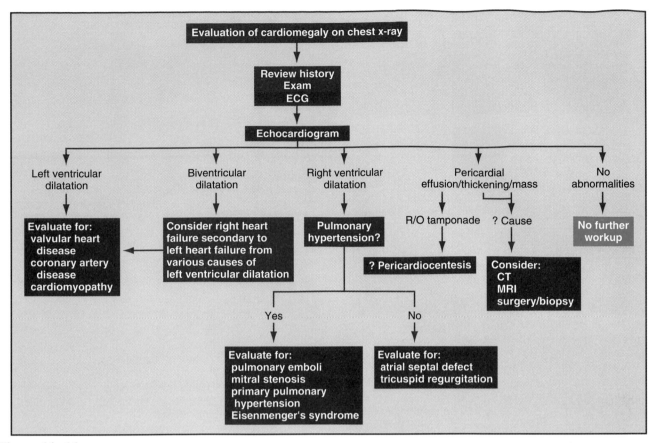

Figure 14–14

Approach to the patient with cardiomegaly. When cardiomegaly is found on the chest radiograph, the history and physical examination should be reviewed and an electrocardiogram (ECG) performed before obtaining a two-dimensional Doppler echocardiographic study. Cardiomegaly may be explained by left ventricular dilatation, biventricular dilatation, right ventricular dilatation, or pericardial abnormalities, or it may be found to be spurious on the echocardiogram. Rarely, isolated abnormalities of the atrium, particularly the left atrium, may cause abnormalities on the chest radiograph but will not cause true cardiomegaly. Depending on the echocardiographic findings, further tests can help elucidate the cause of echocardiographically confirmed cardiomegaly. R/O, rule out; CT, computed tomography; MRI, magnetic resonance imaging.

patients with asymptomatic mitral or aortic regurgitation; and (5) detection of pericardial fluid and assessment of its hemodynamic significance.

The images obtained by transthoracic echocardiography are suboptimal in 10% to 15% of patients because of body habitus or chest wall configuration. In such patients, transesophageal echocardiography is a suitable alternative in assessing the cause of cardiac enlargement. This technique is especially well suited to the study of suspected mitral or aortic valve disease and prosthetic valve function and can be performed safely on outpatients with the aid of light sedation and local anesthesia.

Radionuclide Ventriculography

If the question of the cause of cardiac enlargement focuses exclusively on ventricular size and function (and not valvular morphology), radionuclide ventriculography is an alternative to echocardiography, although it is usually more extensive than transthoracic echocardiography. This technique is safe, accurate, and reproducible in expe-

rienced laboratories, although it does entail a small exposure to ionizing radiation. Left ventricular and right ventricular volumes and ejection fractions and estimates of left ventricular diastolic function can be determined (Fig. 14–15).

Computed Tomography

From a clinical perspective, CT scanning may have only a few specific advantages over echocardiography/Doppler in the assessment of cardiomegaly.[4] It can provide anatomic information pertaining to chamber dimensions and wall thickness, albeit without simultaneous physiologic or valvular detail, but with the disadvantages of requiring exposure to contrast media (to delineate vascular structures) and ionizing radiation. Image quality can be easily affected by patient movement, the presence of intracardiac devices (prosthetic valves, pacemakers), and valvular calcification. Nevertheless, compared with echocardiography, chest CT scanning provides a better assessment of pericardial thickness (Fig. 14–16) and it is a more sensitive test for the detection of pericardial calcifi-

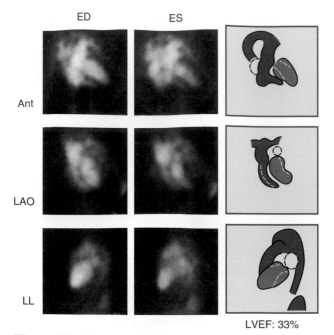

ED   ES

Ant

LAO

LL

LVEF: 33%

Figure 14–15

Equilibrium radionuclide angiocardiogram demonstrating anterior, apical, and septal akinesis in a patient with cardiac enlargement and a left ventricular ejection fraction (LVEF) of 33 percent. End-diastolic (ED) and end-systolic (ES) frames are shown for the anterior (Ant), left anterior oblique (LAO), and left lateral (LL) views. Diagrams of superimposed end-diastolic and end-systolic contours are shown to the right of each image pair. (From Wackers, J.Th., Soufer, R., and Zaret, B.L.: Nuclear cardiology. *In* Braunwald, E. [ed.]: Heart Disease. 5th ed. Philadelphia, W.B. Saunders, 1997, p. 298.)

cation. Its wider field of view and superior spatial resolution enhance its value as an appropriate imaging technique for the assessment of great vessel pathology (e.g., suspected aortic dissection or aneurysm [see Fig. 27–5]) and of other mediastinal structures (tumor, cyst) that may impart the impression of cardiomegaly on chest film. In the majority of patients with cardiac enlargement, chest CT scanning should be pursued only after careful analysis of the data available from the clinical examination, chest radiogram, and echocardiogram and only with a specific question that has been left unanswered, such as pericardial thickness, great vessel appearance, and abnormalities of extracardiac structures.

Magnetic Resonance Imaging

Assessment of cardiac structure and function with MRI is an area of active investigation (Fig. 14–17). Its clinical utility is limited, however, by factors of accessibility and cost.[4] It may be of particular value in patients with cardiac enlargement in whom cross-sectional imaging of the heart, great vessels, or extracardiac structures is important, but in whom contrast media are contraindicated. In addition, MRI can provide information related to tissue and fluid characteristics that may help in the diagnosis. MRI holds great future promise of becoming the single

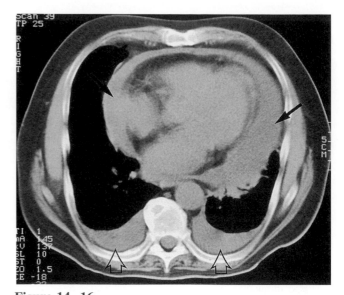

Figure 14–16

This computed tomography chest scan demonstrates a large and circumferential pericardial effusion *(arrows)*.

modality capable of providing critical information regarding myocardial, valvular, pericardial, and coronary arterial anatomy and function in patients with cardiac enlargement.

Exercise Testing

In the patient with left ventricular enlargement, exercise or pharmacologic stress testing is most commonly undertaken to screen for the presence of coronary artery disease or to assess myocardial function in patients with cardiomegaly. The observations made during provocative testing in patients with cardiac enlargement and left ventricular systolic dysfunction (ejection fraction < 0.40) are important determinants of therapy. In particular, the

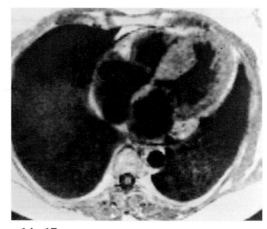

Figure 14–17

Hypertrophic cardiomyopathy. Magnetic resonance imaging displays severe hypertrophy of the entire septum and normal thickness of the lateral wall. (From Higgins, C.B.: Newer cardiac imaging techniques: Magnetic resonance imaging and computed tomography. *In* Braunwald, E. [ed.]: Heart Disease. 5th ed. Philadelphia, W.B. Saunders, 1997, p. 323.)

demonstration of reversible ischemia in such patients argues for surgical revascularization. Myocardial viability and stress-induced ischemia can be assessed by either myocardial perfusion scintigraphy or stress echocardiography.

Cardiopulmonary exercise testing with measurement of oxygen uptake (see Chap. 22) is a standard feature of the assessment and follow-up of patients with cardiac enlargement and severe heart failure who are under consideration for cardiac transplantation. Exercise-related changes in ventricular dimensions or function as assessed by echocardiography may be helpful in the determination of the need for operation in asymptomatic patients with cardiomegaly and mitral or aortic regurgitation.

Coronary Arteriography

The most common indication for coronary arteriography in patients with cardiac enlargement is the need to delineate the coronary anatomy when coronary revascularization is being considered. Coronary angiography is also appropriately undertaken as a late step in the evaluation of patients with dilated cardiomyopathy of uncertain cause and in those who are candidates for cardiac transplantation.

Indications for Hospital Admission or Cardiology Referral

Referral to a cardiac specialist should be driven primarily by the clinical context in which the cardiac enlargement is detected. Early consultation should be considered when uncertainty exists as to the cause or significance of the cardiac enlargement or when an invasive diagnostic (catheterization/angiography/coronary arteriography) or therapeutic (pericardiocentesis) procedure is contemplated. In patients with myocardial ischemia, heart failure, arrhythmias, syncope, valvular heart disease, or hypertension, the indications for cardiology consultation are based on the responsiveness of the clinical syndrome and are no different whether or not cardiomegaly is present.

Long-term follow-up is predicated on the specific diagnosis, the complexity and severity of the patient's illness, and the potential need for cardiac interventions. Once again, the cardiomegaly is usually a reflection of the severity of the underlying condition, and not an indication per se for specific intervention.

References

1. Perloff, J.K.: The movements of the heart—Percussion, palpitation and observation. *In* Perloff, J.K. (ed.): Physical Examination of the Heart and Circulation. 2nd ed. Philadelphia, W.B. Saunders, 1990, pp. 141–180.
2. Steiner, R.M., and Levins, D.C.: Radiology of the heart. *In* Braunwald, E. (ed.): Heart Disease: A Textbook of Cardiovascular Medicine. 5th ed. Philadelphia, W.B. Saunders, 1997, pp. 204–239.
3. Dec, G.W., and Fuster, V.: Idiopathic dilated cardiomyopathy. N. Engl. J. Med. 331:1564, 1994.
4. Higgins, C.B.: Newer cardiac imaging techniques: Magnetic resonance imaging and computed tomography. *In* Braunwald, E. (ed.): Heart Disease: A Textbook of Cardiovascular Medicine. 5th ed. Philadelphia, W.B. Saunders, 1997, pp. 317–348.

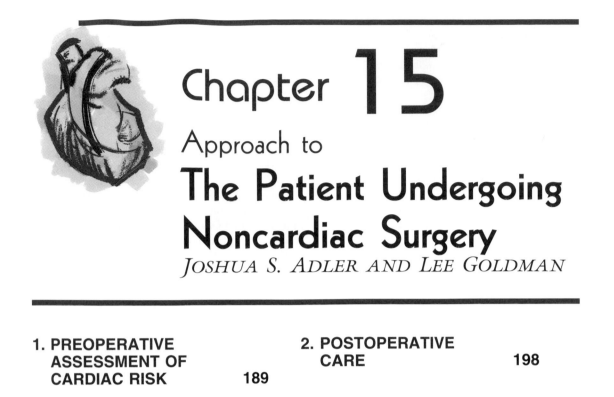

Chapter 15

Approach to

The Patient Undergoing Noncardiac Surgery

JOSHUA S. ADLER AND LEE GOLDMAN

Each year, millions of surgical procedures are performed on adults in the United States. The vast majority of patients do not suffer complications from surgery or the anesthetic. Roughly 3% to 10% do suffer serious complications, approximately half of which are cardiovascular in nature. The cardiovascular complications of surgery are more common in patients with underlying cardiovascular disease. Older patients, at increased risk for cardiovascular disease, make up a disproportionate percentage of patients undergoing surgery. As the population ages, an increasing number of older patients are expected to undergo major noncardiac surgery.

Since the mid-1960s, numerous studies have been published regarding the clinical risk factors associated with perioperative cardiac complications, the utility of preoperative noninvasive cardiac testing, and perioperative management of patients with cardiac disease. There is now substantial consistency in these data with respect to the identification of major risk factors for cardiac complications and the limited role of noninvasive cardiac testing. Several important questions remain, however, regarding the optimal perioperative management of patients with cardiac disease and, in particular, the role of preoperative revascularization.

When the primary care physician's own patient is considered for surgery, collaboration with the surgeon is critical to decide whether the benefits of proceeding with surgery, from both a cardiac and a noncardiac perspective, are outweighed by the risks. In making this decision, the physician must consider not only the morbidity and mortality risks but also the patient's preferences, especially when the surgical procedure is designed to improve quality of life rather than longevity. Much of the needed

preoperative cardiac evaluation may already have taken place even before a surgeon was consulted, but additional evaluation may be required once the scope of the planned surgery is understood. If the primary care physician will not be following the patient personally in the hospital after surgery, arrangements should be made for medical consultation for patients who have any chronic medical problems or who are at high risk for cardiac or noncardiac complications of surgery.

When called as a preoperative medical consultant to aid in the care of a patient whom the primary care physician has not followed longitudinally, the primary care physician must quickly become familiar with the patient to estimate the patient's risk of cardiac and noncardiac complications of surgery, recommend further expeditious testing when appropriate, work in conjunction with the anesthesiologist and surgical team to manage cardiac disease optimally in the perioperative period, and stay in close contact with the patient's usual primary care physician. The preoperative consult must also advise about the timing of surgery, since postponing surgery to address medical problems may reduce the risk of the surgery itself but produce its own risks by delaying a needed operation.

The Urgency and Type of Surgery

The urgency of surgery will dictate the speed and extent of the preoperative evaluation and whether there is any potential to delay surgery in order to perform diagnostic tests or institute new therapy. Multiple studies have

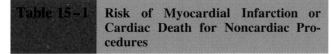

Table 15-1	Risk of Myocardial Infarction or Cardiac Death for Noncardiac Procedures

High Risk (Often >5%)

Aortic surgery
Peripheral vascular surgery
Emergent major operations, particularly in the elderly
Anticipated prolonged surgical procedures associated with larger fluid shifts or blood loss

Intermediate Risk (1%–5%)

Intrathoracic and intraperitoneal surgery
Carotid endarterectomy
Head and neck surgery
Orthopedic surgery
Prostate surgery

Low Risk (Generally <1%)

Endoscopic procedures
Cataract surgery
Superficial procedures and biopsies
Transurethral prostate surgery

Adapted from Guidelines for Perioperative Cardiovascular Evaluation for Noncardiac Surgery. Report of the American College of Cardiology/American Heart Association Task Force on Practice Guidelines. Circulation 93:1278–1317, 1996.

demonstrated that emergency surgery has a two- to five-fold increased risk of complications compared with elective surgery.

The type of surgery is very important in helping to establish a baseline risk of cardiac complications (Table 15–1).[1] Differences in the baseline risk reflect differences in the hemodynamic stress of the individual procedures and differences in the prevalence of preexisting severe cardiovascular disease among patients undergoing the procedure. The complication rates for procedures performed with local anesthetics and minimal sedation (such as cataract extraction) are very low, primarily owing to the short duration and minimal hemodynamic stress during both the procedure and the recovery period. Patients undergoing these procedures generally do not require intensive preoperative evaluation.

At the other extreme, major vascular surgical procedures are associated with the highest risk of complications. This risk is partly attributed to the significant hemodynamic stress of these procedures and partly to a very high prevalence of severe coronary artery disease among patients undergoing them. This latter point is complicated by the fact that many vascular surgery patients have such severe functional limitation due to claudication that the symptoms of coronary ischemia do not become manifest under their normal daily activities.

PREOPERATIVE ASSESSMENT OF CARDIAC RISK

An important principle of risk assessment is that of probabilistic decision-making. Risk assessment using this principle begins with a baseline risk. This will generally be the overall cardiac complication rate for a particular

procedure at a particular institution. This risk can then be modified by considering an individual patient's clinical data: the history, the physical examination, and the resting electrocardiogram (ECG). The focus of this clinical evaluation is an assessment of the stability and severity of known cardiovascular disease and the identification of any symptoms or signs that may represent previously unrecognized cardiovascular disease. In most patients, an accurate estimate of cardiac risk can be made based on these routine clinical data. In only a small subset of patients will noninvasive or invasive cardiac evaluation significantly alter the clinical risk assessment.

An assessment of the cardiac risks for patients undergoing noncardiac surgery can be made using multifactorial indices.[1–3] These indices combine a variety of clinical variables to determine an overall risk of cardiovascular complications including myocardial infarction (MI), cardiac death, pulmonary edema, and important ventricular arrhythmias. The original index of Goldman et al.[4] and the modification of the original index by Detsky et al.[5] are the best-known and most widely used indices in the United States (Table 15–2). The original index has performed well in prospective series of patients undergoing general surgery. The index score is best used not to denote a specific absolute risk of complications but rather to modify the baseline risk (Fig. 15–1).[1–3] A low index score is associated with a decreased risk, whereas a high score is associated with an increased risk. An intermediate score is generally associated with an unchanged risk. An important caution in the use of these indices is that they are relatively insensitive to asymptomatic cardiovascular disease, particularly coronary artery disease, and when used in isolation may underestimate the risk in patients with asymptomatic coronary disease. This is of particular concern in patients undergoing vascular surgery who may have severe coronary artery disease that is clinically silent or underestimated because the patient cannot exercise owing to noncardiac limitations. In patients at risk for important cardiovascular disease, a disease-specific approach to risk assessment is more sensitive to asymptomatic disease than the multifactorial indices. The use of both techniques provides the most comprehensive approach.

Coronary Artery Disease

Coronary artery disease is the most important cardiovascular disorder in the evaluation and assessment of patients in the preoperative period. Coronary artery disease is common in patients undergoing surgery, and the majority of serious cardiac complications are thought to be ischemia-related, particularly MI and cardiac death.[6, 7] Most patients at increased risk for coronary artery disease–related complications can be identified using routine clinical data (Table 15–3). Patients with none of the listed characteristics are at low risk (<0.5%) for ischemic complications during and after surgery. By contrast, patients with one or more of these characteristics are at a 5- to 50-fold increased risk for ischemic cardiac complications. The combination of the absence of known coronary artery disease (i.e., the absence of all characteristics in

Table 15–2 Multifactorial Cardiac Risk Indices

Risk Factor	Points	Interpretation
Goldman et al. (a)		
Age > 70 yr	5	
MI in previous 6 mo	10	Class I 0–5 points } low risk
S₃ gallop or jugular venous distention	11	
Important aortic stenosis	3	Class II 6–12 points } intermediate risk
Rhythm other than sinus or PACs on last preoperative ECG	7	
>5 PVCs/min documented at any time before operation	7	Class III 13–25 points ⎫
		Class IV >26 points ⎭ high risk
PO₂ < 60 or PCO₂ > 50 mm Hg.; K < 3.0 or HCO₃ < 20 mEq/L; BUN > 50 or Cr > 3.0 mg/dl; abnormal AST, signs of chronic liver disease, or bedridden from noncardiac causes	3	
Intraperitoneal, intrathoracic, or aortic operation	3	
Emergency operation	4	
Detsky et al. (b)		
MI in previous 6 mo	10	
MI more than 6 mo previous	5	
Canadian Cardiovascular Society angina		
Class III	10	
Class IV	20	
Unstable angina in previous 6 mo	10	≤15 points = low risk
Alveolar pulmonary edema		
Within 1 wk	10	
Ever	5	>15 points = high risk
Suspected critical aortic stenosis	20	
Rhythm other than sinus or sinus plus PACs on last preoperative ECG	5	
>5 PVCs/min at any time before operation	5	
Poor general medical status	5	
Age > 70 yr	5	
Emergency operation	10	

(a) Data from Goldman, L., Caldera, D.L., Nussbaum, S.R., et al.: Multifactorial index of cardiac risk in noncardiac surgical procedures. N. Engl. J. Med. 297:845–850, 1977.

(b) Data from Detsky, A.S., Abrahms, H.B., McLaughlin, J.R., et al.: Predicting cardiac complications in patients undergoing non-cardiac surgery. J. Gen. Intern. Med. 1: 211–219, 1986.

Abbreviations: MI, myocardial infarction; S₃, third heart sound; PACs, premature atrial contractions; ECG, electrocardiogram; PVCs, premature ventricular contractions; PO₂, partial pressure of oxygen; PCO₂, partial pressure of carbon dioxide; BUN, blood urea nitrogen; Cr, creatinine; AST, aspartate transaminase.

Table 15–1) and a low index score identifies a very low risk group for cardiac complications (see Fig. 15–1).

Patients with known or suspected coronary artery disease, as a group, have a 4% to 5% risk of perioperative cardiac complications and roughly a 1% mortality for major surgery. A risk estimate in these patients can be further refined through an assessment of the stability and severity of ischemic symptoms and the cardiac functional status. Patients with unstable coronary syndromes, including a recent (within 1 month) MI with evidence of persistent ischemia, unstable angina, or accelerated angina are at particularly high risk. Patients with an MI within 6 months before surgery who have evidence of persistent ischemia are likely to be at higher risk than those without persistent ischemia. In patients with stable ischemic symptoms, the severity may be assessed using a standardized approach that estimates functional status (see Chaps.

4 and 18). Patients with class III or IV angina are at substantially increased risk for complications compared with patients with class I or II symptoms. In addition, patients able to exercise to an extent associated with an increase in their heart rate above about 100 beats per minute are at lower risk that those who cannot do so. The majority of patients can be appropriately risk-stratified using this approach and do not require further testing.

For the special case of vascular surgery, the most important independent clinical predictors of cardiac complications have been well defined (Table 15–4).[8] Patients with none of these characteristics are at low risk for cardiac complications (<5%). Patients with three or more of the variables appear to be at high risk (30% to 50%). Patients with one or two of these variables are at intermediate risk, and it is in these patients that further testing is likely to be most useful.

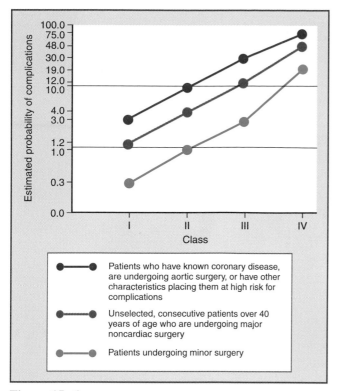

Figure 15–1

Approximate risk of major cardiac complications in different types of patients, according to their prior probability of complications and risk class as determined with the original multifactorial index. The multifactorial index is that described by Goldman et al.[4] The probability of complications is shown on a logarithmic scale. The risks of major complications, defined as pulmonary edema, arrhythmic cardiac arrest, myocardial infarction, and death from cardiac causes, were calculated by multiplying the prior odds of complications by the likelihood ratio for each class. The classes are defined as follows: class I, 0 to 5 points on the index; class II, 6 to 12 points; class III, 13 to 25 points; and class IV, 26 or more points. Points are assigned as shown in Table 15–2. (Redrawn with permission from Mangano, D.T., and Goldman, L.: Current concepts: Preoperative assessment of patients with known or suspected coronary disease. N. Engl. J. Med. 333:1750–1756, 1995. Copyright © 1995 Massachusetts Medical Society. All rights reserved.)

Preoperative Noninvasive Ischemia Testing

In general, noninvasive ischemia testing should be reserved for patients whose functional cardiac status is unknown, those who have intermediate-risk clinical data, and those who have indications for such testing independent of the planned surgery (Fig. 15–2).[1-3, 9]

Exercise Electrocardiography

Exercise electrocardiography has been studied in patients undergoing vascular and general surgery. In patients undergoing vascular surgery, impaired exercise tolerance, manifested by an inability to reach 75% to 85% maximal predicted heart rate and ischemic ECG changes are asso-

Table 15–3	Characteristics Defining Patients with Known or Suspected Coronary Artery Disease

History of myocardial infarction
Prior angiographic evidence of coronary artery disease
Evidence of ischemia on prior noninvasive testing
Typical angina pectoris
Peripheral vascular disease

Adapted from Ashton, C.M., Petersen, N.J., Wray, N.P., et al.: The incidence of perioperative myocardial infarction in men undergoing noncardiac surgery. Ann. Intern. Med. 118:504–510, 1993.

ciated with an increased risk of perioperative cardiac complications. It appears that impaired exercise tolerance is the more important factor.[1] Thus, preoperative exercise testing is likely to be most useful in patients with known or suspected coronary artery disease who are able to exercise but in whom the cardiac functional status cannot be adequately determined from the history.

Dipyridamole-Thallium Scintigraphy

Patients who are unable to exercise because of claudication or orthopedic problems are frequently referred for preoperative dipyridamole-thallium scintigraphy. This test has been used and studied extensively in patients scheduled for vascular surgery (Table 15–5). Early data in patients who were referred for dipyridamole-thallium scintigraphy before vascular surgery demonstrated a sensitivity of at least 90% and a specificity of at least 50% for perioperative cardiac complications. More recent data in unselected patients scheduled for vascular surgery, and especially abdominal aortic aneurysm surgery, found that dipyridamole-thallium scintigraphy was not predictive of cardiac complications. This discrepancy is likely due to a higher prevalence of severe coronary disease among patients referred by their physicians for testing compared with the unselected groups of patients.

Investigators have attempted to identify the subset of patients most likely to benefit from preoperative dipyridamole-thallium scintigraphy, using clinical data as selection criteria for further testing.[8, 10] The results of these studies

Table 15–4	Clinical Predictors of Cardiac Complications in Vascular Surgery Patients

Age > 70 yr
Prior myocardial infarction
Angina pectoris
Symptoms of congestive heart failure
Diabetes mellitus
Ventricular arrhythmias requiring treatment

Based on data from, L'Italien, G.J., Paul, S.D., Hendel, R.C., et al.: Development and validation of a Bayesian model for perioperative cardiac risk assessment in a cohort of 1081 vascular surgical candidates. J. Am. Coll. Cardiol. 27:779–786, 1996.

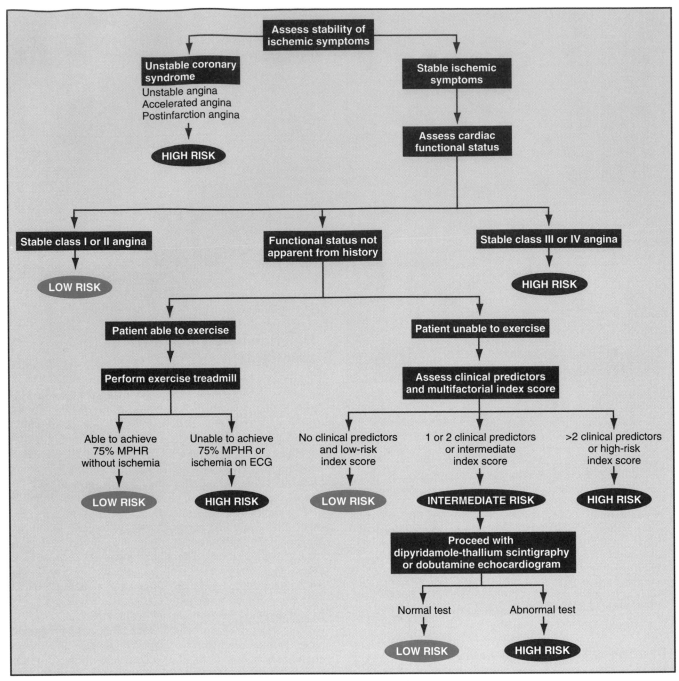

Figure 15–2
Preoperative evaluation of patients with known or suspected coronary artery disease.

have been consistent. In patients found to be at low risk by clinical data, dipyridamole-thallium scintigraphy does not further refine the risk estimate because this test is not sufficiently sensitive to identify truly high-risk patients among those classified as low risk by clinical data. Similarly, dipyridamole-thallium testing is not sufficiently specific to identify truly low-risk patients among those classified as high risk by clinical data. Dipyridamole-thallium scintigraphy appears to be most useful in patients at intermediate clinical risk.[1–3, 9] In these intermediate-risk patients, thallium redistribution is associated with a higher

risk of complications (similar to a high clinical risk), and a normal scan is associated with a lower risk (similar to a low clinical risk).

Data are limited on the use of dipyridamole-thallium scintigraphy in nonvascular surgery. It appears, however, that this test will be most useful in patients found to be at intermediate risk.

In vascular surgery patients, dipyridamole-thallium scintigraphy also appears to predict long-term cardiac morbidity. Patients with a fixed or reversible thallium defect are at substantially higher risk for cardiac morbid-

Table 15–5 Preoperative Dipyridamole-Thallium Scintigraphy as a Predictor of Perioperative Cardiac Complications

Category and Study*	No. of Patients	Thallium Redistribution		Major Cardiac Event		Sensitivity (%)	Specificity (%)	Predictive Value (%)		Relative Risk	Reported P Value
		Yes	No	Yes	No			Pos	Neg		
Selected Patients Referred for Testing											
Eagle et al.	200	82	118	25	5	83	66	30	96	9.9	.0002
Brown and Rowen	231	77	154	15	4	79	71	19	97	9.1	.00001
Hendel et al.	327	167	160	24	5	83	54	14	97	5.2	.0002
Lette et al.	415	182	233	37	2	95	61	20	99	29.5	.00001
Bry et al.	237	110	127	11	3	79	56	10	98	4.6	NS
Total for group	1410	618	792	112	19	85	60	18	98	9.0	—
Unselected, Consecutive Patients											
Mangano et al.	60	22	38	6	7	46	66	27	82	1.5	.43
Baron et al.	457	160	297	31	55	36	65	19	82	1.0	.92

Data from Mangano, D.T., and Goldman, L.: Preoperative assessment of patients with known or suspected coronary artery disease. N. Engl. J. Med. 333:1750–1756, 1995.

*Eagle, K.A., Coley, C.M., Newell, J.B., et al.: Combining clinical and thallium data optimizes preoperative assessment of cardiac risk before major vascular surgery. Ann. Intern. Med. 110:859–866, 1989.

Brown, K.A., and Rowen, M.: Extent of jeopardized viable myocardium determined by myocardial perfusion imaging best predicts perioperative cardiac events in patients undergoing noncardiac surgery. J. Am. Coll. Cardiol. 21:325–330, 1993.

Hendel, R.C., Whitfield, S.S., Villegas, B.J., et al.: Prediction of late cardiac events by dipyridamole thallium imaging in patients undergoing elective vascular surgery. Am. J. Cardiol. 70:1243–1249, 1992.

Lette, J., Waters, D., Cerino, M., et al.: Preoperative coronary artery disease risk stratification based on dipyridamole imaging and a simple three-step, three-segment model for patients undergoing noncardiac vascular surgery or major general surgery. Am. J. Cardiol. 69:1553–1558, 1992.

Bry, J.D.L., Beikin, M., O'Donnell, T.F., Jr., et al.: An assessment of the positive predictive value and cost-effectiveness of dipyridamole myocardial scintigraphy in patients undergoing vascular surgery. J. Vasc. Surg. 19:112–124, 1994.

Mangano, D.T., London, M.J., Tubau, J.F., et al.: Dipyridamole thallium-201 scintigraphy as a preoperative screening test: A reexamination of its predictive potential. Circulation 84:493–502, 1991.

Baron, J.-F., Mundler, O., Bertrand, M., et al.: Dipyridamole-thallium scintigraphy and gated radionuclide angiography to assess cardiac risk before abdominal aortic surgery. N. Engl. J. Med. 330:663–669, 1994.

ity (MI, cardiac death, unstable angina) in the following 3 years compared with those with neither finding.

Dobutamine Stress Echocardiography

Dobutamine stress echocardiography has been studied as a preoperative risk-assessment tool. These analyses have generally been series of patients referred for the test before vascular surgery. Most studies have demonstrated that the presence of one or more regional wall motion abnormalities with stress is associated with an increased risk of cardiac complications (Table 15–6). Patients without this finding seem to be at a much lower risk. In the largest series, 24% of patients with a new regional wall motion abnormality suffered a perioperative MI or cardiac death, compared with none of those who did not demonstrate a new wall motion abnormality.[11] Like dipyridamole-thallium scintigraphy, it appears that dobutamine stress echocardiography does not enhance the risk assessment in low-clinical-risk patients. In contrast, however, dobutamine stress echocardiography may be useful in both intermediate- and high-clinical-risk patients, since the definitive absence of a new segmental wall motion abnormality with stress may be able to identify a very low risk group regardless of the clinical risk stratification. Thus, dobutamine stress echocardiography may be useful in both the intermediate- and the high-clinical-risk groups.

Ambulatory Ischemia Monitoring

Asymptomatic (silent) ischemic ST segment changes are found in roughly 25% of patients with known or suspected coronary artery disease who undergo preoperative 24- or 48-hour ambulatory ECGs. The presence of ischemic changes is associated with an increased risk of perioperative cardiac complications (Table 15–7). The utility of this test is limited, however, by a relatively low sensitivity and thus the inability to reliably define a low-risk group, and because this test cannot be performed in patients with baseline ECG abnormalities. At present, the precise role of preoperative ambulatory ischemia monitoring remains undefined.[3]

In contrast to preoperative asymptomatic ischemia, the presence of intraoperative ischemic ECG changes has not been consistently associated with a major increase in perioperative cardiac complications. Intraoperative ischemia monitoring is not recommended for routine use.

Radionuclide Ventriculography and Echocardiography

Left ventricular systolic dysfunction may be diagnosed by radionuclide ventriculography or standard echocardiography, or both, and valvular abnormalities may be diagnosed by echocardiography. These conditions are associated with increased perioperative morbidity. However, there is no evidence that routine preoperative use of either of these two tests improves on the clinical risk assessment.[12, 13] These tests should generally be reserved for selected patients who have indications for testing independent of surgery, including the evaluation of a previously undiagnosed cardiac murmur and quantitation of known or suspected ventricular dysfunction.

Preoperative Risk Assessment in Patients with Known or Suspected Coronary Artery Disease

(see Fig. 15–2)

The first step is to determine whether a patient is likely to have coronary artery disease. This can be done in nearly all patients with routine clinical data from the history, physical examination, and ECG (see Table 15–2). Patients with none of these characteristics are at low risk for ischemic complications and generally do not require further testing.[1, 2, 9]

Patients with evidence of coronary disease are then subclassified through an assessment of cardiac functional status, the use of multifactorial indices, or in the case of vascular surgery patients, assessment of specific clinical predictors (see Fig. 15–2). Patients with good functional status and low-risk index scores are at low risk and generally do not require further testing. Similarly, in patients found to be at high risk by any method, noninvasive ischemia testing generally does not improve on the clinical risk assessment. Patients found to be at intermediate risk may benefit from noninvasive ischemia testing. The majority of intermediate-risk patients who undergo such testing can then be accurately classified as low or high risk.

Perioperative Management of Patients with Coronary Artery Disease

There are several important issues to consider in the perioperative management of patients with coronary artery disease including: whether to delay surgery, preoperative revascularization, the anesthetic technique and medications, the use of intraoperative and postoperative monitoring, and the use of antianginal medications.

Delaying Surgery

A decision to delay surgery requires careful consideration of the perioperative cardiac risks associated with proceeding as scheduled, the potential reduction in perioperative risk with delayed surgery, and the risk associated with delaying a necessary surgical therapy. In patients who require emergent lifesaving surgery (such as that for a perforated viscus), there is little potential for delay, regardless of the magnitude of the perioperative cardiac risk. In patients with an unstable coronary syndrome, the perioperative cardiac risk is substantial and there is significant potential for reducing the risk by delaying surgery until the coronary status is stable. Thus, when feasible, surgery should be delayed in these patients to allow for stabilization of ischemic symptoms and consideration for revascularization.

Coronary Revascularization

The precise role of preoperative revascularization by either coronary artery bypass graft (CABG) surgery or percutaneous transluminal coronary angioplasty (PTCA) is

---

Table 15–6 Dobutamine Stress Echocardiography to Predict Perioperative Cardiac Complications in Vascular Surgery Patients

Study*	n	Patients with Ischemia (%)	Events MI/Death	Positive Predictive Value (%)	Negative Predictive Value (%)
Lane et al.	38	50	3(8%)	16	100
Lalka et al.	50	50	9(15%)	23	93
Eichelberger et al.	75	36	2(3%)	7	100
Langan et al.	74	24	3(4%)	17	100
Davila-Roman et al.	88	23	2(2%)	10	100
Poldermans et al.	302	72	17(6%)	24	100

Adapted from Guidelines for perioperative cardiovascular evaluation for noncardiac surgery. Report of the American College of Cardiology/American Heart Association Task Force on practice guidelines. Circulation 93:1278–1317, 1996.

Abbreviation: MI, myocardial infarction.

*Lane, R.T., Sawada, S.G., Segar, D.S., et al.: Dobutamine stress echocardiography for assessment of cardiac risk before noncardiac surgery. Am. J. Cardiol. 68:976–977, 1991.

Lalka, S.G., Sawada, S.G., Dalsing, M.C., et al.: Dobutamine stress echocardiography as a predictor of cardiac events associated with aortic surgery. J. Vasc. Surg. 15:831–840, 1992.

Eichelberger, J.P., Schwarz, K.O., Black, E.R., et al.: Predictive value of dobutamine echocardiography just before noncardiac vascular surgery. Am. J. Cardiol. 72:602–607, 1993.

Langan, E.M., III, Yourkey, J.R., Franklin, D.P., et al.: Dobutamine stress echocardiography for cardiac risk assessment before aortic surgery. J. Vasc. Surg. 18:905–911, 1993.

Davila-Roman, V.G., Waggoner, A.D., Sicard, G.A., et al. Dobutamine stress echocardiogrpahy predicts surgical outcome in patients with an aortic aneurysm and peripheral vascular disease. J. Am. Coll. Cardiol. 21:957–963, 1993.

Poldermans, D., Mariarosaria, A., Paolo, M.F., et al: Improved cardiac risk stratification in major vascular surgery with dobutamine-atropine stress echocardiography. J. Am. Coll. Cardiol. 26:648–653, 1995.

Table 15–7	Predictive Value of Preoperative Ambulatory Ischemia Monitoring for Perioperative Myocardial Infarction or Cardiac Death after Major Vascular Surgery					
Study*	n	Patients with Abnormal Test (%)	Sensitivity (%)	Specificity (%)	Positive Predictive Value (%)	Negative Predictive Value (%)
Raby et al.	176	18	75	83	10	99
Pasternack et al.	200	39	78	63	9	98
Mangano et al.	144	18	20	82	4	96
Fleisher et al. '92	67	24	50	78	13	96
McPhail et al.	100	34	56	68	15	94
Kirwin et al.	96	23	7	90	11	94
Fleisher et al. '95	86	23	50	78	10	97

Adapted from Guidelines for perioperative cardiovascular evaluation for noncardiac surgery. Report of the American College of Cardiology/American Heart Association Task Force on practice guidelines. Circulation 93:1278–1317, 1996.

*Raby, K.E., Barry, J., Creager, M.A., et al.: Detection and significance of intraoperative and postoperative myocardial ischemia in peripheral vascular surgery. JAMA 268:222–227, 1992.

Pasternack, P.F., Grossi, E.A., Baumann, F.G., et al.: The value of silent myocardial ischemia monitoring in the prediction of perioperative myocardial infarction in patients undergoing peripheral vascular surgery. J. Vasc. Surg. 10:617–625, 1989.

Mangano, D.T., Browner, W.S., Hollenberg, M., et al.: Association of perioperative myocardial ischemia with cardiac morbidity and mortality in men undergoing noncardiac surgery: The Study of Perioperative Ischemia Research Group. N. Engl. J. Med. 323:1781–1788, 1990.

Fleisher, L.A., Rosenbaum, S.H., Nelson, A.H., et al.: The predictive value of preoperative silent ischemia for postoperative ischemic cardiac events in vascular and nonvascular surgery patients. Am. Heart J. 122:980–986, 1991.

McPhail, N.V., Ruddy, T.D., Barber, G.G., et al: Cardiac risk stratification using dipyridamole myocardial perfusion imaging and ambulatory ECG monitoring prior to vascular surgery. Eur. J. Vasc. Surg. 7:151–155, 1993.

Kirwin, J.D., Ascer, E., Gennaro, M., et al.: Silent myocardial ischemia is not predictive of myocardial infarction in peripheral vascular surgery patients. Ann. Vasc. Surg. 7:27–32, 1993.

Fleisher, L.A., Rosenbaum, S.H., Nelson, A.H., et al.: Preoperative dipyridamole thallium imaging and ambulatory electrocardiographic monitoring as a predictor of perioperative cardiac events and long term outcome. Anesthesiology 83:906–917, 1995.

a subject of controversy, owing in large part to the absence of controlled studies of patients undergoing preoperative revascularization. Patients who have previously undergone CABG surgery are generally at low risk for cardiac complications of subsequent surgery, particularly if the CABG surgery was performed within 5 years of the subsequent surgery. Additional information in patients with angina who have undergone peripheral vascular surgery indicates that those whose angina was treated with CABG surgery had an improved long-term survival compared with those treated with medical therapy.

Results from the Coronary Artery Surgery Study (CASS) demonstrated that patients with coronary artery stenoses of greater than 70% who underwent CABG surgery had a 0.9% mortality with subsequent noncardiac surgery compared with 2.4% for patients treated medically.[14] The data on PTCA are quite limited. In two small series of patients at high risk for cardiac complications, those who survived PTCA were at relatively low risk for cardiac complications with subsequent surgery. Although these data suggest that patients who undergo revascularization with CABG surgery or PTCA are at low risk for complications with subsequent surgery, the magnitude of the risk reduction does not seem to justify the risks of the revascularization procedure itself for low-risk patients, in whom risk is often in the range of about 2% for either approach.

Two decision analyses have attempted to determine the optimal role of angiography and revascularization in high-risk patients undergoing vascular surgery.[15, 16] Both studies concluded that routine angiography and revascularization are not warranted and that the subgroup of patients most likely to benefit from these procedures has not been well defined. Of note, these studies did not evaluate po-

tential long-term mortality benefits of revascularization, which may be particularly important in patients with peripheral vascular disease because this group of patients appears to derive substantial long-term mortality reduction with surgical coronary revascularization compared with medical therapy. Of course, another approach is to reevaluate vascular surgery patients postoperatively to determine whether their status, including the unmasking of coronary symptoms by an improved vascular status, warrants coronary revascularization.

The 1996 AHA guidelines recommend that angiography and revascularization be predominantly limited to patients who meet the indications for these procedures independent of surgery.[1] In such patients, coronary revascularization should generally precede a noncardiac operation, when feasible.

An approach to identifying patients who may benefit from preoperative revascularization is shown in Table 15–8.[3]

Anesthesia

Several studies have evaluated the relative merits of different anesthetic techniques and medications with respect to cardiac outcomes. It appears that there is no ideal technique or medication for the patient with coronary artery disease. Multiple studies have compared the use of different inhalational anesthetic agents and have found no differences in cardiac outcomes. Spinal/epidural anesthesia is associated with peripheral hemodynamic effects similar to those of general anesthesia, and even though spinal anesthesia does not cause the myocardial depression associated with some general anesthetics, it has not

Table 15–8	Recommendations for Perioperative Management of Patients with Coronary Artery Disease

Characteristic of Patient (see Fig. 15–2)	Special Perioperative Treatment
Low risk	Conservative treatment Continue cardiac medications Postoperative ECG on day 1, after any suspicious perioperative event, and again before hospital discharge
High risk	Intensify preoperative medications for coronary artery disease, identify and address cardiac risk factors, and consider re-evaluation of risk status if major changes have been made: if then at low risk, use conservative treatment; if still at high risk, proceed to: a. More intensive perioperative monitoring and medications to control blood pressure and heart rate *or* b. Coronary angiography and revascularization as indicated

Based on recommendations in Mangano, D.T., and Goldman, L.: Preoperative assessment of patients with known or suspected coronary artery disease. N. Engl. J. Med. 333:1750–1756, 1995.

Abbreviation: ECG, electrocardiogram.

been shown to be safer in comparative trials. Finally, opioid-based intravenous anesthetic techniques appear to be associated with greater hemodynamic stability, although they have not been associated with better cardiac outcomes. The choice of anesthetic technique is generally at the discretion of the anesthesiologist and individualized for each patient based on a variety of clinical factors. The medical consultant can provide the anesthesiologist with an accurate cardiac assessment to help the anesthesiologist to choose appropriate individualized anesthesia.

Intraoperative Monitoring

A variety of intraoperative monitoring techniques can be used in patients with coronary artery disease, including pulmonary artery catheterization and transesophageal echocardiography. Trials comparing the routine use of pulmonary artery catheters with selective use for patients who develop clinical indications for such catheters found no differences in perioperative cardiac complications. The limited data on the use of intraoperative transesophageal echocardiography to detect myocardial ischemia suggest that such monitoring does not improve outcomes. Thus, it is prudent to use these monitoring techniques only in high-risk patients, such as those with unstable coronary syndromes or those with stable coronary artery disease undergoing high-risk procedures. In practice, the decision to use these monitoring devices is generally left to the anesthesiologist, although in the rare cases where the use of either technique is of paramount importance, the medical consultant should make such recommendations.

Early identification of postoperative MI may alter management and potentially cardiac outcomes, although this has yet to be demonstrated in clinical studies. Postoperative surveillance for MI using CK-MB isoenzymes or serum troponin I or T levels and the 12-lead ECG has been evaluated in only a few studies. No single best method or ideal patient has been identified. CK-MB isoenzymes may be released from noncardiac tissue during surgery and have been found to have a fairly low specificity for myocardial injury. Electrocardiography has a higher specificity but a lower sensitivity. Serum troponin T levels have been shown to be at least as sensitive and somewhat more specific than CK-MB isoenzymes for perioperative myocardial injury.[17] The AHA guidelines advise limiting routine surveillance for perioperative MI to patients with known or suspected coronary artery disease.[1] An immediate postoperative ECG and one daily for 2 days is the recommended strategy.[3] The use of CK-MB isoenzymes or serum troponin T levels should be reserved for patients at high risk for cardiac complications and for those who experience perioperative events suspicious for an MI.

Antianginal Medications

Patients taking antianginal or other cardiac medications before surgery generally should continue to do so up to and including the day of surgery. Patients with class III or IV angina or those with ischemia on preoperative, noninvasive testing are likely to benefit from optimization of the antianginal regimen followed by a reassessment of functional status or repeat ischemia testing, although this strategy has not yet been proved in clinical trials. By comparison, the institution of new antianginal medications in patients at low risk for ischemic heart disease is unlikely to be of benefit.

In one randomized trial of patients with or at high risk for coronary artery disease, prophylactic atenolol was given as 10 mg intravenously (in two doses of 5 mg each, separated by 10 minutes) just before the induction of anesthesia. This regimen was repeated immediately after surgery and on the morning of the first postoperative day and then continued every 12 hours until the patient could be switched to 50 to 100 mg orally per day. Compared with placebo, 2-year mortality after major noncardiac surgery was reduced by 55%.[18] Although there was no significant difference in cardiac deaths during the hospitalization, significant improvements were evident by 6 months and maintained for an additional 18 months, with an absolute increase of 11 percentage points in overall survival and 15 percentage points in survival free of MI, unstable angina, congestive heart failure, or the need for CABG surgery. Prophylactic intraoperative intravenous nitroglycerin also can decrease myocardial ischemia but has not been demonstrated to improve cardiac outcomes.

Congestive Heart Failure and Left Ventricular Dysfunction

Congestive heart failure and left ventricular systolic dysfunction have been associated with increased perioperative morbidity. A history of congestive heart failure is an independent predictor of cardiac complications, particularly in patients undergoing vascular surgery. Patients with decompensated congestive heart failure, manifested by an audible third heart sound, jugular venous distention, or the presence of pulmonary edema are at substantially increased risk of cardiac morbidity and mortality.

Decreased ventricular function, as measured by radionuclide angiography or echocardiography, is an independent predictor of perioperative pulmonary edema but does not predict other cardiac complications. In vascular surgery patients, the risk of pulmonary edema is three- to fourfold greater in patients with a resting left ventricular ejection fraction of less than 50% compared with patients with an ejection fraction of over 50%.

It is important to determine the underlying cause of heart failure preoperatively because it may have implications for the assessment of risk and for perioperative management (Fig. 15–3). Patients with ischemic cardiomyopathy may be at higher risk than patients with heart failure from hypertension or valvular disease. Furthermore, the perioperative management of medications and intravenous fluids may be different in patients with hypertrophic cardiomyopathy than in those with dilated cardiomyopathy. Thus, preoperative echocardiography is generally recommended for patients with heart failure of unknown cause or in those with heart failure who have not previously had an objective measurement of left ventricular function.

Regardless of cause, a guiding principle in the perioperative management of patients with heart failure is that decompensated patients are at higher risk than well-compensated patients. Thus, efforts should be made in the preoperative period to optimize the medical therapy before surgery, which generally will include diuretics and afterload-reducing agents. Although this strategy is likely to reduce the risk of cardiac morbidity, it has not been studied in randomized clinical trials.

Valvular Heart Disease

The importance of valvular abnormalities in the perioperative period depends largely on the particular valve involved and the severity of the abnormality. In addition, the presence of any valvular abnormality may require the use of antibiotic prophylaxis for endocarditis (see Chap. 16).

Severe aortic stenosis is associated with the greatest risk of perioperative complications. Patients with symptomatic aortic stenosis appear to be at higher risk than asymptomatic patients. It is recommended that noncardiac surgery in patients with severe symptomatic aortic stenosis be delayed until after a valvular procedure—usually valve replacement surgery but occasionally balloon valvuloplasty in very ill or elderly patients in whom only short-term hemodynamic improvement is sought. Limited data suggest that patients with asymptomatic severe aortic stenosis, even those with an aortic valve area less than 1.0 cm^2, may undergo major noncardiac surgery with a complication rate of less than 10%. Nevertheless, noncardiac surgery in these patients should be approached cautiously and may involve the use of intraoperative pulmonary artery catheterization.

Patients with mitral stenosis may be at increased risk for perioperative complications, particularly from atrial arrhythmias and congestive heart failure. These patients may benefit from mitral valve surgery or valvuloplasty before noncardiac surgery. In patients with mild mitral stenosis, preoperative control of the heart rate and congestive heart failure should be ensured.

It is not known whether mitral or aortic valve regurgitation imparts excess perioperative risk independent of those associated with congestive heart failure or coronary artery disease. Preoperative management should focus on controlling congestive heart failure through the use of diuretics and afterload-reducing agents.

In patients on warfarin because of a mechanical heart valve or atrial fibrillation, the medications should be discontinued preoperatively to allow the International Normalized Ratio (INR) to fall to 1.5 or below, and the patient should be treated with subcutaneous heparin beginning about 12 hours after surgery. If needed, small doses (1 mg subcutaneously) of vitamin K can be given to reduce the preoperative INR more rapidly.[19]

Figure 15–3
Preoperative management of congestive heart failure.

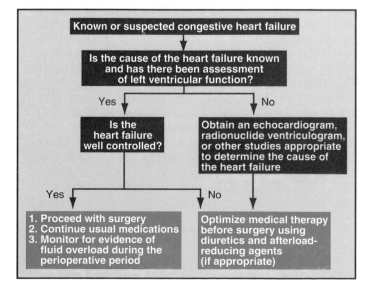

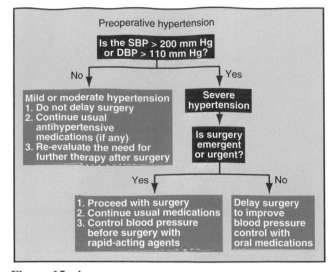

Figure 15–4
Management of preoperative hypertension.

Arrhythmias and Conduction Disease

Atrial and ventricular arrhythmias have been associated with an increased risk of perioperative cardiac complications. Data have demonstrated that these arrhythmias are frequently associated with structural heart disease, particularly coronary artery disease and left ventricular dysfunction. It is likely that much of the perioperative cardiac morbidity in patients with both findings is attributable to the structural heart disease rather than to the rhythm disturbance. Patients with a rhythm disturbance and no evidence of structural heart disease are at very low risk for perioperative cardiac complications. The finding of an arrhythmia on preoperative evaluation should prompt a search for previously unsuspected structural heart disease. This is particularly important if the finding of structural heart disease would alter perioperative management.

Patients with preoperative arrhythmias should receive therapy appropriate for the arrhythmia independent of surgery. Adequate ventricular rate control should be ensured in patients with atrial fibrillation. Symptomatic supraventricular and ventricular arrhythmias should be treated before surgery. Suppression of asymptomatic arrhythmias before surgery is unlikely to reduce the risk of perioperative cardiac morbidity.

Patients who have indications for permanent pacemaker placement independent of the surgery (see Chap. 24) should generally have the pacemaker placed before elective surgery.[9] For urgent surgery, temporary transvenous pacing should be used during surgery and the perioperative period. Patients who do not meet criteria for permanent pacing, such as those with left bundle branch block, generally do not require temporary pacing during or after surgery.[6]

Hypertension

Preoperative hypertension has been associated with intraoperative blood pressure lability and ECG evidence of ischemia. Patients with severe hypertension, defined as a diastolic blood pressure greater than 110 mm Hg, appear to be at increased risk for perioperative MI and congestive heart failure. Patients with mild or moderate hypertension, however, appear to be at no excess risk for important cardiac morbidity.[6]

Antihypertensive medication should be continued up to and including the day of surgery (Fig. 15–4). In patients with severe preoperative hypertension, it is prudent to delay elective surgery to allow for control of blood pressure for several days. When surgery is urgent, blood pressure should be controlled before the induction of anesthesia, using rapidly acting intravenous antihypertensive agents if necessary. Beta blocking agents are useful in this setting (see Chap. 16).

In patients with mild or moderate hypertension, surgery need not be delayed. In these patients, the addition of new antihypertensive agents or dosage changes in existing agents during the immediate preoperative period is not likely to reduce the risk of perioperative cardiac complications. When surgery is not scheduled for several weeks, however, it is prudent to try to improve blood pressure control preoperatively (see Chap. 21).

Role of the Primary Care Physician

The primary care physician should be able to assess and follow his or her own patients through surgery and to serve as a consultant for new patients. The primary care physician should be able to order and evaluate the results of indicated noninvasive tests, but consultation with a cardiologist is recommended when coronary angiography is being considered as a prelude to possible coronary revascularization and for patients whose cardiac problems, such as angina, fail to respond to usual medical treatment.

The primary care physician should not attempt to make recommendations to the anesthesiologist regarding preferred methods for anesthesia, since anesthesiologists are more expert in these decisions and an overwhelming literature reveals no appreciable relationship between anesthetic technique and outcome of common surgical procedures. The medical physician must also be careful not to engage the surgeon in a written debate regarding the advisability of surgery. Any such discussions should be conducted in person or by telephone to be sure that both physicians recognize each other's perspectives.

POSTOPERATIVE CARE

General Considerations

Cardiac disorders in the postoperative period should generally be managed similarly to those in the nonsurgical setting.[6]

Ischemic Heart Disease

Postoperative ischemia or ST segment changes are a potent predictor of postoperative cardiac complications in high-risk patients. There is the potential that early recognition of postoperative ischemia may allow for rapid treatment and prevention of complications. At present, this has not been evaluated in clinical trials. Postoperative ST segment monitoring is of uncertain benefit and thus should be used only in high-risk patients in whom it is likely to alter management.

Patients who sustain a perioperative MI or significant myocardial ischemia are at substantially increased risk for subsequent MI or cardiac death during the following 10 years. The acute management of perioperative MI or ischemia is similar to the treatment in the nonsurgical setting, with the caveat that the recent surgery may make the bleeding risk of anticoagulation or thrombolysis prohibitive. Once stabilized, most of these patients should undergo noninvasive ischemia testing before discharge. Those with persistent ischemia should be considered for angiography and revascularization.

Patients identified during the preoperative evaluation to have stable coronary artery disease should be re-evaluated postoperatively to confirm that medical therapy is optimal and that risk factors for coronary artery disease—including hypertension, hyperlipidemia, and tobacco use—have been addressed. Patients without overt coronary artery disease preoperatively should be considered for screening for and treatment of coronary disease risk factors during the postoperative period.

Arrhythmias

Postoperative arrhythmias, both ventricular and supraventricular, are often due to noncardiac problems including infection, abnormalities in serum electrolyte levels, and hypoxia. Management should focus on the identification of the cause of the arrhythmia, either cardiac or noncardiac, and correction of the underlying disorder. Noncardiac causes of rhythm disorders should generally be corrected before attempting cardioversion because the arrhythmia often resolves spontaneously with correction of the underlying cause. When an arrhythmia is associated with hemodynamic compromise, antiarrhythmic medications or electrical cardioversion may be necessary. Correction of the underlying cause remains essential to prevent recurrence of the arrhythmia.

Hypertension

Brief hypertensive episodes are not uncommon in the immediate postoperative period in patients both with and without hypertension preoperatively. Most episodes occur within 1 hour of the end of anesthesia and resolve in a few hours. These episodes most commonly are precipitated by noncardiac problems such as discomfort from the endotracheal tube, pain, hypoxemia, fluid overload, and hypothermia. Treatment should be directed primarily at these precipitants, which will usually result in adequate control of blood pressure.

Severe or prolonged hypertensive episodes may require specific antihypertensive therapy, although the exact degree or duration of hypertension for which antihypertensive therapy is of benefit has not been evaluated in clinical trials. A reasonable approach is to treat patients with a diastolic blood pressure above 100 mm Hg or a systolic blood pressure above 200 mm Hg, those whose hypertension does not respond to treatment of precipitants, and those with evidence of myocardial ischemia or cerebral dysfunction. Several intravenous medications are effective in rapidly controlling blood pressure in this setting, including sodium nitroprusside, beta blocking agents, and calcium channel blocking agents (see Chap. 16).

Congestive Heart Failure

Postoperative heart failure usually occurs in the first 2 or 3 postoperative days. Excess fluid administration and myocardial ischemia are the most common precipitating factors. In patients who develop heart failure after surgery, it is important to evaluate for myocardial ischemia or infarction with a 12-lead ECG and cardiac enzymes (if appropriate), especially in patients with known coronary artery disease. Diuretic therapy will usually produce rapid improvement, particularly in patients without concomitant myocardial ischemia.

Role of the Primary Care Physician

The primary care physician should participate actively in the postoperative follow-up of the surgical patient. A daily focused history and physical examination should concentrate on the status of chronic medical problems, the development of possible cardiac signs and symptoms, evidence for local infection or other direct surgical complications, the evaluation of possible deep venous thrombosis, and a careful pulmonary examination to exclude postoperative pneumonia. The medical physician should acquire a good sense of the usual pace of recovery after common surgical procedures and recognize that a patient's failure to demonstrate expected improvement may be a nonspecific sign of an impending important cardiac or noncardiac problem. For example, an otherwise unexplained tachycardia or altered mental status may be the first evidence of postoperative hypoxia, myocardial ischemia, or congestive heart failure. The primary care physician should also help guide the patient's transition to posthospital care, including plans for the titration or adjustment of cardiac medications. Consultation with a cardiologist is recommended for patients who develop postoperative MI or who develop myocardial ischemia, arrhythmias, or heart failure that does not respond to usual measures.

References

1. Guidelines for perioperative cardiovascular evaluation for noncardiac surgery. Report of the American College of Cardiology/American Heart Association Task Force on practice guidelines. Circulation 93:1278–1317, 1996.
2. Palda, V.A., and Detsky, A.S.: Perioperative assessment and management of risk from coronary artery disease. Ann. Intern. Med. 127:313–328, 1997.
3. Mangano, D.T., and Goldman, L.: Preoperative assessment of patients with known or suspected coronary artery disease. N. Engl. J. Med. 333:1750–1756, 1995.
4. Goldman, L., Caldera, D.L., Nussbaum, S.R., et al.: Multifactorial

index of cardiac risk in noncardiac surgical procedures. N. Engl. J. Med. 297:845–850, 1977.

5. Detsky, A.S., Abrahms, H.B., McLaughlin, J.R., et al.: Predicting cardiac complications in patients undergoing non-cardiac surgery. J. Gen. Intern. Med 1:211–219, 1986.

6. Goldman, L.: General anesthesia and noncardiac surgery in patients with heart disease. *In* Braunwald, E. (ed.): Heart Disease. 5th ed. Philadelphia, W.B. Saunders, 1997, pp. 1756–1768.

7. Ashton, C.M., Peterson, N.J., Wray, N.P., et al.: The incidence of perioperative myocardial infarction in men undergoing noncardiac surgery. Ann. Intern. Med. 118:504–510, 1993.

8. L'Italien, G.J., Paul, S.D., Hendel, R.C., et al.: Development and validation of a Bayesian model for perioperative cardiac risk assessment in a cohort of 1081 vascular surgical candidates. J. Am. Coll. Cardiol. 27:779–786, 1996.

9 Palda, V.A., and Detsky, A.S., for the American College of Physicians Clinical Efficacy Assessment Subcommittee: Guidelines for assessing and managing the perioperative risk from coronary artery disease associated with major noncardiac surgery. Ann. Intern. Med. 127:309–312, 1997.

10. Shaw, L.J., Eagle, K.A., Gersh, B.J., Miller, D.D.: Meta-analysis of intravenous dipyridamole-thallium-201 imaging (1985 to 1994) and dobutamine echocardiography (1991 to 1994) for risk stratification before vascular surgery. J. Am. Coll. Cardiol. 27:787–798, 1996.

11. Poldermans, D., Mariarosaria, A., Paolo, M.F.: Improved cardiac risk stratification in major vascular surgery with dobutamine-atropine stress echocardiography. J. Am. Coll. Cardiol. 26:648–653, 1995.

12. Baron, J.F., Mundler, O., Bertrand, M., et al.: Dipyridamole-thallium scintigraphy and gated radionuclide angiography to assess cardiac risk before abdominal aortic surgery. N. Engl. J. Med. 330:663–669, 1994.

13. Halm, E.A., Browner, W.S., Tubau, J.R., et al.: Echocardiography for assessing cardiac risk in patients having noncardiac surgery. Study of Perioperative Ischemia Research Group. Ann. Intern. Med. 125:433–441, 1996.

14. Eagle, K.A., Rihal, C.S., Mickel, M.C., et al., for the Coronary Artery Surgery Study (CASS) Investigators and University of Michigan Heart Care Program: Cardiac risk of noncardiac surgery. Influence of coronary disease and type of surgery in 3368 operations. Circulation 96:1882–1887, 1997.

15. Fleisher, L.A., Skolnick, E.D., Holroyd, K.J., Lehmann, H.P.: Coronary artery revascularization before abdominal aortic aneurysm surgery: A decision analytic approach. Anesth. Analg. 79:661–669, 1994.

16. Mason, J.J., Owens, D.K., Harris, R.A., et al.: The role of coronary angiography and coronary revascularization before noncardiac vascular surgery. JAMA 273:1919–1925, 1995.

17. Lee, T.H., Thomas, E.J., Ludwig, L.E., et al.: Troponin T as a marker for myocardial ischemia in patients undergoing major noncardiac surgery. Am. J. Cardiol. 77:1031–1036, 1996.

18. Mangano, D.T., Layug, E.L., Wallace, A., and Tareo, I.: Effects of atenolol on mortality and cardiovascular morbidity after noncardiac surgery. The Multicenter Study of Perioperative Ischemia Research Group. N. Engl. J. Med. 335:1713–1720, 1996.

19. Kearon, C., and Hirsh, J.: Management of anticoagulation before and after elective surgery. N. Engl. J. Med. 336:1506–1511, 1997.

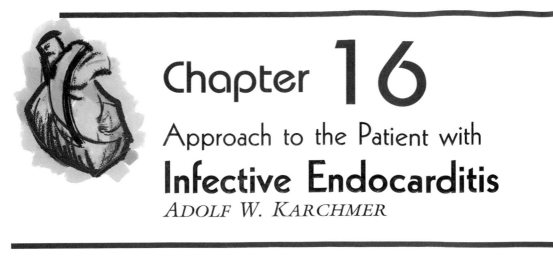

Chapter 16

Approach to the Patient with
Infective Endocarditis

Adolf W. Karchmer

Microbial infection of the endothelial surface of the heart results in the syndrome of infective endocarditis (IE). This infection most commonly involves heart valves but occasionally occurs on the low-pressure side of a septal defect, on a chordae tendineae, or on a patch of mural endocardium that has been injured by an aberrant stream of blood. The actual lesion produced, called a *vegetation,* is an amorphous mass of platelets and fibrin in which is enmeshed the proliferating causative microorganism. In developed countries, IE is a relatively infrequent disease. Its occurrence ranges from 1.7 to 4.2 cases per 100,000 overall population but increases progressively after 30 years of age, so that rates exceed 15 cases per 100,000 population greater than 50 years of age. Among all cases of IE in developed countries, 10% to 20% of infections occur on prosthetic valves (prosthetic valve endocarditis [PVE]). Actuarial estimates suggest that 1.4% to 3.1% of valve recipients develop IE within the initial year after valve surgery and by 5 years 3.2% to 5.7% have developed PVE. Intravenous drug abuse entails an even greater risk for IE than that associated with prosthetic valves or rheumatic heart disease. The rate of IE in this group is 2% to 5% per patient-year.

The morbidity and mortality associated with IE can be significantly reduced by early diagnosis and initiation of effective therapy. Because of the often nonspecific prosaic symptoms associated with IE, patients with this infection are likely to seek initial medical care from their primary care physicians. Accordingly, understanding the clinical presentations of IE, an efficient approach to diagnosis, effective therapy for various forms of IE, and the appropriate role of subspecialty physicians in the management of these patients is essential to achieve an optimal outcome.

CLINICAL FEATURES

The presentation of IE ranges from a syndrome characterized by marked systemic toxicity and rapid progression with intracardiac and extracardiac complications (acute endocarditis) to an indolent prolonged illness with modest fever and toxicity and, in some instances, scant evidence of infection or cardiac disease on examination (subacute endocarditis). The clinical features of IE are primarily nonspecific (Table 16–1). The occurrence of these symptoms and signs, however, in a patient with an underlying cardiac condition or behavior pattern (intravenous drug abuse) known to predispose to endocarditis, particularly in the absence of an overt focal infection, should elicit consideration of IE. Additional important clues to the presence of IE include bacteremia with organisms that commonly cause IE or an embolic event (pulmonary or systemic) that is not attributable to an apparent underlying illness or occurs in the context of a nonspecific feb-

Table 16-1	The Frequency of Signs and Symptoms in Patients with IE		
Symptoms	**%**	**Signs**	**%**
Fever	80–85	Fever	80–90
Chills	40–75	Heart murmur	80–85
Sweats	25	Changing or new murmur	10–40
Anorexia	25–55		
Weight loss	25–35	Systemic emboli	20–40
Malaise	25–40	Splenomegaly	15–50
Cough	25	Clubbing	10–20
Stroke	15–20	Osler's nodes	7–10
Headache	15–40	Splinter hemorrhage	5–15
Myalgia/arthralgia	15–30	Janeway lesions	6–10
Back pain	7–10	Retinal lesions	4–10
Confusion	10–20	(Roth's spots)	

Adapted from Karchmer, A.W.: Infective endocarditis. *In* Braunwald, E. (ed.): Heart Disease. 5th ed. Philadelphia, W.B. Saunders, 1997, p. 1084.
Abbreviation: IE, infective endocarditis.

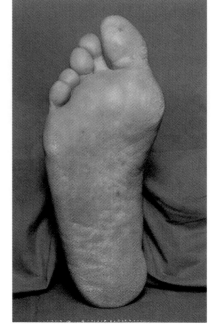

Figure 16–2
Osler's node on the great toe. (From Mir, M.A.: Atlas of Clinical Diagnosis. London, W.B. Saunders, 1995, p. 243.)

rile illness. Similarly, new or rapidly progressive cardiac valvular dysfunction, which is evidence of an active endocardial process, in a patient with unexplained fever may be indicative of IE. Occasionally, patients with indolent IE present with renal dysfunction that is the consequence of immune complex–mediated glomerulonephritis. Some findings on the physical examination are suggestive of IE: *splinter hemorrhages,* i.e., subungual dark red streaks (Fig. 16–1), *Osler's nodes,* i.e., small tender nodules on the finger or toe pads (Fig. 16–2), and *Janeway lesions,* i.e., small hemorrhages on the palms and soles (Fig. 16–3), are characteristic, although not pathognomonic, of IE. A high index of suspicion is required in order to avoid overlooking the diagnosis of IE. This is particularly true when IE occurs in patients without a previously known predisposition to valvular infection or when the cardinal symptom of fever is blunted or absent (the very elderly or those with azotemia, severe debility, or congestive heart failure).

The clinical features of IE among drug abusers and patients with prosthetic heart valves merit special mention. Left-sided IE among intravenous drug abusers is clinically similar to IE among nonaddicts. However, 65% to 75% of IE in this group involves the right heart valves, particularly the tricuspid valve. Right-sided IE, which is often caused by *Staphylococcus aureus,* presents abruptly with cough, dyspnea, hemoptysis, or pleuritic chest pain in addition to the usual features of IE. Chest radiograms in these patients commonly reveal nodular infiltrates due to septic pulmonary infarcts. These infiltrates may subsequently become necrotic, cavitate, and result in a pyopneumothorax. Patients with PVE developing within 60 days of cardiac surgery may have postoperative complications that mask the usual prosaic symptoms of IE. In these patients, as well as in those with later onset of PVE, valve dysfunction with new regurgitant

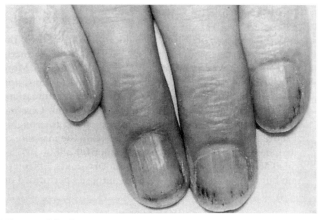

Figure 16–1
Splinter hemorrhages in a patient with infective endocarditis. (From Freeman, R., and Hall, R.J.C.: Infective endocarditis. *In* Julian, D.G., Camm, A.J., Fox, K.M., et al. [eds.]: Diseases of the Heart. 2nd ed. London: W.B. Saunders, 1996, p. 896.)

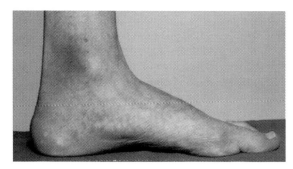

Figure 16–3
Janeway lesion at the medial maleolus. Erythematous lesions in the arch portion of the plantar surface in Figure 16–2 are also Janeway lesions. (From Mir, M.A.: Atlas of Clinical Diagnosis. London, W.B. Saunders, 1995, p. 243.)

murmurs and findings of congestive heart failure are encountered commonly. These features may be due to the impingement of vegetations on the valve parts and orifice or to perivalvular infection with dehiscence of the valve from the annulus and resulting paravalvular leakage. Invasion of the perivalvular tissues and abscess formation complicate approximately 45% of patients with PVE involving mechanical or bioprosthetic valves and are particularly prevalent when PVE occurs within 1 year after cardiac surgery or involves an aortic valve prosthesis.

DIAGNOSIS

The clinical, laboratory, and echocardiographic features of IE have been codified into a scheme, the so-called Duke criteria, that provide a sensitive and specific approach to the clinical diagnosis of IE (Table 16–2). Finding two major criteria, one major and three minor criteria, or five minor criteria allows a definite diagnosis of IE. Occasional patients fall just short of the diagnosis of

Table 16–2 Criteria Used in the Diagnosis of IE

Major Criteria

1. Positive blood culture
   A. Two separate blood cultures yielding organisms typically causing IE: *Viridans* streptococci, *Streptococcus bovis,* or HACEK; community-acquired *Staphylococcus aureus* or enterococci, in the absence of a primary focus of infection
   B. Microorganisms consistent with IE from persistently positive blood cultures: At least two positive cultures of blood drawn >12 hr apart, or all three of three, or a majority of four or more separate blood cultures (first and last cultures drawn at least 1 hr apart)
2. Evidence of endocardial involvement
   A. Positive echocardiogram of IE
      (1) Oscillating intracardiac mass on a valve or supporting structures, in the path of regurgitant jets, or on implanted material in the absence of an alternative anatomic explanation
      (2) Abscess
         or
      (3) New partial dehiscence of a prosthetic valve
   B. New valvular regurgitation (worsening or changing of preexisting murmur not adequate)

Minor Criteria

1. Predisposing heart condition or intravenous drug use
2. Fever: Temperature ≥38.0° C
3. Vascular phenomena: Major arterial emboli, septic pulmonary infarcts, mycotic aneurysm, intracranial hemorrhage, conjunctival hemorrhages, and Janeway lesions
4. Immunologic phenomena: Glomerulonephritis, Osler's nodes, Roth's spots, and rheumatoid factor
5. Microbiologic evidence: Positive blood culture but less than a major criteria (see above)* or serologic evidence of active infection with an organism consistent with IE
6. Echocardiographic findings: Consistent with IE but not meeting a major criterion (see above)

Adapted from American Journal of Medicine, vol. 96, Durack D.T., Lukes, A.S., and Bright, D.K.: New criteria for diagnosis of infective endocarditis: Utilization of specific echocardiographic findings. pp. 200–209, copyright 1994, with permission from Excerpta Medica Inc.
Abbreviations: IE, infective endocarditis; HACEK, *Haemophilus* species, *Actinobacillus actinomycetemcomitans, Cardiobacterium hominis, Eikenella* species, *Kingella kingae.*
* Excludes a single positive blood culture for coagulase-negative staphylococci or organisms that do not cause IE.

definite IE and yet have no alternative diagnosis to explain their febrile illness. These patients should be classified as possibly having IE and should be treated for it. To use as a criterion a positive blood culture for organisms that often contaminate these cultures—that is, coagulase-negative staphylococci or diphtheroids—or that rarely cause IE, such as gram-negative bacilli, requires additional rigor. To do so, blood cultures must be persistently positive or multiple cultures must be positive with a single clone. Also, alternative sites of infection must be ruled out. If the possibility of IE is considered early in the workup of a febrile patient and the evaluation is conducted with care, it is unlikely that the diagnosis of IE will be rejected erroneously when using these guidelines. Alternatively, the diagnosis of culture-negative IE may be accepted erroneously in patients when nonbacterial thrombotic vegetations are detected echocardiographically (e.g., marantic endocarditis, cryptic collagen-vascular disease, and antiphospholipid antibody syndrome).

Blood Cultures

The diagnostic scheme appropriately emphasizes blood cultures and echocardiographic findings. Among patients with IE caused by organisms other than those that are highly fastidious, more than 95% of all blood cultures obtained will be positive. Accordingly, three separate sets of blood cultures, obtained over 24 hours from separate venipunctures, should be sufficient both to identify the causative organism and to demonstrate that the bacteremia is continuous, a finding characteristic of this infection and few others. Each set should utilize two flasks, one of which contains thioglycolate broth (an anaerobic medium), and each flask should receive approximately 10 ml of blood. In spite of technologic advances in microbiology laboratories that enhance the yield of organisms from blood cultures, 5% to 15% of patients with clinically diagnosed IE have negative blood cultures. Of those IE patients with negative blood cultures, approximately 50% have received antibiotics before the cultures were obtained, a factor that likely accounts for the negative cultures. Although the time after cessation of antibiotics that is needed for these patients to develop recrudescent bacteremia is not established, it is a function of the duration of antimicrobial therapy, the antimicrobial agent used, and the susceptibility of the organism to that agent. Given the importance of isolating the causative organism in establishing optimal therapy, as well as the diagnosis of IE, treatment should be delayed for several days when evaluating hemodynamically stable patients with subacute presentations who have received antibiotics within the previous 2 weeks. This delay is not likely to allow otherwise preventable complications to occur and will allow repeat blood cultures to be obtained without further confounding by antimicrobial therapy. When IE is suspected, the microbiology laboratory should be notified so that the blood cultures will be incubated for a prolonged period (3 or more weeks) before they are considered negative.

Echocardiography

Although echocardiographic findings are not required to diagnose definite IE clinically, identification of vegetations or perivalvular complications consistent with IE markedly enhances one's ability to make this diagnosis. The sensitivity of transesophageal echocardiography (TEE) to identify vegetations in patients with clinically diagnosed IE ranges from 90% to 94%; the sensitivity of the transthoracic approach (TTE) is significantly lower (45% to 75%). The false-negative rate with TEE may be as high as 10%. Thus, TEE is likely to confirm the diagnosis, as well as define the anatomy of the process, among patients in whom the suspicion of IE is high and to reasonably exclude the diagnosis when the suspicion is low. Echocardiography is not, however, sufficiently sensitive to rule out IE in a patient in whom the clinical suspicion is high; and hence, negative findings should not dissuade one from treatment. Among patients where there is an intermediate level of suspicion, a negative TEE does not rule out the diagnosis; on the contrary, further evaluation, including another TEE, is required in this situation. Subspecialty consultation may be useful in further assessing these patients.

Other Diagnostic Tests

In most patients, efforts to diagnose IE are not significantly enhanced by tests other than blood cultures and echocardiography. Some of the studies typically obtained, although not diagnostically helpful, are important in the management of patients: complete blood counts, serum creatinine, selected liver function tests, and urinalysis. Other tests that have been obtained often in the past, including circulating immune complex titer, quantitative immunoglobulins, cryoglobulins, C-reactive protein, sedimentation rate, and rheumatoid factor, although often abnormal, are nonspecific, rarely aid in the diagnosis of IE or the assessment of response to treatment, and generally can be omitted. If the diagnosis of IE is made using minor criteria, the sedimentation rate, rheumatoid factor, and circulating immune complex titer may be helpful. Among patients with apparent culture-negative IE that is not attributable to prior antibiotic therapy, serologic tests to identify infection caused by *Brucella* species, *Legionella* species, *Coxiella burnetii* (the causative agent of Q fever), *Chlamydia,* and *Bartonella* species may aid in diagnosing IE. Of note, very fastidious *Bartonella* species have been identified as a cause of IE. These organisms, which are recovered in blood only when special handling is employed, may account for a significant proportion of what previously appeared to be culture-negative IE. Peripheral arterial emboli that occur in patients with apparent culture-negative IE should be extracted surgically and examined microbiologically and histologically to facilitate establishing a causative diagnosis. The sequential evaluation of patients with suspected IE and selected symptoms is outlined in Table 16–3.

Table 16–3	The Evaluation of Patients with Suspected Endocarditis*	
Timing	**Test**	**Comment**
Admission *(before admission if stable)*	CBC, differential, three blood cultures,† urinalysis, ECG, creatinine, bilirubin, AST, alkaline phosphatase, prothrombin time, chest radiograph	Tests, other than blood cultures, do not aid with diagnosis but establish baseline for assessing the complications of IE or treatment
After Admission 24–48 hr Blood culture positive	TTE	TEE is the initial study of choice with suspected prosthetic valve IE
48–72 hr Blood cultures positive, TTE negative, or blood cultures and TTE negative	TEE	See Figure 16–4 and text regarding initiation of therapy
72–96 hr Blood cultures negative	Two blood cultures daily for 2 days†, ESR, rheumatoid factor, circulating immune complex titer	ESR, circulating immune complex titer, and rheumatoid factor add little value if blood cultures and echocardiogram are positive
Days 7–10 Blood cultures remain negative (no antibiotics given)	Serologic tests and special blood cultures for fastidious organisms	See text under Diagnosis of IE and Microbiology of IE; obtain infectious disease consultation and advice of microbiology laboratory director
	Retrieve material embolic to a peripheral artery for culture and histologic examination	
	Repeat TEE if initially negative	Increase the yield for vegetations
Any Time Focal central nervous system symptoms or finding suggesting localized event	Computed tomography (with enhancement); evidence of hemorrhage without mass effect: consider magnetic resonance angiogram or formal angiogram, lumbar puncture	Consider mycotic aneurysm; with acute *Staphylococcus aureus* IE or new focal symptoms without infarct, consider angiography
Left upper quadrant pain (with/without left shoulder pain)	Image spleen (and kidney) for abscess	

Abbreviations: IE, infective endocarditis; CBC, complete blood count; ECG, electrocardiogram; AST, aspartate transaminase; TTE, transthoracic echocardiography; TEE, transesophageal echocardiography; ESR, erythrocyte sedimentation rate.

* For patients who are hemodynamically stable and have a subacute presentation.

† Request that laboratory incubate blood cultures for three weeks (indicate diagnosis of infective endocarditis).

MICROBIOLOGY

A relatively small number of bacterial species cause the majority of cases of IE. This observation is embodied in the major criteria of the Duke diagnostic scheme and enhances the specificity of the scheme. The frequency with which these organisms cause IE varies somewhat among the various clinical subtypes of IE (Table 16–4). Although virtually any bacterial or fungal species can cause IE, understanding the common causes is essential when designing empirical antibiotic therapy for IE or when evaluating the possibility of IE among bacteremic patients. Among patients with community-acquired native valve IE that is unassociated with narcotic addition, *S. aureus* is the predominant cause of the acute endocarditis syndrome. Streptococci, enterococci, coagulase-negative staphylococci, and the HACEK group of organisms (*Haemophilus* species, *Actinobacillus actinomycetemcomitans, Cardiobacterium hominis, Eikenella* species, and *Kingella kingae*) are the major causes of IE presenting in a subacute fashion. Nosocomial IE is an infrequent complication of intravascular device–related bacteremia or bacteremia associated with genitourinary tract manipulations. Nosocomial enterococcal bacteremias, and consequently IE, are increasingly due to strains that are highly resistant to the antibiotics used in the standard treatment of enterococcal IE, for example, vancomycin-resistant *Enterococcus faecium*. *S. aureus* strains causing IE among intravenous drug abusers are frequently methicillin-resistant (also resistant to oxacillin, nafcillin, imipenem, and the cephalosporins). The coagulase-negative staphylococci that cause PVE during the initial year after valve placement are predominantly *Staphylococcus epidermidis,* and 85% of these strains are resistant to methicillin and other beta-lactam antibiotics. Of the coagulase-negative staphylococcal strains causing PVE a year or more after cardiac surgery, 50% are non–*S. epidermidis* species and only 30% are resistant to methicillin.

When, in the absence of confounding prior administration of antibiotics, blood cultures from patients with convincing clinical evidence of IE remain negative after 7 to 10 days of incubation, the causes of culture-negative IE must be evaluated. In addition to the fastidious variants of the common bacterial causes of IE—for example, HACEK group organisms and L-cysteine– or pyridoxal-requiring streptococci (nutritionally deficient streptococci speciated as *Streptococcus defectivus* and *Streptococcus adjacens*)—infection caused by fungi, *Brucella* species, *Legionella* species, *Bartonella* species, *Chlamydia* species, and *Coxiella burnetii* must be considered. Predisposing clinical and epidemiologic circumstances may suggest one of these unusual organisms as the cause of blood culture–negative IE. Special blood culture handling should be requested to isolate these organisms. Additionally, noninfectious causes of fever with associated heart murmur or systemic emboli that mimic IE—including acute rheumatic fever, marantic endocarditis, Libman-Sacks endocarditis, antiphospholipid antibody syndrome, atrial myxoma, carcinoid syndrome, and renal cell cancer—must be considered. The possibility that the heart murmur, which has raised the question of IE, is in fact coincidental and that the presenting syndrome is a "fever of unknown origin" must be considered. (The differential diagnosis of this entity is beyond the scope of this chapter.)

ANTIMICROBIAL THERAPY

Effective antimicrobial therapy requires the use of an agent or combination of agents that is bactericidal for the

Table 16–4	Microbiology of IE in Specific Clinical Situations Number of Cases (%)						
	Native Valve Endocarditis*		Prosthetic Valve Endocarditis† Time of Onset after Valve Surgery			Endocarditis in Drug Addicts†	
Organism	*Community Acquired (n = 603)*	*Nosocomial (n = 82)*	*<2 mo (n = 73)*	*2–12 mo (n = 38)*	*>12 mo (n = 94)*	*Right-Sided (n = 346)*	*Left-Sided (n = 204)*
Streptococci‡	186 (31)	6 (7)	—	2 (5)	31 (33)	17 (5)	31 (15)
Pneumococci	8 (1)	—	—	—	—	—	—
Enterococci	53 (9)	13 (16)	5 (7)	2 (5)	10 (11)	6 (2)	49 (24)
Staphylococcus aureus	217 (36)	45 (55)	10 (14)	5 (13)	12 (13)	267 (77)	47 (23)
Coagulase-negative staphylococci	28 (5)	8 (10)	28 (38)	19 (50)	14 (15)	—	—
Fastidious gram-negative coccobacilli (HACEK group)	18 (3)	—	—	1 (3)	11 (12)	—	—
Gram-negative bacilli	21 (3)	4 (5)	8 (11)		1 (1)	17 (5)	26 (13)
Fungi, *Candida* species	5 (1)	3 (4)	7 (10)	2 (5)	3 (3)	—	25 (12)
Polymicrobial/miscellaneous	36 (6)	1 (1)	3 (4)	2 (5)	1 (1)	28 (8)	20 (10)
Diphtheroids	—	—	9 (12)	1 (3)	2 (2)	—	—
Culture negative	31 (5)	2 (2)	3 (4)	4 (11)	9 (10)	10 (3)	6 (3)

Abbreviation: HACEK, *Haemophilus* species, *Actinobacillus actinomycetemcomitans, Cardiobacterium hominis, Eikenella* species, and *Kingella kingae.*
* Data from Karchmer, A.W.: Treatment of infective endocarditis. *In* Smith, T.W. (ed.): Cardiovascular Therapeutics. Philadelphia, W.B. Saunders, 1996, pp. 718–730.
† Data from Karchmer, A.W.: Infective endocarditis. *In* Braunwald, E. (ed.): Heart Disease. 5th ed. Philadelphia, W.B. Saunders, 1997, pp. 1097–1104.
‡ Includes *Viridans* streptococci, *Streptococcus bovis,* other non-group A, groupable streptococci.

Table 16–5   Recommended Antibiotic Therapy for IE

Infecting Organism	Antibiotic	Dose and Route*	Duration (wk)†	Comments
1. Penicillin-susceptible viridans streptococci, *Streptococcus bovis*, and other streptococci, penicillin MIC ≤ 0.1 µg/ml	A. Penicillin G	12–18 million units IV daily in divided doses q 4 hr	4	
	B. Penicillin G plus gentamicin‡	12–18 million units IV daily in divided doses q 4 hr; 1 mg/kg IM or IV q 8 hr	4; 2	Avoid aminoglycoside-containing regimens when potential for nephrotoxicity or ototoxicity is increased.‡
	C. Penicillin G plus gentamicin‡	Same doses as noted previously	2; 2	See text
	D. Ceftriaxone	2 gm IV or IM daily as single dose	4	Can be used in patients with nonimmediate penicillin allergy. IM administration of ceftriaxone is painful.
	E. Vancomycin§	30 mg/kg IV daily in divided doses q 12 hr	4	Use for patients with immediate or severe penicillin or cephalosporin allergy. Infuse doses over 1 hr to avoid histamine release (red man syndrome).
2. Relatively penicillin-resistant streptococci Penicillin MIC 0.2–0.5 µg/ml	A. Penicillin G plus gentamicin‡	18–24 million units IV daily in divided doses q 4 hr; 1 mg/kg IM or IV q 8 hr	4; 2	
Penicillin MIC > 0.5 µm/ml	B. Penicillin G plus gentamicin‡	See regimens recommended for enterococcal endocarditis	4	Preferred for nutritionally variant (pyridoxal- or cysteine-requiring) streptococci.
3. Enterococci (in vitro evaluation for MIC to penicillin and vancomycin, beta-lactamase production, and high-level resistance to gentamicin and streptomycin required)	A. Penicillin G plus gentamicin‡	18–30 million units IV daily in divided doses q 4 hr; 1 mg/kg IM or IV q 8 hr	4–6	See text for use of streptomycin instead of gentamicin in these regimens. Four wk of therapy recommended for patients with shorter history of illness (<3 mo) who respond promptly to treatment.
	B. Ampicillin plus gentamicin‡	12 gm IV daily in divided doses q 4 hr; Same dose as noted previously	4–6; 4–6	
	C. Vancomycin§ plus gentamicin‡	30 mg/kg IV daily in divided doses q 12 hr; Same dose as noted previously	4–6; 4–6	Use for patients with penicillin allergy. Do not use cephalosporins.

Organism	Regimen	Dose	Duration (wk)	Comments
4. Staphylococci infecting native valves (assume penicillin resistance), methicillin-susceptible	A. Nafcillin or oxacillin plus optional addition of gentamicin‡	12 gm IV daily in divided doses q 4 hr	4–6	Penicillin—18–24 million units daily in divided doses q 4 hr can be used instead of nafcillin, oxacillin, or cefazolin if strains do not produce beta-lactamase.
	gentamicin‡	1 mg/kg IM or IV q 8 hr	3–5 days	
	B. Cefazolin plus optional addition of gentamicin‡	2 gm IV q 8 hr	6	Cephalothin or other first-generation cephalosporin in equivalent doses can be used.
	gentamicin‡	Same dose as previously	3–5 days	
	C. Vancomycin§	30 mg/kg IV in divided doses q 12 hr	6	Use for patients with immediate penicillin allergy.
5. Staphylococci infecting native valves, methicillin-resistant	A. Vancomycin§	30 mg/kg IV in divided doses q 12 hr	6	
6. Staphylococci infecting prosthetic valves, methicillin-susceptible (assume penicillin resistance)	A. Nafcillin or oxacillin plus gentamicin‡ plus rifampin§	12 gm IV daily in divided doses q 4 hr	6	First-generation cephalosporin or vancomycin could be used in penicillin-allergic patients. Use gentamicin during initial 2 wk. See text for alternatives to gentamicin. For patients with immediate penicillin allergy, use regimen 7.
	gentamicin‡	1 mg/kg IV or IM q 8 hr	2	
	rifampin§	300 mg orally q 8 hr	6	
7. Staphylococci infecting prosthetic valves, methicillin-resistant	A. Vancomycin§ plus gentamicin‡ plus rifampin¶	30 mg/kg IV in divided doses q 12 hr	6	Use gentamicin during the initial 2 wk of therapy. See text for alternatives to gentamicin. Do not substitute a cephalosporin or imipenem for vancomycin.
	gentamicin‡	1 mg/kg IV or IM q 8 hr	2	
	rifampin¶	300 mg orally q 8 hr	6	
8. HACEK organisms**	A. Ceftriaxone	2 gm IV or IM daily as a single dose	4	Cefotaxime or other third-generation cephalosporin in comparable doses may be used
	B. Ampicillin plus gentamicin‡	12 gm IV daily in divided doses q 4 hr	4	Test organism for beta-lactamase production. Do not use this regimen if beta-lactamase is produced.
	gentamicin‡	1 mg/kg IV or IM q 8 hr	4	

From Karchmer, A.W.: Treatment of infective endocarditis. *In* Smith, T.W. (ed.): Cardiovascular Therapeutics. Philadelphia, W.B. Saunders, 1996, pp. 722–723.

Abbreviations: IE, infective endocarditis; MIC, minimal inhibitory concentration; IV, intravenous; IM, intramuscular.

* Recommended doses are for adults with normal renal and hepatic function. Doses of gentamicin, streptomycin, and vancomycin must be adjusted in patients with renal dysfunction. Use ideal body weight to calculate doses (men = 50 kg + 2.3 kg per inch over 5 ft; women = 45.5 kg + 2.3 kg per inch over 5 ft).

† All durations in weeks except where specifically noted (4.A and B with gentamicin).

‡ Aminoglycosides should not be administered as a single daily dose in patients with normal renal function.

§ Peak levels obtained 1 hr after completion of the infusion should be 30–45 μg/ml.

¶ Rifampin increases the dose of warfarin or dicumarol required for effective anticoagulation.

** HACEK organisms include *Haemophilus species, Actinobacillus actinomycetemcomitans, Cardiobacterium hominis, Eikenella corrodens,* and *Kingella kingae.*

organism causing IE. The regimens recommended for therapy are based on the precise susceptibility of the causative organism and prior clinical experience in the treatment of IE caused by the organism. Selection of treatment must also consider limitations unique to the individual patient, including existing allergies, renal and hepatic dysfunction, potential interactions with other required therapy, and the risk of adverse events. The regimens generally recommended for the treatment of the common bacterial causes of IE are similar for patients with infection of native and prosthetic valves (Table 16–5). Treatment of PVE is, however, usually several weeks longer than that used for native valve IE, and staphylococcal PVE is treated, where possible, with a combination regimen that includes rifampin.

Initiating Therapy

The optimal sequence of evaluation and treatment of a patient with suspected IE begins with a careful history and physical examination, with particular attention focused on the clinical manifestations and possible complications of IE (Fig. 16–4). Baseline laboratory tests should include complete blood counts, platelet count, serum creatinine, liver function tests, chest radiogram, electrocardiogram, and three blood cultures. An echocardiogram should also be obtained. In patients with significantly increased anteroposterior chest dimension or those with suspected PVE, the initial study should be performed transesophageally. Otherwise, a transthoracic approach can be used initially and the TEE can be reserved for use when the TTE is inadequate. If focal extracardiac complications are suspected, the area in question should be studied with appropriate imaging techniques.

The timing for initiating antimicrobial therapy may be critical. Pressures to contain medical cost often cause physicians to begin empirical antimicrobial therapy for suspected IE immediately after blood cultures have been obtained. This practice is appropriate when patients present with highly toxic, acute endocarditis, which may rapidly destroy cardiac valves, or with severe hemodynamic decompensation for which emergency valve surgery will be required (see Fig. 16–4). Prompt initiation of therapy to these patients may forestall valve damage or may quench infection and reduce the risk of reinfection after emergency valve replacement. However, among he-

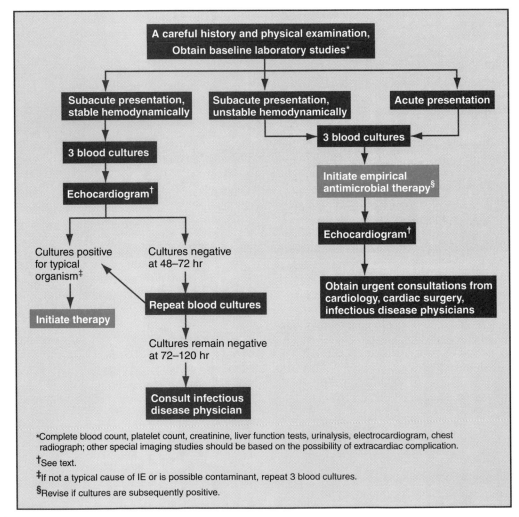

Figure 16–4
Diagnostic evaluation and the initiation of therapy in patients with suspected endocarditis. IE, infective endocarditis.

modynamically stable patients with suspected subacute endocarditis, precipitous initiation of therapy before blood cultures have yielded an isolate may be counterproductive. When initial blood cultures are negative because the patient has taken antibiotics, this precipitous therapy compromises the opportunity to obtain additional cultures that are not confounded by antibiotic therapy (see Diagnosis of IE). It is prudent to delay therapy for several days in the hemodynamically stable patient while waiting for the results of the initial blood cultures. It is unlikely that empirical therapy initiated a few days earlier will prevent complications.

Selecting Therapy

Consensus regimens have been developed for treatment of patients with commonly encountered forms of IE (see Table 16–5). Where choices among regimens are offered, they address variations in the antibiotic susceptibility of the particular organism, opportunities to avoid toxicities anticipated with some antibiotics, and alternative treatment when there is hypersensitivity to a recommended antibiotic. It is prudent to administer the regimen as it is specified. Compromises in the agent selected, dose, route of administration, and duration of therapy, in general, should be avoided, and if compromises seem necessary, they should be approached with the assistance of an infectious disease consultant.

Outpatient Therapy

Home health care systems with well-trained staff combined with technical advances in infusion therapy enable physicians to safely administer antibiotic therapy for IE in an outpatient setting. Even multiple daily dose regimens, including regimens using two antibiotics, can be administered to outpatients using portable, programmable computer-driven pumps. Physicians must exercise clinical judgment in identifying appropriate patients for outpatient antibiotic therapy. The patient must be reliable and compliant regarding treatment. Underlying conditions must not impair management outside of the hospital setting. The home setting, including the family and professional support services, must be capable of managing the complexities of parenteral therapy—suitable storage of antibiotic solutions and infusion materials, the sterile initiation and discontinuation of intravenous infusions, and the maintenance of intravenous access. Finally, the symptoms of IE should have abated before embarking on outpatient treatment. In particular, the patient should have been afebrile for 3 to 4 days and free of clinical evidence suggesting impending complications. To this end, echocardiographic assessment of the site of infection and cardiac function should be obtained before discharge, and blood cultures, although not routinely monitored during therapy, should have become negative.

Careful physician and laboratory monitoring for complications of IE or therapy are necessary during outpatient therapy. Patients should be examined at intervals of 3 to 7 days, the frequency depending on the duration of prior therapy and the patient's clinical stability. Laboratory tests are monitored to detect early antibiotic toxicities and

thus vary with the regimen used (see Monitoring during Antimicrobial Therapy). The ability of the home health care system to assist with monitoring, including the maintenance of intravenous access and obtaining periodic laboratory tests, is an important variable in the decision to administer antimicrobial therapy in the outpatient setting.

Therapy in the outpatient setting can significantly reduce total cost of therapy, although at times, because of payor policies, it shifts cost burdens to the patient. Before being discharged to outpatient treatment, patients should be advised that unpredictable complications may occur in either the outpatient or the hospital setting and that continued hospitalization will not prevent these complications. Patients should be instructed to report untoward events promptly. Lastly, outpatient therapy must not result in compromised suboptimal antimicrobial therapy.

Specific Treatment Regimens

Streptococcal IE (Fig. 16–5)

The vast majority of the streptococci that cause IE are highly susceptible to penicillin (minimal inhibitory concentration [MIC] ≤ 0.1 μg/ml) and can be effectively treated with any of the recommended regimens (see Table 16–5, 1.A–E). The 2-week regimen (see Table 16–5, 1.C), although effective for uncomplicated streptococcal IE, should not be used to treat IE caused by pyridoxal- or L-cysteine–requiring strains, streptococcal PVE, or IE complicated by myocardial abscess, mycotic aneurysm, or focal extracardiac infection. The ceftriaxone regimen (see Table 16–5, 1.D) is easily administered in an outpatient setting and can usually be given to patients with a history of penicillin allergy that does not suggest an immediate allergic reaction (urticaria, angioedema, or symptoms suggestive of anaphylaxis). Vancomycin (see Table 16–5, 1.E) is recommended for patients with a history of an immediate allergic reaction to a penicillin or a cephalosporin. Patients with PVE caused by penicillin-susceptible streptococci should be treated for 6 weeks with penicillin or ceftriaxone (see Table 16–5, 1.A or D); gentamicin 1 mg/kg every 8 hours (adjusted for decreased renal function) should be given intravenously during the initial 2 weeks.

Relative resistance to penicillin (MIC ≥ 0.2 μg/ml) is detected in 15% of streptococci that cause IE. IE caused by these organisms, as well as that caused by the potentially more virulent Lancefield group B streptococci (S. agalactiae), is optimally treated with a regimen that includes gentamicin (see Table 16–5, 2.A and B). Vancomycin alone (see Table 16–5, 1.E) provides effective therapy for patients with a penicillin allergy who have IE caused by streptococci with a penicillin MIC between 0.2 and 0.5 μg/ml. Alternatively, those patients with a non-immediate penicillin allergy could be treated with ceftriaxone (see Table 16–5, 1.D) plus gentamicin during the initial 2 weeks. IE caused by streptococci with a penicillin MIC > 0.5 μg/ml or by pyridoxal- or L-cysteine–requiring strains is treated with a regimen used for enterococcal IE (see Table 16–5, 3.A–C).

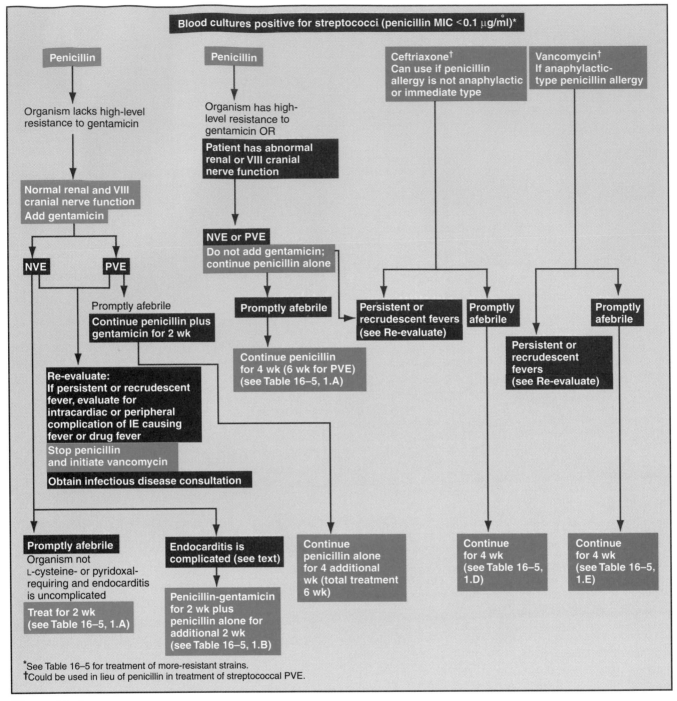

Figure 16–5

Treatment of streptococcal endocarditis. MIC, minimal inhibitory concentration; NVE, native valve endocarditis; PVE, prosthetic valve endocarditis; IE, infective endocarditis.

Enterococcal IE

Enterococcus faecalis and *Enterococcus faecium* cause 85% and 10% of the episodes of enterococcal IE, respectively. In contrast to streptococci, enterococci are inhibited rather than killed by penicillin, ampicillin, and vancomycin and are not susceptible to cephalosporins or the antistaphylococcal penicillinase-resistant penicillins (nafcillin and oxacillin). The bactericidal antibiotic effect

needed for optimal treatment of enterococcal IE requires the synergistic interaction of a cell wall–active antibiotic (penicillin, ampicillin, or vancomycin) that inhibits the organism at concentrations achievable clinically and an aminoglycoside (primarily gentamicin or streptomycin) that, in the presence of the cell wall–active agent, is able to exert a lethal effect. The ability of an enterococcus to grow in the presence of high concentrations of streptomycin (2000 μg/ml) or gentamicin (500 to 2000 μg/ml) is indicative of the inability of the aminoglycoside to exert a lethal effect and thus to participate in the bactericidal synergistic interaction. This degree of aminoglycoside resistance is referred to as *high-level resistance*. Additionally, high-level resistance to gentamicin predicts the resistance of the organism to all other aminoglycosides (except streptomycin, which must be tested individually) as well as the inability of these aminoglycosides to interact synergistically with a cell wall–active agent to kill the enterococcus. Even in the absence of high-level resistance, other aminoglycosides cannot be assumed to be effective agents for synergistic therapy and should not be used in lieu of streptomycin or gentamicin.

The standard regimens recommended for the treatment of enterococcal IE (see Table 16–5, 3.A–C) provide synergistic bactericidal therapy if, as noted previously, the organism is inhibited by clinically achievable concentrations of the cell wall–active agent and does not exhibit high-level resistance to the aminoglycoside. Treatment of enterococcal IE with a nonbactericidal cell wall–active agent alone, that is, ampicillin, penicillin, and vancomycin, is successful in only 30% to 40% of patients. Accordingly, optimal therapy for enterococcal IE requires a synergistic bactericidal combination of antibiotics. If selected and used appropriately, these combination regimens achieve a bacteriologic cure in 85% of patients. Streptomycin, 9.5 mg/kg given intramuscularly or intravenously every 12 hours to achieve peak serum concentrations of approximately 20 μg/ml, can be used instead of gentamicin if the causative strain does not possess high-level resistance to streptomycin. Cephalosporins are never used to treat enterococcal IE. Patients with enterococcal IE who are allergic to penicillins must be treated with either the vancomycin regimen (see Table 16–5, 3.C) or with a penicillin or ampicillin regimen (see Table 16–5, 3.A and B) after being cautiously desensitized to penicillin.

Antimicrobial resistance among enterococci is increasingly common and complex. It cannot be predicted without in vitro testing. Thus, enterococci causing IE must always be tested for susceptibility to ampicillin and vancomycin, for beta-lactamase production, and for high-level resistance to streptomycin and gentamicin. If IE is caused by a strain that is resistant to the cell wall–active agents or that possesses high-level resistance to both streptomycin and gentamicin, so that synergistic bactericidal therapy (see Table 16–5, 3.A–C) is not possible, consultation from an infectious disease specialist should be sought. Administration of an aminoglycoside when IE is caused by a strain with high-level resistance to streptomycin and gentamicin exposes the patient to potential aminoglycoside toxicity without clinical benefit. The complexity of the regimens for treatment of enterococcal IE, their potential toxicity, and the evolving resistance among enterococci suggest that patients with enterococcal IE should be seen by an infectious disease consultant to aid in the selection of optimal therapy.

Staphylococcal IE (Fig. 16–6)

Plasmids that produce penicillinase are present in the overwhelming majority of coagulase-negative staphylococci and *S. aureus* and render these organisms resistant to penicillin and ampicillin. Many coagulase-negative staphylococci, particularly those causing nosocomially acquired IE, and some *S. aureus* are resistant to methicillin and to all other currently available beta-lactam antibiotics. Fortunately, the vast majority of methicillin-resistant strains remain susceptible to vancomycin.

Nafcillin, oxacillin, and cefazolin are the primary agents recommended for the treatment of native valve IE caused by methicillin-susceptible staphylococci. Gentamicin is often given concurrently during the initial 3 to 5 days of therapy in an attempt to accelerate control of the infection through the synergistic interaction of the beta-lactam antibiotic and the aminoglycoside (see Table 16–5, 4.A and B). Longer courses of gentamicin are not advocated because of potential nephrotoxicity. If beta-lactams cannot be used because of hypersensitivity, treatment with vancomycin is recommended (see Table 16–5, 4.C). An aminoglycoside is not routinely combined with vancomycin because of the potential enhanced nephrotoxicity of this combination. Vancomycin is not as bactericidal for methicillin-susceptible staphylococci as are beta-lactam agents and should not be used to treat staphylococcal IE for convenience only (reduced doses per day facilitating administration) reasons. Optimal treatment of native valve IE caused by methicillin-resistant staphylococci requires vancomycin (see Table 16–5, 5.A). Rifampin is not routinely used in the treatment of staphylococcal native valve IE.

If IE caused by methicillin-susceptible *S. aureus* is limited to the right-sided valves (a situation encountered mainly among drug addicts), 2 weeks of therapy using a semisynthetic penicillinase-resistant penicillin plus gentamicin (1 mg/kg every 8 hours) is highly effective among those patients who promptly become afebrile and do not have focal extracardiac infection detected on subsequent evaluations during treatment. Vancomycin does not appear to be an effective alternative to the beta-lactam agent in this abbreviated regimen.

Staphylococcal infection involving prosthetic valves or other intracardiac foreign material is optimally treated with a multidrug regimen (see Table 16–5, 6.A and 7.A). In this setting, rifampin plays a pivotal role in the killing of staphylococci that are adherent to foreign material. Because resistance to rifampin emerges easily in this setting, an additional agent that is known to be effective against the staphylococcus should be added to the beta-lactam antibiotic or vancomycin that serves as primary treatment. Gentamicin is the preferred agent; however, some strains will be resistant to gentamicin. In that case, an effective alternative aminoglycoside or fluoroquinolone should be used. Treatment with rifampin ideally should be delayed until the two agents have been used for a few days. Staphylococcal PVE is treated for a minimum of 6, and often 8, weeks.

IE Caused by HACEK and Other Organisms

Some HACEK organisms produce beta-lactamase and are resistant to ampicillin. Accordingly, ceftriaxone has become the treatment of choice for HACEK IE (see Table 16–5, 8.A).

Consensus recommendations for treatment of patients with IE caused by the broad array of bacteria and fungi that cause infrequent sporadic episodes of valve infection are not available. In many instances, clinical experience with the species encountered is limited, susceptibility testing may be difficult, and complex, potentially toxic regimens may be warranted. Accordingly, physicians are urged to seek assistance from experienced infectious disease consultants when treating IE caused by atypical organisms or when planning IE treatment for patients with negative blood cultures.

Monitoring during Antimicrobial Therapy

Careful clinical monitoring during antibiotic treatment, especially during the initial 2 weeks, to assess the response to therapy and to detect complications of IE is essential. Persistent fever beyond 7 to 10 days may indicate a failure of antimicrobial treatment or the presence of a myocardial abscess, focal extracardiac infection (splenic or renal abscess), emboli, hypersensitivity to an antimicrobial agent, or an infusion device–related complication

(catheter-related infection, thrombophlebitis). Prompt detection of these events or other complications of IE (hemodynamic decompensation or neurologic event) may allow lifesaving revisions of therapy or initiation of adjunctive therapy.

Proper selection of antibiotic therapy requires reliable antimicrobial susceptibility testing of the causative organism. The recommended organism-specific consensus regimens (see Table 16–5) result in predictably high bactericidal antimicrobial activity in the patient's serum from dose to dose. As a result, measurement of the serum bactericidal titer, the highest dilution of the patient's blood at a given time that kills 99.9% of a standard inoculum of the infecting organism, is no longer recommended. It is, however, appropriate to monitor serum concentrations of vancomycin and aminoglycosides when they are used. This allows dose adjustments, which ensures optimal therapy and reduces adverse events. Serum creatinine must be monitored when treatment employs vancomycin or an aminoglycoside. Complete blood counts should be checked weekly in patients receiving a beta-lactam antibiotic or vancomycin, and liver function tests should be monitored every 7 to 10 days in those receiving oxacillin or nafcillin.

Routine blood cultures in patients on therapy who no

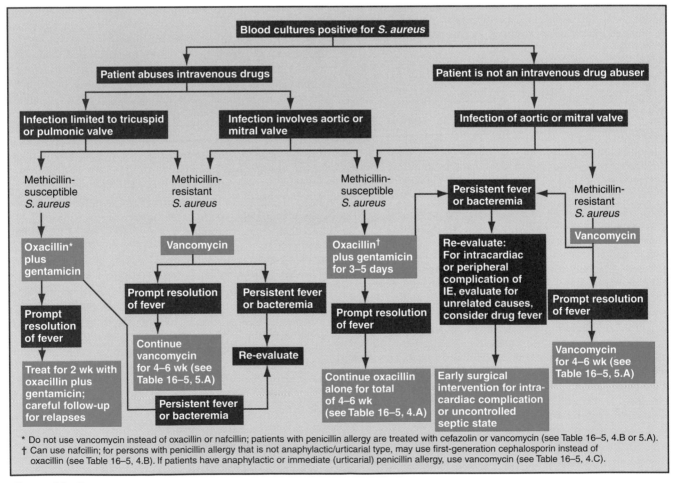

Figure 16–6

Treatment of native valve endocarditis caused by *Staphylococcus aureus*. IE, infective endocarditis.

Table 16–6	Indications for Cardiac Surgery in Patients with IE

Indications*

Moderate to severe congestive heart due to valve dysfunction
Partially dehisced unstable prosthetic valve
Persistent bacteremia in the face of optimal antimicrobial therapy
Absence of effective, bactericidal therapy
Fungal endocarditis
Relapse of PVE after optimal antimicrobial therapy
Persistent unexplained fever (≥ 10 days) in culture-negative PVE
Staphylococcus aureus PVE

Relative Indications†

Perivalvular extension of infection (myocardial, septal, or annulus abscess, intracardiac fistula)
Poorly responsive *Staphylococcus aureus* endocarditis involving the aortic or mitral valve
Relapse of native valve IE after optimal antimicrobial therapy
Large (> 10 mm diameter) hypermobile vegetations
Persistent unexplained fever (≥ 10 days) in culture-negative native valve IE
Endocarditis due to highly antibiotic-resistant enterococci or gram-negative bacilli

Abbreviations: IE, infective endocarditis; PVE, prosthetic valve endocarditis.
* Cardiac surgery required for optimal outcome.
† Surgery, although not always required, must be carefully considered.

longer have fever are not indicated. However, persistence or recrudescence of fever during therapy should be evaluated with blood cultures. Doing so may detect breakthrough bacteremia or new infections. Several blood cultures to document cure of IE are often obtained 2 to 8 weeks after completion of treatment. Recurrence of fever during this period after treatment demands blood cultures to assess the possibility of relapsed IE.

SURGICAL TREATMENT OF INTRACARDIAC COMPLICATIONS

The mortality rates for various forms of IE continue to range from 10% to 50% in spite of treatment with increasingly potent antimicrobial regimens. Although mortality, in part, relates to the increased age and underlying diseases of patients with IE, intracardiac and central nervous system complications are important additional causes of death due to IE. Some life-threatening intracardiac complications, although not responsive to antimicrobial therapy, are amenable to surgical treatment. The unacceptably high mortality rates encountered among medically treated patients with these complications are reduced when treatment includes antibiotics and surgical intervention. As a result, these intracardiac complications and other instances of failed antimicrobial therapy have become indications for cardiac surgery (Table 16–6). Occasionally, the occurrence of one of these events is an unequivocal indication for surgery. More commonly, the event evokes consideration of surgical intervention, whereupon the risk-benefit ratio and timing of surgery must be weighed. When these circumstances arise, patients should be hospitalized in a setting where urgent

cardiac surgery is available, if needed. At this juncture, multiple specialists—including cardiologists, cardiac surgeons, and infectious disease physicians—should be involved in the care of the patient.

Specific Indications

Valvular Dysfunction and Heart Failure

Patients with moderate to severe heart failure (New York Heart Association class III or IV) resulting from IE-induced valve dysfunction who are treated medically experience a mortality rate of 50% to 90% during hospitalization and over the ensuing 6 months. Among patients with comparable hemodynamic disability who undergo valve surgery, survival rates of 60% to 80% and 45% to 65% are achieved for native valve IE and PVE, respectively. Patients with aortic valve regurgitation deteriorate more rapidly than those with mitral valve regurgitation and require earlier surgical intervention. Occasionally, large vegetations significantly obstruct the orifice of the valve, particularly prosthetic mitral valves, necessitating surgery to relieve valve stenosis.

Perivalvular Extension of Infection

Extension of infection beyond the valve into adjacent tissues complicates 10% to 15% of patients with native valve IE and 45% to 60% of cases of PVE. This complication is suggested by persistent unexplained (by an extracardiac source) fever in spite of appropriate antibiotic therapy. Pericarditis in patients with infection at the aortic valve site suggests extension through the annulus into the pericardial space. New onset and persistent electrocardiographic conduction abnormalities (otherwise unexplained), especially with aortic valve IE, although not sensitive, are a highly specific indicator of paravalvular infection. The most sensitive evaluation for this complication utilizes TEE and includes Doppler and color-flow Doppler evaluation. The TTE is not sufficiently sensitive for use in this assessment, particularly when investigating patients with PVE. Persistent unexplained fever in spite of 10 days or more of appropriate antibiotic therapy for PVE and relapse of PVE after appropriate therapy are unusually indicative of invasive infection and the need for surgical intervention. Although occasional patients with invasive infection will be cured with antibiotics alone, most appear to require surgical intervention to débride abscesses and repair structural damage.

Uncontrolled Infection

Failure to control infection, which manifests by persistent fever or continued positive blood cultures, may be the result of anatomic situations (undébrided abscess), resistant infecting organisms (highly resistant enterococci, *Pseudomonas aeruginosa,* gram-negative facultative bacilli), or inadequate antimicrobial agents (fungi, *Brucella* species, *C. burnetii*). Before ascribing persistent fever to antibiotic failure, the susceptibility of the infecting organism to current therapy must be reassessed, extracardiac foci of infection must be excluded, and noninfectious causes of fever, including drug fever, must be evaluated. Scattered reports of medical cure of *Candida* species IE with prolonged antifungal therapy have been published. Although it may be possible to chronically suppress *Candida* IE with prolonged (over years) fluconazole treatment, medical cure of this entity remains unlikely.

S. aureus IE

S. aureus infection of the mitral or aortic valve is a common cause of death. Patients with these infections whose course suggest invasive infection or who remain septic during the initial week of therapy, with or without bacteremia, are more likely to survive with surgical intervention than with continued antibiotics alone. The likelihood of curing patients with *S. aureus* PVE is markedly improved if these patients, both those with and those without intracardiac complications, are treated surgically. In contrast, intravenous drug addicts with *S. aureus* IE restricted to the right heart valves can usually be cured with continued antibiotic therapy, even in the face of persisting fever (14 or more days). It is likely that these patients will return to drug abuse and be at risk for recurrent IE; hence, it is prudent to avoid valve replacement, when possible.

Culture-Negative IE

Persistence of fever during empirical antimicrobial therapy in patients with echocardiographically confirmed, blood culture–negative IE suggests that either antibiotic therapy is inadequate or invasive infection is present. Accordingly, after excluding extracardiac infection and noninfectious causes of fever, these patients should be considered for surgery.

Large, Hypermobile Vegetations

The risk of arterial embolization appears greater among patients with large vegetations (>10 mm), particularly when these are pedunculated or hypermobile, than among patients with smaller or no echocardiographically demonstrable vegetations. Central nervous system emboli remain an important source of morbidity and mortality in patients with IE. Nevertheless, that large vegetations in and of themselves are an indication for cardiac surgery to prevent emboli is not established. Importantly, the risk of embolism decreases significantly after 2 weeks of effective antimicrobial therapy; hence, timing is an important variable. The role of surgery in the management of patients with large vegetations remains controversial. When vegetations are exceptionally large, size alone may serve as an indication to proceed with surgery. More often, however, vegetation characteristics should be one of multiple clinical and echocardiographic observations weighed when considering surgery.

Timing of Cardiac Surgery

If the potential for cardiac surgical intervention to reduce mortality and morbidity in patients with IE is to be realized, primary care physicians must not only recognize the indications for surgery but also understand the optimal timing of surgery for each indication. Preventable morbidity or mortality may occur when tardily placed requests for surgical consultation result in delayed surgery. Surgery to correct valve dysfunction that has caused congestive heart failure must be performed before intractable hemodynamic deterioration occurs, regardless of the duration of prior antibiotic therapy. It is clear that survival after surgery is inversely proportional to the severity of the preoperative hemodynamic disability. Uncontrolled infection also requires early surgical intervention. Delaying surgery in order to administer additional antibiotic therapy to patients who are failing antibiotic therapy does not improve outcome. In contrast, if the hemodynamic status is stable and infection is controlled, other considerations should determine the timing of surgery. For example, in a patient with valve dysfunction that requires surgery but who is hemodynamically stable and in whom infection is controlled, surgery can be delayed until nearing the completion of the planned antibiotic regimen. In a patient who ultimately requires surgery because of valve dysfunction, detection of a very large vegetation may prompt surgery earlier than originally planned in an effort to reduce emboli. The high likelihood of severe neurologic deterioration is offered as a contraindication to cardiac surgery in patients with central nervous system embolic infarcts or hemorrhage. In fact, the risk of neurologic deterioration decreases to 15% and 10% 2 and 3 weeks after an infarct, respectively. Thus, if cardiac surgery is considered lifesaving, it can be performed with acceptable neurologic risk at this time. Worsening of preexisting cerebral hemorrhage during cardiac surgery, however, remains a risk for at least 1 month after the original hemorrhage and makes surgical intervention hazardous throughout the period of active IE.

Table 16–7	Situations Warranting Subspecialty Consultation in the Treatment of IE

Uncertain diagnosis
Apparent culture-negative endocarditis
Patient allergic to or intolerant of recommended therapy
Endocarditis caused by an unusual organism or an unusually resistant organism
Enterococcal endocarditis
Staphylococcus aureus left-sided endocarditis
PVE
Relapse after appropriate therapy
Persistent bacteremia or fever during therapy
An indication or relative indication for cardiac surgical intervention (see Table 16–6)
Neurologic complication
Arterial embolic event
Cerebral or peripheral mycotic aneurysm

Abbreviations: IE, infective endocarditis; PVE, prosthetic valve endocarditis.

Table 16–8	Risk of IE Associated with Cardiac Abnormalities	
High Risk	**Moderate Risk**	**Low or Negligible Risk**
Prosthetic heart valves	Congenital cardiac malformations (other than high-/low-risk lesions)	Isolated ostium secundum atrial septal defect
Prior bacterial endocarditis	Acquired valvular dysfunction	Surgically repaired atrial or ventricular septal defect or patent ductus arteriosus
Complex cyanotic congenital heart disease	Hypertrophic cardiomyopathy	Prior coronary artery bypass surgery
Surgically constructed systemic-pulmonary shunts	Mitral valve prolapse with valvular regurgitation or thickened leaflets	Mitral valve prolapse without valvular regurgitation
		Physiologic, functional, or innocent heart murmurs
		Prior Kawasaki's disease or rheumatic fever without valvular dysfunction
		Cardiac pacemakers and implanted defibrillators

Adapted from Dajani, A.S., Taubert, K.A., Wilson, W., et al.: Prevention of bacterial endocarditis: Recommendations by the American Heart Association, from the Committee on Rheumatic Fever, Endocarditis, and Kawasaki Disease, Council on Cardiovascular Diseases in the Young. JAMA 277:1794–1801, 1997.
Abbreviation: IE, infective endocarditis.

EXTRACARDIAC COMPLICATIONS

Focal extracardiac septic complications occasionally require treatment that differs significantly from that given for IE alone. Unique treatment may entail a longer duration of antibiotic therapy or drainage of a localized abscess. Splenic abscess, which complicates 3% to 5% of cases of IE, can be identified by ultrasound or computed tomography. Successful therapy almost always requires drainage percutaneously or splenectomy. Effective therapy for vertebral osteomyelitis may require a longer course of therapy than that for IE itself.

Mycotic aneurysms complicate 2% to 10% of cases of IE, and half of these aneurysms are located intracranially. Focal neurologic symptoms, persistent headache, or embolic events may be a harbinger of an aneurysm. Intracranial mycotic lesions that hemorrhage should be resected, if possible, to avoid further bleeding. Unruptured aneurysms may resolve with antibiotic therapy. Thus, these

are followed angiographically. Failure to resolve or progressive enlargement during therapy is an indication for resection if technically feasible.

CONSULTATIVE SERVICES

The high cure rates for uncomplicated, subacute, viridans streptococcal and enterococcal IE suggest to the inexperienced physician that patients with IE are easily managed. In fact, IE is a treacherous disease, in part because the site of infection, the vegetation, cannot be examined directly to assess progress. In addition, life-threatening complications—for example, arterial emboli, rupture of a mycotic aneurysm, valve destruction, and congestive heart failure—may occur without warning. As a result, it is prudent to seek infectious disease and other subspecialty consultative assistance when treating any pa-

Table 16–9	Dental Procedures for Which IE Prophylaxis Is Considered	
Prophylaxis Recommended		**Prophylaxis Not Recommended**
Dental extractions		Restorative dentistry (operative and prosthodontic) with/without retraction cord
Periodontal procedures (surgery, scaling, root planing, probing)		Local anesthetic injection (not intraligamentary)
Dental implant placement, reimplantation of avulsed teeth		Intracanal endodontic treatment (postplacement and buildup)
Endodontic instrumentation (root canal) or surgery beyond the apex		Placement of rubber dams
Subgingival placement of antibiotic fibers/strips		Suture removal
Initial placement of orthodontic bands (not brackets)		Placement of removable prosthodontic/orthodontic appliances
Intraligamentary local anesthetic injections		Taking oral impressions or radiographs
Prophylactic cleaning of teeth or implants where bleeding is anticipated		Orthodontic appliance adjustment
		Shedding primary teeth

Adapted from Dajani, A.S., Taubert, K.A., Wilson, W., et al.: Prevention of bacterial endocarditis: Recommendations by the American Heart Association, from the Committee on Rheumatic Fever, Endocarditis, and Kawasaki Disease, Council on Cardiovascular Diseases in the Young. JAMA 277:1794–1801, 1997.

Table 16–10	Procedures for Which IE Prophylaxis Is Considered

Prophylaxis Recommended	Prophylaxis Not Recommended
Respiratory Tract	
Surgical operation involving mucosa	Endotracheal intubation
Bronchoscopy with rigid bronchoscope	Bronchoscopy with flexible bronchoscope with or without biopsy*
	Tympanostomy tube insertion
Gastrointestinal Tract†	
Sclerotherapy for esophageal varices	Transesophageal echocardiography
Dilatation of esophageal stricture	Endoscopy with or without biopsy*
Endoscopic retrograde cholangiography with biliary obstruction	
Biliary tract surgery	
Surgery involving intestinal mucosa	
Genitourinary Tract	
Prostate surgery	Vaginal hysterectomy*
Cytoscopy	Vaginal delivery*
Urethral dilatation	Cesarean section
	In the absence of infection:
	Urethral catheterization, uterine dilatation and curettage, therapeutic abortion, sterilization, insertion/removal of intrauterine device
Other	
	Cardiac catheterization, coronary angioplasty
	Implantation of pacemakers, defibrillators, coronary stents
	Clean surgery
	Circumcision

Adapted from Dajani, A.S., Taubert, K.A., Wilson, W., et al.: Prevention of bacterial endocarditis: Recommendations by the American Heart Association, from the Committee on Rheumatic Fever, Endocarditis, and Kawasaki Disease, Council on Cardiovascular Diseases in the Young. JAMA 277:1794–1801, 1997.
Abbreviation: IE, infective endocarditis.
* Prophylaxis is optional for high-risk patients.
† Recommended for high-risk patients; optional for moderate-risk group.

tient with IE except those with forms that are caused by typical bacterial organisms and are totally uncomplicated (Table 16–7). Because of the high mortality rates and the high frequency of invasive infection, patients with left-sided *S. aureus* IE and all patients with PVE should be seen in consultation by an infectious disease specialist. If these patients have been admitted to a hospital where cardiac surgery cannot be performed, provisional arrangements for urgent transfer to such a facility should be made at the time of diagnosis. Additionally, interpretation of enterococcal susceptibility tests and design of optimal therapy may require subspecialty consultation.

PREVENTION

The rationale and regimens for prophylaxis of IE are based on the recognition of the lesions that predispose to IE, the bacteria (and their antibiotic susceptibility) that cause IE, and the procedures that generate a moderately high frequency of transient bacteremia with these organisms. Although experimental models of the pathogenesis and prophylaxis of IE support the concept of antibiotic prophylaxis to prevent IE, no randomized, controlled human trial has established the efficacy of chemoprophylaxis. Furthermore, most episodes of IE arise in patients unrelated to events for which prophylaxis is indicated. Although it is likely that optimal prophylaxis prevents

only a small fraction of IE episodes, efforts to provide prophylaxis remain the standard of care. An American Heart Association expert committee has identified the patients likely to benefit from prophylaxis and the procedures warranting prophylaxis (Tables 16–8 through 16–10) and has suggested regimens for use to prevent IE (Tables 16–11 and 12). By recognizing the cardiac lesions at risk for IE, repetitively reminding patients that they are at risk, and prescribing appropriate antibiotic prophylaxis, the primary care physician is ideally positioned to prevent IE. In addition to prevention of IE by antibiotic prophylaxis, the primary care physician can reduce the risk of IE by encouraging patients to maintain good oral hygiene through regular dental care and by directing patients to have dental disease treated before undergoing cardiac valve surgery.

Patients with cardiac abnormalities can be divided into those at high, moderate, and low or negligible risk for developing IE (see Table 16–8). Prophylaxis is not recommended for those at low or negligible risk. By 6 months after complete repair, the moderate risk for IE associated with patent ductus arteriosus, ventricular septal defect, ostium primum atrial septal defect, and coarctation of the aorta is eliminated. Mitral valve prolapse (MVP) is a common finding in patients. The need for prophylaxis for this abnormality is controversial. The risk for IE in patients with MVP appears to be 5 to 10 times higher than in the general population but 100 times lower than that in patients with rheumatic valvular disease. The risk for IE relates to regurgitant blood flow across the mitral valve, therefore prophylaxis is recommended for patients with clinical evidence of MVP (systolic click) and a murmur of mitral regurgitation. Among patients over 45 years of age who on prior echocardiography have evidence of MVP and thickened leaflets, prophylaxis is warranted even in the absence of regurgitation at rest. However, routine echocardiographic screening for MVP to identify candidates for prophylaxis is not recommended.

The procedures likely to induce bacteremia with IE-prone bacteria are those for which prophylaxis is advised (see Tables 16–9 and 16–10). When multiple dental procedures are required in close sequence, it may be desirable to separate them by 1 to 3 weeks to lessen the potential for selecting antibiotic-resistant oral flora. When surgery is to be performed on the genitourinary tract, cultures should be obtained preoperatively and infection eradicated before proceeding with surgery. This will reduce the frequency of bacteremia with the subsequent procedure.

The regimens recommended for use as prophylaxis are targeted to the IE-prone bacteria likely to be encountered in the manipulated areas (see Tables 16–11 and 16–12). Antibiotic regimens to prevent recurrence of acute rheumatic fever are not adequate for prophylaxis of IE. Because patients receiving these regimens may have oral cavity flora that are resistant to penicillins, clindamycin or clarithromycin should be used for prophylaxis of IE. Surgical procedures on infected tissues, including incision and drainage, may induce bacteremia; consequently, prophylaxis should be considered when IE-prone patients un-

dergo these procedures. When *S. aureus* is the likely infecting organism, prophylaxis regimens should use an antistaphylococcal penicillin, a first-generation cephalosporin, or if methicillin-resistant *S. aureus* is anticipated, vancomycin.

Table 16–12 Regimens for IE Prophylaxis in Adults: Genitourinary and Gastrointestinal* Tract Procedures

Setting	Antibiotic	Regimen†
High-risk patients	Ampicillin plus gentamicin	Ampicillin 2.0 gm IV/IM plus gentamicin 1.5 mg/kg within 30 min of procedure, repeat ampicillin 1.0 gm IV/IM or amoxicillin 1.0 gm po 6 hr later
High-risk, penicillin-allergic patients	Vancomycin plus gentamicin	Vancomycin 1.0 gm IV over 1–2 hr plus gentamicin 1.5 mg/kg IM/IV infused or injected 30 min before procedure; no second dose recommended
Moderate-risk patients	Amoxicillin or ampicillin	Amoxicillin 2.0 gm po 1 hr before procedure or ampicillin 2.0 gm IM/IV 30 min before procedure
Moderate-risk, penicillin-allergic patients	Vancomycin	Vancomycin 1.0 gm IV infused over 1–2 hr and completed within 30 min of procedure

Adapted from Dajani, A.S., Taubert, K.A., Wilson, W., et al.: Prevention of bacterial endocarditis: Recommendations by the American Heart Association, from the Committee on Rheumatic Fever, Endocarditis, and Kawasaki Disease, Council on Cardiovascular Diseases in the Young. JAMA 277:1794–1801, 1997.
Abbreviation: IE, infective endocarditis; IV, intravenous; IM, intramuscular; po, by mouth.
* Excludes esophageal procedures (see Table 16–11).
† Dosing for children: Ampicillin 50 mg/kg IV/IM, vancomycin 20 mg/kg IV, gentamicin 1.5 mg/kg IV/IM (children's doses should not exceed adult doses).

Table 16–11 Regimens for IE Prophylaxis in Adults: Oral, Respiratory Tract, or Esophageal Procedures

Setting	Antibiotic	Regimen*
Standard	Amoxicillin	2.0 gm po 1 hr before procedure
Unable to take oral medication	Ampicillin	2.0 gm IM or IV within 30 min of procedure
Penicillin-allergic patients	Clindamycin	600 mg po 1 hr before procedure or IV 30 min before procedure
	Cephalexin†	2.0 gm po 1 hr before procedure
	Cefazolin†	1.0 gm IV or IM 30 min before procedure
	Cefadroxil†	2.0 gm po 1 hr before procedure
	Clarithromycin	500 mg po 1 hr before procedure

Adapted from Dajani, A.S., Taubert, K.A., Wilson, W., et al.: Prevention of bacterial endocarditis: Recommendations by the American Heart Association, from the Committee on Rheumatic Fever, Endocarditis, and Kawasaki Disease, Council on Cardiovascular Diseases in the Young. JAMA 277:1794–1801, 1997.
Abbreviations: IE, infective endocarditis; po, by mouth; IM, intramuscular; IV, intravenous.
* For patients in the high-risk group, administer half the dose 6 hr after the initial dose; dosing for children: amoxicillin, ampicillin, cephalexin, or cefadroxil use 50 mg/kg po; cefazolin IV 25 mg/kg; clindamycin 20 mg/kg po, 25 mg/kg IV; clarithromycin 15 mg/kg po.
† Do not use cephalosporins in patients with immediate hypersensitivity (urticaria, angioedema, anaphylaxis) to penicillin.

Suggested Reading

Aragam, J.R., and Weyman, A.E.: Echocardiographic findings in infective endocarditis. *In* Weyman, A.E. (ed.): Principles and Practice of Echocardiography. 2nd ed. Philadelphia, Lea & Febiger, 1994, pp. 1178–1197.

Dajani, A.S., Taubert, K.A., Wilson, W., et al.: Prevention of bacterial endocarditis: Recommendations by the American Heart Association, from the Committee on Rheumatic Fever, Endocarditis, and Kawasaki Disease, Council on Cardiovascular Diseases in the Young. JAMA 277:1794–1801, 1997.

Daniel, W.G., Mugge, A., Martin, R.P., et al.: Improvement in the diagnosis of abscesses associated with endocarditis by transesophageal echocardiography. N. Engl. J. Med. 324:795–800, 1991.

Durack, D.T.: Prevention of infective endocarditis. N. Engl. J. Med. 332:38–44, 1995.

Durack, D.T., Lukes, A.S., and Bright, D.K.: New criteria for diagnosis of infective endocarditis: Utilization of specific echocardiographic findings. Am. J. Med. 96:200–209, 1994.

Karchmer, A.W.: Infective endocarditis. *In* Braunwald, E. (ed.): Heart Disease. 5th ed. Philadelphia, W.B. Saunders, 1997, pp. 1097–1104.

Karchmer, A.W.: Treatment of infective endocarditis. *In* Smith, T.W. (ed.): Cardiovascular Therapeutics. Philadelphia, W.B. Saunders, 1996, pp. 718–730.

Karchmer, A.W., and Gibbons, G.W.: Infections of prosthetic heart valves and vascular grafts. *In* Bisno, A.L., and Waldvogel, F.A.

(eds.): Infections Associated with Indwelling Devices. 2nd ed. Washington, DC, American Society for Microbiology, 1994, pp. 213–249.

Kaye, D.: Infective endocarditis. *In* Fauci, A.S., Braunwald, E., Isselbacher, K.J., et al. (eds.): Harrison's Principles of Internal Medicine. 14th ed. New York, McGraw-Hill, 1998, pp. 785–791.

Ojemann, R.G.: Surgical management of bacterial intracranial aneurysms. *In* Schmidek, H.H., and Sweet, W.H. (eds.): Operative Neurosurgical Techniques. 2nd ed. Orlando, FL, Grune & Stratton, 1988, pp. 997–1001.

Scheld, W.M., and Sande, M.A.: Endocarditis and intravascular infections. *In* Mandell, G.L., Bennett, J.E., and Dolin, R. (eds.): Mandel, Douglas and Bennett's Principles and Practice of Infectious Diseases. 4th ed. New York, Churchill Livingstone, 1995, pp. 740–783.

Steckelberg, J.M., Murphy, J.G., and Wilson, W.R.: Management of complications of infective endocarditis. *In* Kaye. D. (ed.): Infective Endocarditis. 2nd ed. New York, Raven Press, 1992, pp. 435–453.

Torres-Tortosa, M., de Cueto, M., Vergara, A., et al.: Prospective evaluation of a two-week course of intravenous antibiotics in intravenous drug addicts with infective endocarditis. Eur. J. Clin. Microbiol. Infect. Dis. 13:559–564, 1994.

Wilson, W.R., Karchmer, A.W., Bisno, A.L., et al.: Antibiotic treatment of adults with infective endocarditis due to viridans streptococci, enterococci, other streptococci, staphylococci, and HACEK microorganisms. JAMA 274:1706–1713, 1995.

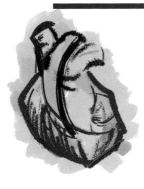

Chapter 17

Approach to

Cardiovascular Emergencies

ROBERT A. BARISH AND
JEROME F. X. NARADZAY

PRIMARY CARE PHYSICIANS' ROLES IN THE CHAIN OF SURVIVAL

The *chain of survival* once referred to the sequence of events surrounding an out-of-hospital cardiac arrest; however, with a shift in health care management from hospital-based to office-based, the primary care physician has become a key link in the chain of survival for a patient with a cardiovascular emergency. With the increasing limitations on health care resources and dollars, physicians' offices are more likely than emergency departments to be treatment sites for patients with nonurgent cardiovascular conditions. Concomitantly, because of the nature of cardiovascular disease and because of patients' decisions about where to seek medical help, primary care physicians will encounter increasing numbers of true cardiovascular emergencies in their offices. The physician must be able not only to recognize and treat nonurgent cases but also to initiate triage of patients with tenuous or life-threatening conditions to a hospital. The primary care physician must communicate with the emergency department physician to avoid redundant costs and penalties for inappropriate triage. It is the primary care physician who can identify the high-risk patient, activate the emergency medical services system, and transfer care to the emergency physician.

Patient Education

One effect of changes in the health care system is evident in patients' decisions about where to seek help in a real or perceived cardiovascular emergency. Financial concerns, demographic variables, proximity to emergency departments, accessibility of a primary care physician, and behavior associated with an acute illness influence patients' choice of a primary care physician's office or an emergency department.

A patient's decision to seek medical care will progress through three phases: self-evaluation, lay evaluation, and medical evaluation. The self-evaluation phase is the longest. During this phase, the patient has symptoms but keeps them secret and is influenced by available medical resources and reluctance to impose on supporters.[3] In the lay evaluation phase, the patient reveals the presence of symptoms by seeking the opinions of others. The medical evaluation phase begins when the patient arrives at a physician's office or emergency department for professional evaluation.

The patient must make a conscious choice regarding treatment site. The two best predictors of facility choice are the patient's type of insurance and his or her problem-solving abilities. The primary care physician must influence this decision-making process by educating the patient about the illness, maintaining compliance with medications, developing problem-solving skills so that the patient knows how to deal with symptoms of the disease, and distinguishing between serious and not-so-serious symptoms. Patients must be very well informed about their medical history, cardiac history, medications, surgery, angioplasty, and the like. Ultimately, the patient must know when to seek medical advice or attention before symptoms progress to critical levels. For example, a patient's delay in seeking medical attention represents two-thirds of the total time from symptom onset to initiation of thrombolytic therapy. Unfortunately, public education has not significantly reduced patient-related delays.[1]

It is imperative that the primary care physician inform the patient about situations that warrant medical attention. Discussion should focus on the meaning of recurrent symptoms, problem-solving techniques, and guidelines for seeking information about symptoms. Presenting the patient with a summary of her or his medical history, a list of medications, diagnostic evaluation results, and a method for contacting the primary care physician enhances patient understanding and can help overcome knowledge deficits that contribute to delays in seeking care and receiving treatment.

A patient who calls a primary care physician and describes symptoms of a cardiovascular emergency should be encouraged to access the emergency medical service system immediately from his or her location. Then the physician should notify the emergency department of the impending arrival. If possible, the primary care physician should provide the emergency department with relevant medical history, medications, facsimiles of electrocardiograms (ECGs), results of diagnostic tests, and information about the patient's health care proxy. Hospitals, emergency departments, and primary care physicians' offices should work together to form "seamless," integrated patient information systems.

Stabilization in the Primary Care Physician's Office

The primary care physician's office should stock the supplies and medications necessary to stabilize a patient with a suspected cardiovascular emergency while transport arrangements are being made (Table 17–1). Commercially available code carts contain medications necessary to stabilize the patient with a cardiovascular emergency. Direct communication with the emergency department physician is the hallmark of continuity of care. For example, a telephone call from the primary care physician stating that a left bundle branch block is new

or that the patient has evidence of digoxin toxicity can facilitate immediate management in the emergency department. In addition, prehospital ECGs, performed on all patients with chest pain, reduce the time required for emergency department evaluation and thus the time to treatment.[4]

Contacting the Emergency Medical Service System

Early access to the emergency medical service system is essential for reducing mortality. Prehospital care is provided at several levels, each with unique capabilities and levels of intervention. Interventions by emergency medical service system personnel differ from state to state and even among regions within a state, so the primary care physician should be familiar with interventions and protocols unique to basic life support, advanced life support, and critical care providers. At all levels, prehospital care personnel are trained in emergency interventions only (Table 17–2).

After accessing the emergency medical service system, the primary care physician should notify the emergency medical dispatcher of the nature of the emergency, and together they should decide on the most appropriate means of transport. The relationship of primary care physicians, emergency medical service system technicians, and emergency physicians contributes to the overall success of treating the patient with a cardiovascular emergency.

The foundation for safe and effective patient transfer from the primary care physician's office is a secure communication system with the receiving emergency department. The primary care physician should be familiar with the staff and services available in the local emergency department (see Table 17–2). Before transferring, or referring, a patient to the emergency department, the primary care physician should either know or ascertain key characteristics of the hospital to which the patient is referred. Does the emergency department have a chest pain evaluation center? Can the hospital initiate thrombolytic therapy only or should the patient go to a facility that can perform percutaneous transluminal coronary angioplasty? Is echocardiography available on an emergency basis?

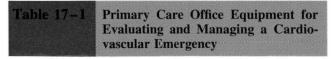

Table 17–1 Primary Care Office Equipment for Evaluating and Managing a Cardiovascular Emergency

Supplemental oxygen and delivery systems: nasal cannula, bag-valve-mask, intubation equipment
12-lead electrocardiogram
Transcutaneous pacemaker
Defibrillator
Intravenous supplies
"Code cart" with medications needed to treat cardiac emergencies

---

Table 17–2 Types of EMS Providers

EMS Level	Intervention
EMT—basic	Field stabilization of fractures; extrication techniques; administration of oxygen, CPR
EMT—intermediate	Possible: intubation, defibrillation, medications, and intravenous therapy
EMT—paramedic	Intravenous medications and fluid, intubation, lifesaving surgical procedures, defibrillation, transcutaneous cardiac pacing
Aeromedical transport	Intravenous medications and fluid, intubation, lifesaving surgical procedures, defibrillation, transcutaneous cardiac pacing

Abbreviations: EMS, emergency medical services; EMT, emergency medical technician; CPR, cardiopulmonary resuscitation.

Can patients be stabilized for emergency cardiac bypass or intra-aortic balloon pump insertion? Knowledge of services available facilitates patient transfer to the most suitable facility. For example, in a community hospital, a patient with an acute myocardial infarction is best treated with thrombolytic therapy, and emergency departments are best suited to deliver this treatment rapidly and safely. On the other hand, a patient with a known aortic dissection is best treated in an operating room and should be transferred directly to the care of a cardiovascular surgeon, omitting transfer to an emergency department.

Advance Directives

A recent multicenter study found that resuscitation orders are not stated for nearly half of the patients requesting such orders.[2] A large problem identified in this study is related to the lack of communication about health care directives among patients, families, and health care providers. Explicit resuscitation directives are humane and must replace vague terms such as "do not resuscitate," "comfort care only," and "conservative care only." These philosophic expressions should be replaced with directions such as "In the case of a cardiac arrest, do not provide mechanical ventilation support, defibrillation, or chest compressions," "Do not provide medication, including blood products, to support blood pressure," "Do not attempt intravenous access," "The only medication I authorize is for analgesia, given intramuscularly or orally," and "Fluid therapy and antibiotics are not to be used except if they can be administered orally." Resuscitation directives can be customized to the patient's medical condition. For example, if a patient has an abdominal aortic aneurysm, the directive can state: "I have an abdominal aortic aneurysm. I do not want resuscitation attempted in any form if doctors diagnose abdominal aortic aneurysm rupture."

Primary care physicians may be responsible for patients in a nursing home, retirement village, hospice, or rehabilitation center and may receive a call from staff at one of these centers reporting a change in the patient's condition that warrants a medical evaluation. Before the primary care physician reflexively orders that the patient be sent to the emergency department for "evaluation," consideration must be given to the sequence of events that will happen when the patient reaches the emergency department. If the primary care physician and the emergency department physician do not present explicit health care directives, the patient may be subjected to full resuscitation. The emergency department physician is trained to provide medical and surgical interventions aggressively to stabilize critically ill patients. Interventions deemed "extraordinary" to the internist or primary care physician are probably routine for the emergency department physician. For example, intubation and intravenous therapeutic medications are *ordinary* treatment for a patient in respiratory distress with evidence of florid pulmonary edema. If such a patient is sent to the emergency department for "evaluation," and the emergency department physician does not receive health care directives, the patient may be intubated and resuscitated even though a health care proxy prohibits resuscitation. The primary care physician should

seriously ask, Does this patient truly need to go to the emergency department, or can this patient remain where she or he is even though it may result in death?

TREATING THE PATIENT WITH A CARDIOVASCULAR EMERGENCY

The history and physical examination of the patient with suspected cardiovascular emergency are directed toward rapidly generating a differential diagnosis that gives preference to the most life-threatening causes of the patient's symptoms and signs (Table 17–3).[3] Symptoms or findings may be attributable to noncompliance with medication as well as with progression of an underlying disease or appearance of a new problem. Essentially, the primary care physician is generating a differential diagnosis, with life-threatening causes of the patient's symptoms or signs at the top. The following section presents the directed approach to cardiovascular emergency, via algorithms, to manage life-threatening cardiovascular conditions. During early evaluation, the primary care physician should anticipate the most lethal diagnosis and initiate universal treatment.

The Adult Patient in Cardiac Arrest

For the adult patient in cardiac arrest, the primary care physician should initiate treatment delineated by the universal algorithm[4] (Fig. 17–1). The tenets of treatment are
- Activate the emergency medical service system.
- Prepare the code cart.
- Initiate ECGs and treatment for malignant arrhythmia.
- Assist breathing and circulation.

Table 17–3	Cardiovascular Diagnoses Requiring Immediate Care

Acute myocardial infarction
Acute ischemic heart disease
Symptomatic dysrhythmia
   Atrial arrhythmia: atrial fibrillation, atrial flutter
   Bradyarrhythmias: sinus arrest, second-degree heart block, third-degree heart block
   Ventricular arrhythmias
Acute congestive heart failure
Pulmonary edema
Pericardial tamponade
Hypertensive crisis related to
   Pregnancy
   Aortic dissection
   Intracerebral event
   Renal failure
   Drug withdrawal
   Sympathomimetic use (e.g., cocaine, stimulants)
Pacemaker failure
Pulmonary embolism
Acute vascular occlusion

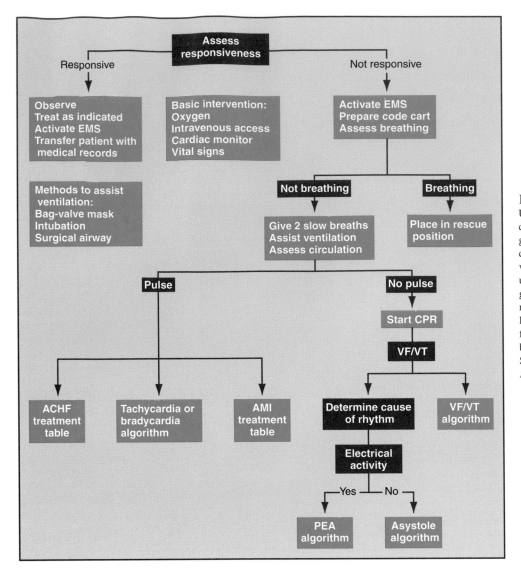

Figure 17–1

Universal algorithm for adult cardiovascular emergency. EMS, emergency medical services; CPR, cardiopulmonary resuscitation; VF, ventricular fibrillation; VT, ventricular tachycardia; ACHF, acute congestive heart failure; AMI, acute myocardial infarction; PEA, pulseless electrical activity. (Modified from Cummins, R.O. [ed.]: Textbook of Advanced Cardiac Life Support. Dallas, American Heart Association, 1994.)

• Notify the emergency department of impending transfer.

Conditions with the potential for deterioration to cardiac arrest, or a lethal outcome, must be identified and basic care initiated in the primary care physician's office. Specific interventions are based on the cause (e.g., arrhythmia, pulmonary embolism) of the arrest and can be found in their respective algorithms.

Life-Threatening Arrhythmias

The precipitating event for malignant dysrhythmia can be noncompliance with medication or progression of an underlying nonreversible disease. Many life-threatening rhythms occur in the peri-infarct period, but they can also be associated with acute pulmonary disease, acute congestive heart failure, aortic dissection, metabolic disorders (e.g., serum electrolyte abnormality), pulmonary embolism, and stroke. The emergent management of serious arrhythmias such as ventricular tachycardia and ventricular fibrillation emphasizes rapid recognition and treatment (Figs. 17–2 through 17–4) (see Chaps. 23 and 24 for diagnosis of arrhythmias).

Acute Myocardial Infarction (see Chap. 19)

The keys to reducing the extent of an acute myocardial infarction are early diagnosis and rapid restoration of myocardial perfusion. Rapid diagnosis of an acute myocardial infarction depends on collating data from high-risk combinations of history, symptoms, signs, risk factors, and diagnostic test results (see Chaps. 7 and 19). The cornerstone to therapy is rapid transfer to a well-equipped emergency setting, although in the absence of known allergy or sensitivity, aspirin should be administered even as this process is being started.

Outside the United States, in countries with different health care delivery systems, varied success has been achieved by media education to reduce patient-related de-

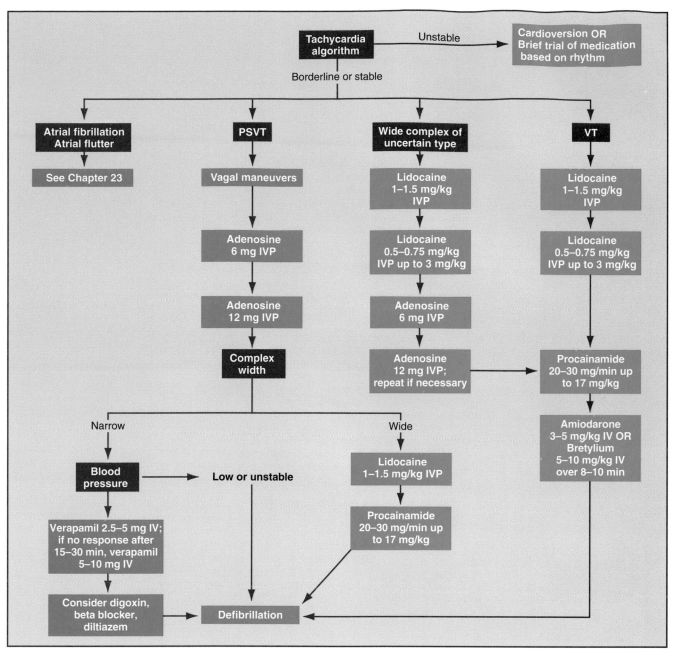

Figure 17–2

Tachycardia algorithm. PSVT, paroxysmal supraventricular tachycardia; VT, ventricular tachycardia; IVP, intravenous push; IV, intravenous. (Modified from Emergency Cardiac Care Committee and Subcommittees, American Heart Association: Guidelines for cardiopulmonary resuscitation and emergency cardiac care: Part III, Adult advanced cardiac life support. JAMA 268:2199–2240, 1992. Copyright 1992, American Medical Association.)

lays.[1, 5] Mass media education in the United States has not reduced the time between the emergence of symptoms and the patient's arrival at an emergency department. The primary care physician must educate the patient adequately about symptoms of cardiac disease. The patient must be well versed about angina and infarction symptoms. Hospital-related delays can be reduced by preparing a summary for the emergency department physicians containing the patient's medical history, list of medications, ECG tracings, and other data that can expedite treatment when the clinician is unfamiliar with the patient.

Once myocardial infarction is diagnosed, the next hurdle to overcome is delivering thrombolytic therapy within 6 hours of symptom onset. The goal of every emergency physician should be to deliver reperfusion therapy as soon as possible.

In the future, emergency medical service system paramedics and prehospital care providers (including primary care physicians) may administer thrombolytic therapy, thereby further reducing prehospital delay (Table 17–4). A 17% reduction in the 30-day mortality rate has been reported when prehospital treatment is administered by capable providers in consultation with remote physicians.[5] Use of highly specific immunoassay kits may allow iden-

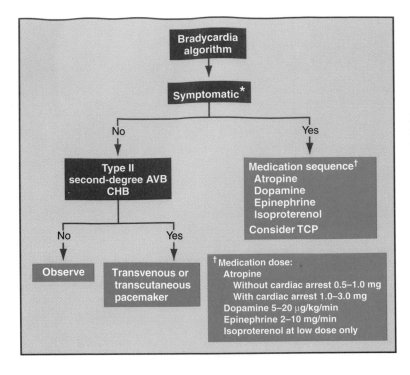

Figure 17–3
Bradycardia algorithm. The transcutaneous pacemaker is a temporary device until the rhythm is stable or an implantable pacemaker is inserted. AVB, atrioventricular block; CHB, complete heart block; TCP, transcutaneous pacemaker; *chest pain, hypotensive, altered mental status. (Modified from Emergency Cardiac Care Committee and Subcommittees, American Heart Association: Guidelines for cardiopulmonary resuscitation and emergency cardiac care: Part III, Adult advanced cardiac life support. JAMA 268:2199–2240, 1992. Copyright 1992, American Medical Association.)

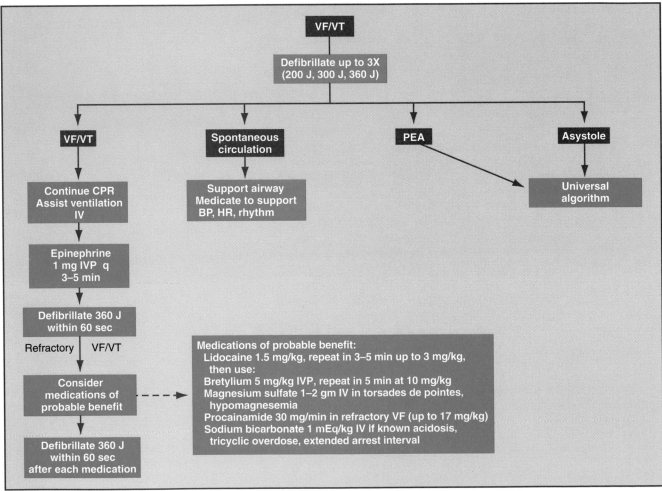

Figure 17–4
Algorithm for ventricular fibrillation/ventricular tachycardia (VF/VT). PEA, pulseless electrical activity; CPR, cardiopulmonary resuscitation; IV, intravenous; BP, blood pressure; HR, heart rate; IVP, intravenous push; VF, ventricular fibrillation. (Modified from Emergency Cardiac Care Committee and Subcommittees, American Heart Association: Guidelines for cardiopulmonary resuscitation and emergency cardiac care: Part III, Adult advanced cardiac life support. JAMA 268:2199–2240, 1992. Copyright 1992, American Medical Association.)

Table 17-4	Recommended Therapy in the Office for Acute Myocardial Infarction Pending Transfer to an Emergency Department or Hospital

Therapy	Dose
Place IV line if possible while arranging transport	
Nitrates	0.4 mg every 5 min × 3 sublingual or 0.5–2 inches of paste
Aspirin	160–325 mg orally
Beta blockers	
Metoprolol	5 mg IV every 5 min × 3, then 50 mg every 6 hr po
Atenolol	5 mg IV every 5 min × 2, then 100 mg/day po
Morphine sulfate	2–5 mg IV every 5–15 min
Consider reperfusion therapy	Thrombolytic therapy in office or during transport

Abbreviations: IV, intravenous; po, by mouth.

Table 17-5	Evaluation of the Patient with Hypertensive Crisis: Uncovering Reversible Causes and Evidence of End-Organ Injury

History of Present Hypertensive Episode	Physical Examination
Onset and duration of hypertensive episode	Vital signs
Onset and duration of symptoms	BP in each arm with appropriately sized cuff
Pain symptoms	Repeat BP following a rest period
Chest	General appearance
Back	Level of consciousness
Abdomen	Level of distress
Neurologic symptoms	Head
Headache	Superficial artery palpation
Change in mental status or speech	Intraocular pressure
Extremity weakness	Funduscopic examination
Seizure	Neck
Medications	Jugular venous distention
History of noncompliance or sudden cessation	Carotid/vertebral bruit
Review of systems	Pain/meningismus
Coronary artery disease	Respiratory
Aneurysm	Auscultory findings: rales, wheezes
Stroke	Cardiac
Pheochromocytoma	S_3 gallop
Thyroid disease	Aortic murmur
Renal disease	Abdomen
Pregnancy	Appearance (flat, distended)
Surgery	Tenderness
Social	Gravid uterus
Cigarette smoking	Bruit
Cocaine exposure	Extremity
Diet pills	Comparative peripheral pulses
Stimulants	Peripheral arterial bruit
	Edema
	Neurologic
	Complete system examination
	Visual field by confrontation
	Language

Abbreviations: BP, blood pressure; S_3, third heart sound.

tification of acute myocardial infarction within 4 hours of infarct.[6] Rapid diagnosis can allow the primary care physician to initiate thrombolytic therapy before transfer.

Ischemic Heart Disease

Errors in the diagnosis of chest pain account for more than 20% of medical malpractice judgments against emergency physicians. When evaluating a patient with chest pain, the clinician should separate life-threatening and non–life-threatening causes and be sure that patients with possible or probable ischemic heart disease are rapidly treated to alleviate pain, monitored for cardiac rhythm disturbances, and transported to an emergency department setting (see Chap. 7). Those with unstable angina may receive oxygen, morphine, nitroglycerin (topical, sublingual, and intravenous for persistent chest pain), beta blocker therapy, and anticoagulation with heparin (see Chap. 20).

Hypertensive Crisis

(see Chap. 21)

The overwhelming majority of patients with elevated blood pressure have *essential hypertension* with no underlying cause; the remaining patients have *secondary hypertension* with a reversible cause. Elevated blood pressure must be evaluated carefully before initiating treatment (Table 17–5). A hypertensive emergency can be associated with a rapid deterioration of organ function owing to inappropriately elevated blood pressure. The condition may require immediate therapeutic intervention (Fig. 17–5; Table 17–6). Conversely, it may not require any intervention at all, and acutely lowering the blood pressure may have a deleterious effect (e.g., acute cerebral ischemia). For less severe elevation in blood pressure or for markedly elevated blood pressures (above about 220 mm Hg systolic or 120 mm Hg diastolic) without evidence of end-organ abnormalities, oral medications can be used to treat the blood pressure (Table 17–7) and the underlying cause. Sublingual nifedipine is no longer recommended because of its poor efficacy and potential side effects.

Acute Pulmonary Edema

(see Chap. 22)

Pulmonary edema can be associated with primary cardiac disease or noncardiac disease. At the same time that the cause of a patient's heart failure is being sought, treatment must be started. Common errors in diagnosis and treatment include not evaluating the patient for noncardiac causes of dyspnea or peripheral edema, attributing respiratory symptoms to chronic obstructive pulmonary disease, not identifying reversible causes of heart failure, failing to measure left ventricular function, and not properly evaluating the patient for myocardial ischemia. The majority of patients in acute congestive heart failure have

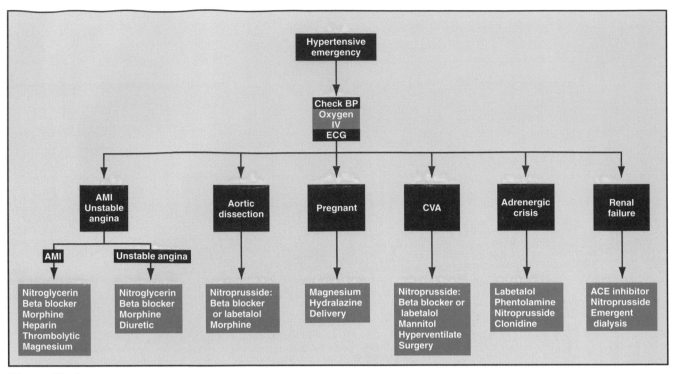

Figure 17–5

Emergency management of hypertension. Refer to text for medication dose and route of administration. BP, blood pressure; IV, intravenous; ECG, electrocardiogram; AMI, acute myocardial infarction; CVA, cerebrovascular accident, intracranial hemorrhage, ischemic stroke; adrenergic crisis, drug withdrawal, cocaine toxicity, pheochromocytoma; ACE, angiotensin-converting enzyme.

a progression of underlying heart disease or myocardial ischemia.

Acute alveolar congestion and pulmonary edema can occur when there is increased pulmonary capillary hydrostatic pressure (cardiogenic pulmonary edema) or altered alveolar or pulmonary capillary permeability (noncardiac pulmonary edema). Regardless of cause, the impressive symptoms are shortness of breath and respiratory distress (Table 17–8). The treatment of acute pulmonary edema should emphasize the reduction of fluid return to the right heart via both venous pooling and diuresis. The patient should be kept in a sitting position, preferably with the legs hanging over the bed to decrease venous return. Intravenous morphine in repetitive doses of 2 to 6 mg up to every 5 to 10 minutes can diminish anxiety and increase venous pooling, hence reducing pulmonary congestion (Table 17–9). Intravenous diuretics, commonly furosemide in doses of 40 to 100 mg or bumetanide in doses of 1 to 2 mg, not only cause diuresis but also have an acute effect to increase venous capacity and hence decrease blood return to the heart and lungs. Oxygen should be given by mask, commonly at 100% concentrations and under positive pressure if possible.

In more refractory cases, afterload reduction with intravenous nitroprusside should be seriously considered, especially if the systolic blood pressure is above about 100 mm Hg. When the pulmonary edema is associated with marked myocardial ischemia, nitroglycerin may be preferable to nitroprusside because of its less deleterious effects on coronary blood flow despite its lesser effects

on peripheral arterial resistance. Intravenous angiotensin-converting enzyme inhibitors may be beneficial but are more difficult to titrate. Digoxin is sometimes begun in patients not already on it, but its inotropic effects will not be seen for several hours and are usually not essential for emergency treatment. When pulmonary edema is associated with hypotension, inotropic agents may be required. After a brief aggressive trial of medications to improve oxygenation and cardiac output, mechanical ventilatory support is required for the patient with signs of impending respiratory collapse, shock, or worsening hypoxemia.

Pericardial Emergencies

(see Chap. 28)

Disorders of the pericardium and pericardial space include acute pericarditis, constrictive pericarditis, and pericardial tamponade. Chest pain is common in pericardial disease, but distinction between the pain of pericarditis and other causes of pain can be difficult (see Chap. 7).

The acute evaluation requires the accurate distinction between possible tamponade, as compared with constrictive or simple inflammatory pericarditis, and a decision as to whether emergent pericardiocentesis or hospitalization, or both, is required (Fig. 17–6).

Tamponade is commonly associated with hypotension, tachycardia, pulsus paradoxus, elevated jugular venous pressure, and sometimes pulmonary congestion. It may present with or progress to total cardiovascular collapse.

Table 17–6 | **Parenteral Treatment for Hypertensive Emergencies**

Hypertensive Emergency	Indications for Treatment	Treatment Options	Goal/Comments
Malignant/accelerated	Persistent elevation of BP with evidence of end-organ damage DBP > 130 mm Hg Nonspecific symptoms: H/A, visual changes, nocturia, weakness, weight loss Retinopathy: flame hemorrhages, soft exudates, papilledema Proteinuria, hematuria, progressive azotemia, oliguria Progression to encephalopathy Hypokalemia DIC	1. IV nitroprusside, initial dose 0.2–0.5 μg/kg/min, titrate to effect every 5 min up to 8 μg/kg/min 2. IV labetalol, 20–80 mg/min, additional bolus after 30 min as needed 3. IV nicardipine, 5–15 mg/hr 4. IV enalaprilat, 1.25 mg/6 hr	Lower BP over 1 hr Contraindicated in pregnancy Switch to a different drug when BP is controlled Combined alpha- and beta-blockade contraindicated in beta blocker–sensitive patients Calcium antagonist Onset of action 5–15 min Allows smooth reduction in BP ACE inhibitor Onset of action 15 min Choice for CHF, high renin states
Aortic dissection	Clinical evidence, including symptoms of rupture, leak, or dissection	IV morphine, 2 mg titrated to relieve pain IV nitroprusside, 0.2–0.5 μg/kg/min *or* IV esmolol, 500 μg/kg over 1 min *or* IV labetalol, 20–40 mg, increasing dose every 10 min	Reduce shear force by reducing peripheral resistance and ventricular contractions The goal is an SBP < 120 mm Hg.
Renal failure	Marked increase in BP, complications related to fluid overload such as ACHF, IHD Acutely elevated creatine	Emergent dialysis IV nitroprusside, 0.2–0.5 mg/kg/min	Treat ACHF, IHD pending dialysis
IHD	Chest pain, evidence of ischemia or infarction	SL or topical NTG IV nitroprusside, 0.2 to 8 μg/kg/min IV morphine, 2 mg	Treat the underlying disease
Acute CHF	Respiratory distress, hypoxemia, IHD, pulmonary edema, complicating medical illness (i.e., AMI, CVA)	IV furosemide, 40–100 mg over 2 min *or* IV bumetanide, 0.5–2.0 mg SL NTG 0.3 mg Transdermal NTG, 1–2 inches IV morphine, 2 mg (titrate to effect, up to 8 to 10 mg)	Evaluate for precipitating event
Drug withdrawal Cocaine toxicity	Persistently elevated BP with evidence of end-organ damage	Reinstitute antihypertensive medication Benzodiazepine sedation	

Abbreviations: BP, blood pressure; IV, intravenous; DBP, diastolic blood pressure; H/A, headache; DIC, diffuse intravascular coagulation; ACE, angiotensin-converting enzyme; CHF, congestive heart failure; SBP, systolic blood pressure; ACHF, acute congestive heart failure; IHD, ischemic heart disease; SL, sublingual; NTG, nitroglycerin; AMI, acute myocardial infarction; CVA, cerebrovascular accident.

If time permits, an echocardiogram is diagnostic. Supportive therapy for tamponade should emphasize intravenous fluids to support the blood pressure, if pulmonary congestion is not also present, and the judicious use of inotropic agents before percardiocentesis, if both hypotension and pulmonary congestion are present. Pericardiocentesis should be performed under controlled conditions by an experienced cardiologist, preferably in a catheterization laboratory, if time permits. In the presence of cardiovascular collapse or severe hypotension, however, emergent bedside pericardiocentesis may be lifesaving (Fig. 17–7).

Acute Vascular Occlusion

Sudden loss of a peripheral pulse combined with severe, steady pain and diminished or absent sensation and motor function of an extremity are cardinal signs of arterial insufficiency or frank arterial occlusion. Patients who present within 6 hours with symptoms and signs are considered to have an acute occlusion; their treatment differs from that of patients who present later than 6 hours with signs of occlusion.

Table 17–7 | **Oral Medications for Hypertensive Emergencies**

Medication	Dose	Onset
Labetalol	200–400 mg	30 min–2 hr
Clonidine	0.1–0.2 mg	30–60 min
Captopril	25 mg	15–30 min

Adapted from Gales, M.A.: Oral antihypertensive urgencies. Ann. Pharmacother. 28:352–358, 1994.

Table 17–8 **Signs Associated with Acute Pulmonary Edema**

Signs
Ascites
Diaphoresis
Decreased peripheral perfusion: cool, clammy skin
Hepatomegaly
Hepatojugular reflux
Hypertension*
Jugular venous distention
Peripheral edema
Rales
S_3, S_4
Tachypnea, labored conversation and respiratory pattern
Wheezing

Laboratory Findings

Abnormal ECG: dysrhythmia, low-voltage QRS, inverted T-wave, left atrial enlargement, left ventricular hypertrophy, myocardial ischemia, myocardial infarction
Abnormal arterial blood gas: hypoxemia, hypercapnia, mixed acidosis
Abnormal chest radiograph: alveolar consolidation, bilateral pulmonary infiltrates, cardiomegaly, pulmonary vascular redistribution, Kerley-A lines, Kerley-B lines

Abbreviations: S_3, third heart sound; S_4, fourth heart sound; ECG, electrocardiogram.
* Patients with cardiac ischemia or infarction can be hypotensive.

Table 17–9 **Medications for Acute Pulmonary Edema***

Medication	Dosage
Morphine sulfate	2–6 mg IV every 5–100 min
Diuretics	
Furosemide	40–100 mg IV
Bumetanide	1–2 mg IV
Torsemide	10–20 mg IV
Nitrates	
Nitroprusside	0.5–8.0 μg/kg/min IV infusion†
Nitroglycerin	0.4 mg SL
	1 to 2 mg inches topical paste
	10–500 mg/kg/min IV infusion†
ACE inhibitor	
Enalaprilat	1.25 mg IV over several min
Digoxin	0.25–1.0 mg IV loading dose followed by 0.125–0.25 mg/day
Inotropic catecholamines‡	
Dopamine	1–2 mg/kg/min IV infusion
Dobutamine	0.5–20.0 mg/kg/min IV infusion

Abbreviations: IV, intravenous; SL, sublingual; ACE, angiotensin-converting enzyme
* Treatment should occur concurrently with the search for the underlying cause. Early intervention includes supplemental oxygen, IV access, and continuous cardiac monitoring.
† Infusion is titrated to improve clinical response.
‡ Pulmonary edema associated with hypotension.

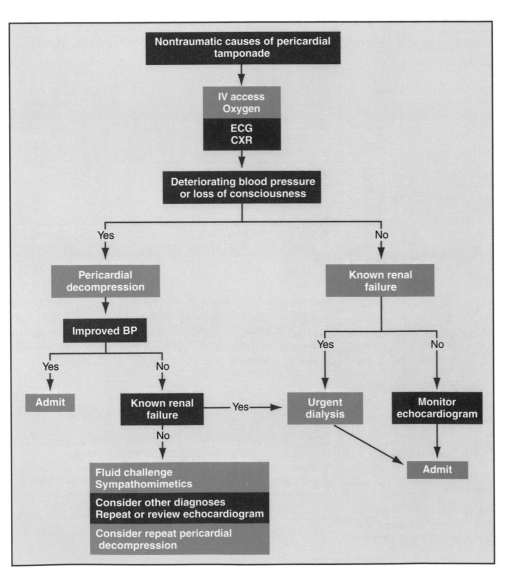

Figure 17–6
Emergency treatment of pericardial tamponade. IV, intravenous; ECG, electrocardiogram; CXR, chest radiograph; BP, blood pressure.

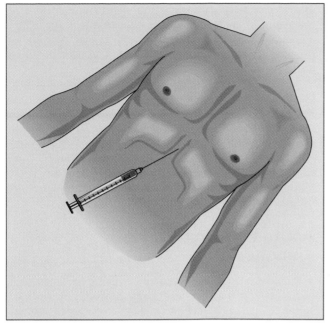

Figure 17–7
Subxiphoid approach for pericardiocentesis. With the torso flexed 45 degrees, the needle is inserted under the xiphoid, directing it to the left of the sternum while maintaining (approximately) a 45-degree angle between the needle and the skin surface. Constant aspiration of the plunger will produce a rapid return of blood when pericardial penetration has occurred.

Cause

The differential diagnosis of acute arterial occlusion includes arterial embolic phenomena (thromboembolism and atheroembolism [microemboli]), arterial thrombosis, arterial inflammation (drug-induced, arterial vasculitis, infectious arteritis), vasospasm, peripheral arteriovenous fistula, and arterial trauma (Table 17–10). Life-threatening causes such as acute aortic dissection, shock, and sepsis are included in the evaluation of a suddenly pale, painful, pulseless extremity.

The physical examination should assess temperature demarcation, pulse, sensory status, motor function, evidence of tissue ischemia (e.g., appearance of skin and skin appendages, ulcers, mottling). In the case of acute arterial occlusion, limb survival depends on restoring blood flow within 6 hours (Fig. 17–8). When limb ischemia has been present for more than 6 hours, or if reperfusion is achieved (spontaneously or owing to intervention) after prolonged ischemia, a rapid metabolic acidosis can occur, leading to hyperkalemia, declining cardiac function, dysrhythmia, myoglobinuria, myoglobin precipitation–induced renal failure, and death.

Emergency Treatment

Evaluation is directed toward diagnosing the cause and extent of the vascular occlusion (Table 17–11), but treatment should begin without delay. To reduce tissue ische-

Table 17–10	**Clinical Features of Acute Arterial Occlusion**		
Diagnosis	**Cause and Source of Occlusion**	**Location of Occlusion**	**Treatment**
Arterial embolism			
Thromboembolism	85% originate in the heart 60%–70% are due to left ventricular thrombus post-MI Mitral stenosis Rheumatic valve disease Atrial fibrillation	Femoral and popliteal arteries	1. Fogarty's catheter thrombectomy 2. Heparinization 3. Treat underlying rhythm
Atheroembolism	Microemboli composed of cholesterol, calcium, and platelets from proximal atherosclerotic plaques	Cortical vessels Lower extremity digits ("blue toe syndrome")	1. Treat underlying cause 2. Local and conservative care 3. Anticoagulation is contraindicated
Arterial thrombosis	In situ blood clot formation due to endothelial injury, altered arterial blood flow, acute vasculitis, trauma, severe atherosclerosis	Based on mechanism	1. Heparinization 2. Direct arterial thrombolytic therapy 3. Surgical thromboembolectomy/ bypass
Inflammation			
Miscellaneous	Drugs, irradiation, trauma, infectious, necrotizing (noninfectious)	Peripheral extremities	1. Reduce exposure to drug 2. Treat underlying infection 3. NSAIDs
Vasculitides	Possible immune complex mediated	Small vessels, retina, kidney, multiple organ dysfunction	1. Immunosuppression
Vasospasm	Mechanism unknown, possible autonomic dysfunction	Distal small arteries	1. Vasodilator* 2. Sympathectomy†
Trauma	In situ blood clot formation due to endothelial injury, altered arterial blood flow, acute vasculitis	Location of trauma	1. Thromboembolectomy/bypass

Abbreviations: MI, myocardial infarction; NSAIDs, nonsteroidal anti-inflammatory drugs.
* Recommended agents: prazosine, nifedipine, reserpine, phenoxybenzamine, and pentoxifylline.
† Limited to Buerger's disease.

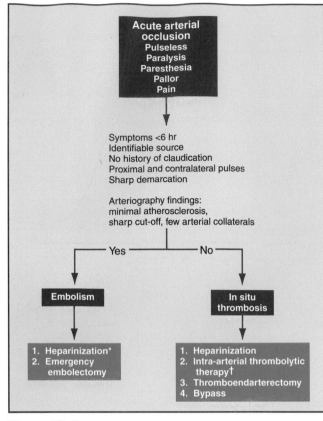

Figure 17–8

Algorithm for the treatment of acute arterial occlusion. The presence of paresthesia and the absence of a pulse are sufficient to warrant emergent embolectomy. *Heparinization can be initiated if embolectomy is delayed. †Thrombolytic therapy in consultation with the vascular surgeon.

Table 17–11	Differentiating Arterial Embolus from Thrombosis	
Character	**Embolus**	**Thrombosis**
Patient age	Not dependent on age	Older
Onset	Sudden	Gradual
Risk factor for embolus	Common	Uncommon
History of claudication	Uncommon	Common
Physical examination findings of vascular disease	Uncommon	Common
Skin temperature demarcation	Sharp	Poorly demarcated
Arteriogram	Minimal atherosclerosis, few collaterals	Diffuse atherosclerosis, well-developed collaterals
Ideal emergent treatment*	Embolectomy	Heparinization Thromboembolectomy Bypass

Modified from Brewster, D.C.: How you can best identify and treat arterial embolism. J. Cardiovasc. Med. 7:354–369, 1982.
* Symptoms present <6 hr.

mia, the primary care physician should initiate treatment immediately, including alkalization of the urine with an ampule of sodium bicarbonate and forced diuresis with intravenous saline solution and added intravenous diuretics as needed.

A vascular surgeon must be consulted immediately if the patient has evidence of acute ischemia with a cool, pulseless limb, even if motor and sensory function are not yet compromised. Intravenous heparin is usually begun in the meantime, but even a transient improvement does not obviate the need for rapid evaluation, commonly with angiography, so that the potential benefit of thrombolysis, thrombectomy, and catheter or surgical revascularization can be addressed.

Acute Pulmonary Embolism

Pulmonary embolism can be difficult to diagnose because many of its signs and symptoms are not specific. In addition, making a definitive diagnosis carries morbidity and health care costs that most physicians would rather avoid. It is estimated that the diagnosis of pulmonary embolism is missed more than 400,000 times a year. Not making a correct diagnosis is associated with high cost: a 30% mortality rate for undiagnosed pulmonary embolism, equivalent to more than 100,000 deaths per year.[7]

As described in detail in Chapter 30, the primary care physician should have a low threshold for suspecting pulmonary embolism in patients with unexplained dyspnea or pleuritic chest pain. Rapid transfer to an emergency department is needed for definitive evaluation.

In the meantime, basic therapeutic interventions for the patient with suspected pulmonary embolism include supplemental oxygenation and analgesia. If the clinical presentation and chest radiograph raise a sufficiently high probability of pulmonary embolism, anticoagulation with heparin (bolus injection of 5000 to 10,000 units, followed by an infusion of 1000 to 1250 units per hour) may sometimes be indicated even before the definitive diagnosis is established by lung perfusion scintigraphy or pulmonary angiography.

Aortic Aneurysm

ABDOMINAL AORTIC ANEURYSMS. These generally expand asymptomatically, but they also can present acutely with pain, peripheral emboli from clot within the aneurysm, leaking, or frank rupture (Table 17–12). In patients with rapidly expanding or leaking aneurysms, pain is commonly in the midabdomen, flank, or lower back, and it may range from mild to very severe. Patients commonly have tenderness on physical examination, often in the presence of a palpable, pulsatile mass. Lower extremity ischemia, spinal cord ischemia, or renal ischemia and failure may develop. In the presence of a slow leak, anemia and relative hypotension may be present; with acute rupture, shock and cardiovascular collapse develop rapidly. Diagnosis is based on clinical suspicion, suggestive clinical examination, and abdominal ultrasound. Preoperative evaluation to localize the site of the aneurysm

Table 17-12	Symptoms and Signs of Aortic An-eurysm Leaking, Rupture, and Dis-section

Abdominal aortic aneurysm—leaking but unruptured
  Back or abdominal pain
  Pulsatile abdominal mass
  Ischemic lower extremity
  Spinal cord ischemia with signs of paralysis
  Anemia
  Acute renal failure
Abdominal aortic aneurysm rupture
  Mid-diffuse abdominal pain
  Pulsatile abdominal mass
  Shock
Thoracic aneurysm dissection
  Severe chest or back pain of sudden onset
  Discordant upper extremity blood pressures
  Stroke/TIA/mental status change
  Ischemic upper extremity
  Myocardial infarction, especially of inferior wall from occlusion of
    right coronary artery
  Acute aortic insufficiency from dissection back into valve ring
  Pericardial tamponade from dissection back into the pericardium

Abbreviation: TIA, transient ischemic attack.

may include computed tomography scanning, magnetic resonance imaging, or aortography. Painful expansion of a previously asymptomatic abdominal aortic aneurysm is commonly a sign of impending leak or rupture and should prompt immediate surgical consultation. If there is evidence of leaking, acute stabilization should be attempted and the patient should be prepared for emergency surgery (Table 17–13). For frank rupture, survival rates will be only about 10% to 20%.

THORACIC AORTIC ANEURYSMS. These are most commonly caused by atherosclerosis, although Marfan's syndrome and other vasculitic processes can also result in thoracic aneurysms[8] (see Chap. 27). Syphilis,

Table 17-13	Treatment of Unstable Aortic An-eurysm

Large-bore IV access; avoid groin lines
IV nitroprusside 0.5 to 8.0 μg/kg/min to achieve systolic pressure of about 110–120 mm Hg for abdominal aortic aneurysm and about 100 mm Hg for thoratic aortic dissection
IV beta-blockade with esmolol 500 mg/kg/min, followed by continuous infusion at a rate of 50 μg/kg/min for 3–5 min. Repeat bolus and titrate infusion to achieve effect; propranolol 1 mg, or labetalol, 5–10 mg, titrated to achieve a heart rate of about 60 beats/min
Upright chest and abdominal flat plate radiograph
Fluid resuscitation and PASG to treat hypotension
Right radial artery cannulation for pressure monitoring
Contact surgical service based on clinical findings
Type and cross-match 10 units of packed cells
Type and cross-match 4 units of fresh frozen plasma
Avoid hypothermia
Urethral catheter
Nasogastric tube

Do not delay transfer to an operating room to complete resuscitation or diagnostic tests.

Abbreviations: IV, intravenous; PASG, pneumatic antishock garment.

previously the most common cause, is now very unusual. Thoracic aneurysms oftentimes present as expanding masses with pressure on surrounding structures. As a result, patients may develop hoarseness, cough, dysphasia, or the superior vena cava syndrome. Patients with thoracic aortic aneurysms should be evaluated by a cardiologist to evaluate whether they are possible operative candidates. Once thoracic aneurysms begin to leak or rupture, cardiovascular collapse ensues rapidly and surgical treatment is unlikely to be beneficial.

Aortic Dissection
(see also Chap. 27)

Aortic dissection may be caused by a tear in the aortic intima or by bleeding into the media of the arterial wall itself.[9] Proximal dissections of the ascending aorta, also called *type A dissections,* may progress antegrade down the aortic arch or retrograde into the coronary ostium, especially the ostium of the right coronary, and the pericardium. Distal aortic aneurysms, also called *type B,* begin after the great vessels and may extend well into the abdomen (Fig. 17–9). Aortic dissections are usually preceded by hypertension, Marfan's syndrome, or severe atherosclerosis of the aorta. However, pregnancy, annuloec-

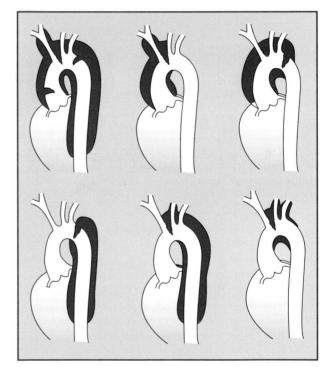

Figure 17–9

Classification of aortic dissections. Stanford classification: Type A dissections *(top panels)* involve the ascending aorta independent of site of tear and distal extension. Type B dissections *(bottom panels)* involve transverse or descending aorta without involvement of the ascending aorta. DeBakey classification: Type I dissection involves ascending to descending aorta *(top left)*; type II dissection is limited to ascending or transverse aorta, without descending aorta *(top center + top right)*; type III dissection involves descending aorta only *(bottom left)*. (Redrawn from Miller, D.C. *In* Doroghazi, R.M., and Slater, E.E. [eds.]: Aortic Dissection. New York, McGraw-Hill, 1983.)

tasia of the aorta, and even a bicuspid aortic valve have been associated with an increased risk of the aortic dissection.

Patients commonly present with the sudden onset of severe chest discomfort (see Table 17–12), which is more likely to be in the anterior chest for ascending aortic dissections and in the back and even in the abdomen for descending aortic dissections. If the dissection compromises flow in the great vessels, there will be evidence of delayed or decreased pulses or reduced blood pressure in the carotid, brachial, radial, or femoral arteries. In more severe cases, blood flow in the great vessels may be sufficiently compromised to cause ischemic signs and symptoms. Retrograde dissection may involve the right coronary ostium to cause acute inferior wall myocardial infarction or the aortic annulus to cause acute aortic regurgitation; dissections back into the pericardium may cause pericardial tamponade.

The ECG is nonspecific in acute aortic dissection. Many patients have underlying hypertension and may therefore have left ventricular hypertrophy by ECG. Involvement of the right coronary artery may result in an acute inferior wall myocardial infarction.

The chest x-ray may show a widened mediastinum, tortuous aorta, or even left pleural effusion indicative of leaking into the pleural space. Transesophageal echocardiography is the recommended next diagnostic test because of its high sensitivity. Preoperative confirmation may be obtained by magnetic resonance imaging or angiography. Once aortic dissection is seriously considered, urgent cardiovascular surgery consultation is required. Unless hypotension is present, emergent treatment for both types of dissections should be aimed at reducing systolic blood pressure and pulse pressure, commonly with a combination of nitroprusside to titrate systolic blood pressure to about 100 mm Hg and intravenous beta-adrenergic antag-

onists to maintain a target pulse rate of about 60 beats per minute or less.

Patients with proximal aortic dissections usually require emergency surgery. Uncomplicated distal dissections are commonly managed medically, with surgery reserved for patients with continuing pain, extension of the dissection despite treatment, or vascular compromise. Even with distal dissections, however, all patients should also be treated aggressively so that emergent surgery can be performed if necessary (see Table 17–13).

References

1. Blohm, M., Herlitz, J., Hartford, M., et al.: Consequences of a media campaign focusing on delay in acute myocardial infarction. Am. J. Cardiol. 69:411–413, 1992.
2. Knaus, W.A., Harrell, F.E., Jr., Lynn, J., et al.: The SUPPORT prognostic model: Objective estimates of survival in seriously ill hospitalized adults. Ann. Intern. Med. 122:191–203, 1995.
3. Handley, A.J., Becker, L.B., Allen, M., et al.: Single-rescuer adult basic life support: An advisory statement from the Basic Life Support Working Group of the International Liaison Committee on Resuscitation. Circulation 95:2174–2179, 1997.
4. Kloeck, W., Cummins, R.O., Chamberlain, D., et al.: The Universal Advanced Life Support Algorithm: An advisory statement from the Advanced Life Support Working Group of the International Liaison Committee on Resuscitation. Circulation 95:2180–2182, 1997.
5. Weaver, W.D.: Time to thrombolytic treatment: Factors affecting delay and their influence on outcome. J. Am. Coll. Cardiol. 25(Suppl):3S–9S, 1995.
6. Ravkilde, J., Nissen, H., Horde, M., et al.: Independent prognostic value of serum creatinine kinase isoenzyme MB mass, cardiac troponin T and myosin light chain levels in suspected acute myocardial infarction. J. Am. Coll. Cardiol. 25:574–581, 1995.
7. Feied, C.: Pulmonary embolism. In Rosen, P., and Barkin, R.M. (eds.): Emergency Concepts and Clinical Practice. St. Louis, Mosby–Year Book 1992; pp. 1285–1311.
8. Kouchoukos, N., and Dougenis, D.: Surgery of the thoracic aorta. N. Engl. J. Med 336:1876–1888, 1997.
9. Pretre, R., Von Segesser, L. K.: Aortic dissection. Lancet 349:1461–1464, 1997.

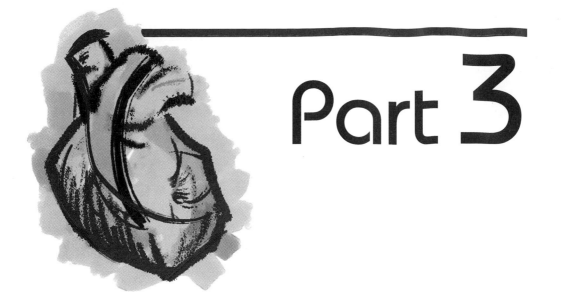

Part 3

Recognition and Management of Patients with Specific Cardiac Problems

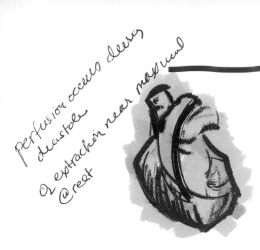

perfusion occurs during diastole Q extraction near maximal @ rest

Chapter 18

Recognition and Management of Patients with

Stable Angina Pectoris

KANU CHATTERJEE

Definition and Clinical Presentations

Angina pectoris is defined as chest discomfort or other related symptoms caused by myocardial ischemia. Angina is a *clinical diagnosis* that can be established only by a careful history (Table 18–1). Although a number of non-invasive and invasive investigations are performed in clinical practice in patients with suspected or established angina, these investigations usually suggest or establish only the presence or absence of myocardial ischemia or coronary artery disease (CAD) but not *angina.*

Angina pectoris is typically a heaviness, pressure, squeezing, constriction, or pain, but some patients have difficulty describing the discomfort or deny that their discomfort is truly pain (see Chap. 5). The most frequent initial location of angina is in the central chest and retrosternal area, but the left pectoral region, arms and hands, root of the neck, epigastrium, and even the right side of the chest may be initial sites. Occasionally, patients may complain of only interscapular or left infrascapular back pain. Discomfort that is located below the umbilicus or above the mandible is unlikely to be angina. The duration of angina is variable but it usually lasts 2 to 5 minutes. Very brief (<60 sec), or prolonged (>30 min) discomfort occurs uncommonly in stable angina.

Angina is considered to be stable when it remains reasonably constant and predictable in terms of severity, presentation, character, precipitants, and response to therapy. Patients with progressively worsening angina (accelerated angina), one or more episodes of rest angina, or new-onset angina have *unstable* angina (see Chap. 20).

Exertional angina, which is the most common clinical presentation of patients with stable angina, is precipitated by an increase in myocardial oxygen demand above the limits of myocardial oxygen supply. In some patients, however, myocardial ischemia is partially or totally consequent to a spontaneous decrease in coronary blood flow.

Pathophysiology

Myocardial ischemia, whether silent or symptomatic, results from an imbalance between myocardial oxygen demand (consumption) and myocardial oxygen supply (Fig. 18–1). Ventricular wall tension, heart rate, and myocardial contractility are the major determinants of myocardial consumption. Intraventricular systolic pressure, ventricular volume, and wall thickness are the major determinants of left ventricular wall tension. Adrenergic stimulation of the heart and tachycardia are the major determinants of contractility. Tachycardia also increases myocardial oxygen consumption and reduces myocardial perfusion by decreasing the duration of diastole, during which left ventricular perfusion occurs. Reduction of heart rate is associated with a decrease in myocardial oxygen demand and improved left ventricular perfusion.

Oxygen extraction by the myocardium is near maximum at rest, and arterial oxygen content is usually stable, except with anemia or marked hypoxia; therefore, myocardial oxygen supply is determined primarily by coronary blood flow. Coronary blood flow is a function of myocardial perfusion pressure (aortic diastolic pressure) and the duration of diastole and is inversely proportional to the coronary vascular resistance. Coronary vascular resistance, in turn, is determined by the severity of epicardial coronary artery stenoses, by changes in epicardial

Table 18–1	The Clinical Presentations of Stable Angina Syndromes with Potential Mechanisms of Myocardial Ischemia
Angina of effort	Angina during predictable level of physical activity or during emotional stress (demand ischemia)
Walk-through angina	Angina at the onset of exercise, relieved during continued exercise (supply ischemia)
Vasospastic angina	Spontaneous angina at rest, usually not provoked by exercise (supply ischemia)
Nocturnal angina	Occurs soon after retiring, assuming recumbent position (demand ischemia)
	Occurs many hours after retiring (supply ischemia)
Postprandial angina	Angina during or soon after eating meals (supply and demand ischemia)
Syndrome X	Exertional angina (abnormal coronary vasodilatation during exercise) or vasoconstriction in response to certain stimuli in the presence of angiographically normal epicardial coronary arteries

coronary artery tone, and by coronary arteriolar resistance; the latter is regulated by metabolic, neural, humoral, and autonomic activity. Increased myocardial oxygen demand occurs during physical exertion; normally, this reduces coronary arteriolar resistance, which allows coronary blood flow to rise (autoregulatory reserve). With increasing severity of epicardial coronary arterial stenosis, this autoregulatory reserve diminishes progressively. When coronary artery stenosis reaches about 90% of the luminal diameter, the coronary arteriolar bed is maximally

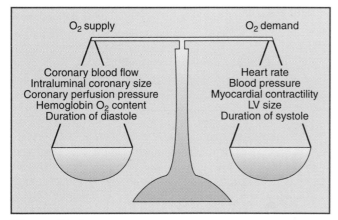

Figure 18–1

Balance of myocardial oxygen supply and demand. Transient ischemic episodes arise from imbalanced myocardial oxygen supply and demand. Determinants of myocardial oxygen supply include coronary blood flow, intraluminal coronary artery size, coronary perfusion pressure, hemoglobin oxygen content, and duration of diastole. Determinants of myocardial oxygen demand include heart rate, blood pressure, myocardial contractility, left ventricular (LV) size, and duration of systole. Any imbalance between supply and demand may induce ischemia. (Redrawn from Bertolet, B.D., and Pepine, C.J.: Silent myocardial ischemia. *In* Beller, G.A. [vol. ed.]: Chronic Ischemic Heart Disease. Braunwald, E. [ser. ed.]: Atlas of Heart Diseases. Vol. 5. Philadelphia, Current Medicine, 1995, p. 8.18.)

dilated and coronary blood flow becomes dependent on perfusion pressure. Under these conditions, reduction of arterial pressure may induce ischemia, even though myocardial oxygen demand also decreases concomitantly.

DIAGNOSIS

History

Presentation

Angina of effort or classic angina is characteristically induced by physical activity and is often precipitated more easily in cold weather or after eating. Some patients experience angina more frequently in the morning than during the remainder of the day despite less physical activity at this time. Exercising the upper extremities above the head precipitates angina more readily than exercising the lower extremities. Angina may also be precipitated by emotional stress.

The relief of angina usually occurs within several minutes after cessation of exertion. Prompt relief is also achieved with the use of sublingual nitroglycerin. The hemodynamic effects of sublingual nitroglycerin usually begin within 1 minute, and the angina is generally relieved within 2 or 3 minutes. Chest discomfort that is *instantaneously* relieved by nitroglycerin is unlikely to be angina pectoris.

In some patients, dyspnea, not chest discomfort, during activity is a manifestation of exercise-induced myocardial ischemia and is termed an *angina equivalent*. Both ischemic cardiac discomfort and cardiac dyspnea are worse during physical activity than at rest, and if patients are relieved of these symptoms during activity it is unlikely that the symptoms are related to myocardial ischemia.

Severity

During the initial evaluation of patients with suspected or established angina, it is desirable to assess its severity as a guide to therapy. A number of methods have been proposed to assess functional impairment by history, based on the degree of physical activity that precipitates angina. The New York Heart Association functional classification has largely been replaced by the Canadian Cardiovascular Society functional classifications or by classification systems based on the activity levels that can be related to the metabolic equivalents during treadmill exercise tests (see Chap. 3).[1]

After an episode of severe, *transient* ischemia, the myocardium may be temporarily stunned, which means that it remains transiently dysfunctional after the ischemia has resolved. When an area of the myocardium is *chronically hypoperfused*, it may not show evidence of ischemia electrocardiographically but may be dysfunctional or even akinetic. It is important to distinguish this so-called hibernating myocardium from myocardium that is dysfunctional secondary to infarction because hibernating myocardium may regain normal function when perfusion is restored.

[handwritten margin note: hibernating myocardium]

Risk Factors

During initial evaluation of the patient with possible angina, the physician should determine whether risk factors for atherosclerotic CAD—including hyperlipidemia, diabetes mellitus, hypertension, cigarette smoking, obesity, and a family history of premature CAD—are present, since these risk factors not only increase the likelihood that the patient has underlying coronary disease but also serve as potential targets for intervention. In women, the menstrual status as well as hormone replacement therapy should be assessed, since the risk of CAD rises in postmenopausal women who are not receiving estrogen (or estrogen/progesterone) replacement (see Chap. 6). Inquiries should be made for a history of peripheral vascular disease, or symptoms thereof, such as leg claudication and transient ischemic attacks, because the prevalence of CAD is substantially higher in patients with peripheral vascular disease, carotid artery disease, and thoracoabdominal aortic aneurysms.

Although CAD is, by far, the most frequent cause of angina, in the absence of atherosclerotic obstructive CAD, typical angina can be a symptom of hypertrophic cardiomyopathy, ischemic and nonischemic dilated cardiomyopathy, restrictive cardiomyopathy, and pulmonary hypertension. Clinical evaluation and appropriate investigations establish the diagnosis in such patients (see Chaps. 7, 30, and 31).

Recognition of Clinical Subsets

WALK-THROUGH ANGINA. In the majority of patients with obstructive atherosclerotic CAD, the intensity of angina increases with continued physical activity. A subset has so-called walk-through angina. In this syndrome, the patient experiences angina at the beginning of physical activity (e.g., walking) but the angina then disappears despite continuation of the activity. The precise pathophysiologic mechanism of walk-through angina remains unclear, although an increase in coronary vascular tone and therefore a spontaneous reduction in coronary blood flow at the beginning of the exercise have been implicated.

MIXED (VARIABLE THRESHOLD) ANGINA. The essential clinical feature of mixed angina is a substantial variation in the degree of physical activity that induces angina. These patients may also experience rest or nocturnal angina on certain occasions. Angina may also occur on exposure to cold, during emotional stress, or after meals. Dynamic vasoconstriction superimposed on fixed atherosclerotic coronary artery obstructions has been postulated as the mechanism for the variable exercise threshold.

NOCTURNAL ANGINA. In clinical practice, two types of nocturnal angina are encountered. Some patients experience angina within an hour or two after retiring. The mechanism of angina in this group of patients is likely to be an increase in venous return and hence increased intracardiac volume with a resulting increase in myocardial oxygen requirements. Other patients with nocturnal angina experience chest discomfort much later, in the early hours of the morning. In these patients, a primary reduction in coronary blood flow owing to increased coronary vascular tone, perhaps related to different stages of sleep, has been postulated as the potential mechanism.

POSTPRANDIAL ANGINA. Angina can occur after meals without any physical activity because of increased coronary vascular tone and a primary decrease in coronary blood flow. However, postprandial angina may occur only during physical activity after meals because of an associated increase in myocardial oxygen demand. Postprandial angina is almost always associated with significant atherosclerotic CAD.

SYNDROME X. *Syndrome X* is defined as the presence of typical anginal chest pain with angiographically normal coronary arteries. Although the syndrome originally referred to patients in whom the chest pain was due to noncoronary causes, the current, stricter definition limits it to those patients who appear to have true myocardial ischemia despite epicardial coronary arteries that are normal or nearly so on coronary angiography. To establish the diagnosis, patients must have evidence of myocardial ischemia by exercise electrocardiography, stress scintigraphy, or stress echocardiography in conjunction with anginal chest discomfort. Some of these patients have documented reductions in coronary vasodilator reserve presumably due to abnormalities in the coronary microcirculation and can be shown to have true ischemia because their myocardium produces rather than removes lactate during stress. The syndrome may be more common in patients with hypertrophied myocardium of any cause. Although the symptoms of syndrome X do not respond well to medical management, the prognosis in terms of major coronary events appears to be benign.

Clinical Evaluation

The physical examination may be entirely normal in patients with stable angina, although hypertension, a major risk factor for CAD, may be present. The cardiovascular examination *during* ischemia, however, may reveal transient third and fourth heart sounds, a sustained outward (dyskinetic) systolic movement of the left ventricular apex, a murmur of mitral regurgitation, and paradoxical splitting of the second heart sound. The physical examination should also focus on the detection of abnormal findings suggestive of left-sided and right-sided heart failure and of nonischemic causes of angina, that is, valvular or aortic stenosis, cardiomyopathy, and pulmonary hypertension. Cardiovascular assessment should also include an examination of the peripheral pulses, fundoscopic evaluation, and screening for risk factors for CAD, such as tendon xanthomas, xanthelasma, and corneal arcus, particularly in patients under the age of 50 years. Palpation of peripheral arterial pulses, examination of the carotid arteries for bruits, and palpation of the abdomen for aneurysm are important, since the presence of noncoronary atherosclerotic disease increases the likelihood of the presence of coronary disease.

Diagnostic Testing

Electrocardiography

The electrocardiogram (ECG) at rest is normal in approximately half of patients with chronic stable angina without a history of previous myocardial infarction. In the others, a variety of ECG findings may suggest ischemic heart disease. Q-waves suggest prior myocardial infarction, but in the absence of a clinical history of previous myocardial infarction or CAD, Q-waves may also be caused by other conditions, including hypertrophic cardiomyopathy, left ventricular hypertrophy, dilated nonischemic cardiomyopathy, and accessory atrioventricular pathways. ST segment depression and T-wave inversions in the resting ECG, left bundle branch block, and left anterior hemiblock are compatible with, but are not specific for, CAD, although these abnormal findings should be considered as indications for further evaluation. Giant T-wave inversion in the precordial leads is sometimes an important indicator of severe left anterior descending coronary artery stenosis.

Exercise Electrocardiography

The exercise ECG is more useful than the resting ECG in detecting myocardial ischemia and evaluating the cause of chest pain. Downsloping or horizontal ST segment depressions are very suggestive of myocardial ischemia (see Chap. 4), particularly when these changes occur at a low workload, during early stages of exercise, persist for more than 3 minutes after exercise, or are accompanied by chest discomfort that is compatible with angina (Table 18–2; Fig. 18–2). Upsloping ST segments are much less specific indicators of CAD.

An abnormal resting ECG associated with left ventricular hypertrophy, intraventricular conduction abnormalities, a pre-excitation syndrome, electrolyte imbalance, or therapy with digitalis increases the probability that an exercise ECG will yield a false-positive result. In women, the lower prior probability of CAD is associated with more false-positive results on exercise ECG (see Chaps. 4 and 6). On the other hand, a fall in systolic pressure of 10 mm Hg or more during exercise or the appearance of a murmur of mitral regurgitation during exercise increases the probability that an abnormal stress ECG is a true-positive test result.

Treadmill exercise is generally preferable to bicycle exercise for detecting myocardial ischemia. In patients who cannot perform treadmill exercise, pharmacologic stress scintigraphy or echocardiography (see later) is preferable to upper body arm exercise. Exercise electrocardiography has a sensitivity of about 70% for detecting CAD and a specificity of about 75% for excluding it (see Table 4–1).[2] To assess the probability of CAD in an individual patient, the exercise ECG result must be integrated with the patient's clinical presentation (see Chap. 4 and Figs. 2–5 through 2–7).

Perfusion Scintigraphy

Myocardial perfusion scintigraphy with thallium-201 is frequently employed as a noninvasive test to evaluate abnormalities of myocardial perfusion in patients with established or suspected CAD.[3] Myocardial uptake of thallium-201 chloride is proportional to regional myocardial blood flow and is dependent on the presence of viable myocardium. During exercise, the magnitude of the increase in blood flow to the nonischemic myocardial zones is greater than to the zones supplied by stenotic coronary arteries. Owing to this heterogeneous distribution of blood flow, the relative extraction of thallium by nonischemic myocardium is greater than that by ischemic myocardium (see Fig. 4–2).

During exercise thallium testing, the isotope is administered intravenously during peak exercise, and stress images are obtained immediately after discontinuation of exercise. These images reveal a decreased uptake by the ischemic myocardium, creating a perfusion defect. Redistribution images are obtained after 4 hours. Myocardium that was ischemic during stress but that is not ischemic at rest now extracts the isotope. Therefore, the perfusion defects during stress images are not observed in the rest

Table 18–2	Common Exercise Test Protocols					
Protocol	Stage	Duration (min)	Grade (%)	Rate (mph)	Metabolic Equivalents at Completion	Functional Class
Modified	1	3	0	1.7	2.5	III
Bruce protocol*	2	3	10	1.7	5	II
	3	3	12	2.5	7	I
	4	3	14	3.4	10	I
	5	3	16	4.2	13	I
Naughton protocol†	0	2	0	2	2	III
	1	2	3.5	2	3	III
	2	2	7	2	4	III
	3	2	10.5	2	5	II
	4	2	14	2	6	II
	5	2	17.5	2	7	I

* Commonly used in ambulatory patients.
† Commonly used in patients with recent myocardial infarction, unstable angina, or other conditions that are expected to limit exercise.

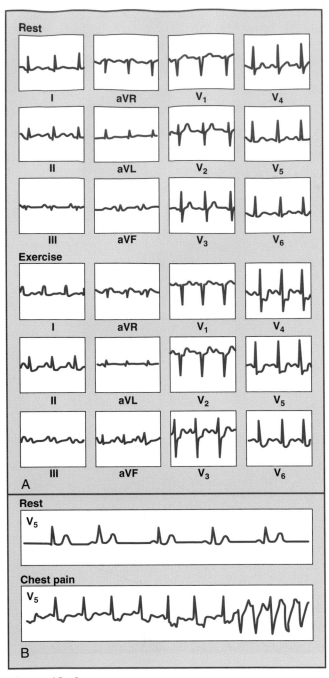

Figure 18–2

Diagnostic approaches for documenting myocardial ischemia in patients believed to have angina pectoris. *A*, Positive exercise test. Note the development of ST segment depression with exercise-associated angina. *B*, ST segment depression during ambulatory monitoring. Ambulatory (Holter) recordings in patients with angina and myocardial ischemia often demonstrate transient ST segment depression throughout the day. Most (>70%) such episodes are asymptomatic, but in patients with stable angina, symptomatic attacks are often recorded, as in this case. Note that the transient ischemic episode is accompanied by a brief burst of ventricular tachycardia. Patients who have positive electrocardiogram (ECG) exercise tests are far more likely to have demonstrable asymptomatic (or silent) ischemia on monitoring than are individuals with normal exercise tests. Episodes of angina can also occur without ECG abnormalities. (*A* and *B*, Redrawn from Abrams, J.: Medical therapy of stable angina pectoris. *In* Beller, G.A. [vol. ed.]: Chronic Ischemic Heart Disease. Braunwald, E. [ser. ed.]: Atlas of Heart Disease. Vol. 5. Philadelphia, Current Medicine, 1995, p. 7.5.)

images, and these reversible perfusion defects indicate the presence of viable myocardium. If the perfusion defects in stress images persist in the rest images, that is, if the perfusion defects are fixed, the myocardium is usually necrotic or fibrotic. A repeat injection of thallium and scanning 24 hours after stress can distinguish severely ischemic from viable myocardium.

Thallium images may be planar or tomographic (single-photon emission computed tomography). The latter are more accurate and are therefore used more frequently to assess the presence and extent of ischemic and infarcted myocardium. In pooled analyses from multiple studies, exercise treadmill thallium myocardial scintigraphy has a sensitivity for detecting CAD and a specificity for excluding it of about 84% and 88%, respectively (see Table 4–1). The sensitivity approaches 90% with a quantitative computer-assisted analysis of the images without loss of specificity.

Considerable experience is required for the performance and interpretation of exercise thallium scintigraphy to achieve these high degrees of specificity and sensitivity. Exercise thallium scintigraphy is less likely than exercise electrocardiography to provide false-positive results in women, but it may give false-positive results in patients with hypertrophic, dilated, and infiltrative cardiomyopathies. Like the exercise ECG, thallium stress scintigraphy is less sensitive in the diagnosis of ischemia owing to single-vessel CAD, particularly of circumflex coronary artery stenosis, than multivessel disease.

Technetium-99m, a calcium analog with a higher photon energy and a shorter half-life than thallium chloride, can be linked to a variety of agents and used as a marker of myocardial perfusion. Technetium-99m-sestamibi is an isonitrile compound that, like thallium, is taken up by the myocardium proportional to blood flow but in contrast to thallium does not undergo redistribution. Tomographic images with technetium-99m-sestamibi provide better resolution and are now replacing thallium for assessment of myocardial perfusion in many laboratories.[4] The physical properties of technetium-99m also allow images to be acquired on the first pass through the ventricle and can be used to assess the ventricular ejection fraction. However, less-expensive noninvasive tests such as echocardiography are usually preferable for this purpose.

Perfusion Scintigraphy with Pharmacologic Stress

Many patients with known or suspected angina are unable to perform adequate exercise tests owing to peripheral vascular disease, musculoskeletal disorders, diseases of the lower extremities, severe obesity, or deconditioning. Myocardial perfusion scintigraphy during pharmacologic stress can be employed in these patients. Non–endothelium-dependent coronary vasodilators such as dipyridamole or adenosine can be used to increase flow to the nonischemic myocardial segments and thus produce perfusion defects in ischemic areas that can be detected by scintigraphy. Alternatively, dobutamine can be used to increase heart rate and contractility, which increases myocardial oxygen demand, and this too may compromise perfusion of ischemic areas; the resultant ischemia can be detected by perfusion scintigraphy. Dobutamine may cause true myocardial ischemia, not simply a relative increase in flow to nonischemic myocardium. Hence, it must be administered carefully with close monitoring and rapid cessation for potential symptomatic ischemia. All three of these pharmacologic stress tests have diagnostic accuracies (sensitivity, specificity, and predictive values) comparable with those of exercise perfusion scintigraphy.

Both dipyridamole and adenosine produce similar side effects, which consist of bronchospasm, flushing, dizziness, headaches, nausea, atypical chest pain, and throat or jaw pain. Dipyridamole infusion has been reported to induce severe myocardial ischemia and, rarely, myocardial infarction. Adenosine, on the other hand, can produce significant bradyarrhythmias. Adenosine stress tests are therefore contraindicated in patients with atrioventricular block and sick sinus syndrome.

Echocardiography

Echocardiography is useful in the detection of ischemia-induced regional wall motion abnormalities that occur at rest (Fig. 18–3), during exercise, or with pharmacologic stress testing (Fig. 18–4). Upright treadmill exercise and supine bicycle ergometry, pacing, and pharmacologic stress, particularly with dobutamine, have been used in conjunction with two-dimensional echocardiography to detect regional wall motion abnormalities that most frequently occur during induced myocardial ischemia associated with CAD. Exercise echocardiography has been reported to have a sensitivity of 74% to 100% and a specificity of 64% to 93% for detecting CAD. Exercise echocardiography appears to be more sensitive and more specific and to have a higher predictive value than exercise electrocardiography.

Good agreement has also been reported between stress echocardiography and stress scintigraphy. With the usual high dose of dobutamine (up to 50 gm/kg/min), dobutamine stress echocardiography has been reported to have a sensitivity of 86% to 96% and a specificity of 66% to 95%. Lower-dose dobutamine can also be used to detect hibernating myocardium. Areas of hibernating myocardium exhibit poor or absent contraction at rest but normal contraction during dobutamine infusion. By comparison, areas damaged by myocardial infarction or fibrosis exhibit no improvement with dobutamine.

Positron Emission Tomography

Positron emission tomography can also assess regional coronary blood flow reserve, myocardial perfusion, and the presence and extent of hibernating myocardium. Rubidium-82 or ammonia (N13) are used for assessment of myocardial perfusion, whereas labeled carbohydrates such as fludeoxyglucose F-18, lipids, and some amino acids can be used to assess myocardial metabolism and viable ischemic myocardium. With combined assessment of myocardial perfusion and metabolism, the sensitivity and specificity for the detection of CAD may approach 95%. However, positron emission tomography is a very expensive noninvasive test. Its added value is principally in difficult situations in which myocardial perfusion by thallium scintigraphy and assessment of left ventricular systolic function by echocardiography or radionuclide ventriculography do not reveal the extent of hibernating myocardium.[5]

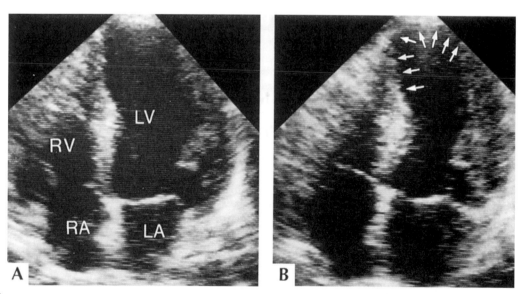

Figure 18–3

Resting wall motion abnormality. *A*, Two-dimensional echocardiographic apical four-chamber view at end diastole. *B*, Two-dimensional echocardiographic apical four-chamber view at end systole. The right ventricle (RV) and the septal and lateral walls at the base of the left ventricle (LV) demonstrate normal inward motion from diastole through systole; however, the distal septum and apex demonstrate akinesis (*arrows* in *B*). The wall motion abnormality demonstrated in this frame was caused by ischemia from a lesion in the mid-left anterior descending artery. LA, left atrium. RA, right atrium. (*A* and *B*, From Picard, M.H., and Weyman, A.E.: Echocardiography in chronic ischemic heart disease. *In* Beller, G.A. [vol. ed.]: Chronic Ischemic Heart Disease. Braunwald, E. [ser. ed.]: Atlas of Heart Diseases. Vol. 5. Philadelphia, Current Medicine, 1995, p. 4.2.)

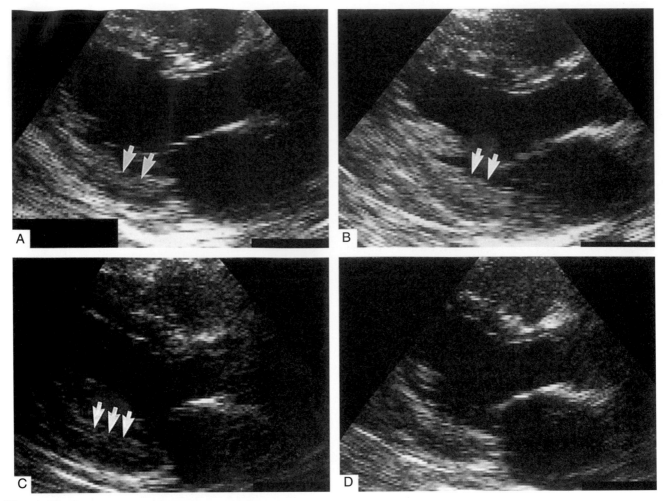

Figure 18–4

A, Stage 1 image of the patient at rest. Note severe hypokinesis (*arrows*). *B,* Stage 2 image at low dose (5 μg/kg/min). Note augmentation of wall motion of the previously hypokinetic zone (*arrows*). *C,* Stage 3 at peak dose (40 μg/kg/min). Note akinesis (*arrows*). *D,* Stage 4 image at recovery. An initial improvement in inferoposterior wall motion was observed with low-dose dobutamine. The improvement deteriorates at high doses, however, suggesting that there is viable myocardium in the infarct zone that is supplied by a stenotic right coronary artery. Subsequent coronary angiography demonstrated 75% lesions in both the left circumflex and the posterior descending coronary arteries. (*A–D,* From Picard, M.H., and Weyman, A.E.: Echocardiography in chronic ischemic heart disease. *In* Beller, G.A. [vol. ed.]: Chronic Ischemic Heart Disease. Braunwald, E. [ser. ed.]: Atlas of Heart Diseases. Vol. 5. Philadelphia, Current Medicine, 1995, p. 4.13.)

Ambulatory ST Segment Monitoring

Many patients with CAD experience episodes of asymptomatic myocardial ischemia detectable by ST segment monitoring whether or not they have angina pectoris (Fig. 18–5). Patients with symptomatic angina also often have multiple additional episodes of asymptomatic ischemia, and the frequency and severity of these episodes correlate with prognosis. Although exercise or pharmacologic stress electrocardiography, perfusion scintigraphy, or echocardiography is generally preferable to ambulatory ST segment monitoring in patients with effort angina, ambulatory ST segment monitoring is an alternative for patients who cannot exercise and is the preferred test in patients with suspected vasospastic angina that may not be provoked by effort or by pharmacologic agents such as dipyridamole, adenosine, or dobutamine.

Ultrafast Computed Tomography

Ultrafast computed tomography can be used to detect coronary calcifications, which often precede symptomatic coronary artery stenoses. However, coronary calcification is also observed in patients without important coronary disease at angiography. Although this test has generated substantial interest and publicity, its cost and the current lack of information from large-scale assessments make it premature to recommend its use in routine clinical care.

Selecting the Best Test for the Individual Patient

(Table 18–3)

The exercise ECG is the test of choice in patients with typical exertional angina with a normal resting ECG who

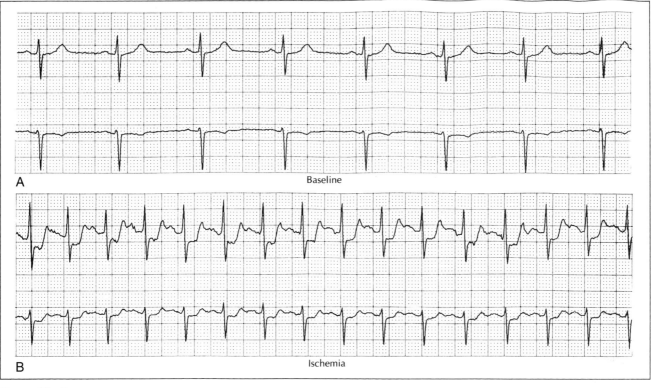

Figure 18–5

A and B, Detection of silent myocardial ischemia by ambulatory electrocardiographic monitoring. A, Baseline recording from an ambulatory electrocardiographic monitor. B, The same two leads showing 2 mm of ischemic-type ST segment depression while the patient, who had not experienced symptoms, was walking home. (A and B, From Bertolet, B.D., and Pepine, C.J.: Silent myocardial ischemia. In Beller, G.A. [vol. ed.]: Chronic Ischemic Heart Disease. Braunwald, E. [ser. ed.] Atlas of Heart Diseases. Vol. 5. Philadelphia, Current Medicine, 1995, p. 8.12.)

are able to exercise. Even when the exercise ECG is not necessary to establish the diagnosis of CAD, it is very helpful in assessing its severity. If evidence for ischemia (by electrocardiography or by perfusion scintigraphy or echocardiography) is detected during the first stage of exercise, the likelihood of the presence of three-vessel disease or left main coronary artery stenosis is greater than if more exercise is required to provoke a positive test.

Exercise electrocardiography in patients with suspected or established stable angina is also useful to decide about nonpharmacologic and pharmacologic therapeutic interventions. In patients with stable angina, mixed angina, walk-through angina, or postprandial angina with or without prior myocardial infarction, exercise electrocardiography is usually adequate for assessing the presence and severity of myocardial ischemia, provided the patient does not have changes on the resting ECG—such as a left bundle branch block or paced rhythm—that will obscure ischemia and does not have a condition such as a pre-excitation syndrome or digitalis use that predisposes to a false-positive test. The diagnosis of syndrome X is established by the presence of typical anginal discomfort that is accompanied by ischemic changes on exercise electrocardiography (or exercise or stress scintigraphy) with subsequent demonstration of the absence of critical coronary artery obstruction on coronary arteriography.

In women with typical angina, exercise electrocardiog-

raphy is also usually adequate. However, because of the higher incidence of false-positive results with stress electrocardiography in women, exercise perfusion scintigraphy or echocardiography is a reasonable alternative and should also be considered (see Chaps. 4 and 6).

Exercise perfusion scintigraphy should be considered the test of choice when stress ECGs are uninterpretable, as in patients with bundle branch block, intraventricular conduction defects, left ventricular hypertrophy with baseline ST segment or T-wave abnormalities, pre-excitation syndromes, or ST segment changes owing to electrolyte imbalance or digitalis therapy. Stress perfusion scintigraphy also is more accurate than stress electrocardiography to determine the *extent* and *distribution* of ischemia.

Adenosine or dipyridamole perfusion scintigraphy and dobutamine echocardiography are the preferred noninvasive tests to assess the presence and extent of myocardial ischemia in patients who are unable to exercise, and these are often recommended in patients with a blunted heart rate response because of antianginal therapy. In patients with moderate or severe bronchospastic airway disease and poor exercise tolerance, dobutamine echocardiography is preferable to dipyridamole or adenosine scintigraphy.

Not all noninvasive or invasive tests that are available for the diagnosis of CAD and myocardial ischemia are applicable to all clinical subsets of patients with stable angina. For patients with stable exertional angina, mixed angina, postprandial angina, walk-through angina, and

Table 18–3	Suggested Noninvasive Tests According to Clinical Presentations of Patients with Stable Angina

Exertional angina, mixed angina, walk-through angina, postprandial angina with or without prior myocardial infarction
  A. Normal resting ECG: treadmill exercise ECG test
  B. Abnormal uninterpretable resting ECG: exercise myocardial perfusion scintigraphy (thallium-201-sestamibi)
  C. Unsuitable for exercise, unable to exercise adequately: dipyridamole or adenosine myocardial perfusion scintigraphy, dobutamine stress echocardiography

Atypical chest pain with normal or borderline abnormal resting ECG or with nondiagnostic stress ECG, particularly in women: exercise myocardial perfusion scintigraphy

Vasospastic angina: ECG during chest pain, ST segment depressed during ambulatory ECG

Dilated ischemic cardiomyopathy with typical angina or for assessment of the extent of hibernating myocardium: assessment of regional and global ejection fraction by radionuclide ventriculography or two-dimensional echocardiography, radionuclide myocardial perfusion scintigraphy; in selected patients, flow and metabolic studies with positron emission tomography

Syndrome X: initially treadmill exercise stress ECG (after demonstration of presence of normal coronaries; coronary blood flow reserve can be assessed noninvasively by positron emission tomography)

Known severe aortic stenosis or severe hypertrophic cardiomyopathy with stable angina: exercise stress tests are contraindicated; dipyridamole or adenosine myocardial perfusion scintigraphy in selected patients

Mild aortic valvular disease or hypertrophic cardiomyopathy with typical exertional angina: treadmill myocardial perfusion scintigraphy under strict supervision or dipyridamole or adenosine myocardial perfusion scintigraphy

Abbreviation: ECG, electrocardiogram.

Table 18–4	Other Laboratory Tests Suggested in Patients with Stable Angina

LDL and HDL cholesterol
Triglyceride level
Fasting glucose
Homocysteine level in patients with strong family history, especially if not explained by other risk factors
Hematocrit
Test of thyroid function (T_4 level)

Abbreviations: LDL, low-density lipoprotein; HDL, high-density lipoprotein; T_4, thyroxine.

nocturnal angina within 1 to 2 hours after retiring, it is desirable to select tests that are likely to induce myocardial ischemia by increasing myocardial oxygen requirements. In these patients, exercise electrocardiography, exercise or stress perfusion scintigraphy, and echocardiography are designed to provoke ischemia. On the other hand, in patients with suspected vasospastic (Prinzmetal's) angina (see Chap. 20) or with delayed nocturnal angina, a negative exercise or pharmacologic stress test is not as useful as is ST segment ambulatory Holter monitoring, which may demonstrate spontaneous ST segment shifts with or without associated chest pain.

In patients with stable angina, particularly those with documented prior myocardial infarction, assessment of left ventricular systolic function is necessary for selecting the appropriate therapy. In such patients, assessment for myocardial ischemia and ventricular function can be performed by the combination of a test for ischemia, such as exercise electrocardiography, and a test of left ventricular function, such as resting echocardiography, or by use of a single test such as resting and stress echocardiography.

Laboratory Tests (Table 18–4)

Hyperlipidemia and carbohydrate intolerance are established risk factors for CAD. Furthermore, the correction of hyperlipidemia in patients with established CAD may reduce the incidence of death or nonfatal myocardial infarction (see Chap. 29). Thus, a fasting glucose level as well as low-density lipoprotein and high-density lipoprotein cholesterol measurements should be performed in all patients with suspected or documented ischemic heart disease. Routine hematologic and thyroid function tests should also be performed to exclude significant anemia or abnormal thyroid function, which can be associated with worsening angina.

Homocysteinemia has been found to be a risk factor for CAD, and folate, vitamin B_{12}, and vitamin B_6 can lower the homocysteine level. Although the therapeutic implications of lowering homocysteine levels have not been fully defined, homocysteine concentrations should be measured in patients with a strong family history of coronary disease, especially if it is not explained by traditional risk factors. Elevated fibrinogen levels are also associated with higher risks of coronary disease, but in practice, coagulation studies are not recommended.

Coronary Arteriography

(Table 18–5)

The principal indication for coronary angiography in patients with stable angina pectoris, with or without previous myocardial infarction, is the consideration of coronary revascularization (see later). Occasionally, coronary arteriography is recommended for diagnostic purposes be-

Table 18–5	Indications for Coronary Angiography

When revascularization surgery or angioplasty is contemplated because of symptoms or because stress ECG or thallium myocardial perfusion scintigraphy suggests high-risk coronary artery disease for which revascularization will improve prognosis
Patients with atypical chest pain, when other diagnostic tests have failed to clarify the diagnosis
Suspected syndrome X
In patients with stable angina and valvular heart disease to delineate the coronary anatomy and to establish the mechanism of angina
In patients with known vasospastic angina to determine whether there are fixed coronary stenoses and in patients with suspected vasospastic angina to determine whether spasm can be provoked pharmacologically

Abbreviation: ECG, electrocardiogram.

cause the patient's clinical presentation and noninvasive test results are inconclusive. When the diagnosis of vasospastic angina is strongly suspected but cannot be documented by noninvasive studies, coronary angiography with ergonovine provocation is indicated (see Chap. 20). Even when vasospastic angina can be diagnosed by noninvasive studies, coronary arteriography is indicated to determine whether fixed coronary artery stenoses are present in addition to the spasm.

The indications for coronary arteriography in patients with walk-through angina, mixed angina, and postprandial angina are similar to those in patients with stable exertional angina. It should be appreciated, however, that the demonstration of the presence of one or more critical coronary artery stenoses does not necessarily indicate that they are the cause of a chest pain syndrome. Furthermore, typical angina pectoris can occur in the absence of obstructive atherosclerotic CAD, thus raising the question of the presence of vasospastic angina, syndrome X, or nonischemic causes of chest pain. In general, a stenosis of 70% or more of the luminal diameter, which corresponds to a reduction of 50% or more of the cross-sectional area, is considered significant CAD, since stenosis of this severity reduces coronary blood flow with exercise even though more severe stenoses are required to reduce flow at rest. The extent of CAD is often expressed in terms of the number of major epicardial coronary arteries with 70% or greater-diameter stenosis.

PROGNOSIS

Extent of Coronary Disease and Degree of Left Ventricular Dysfunction

Approximately half of all patients with documented or suspected CAD present initially with stable angina pectoris. The average annual mortality rate associated with stable angina in patients with documented CAD ranges from 1% to 4%, but the prognosis varies widely depending on several factors, especially the extent and severity of CAD and the state of left ventricular function (Fig. 18–6). Left main coronary artery stenosis with or without associated lesions of the other major coronary arteries carries a much worse prognosis, and the 4-year mortality in medically treated patients has been reported to be as high as 25%. The annual mortality rate in patients with one- and two-vessel disease is about 1.5%, but it is approximately 7% for those with three-vessel disease.

The severity of symptoms and exercise capacity also influence the prognosis. The annual mortality rate of patients with three-vessel disease and with good exercise capacity documented by exercise testing is about 4%, but it is approximately 10% in patients with poor exercise capacity.

Impairment of left ventricular systolic function also adversely influences the long-term prognosis of patients

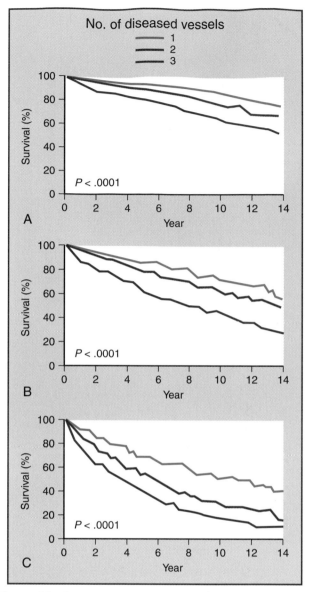

Figure 18–6

Graphs showing survival for medically treated Coronary Artery Surgery Study (CASS) patients. *A,* Patients with one-, two-, or three-vessel disease and ejection fraction 50% to 100% by number of diseased vessels. *B,* Patients with one-, two-, or three-vessel disease and ejection fraction 35% to 49% by number of diseased vessels. *C,* Patients with one-, two-, or three-vessel disease and ejection fraction 0% to 34% by number of diseased vessels. (*A–C,* Redrawn from Emond, M., Mock, M.B., Davis, K.B., et al.: Long-term survival of medically treated patients in the Coronary Artery Surgery Study [CASS] Registry. Circulation 90:2645, 1994. Copyright American Heart Association.)

with chronic stable angina. In patients with three-vessel CAD, an ejection fraction less than 50% or evidence of clinical heart failure is associated with a mortality almost three times as high as the mortality in patients with normal ventricular function and a similar extent of CAD. The 5-year mortality rate may be as high as 90% in patients with three-vessel CAD, diffuse left ventricular systolic dysfunction, and ejection fraction less than 25%.

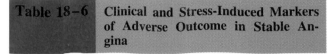

Table 18-6 | **Clinical and Stress-Induced Markers of Adverse Outcome in Stable Angina**

Clinical Markers

Prior myocardial infarction
Hypertension
Severe angina (class III or IV)
Cardiomegaly on chest x-ray
ST segment depression in the resting ECG
Peripheral vascular disease

Stress-Induced Markers

Failure to complete Bruce stage 1 or equivalent workload with >1 mm ST segment depression in the stress ECG
2 mm or greater ST segment depression in the stress ECG irrespective of level of exercise achieved
>10 mm Hg decrease in blood pressure or failure to increase blood pressure to >130 mm Hg
Left ventricular dysfunction with ST segment depression
Increased lung uptake in poststress thallium images
Multisegmental thallium-201 or technetium-99m-sestamibi defects or multiple new echocardiographic wall motion abnormalities with or without associated depressed left ventricular systolic function

Abbreviation: ECG, electrocardiogram.

Clinical Factors and Noninvasive Tests

(Table 18-6)

Clinical markers of adverse outcome include previous myocardial infarction, peripheral vascular disease, hypertension, cardiomegaly on chest x-ray, and ST segment depression on the resting ECG. Patients with more severe ischemia, manifested by either a low threshold for the induction of ischemia or evidence for more extensive is-

chemia by electrocardiography, perfusion scintigraphy, or echocardiography, have a poorer prognosis.

Noninvasive stress tests can also identify patients at higher risk of adverse outcome. These markers of high risk include failure to complete Bruce stage 1 or an equivalent workload with greater than 1 mm ST segment depression, and a downsloping or horizontal ST segment depression greater than 2 mm at any stage of the treadmill exercise test (Fig. 18-7). Multiple or large myocardial perfusion defects or increased lung uptake during myocardial perfusion scintigraphy and thallium images, as well as ECG evidence of silent ischemia at a low level of physical activity, usually indicates a poor prognosis (Figs. 18-8 and 18-9).

Syndrome X

The prognosis of patients with syndrome X is excellent, and myocardial infarction and cardiac death are extremely rare. Similarly, the natural history of atypical chest pain that is often confused with angina pectoris in patients who have normal coronary arteriograms appears to be benign.

Approach to the Patient

The evaluation of the patient with known or suspected stable angina is designed to guide medical therapy and determine the potential indications for coronary revascularization.[6,7] Coronary revascularization is indicated to improve the quality or the duration of life, or both. Thus, it is used for the relief of symptoms that cannot be controlled to the satisfaction of the patient by medical therapy and in patients in whom the prognosis is likely to be improved. In making these decisions, the physician must consider not only the patient's clinical response to medi-

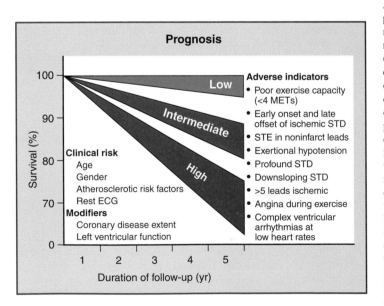

Figure 18-7

Actuarial survival curves of patients with normal or mildly impaired left ventricular function who have prognostic low-, intermediate-, and high-risk mortality estimates based on exercise test results. Patients able to exercise to at least 7 metabolic equivalents (METs) with a normal exercise electrocardiogram (ECG) have an excellent 5-year prognosis for survival, even in the presence of obstructive coronary disease. The presence of several adverse indicators, such as poor exercise capacity and early onset and late offset of myocardial ischemia on the exercise ECG, places the patient into a prognostic high-risk group. Patients in the intermediate category, who have less marked adverse indicators than individuals in the higher-risk group, fall into a subgroup for which myocardial perfusion imaging or exercise ECG would significantly enhance the prognostic information used to guide the decision for coronary angiography and revascularization. The survival curves shift downward for patients with moderate or severe left ventricular dysfunction. STD, ST segment depression, STE, ST segment elevation. (Redrawn from Chaitman, B.R.: Exercise electrocardiographic stress testing. *In* Beller, G.A. [vol. ed.]: Chronic Ischemic Heart Disease. Braunwald, E. [ser. ed.]: Atlas of Heart Diseases. Vol. 5. Philadelphia, Current Medicine, 1995, p. 2.19; adapted from Chaitman, B.R.: Exercise ECG testing. *In* Iskandrian, A.S. [ed.]: Myocardial Perfusion Imaging (Part I): Diagnosis of Ischemic Heart Disease. New York, Cahners Healthcare Communications, 1993, pp. 3-9.)

cal therapy but also the patient's overall medical condition, prognosis, and preferences.

As part of the initial evaluation of patients with established or suspected stable angina, the physician should assess the severity of myocardial ischemia, the exercise capacity, and the status of left ventricular systolic function. Thus, every patient with stable angina who is able to exercise and in whom coronary revascularization is not excluded should have a noninvasive test of functional capacity and some test to assess the severity of ischemia and of left ventricular function. The evaluation must be sufficient to serve as a baseline functional evaluation and to determine whether the patient has disease that is severe enough that coronary revascularization will result in an improved prognosis, independent of symptom relief. For patients whose function is not at the level desired by the patient or physician, repeat functional assessment after medical management is helpful.

The noninvasive evaluation is especially important for identifying patients with reversible ischemia in whom angiography should be recommended to determine whether the severity of the disease is sufficient to advise revascularization to improve prognosis even if the patient's symptoms do not otherwise warrant it. Since the various tests are reasonably similar in accuracy, the choice among them should be based not only on the patient's characteristics but also on local availability and expertise. Coronary angiography is generally recommended in patients with a positive stress test for ischemia and heart failure or impaired ventricular function in whom the presence of three-vessel disease would be an indication for revascularization to improve prognosis (see later). Similarly, angi-

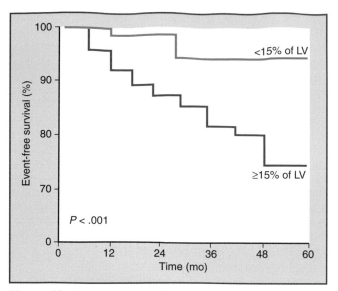

Figure 18–9

The correlation between event-free survival and the size of exercise-induced myocardial perfusion defects. A 2.5-year follow-up in 316 patients demonstrated a significant difference in event-free survival between the two groups. (Redrawn from Wackers, F.J.Th.: Stress radionuclide imaging for detecting and assessing prognosis of coronary artery disease. *In* Beller, G.A. [vol. ed.]: Chronic Ischemic Heart Disease. Braunwald, E. [ser. ed.]: Atlas of Heart Diseases. Vol. 5. Philadelphia, Current Medicine, 1995, p. 3.17.)

ography is recommended in patients with a high-risk noninvasive stress test as well as those in whom symptoms are not adequately controlled by medical therapy.

MANAGEMENT

Risk Factor Modification
(Table 18–7)

Modification of coronary risk factors is essential in patients with chronic stable angina due to atherosclerotic obstructive CAD. Angina can be precipitated by the inhalation of tobacco smoke (tobacco angina). Smoking can precipitate angina by causing a rise in heart rate as well as an increase in both systemic and coronary vascular resistance. Tobacco smoking can interfere with the efficacy of antianginal drugs, and continued smoking wors-

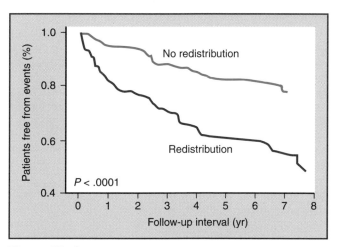

Figure 18–8

The significant difference in event-free survival in patients who had angiographic coronary artery disease with and without evidence of thallium-201 redistribution. *Event-free* indicates freedom from death, nonfatal myocardial infarction, coronary bypass surgery, or angioplasty for 3 months or longer after completion of the study. Five-year event-free survival was 82% for patients with no redistribution and 60% for patients with redistribution. (Redrawn from Wackers, F.J.Th.: Stress radionuclide imaging for detecting and assessing prognosis of coronary artery disease. *In* Beller, G.A. [vol. ed.]: Chronic Ischemic Heart Disease. Braunwald, E. [ser. ed.] Atlas of Heart Diseases. Vol. 5. Philadelphia, Current Medicine, 1995, p. 3.16.)

Table 18–7	Risk Factor Modifications Recommended for Patients with Stable Angina
	Cease smoking
	Control blood pressure
	Reduce LDL cholesterol to below 120 mg/dl
	Take aspirin
	Exercise as prescribed

Abbreviation: LDL, low-density lipoprotein.

ens the long-term prognosis of patients with coronary disease. Of all of the interventions to reduce coronary risk, none has more potential to improve life expectancy than smoking cessation, and multiple studies have demonstrated that persons with coronary disease have significantly fewer coronary events if they discontinue smoking.

Twenty percent or more of cigarette smokers will discontinue smoking after an event such as a myocardial infarction, percutaneous transluminal coronary angioplasty (PTCA), or coronary artery bypass grafting (CABG). Although only about 5% of cigarette smokers discontinue based on their physician's advice alone, these rates can be doubled using nicotine replacement therapy with gum or transdermal patches. Both the physician's firm and consistent advice and nicotine replacement therapy have been estimated to be cost-effective, with costs between $6,000 and $15,000 per year of life saved. Group counseling and nurse-managed interventions are also cost-effective.[8]

Control of hypertension is an important goal in the management of angina pectoris (see Chap. 21). Although diabetes mellitus and obesity are important risk factors for coronary heart disease, the impact of the rigid control of diabetes and the treatment of obesity on the prognosis of patients with established stable angina remains unclear. However, because insulin resistance has been implicated not only in the genesis of atherosclerosis but also as a contributing factor in the pathogenesis of plaque instability, adequate control of diabetes appears to be highly desirable.

Control of hyperlipidemia should be considered as an important therapy for management of patients with stable angina due to atherosclerotic CAD.[9-11] It is now established that in patients with documented CAD (i.e., in those with previous myocardial infarction, CABG, or PTCA and in those with typical exertional angina) and with average cholesterol levels or with mild to moderate hyperlipidemia or in those with severe hyperlipidemia who do not yet have clinical coronary disease, the use of 3-hydroxy-3-methylglutaryl coenzyme A (HMG CoA) reductase inhibitors (statins) is associated with a substantial decrease in cardiovascular events and mortality (see Chap. 29).

In the absence of contraindications, all patients with angina should receive 75 to 160 mg aspirin daily. Observational studies suggest that flavonoids, vitamin E, and other antioxidants inhibit the development and progression of CAD. In two major randomized trials, however, neither vitamin E nor beta-carotene was found to be beneficial when used for secondary prevention of coronary events in patients with existing CAD.[12,12a] The strong correlation between homocysteine levels and coronary disease, coupled with the known ability of folate and vitamins B_{12} and B_6 to lower homocysteine levels, makes supplementation with these substances a potentially attractive intervention.

Exercise

Although moderate isotonic exercise should be encouraged,[13] improved exercise tolerance appears to be related to a reduction in the myocardial oxygen demand for a given workload. Patients should be discouraged from performing very strenuous, vigorous exercise that can be expected to cause angina, but instead they should be encouraged to engage in regular, moderate exercise. Isotonic exercise, such as walking, is associated with peripheral vasodilatation and is preferable to isometric exercise, such as weight lifting, which is associated with an increase in peripheral vasoconstriction. Patients should also be advised to avoid arm exercise, which is associated with a lower threshold for angina compared with leg exercise. Patients should also be cautioned about exercising at cold or hot temperatures, which brings on angina more frequently than exercising at moderate temperatures.

Exercise programs should be guided by the results of the exercise testing. It is desirable not to exceed 75% of the heart rate shown to induce ischemia determined during the treadmill test.

Mean maximal heart rate during sexual intercourse usually does not exceed 70% of the maximal predicted heart rate. Thus, if patients can achieve a heart rate of up to 120 beats per minute on an exercise tolerance test without angina, it is unlikely that sexual activity will precipitate symptoms. Patients should *not be* advised against sexual activity and, if necessary, should be encouraged to use nitrates prophylactically.

Pharmacologic Treatment for Ischemia

Nitroglycerin and Nitrates

Nitroglycerin and other nitrates are endothelium-independent vasodilators that produce their beneficial effects both by decreasing myocardial oxygen requirements and by improving myocardial perfusion.[14,15] It has been postulated that nitrates, after entering the vessel wall, are converted to nitric oxide, which stimulates guanylate cyclase to produce cyclic guanosine monophosphate, the substance that is responsible for vasodilatation.

Nitrates dilate large coronary arteries and collateral vessels, relieve coronary vasospasm, and decrease the degree of coronary artery stenosis produced by an eccentric atherosclerotic plaque. Nitrates, therefore, have the potential to improve myocardial perfusion by coronary vasodilatation, by decreasing the degree of epicardial coronary artery stenosis, and by increasing collateral blood flow to the ischemic myocardium. Nitrates also decrease myocardial oxygen requirements by decreasing intracardiac volumes consequent to reduced venous return resulting from peripheral venous dilatation and by reducing arterial pressure. These beneficial effects may be offset partly by a reflex increase in heart rate, which can be prevented by simultaneous beta-adrenergic blockade.

Nitrates are effective for the management of various clinical subsets of stable angina. In patients with exertional angina, nitrates improve exercise tolerance, the time to the onset of angina, and ST segment depression during the treadmill exercise test. In patients with vasospastic angina, nitrates relax the smooth muscles of the epicardial coronary arteries and thereby relieve coronary artery spasm. In patients with mixed angina and postprandial

Table 18–8	Nitroglycerin and Nitrates in Angina		
Compound	**Route**	**Dose**	**Duration of Effects**
Nitroglycerin	Sublingual tablets	0.3–0.6 mg up to 1.5 mg	1.5–7 min
	Spray	0.4 mg, as needed	Similar to sublingual tablets
	Ointment	2% 6 × 6 inches	Effects up to 7 hr
		15 × 15 cm	
		7.5–40 mg	
	Transdermal patches	0.2–0.8 mg/hr every 12 hr	8–12 hr during intermittent therapy
	Oral—sustained released	2.5–13 mg	4–8 hr
		1–2 tablets 3 times daily	
	Buccal	1–3 mg 3 times daily	3–5 hr
	Intravenous	5–200 mg/min	Tolerance in 7–8 hr
Isosorbide dinitrate	Sublingual	2.5–15 mg	Up to 60 min
	Oral	5–80 mg 2–3 times daily	Up to 8 hr
	Spray	1.25 mg	2–3 min
	Chewable	5 mg	2–2½ hr
	Oral—slow release	40 mg 1–2 times daily	Up to 8 hr
	Intravenous	1.25–5.0 mg/hr	Tolerance in 7–8 hr
	Ointment	100 mg/24 hr	Not effective
Isosorbide mononitrate	Oral	20 mg twice daily	12–24 hr
		60–240 mg, once daily	
Pentaerythritol tetranitrate	Sublingual	10 mg as needed	Not known
Erythrityl tetranitrate	Sublingual	5–10 mg as needed	Not known
	Oral	10–30 mg, 3 times daily	Not known

Adapted from Thadani, U., and Opie, L.H.: Nitrates. *In* Opie, L.H. (ed.): Drugs for the Heart. 4th ed. Philadelphia, W.B. Saunders, 1995, pp. 31–48.

angina, nitrates reduce myocardial oxygen demand and promote coronary vasodilatation.

A variety of nitrate preparations are currently available (Table 18–8). The onset of action of sublingual nitroglycerin tablets or nitroglycerin spray is within 1 to 3 minutes, making these the preferred agents for the acute relief of effort or rest angina. Nitroglycerin is also very useful for prophylaxis when used several minutes before planned exertion. However, its short duration of action (20 to 30 min) makes it less practical for long-term prevention of ischemia in patients with stable angina.

For angina prophylaxis, long-acting nitrate preparations such as isosorbide dinitrate, mononitrates, transdermal nitroglycerin patches, and nitroglycerin paste are preferable (see Table 18–8). However, the major clinical problem for long-term continued nitrate therapy is nitrate tolerance (Table 18–9). The most reliable method for the prevention of nitrate tolerance is to ensure a nitrate-free period of approximately 10 hours, usually including sleeping

hours, in patients with effort angina. Isosorbide dinitrate should not be used more frequently than three times a day, or a transdermal patch more often than every 12 hours.

The most common side effect of nitrate therapy is a throbbing headache, which tends to decrease with continued use (Table 18–10). Although postural dizziness and weakness occur in some patients, frank syncope due to hypotension is relatively uncommon. Nitrates do not worsen glaucoma, once thought to be a contraindication to their use, and they can be used safely in the presence of increased intraocular pressure.

Beta-Adrenergic Blocking Agents (Table 18–11)

In general, beta blocking drugs decrease heart rate, blood pressure, and contractility and, as a result, reduce myocardial oxygen consumption (Fig. 18–10).[16] A slowing of heart rate is associated with an increased left ventricular perfusion time. Exercise-induced increases in heart rate and blood pressure are also blunted. In patients with stable angina, beta-adrenergic blocking agents increase exercise duration and the time to the onset of angina and of ST segment depression, although the double-product threshold (heart rate multiplied by blood pressure) at which ischemia occurs remains unchanged.

Beta blocking agents with beta$_1$ selectivity (such as metoprolol and atenolol) are preferable in patients with mild asthma, chronic obstructive pulmonary disease, insulin-dependent diabetes, or intermittent claudication. However, with increased doses of such agents, selectivity is lost and both types of beta receptors are blocked.

The major side effects of beta blocker therapy (see Table 18–10) include fatigue, impaired exercise toler-

Table 18–9	Proposed Mechanisms of Nitrate Tolerance

Decreased availability of intracellular sulfhydryl groups involved in the conversion of the parent organic nitrate to nitric oxide; this mechanism may involve the enzyme responsible for nitrate bioconversion to nitric oxide

Neurohormonal activation with increased circulating catecholamines, renin, angiotensin, and vasopressin, which results in enhanced systemic vasoconstrictor activity

Plasma volume expansion

Deranged enzymatic conversion of nitrate to nitric oxide

From Abrams, J.: Medical therapy of stable angina pectoris. *In* Beller, G.A. (vol. ed.): Chronic Ischemic Heart Disease. Braunwald, E. (ser. ed.): Atlas of Heart Diseases. Vol. 5. Philadelphia, Current Medicine, 1995, p. 7.17.

Table 18–10 Side Effects of Antianginal Drugs*

	Hypotension Flushing, Headache	Left Ventricular Dysfunction	Decreased Heart Rate Atrioventricular Block†	Gastrointestinal Symptoms	Bronchoconstriction‡	Edema
Beta blockers	0	++	+++	+	+++	0
Nitrates	+++	0	0	0	0	0
Diltiazem	+	+	+	0	0	+
Nifedipine	+++	0	0	0	0	+++
Verapamil	+	+	++	++	0	+
Amlodipine	+	0	0	0	0	+++

Adapted from Braunwald, E.: Mechanism of action of calcium channel blocking agents. N. Engl. J. Med. 307:1618, 1982. Copyright 1982 Massachusetts Medical Society. All rights reserved.

* 0, absent; +, mild; ++, moderate; +++, sometimes severe.

† In patients with sick sinus node syndrome or conduction system disease.

‡ In patients with obstructive lung disease.

ance, depression, insomnia, nightmares, and worsening claudication and bronchospasm. Severe bradycardia, episodes of second- or third-degree heart block, poorly controlled left ventricular failure, severe depression of left ventricular function, and severe peripheral vascular disease are contraindications to the use of beta blockers. Beta blockers may increase the blood sugar level and impair insulin sensitivity, particularly when used concurrently with diuretics. They may decrease the reaction to hypoglycemia in insulin-dependent diabetics and may exert unfavorable effects on the blood lipid profile with an increase in triglycerides and reduction in high-density lipoprotein cholesterol. However, the clinical significance of these adverse changes in the lipid profile with beta blockers has not yet been defined.

The effective dose of any beta blocking drug varies considerably from patient to patient. Resting heart rate should be reduced to between 45 and 60 beats per minute, and heart rate during moderate exercise, such as climbing two flights of stairs at a normal pace, should be below 90 beats per minute. If beta blockers induce symptomatic heart failure, they should be discontinued or the dose reduced. For maintenance therapy of stable angina,

beta blocking drugs with a relatively long half-life are preferable. The sudden withdrawal of beta blocker therapy may result in worsening of angina and precipitation of acute ischemic episodes; it is preferable to taper these medications gradually over 2 to 3 weeks.

Calcium Channel Blockers

These agents reduce the transmembrane flux of calcium via the slow calcium channel (Table 18–12). The dihydropyridines, for example, nifedipine, exert a greater inhibitory effect on vascular smooth muscle than on the myocardium. Thus, the major therapeutic effect can be expected to be peripheral or coronary vasodilatation. These agents, however, also exert a negative inotropic effect and therefore can produce myocardial depression, which is less pronounced with amlodipine and nisoldipine. The peripheral vasodilatation caused by the dihydropyridines also can cause reflex adrenergic activation, tachycardia, and stimulation of the renin-angiotensin system. These agents increase coronary blood flow owing to vasodilatation of both conductance and resistance coronary vessels. Intermittent adrenergic activation with short-

Table 18–11 Properties of Beta-Receptor Blocking Drugs in Clinical Use

Drugs	Selectivity	Partial Agonist Activity	Local Anesthetic Action	Lipid Solubility	Elimination Half-Life
Propranolol	None	No	Yes	High	Immediate release: 3½–6 hr
Metoprolol	Beta₁	No	Yes	Moderate	Immediate release: 3–4 hr
Atenolol	Beta₁	No	No	Low	6–9 hr
Nadolol	None	No	No	Low	14–24 hr
Timolol	None	No	No	Moderate	4–5 hr
Acebutolol	Beta₁	Yes	Yes	Low	3–4 hr
Betaxolol	Beta₁	No	Slight	Low	14–22 hr
Bisoprolol	Beta₁	No	No	Low	9–12 hr
Carteolol	None	Yes	No	Low	6 hr
Esmolol (intravenous)	Beta₁	No	No	Low	10 min
Labetalol†	None	Yes*	Yes	Moderate	5 hr
Pindolol	None	Yes	Yes	Moderate	3–4 hr
Sotalol‡	None	No	No	Low	12 hr

Adapted from Hoffman, B.B.: Adrenoreceptor-blocking drugs. *In* Katzung, B.G. (ed.): Clinical Pharmacology. Norwalk, CT, Appleton & Lange, 1994, pp. 131–146.

* Partial agonist effects at beta₂ receptors.

† Also causes alpha₁-selective blockade.

‡ Also type III antiarrhythmic agent and primarily used as an antiarrhythmic drug.

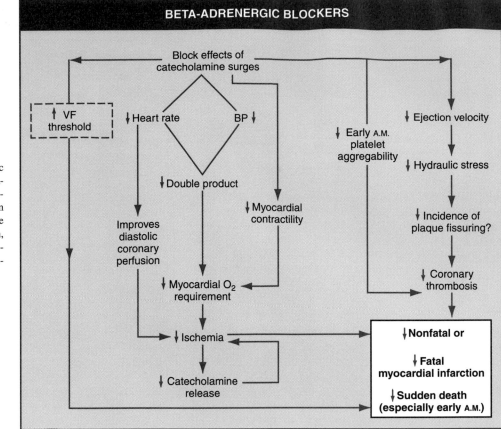

Figure 18–10

Salutary effects of beta-adrenergic blockade. VF, ventricular fibrillation; BP, blood pressure; ⬦, increase; ⬦, decrease. (Redrawn from Khan, M.G., and Topol, E.J.: Acute myocardial infarction. *In* Khan, M.G. [ed.]: Heart Disease: Diagnosis and Therapy. Baltimore, Williams & Wilkins, 1996, p. 2.)

Table 18–12 Properties of Calcium Channel Blocking Drugs in Clinical Use

Drugs	Vascular Selectivity*	Usual Dose	Plasma Half-Life	Side Effects
Dihydropyridines				
Nifedipine	3.1	Immediate release: 20–40 mg 3 times daily Slow release: 30–180 mg once daily	4 hr	Hypotension, dizziness, flushing, nausea, constipation, edema
Amlodipine	†	5–10 mg once daily	30–50 hr	Headache, edema
Felodipine	5.4	5–10 mg once daily	11–16 hr	Headache, dizziness
Isradipine	7.4	2.5–10 mg twice daily	8 hr	Headache, fatigue
Nicardipine	17.0	20–40 mg three times daily	2–4 hr	Headache, dizziness, flushing, edema
Nisoldipine	†	20–40 mg once daily	2–6 hr	Similar to nifedipine
Nitrendipine	14.4	20 mg once or twice daily	5–12 hr	Similar to nifedipine
Other				
Bepridil	‡	200–400 mg once daily	24–40 hr	Arrhythmias, dizziness, nausea
Diltiazem	0.3	Immediate release: 30–80 mg 4 times daily Slow release: 120–320 mg once daily	3–4 hr	Hypotension, dizziness, flushing, bradycardia
Verapamil	1.3	Immediate release: 80–160 mg three times daily Slow release: 120–480 mg once daily		Hypotension, myocardial depression, heart failure, edema
Mibefradil	—	50–100 mg once daily	17–25 hr	Bradycardia, atrioventricular block, headache, dizziness, hypotension

Adapted from Katzung, B.G., and Chatterjee, K.: Vasodilators and the treatment of angina. *In* Katzung B.G. (ed.): Clinical Pharmacology. Norwalk, CT, Appleton & Lange, 1994, pp. 171–187.

*Numerical data give the ratio of vascular potency to cardiac potency; higher numbers indicate greater vascular, less cardiac potency.

†Significant degree of vasodilatation greater than myocardial depression.

‡Myocardial depression greater than vasodilatation.

acting dihydropyridines has been implicated as the mechanism for the potentially adverse cardiovascular effects.[17]

The nondihydropyridine calcium channel blockers such as verapamil and diltiazem cause slowing of the sinus node and hence may potentiate the bradycardia of beta blockers. However, they are less potent peripheral vasodilators than the dihydropyridines and less likely to cause hypotension, flushing, and dizziness.

Epicardial coronary artery spasm is effectively relieved and prevented by calcium channel blockers, so that these are the agents of choice (along with nitrates) for the treatment of vasospastic angina (see Chap. 20). With some calcium channel blockers, such as verapamil and diltiazem, heart rate may also decrease, associated with a reduced myocardial oxygen requirement. In patients with mixed, walk-through, postprandial, and late nocturnal angina, in which increased coronary vascular tone appears to contribute to the pathogenesis of the ischemia, the use of calcium channel blockers may be of benefit, particularly when nitrate therapy alone is inadequate.

In patients with stable exertional angina, calcium channel blockers improve exercise tolerance and time to the onset of angina and to ST segment depression during treadmill exercise tests. The mechanism of these beneficial effects is primarily decreased myocardial oxygen consumption. Calcium channel blockers and beta-adrenergic blocking drugs in combination can produce synergistic beneficial effects in stable angina.

Controversy exists for the use of calcium channel blockers for the long-term treatment of stable exertional angina, since the short-acting, immediate-release dihydropyridines, such as nifedipine, may increase the risk of myocardial infarction and mortality. Worsening congestive heart failure and increased mortality has also been observed with diltiazem in postinfarction patients with depressed left ventricular ejection fraction. However, second-generation vasoselective dihydropyridine calcium channel blockers, such as amlodipine and felodipine, are well tolerated by patients with left ventricular dysfunction and even overt clinical heart failure, and no increase in the risk of mortality has been described. Furthermore, vasoselective long-acting dihydropyridines (such as amlodipine) and extended-release nifedipine and slow-release verapamil and diltiazem have all been shown to reduce angina. Thus, if necessary, these agents can be used for treatment of stable exertional angina. The new T-channel type of calcium blockers are also effective in controlling hypertension and angina. They appear to possess little negative inotropic effect and produce little or no edema or constipation.

The general side effects of calcium channel blockers are constipation, peripheral edema, dizziness, and occasionally, headache (see Table 18–10). With dihydropyridines, a reflex tachycardia may produce palpitation. With diltiazem and verapamil, sinus bradycardia and atrioventricular block may occur. In choosing a particular calcium channel blocker in a given patient, the hemodynamic profile should be considered. Dihydropyridines are preferable in the presence of sinus bradycardia, sinus node dysfunction, or atrioventricular block, particularly when the blood pressure is not adequately controlled. Diltiazem or verapamil is preferable in patients with relative tachycardia.

Choices among Pharmacologic Agents for Angina (Table 18–13)

In patients with stable exertional angina, beta blocker therapy is the preferred initial treatment. These agents reduce or prevent ischemia with a single daily dose, and their known long-term prognostic benefit after acute myocardial infarction (see Chap. 19) may also be generalizable to other patients with ischemic heart disease. All patients should also be given nitroglycerin and instructions about its therapeutic and prophylactic use.

Calcium channel blockers are *not* preferred initial therapy for the management of patients with stable exertional angina. In patients with special circumstances or concomitant diseases, specific medications or combinations of medications are preferable (see Table 18–13). For most patients, however, the initial therapy should consist of use of beta-adrenergic blocking agents, and nitrates should be added if the response to beta blocker therapy is inadequate. Calcium channel blockers should be considered in patients who cannot tolerate beta blockers or nitrates or who respond inadequately to these drugs. Extended-release nifedipine, second-generation vasoselective calcium channel blockers, and extended-release verapamil or diltiazem are the calcium blockers of choice.

Approach to the Patient with Possible Asymptomatic Ischemia

In some patients, angina may not be present but asymptomatic (silent) ischemia may be suspected. Unlike patients with an angina equivalent, such as exertional dyspnea, in whom the symptom can be used as a guide to therapy, the patient with possible asymptomatic ischemia requires a distinctive approach. In most cases, the asymptomatic ischemia is detected by a screening test (see Chap. 5) or by electrocardiographic monitoring during surgery or an unrelated illness.

Determining Whether a Positive Screening Test Is a True Positive or a False Positive

Since the prevalence of asymptomatic CAD varies by age, gender, and risk factors, the interpretation of a positive screening test result varies among different types of patients. Assuming an overall presence of asymptomatic coronary disease of about 5% in the adult American population, an exercise ECG that shows 2 mm or more of ST depression (in the absence of underlying ST abnormalities or medications or conditions that are known to cause false-positive results) or a clearly positive result on a myocardial perfusion scan increases the probability of

[handwritten annotation at top: strongly pos stress + strong ⊕ perfusion scan ~ 90% prob / ♂ < 40 ♀ < 50 ~ 80%]

Table 18-13	Choice of Drug Therapy for Special Cases of Angina

Concomitant Disease or Clinical Status	Drug of Choice
Hypertension	Beta blocker
	Calcium antagonist* or combination
Asthma or COPD	Calcium antagonist: Verapamil
Class III or IV angina awaiting angioplasty or CABG	Triple therapy†
Heart failure or EF <30%	Nitrates ± amlodipine
Left ventricular dysfunction‡	
Moderate: EF 30%–40%§	Nitrates + beta blockers ± amlodipine
Severe: EF 20%–30%	Nitrates + small-dose beta blockers
Tendency to bradycardia	Nifedipine ER or amlodipine + nitrates or acebutolol + nitrates
Diabetic	
Mild	Beta blocker + nitrates
Brittle, on insulin	Calcium antagonist
Hypertrophic cardiomyopathy	Beta blocker or verapamil
Mitral valve prolapse	Beta blocker
Peripheral vascular disease	
Mild	Beta blocker
Severe	Calcium antagonist + nitrate
Abdominal aortic aneurysm	Beta blocker
Heavy smoker (will not quit)	Timolol, acebutolol, atenolol, metoprolol
Cocaine : ischemia	Nitroglycerin IV + calcium antagonist

From Khan, M.G.: Angina. *In* Khan, M.G. (ed.): Heart Disease: Diagnosis and Therapy. Baltimore, Williams & Wilkins, 1996, pp. 133–186.
Abbreviations: COPD, chronic obstructive pulmonary disease; CABG, coronary artery bypass grafting; EF, ejection fraction; IV, intravenous.
* Second choice, amlodipine or diltiazem (Cardizem CD), nifedipine extended release.
† Beta blocker, nitrate + calcium antagonist.
‡ No overt heart failure.
§ Diltiazem or verapamil contraindicated.

coronary disease to about 50% (see Fig. 2–7). The combination of a strongly positive exercise ECG and a strongly positive myocardial perfusion scan raises the probability to about 90% and may be considered sufficient to make the clinical diagnosis of presumptive asymptomatic ischemia (Fig. 18–11). However, in asymptomatic men under the age of 40 years and asymptomatic women under the age of 50 years, in whom the prevalence of coronary disease is less than 5%, the combination of two positive test results predicts a probability of coronary disease of 80% or less. Similarly, when the results of the exercise ECG, myocardial perfusion scan, or exercise or stress echocardiogram are less indicative of ischemia—such as an exercise ECG showing less than 2 mm of ST segment depression at a high workload—the presence of asymptomatic myocardial ischemia is suggested but cannot be considered to be presumptive.

In other situations with a lower pretest probability (prevalence) of coronary disease, coronary arteriography is required to make a definitive diagnosis. In addition, for determining whether the observed coronary artery stenosis is truly causing ischemia, correlation between the anatomic distribution of the coronary disease and the evidence for ischemia on noninvasive testing is helpful.

A strongly positive exercise ECG in an asymptomatic person cannot be neutralized by a negative result on a myocardial perfusion scan or exercise or stress echocardiogram. For example, in an individual with a 5% pretest probability (prevalence) of CAD, the probability of coronary disease in the presence of a strongly positive exercise ECG but a negative myocardial perfusion scan is still

about 20% (see Fig. 2–7). To exclude CAD in such a patient, coronary arteriography is required (see Fig. 18–11).

Approach to the Patient with a Clinical Diagnosis of Presumptive Asymptomatic Myocardial Ischemia by Noninvasive Testing

(Fig. 18–12)

In patients with presumptive asymptomatic ischemia, the physician must determine whether other high-risk characteristics are present to suggest that the patient may have such severe CAD that coronary revascularization is warranted from a prognostic standpoint (see Fig. 18–12). In the absence of such high-risk characteristics, or in patients in whom there are other contraindications to coronary revascularization, medical management follows many of the same approaches used in patients with stable angina. Patients should be fully evaluated for coronary risk factors as well as for other abnormalities that may precipitate or exacerbate myocardial ischemia. Current therapeutic recommendations include routine aspirin therapy unless there are contraindications, aggressive control of hypertension (see Chap. 21), treatment of hyperlipidemia as indicated for secondary prevention (see Chap. 29), smoking cessation, and appropriate exercise prescriptions. The principal exception is that symptomatic control, which is so useful in the management of patients with

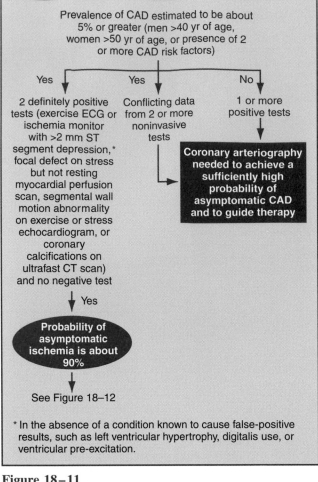

Figure 18–11

Making the clinical diagnosis of presumptive asymptomatic myocardial ischemia. CAD, coronary artery disease; ECG, electrocardiogram; CT, computed tomography.

stable angina, cannot be used effectively to monitor and treat the patient with a clinical diagnosis of presumptive asymptomatic ischemia.

In patients with asymptomatic ischemia, treatment with beta blockers reduces the frequency and duration of episodes of asymptomatic ischemia. In patients with asymptomatic or minimally symptomatic ischemia, 100 mg/day of atenolol reduces the risk of subsequent symptomatic coronary events. Beta blockers also aid in maintaining a blood pressure and heart rate below the individual's ischemia threshold as determined by formal exercise testing. Ambulatory electrocardiographic (Holter) monitoring should be used to adjust anti-ischemic therapy.

Although patients with totally asymptomatic ischemia may have a somewhat more favorable prognosis than do symptomatic patients, those with asymptomatic ischemia also appear to benefit from coronary revascularization if their anatomy is suitable (and would warrant revascularization if the ischemia were symptomatic). In such situations, revascularization can reduce ischemia, improve ischemia-free survival, and probably reduce coronary events. Thus, the invasive approach to patients with diagnosed asymptomatic ischemia closely parallels what is

recommended in symptomatic patients with ischemia and anatomy of similar severity.

Myocardial Revascularization

Two proven forms of myocardial revascularization have been developed for the treatment of chronic stable angina: catheter-based techniques (principally PTCA, coronary stenting, directional or rotational atherectomy) and CABG. Excimer laser angioplasty has no apparent benefit compared with these other, more standard catheter-based techniques.[18] Endomyocardial laser revascularization, by which it is hoped new coronary vessels will be formed in situations in which PTCA and CABG are not feasible, remains experimental at the present time.

Catheter-Based Revascularization

The principal indication for catheter-based revascularization is angina pectoris that fails to respond adequately to medical management in a patient with coronary artery lesions that are amenable to the procedure. The definition of an inadequate response to medical management is quite variable among patients and depends on the patient's lifestyle, occupation, and expectations. At one extreme are patients who are disabled by angina pectoris despite treatment with maximally tolerated doses of triple therapy (beta-adrenergic blockers, long-acting nitrates, and calcium antagonists) after lifestyle modifications, including achievement of optimal weight and cessation of smoking. At the other end of the spectrum are patients

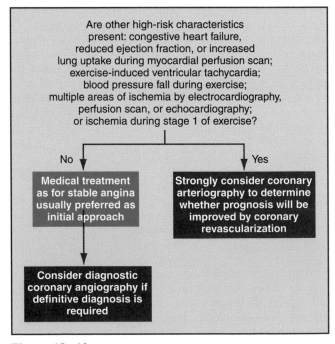

Figure 18–12

Approach to the patient with a clinical diagnosis of presumptive asymptomatic myocardial ischemia by noninvasive testing.

who consider medical therapy to have failed if control of angina pectoris requires doses of antianginal medications that cause side effects such as insomnia, fatigue, and sexual dysfunction. The usual candidate for a catheter-based intervention is somewhere between the extremes of this spectrum—that is, the patient who, although not totally disabled by angina, continues regularly to experience angina when engaging in activities of importance to him or her, such as recreational sports.

In a randomized trial of medical therapy versus PTCA for patients with class II or III angina, medical therapy was associated with a decreased risk of death or nonfatal MI but PTCA provided better relief of angina. These results emphasize the need to tailor therapy for the individual patient.[17a]

Ideal candidates for catheter-based revascularization have stable angina, are under 75 years of age, male, with single-vessel, single-lesion CAD, without a history of diabetes. Lesions that are optimal for these procedures are short (<10 mm), concentric, discrete, and readily accessible. Catheter-based interventions are by no means excluded in patients without these features, but the risk of morbidity and mortality from the procedure is increased, particularly in patients with long (>20 mm), tortuous, irregular, angulated, calcified, severely stenotic (>90% stenosis) lesions and particularly when more than one such lesion is present in an artery. Angiographic criteria are changing as additional experience is obtained with newer devices, including directional atherectomy and particularly stents.

Primary success of catheter-based interventions is generally defined as an absolute increase of 20 percentage points in luminal diameter and a final diameter obstruction less than 50%. Such angiographic success can be anticipated in more than 90% of properly selected patients.

The major complication of coronary angioplasty is abrupt closure, recognized angiographically before the patient leaves the laboratory, and is usually accompanied by manifestations of acute ischemic chest pain and ECG changes. The incidence of abrupt closure is approximately 5%, and it occurs more commonly in patients over the age of 75 years, in women, in the presence of unstable angina, diabetes, and recent thrombolytic therapy, and with the angiographic features described previously. The mortality of catheter-based coronary revascularization in patients with stable angina is approximately 1% and usually occurs after abrupt closure. The frequency of this complication can be reduced by pretreatment with the platelet glycoprotein IIb/IIIa receptor blockers. It may be treated by the insertion of a coronary stent and, if this procedure does not restore adequate flow, by emergency CABG.

Restenosis is usually defined as a greater than 50% diameter stenosis and a greater than 50% late loss of the acute luminal diameter. The incidence of this complication is approximately 30% to 40% after PTCA or atherectomy but appears to be reduced to about 20% after stenting; newer techniques, which are currently under investigation, such as irradiation, may reduce it further. Restenosis appears to occur more frequently in older patients, diabetics, and cigarette smokers and when lesions

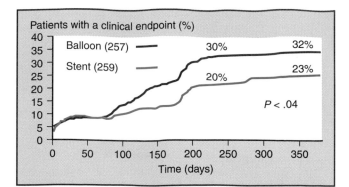

Figure 18–13

Balloon angioplasty versus coronary stenting. Cumulative frequency distribution curve for two study groups showing percentage of patients with primary clinical endpoints (death, cerebrovascular accident, myocardial infarction, bypass surgery, a repeat percutaneous procedure at the site of the previously treated lesion) at follow-up. Significant differences in the incidence of major clinical events appearing in the first 6 months are maintained at 1-year follow-up. (Redrawn from *Journal of the American College of Cardiology,* Vol. 27, Macaya, C., Serruys, P.W., Ruygrok, P., et al.: Continued benefit of coronary stenting versus balloon angioplasty: One-year clinical follow-up of Benestent trial. Benestent Study Group, pp. 255–261, Copyright 1996, with permission from the American College of Cardiology.)

cause total coronary occlusion, involve the left anterior descending coronary artery, include thrombosis as well as plaque, or were complicated by severe dissection during the course of the procedure. Restenosis commonly occurs within 6 months after the procedure and is less common when the postprocedure lumen is larger. Recurrent severe angina occurs in approximately half of the patients who develop angiographic restenosis and usually responds to repeat angioplasty (or stenting). The higher overall success rate of stenting—both at the time of the procedure (about 96% vs. 90% for balloon angioplasty) and at least 1 year after the procedure (Fig. 18–13)—appears to be worth the cost, especially if PTCA alone does not give an adequate angiographic result or if restenosis occurs.[19, 20] Atherectomy provides a larger postprocedure coronary lumen than PTCA and may be preferred over PTCA for certain types of coronary lesions, but it has been associated with no better, and perhaps somewhat worse, results at 6 months when compared with PTCA in randomized studies of patients who are felt to be candidates for either procedure.[18]

Coronary Artery Bypass Surgery

In this procedure, which is generally carried out after sternotomy and on cardiopulmonary bypass, coronary obstructions (usually >70% narrowing of the luminal diameter) are bypassed with an internal mammary (arterial) or saphenous vein graft. Arterial grafts have excellent long-term patency rates (90% at 10 years), whereas saphenous vein grafts show accelerated atherosclerosis with approximately 50% patency at 10 years. Therefore, it is not surprising that internal mammary artery grafts are associated with a 27% reduction in 15-year mortality compared with saphenous vein grafts.[21] When it is technically feasible, an arterial conduit, usually involving one or both internal mammary arteries, is recommended. For technical reasons, the left internal mammary artery is most conducive to a graft to the left anterior descending coronary artery and the right internal mammary artery is most applicable to graft to the right coronary artery. Patients who require more than two grafts generally receive a combination of arterial and venous grafts. Newer, minimally invasive CABG via a smaller thoracotomy incision or a thorascopic approach may reduce the morbidity and hospital length-of-stay.

The operative mortality of CABG has stabilized at approximately 2%, with rates of 1% to 1.5% for uncomplicated patients with stable angina. The steady improvements in perioperative care have been offset by the progressively sicker patients who are referred for this procedure. With the widespread use of catheter-based interventions, an increasing fraction of those undergoing CABG are elderly patients who in the past would not have undergone such a procedure or who are poor candidates for any procedure because of advanced serious multivessel, multilesion disease. An increasing number of patients are undergoing repeat CABG because of atherosclerosis in venous bypass grafts, and these patients too are at higher risk.

Angina pectoris is relieved in more than 90% of patients who undergo CABG. Severe (Canadian class III or IV) angina occurs in 5% to 10% of patients at 3 years and increases gradually thereafter. The recurrence of angina is due to graft stenosis or progression of disease in nongrafted vessels. Therefore, it is essential for the revascularization to be as complete as possible.

INDICATIONS. CABG should be carried out to prolong life[22] or improve its quality. Prolongation of life has been demonstrated in patients with more than 50% luminal diameter obstruction of the left main coronary artery and in those with impaired left ventricular function (left ventricular ejection fraction <40%) and critical obstruction (>70% stenosis) in all three major coronary arteries or in two arteries, one of which is the proximal left anterior descending artery. The presence of a high-risk result on a noninvasive test also increases the relative

benefit of surgery. Patients with severe left ventricular dysfunction or failure obtain a survival benefit from CABG if the myocardium with impaired contractile function is viable, that is, is hibernating rather than necrotic.

The Choice between Catheter-Based Interventions and CABG

In patients with single-vessel disease who require revascularization for symptoms and who are suitable for *either* procedure by angiography, both percutaneous procedures and CABG provide a substantial symptomatic benefit, but neither has been shown to prolong survival.[18] In patients with multivessel disease, several clinical trials comparing these methods of revascularization have shown that in nondiabetic patients the occurrence of death and myocardial infarction in 3 to 5 years is somewhat but not significantly higher with PTCA than with CABG[23, 24] (Table 18–14), although patients return to work sooner after PTCA. Initially, CABG provides better symptomatic relief and exercise tolerance. By 3 to 5 years later, however, these differences tend to narrow because of repeated procedures in patients originally treated with PTCA and a decline in benefit from CABG, but overall they still are in favor of CABG.[25]

Because of the high incidence of restenosis, the need for repeat revascularization is much higher in PTCA patients, reaching approximately 50% at 5 years compared with 5% to 10% after CABG. In diabetic patients with multivessel disease, survival is superior with CABG.[24]

Although the cost of catheter-based revascularization is lower than that of CABG initially, PTCA is associated with a greater need for repeat hospitalization, medical attention, and repeat revascularization. Therefore, the long-term costs of the two approaches are approximately equal.

Based on these considerations, patients with single-vessel disease who require revascularization are usually referred for a catheter-based intervention if they are deemed suitable arteriographically (Table 18–15). On the other hand, patients with left main CAD should undergo sur-

Table 18–14	Comparison of Surgical Therapy and Coronary Angioplasty			
	Pocock et al.*		BARI Study†	
End Point	*CABG (n = 1303)*	*PTCA (n = 1336)*	*CABG (n = 914)*	*PTCA (n = 915)*
	Percentage of Patients			
Death	2.8	3.1	10.7	13.7
Death or MI	8.5	8.1	19.6	21.3
Repeated CABG	0.8	18.3‡	0.7	20.5‡
Repeated CABG or PTCA	3.2	34.5‡	8.0	54.0‡
More than mild angina	12.1	17.8‡	—	—

Adapted from Bittl, J.A.: Advances in coronary angioplasty. N. Engl. J. Med. 335:1290–1302, 1996. Copyright 1996 Massachusetts Medical Society. All rights reserved.
Abbreviations: BARI, Bypass Angioplasty Revascularization Investigators; CABG, coronary artery bypass grafting; PTCA, percutaneous transluminal coronary angioplasty; MI, myocardial infarction.
* This study[23] was a meta-analysis of the results of six trials at 1 year. Patients with multivessel disease were studied.
† Data were obtained from the BARI investigators.[24] Patients with multivessel disease were studied. The results reported are for the 5-year follow-up.
‡ $P < .05$.

Table 18–15	Therapeutic Approach for Stable Angina

General medical therapy—cessation of smoking; control of hypertension, diabetes, and hyperlipidemia; regular exercise and reduction of weight; aspirin if not contraindicated

Medical therapy in patients with stable angina in the absence of specific indications for revascularization to improve prognosis and prevent symptoms (beta blockers); pre-exercise prophylaxis (nitroglycerin); add long-acting nitrates and then calcium channel blockers as needed; goal is acceptable exercise capacity and quality of life and prevention of frequent or severe ischemia; revascularization therapy (catheter-based revascularization or surgical revascularization procedure depending on anatomic considerations) unless contraindications of refractory angina, frequent or severe symptomatic ischemia, unacceptable quality of life, or intolerable side effects of medications

Indications for revascularization therapy to improve prognosis in the absence of other major life-limiting diseases

  Significant left main coronary artery stenosis → coronary artery bypass surgery

  Significant three-vessel coronary artery disease with or without associated left main coronary artery stenosis and with or without normal left ventricular ejection fraction → coronary artery bypass surgery, including internal mammary arteries as conduits

  Double-vessel coronary artery stenosis, including proximal left anterior descending coronary artery stenosis → coronary artery bypass surgery or catheter-based revascularization

  Other single- or double-vessel coronary artery stenosis → catheter-based revascularization or coronary artery bypass surgery

In elderly (above age 75 years) patients, patients with other life-limiting diseases, or patients needing urgent noncardiac surgery, catheter-based revascularization may be preferable when either type of revascularization is reasonable from a coronary perspective

In patients with moderately to severely depressed left ventricular ejection fraction with angina or angina equivalent with or without signs of heart failure → surgical revascularization if feasible

---

gery, as should patients with three-vessel, multilesion disease who have left ventricular failure or dysfunction (left ventricular ejection fraction <40%). In patients who fall between these two extremes and who, on the basis of the findings on coronary arteriography, are suitable for both CABG and catheter-based interventions, either approach may be employed with the following caveats: (1) surgical treatment is superior in diabetics with multivessel disease; (2) catheter-based interventions may be more desirable in nondiabetic patients with two-vessel disease that does not involve the proximal left anterior descending coronary artery and in whom ventricular function is normal or near-normal.

In practice, catheter-based revascularization is especially attractive in situations in which the risks of CABG are higher either in terms of overall mortality or in terms of neurologic side effects, each of which increases in the elderly, especially above age 75 years. In patients with life-limiting noncoronary diseases, the approach must be tempered by a careful consideration of the patient's overall prognosis. In those who need an urgent noncardiac operation, a catheter-based approach is generally preferable, so that the patient can proceed to the noncardiac surgery without the morbidity of a thoracotomy.

In any case, the experience and skill of the operators available should be given strong consideration in the choice. The advantages and disadvantages of the two approaches should be explained to the patients who fall into the middle groups, and the personal preferences of the patient and the family should be respected.

References

1. Goldman, L., Hashimoto, B., Cook, E.F., et al.: Comparative reproducibility and validity of systems for assessing cardiovascular functional class: Advantages of a new specific activity scale. Circulation 64:1227, 1981.
2. Gianrossi, R., Detrano, R., Mulvihill, D., et al.: Exercise-induced ST depression in the diagnosis of coronary artery disease—A meta-analysis. Circulation 80:87–98, 1989.
3. Beller, G.A.: Myocardial perfusion imaging with thallium-201. J. Nucl. Med. 35:674–680, 1994.
4. Berman, D.S., Hachamovitch, R., Kiat, H., et al.: Incremental value of prognostic testing in patients with known or suspected ischemic heart disease: A basis for optimal utilization of exercise technetium-99m sestamibi myocardial perfusion single-photon emission computed tomography. J. Am. Coll. Cardiol. 26:639–647, 1995.
5. Bonow, R.O., Bernan, D.S., Gibbons, R.J., et al.: Cardiac positron emission tomography—A report for health professionals from the Committee on Advanced Cardiac Imaging and Technology of the Council on Clinical Cardiology, American Heart Association. Circulation 84:447–454, 1991.
6. Ardissino, D., Savonitto, S., Egstrup, K., et al.: Selection of medical treatment in stable angina pectoris: Results of the International Multicenter Angina Exercise (IMAGE) study. J. Am. Coll. Cardiol. 25:1516–1521, 1995.
7. Younis, L.T., and Chaitman, B.R.: Management of stable angina pectoris. Cardiology (special ed.) 1:61–64, 1995.
8. Goldman, L.: Cost-effective strategies in cardiology. In Braunwald, E. (ed.): Heart Disease. 5th ed. Philadelphia, W.B. Saunders, 1996, pp. 1741–1755.
9. Byington, R.P., Jukema, J.W., Salonen, J.T., et al.: Reduction in cardiovascular events during pravastatin therapy. Pooled analysis of clinical events of the Pravastatin Atherosclerosis Intervention Program. Circulation 92:2419–2425, 1995.
10. Scandinavian Simvastatin Survival Study Group: Randomised trial of cholesterol lowering in 4,444 patients with coronary heart disease: The Scandinavian Simvastatin Survival Study (4S). Lancet 344:1383–1389, 1994.
11. Sacks, F.M., Pfeffer, M.A., Moye, C.A., et al., for the Cholesterol and Recurrent Events Trial Investigators: The effect of pravastatin on coronary events after myocardial infarction in patients with average cholesterol levels. N. Engl. J. Med. 335:1001–1009, 1996.
12. Stephens, N.F., Parsons, A., Schofield, P.M., et al.: Randomised controlled trial of vitamin E in patients with coronary disease: Cambridge Heart Antioxidant Study (CHAOS). Lancet 347:781–786, 1996.
12a. Rapola, J.M., Virtamo, J., Ripatti, S., et al.: Randomised trial of α-tocopherol and β-carotene supplements on incidence of major coronary events in men with previous myocardial infarction. Lancet 349:1715–1720, 1997.
13. Curfman, G.D.: Is exercise beneficial or hazardous to your heart? N. Engl. J. Med. 329:1730–1731, 1993.
14. Katzung, B.G., and Chatterjee, K.: Vasodilators and the treatment of angina pectoris. In Katzung, B.G. (ed.): Clinical Pharmacology. Norwalk, CT, Appleton & Lange, 1994, pp. 171–187.
15. Thadani, U., and Opie, L.H.: Nitrates. In Opie, L.H. (ed.): Drugs for the Heart. 4th ed. Philadelphia, W.B. Saunders, 1995, pp. 31–48.
16. Hoffman, B.B.: Adrenoreceptor-blocking drugs. In Katzung, B.G. (ed.): Clinical Pharmacology. Norwalk, CT, Appleton & Lange, 1994, pp. 131–146.
17. Yusuf, S.: Calcium antagonists in coronary artery disease and hypertension: Time for re-evaluation. [Editorial.] Circulation 92:1079–1082, 1995.
17a. RITA-2 Trial Participants: Coronary angioplasty versus medical therapy for angina: The second Randomised Intervention Treatment of Angina (RITA-2). Lancet 350:461–468, 1997.
18. Bittl, J.A.: Advances in coronary angioplasty. N. Engl. J. Med. 335:1290–1302, 1996.

19. Pepine, C.J., Holmes, D.R., Block, P.C., et al.: Coronary artery stents. J. Am. Coll. Cardiol. 28:782–794, 1996.

20. Macaya, C., Serruys, P.W., Ruygrok, P., et al.: Continued benefit of coronary stenting versus balloon angioplasty: One-year clinical follow-up of Benestent trial. J. Am. Coll. Cardiol. 27:255–261, 1996.

21. Cameron, A., Davis, K.B., Green, G., and Schaff, H.V.: Coronary bypass surgery with internal thoracic artery grafts: Effects on survival over a 15-year period. N. Engl. J. Med. 334:216–219, 1996.

22. Yusuf, S., Zucker, D., Peduzzi, P., et al.: Effect of coronary artery bypass graft surgery on survival: Overview of 10-year results from randomised trials by the Coronary Artery Bypass Graft Surgery Trialists Collaboration. Lancet 344:563–570, 1994.

23. Pocock, S.J., Henderson, R.A., Rickards, A.F., et al.: Meta-analysis of randomised trials comparing coronary angioplasty with bypass surgery. Lancet 346:1184–1189, 1995.

24. The Bypass Angioplasty Revascularization Investigators (BARI): Comparison of coronary bypass surgery with angioplasty in patients with multivessel disease. N. Engl. J. Med. 335:217–225, 1996.

25. Hlatky, M.A., Rogers, W.J., Johnstone, I., et al.: Medical care costs and quality of life after randomization to coronary angioplasty or coronary artery bypass surgery. N. Engl. J. Med. 336:92–99, 1997.

Chapter 19

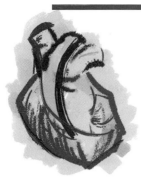

Recognition and Management
of Patients with

Acute Myocardial Infarction

EUGENE BRAUNWALD

Acute myocardial infarction (AMI) occurs in approximately 900,000 persons in the United States each year, and it is fatal in about one-fourth of these.[1] Approximately half of these fatalities occur within 1 hour of the onset of symptoms and before the patient reaches the hospital; these fatalities account for a large percentage of all sudden cardiac deaths.

PATHOLOGY

On pathologic examination, AMI may be divided into full-thickness (i.e., transmural infarction) or subendocardial (i.e., nontransmural infarction). The former usually occurs consequent to a platelet-fibrin thrombus on a ruptured plaque that had *not* been critically stenotic before the acute event, did not cause ischemia, and therefore did not lead to the formation of extensive protective collateral vessels. Nontransmural infarctions are seen most commonly in the presence of severely narrowed coronary arteries that do not become totally occluded, become occluded only transiently, or become occluded for longer periods in the presence of abundant protective collaterals.

Pathogenesis

In almost all instances, AMI is a complication of coronary atherosclerosis. Atherosclerotic plaques can be classified in terms of severity (i.e., percentage diameter stenosis) and susceptibility to rupture or fissure.[2] Unstable (i.e., "vulnerable") coronary atherosclerotic plaques (Fig. 19–1) are usually characterized by a relatively large lipid core that is separated from the circulating blood by a thin fibrous cap. Endothelial injury, which may be precipitated by stimuli such as flow shear stress, hypertension, hyperlipidemia, or their combination, may cause plaque fissuring or rupture, exposing the thrombogenic core of collagen and lipids. In addition, activated macrophages in the atheroma destabilize the plaque by (1) secreting metalloproteinase enzymes, which degrade the interstitial matrix and contribute to plaque rupture, and (2) elaborating cytokines that inhibit vascular smooth muscle from forming plaque-stabilizing collagen. Exposure of the thrombogenic core causes platelet aggregation and the formation of a fibrin clot, resulting in total or subtotal arterial obstruction (Fig. 19–2). Platelet aggregation also causes coronary vasoconstriction, which contributes to luminal narrowing.

Relatively stable plaques may have no distinct lipid core or only a small one, but even if their core is large, it

full thickness MI more likely to occur in absence of previously occluded vessel

257

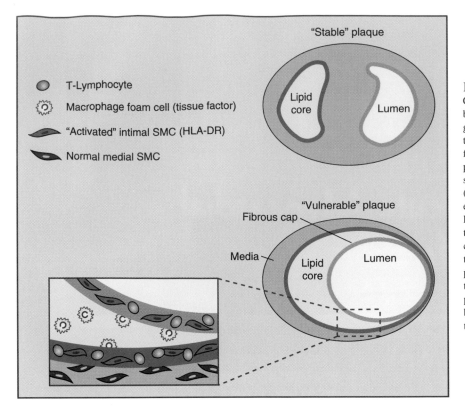

Figure 19–1

Comparison of the characteristics of "vulnerable" and "stable" plaques. Vulnerable plaques grow outward initially. The vulnerable plaque typically has a substantial lipid core and a thin fibrous cap separating the thrombogenic macrophages bearing tissue factor from the blood. At sites of lesion disruption, smooth muscle cells (SMCs) are often activated, as detected by their expression of the transplantation antigen human leukocyte antigen–DR (HLA-DR). In contrast, the stable plaque has a relatively thick fibrous cap protecting the lipid core from contact with the blood. Clinical data suggest that stable plaques more often show luminal narrowing detectable by angiography than do vulnerable plaques. (Redrawn from Libby, P.: Molecular bases of the acute coronary syndromes. Circulation 91:2844, 1995.)

is covered by a relatively thick fibrous cap separating it from contact with the blood (see Fig. 19–1); therefore, these plaques are unlikely to rupture. However, as stable plaques grow, they may produce very severe luminal narrowing and these are typically responsible for progressive exertional angina. Their gradual progression may lead to total occlusion, which may cause infarction. In many such cases, however, the presence of collateral vessels, developed over months and years of plaque growth, prevents infarction despite complete occlusion.

In the absence of adequate collateral vessels, *acute coronary obstruction* causes severe transmural myocardial ischemia and, if the latter is sustained for more than 20 to 30 minutes, infarction occurs. Non–Q-wave infarction is most commonly caused by the development of a nonocclusive thrombus on a vulnerable plaque or by lysis

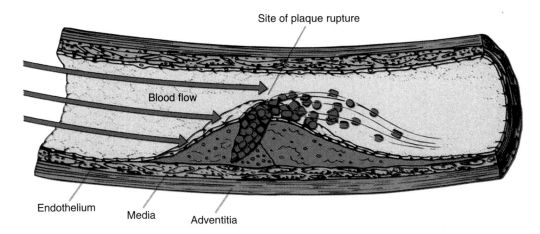

Figure 19–2

Diagram of arterial thrombus responsible for acute myocardial infarction (MI). Platelet adhesion and aggregation occur at the site of plaque rupture ("white thrombus"). Activated platelets exert procoagulant effects and the soluble coagulation cascade is activated. Fibrin strands and erythrocytes predominate within the lumen of the vessel and downstream in the "body" and "tail" of the thrombus. (Redrawn from Califf, R.M.: Acute myocardial infarction and other acute ischemic syndromes. *In* Braunwald, E. [ed.-in-chief]: Essential Atlas of Heart Diseases. Philadelphia: Current Medicine, 1997, p. 2.21.)

Table 19-1	**Conditions Other than Coronary Atherosclerosis that May Cause Acute Myocardial Infarction**
Coronary emboli	Causes include aortic or mitral valve lesions, left atrial or ventricular thrombi, prosthetic valves, fat emboli, intracardiac neoplasms, infective endocarditis, and paradoxical emboli
Thrombotic coronary artery disease	May occur with oral contraceptive use, sickle cell anemia and other hemoglobinopathies, polycythemia vera, thrombocytosis, thrombotic thrombocytopenic purpura, disseminated intravascular coagulation, antithrombin III deficiency and other hypercoagulable states, macroglobulinemia and other hyperviscosity states, multiple myeloma, leukemia, malaria, and fibrinolytic system shutdown secondary to impaired plasminogen activation or excessive inhibition
Coronary vasculitis	Seen with Takayasu's disease, Kawasaki's disease, polyarteritis nodosa, lupus erythematosus, scleroderma, rheumatoid arthritis, and immune-mediated vascular degeneration in cardiac allografts
Coronary vasospasm	May be associated with variant angina, nitrate withdrawal, cocaine or amphetamine abuse, and angina with "normal" coronary arteries
Infiltrative and degenerative coronary vascular disease	May result from amyloidosis, connective tissue disorders such as pseudoxanthoma elasticum, lipid storage disorders and mucopolysaccharidoses, homocystinuria, diabetes mellitus, collagen vascular disease, muscular dystrophies, and Friedreich's ataxia
Coronary ostial occlusion	Associated with aortic dissection, luetic aortitis, aortic stenosis, and ankylosing spondylitis syndromes
Congenital coronary anomalies	Including Bland-White-Garland syndrome of anomalous origin of the left coronary artery from the pulmonary artery, left coronary artery origin from the anterior sinus of Valsalva, coronary arteriovenous fistula or aneurysms, and myocardial bridging with secondary vascular degeneration
Trauma	Associated with and responsible for coronary dissection, laceration, or thrombosis (with endothelial cell injury secondary to trauma such as angioplasty); radiation; and cardiac contusion
Augmented myocardial oxygen requirements exceeding oxygen delivery	Encountered with aortic stenosis, aortic insufficiency, hypertension with severe left ventricular hypertrophy, pheochromocytoma, thyrotoxicosis, methemoglobinemia, carbon monoxide poisoning, shock, and hyperviscosity syndromes

From Sobel, B.E.: Acute myocardial infarction. *In* Bennett, J.C., and Plum, F. (eds.): Cecil Textbook of Medicine. 20th ed. Philadelphia, W.B. Saunders, 1996, p. 302.

(pharmacologically induced or spontaneous) of an occlusive thrombus. Non–Q-wave infarction may also occur when—in the presence of a severely stenotic, flow-limiting atherosclerotic lesion—blood flow is further reduced by the development of hypotension, as may occur during surgery or severe infection. Alternatively, non–Q-wave myocardial infarction (MI) can be caused by an increase in myocardial oxygen requirements, produced by tachycardia or fever, or both, in the presence of stable, severe coronary obstruction. Rarely, severe persistent coronary vasospasm, as occurs in Prinzmetal's angina, may cause severe persistent ischemia and ultimately MI (see Chap. 20).

A number of pathologic processes other than atherosclerosis may also cause MI.[2] These include coronary emboli, congenital malformations of the coronary vessels, and a variety of inflammatory abnormalities of the coronary arteries (Table 19–1).

Pathophysiology

Severe ischemia or necrosis acutely impairs myocardial contraction and relaxation. If the mass of acutely ischemic or necrotic myocardium is relatively small—less than 15% to 20% of the left ventricle—global ventricular function is usually maintained by increased contractile activity of the nonischemic myocardium. However, if the affected myocardium comprises a larger fraction of the left ventricle—more than 20% to 25%—global ventricular function becomes depressed, and this may lead to acute congestive heart failure, secondary to impaired ventricular emptying or filling, that is, systolic or diastolic heart failure, or both. When infarction is massive and involves more than approximately 35% of the left ventricle, cardiogenic shock due to left ventricular pump failure may develop. In the case of transmural infarction, especially involving the anterior wall or apex, infarct expansion, a process consisting of dilatation and thinning of the area of infarction caused by a slippage between the muscle bundles, is common. This may lead to dyskinesia, that is, paradoxical systolic expansion, of the affected wall. Such areas of abnormal wall motion further increase the burden placed on the remaining viable myocardium and the likelihood of acute heart failure.

CLINICAL MANIFESTATIONS

History

A precipitating factor such as severe emotional stress, unusually vigorous exercise, or a serious illness is present in about 50% of patients experiencing MI (Figs. 19–3 and 19–4). Approximately half of patients with AMI describe prodromal symptoms such as intermittent periods of rest pain not present previously or increasing intensity or frequency of preexistent angina (see Chap. 7). A higher frequency of onset of AMI occurs in the early morning hours, shortly after awakening, than at other times of the day or night. In a minority of patients, one of several factors that increase the imbalance between myocardial oxygen supply and demand can be identified. These include unusually heavy exercise, fever, tachycardia, emotional stress, hypoxemia, pulmonary embolism, or a surgical procedure associated with hypotension.

CHEST PAIN (see Chap. 7). The majority of patients who are experiencing an AMI complain of prolonged (>30 min) chest pain characterized as "oppressive," "crushing," "constricting," "choking," or "viselike," and that is sometimes described with a clenched fist held

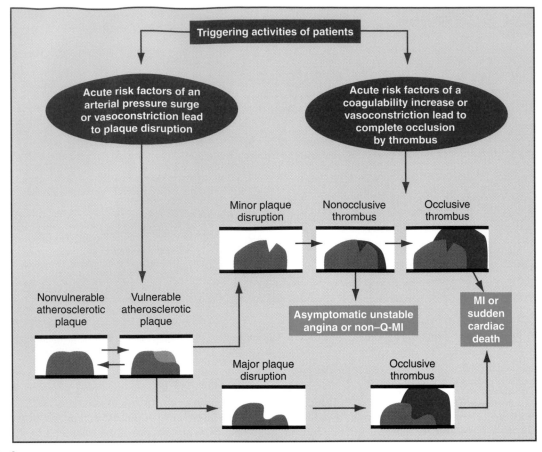

Figure 19–3

Hypothetical steps in the triggering of coronary thrombosis. Plaque disruption with thrombus formation occurs at a critical moment when a threshold combination of hemodynamic, prothrombotic, and vasoconstrictive forces (acute risk factors) is rapidly generated by external stressors (triggers) during a period of plaque vulnerability. MI, myocardial infarction. (Redrawn from Waxman, S., and Muller, J.E.: Risk factors for an acute ischemic event. *In* Califf, R.M. [vol. ed.]: Acute Myocardial Infarction and Other Acute Ischemic Syndromes. Braunwald, E. [ser. ed.]: Atlas of Heart Diseases. Vol. 8. Philadelphia, Current Medicine, 1996, p. 2.11.)

against the sternum. Typically, the pain is retrosternal in location and spreads to the anterior chest, more commonly the left side; it often radiates down the arms, especially the ulnar aspect of the left arm, to the shoulders, upper extremities, jaw, neck, interscapular regions, and epigastrium. The pain is similar to that of angina pectoris but more severe. Nausea, vomiting, and epigastric pain are common symptoms and may result in confusion with gastrointestinal disturbances such as esophagitis, gastritis, peptic ulcer, or acute cholecystitis. Indeed, patients with AMI may refer to their distress as "acute indigestion" or "heartburn." In some patients, only a dull ache or numbness is noted, and in others, perhaps as many as a third of patients, especially elderly patients or those with diabetes, AMI may be painless and is discovered only by an incidental electrocardiogram (ECG). Approximately half of these painless infarcts are not accompanied by *any* symptoms that the patient can recall, whereas in the others the history of an episode characterized by dyspnea, lightheadedness, a confusional state, gastrointestinal upset, or chest pain not sufficiently intense to induce the patient to seek medical attention can be elicited.

OTHER SYMPTOMS. These include dizziness, weakness, dyspnea, lightheadedness, palpitations, and fatigue, which may be profound, especially in the elderly, and they may occur with or without chest pain. In a small fraction of patients, syncope is the presenting or an early complaint. Nervousness and apprehension, sometimes described as a feeling of impending doom, are also frequently described.

Physical Examination

Patients experiencing an AMI often appear restless, anxious, and in obvious distress and sit up in bed clutching the chest. Pallor of the skin and perspiration may be prominent. Indeed, severe chest pain accompanied by diaphoresis points strongly to the diagnosis of AMI. Large infarctions may cause pulmonary edema, with frothy pink sputum and a feeling of suffocation. Massive infarction causing cardiogenic shock (see p. 274) results in cool and clammy skin, facial pallor, and cyanosis of the lips and nail beds. Although a variety of arrhythmias may occur in MI (see later), mild sinus tachycardia at a rate of 100 to

[handwritten margin notes: Silent AMI / ~55%: NC sx / ~50%: episode of / most common rhythm / ST & PVC's]

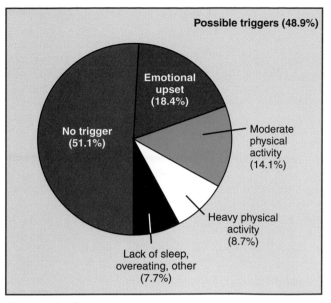

Figure 19–4

Possible triggers of myocardial infarction. (Redrawn from Waxman, S., and Muller, J.E.: Risk factors for an acute ischemic event. *In* Califf, R.M. [vol. ed.]: Acute Myocardial Infarction and Other Acute Ischemic Syndromes. Braunwald, E. [ser. ed]: Atlas of Heart Diseases. Vol. 8. Philadelphia, Current Medicine, 1996, p. 2.5; adapted from American Journal of Cardiology, vol 66, Tofler, G.H., Stone, P.H., Maclure, M., and the MILIS Study Group: Analysis of possible triggers of acute myocardial infarction [the MILIS study], pp 22–27, Copyright 1990, with permission from Excerpta Medica Inc.)

110 beats per minute with frequent ventricular premature beats is the most common rhythm observed. Large infarctions, even when uncomplicated, usually lower both systolic and diastolic pressures by 10 to 20 mm Hg. Therefore, previously hypertensive patients often become normotensive, and previously normotensive persons may exhibit borderline hypotension, with systolic pressures between 90 and 110 mm Hg. A narrow pulse pressure (< 30 mm Hg) reflects a depressed stroke volume in patients with more extensive infarctions. Patients with massive infarction and cardiogenic shock have, by definition, systolic pressures below 80 mm Hg (see Cardiogenic Shock). Hypotension secondary to left ventricular dysfunction or pump failure is generally associated with sinus tachycardia and should be distinguished from the hypotension accompanied by bradycardia due to activation of vagal receptors and resultant excess parasympathetic stimulation; excess parasympathetic stimulation is seen most commonly in patients with inferior wall MI. Low-grade fever (to 38° C) develops within 24 hours of the onset of a large infarction.

The jugular venous pulse is normal except in patients with severe left ventricular or right ventricular failure, or both, in whom it is elevated, with prominent A- or V-waves (see Chap. 3). The carotid pulse is usually normal in contour, but it may be reduced in volume, suggesting a reduced stroke volume. Patients with systolic or diastolic failure may present with moist rales over more than half of the lung fields, which do not clear on coughing. In patients with right ventricular infarction and resultant acute right ventricular failure, a positive hepatojugular reflux can often be elicited.

The coronary atherosclerosis responsible for AMI may be associated with peripheral vascular disease and diminished or absent popliteal, dorsalis pedis, and posterior tibial pulses and an ankle/brachial artery index less than 0.8. Funduscopic examination may show the findings characteristic of hypertension or diabetes (see Chap. 3).

Cardiovascular Examination

AMI often acutely reduces stroke volume. As a consequence, precordial movements are reduced or even imperceptible on inspection and palpation and the peripheral pulses are weak. In patients with large transmural infarctions, the only precordial pulsations may be presystolic instead of systolic. An outward movement in early diastole, synchronous with the third heart sound (S_{3}), is also sometimes palpable in patients with left ventricular failure.

AUSCULTATION. The heart sounds are usually normal in patients with small infarcts, but in patients with large infarcts the first heart sound (S_{1}) may be soft or indistinct and the second heart sound (S_{2}) accentuated. Severe left ventricular failure or left bundle branch block may cause paradoxical splitting of the S_{2} (see Chap. 3). An S_{3}, most easily audible at the apex, reflects *severe* ventricular dysfunction or heart failure. A fourth heart sound (S_{4}), best heard between the left sternal border and the apex, is a common finding in AMI and is of little prognostic significance. New, soft (grade 1 to 2/6) systolic murmurs are frequently audible at the apex and may be caused by mitral regurgitation secondary to papillary muscle dysfunction. A new, loud (grade ≥ 3/6) systolic murmur, accompanied by a thrill at or medial to the apex, suggests mitral regurgitation secondary to rupture of the head of a papillary muscle or a ventricular septal defect caused by perforation of the ventricular septum (see p. 274). Pericardial friction rubs are heard along the left sternal border in approximately 15% of patients with AMI. They are usually evanescent and occur most commonly on the second or third day.

LABORATORY FINDINGS

Serum Markers

With myocyte death, intracellular macromolecules pass through the damaged cell membrane and the appearance of these substances in the blood stream signifies the presence of infarction.[3] The pattern of rise is helpful diagnostically, with both peak creatine kinase (CK) and the MB isoenzyme of creatine kinase (CK-MB) beginning to rise above normal levels approximately 4 to 6 hours after the onset of symptoms, reaching a peak in approximately 24 hours and returning to baseline within 3 or 4 days, unless reinfarction occurs. Although CK-MB has been the most widely used serum marker for confirming the diagnosis of AMI, its clinical value is limited by its lack of

BP drops 10-20

↓BP + pump failure --> ↑ ST
↑BP + ↓HR ~ inferior wall MI

appearance during the first few hours of infarction and by its lack of total specificity, that is, its release with marked skeletal muscle damage. These limitations have spurred the search for other markers.

Cardiac-specific troponin T (cTnT) and I (cTnI) are absent in extracardiac tissue, and their presence in the serum at *any* detectable concentration is highly specific for myocardial necrosis. The kinetics of the *initial* release of the cardiac-specific troponins are similar to those of CK and CK-MB, beginning to rise at 4 to 6 hours after the onset of infarction and reaching a peak at approximately 24 hours. However, since they are components of the structural apparatus of myocytes, the troponins are released continuously for as long as 10 to 14 days from deteriorating cells, allowing the late diagnosis of infarction. The release of cTnT and cTnI is enhanced by reperfusion of the infarction, whether it is induced therapeutically or occurs spontaneously, causing an earlier and higher peak value in serum. The assays for the troponins are becoming widely available and are replacing CK and CK-MB. Hand-held devices that can provide a semiquantitative bedside measure of the troponins at the point of care, generally in the emergency department, are proving to be increasingly valuable in the rapid recognition of myocardial necrosis.

The CK isoform MB_2, a subtype of the isoenzyme, may be released into the circulation by 2 to 3 hours after the onset of infarction. This assay may permit earlier diagnosis. Myoglobin is a relatively small molecule that is rapidly excreted into the urine, and therefore, its duration of elevation after infarction is usually less than 24 hours, unlike CK-MB and the troponins, which remain elevated for longer periods. Although myoglobin is a very sensitive marker of muscle necrosis, it is nonspecific because it is a constituent of skeletal muscle and may be released from this tissue with even slight damage. Diagnosis or triage decisions based on myoglobin are therefore not recommended at this time.

An electrocardiogram (ECG) should be obtained and CK-MB, cTnT, or cTnI should be measured at the time of presentation and again 6 to 8 hours later in patients with suspected infarction. Since values of serum CK, CK-MB, cTnT, and cTnI usually remain normal during the first 4 hours after the onset of infarction, patients with a history consistent with possible AMI should not be discharged from the emergency department without several hours of observation. In patients with a low (<5%) clinical suspicion of AMI and no recurrent symptoms, the absence of new ischemic ECG changes or enzyme elevations during a 6- to 12-hour observation period is adequate to exclude AMI with about a 99% certainty. In patients with a more classic history or with ECG changes suggestive of ischemia on presentation, 24 hours of negative serial ECGs and enzymes (every 6 to 8 hr) is required to reach a similar level of certainty.

Unless patients have other conditions requiring intensive care, this "rule out MI" care can be provided in a chest pain evaluation unit or stepdown unit (see Chap. 7).

Electrocardiography

Often, the first ECG sign of acute transmural ischemia is the development of transient, giant, so-called hyper-

acute, T-waves overlying the affected myocardium (Fig. 19–5). ST segment elevation is also observed in leads overlying the ischemia when the latter involves the epicardium (Fig. 19–6), whereas ST segment depression occurs in the presence of subendocardial ischemia.[2] Hyperacute T-wave changes and ST segment deviations are followed by T-wave inversions and sometimes by loss of the height of R-waves and the development of Q-waves. In contrast, non–Q-wave infarctions are often accompanied by ST depression and T-wave inversion; the latter occurs early in the course of the infarction and may persist after the depressed ST segments have returned to isoelectricity (Fig. 19–7). In patients who do not receive reperfusion therapy, ST segment elevations typically persist for 6 to 18 hours after the onset of chest pain, and as the ST segments become isoelectric, the T-waves become inverted and Q-waves develop in the same leads.

For many years, infarcts with Q-waves were referred to as *transmural infarcts,* and non–Q-wave infarcts as *nontransmural infarcts.* However, pathologic-ECG correlations do not support such terminology and the preferred designations now are simply *Q-wave* and *non–Q-wave infarctions.*

The infarction can be localized to the anterior septal region of the left ventricle if the aforementioned ECG

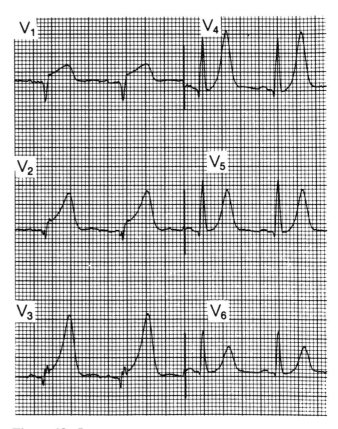

Figure 19–5

Hyperacute phase of anteroseptal myocardial infarction (MI). Note the tall positive T-waves (V_2 to V_3) along with ST segment elevations and Q-waves (V_1 to V_3). (From Goldberger, A.L.: Electrocardiography. *In* Fauci, A., Braunwald, E., Isselbacher, K.J., et al. [eds.]: Harrison's Principles of Internal Medicine. 14th ed. New York, McGraw-Hill, 1998, p. 1243.)

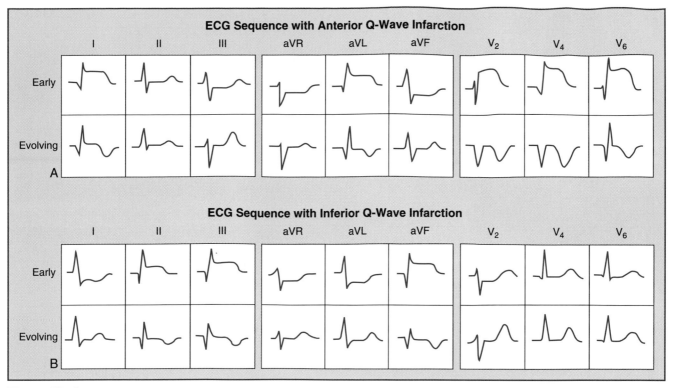

Figure 19–6

Sequence of depolarization and repolarization changes with acute anterior *(A)* and acute inferior *(B)* Q-wave infarctions. With anterior infarcts, ST elevation in leads I, aVL (augmented voltage, unipolar left arm lead), and the precordial leads may be accompanied by reciprocal ST depressions in leads II, III, and aVF (augmented voltage, unipolar left leg lead). Conversely, acute inferior (or posterior) infarcts may be associated with reciprocal ST depressions in leads V$_1$ to V$_3$. aVR, augmented voltage, unipolar right arm lead. *(A and B,* Redrawn from Goldberger, A.L.: Electrocardiography. *In* Fauci, A., Braunwald, E., Isselbacher, K.J., et al. [eds.]: Harrison's Principles of Internal Medicine. 14th ed. New York, McGraw-Hill, 1998, p. 1244; modified from Goldberger, A.L., and Goldberger, E. [eds.]: Clinical Electrocardiography: A Simplified Approach. 4th ed. St. Louis, Mosby–Year Book, 1990, pp. 89, 90.)

changes occur in leads V$_1$ to V$_3$; to the apex of the left ventricle if they occur in leads V$_4$ to V$_6$; to the lateral wall with changes in leads V$_5$, V$_6$, and aVL; and to the inferior wall with changes in leads II, III, and aVF. Posterior wall infarction may cause reciprocal ST segment depression and paradoxical R-wave elevation in leads V$_1$ to V$_4$. Right ventricular infarction causes ST segment deviation and QS patterns in right-sided leads (V$_1$, V$_{3R}$, V$_{4R}$) and is usually accompanied by inferior wall infarction.

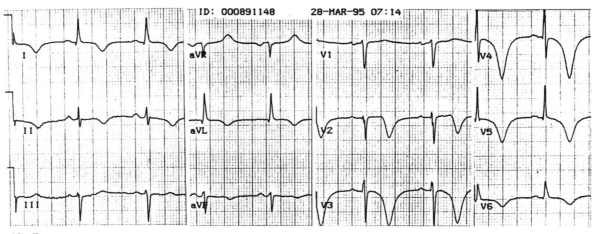

Figure 19–7

Non–Q-wave myocardial infarction. There is deep broad-based T-wave inversion. (Redrawn from Andreoli, T.E., Bennett, J.C., Carpenter, C.C.J., and Plum, F.: Special tests and procedures in the patient with cardiovascular disease. *In* Cecil Essentials of Medicine. 4th ed. Philadelphia, W.B. Saunders, 1997, p. 26.)

In the minority of patients with AMI, the ECG is entirely normal or shows only minor ST- and T-wave changes.

Cardiac Imaging

Echocardiography

The *two-dimensional echocardiogram* is useful in the evaluation of patients with acute chest pain. Typically, patients with AMI, especially transmural infarction, exhibit a regional wall motion disorder (akinesis or dyskinesis of the involved myocardium), which is readily recognized by means of transthoracic two-dimensional echocardiography. Echocardiography is particularly useful when the ECG is atypical or nondiagnostic, as when a conduction disturbance, particularly left bundle branch block, is present. It is useful in assessing left ventricular function and in the identification of right ventricular infarction and pericardial effusion as well as left ventricular aneurysm and thrombus. However, this technique does not differentiate among old infarction, acute infarction, acute ischemia, or myocardial stunning (postischemic ventricular dysfunction).

Doppler echocardiography is helpful in the evaluation of patients with AMI and systolic heart murmurs, particularly in detecting and assessing the severity of tricuspid valvular regurgitation and in estimating right ventricular systolic pressure. It is especially useful in patients with cardiogenic shock or severe heart failure and new systolic murmurs, since it allows the detection of complications that may be surgically correctable (mitral regurgitation or ventricular septal defect), as well as ventricular aneurysm, pericardial effusion, and right ventricular infarction. Color Doppler echocardiography is also helpful in patients with a nondiagnostic ECG suspected of having an aortic dissection (see Chap. 27) in which it frequently demonstrates an intimal flap.

Nuclear Imaging

A variety of nuclear imaging techniques—radionuclide angiography, myocardial perfusion imaging, infarct avid scintigraphy, and positron emission tomography—show characteristic changes in AMI. However, the ease with which echocardiography can be performed compared with the necessity of moving a critically ill patient from the emergency department to a nuclear medicine department generally limits the applicability of these other methods.

Differential Diagnosis

A typical history and ECG and release into the serum of a macromolecular marker such as CK-MB or cTn are the three cornerstones to establishing the diagnosis of AMI. The World Health Organization requires the presence of two of these three findings for the diagnosis of AMI. Although patients with unstable angina may have symptoms and ECG ST- and T-wave changes similar to those with AMI, they can subsequently be distinguished by the *absence* of development of new Q-waves and failure to release macromolecular markers into the serum.

Differentiation of AMI from acute pericarditis (see Chap. 28) may be challenging because the pain and ST segment elevations may be similar and serum markers sometimes rise slightly in pericarditis because of the associated epicardial injury. However, in pericarditis, the pain often persists for several days, ST segment elevations typically are more persistent and widespread than in AMI and occur in many (generally ≥6 of the 12) ECG leads, the ST segments often remain elevated for several days *after* the T-waves have become inverted, and Q-waves fail to develop.

MANAGEMENT

Prehospital Management

(see also Chap. 17)

The risk to life is highest during the first minutes after coronary occlusion and declines progressively in the hours, days, weeks, and years thereafter. Indeed, approximately half of all deaths associated with AMI occur during the first hour after its onset, and these are usually due to ventricular fibrillation. Therefore, the overarching principle in the management of AMI is to shorten the time between the onset of symptoms and treatment to an absolute minimum.[4, 5] The three components of delay in the onset of treatment are (1) patient delay in seeking medical attention, (2) prehospital evaluation and transportation, and (3) evaluation and initiation of treatment in the hospital. Attention must be directed to reducing all three of these components.[4, 5]

The general public and especially patients known to be at high risk of MI or reinfarction must be educated about the symptoms of AMI. They should be encouraged to seek urgent medical attention for chest discomfort, especially if it is accompanied by fatigue or dyspnea. It is useful for patients at especially high risk, such as those who have previously experienced an acute coronary syndrome (AMI or unstable angina), to have a copy of their resting ECG with them at all times to serve as a basis for possible future comparisons. Patients at high risk should be instructed to call emergency services through 911 with the onset of ischemic-type discomfort or to be taken directly to the nearest hospital that offers 24-hour emergency cardiac care. They should *not* be transported to the physician's office. While making arrangements for transportation, they should take one tablet of nitroglycerin sublingually, which may, if necessary and tolerated, be repeated twice at 5-minute intervals.

CARE IN THE AMBULANCE. Patients who are recognized in the field by emergency medical services as having signs of pulmonary congestion, tachycardia, and systolic blood pressure less than 90 mm Hg should, whenever possible, be transported to facilities in which cardiac catheterization and coronary revascularization can be carried out, so that the subsequent transfer to a tertiary hospital may be avoided.

It is highly desirable for emergency medical services to be upgraded to provide ventricular defibrillation, since it is lifesaving and if patients with AMI are immediately defibrillated, their survival and recovery are excellent.[6] Whenever possible, emergency medical personnel should also be capable of providing advanced cardiac life support, including intubation. Paramedics have been trained to provide such therapy, but basic emergency medical technicians have not and cannot provide defibrillation (see Chap. 17).

Use of a checklist (Table 19–2) and a 12-lead ECG during prehospital evaluation is helpful. Prehospital care should include establishing venous access, early relief of pain with morphine sulfate 5 mg every 5 minutes three

Table 19–2	Chest Pain Checklist for Use by EMT/Paramedic for Diagnosis of Acute Myocardial Infarction and Thrombolytic Therapy Screening

Check each finding below. If all [yes] boxes are checked and ECG indicates ST elevation or new BBB, reperfusion therapy with thrombolysis or primary PTCA may be indicated. Thrombolysis is generally not indicated unless all [no] boxes are checked and BP ≤ 180/110 mm Hg.

	Yes	No
Ongoing chest discomfort (≥20 min and <12 hr)	☐	—
Oriented, can cooperate	☐	—
Age >35 yr (>40 yr if female)	☐	—
History of stroke or TIA	—	☐
Known bleeding disorder	—	☐
Active internal bleeding in past 2 wk	—	☐
Surgery or trauma in past 2 wk	—	☐
Terminal illness	—	☐
Jaundice, hepatitis, kidney failure	—	☐
Use of anticoagulants	—	☐

Systolic/diastolic BP
Right arm: ___/___
Left arm: ___/___

	Yes	No
ECG done	☐	—

High-risk profile*	Yes	No
Heart rate ≥ 100 bpm	☐	—
BP ≤ 100 mm Hg	☐	—
Pulmonary edema (rales greater than halfway up)	☐	—
Shock	☐	—

* Transport to hospital capable of angiography and revascularization if needed.

Pain began	——	A.M./P.M.
Arrival time	——	A.M./P.M.
Begin transport	——	A.M./P.M.
Hospital arrival	——	A.M./P.M.

Reprinted from *Journal of the American College of Cardiology*, Vol. 28, Ryan, T.J., Anderson, J.L., Antman, E.M., et al.: ACC/AHA guidelines for the management of patients with acute myocardial infarction, pp. 1328–1428, Copyright 1996, with permission from the American College of Cardiology; adapted from the Seattle/King County EMS Medical Record.

Abbreviations: EMT, emergency medical technician; ECG, electrocardiogram; BBB, bundle branch block; PTCA, percutaneous transluminal coronary angioplasty; BP, blood pressure; TIA, transient ischemic attack.

times if necessary, the administration of nitroglycerin, and treatment of ventricular tachycardia with lidocaine (75 to 100 mg bolus followed by an infusion of 1 to 2 mg/min).

PREHOSPITAL THROMBOLYSIS. Since the earliest possible re-establishment of coronary reperfusion is of great importance, thrombolytic therapy should be begun as soon as possible in appropriate patients (see Myocardial Reperfusion: Thrombolytic Therapy). When treatment in the field allows initiation of thrombolytic therapy by more than 1 hour earlier than in the hospital, prehospital-initiated thrombolytic therapy can reduce relative mortality by 15% to 20% below that achieved by standard hospital-initiated treatment. Prehospital thrombolytic therapy may be especially useful in communities with transport delays of 90 minutes or longer.[7] Prehospital thrombolysis, however, requires physicians or, more commonly, very well trained and experienced emergency medical technicians in the ambulances as well as the capacity to transmit the ECG to the receiving hospital electronically. Without these, it is better to emphasize rapid transportation and shortening of the "door-to-needle" time once the patient reaches the emergency department.[4]

Management in the Emergency Department
(see also Chap. 17)

A clear plan for rapidly assessing the patient for reperfusion therapy is mandatory (Fig. 19–8). On arrival in the emergency department, patients with suspected AMI should immediately have a targeted cardiovascular history and physical examination and intravenous access should be established. A 12-lead ECG should be obtained, and the rhythm should be monitored continuously (Fig. 19–9). Aspirin, at a dose of 160 or 325 mg, should be given to all patients with suspected AMI (regardless of whether thrombolytic therapy will be used and irrespective of the thrombolytic agent) unless true aspirin allergy is present.[5, 8] If the first dose is chewed, a blood level is achieved more rapidly than if it is swallowed. Patients who have a true aspirin allergy may receive ticlopidine 250 mg instead, but this drug does not act for 24 to 48 hours. If possible, this initial evaluation should be completed within 15 minutes of arrival. The three principal goals of care in the emergency department are (1) stabilization, (2) triage, and (3) initiation of myocardial reperfusion.

Stabilization

Patients with acute chest pain thought to be due to ischemia should receive one sublingual nitroglycerin tablet (0.3 or 0.4 mg), unless the initial systolic blood pressure is less than 90 mm Hg, the heart rate less than 50 beats per minute or greater than 100 beats per minute. The nitroglycerin, which may be repeated twice at 5-minute intervals if the pain persists, also often improves hemodynamics in patients with MI by dilating systemic and coronary arteries as well as systemic veins. Nitroglycerin should be avoided in patients suspected of hav-

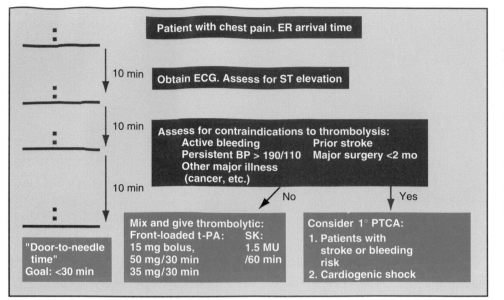

Figure 19–8

Algorithm for rapid triage of patients in the emergency room (ER) to provide thrombolysis with the shortest possible "door-to-needle" time. The time of each key event should be noted. ECG, electrocardiogram; BP, blood pressure; t-PA, tissue-type plasminogen activator; SK, streptokinase; MU, million units; PTCA, percutaneous transluminal coronary angioplasty. (Redrawn from Cannon, C.P., Antman, E.M., Walls, R., and Braunwald, E.: Time as an adjunctive agent to thrombolytic therapy. J. Thromb. Thrombolysis 1:31, 1994.)

ing right ventricular infarction (see Right Ventricular Infarction) because of the potential for excessive reduction of preload. This drug often relieves ischemic pain in patients with unstable angina (see Chap. 20) or esophageal spasm, so that response to nitroglycerin should not be interpreted as a specific diagnostic intervention in the setting of acute chest pain.

Effective *analgesia* should be established with intravenous morphine (5 mg boluses given intravenously every 5 to 15 min) until severe pain has been relieved. Respiratory depression secondary to morphine is unusual in patients with AMI and can be treated with naloxone (0.4 mg intravenously up to three times).

It is important to measure *blood pressure* repeatedly in patients receiving nitroglycerin or morphine. If systolic arterial pressure declines below 100 mm Hg, and the patient does not have pulmonary congestion, the lower extremities should be elevated. If sinus bradycardia accompanies hypotension, atropine (0.5 to 1.0 mg intravenously repeated every 5 min to a total dose of 2.5 mg) is often helpful. Atropine is particularly effective in hypotensive patients with (1) sinus bradycardia or frequent premature contractions, (2) inferior infarction and atrioventricular (AV) block with narrow QRS complexes, (3) after the administration of nitroglycerin, (4) nausea and vomiting after the administration of morphine, and (5) type I second-degree AV block (see Chap. 24).

Oxygen saturation should be monitored with an oximeter in patients believed to have ongoing acute ischemic discomfort, and oxygen should be administered, usually by nasal prongs, in those with saturation under 90%. In patients in whom severe hypoxemia cannot be corrected by supplemental inspired oxygen, intubation and mechanical ventilation may be necessary.

Triage

After initial stabilization in the emergency department, patients should be triaged into three groups:

1. Patients with probable infarction who require reperfusion therapy. If reperfusion is to be by means of thrombolytic therapy, this should be begun immediately in the emergency department *before* transfer to the coronary care unit (CCU). Alternatively, if reperfusion via percutaneous transluminal coronary angioplasty or other catheter-based intervention is selected and the laboratory and team are available, the patient should be transferred immediately to the cardiac catheterization laboratory.
2. Patients with probable infarction who are not candidates for reperfusion therapy and who are not low-risk patients (see later) should be transferred to the CCU.
3. Patients considered to be at low risk may be admitted to a coronary observation (intermediate-care or stepdown) unit, which has the capability for continuous ECG monitoring and ventricular defibrillation. These include stable patients with typical or atypical symptoms, but without ECG changes or with only minor ST–T-wave changes, as well as patients who are pain-free, hemodynamically stable, and without co-morbid illness.

The ECG obtained in the ambulance or emergency department is at the center of the decision pathway for management because ST segment elevation in patients with typical clinical findings identifies those who may benefit from reperfusion therapy (Fig. 19–10; see also Fig. 19–9). Exceptions include patients in the very early phase of AMI, with hyperacute T-waves before the development of ST segment elevation (see Fig. 19–5), those with posterior infarction who have ST segment depression in leads V_1 through V_3, as well as those with presumably new left bundle branch block, all of whom may benefit from acute myocardial reperfusion. Some patients without ST segment elevations on admission subsequently develop such elevation and become candidates for acute reperfusion therapy. Therefore, serial tracings should be obtained

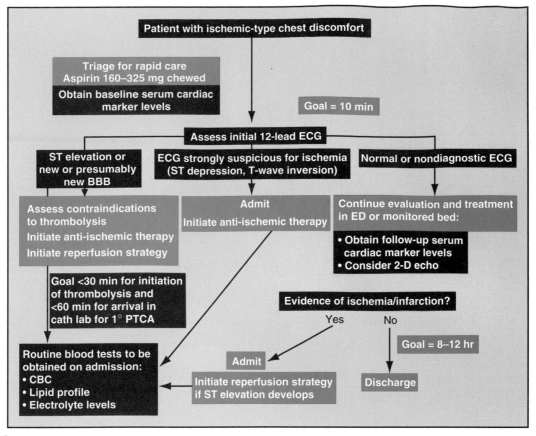

Figure 19–9

Algorithm for management of patients with suspected acute myocardial infarction in the emergency department (ED). All patients with ischemic-type chest discomfort should be evaluated rapidly and receive aspirin. The initial 12-lead electrocardiogram (ECG) is used to define the acute management strategy. Patients with ST segment elevation or new or presumably new bundle branch block (BBB) should be considered candidates for reperfusion; those without ST segment elevation but with an ECG and clinical history that are strongly suspicious for ischemia should be admitted for initiation of anti-ischemic therapy. Patients with a normal or nondiagnostic ECG should undergo further evaluation in the ED or short-term observation until results of serial serum cardiac marker levels are obtained. The following routine blood tests should be obtained in all patients admitted: a complete blood count (CBC), lipid profile, and electrolyte levels. 2-D, two-dimensional; 1°, primary; PTCA, percutaneous transluminal coronary angioplasty. (Redrawn from Ryan, T.J., Anderson, J.L., Antman, E.M., et al.: ACC/AHA guidelines for the management of patients with acute myocardial infarction. J. Am. Coll. Cardiol. 28:1328–1428, 1996; modified from Antman, E.M., and Braunwald, E.: Acute myocardial infarction. *In* Braunwald, E. [ed.]: Heart Disease. 5th ed. Philadelphia, W.B. Saunders, 1997.)

in patients with a history that suggests AMI and a nondiagnostic ECG.

Potential candidates for thrombolytic therapy should be screened immediately for contraindications (Table 19–3). Approximately half of all patients with AMI do not qualify for thrombolysis because the admission ECG does not show ST segment elevations (or new left bundle branch block), because they present more than 12 hours after the onset of symptoms, or because of contraindications to thrombolysis.

Myocardial Reperfusion: Thrombolytic Therapy

Since coronary thrombosis is the proximate cause of MI, it is not surprising that relief of the thrombotic obstruction—by either coronary thrombolysis or a catheter-based intervention—is effective therapeutically if it is carried out *before* the infarct is completed. There is strong evidence that the beneficial effect of thrombolytic

therapy, expressed as the number of lives saved per thousand patients treated, is dependent on the time from symptom onset to initiation of therapy (see Fig. 19–11).[9] Although there is no definitive evidence of benefit in patients reperfused more than 12 to 24 hours after the onset of chest pain, thrombolytic therapy may nonetheless still be considered in those who have ongoing ischemic pain and extensive, persistent ST segment elevation, even at this time. Because of the time dependency of the effectiveness of thrombolytic therapy, the overall strategy must focus on reducing the "door-to-needle" time for the administration of thrombolytic agents to 30 minutes or less.

The relative benefit of thrombolytic therapy has been demonstrated in both men and women and in patients with or without a history of previous MI; it is greater in patients with ST segment elevation in anterior as compared with inferior leads, as well as in patients with diabetes mellitus, hypotension, or tachycardia (Fig. 19–11). The major complications are related to hemorrhage, with intracranial hemorrhage the most serious complica-

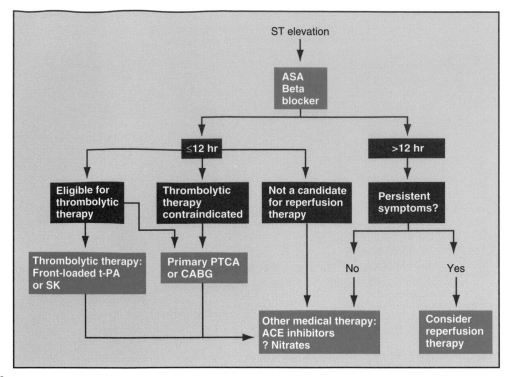

Figure 19–10

Recommendations for management of patients with ST elevation. All patients with ST segment elevation on the electrocardiogram should receive aspirin (ASA), beta-adrenergic blocking agents (in the absence of contraindications), and heparin (particularly if tissue-type plasminogen activator [t-PA] is used for thrombolytic therapy). Whether heparin is required in patients receiving streptokinase (SK) remains a matter of controversy; the small additional risk for intracranial hemorrhage may not be offset by any survival benefit afforded by adding heparin to SK therapy. Patients treated within 12 hours who are eligible for thrombolytics should expeditiously receive either front-loaded t-PA or SK or should be considered for primary percutaneous transluminal coronary angioplasty (PTCA). Primary PTCA is also to be considered when thrombolytic therapy is absolutely contraindicated. Coronary artery bypass grafting (CABG) may be considered if the patient is less than 6 hours from onset of symptoms. Patients treated after 12 hours should receive the initial medical therapy noted previously and, on an individual basis, may be candidates for reperfusion therapy or angiotensin-converting enzyme (ACE) inhibitors (particularly if left ventricular function is impaired). (Redrawn from Ryan, T.J., Anderson, J.L., Antman, E.M., et al: ACC/AHA guidelines for the management of patients with acute myocardial infarction. J. Am. Coll. Cardiol. 28:1328–1428, 1996; modified from Antman, E.M.: Medical therapy for acute coronary syndromes: An overview. *In* Califf, R.M. [vol. ed.]: Acute Myocardial Infarction and Other Acute Ischemic Syndromes. Braunwald, E. [ser. ed.]: Atlas of Heart Diseases. Vol. 8. St. Louis, Mosby–Year Book, 1996, pp. 10.1–10.25.)

tion. The risk of intracranial hemorrhage with thrombolytic therapy is increased by advanced age (>75 years), low body weight (<70 kg), hypertension (>180/100 mm Hg) and the use of tissue plasminogen activator (t-PA) (as opposed to streptokinase).[10] Although the *relative* benefit appears to be reduced in patients 75 years or older, an effort to achieve myocardial reperfusion should still be made in such patients unless specific contraindications exist. Thrombolytic therapy is *not* advised in patients without ST segment elevation (except for the subgroup with posterior infarction with ST segment depression limited to leads V_1 and V_2).

CHOICE OF THROMBOLYTIC AGENT. There has been considerable debate concerning the choice of thrombolytic agent.[11, 12] Four such drugs, streptokinase, t-PA (Activase), r-PA (reteplase), and anisoylated plasminogen streptokinase activator complex (APSAC) have been approved at the time of this writing. The first two have received the most intensive study. The advantage of t-PA over streptokinase is that it establishes earlier patency of the infarct-related artery, is associated with

slightly better ventricular function, and in the large GUSTO (Global Utilization of Streptokinase and Tissue Plasminogen Activator for Occluded Coronary Arteries) I trial, has a 1% lower absolute 30-day mortality (6.3% vs. 7.3%).[13] The usual front-loaded, accelerated regimen of t-PA is a 15-mg bolus, followed by 0.75 mg/kg over 30 minutes (maximum 50 mg) then 0.50 mg/kg over 60 minutes (maximum 35 mg). It requires cotherapy with heparin. The disadvantages of t-PA are a slightly greater risk of intracranial hemorrhage compared with streptokinase (0.6% vs. 0.3%). However, a 30-day mortality or nonfatal stroke composite clinical endpoint, which considered this serious complication, was shown in the GUSTO I trial to be slightly but statistically lower with t-PA (7.2%) than with streptokinase (8.1%). The other disadvantage of t-PA is its much greater cost than streptokinase.

The usual dose of streptokinase is 1.5 million units/100 ml given as a continuous infusion over 60 minutes. The major complications of this thrombolytic agent are fever, rash, hypotension, and very rarely, anaphylactic reaction.

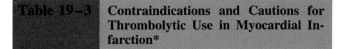

Table 19–3 Contraindications and Cautions for Thrombolytic Use in Myocardial Infarction*

Contraindications

Previous hemorrhagic stroke at any time; other strokes or cerebrovascular events within 1 yr
Known intracranial neoplasm
Active internal bleeding (does not include menses)
Suspected aortic dissection

Cautions/Relative Contraindications

Severe uncontrolled hypertension on presentation (blood pressure > 180/110 mm Hg)†
History of prior cerebrovascular accident or known intracerebral pathology not covered in Contraindications
Current use of anticoagulants in therapeutic doses (INR ≥ 2–3); known bleeding diathesis
Recent trauma (within 2–4 wk), including head trauma or traumatic or prolonged (>10 min) CPR or major surgery (<3 wk)
Noncompressible vascular punctures
Recent (within 2–4 wk) internal bleeding
For streptokinase/anistreplase: prior exposure (especially within 5 days–2 yr) or prior allergic reaction
Pregnancy
Active peptic ulcer
History of chronic severe hypertension

Reprinted from *Journal of the American College of Cardiology,* Vol. 28, Ryan, T.J., Anderson, J.L., Antman, E.M., et al.: ACC/AHA guidelines for the management of patients with acute myocardial infarction, pp. 1328–1428, Copyright 1996, with permission from the American College of Cardiology.

Abbreviations: INR, International Normalized Ratio; CPR, cardiopulmonary resuscitation.

* Viewed as advisory for clinical decision-making and may not be all-inclusive or definitive.

† Could be an absolute contraindication in low-risk patients with myocardial infarction.

A disadvantage of streptokinase is that it may be ineffective in patients with antistreptococcal antibodies, which includes patients who have ever received the drug and those who have suffered a streptococcal infection during the preceding year.

r-PA (reteplase) is a new thrombolytic agent whose efficacy, risk of intracranial hemorrhage, and price are similar to those of t-PA. However, it has the advantage of simpler administration; two bolus injections of 10 million units are administered 30 minutes apart.

One approach to choosing among these agents is to use t-PA or r-PA in those patients in whom the accelerated opening of the infarct-related coronary artery accomplished by these relatively expensive agents is likely to be of the greatest benefit. This includes patients at high risk: for example, those with prior MI, depressed left ventricular function, anterior MI, diabetes mellitus, systolic pressure less than 100 mm Hg, those presenting in the first 4 hours after the onset of symptoms in whom the speed of reperfusion is of paramount importance, and those in whom there is a contraindication to streptokinase (most commonly those who have received the drug in the past). Streptokinase, on the other hand, may be preferable in patients in whom the speed of reperfusion of the infarct-related artery is of lesser importance, for example, patients presenting more than 4 hours after the onset of chest pain, those who are at lower risk of death (e.g., patients with inferior wall MI without hemodynamic dis-

turbance), or whose risk of intracranial hemorrhage is high, that is, patients older than 75 years or with moderate hypertension (not severe enough to serve as an absolute contraindication) (see Table 19–3).

Irrespective of which agent is used, unnecessary venous or arterial interventions should be avoided in patients treated with thrombolysis.

Patients who receive t-PA or r-PA should receive intravenous heparin (a bolus of 60 to 70 U/kg followed by an infusion of 12 to 15 U/kg/hr) for approximately 48 hours. The activated partial thromboplastin time (aPTT) should initially be measured 6 hours after the start of thrombolysis and then at least once every 24 hours, with adjustments to maintain an aPTT of 50 to 75 seconds (Table 19–4). In patients who receive streptokinase, heparin should be added if there is a large anterior wall infarction, heart failure, or a mural thrombus visible on echocardiography. Heparin use is optional in other patients who receive streptokinase.

Emergency Catheter-Based Reperfusion

Emergency catheter-based interventions (primary angioplasty or stenting) are gaining increasing popularity as an effective means of achieving myocardial reperfusion in AMI.[14] The advantages of this approach are (1) achievement of reperfusion without the risk of hemorrhage, especially intracranial bleeding, that accompanies thrombolytic therapy, (2) higher full-patency rates (approximately 90% compared with 60% for thrombolytics), and (3) more complete opening of the infarct-related artery, with less residual stenosis, lower reocclusion rates, less recurrent ischemia, and a lower likelihood of requiring coronary revascularization compared with thrombolytic therapy. However, the applicability of this strategy as a primary therapy for AMI is currently limited to less than 10% of hospitals in the United States that have the skilled team and catheterization laboratory available around the clock and 7 days a week required for primary angioplasty.

The success of emergency catheter-based myocardial revascularization is highly operator-dependent. In general, it should be limited to centers that perform more than 200 catheter-based revascularization procedures per year and to operators who perform more than 75 such procedures per year. Since patients with AMI who have failed angioplasty with evidence of persistent ischemia or hemodynamic instability should be considered for urgent coronary bypass surgery, catheter-based reperfusion therapy for AMI should, in general, be limited to centers that have the capability for such procedures. Coronary bypass surgery is also recommended in patients with AMI who have persistent ischemia that is refractory to medical therapy and who are not candidates for thrombolysis or catheter-based interventions.

Even in hospitals with the available staff and facilities, valuable time may be lost between the patient's arrival in the emergency department and the opening of the occluded artery, thereby negating the potential advantage of this approach. Even more time can be lost if patients are transferred from one hospital's emergency department to a second hospital that can perform the emergency inter-

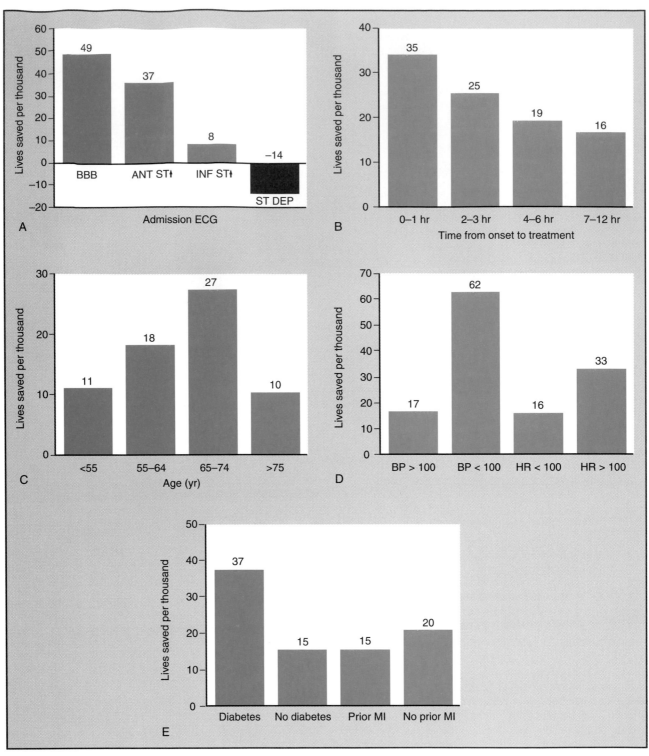

Figure 19–11

The effect of thrombolytic therapy on mortality in various patient subsets classified according to the admission electrocardiogram (ECG) *(A)*, the time from symptom onset to treatment *(B)*, age *(C)*, the blood pressure (BP) and heart rate (HR) *(D)*, and the presence or absence of diabetes or prior myocardial infarction (MI) *(E)*. Patients with bundle branch block (BBB) and anterior ST segment elevation (ANT ST) derive the most benefit from thrombolytic therapy; effects in patients with inferior ST segment elevation (INF ST) are much less; and patients with ST segment depression (ST DEP) do not benefit. Patients treated early derive the most benefit. Despite a higher overall risk of death, patients over the age of 75 years do not derive a greater absolute benefit than do younger patients. Patients with hypertension or tachycardia benefit the most, and patients with diabetes are more likely to benefit than nondiabetic patients. The presence of prior infarction does not predict a greater benefit. *(A–E,* Redrawn from Martin, G.V., and Kennedy, J.W.: Choice of thrombolytic agent. *In* Julian, D.G., and Braunwald, E. [eds.]: Management of Acute Myocardial Infarction. London, W.B. Saunders, 1994, pp. 90–91.)

| Table 19–4 | Heparin Adjustment Nomogram for Standard Laboratory Reagents with a Mean Control aPTT of 26–36 sec* |||||

aPTT (sec)	Bolus Dose (U)	Stop Infusion (min)	Rate Change (ml/hr)	Repeat aPTT
<40	3000	0	+2	6 hr
40–49	0	0	+1	6 hr
50–75	0	0	0 (no change)	Next A.M.
76–85	0	0	−1	Next A.M.
86–100	0	30	−2	6 hr
101–150	0	60	−3	6 hr
>150	0	60	−6	6 hr

Reprinted from *Journal of the American College of Cardiology,* Vol. 28, Ryan, T.J., Anderson, J.L., Antman, E.M., et al.: ACC/AHA guidelines for the management of patients with acute myocardial infarction, pp. 1328–1428, Copyright 1996, with permission from the American College of Cardiology; adapted with permission from Hirsh, J., Raschke, R., Warkentin, T.E., et al.: Heparin: Mechanism of action, pharmacokinetics, dosing considerations, monitoring, efficacy, and safety. Chest 108:258S–275S, 1995.

Abbreviation: aPTT, activated partial thromboplastin time.

* Heparin infusion concentration = 50 U/ml; target aPTT = 50–75 sec. For aPTTs obtained before 12 hr after initiation of thrombolytic therapy: (1) Do *not* discontinue or decrease infusion unless significant bleeding or aPTT > 150 sec. (2) Adjust infusion upward if aPTT < 50 sec. For aPTTs obtained ≥12 hr after initiation of thrombolytic therapy, use entire nomogram: Deliver bolus, stop infusion, and/or change rate of infusion based on aPTT, as noted on appropriate line of nomogram.

vention, and this strategy is usually not advisable. Registries of patients with AMI have shown a greater time delay between the onset of chest pain and reperfusion when primary angioplasty is performed than when thrombolytic therapy is administered.

When available without time delay, and when it can be performed by a skilled operator and trained team, emergency catheter-based reperfusion should be employed within 6 hours of the onset of symptoms in patients with AMI and ST segment elevation who are not eligible for thrombolysis (see Table 19–3), and in those who are at relatively high risk of intracranial hemorrhage (age >75 years or hypertension, or both) as a consequence of thrombolysis. It can also be used as an alternative to thrombolysis in candidates for this therapy, but its superiority in this group has not been established definitively. Some also recommend emergency catheter-based reperfusion in patients with cardiogenic shock, but the value of this approach has not been established in a randomized trial at the time of this writing.

Patients who have received thrombolytic therapy should undergo coronary arteriography and, if the anatomic findings are appropriate, catheter-based revascularization if there is persistent chest pain and ST segment elevation 90 minutes after the onset of this therapy or if chest pain recurs and the ST segments become re-elevated.

Patients with AMI *without* ST segment elevations are not candidates for thrombolytic therapy or emergency (primary) angioplasty.[15] Other patients believed to have AMI who do not qualify for reperfusion therapy because of late arrival in the emergency department, nondiagnostic ECG changes, and contraindications to thrombolytic therapy should receive aspirin, heparin, and intravenous beta blockers, unless there are contraindications to these drugs (Fig. 19–12).

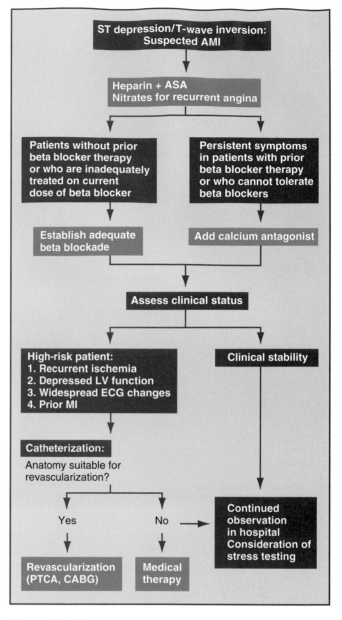

Figure 19–12

Recommendations for management of patients with acute myocardial infarction (AMI) without ST elevation. All patients without ST elevation should be treated with an antithrombin and aspirin (ASA). Nitrates should be administered for recurrent episodes of angina. Adequate beta-adrenoceptor blockade should then be established; when this is not possible or contraindications exist, a calcium antagonist can be considered. High-risk patients should be triaged to cardiac catheterization with plans for revascularization if they are clinically suitable; patients who are clinically stable can be treated more conservatively, with continued observation in the hospital and consideration of a stress test to screen for myocardial ischemia that can be provoked. LV, left ventricular; ECG, electrocardiogram; MI, myocardial infarction; PTCA, percutaneous transluminal coronary angioplasty; CABG, coronary artery bypass graft. (Redrawn from Ryan, T.J., Anderson, J.L., Antman, E.M., et al: ACC/AHA guidelines for the management of patients with acute myocardial infarction. J. Am. Coll. Cardiol. 28:1328–1428, 1996; modified from Antman, E.M.: Medical therapy for acute coronary syndromes: An overview. *In* Califf, R.M. [ed.]: Acute Myocardial Infarction and Other Acute Ischemic Syndromes. Braunwald, E. [ser. ed.]: Atlas of Heart Diseases. Vol. 8. St. Louis, Mosby–Year Book, 1996, pp. 10.1–10.25.)

Hospital Management

The CCU

The CCU should have a skilled, experienced staff and equipment for the monitoring of multiple ECG leads for cardiac rhythm and ST segment deviation, arterial oxygen saturation, and the invasive measurement of arterial pressure through an intra-arterial line and pulmonary artery pressure through a balloon flotation catheter. Equipment should also be available for defibrillation, standby percutaneous cardiac pacing, insertion of transvenous pacemakers, placement of an intra-aortic counterpulsation balloon, and noninvasive automatic monitoring of arterial pressure using a sphygmomanometric cuff.

General Measures

For the first 12 hours, patients should receive either nothing by mouth or a clear liquid diet and should be placed at bedrest (Table 19–5). Arterial oxygen saturation should be measured (usually with an oximeter), and hypoxemia should be corrected.[16] Disturbances of acid-base balance or of electrolytes should be corrected, and in some instances, antianxiety agents (such as oral diazepam [2 to 10 mg] or oxazepam [15 to 30 mg] two to four times daily for 48 hours) may be helpful. Docusate sodium (200 mg daily) is useful as a stool softener. Patients who have no complications may use a bedside commode shortly after admission and should commence physical activity as shown in Table 19–6.

Patients with AMI can be discharged from the CCU after 24 hours if there are no complications (heart failure,

Table 19-5	Sample Admitting Orders
Condition	Serious
IV	NS or D$_5$W to keep vein open.
Vital signs	q ½ hr until stable, then q 4 hr and prn. Notify if HR < 60 or > 110: BP < 90 or > 150; RR < 8 or > 22. Pulse oximetry × 24 hr.
Activity	Bedrest with bedside commode and progress as tolerated after approximately 12 hr.
Diet	NPO until pain-free, then clear liquids. Progress to a heart-healthy diet (complex carbohydrates = 50%–55% of kilocalories, monounsaturated and unsaturated fats ≤30% of kilocalories), including foods high in potassium (e.g., fruits, vegetables, whole grains, dairy products), magnesium (e.g., green leafy vegetables, whole grains, beans, seafood), and fiber (e.g., fresh fruits and vegetables, whole-grain breads, cereals).
Medications	Nasal O$_2$ 2 L/min × 3 hr. Enteric-coated ASA daily (165 mg). Stool softener daily. Beta blockers? Consider need for analgesics, nitroglycerin, anxiolytics.

Reprinted from *Journal of the American College of Cardiology*, Vol. 28, Ryan, T.J., Anderson, J.L., Antman, E.M., et al.: ACC/AHA guidelines for the management of patients with acute myocardial infarction, pp. 1328–1428, Copyright 1996, with permission from the American College of Cardiology.

Abbreviations: IV, intravenous; NS, normal saline solution; D$_5$W, 5% dextrose in water; prn, as required; HR, heart rate; BP, blood pressure; RR, respiratory rate; NPO, nothing by mouth; ASA, acetylsalicylic acid.

Table 19-6	Activity Progression after Myocardial Infarction

General Guidelines

When progressing through the stages noted below, specific activities should be stopped for increasing shortness of breath or the patient's perception of fatigue or detection of an increase in the heart rate of >20–30 beats/min^{-1}. Vital signs should be monitored before and after progression from one stage to the next and also from one level to the next within each stage. Energy-conserving techniques should be emphasized and the use of prophylactic nitroglycerin should be reviewed with the patient.

Stage I (Days 1–2)

Use a bedpan/commode. Feed self-prepared tray with arm and back support. Complete assistance with bathing. Passive ROM to all extremities. Active ankle motion (with footboard if available). Emphasis on relaxation and deep breathing.
Partially bathe upper body with back support. Bed to chair transfers for 1–2 hr per day. Active ROM to all extremities 5–10 times (sitting or supine).

Stage II (Days 3–4)

Bathe, groom, self-dress sitting on bed or chair. Bed to chair transfers ad lib. Ambulate in room with gradual increase in duration and frequency.
May shower or stand at sink to bathe. May dress in own clothes. Supervised ambulation outside of room (100–600 ft several times per day) (33–200 m).
Partially bathe upper body with back support. Bed to chair 20–30 min daily. Active assisted to active ROM all extremities: 5–10 times (sitting or supine).

Stage III (Days 5–7)

Ambulate 600 ft (200 m) 3 times per day. May shampoo hair (e.g., activity with arms over head).
Supervised stair walking.
Predischarge exercise tolerance test.

From Antman, E.M.: General hospital management. *In* Julian, D., and Braunwald, E. (eds.): Management of Acute Myocardial Infarction. London, W.B. Saunders, 1994, p. 34.

Abbreviations: ROM, range of motion; ad lib., as desired.

hypotension, other hemodynamic instability, severe ventricular tachyarrhythmias, advanced AV block, large pericardial effusion, atrial fibrillation, persistent ischemic pain) or when they have been stable for 24 hours after successful treatment of a complication. After discharge from the CCU, patients should be followed in an intermediate CCU, where continuous monitoring of the ECG allows prompt, effective treatment of ventricular fibrillation and other serious arrhythmias.

The rate of progression from the CCU to the intermediate CCU, to a regular hospital floor, and to hospital discharge is governed by the patient's risk and clinical course.[17] Patients without complications and not at high risk (see earlier) can generally be moved from the CCU to the intermediate CCU after 24 to 36 hours. If no complication supervenes during an additional 24 to 36 hours in the intermediate CCU, they can be moved to a regular hospital bed and discharged from the hospital by 4 to 6 days. Patients at higher risk may be moved from the CCU to the intermediate CCU after 2 or 3 days if their course has been stable. These patients may also benefit from longer observation (2 to 4 days) in the intermediate CCU and an equal time in a regular hospital bed. Unless complications occur or recur, even such higher-

Table 19–7	Hemodynamic Classifications of Patients with Acute Myocardial Infarction

A. Based on Clinical Examination		B. Based on Invasive Monitoring	
Class	Definition	Subset	Definition
I	Rales and S₃ absent	I	Normal hemodynamics PCWP <18, CI >2.2
II	Rales over <50% of lung	II	Pulmonary congestion PCWP >18, CI <2.2
III	Rales over >50% of lung fields (pulmonary edema)	III	Peripheral hypoperfusion PCWP <18, CI >2.2
IV	Shock	IV	Pulmonary congestion and peripheral hypoperfusion PCWP >18, CI <2.2

A and *B*, From Antman, E.M., and Braunwald, E.: Acute myocardial infarction. *In* Braunwald, E. (ed.): Heart Disease. 5th ed. Philadelphia, W.B. Saunders, 1997, p. 1234; *(A)* modified from *American Journal of Cardiology,* Vol. 20, Killip, T., and Kimball, J.: Treatment of myocardial infarction in a coronary care unit. A two-year experience with 250 patients, pp. 457, Copyright 1967, with permission from Excerpta Medica Inc; and *(B)* data from Forrester, J., Diamond, G., Chatterjee, K., et al.: Medical therapy of acute myocardial infarction by the application of hemodynamic subsets. N. Engl. J. Med. 295:1356, 1976.
Abbreviations: S₃, third heart sound; PCWP, pulmonary capillary wedge pressure; CI, cardiac index.

risk patients can generally be discharged by 8 to 10 days after admission.

EDUCATION. Efforts should be made to educate the patient about his or her illness while in the hospital.[18] The nature of coronary artery disease, its risk factors, and the importance of diet, exercise, rehabilitation, smoking cessation, medication, and return to work and other life activities should be explained. This can be carried out by the primary care physician, nurses, and other health care professionals. Group instruction and videotaped programs may be useful, but these should be considered adjuncts and cannot take the place of one-on-one contact with a caregiver.

COMPLICATIONS

Hemodynamic Disturbances

Based on clinical examination, patients can be divided into four groups based on the Killip classification (Table 19–7A). Invasive monitoring, with a pulmonary artery flotation (Swan-Ganz) catheter and an intra-arterial line, is indicated in patients in class IV with a systolic pressure below 80 mm Hg and pulmonary rales, as well as in patients with pulmonary edema that is not corrected by intravenous furosemide (see later), and in patients with hypotension that is not readily corrected with fluid administration, leg raising, or atropine. Although there should be no hesitation to insert a pulmonary artery catheter in appropriate patients, this procedure should be carried out by an experienced operator. Complications of inserting a pulmonary artery catheter occur in approximately 4% of cases and include sepsis, pulmonary infarction, and very rarely, pulmonary artery rupture. Cardiac output should be measured in these patients with the indicator dilution technique with injection of the indicator (cool saline) into the right atrium and sampling (with a thermistor) in the pulmonary artery.

Table 19–8	Therapy by Hemodynamic Subset*

I. No treatment other than standard (aspirin, beta blockers, ACE inhibitors, heparin)
II. Diuretic therapy to lower PAWP to 18 mm Hg (also consider nitroglycerin given intravenously and afterload reduction with ACE inhibitors)
III. Volume expansion to a PAWP of 18 mm Hg (also consider dobutamine)
IV. Afterload reduction with nitroglycerin given intravenously, nitroprusside, or ACE inhibitors with or without an inotrope such as dobutamine or dopamine (search for correctable complication of infarction)

From Reeder, G.S., and Gersh, B.J.: Acute myocardial infarction. *In* Stein, J.H. (ed.): Stein's Internal Medicine. St. Louis, Mosby–Year Book, 1994, pp. 169–189.
Abbreviations: ACE, angiotensin-converting enzyme; PAWP, pulmonary artery wedge pressure.
* *Hemodynamic subset* is defined in Table 19–7B.

Hemodynamic assessment allows patients to be classified as shown in Table 19–7B and treated as shown in Table 19–8. Hypoperfusion is identified by a cardiac index below 2.2 L/min/m², whereas pulmonary congestion is reflected by a pulmonary capillary wedge pressure (PCWP) above 18 mm Hg. Patients who are hypotensive or have hypoperfusion but a PCWP below 18 mm Hg may be suffering from hypovolemia and should receive a bolus of 100 ml normal saline solution, followed by 50-ml increments every 5 minutes until the systolic arterial pressure reaches 110 mm Hg or the PCWP exceeds 18 mm Hg. Patients with pulmonary congestion or rales involving more than one-third of the lung fields that do not clear on coughing, and with a systolic arterial pressure exceeding 100 mm Hg should receive a diuretic (e.g., furosemide, 20 to 40 mg intravenously repeated every 4 hr). Normotensive patients with pulmonary congestion despite diuretics should receive vasodilator therapy. The vasodilator of choice is intravenous nitroglycerin given in a dose of 5 μg/min, with the dose increased by 10 μg/min every 5 minutes to a maximum of 200 μg/min until the hemodynamics have been optimized or until the systolic arterial pressure has declined to 90 mm Hg. In patients with persistent heart failure, oral vasodilators, especially angiotensin-converting enzyme (ACE) inhibitors, should be used.

Cardiogenic Shock

This severe form of ventricular failure is characterized by markedly elevated ventricular filling pressure (PCWP > 20 mm Hg), very low cardiac index (< 1.8 L/min/m²), persistent severe systemic hypotension (systolic arterial pressure < 80 mm Hg), and evidence of organ hypoperfusion such as a clouded sensorium, cool extremities, oliguria, or metabolic acidosis.[19] Cardiogenic shock is most commonly due to extensive damage to the left or right ventricular myocardium or to a mechanical defect (ventricular septal rupture or papillary muscle rupture). Cardiogenic shock occurs in approximately 10% of patients with AMI and usually is not present at the time of admission but develops during the course of hospitalization.

MANAGEMENT. In the patient with cardiogenic shock due to left ventricular dysfunction but without a mechanical defect (ventricular septal defect or mitral regurgitation), continuous hemodynamic assessment is essential. Inotropic stimulation with a sympathomimetic agent is usually indicated. When systolic arterial pressure is very low (< 70 mm Hg), norepinephrine 2 to 10 μg/kg/min is the drug of choice. In patients with moderate hypotension (systolic arterial pressure 70 to 90 mm Hg), dopamine (5–20 μg/kg/min) is used. When the systolic arterial pressure is higher (≥ 90 mm Hg), dobutamine (2–20 μg/kg/min) may be the optimal agent (Table 19–9).

In patients in whom cardiogenic shock persists despite inotropic support as outlined previously, intra-aortic balloon counterpulsation, with insertion of the balloon percu-

taneously or via an arterial cutdown in the femoral artery, is indicated.[20] The balloon is inflated during early diastole and deflated just before the onset of systole. This augments coronary blood flow and lowers the pressure against which the left ventricle ejects and results in a small (approximately 15%) increase in cardiac output and moderate (approximately 5 mm Hg) lowering of PCWP.

Despite the favorable hemodynamic effects of the combination of the administration of sympathomimetic amines and intra-aortic balloon counterpulsation, these therapies have only a minor beneficial effect on mortality. Therefore, after stabilization with inotropic agents and intra-aortic balloon counterpulsation, cardiac catheterization and coronary arteriography should be carried out unless myocardial revascularization is contraindicated or not feasible. Coronary revascularization—either via a catheter-based technique or by means of coronary bypass grafting—is performed whenever possible. Although the mortality in patients with cardiogenic shock treated by revascularization is approximately 50%, compared with 80% in those who are not revascularized, it is not clear whether this is due to the selection of less sick patients for revascularization or to the effects of the procedure itself.

A New Systolic Murmur

The presence of a new loud systolic heart murmur suggests the presence of a mechanical complication (Table 19–10), an interventricular septal defect due to rupture of the ventricular septum, or massive mitral regurgitation secondary to rupture of the head of a papillary muscle. These complications, which may accompany cardiogenic shock, can be recognized and differentiated by two-dimensional echocardiography (Fig. 19–13) with

Table 19–9	Choice of Pharmacologic Agents in Patients with Acute Myocardial Infarction Based on Hemodynamic Parameters				
Drug Effect	**Furosemide**	**IV Nitrates**	**Dobutamine**	**Dopamine**	**ACE Inhibitors**
Preload	↓	↓	—	↑	↓
Afterload	—	Minimal ↓	Minimal ↓	↑	↓
Sinus tachycardia	No	Yes	Minimal	Yes	No, minimal
Parameters					
Moderate heart failure, PCWP ≥ 20 > 24	Yes	Yes	Yes, if BP > 70	Yes, if BP < 70 and oliguria (on dobutamine)	Oral maintenance weaning nitroprusside
Severe heart failure, PCWP > 24, cardiac index > 2.5 L/min/m²	Yes	Yes, if BP > 95	Yes, if BP > 70	Yes, if BP < 70	Yes
Cardiogenic shock if BP < 95 PCWP > 18, cardiac index < 2.5 L/min/m²	CI	CI	Yes	Yes IABP	RCI
Right ventricular infarction, JVP ↑	CI	CI	Useful with titrated volume infusion	Relative CI ↑ PA pressure	CI

Modified from Khan, M.G.: Complications of myocardial infarction and postinfarction care. *In* Khan, M.G. (ed.): Heart Disease: Diagnosis and Therapy. Baltimore, Williams & Wilkins, 1996, p. 66.
Key: Yes, useful; ↓, decrease; —, no change; ↑, increase.
Abbreviations: ACE, angiotensin-converting enzymes; BP, systolic blood pressure (mm Hg); PCWP, pulmonary capillary wedge pressure; CI, contraindication; IABP, intra-aortic balloon pump; RCI, relative contraindication; JVP, jugular venous pressure; PA, pulmonary artery.

Table 19–10	Acute Myocardial Infarction—Mechanical Complications, Incidence, Timing, and Mortality				
	% of Total Acute Infarcts	Incidence and Timing	% of Total Rupture	% of Total In-Hospital Mortality	Type of Infarct
Cardiac rupture	3–10	Up to 40%; day 1 Up to 50%; days 2–3		8–17*	
Free wall	2–6*†	25%; day 1 10%; days 4–7	85	7–14	Lateral
Papillary muscle rupture	1	25%; days 1–2 or 6–10 75%; days 3–5	5	1	Commonly inferoposterior
Ventricular septal rupture	1–2	25%; days 1–2 or 6–14 75%; days 3–5	10	1–2	60% anterior 40% inferior
Severe mitral regurgitation	<2%	days 1–5			
LV aneurysm	7–12	3 mo			90% anterior 10% inferior

Modified from Khan, M.G.: Complications of myocardial infarction and postinfarction care. *In* Khan, M.G. (ed.): Heart Disease: Diagnosis and Therapy. Baltimore, Williams & Wilkins, 1996, p. 83.
Abbreviation: LV, left ventricular.
* Am. Heart J. 117:809, 1989.
† Am. J. Cardiol. 68:961, 1991.

Doppler flow imaging. Alternatively, they may be recognized by means of a balloon flotation catheter, in which an oxygen step-up is observed as the catheter is advanced from the right atrium into the right ventricle in the presence of a ventricular septal defect, or a tall V-wave is observed in the PCWP in the presence of mitral regurgitation.

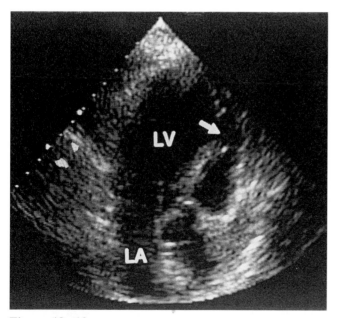

Figure 19–13
Two-dimensional echocardiographic view from the apical position demonstrating a ventricular septal defect *(arrow)* seen as a dropout in the area of the ventricular septum. LV, left ventricle; LA, left atrium. (From Nishimura, R.A.: The role of echocardiography. *In* Fuster, V., Ross, R., and Topol, E.J. [eds.]: Atherosclerosis and Coronary Artery Disease. Philadelphia, Lippincott-Raven, 1996, p. 869.)

MANAGEMENT. If one of the previously mentioned mechanical defects is suspected, and after aggressive therapy has been agreed on following discussion with the patient or relatives, the diagnosis should be confirmed by cardiac catheterization and coronary angiography. Intra-aortic balloon counterpulsation is often useful for stabilizing the patient before operation.[20] Surgical correction of the defect is commonly combined with coronary revascularization.

Right Ventricular Infarction

This usually is seen in patients with coexistent inferior left ventricular infarction and rarely (<5%) occurs in an isolated form.[21] Right ventricular infarction should be suspected in patients with inferior left ventricular infarction with unexplained, persistent hypotension, clear lung fields, and elevated jugular venous pressure. Right atrial pressure is elevated, right ventricular pulse pressure is reduced, and PCWP is usually normal or only slightly raised. The ECG shows ST segment elevations in right precordial leads, especially V_{4R} (the right precordial lead in the V_4 position). The right atrial pressure pulse usually reveals a prominent Y descent, whereas the right ventricular pressure tracing shows an early diastolic drop and plateau, that is, a "square root sign" similar to that observed in constrictive pericarditis (see Chap. 28). Kussmaul's sign—an increase in jugular venous pressure with inspiration—in the presence of an inferior wall AMI, suggests right ventricular involvement. Echocardiography often reveals right ventricular dilatation. The reduction of preload (hypovolemia, diuretic use, nitroglycerin) intensifies hypotension.

Treatment consists of the expansion of plasma volume with saline solution and, if this is insufficient, the addition of dobutamine. Pulmonary artery pressure monitoring is needed if the patient does not respond to fluids or develops signs suggestive of left ventricular failure. It is especially important to maintain AV synchrony in patients with right ventricular infarction, and AV sequential pacing is highly desirable in such patients who have heart block and hypotension.

Arrhythmias

(see Chaps. 23 and 24)

The majority of patients with AMI develop one or more cardiac arrhythmias.[22] Many of these are transient and benign and do not require specific therapy. Others are more serious and life-threatening and require prompt treatment.

Tachyarrhythmias

SUPRAVENTRICULAR TACHYARRHYTHMIAS. *Sinus tachycardia* is a common arrhythmia in AMI and is typically associated with increased sympathetic activity, hypertension or hypotension, left ventricular failure, and anxiety. Treatment consists of correction of the underlying disorder and the use of beta-adrenergic blockers unless there is a contraindication to the use of these drugs (see later).

Atrial fibrillation occurs in approximately 15% of patients with AMI. It is seen most often during the first 24 hours, may be transient, and is more frequent in patients with left ventricular failure, with large anterior wall MIs, or with AV block, and in the elderly.[23] In the *absence* of heart failure, a beta-adrenergic blocker (e.g., metoprolol 5 mg by intravenous bolus every 5 to 10 min for three doses followed by 25 or 50 mg orally every 6 hr) is often effective. In patients with atrial fibrillation and left ventricular failure in whom beta blockers are contraindicated, and who are not receiving maintenance digitalis therapy, digoxin 0.4 mg intravenously followed 4 hours later by another 0.2 to 0.4 mg is useful. In patients with severe hemodynamic compromise or ongoing ischemia, electrocardioversion beginning with 50 joules, with the energy gradually increased if the first shock is not successful, is indicated. Amiodarone, 200 mg/day for 6 weeks, is useful for suppressing recurrence of atrial fibrillation. Patients with recurrent atrial fibrillation should receive oral anticoagulants to prevent thromboembolism.

VENTRICULAR PREMATURE BEATS. These are detectable by monitoring in the vast majority of patients with AMI. Even if these beats are frequent, that is, more than 5 per minute of multiform configuration, occur in bigeminal rhythm, or if they occur early ("R on T"), prophylactic suppression with antiarrhythmic agents such as lidocaine or procainamide is not necessary when patients are closely monitored. Indeed, such prophylaxis may even be harmful. It is now considered best to treat such premature beats with intravenous beta blockers and to screen for and correct electrolyte or acid-base disturbances, hypoxemia, or heart failure.

ACCELERATED IDIOVENTRICULAR RHYTHM. A ventricular rhythm with a rate of 60 to 120 beats per minute (sometimes termed *slow ventricular tachycardia*) occurs during the first 2 days in 10% to 20% of patients with AMI. Accelerated idioventricular rhythm is especially common after successful reperfusion. Treatment with atropine or atrial pacing is indicated when the AV dissociation causes hemodynamic compromise.

VENTRICULAR TACHYCARDIA. This arrhythmia is classified as either nonsustained (<30 sec) or sustained (>30 sec) and as monomorphic or polymorphic. Sustained ventricular tachycardia, with a ventricular rate above 150 beats per minute that causes hypotension or other hemodynamic compromise, requires immediate therapy with electric countershock. When the tachycardia is polymorphic, it should be treated with an unsynchronized discharge of 200 joules, whereas monomorphic ventricular tachycardia should be treated with a synchronized discharge of 100 joules. The energy should be increased in 50-joule increments if the patient does not respond to the first shock. When the ventricular rate is slower than 150 beats per minute and the ventricular tachycardia is well tolerated hemodynamically, the following pharmacologic regimens may be employed:

1. **Lidocaine:** A bolus of 1.0 to 1.5 mg/kg followed by supplemental bolus injections of 0.5 to 0.75 mg/kg every 5 to 10 minutes to a maximum of 3 mg/kg followed by a maintenance infusion of 20 to 50 μg/kg/min. The dose should be reduced in older patients (>70 years). Patients with heart failure and hepatic dysfunction should have slower infusion rates of 10 to 20 μg/kg/min.
2. **Procainamide**: A loading infusion of 12 to 30 mg/min should be followed by a maintenance infusion of 1 to 4 mg/min.
3. **Amiodarone**: 75 to 150 mg infused over 10 minutes followed by an infusion of 1.0 mg/min for 6 hours and then reduced to 0.5 mg/min.

VENTRICULAR FIBRILLATION. Three major forms of ventricular fibrillation occur in patients with AMI. *Primary* ventricular fibrillation occurs early (<48 hr from the onset), suddenly, and unexpectedly in the absence of left ventricular failure. The incidence of this arrhythmia has declined strikingly during the past two decades. *Secondary* ventricular fibrillation usually also occurs early, but it is associated with (and secondary to) left ventricular failure and cardiogenic shock. *Late* ventricular fibrillation occurs more than 48 hours after MI and also frequently accompanies ventricular dysfunction. Primary ventricular fibrillation, even when treated successfully, may increase mortality during the hospital course, but the postdischarge prognosis is not altered. On the other hand, both secondary and late ventricular fibrillation are associated with a worse prognosis because they are associated with extensive myocardial damage.

Ventricular fibrillation should be treated as rapidly as possible with an unsynchronized electric shock of 200 to 300 joules. If unsuccessful, 300 to 400 joules should be used. If ventricular fibrillation persists, epinephrine (5 to 10 ml/1-1:10,000 intracardiac or 1 mg intravenously) is indicated. Additional adjunctive treatment includes intravenous lidocaine (1.5 mg/kg), bretylium (5 to 10 mg/kg), or amiodarone (75 to 150 mg bolus), or a combination. After defibrillation, patients should receive an intravenous beta blocker and infusion of an antiarrhythmic drug (lidocaine 2 mg/min, procainamide 1 to 4 mg/min, or amiodarone 1.0 mg/min for 6 hours followed by 0.5 mg/min) for 12 to 24 hours and then should be reassessed for the need for future therapy. Serum electrolytes should be measured; hypokalemia and hypomagnesemia should be treated as well.

Bradyarrhythmias

SINUS BRADYCARDIA. This arrhythmia occurs early in the course of infarction in about one-third of patients, and it is more common in patients with inferior or posterior infarction. Intravenous atropine should be administered if the heart rate is below 50 beats per minute, or if the heart rate is between 50 and 60 beats per minute and the patient is hypotensive or exhibits frequent ventricular ectopic beats. If the bradycardia persists despite atropine and the patient remains symptomatic or hypotensive, electric pacing is indicated.

FIRST-DEGREE AV BLOCK AND MOBITZ TYPE I SECOND-DEGREE AV BLOCK. Each of these arrhythmias occurs in approximately 10% of patients with AMI and generally does not require treatment, except for the discontinuation of drugs which interfere with AV conduction (digitalis, beta blockers, verapamil, diltiazem). Atropine is indicated in patients with Mobitz type I second-degree AV block and bradycardia (<50 beats/min) or hypotension.

MOBITZ TYPE II SECOND-DEGREE BLOCK AND THIRD-DEGREE AV BLOCK. When associated with anterior wall MI, these forms of heart block are usually characterized by wide QRS complexes. These patients are at high risk and should be treated with temporary transvenous pacing. AV sequential pacing should be employed when there is left ventricular failure (Table 19–11). When these forms of block are associated with inferior infarction, they are usually accompanied by ventricular rates above 40 beats per minute and narrow QRS complexes and are secondary to an intranodal lesion.[24] This latter form of block is usually transient and should be treated with atropine. If it fails to respond, temporary transvenous pacing should be employed.[25]

INTRAVENTRICULAR BLOCK. Block in a single division of the conduction system (left anterior divisional block, left posterior divisional block, or right bundle branch block) is associated with large infarcts and therefore with a higher mortality. Patients with such blocks require careful observation for the development of more advanced forms of block but no specific therapy. Bifascicular block (right bundle branch block with either left anterior or posterior divisional block or left bundle branch block) is usually secondary to extensive myocardial necrosis and should be managed initially with the application of transcutaneous pacing electrodes in a standby mode that will be activated if ventricular rate drops below a preset threshold. Although transcutaneous external temporary pacing is associated with discomfort, it can be employed for brief periods in patients at risk of developing high-degree AV block before a transvenous pacemaker is inserted.

Temporary transvenous ventricular pacing is carried out by inserting a pacing catheter percutaneously through the jugular, subclavian, or femoral veins and advancing it to the right ventricular apex. AV dual-chamber pacing is required in some patients to achieve hemodynamic compensation and requires insertion of a second catheter into the right atrial appendage. In patients with persistent third-degree or Mobitz type II second-degree AV block, permanent pacing is indicated.

Recurrent Chest Pain

Recurrent ischemia and acute pericarditis are the most important causes of recurrent chest discomfort. The first task is to distinguish between these two causes.

Recurrent Ischemia or Reinfarction

Recurrent ischemia or reinfarction occurs in approximately 25% of patients and is the most important cause of recurrent pain during the first 18 hours of AMI. This diagnosis is aided by the development or recurrence of ST segment and T-wave changes, usually in the same leads in which Q-waves appeared, and sometimes by re-elevation of CK-MB or other biochemical markers of myocardial necrosis.

Patients with recurrent ischemia should receive intravenous nitroglycerin and intravenous beta blockers, heparin, and aspirin (if they are not already receiving these drugs). Unless there are obvious contraindications to revascularization, such as a serious co-morbid condition, they should undergo urgent coronary arteriography and, depending on the anatomic findings, catheter-based or surgical revascularization.

Pericarditis (see Chap. 28)

This complication is observed most frequently 24 hours to 6 weeks after Q-wave MI and occurs in approximately 20% of patients.[26] Although the discomfort may resemble post-MI angina, it frequently radiates to the trapezius ridge and the left shoulder and becomes worse during deep inspiration. It is often but not uniformly associated with a pericardial friction rub, concave upward ST segment elevation and PR segment depression, and a pericardial effusion that can be detected by two-dimensional transthoracic echocardiography. The treatment of choice is aspirin, up to 650 mg four times daily.[2, 5] Corticosteroids and nonsteroidal anti-inflammatory drugs should be avoided, since these agents may interfere with myocardial healing. Patients with pericarditis receiving anticoagulants should be observed carefully for increasing pericardial effusion due to bleeding into the pericardial sac.

Cardiac Rupture

Rarely, recurrent pain may also be caused by cardiac rupture.[27] The risk factors for this catastrophic complication are infarcts that are first infarcts, anterior in location, and occurring in older patients (>70 years), in women, and in patients with a history of hypertension (see Table 19–10). This event is associated with cardiac tamponade and requires immediate pericardiocentesis and emergency surgical repair (see Chap. 28).

Table 19–11	Acute MI: Nonmedical Therapies	
Modality	**Indications**	**Comments**
Pulmonary artery (Swan-Ganz) catheterization	Hypotension unresponsive to fluids Unexplained tachycardia, tachypnea, hypoxemia, or acidosis Suspicion of ventricular septal rupture or acute mitral regurgitation Refractory pulmonary edema	Swan-Ganz allows determination of wedge pressure, cardiac output, and systemic vascular resistance, which can be used to distinguish cause of hypotension Selected hemodynamic subsets: RV infarction: ↑ RA pressure, RA/PCW pressure ratio > 0.9, ↓ CO Cardiogenic shock: ↓ BP, ↓ CO, ↑ PCW pressure, ↑ SVR Acute MR: ↑ PCW pressure (prominent V-wave may be seen); CO usually ↓ Acute VSD: ≥8% oxygen step-up from RA → RV and PA. CO calculations are falsely elevated (reflecting L → R shunting with ↑ pulmonary flow) Acute tamponade: ↓ BP, paradoxical pulse, RA ~ PCW pressure, ↓ CO; prominent X-descent may be seen on RA tracing. May need echo to distinguish from RV infarct Massive pulmonary embolism: ↓ BP, ↓ CO, ↑ PA pressure and PVR, normal PCW pressure
Temporary pacemaker Prophylactic	New LBBB Bifascicular block: RBBB with left anterior or left posterior fascicular block Alternating LBBB and RBBB	Prophylactic pacing (usually for 48–72 hr) is recommended to prevent hemodynamic collapse in the event that conduction delay progresses to 3° AV block Transcutaneous or transvenous leads are acceptable; transcutaneous leads are quickly placed and avoid bleeding complications if thrombolytics or anticoagulants have been given
Therapeutic	Asystole Mobitz II 2° AV block 3° AV block Bradycardia with hypotension	Transvenous lead is recommended; a transcutaneous lead may be needed until the transvenous lead is in place when hemodynamic or clinical instability is present Temporary pacing may not be required if bradycardia or 3° AV block occurs with inferior MI and resolves with atropine AV sequential pacing may be preferred over ventricular pacing in severe LV dysfunction/hypertrophy and RV infarction; optimization of AV synchrony ("atrial kick") may facilitate cardiac output

Modified from Grines, C.L.: Myocardial infarction. *In* Freed, M., and Grines, C. (eds.): Essentials of Cardiovascular Medicine. Birmingham, MI: Physicians' Press, 1994, pp. 112–113.

Abbreviations: MI, myocardial infarction; RV, right ventricular; RA, right atrial; PCW, pulmonary capillary wedge; CO, cardiac output; BP, blood pressure; SVR, systemic vascular resistance; MR, mitral regurgitation; VSD, ventricular septal defect; PA, pulmonary artery; L → R, left-to-right; PVR, pulmonary vascular resistance; LBBB, left bundle branch block; RBBB, right bundle branch block; 3°, third-degree; AV, atrioventricular; 2°, second-degree; LV, left ventricular.

PHARMACOTHERAPY

Beta-Adrenergic Blockers

These drugs diminish myocardial oxygen consumption by reducing heart rate, arterial blood pressure, and myocardial contractility. Several multicenter trials have shown the benefits of early treatment, that is, less than 4 hours after onset of pain, with intravenous beta blockade followed by oral therapy. Patients who present later can be begun on oral therapy that is usually continued for an indefinite period (Fig. 19–14).

When given intravenously in the acute stage, beta blocker therapy has been shown to reduce the rate of development of definite MI, infarct size, and the incidence of tachyarrhythmias, sudden death, and total mortality.[28] When administered chronically, these drugs reduce the incidence of reinfarction, sudden death, and total mortality. Contraindications to beta blockers are shown in Table 19–12. If complications such as heart failure, heart block, or bronchospasm develop, beta blockers should be withdrawn or their dose decreased until complications resolve.

Two useful regimens are intravenous atenolol 5 to 10 mg followed by oral atenolol 100 mg daily, or metoprolol 15 mg intravenously in three divided doses, followed by 100 mg orally twice a day.

ACE Inhibitors

By lowering ventricular afterload and preload, ACE inhibitors reduce the incidence of congestive heart failure, ventricular dilatation, and remodeling. These drugs appear to be useful when administered for 1 month, beginning as early as 1 day after infarction.[29] When continued for several years, they improve clinical outcome in patients with left ventricular dysfunction and heart failure.[30]

In the absence of contraindications (hypotension, known hypersensitivity, bilateral renal artery stenosis, and possible pregnancy), an oral ACE inhibitor should be

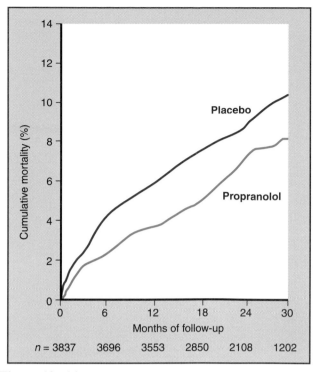

Figure 19-14

Survival after acute myocardial infarction: The BHAT trial. Life-table cumulative mortality curves for propranolol hydrochloride and placebo groups. n, total number of patients followed-up through each time point. (Redrawn from β-Blocker Heart Attack Study Group. The β-blocker heart attack trial. JAMA 246:2073–2074, 1981.)

given to all hemodynamically stable AMI patients with ST segment elevation. ACE inhibitor therapy should be begun within the first 24 hours, after reperfusion therapy has been completed and the blood pressure has stabilized. Left ventricular function should be evaluated before hospital discharge, and ACE inhibition should be continued for an indefinite period in patients with heart failure, with prior infarction, with evidence of a reduced ejection fraction (< 40%), or with large regional wall motion abnormalities. In patients without any of these features at the

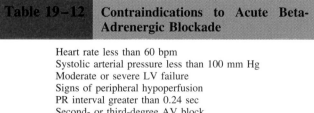

Table 19-12	Contraindications to Acute Beta-Adrenergic Blockade

Heart rate less than 60 bpm
Systolic arterial pressure less than 100 mm Hg
Moderate or severe LV failure
Signs of peripheral hypoperfusion
PR interval greater than 0.24 sec
Second- or third-degree AV block
Severe chronic obstructive pulmonary disease
History of asthma
Severe peripheral vascular disease
Insulin-dependent diabetes mellitus

Reprinted from *Journal of the American College of Cardiology*, Vol. 28, Ryan, T.J., Anderson, J.L., Antman, E.M., et al.: ACC/AHA Guidelines for the Management of Patients with Acute Myocardial Infarction, pp. 1328–1428, Copyright 1996, with permission from the American College of Cardiology.
Abbreviations: LV, left ventricular; AV, atrioventricular.

time of hospital discharge, the ACE inhibitor may be discontinued. A number of regimens—such as lisinopril 5 mg/day for 2 days and then 10 mg daily, or trandolapril 2 mg/day for 2 days followed by 4 mg/day—may be employed.

Nitroglycerin

This drug exerts favorable pharmacologic actions by reducing right and left ventricular preload and afterload and causes coronary vasodilatation. There is no clear-cut evidence that the routine administration of nitroglycerin is beneficial in patients with uncomplicated MI who receive thrombolytic therapy. However, intravenous nitroglycerin (5 to 10 μg/min, up to 150 μg/min as long as hemodynamic stability is maintained) is the drug of choice with the recurrence of angina. It is especially useful in nonhypotensive patients with left ventricular failure and may be used for 24 to 48 hours in patients with large Q-wave anterior wall MIs to reduce ventricular remodeling and dilatation. It may then be continued orally or topically for 4 to 6 days in these patients.

Calcium Antagonists

These drugs have not been shown to reduce mortality in AMI.[28] Indeed, since it has been suggested that immediate-release nifedipine is associated with a dose-related increased risk of in-hospital mortality, this drug should *not* be used in patients with AMI. Verapamil (240 to 480 mg/day in divided doses or once daily with sustained release) or diltiazem (120 to 360 mg daily in three or four doses or once daily with sustained release) may be useful in controlling attacks of recurrent ischemia or atrial fibrillation in patients without heart failure or AV block.

POST-MI RISK STRATIFICATION

Risk stratification before hospital discharge is an important aspect of management and determines whether coronary angiography is indicated.[31] The first step is to determine whether the *clinical* variables indicating a relatively high risk for future cardiac events are present (Fig. 19-15A). Patients who have had recurrent ischemia at rest or with mild activity, who have had evidence of congestive heart failure, or who are known to have an ejection fraction below 40%, and in whom there are no contraindications for revascularization, should undergo cardiac catheterization and coronary arteriography. Revascularization should then be carried out if the coronary anatomy is suitable and there are no contraindications. Patients who have had an episode of ventricular fibrillation or sustained ventricular tachycardia more than 48 hours after AMI should be considered for electrophysiologic study or amiodarone therapy, or both. Coronary angiography is often performed routinely 1 to 2 days after admission in patients with non-Q-wave MI or unstable angina (see Chap. 20) who appear on clinical grounds to be candidates for coronary revascularization, and who are cared for in cardiac centers. Revascularization may then

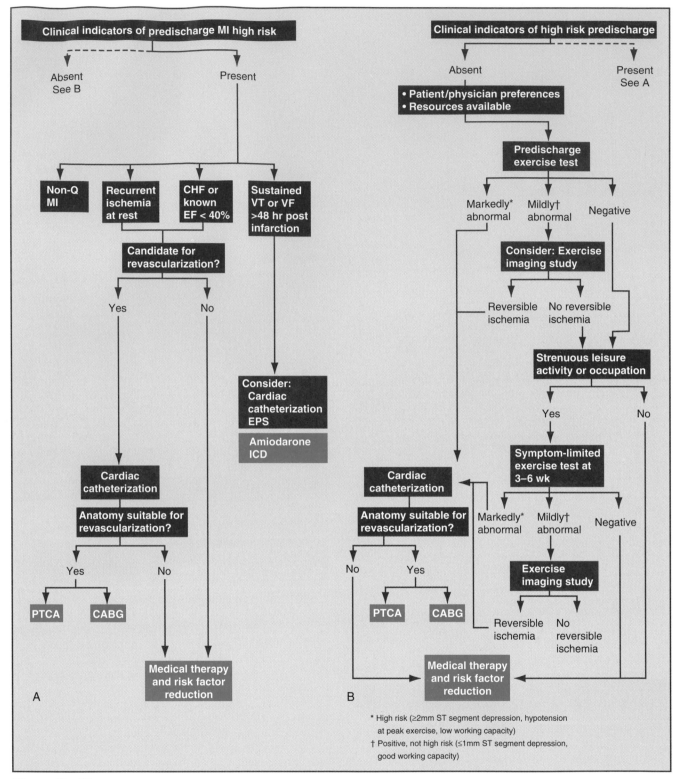

Figure 19–15

Management algorithm for risk stratification after acute myocardial infarction (MI). *A,* Patients with clinical indicators of high risk at hospital discharge, such as recurrent ischemia at rest or depressed left ventricular function, should be considered candidates for revascularization and referral to cardiac catheterization for ultimate triage to either percutaneous transluminal coronary angioplasty (PTCA)/coronary artery bypass graft surgery (CABG) or medical therapy and risk factor reduction. Patients with life-threatening arrhythmias, such as sustained ventricular tachycardia (VT) or ventricular fibrillation (VF), should be considered for diagnostic cardiac catheterization, electrophysiology study (EPS), and management with either amiodarone or an implantable cardioverter-defibrillator (ICD), or both. CHF, congestive heart failure; EF, ejection fraction. *B,* Patients without indicators of high risk at hospital discharge can be evaluated either with a submaximal exercise test prior to discharge (at 5 to 7 days) or with a symptom-limited exercise test at 14 to 21 days. Patients with either a markedly abnormal exercise test or no evidence of reversible ischemia on an exercise imaging study can be managed with medical therapy and risk factor reduction. (*A* and *B,* From Antman, E.M., and Braunwald, E.: Acute myocardial infarction. *In* Braunwald, E. [ed.]: Heart Disease. 5th ed. Philadelphia, W.B. Saunders, 1997, p. 1262.)

be carried out if the coronary anatomy is appropriate. Although this approach has not been shown to reduce mortality, it does reduce the incidence of postdischarge ischemia and the subsequent need for antianginal medications. Other high-risk patients should receive medical therapy (see later) and risk factor reduction.

Patients without these clinical indicators of high risk should undergo an assessment of left ventricular function (echocardiogram or radionuclide angiogram and submaximal stress test) before hospital discharge (see Fig. 19–15B). In patients who have an interpretable ECG and who can exercise, a submaximal exercise test (see Chap. 4) is suitable. If the test is negative, they may return for a symptom-limited exercise test at 3 to 6 weeks. If that too is negative, they can remain on medical therapy and risk factor reduction. On the other hand, if the resting ejection fraction is under 40% or the stress test is markedly abnormal (>2 mm ST segment depression, hypotension at peak exercise, or low working capacity) (see Chap. 4), and there are no obvious contraindications to revascularization, coronary angiography should be carried out. In patients in whom the ECG is uninterpretable because of resting ST–T-wave abnormalities, digitalis therapy, or left bundle branch block, rest and exercise radionuclide myocardial perfusion scintigraphy (with thallium or sestamibi) or rest and exercise echocardiography should be performed. Patients who cannot exercise should undergo a pharmacologic stress imaging study such as adenosine or dipyridamole myocardial perfusion scintigraphy or echocardiography with dobutamine or dipyridamole stress.[32] A marked abnormality in any of these tests, or a resting ejection fraction below 40%, measured by echocardiography or a radionuclide technique, should be followed by coronary angiography.

Ambulatory ECG monitoring (Holter monitoring) for ischemia or arrhythmia was widely employed in the past, but it is not recommended for routine management. It may be useful in patients who have experienced symptomatic arrhythmias.

POSTDISCHARGE CARE

The primary care physician plays a critical role in postdischarge care and in the prevention of reinfarction. Perhaps most important is education regarding the nature of coronary artery disease and the risk factors for recurrent infarction. Lifestyle modifications are of paramount importance. These include smoking cessation; it should be emphasized to the patient that within 2 years of discontinuing smoking, the risk of a nonfatal recurrent MI falls to the level observed in patients who never smoked.

Cardiac Rehabilitation

This includes an organized program of exercise training and education about coronary risk factor modification, an American Heart Association step I diet, smoking cessation, and weight optimization. These measures have been shown to improve the quality of life, reduce ischemic symptoms, and lower the incidence of subsequent coro-

nary events.[33, 34] Because mortality is higher in patients after AMI without social support, every effort should be made to provide such support. This includes not only strengthening family ties but also encouraging participation in group activities and, whenever possible, return to work. Unless the patient is limited by symptoms of ischemia or heart failure, physical activity should be encouraged on hospital discharge. Physical conditioning programs should be undertaken; level walking, biking, and light calisthenics should be increased progressively. A negative, symptom-limited stress test at 3 to 6 weeks after discharge can be taken as a signal to increase physical activities to include swimming, rapid walking, and jogging. It is useful for the exercise to be undertaken as part of an organized rehabilitation program that includes instruction in diet, achievement of optimal weight, and smoking cessation. In patients with a mildly abnormal symptom-limited exercise test at 3 to 6 weeks, physical activity should be encouraged, but not to the level that will regularly provoke symptoms of ischemia.

Hypertension

It is imperative to treat post-MI hypertension. In view of the long-term benefits of ACE inhibitors and beta blockers in these patients, this combination of antihypertensive drugs is preferred. A third agent, usually a diuretic, is added if hypertension persists despite treatment with the combination. The major long-term side effect of ACE inhibitors is cough, and if it develops, the dose may be reduced (e.g., lisinopril 10 mg to 5 mg). The major side effects of long-term beta-adrenergic blockers are fatigue, depression, and sexual dysfunction.

Lipid-Lowering Therapy

(see Chap. 29)

A lipid profile should be obtained on all patients with MI. Since cholesterol levels may fall after 24 to 48 hours, it is important that these measurements be obtained on admission, otherwise a 6-week wait is necessary for the cholesterol to reach pre-MI levels. It is desirable to fractionate the cholesterol, and in patients who have a low-density lipoprotein (LDL) cholesterol exceeding 125 mg/dl, treatment with cholesterol-lowering therapy should be employed. The National Cholesterol Education Program has suggested that the target LDL be below 100 mg/dl.[35] Diet is a mandatory component of cholesterol lowering with the American Heart Association step I diet. Two large randomized trials, the Scandinavian Simvastatin Survival Study (4S)[36] and the Cholesterol and Recurrent Events (CARE)[37] trials have shown that the incidence of recurrent coronary events can be reduced with statin therapy in post-MI patients and these drugs are very helpful in achieving reductions of cholesterol in patients with LDL levels exceeding 125 mg/dl.

Medical Therapy

The greatest mortality benefit from chronic beta blockade is observed in patients with impaired ventricular function and ventricular arrhythmias. In the absence of contraindications (Table 19–12), beta blockers should be continued indefinitely in patients with confirmed MI. Aspirin 160 or 325 mg/day should also be continued indefinitely. Treatment with an ACE inhibitor for an indefinite period is recommended in patients with evidence of congestive heart failure, an ejection fraction below 40%, or a large regional wall motion abnormality.

Although epidemiologic studies suggest that increased intake of vitamin E is associated with a reduction in cardiovascular events, there is not sufficient evidence at this point to recommend vitamin E supplementation in patients post-MI.

The widespread use of aspirin has greatly diminished the need for warfarin in the post-MI patient. At the present time, the latter is limited to secondary prevention of infarction in patients who are unable to take aspirin, to those with persistent or paroxysmal atrial fibrillation or a documented left ventricular thrombus, or to those with extensive wall motion abnormality.

Estrogen replacement should be considered in postmenopausal women after MI *without* greater than usual risks of breast cancer (a family history of breast cancer). Such therapy improves the lipid profile, and epidemiologic observational studies have shown a reduction in coronary events.[38] Postmenopausal women who have had a hysterectomy are usually treated with 0.625 mg oral conjugated estrogen daily. In those who have a uterus, a combination of estrogen and progestin therapy is employed.

Class I *antiarrhythmic drugs* should *not* be used routinely prophylactically in post-MI patients with frequent and complex ventricular ectopy. Patients with severe *symptomatic* ventricular tachyarrhythmias should be treated with beta blockers, undergo screening for provokable ischemia, and be considered for specialized procedures such as implantation of antitachycardia devices or ablation of arrhythmogenic foci (see Chap. 23).

References

1. Heart and Stroke Facts. 1997 Statistical Supplement. Dallas, American Heart Association.
2. Antman, E.M., and Braunwald, E.: Acute myocardial infarction. *In* Braunwald, E. (ed.): Heart Disease. 5th ed. Philadelphia, W.B. Saunders, 1997, pp. 1184–1288.
3. Adams, J., Abendschein, D., and Jaffe, A.: Biochemical markers of myocardial injury: Is MB creatine kinase the choice for the 1990s? Circulation 88:750, 1993.
4. National Heart Attack Alert Program Coordinating Committee, 60 minutes to Treatment Working Group: Emergency department: Rapid identification and treatment of patients with acute myocardial infarction. Ann. Emerg. Med. 23:311, 1994.
5. Ryan, T.J., Anderson, J.L., Antman, E.M., et al.: ACC/AHA guidelines for the management of patients with acute myocardial infarction. J. Am. Coll. Cardiol. 28:1328, 1996.
6. Weaver, W.D., Hill, D., Fahrenbruch, C.E., et al.: Use of the automatic external defibrillator in the management of out-of-hospital cardiac arrest. N. Engl. J. Med. 319:661, 1988.
7. The European Myocardial Infarction Project Group: Prehospital thrombolytic therapy in patients with suspected acute myocardial infarction. N. Engl. J. Med. 329:383, 1993.
8. Fuster, V., Dyken, M.L., Vokonas, P.S., and Hennekens, C.: Aspirin as a therapeutic agent in cardiovascular disease. Circulation 87:659, 1993.
9. Fibrinolytic Therapy Trialists (FTT) Collaborative Group: Indications for fibrinolytic therapy in suspected acute myocardial infarction: Collaborative overview of early mortality and major morbidity results from all randomised trials of more than 1000 patients. Lancet 343:311, 1994.
10. Simoons, M.L., Maggioni, A.P., Knatterud, G., et al.: Individual risk assessment for intracranial hemorrhage during thrombolytic therapy. Lancet 342:1523, 1993.
11. Martin, G.V., and Kennedy, J.W.: Choice of thrombolytic agent. *In* Julian, D.G., and Braunwald, E. (eds.): Management of Acute Myocardial Infarction. London, W.B. Saunders, 1994, p. 71.
12. White, H.D.: Selecting a thrombolytic agent. Cardiol. Clin. 13:347, 1995.
13. The GUSTO Investigators: An international randomized trial comparing four thrombolytic strategies for acute myocardial infarction. N. Engl. J. Med. 329:673, 1993.
14. Michels, K.B., and Yusuf, S.: Does PTCA in acute myocardial infarction affect mortality and reinfarction rates? A quantitative overview (meta analysis) of the randomized clinical trials. Circulation 91:476, 1995.
15. Libby, P.: Atherosclerosis. *In* Fauci, A., Braunwald, E., Isselbacher, K., et al. (eds.): Harrison's Principles of Internal Medicine. 14th ed. New York, McGraw-Hill, 1998, pp. 1345–1352.
16. Antman, E.M.: General hospital management. *In* Julian, D.G., and Braunwald, E. (eds.): Management of Acute Myocardial Infarction. London, W.B. Saunders, 1994, p. 42.
17. Parsons, R.W., Jamrozik, K.D., Hobbs, M.S., and Thompson, P.L.: Early identification of patients at low risk of death after myocardial infarction and potentially suitable for early hospital discharge. BMJ 308:1006, 1994.
18. Duryee, R.: The efficacy of inpatient education after myocardial infarction. Heart Lung 21:217, 1992.
19. Hochman, J.S., Boland, J., Sleeper, L.A., et al.: Current spectrum of cardiogenic shock and effect of early revascularization on mortality: Results of an international registry. SHOCK Registry Investigators. Circulation 91:873, 1995.
20. Weber, K.T., and Janicki, J.S.: Intraaortic balloon counterpulsation: A review of physiologic principles, clinical results and device safety. Ann. Thorac. Surg. 17:602, 1994.
21. Kinch, J.W., and Ryan, T.J.: Right ventricular infarction. N. Engl. J. Med. 330:1211, 1994.
22. Campbell, R.W.F.: Arrhythmias in acute myocardial infarction. *In* Julian, D.G., and Braunwald, E. (eds.): Management of Acute Myocardial Infarction. London, W.B. Saunders, 1994, p. 223.
23. Behar, S., Zahavi, Z., Goldbourt, U., and Reicher-Reiss, H.: Long-term prognosis of patients with paroxysmal atrial fibrillation complicating acute myocardial infarction. SPRINT Study Group. Eur. Heart J. 13:45, 1992.
24. Berger, P.B., Ruocco, N.A., Jr., Ryan, T.J., et al.: Incidence and prognostic implications of heart block complicating inferior myocardial infarction treated with thrombolytic therapy: Results from TIMI 11. J. Am. Coll. Cardiol. 20:533, 1992.
25. Wood, M.A.: Temporary transvenous pacing. *In* Ellenbogen, K.A., Kay, G.N., and Wilkoff, B.L. (eds.): Clinical Cardiac Pacing. Philadelphia, Lippincott-Raven, 1996.
26. Tofler, G.H., Muller, J.E., Stone, P.H., et al.: Pericarditis in acute myocardial infarction: Characterization and clinical significance. Am. Heart J. 117:86, 1989.
27. Becker, R.C., Gore, J.M., Lambrew, C., et al.: A composite view of cardiac rupture in the United States National Registry of Myocardial Infarction. J. Am. Coll. Cardiol. 27:1321, 1996.
28. Held, P.H., and Yusuf, S.: Effects of beta-blockers and calcium channel blockers in acute myocardial infarction. Eur. Heart J. 14(Suppl F):18, 1993.
29. Latini, R., Maggioni, A.P., Flather, M., et al.: ACE inhibitor use in patients with myocardial infarction: Summary of evidence from clinical trials. Circulation 92:3132, 1995.
30. Pfeffer, M.A., Braunwald, E., Moye, L.A., et al.: Effect of captopril on mortality and morbidity in patients with left ventricular dysfunction after myocardial infarction: Results of the Survival and Ventricular Enlargement trial—The SAVE Investigators. N. Engl. J. Med. 327:669, 1992.
31. Peterson, E.D., Shaw, L.J., Califf, R.M.: Risk stratification after myocardial infarction. Ann. Intern. Med. 126:561, 1997.
32. van Daele, M.E., McNeil, A.J., Fioretti, P.M., et al.: Prognostic value of dipyridamole sestamibi single-photon emission computed tomography and dypyridamole stress echocardiography for new cardiac events after an uncomplicated myocardial infarction. J. Am. Soc. Echocardiogr. 7:370, 1994.
33. Oldridge, N.B., Guyatt, G.H., Fischer, M.E., and Rimm, A.A.:

Cardiac rehabilitation after myocardial infarction: Combined experience of randomized clinical trials. JAMA 260:945, 1988.

34. Dennis, C.: Rehabilitation of patients with coronary artery disease. *In* Braunwald, E. (ed.): Heart Disease. 5th ed. Philadelphia, W.B. Saunders, 1997, pp. 1392–1403.

35. National Cholesterol Education Program: Second report of the Expert Panel on Detection, Evaluation, and Treatment of High Blood Cholesterol in Adults. Adult Treatment Panel II. Circulation 89:1329, 1994.

36. Scandinavian Simvastatin Survival Study Group: Randomised trial of cholesterol lowering in 4444 patients with coronary heart disease: The Scandinavian Simvastatin Survival Study (4S). Lancet 344:1383, 1994.

37. Sacks, F.M., Pfeffer, M.A., Moye, L.A., et al., for the CARE Investigators: The effect of pravastatin on coronary events after myocardial infarction in patients with average cholesterol levels. N. Engl. J. Med. 335:1001, 1996.

38. Kafonek, S.D.: Postmenopausal hormone replacement therapy and cardiovascular risk education: A review. Drugs 47(Suppl 2):16, 1994.

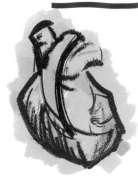

Chapter 20

Recognition and Management of Patients with

Unstable Angina

EUGENE BRAUNWALD

CLINICAL MANIFESTATIONS

Clinical coronary artery disease includes a wide spectrum of conditions, ranging from acute, Q-wave myocardial infarction at one end to chronic stable angina at the other. Unstable angina is at the center of this spectrum.[1] This condition has features common to both acute infarction and chronic angina and was previously termed the *intermediate coronary syndrome*. Since acute myocardial infarction is frequently preceded by a prodrome of unstable angina, the latter has also been referred to as *preinfarction angina*.

Patients with unstable angina represent an increasing fraction of those hospitalized with acute coronary syndrome (unstable angina plus acute myocardial infarction). Unstable angina is responsible for approximately 600,000 hospital admissions and more than 3 million patient-days in the United States each year. Patients with this diagnosis are characterized by one or more of three features (Table 20–1): (1) angina at rest; (2) increasing or crescendo angina—angina that is more severe, prolonged, or frequent—superimposed on a pattern of chronic stable angina; and (3) angina of new onset (<2 months) that is severe (Canadian Classification III or IV) and brought on by minimal exertion.

Ischemic pain at rest also occurs in Prinzmetal's variant angina, but this condition is pathogenetically and clinically distinct from the usual forms of unstable angina and is discussed separately (see p. 294). As noted previously, new onset of angina qualifies as unstable angina only if it is severe; the new onset of chronic angina that is mild to moderate in severity (Canadian Classification I or II) is *not* considered to be unstable angina.

Since unstable angina is a heterogeneous condition, a classification based on four important features (Table 20–2) has been devised:[2] (1) the severity of the clinical manifestations, ranging from new-onset or accelerated angina (the mildest) to acute angina at rest (the most severe); (2) the clinical circumstances that have precipitated the unstable angina, ranging from unstable angina secondary to an extracardiac cause (the mildest) to post–myocardial infarction angina (the most serious); (3) the presence or absence of transient electrocardiographic changes during the ischemic episodes; and (4) the intensity of anti-ischemic therapy at the time that the unstable angina occurs. A number of prospective studies have shown that both the incidence of adverse outcomes (death or myocardial infarction) and the severity of obstructive disease found at coronary arteriography correlate with the higher classes of severity and clinical circumstances.[3] Patients in class IIIC (post–myocardial infarction patients with rest pain) who develop transient ST segment changes despite intensive anti-ischemic therapy have the worst prognosis, whereas those in class IA (patients with an extracardiac condition that leads to accelerated angina but who have no rest pain) who are not receiving anti-ischemic therapy and without electrocardiographic changes have the best outlook.

Pathophysiology

A large majority of patients with unstable angina have obstructive coronary artery disease, with the unstable state

Table 20–1	Principal Presentations of Unstable Angina
Rest angina	Angina occurring at rest and within a week of presentation for medical care; usually lasts >20 min
New-onset angina	Angina of at least CCSC III severity with onset within 2 mo of initial presentation
Increasing angina	Previously diagnosed angina that is distinctly more frequent, longer in duration, or lower in threshold (i.e., increased by at least one CCSC class within 2 mo of initial presentation to at least CCSC III severity)

From Archibald, N.D., and Jones, R.H.: Guidelines for treatment of unstable angina. *In* Califf, R.M. (vol. ed.): Acute Myocardial Infarction and Other Ischemic Syndromes. Braunwald, E. (ser. ed.): Atlas of Heart Diseases. Vol. 8. Philadelphia, Current Medicine, 1996.
Abbreviation: CCSC, Canadian Cardiovascular Society Classification.

usually precipitated by an increase in coronary obstruction and, therefore, a reduction in oxygen supply. The increase in obstruction may be caused by greater encroachment on the coronary lumen by the gradual enlargement of atherosclerotic plaques, but more commonly, one or more of three other processes are operative:[1, 4]

1. Fissuring of an atherosclerotic plaque causing exposure of the subendothelium to platelets (Figs. 20–1 and 20–2). Glycoprotein receptors IIa/IIb on plate-

Table 20–2	Classification of Unstable Angina

Severity

Class I	New-onset, severe, or accelerated angina
	Patients with angina of less than 2 months' duration, severe or occurring three or more times per day, or angina that is distinctly more frequent and precipitated by distinctly less exertion; no rest pain in the last 2 mo
Class II	Angina at rest; subacute
	Patients with one or more episodes of angina at rest during the preceding month but not within the preceding 48 hr
Class III	Angina at rest; acute
	Patients with one or more episodes at rest within the preceding 48 hr

Clinical Circumstances

Class A	Secondary unstable angina
	A clearly identified condition extrinsic to the coronary vascular bed that has intensified myocardial ischemia, e.g., anemia, infection, fever, hypotension, tachyarrhythmia, thyrotoxicosis, hypoxemia secondary to respiratory failure
Class B	Primary unstable angina
Class C	Postinfarction unstable angina (within 2 wk of documented myocardial infarction)

Electrocardiogram

Without/with transient ST segment deviations or T-wave changes

Intensity of Treatment

1. Absence of treatment or minimal treatment
2. Occurring in presence of standard therapy for chronic stable angina (conventional doses of oral beta blockers, nitrates, and calcium antagonists)
3. Occurring despite maximally tolerated doses of all three categories of oral therapy, including intravenous nitroglycerin.

Adapted from Braunwald, E.: Unstable angina: A classification. Circulation 80:410, 1989.

lets bind them to fibrinogen and cause their aggregation.
2. An active thrombotic process caused by the coagulation cascade that is triggered by thrombin and that leads to fibrin formation.[5] Thrombi are recognized as typical filling defects at coronary arteriography in approximately one-third of patients with unstable angina (Fig. 20–3).[6] Thrombi have also been noted at coronary angioscopy in a large fraction of the remainder.[7]
3. Coronary vasoconstriction caused by an increase in neurogenically mediated coronary vascular tone or endothelial dysfunction that prevents the release of coronary vasodilators such as prostacyclin or nitric oxide.

Since inhibition of platelet aggregation by aspirin, interference with clot formation by heparin, and the administration of coronary vasodilators, such as nitrates and calcium antagonists, are all effective therapeutic measures in unstable angina,[8] it is likely that all three factors are involved.

The culprit lesion in a coronary artery responsible for the development of unstable angina is usually a subtotal coronary occlusion that causes severe ischemia but not necrosis;[6] alternatively, unstable angina may be caused by coronary occlusion, but the presence of collateral vessels may prevent the development of infarction. It has been postulated that vasoconstriction, most likely of the coronary microvasculature, is responsible for ischemia in the approximately 15% of patients with unstable angina without obstructive epicardial coronary artery disease.

Clinical and Laboratory Findings

Like chronic stable angina, unstable angina occurs in both women and men, most often in the sixth to eighth decades of life, who have one or more of the major risk factors for coronary atherosclerosis (hypertension, hyperlipidemia, cigarette smoking, or diabetes mellitus). In unstable angina, the chest discomfort resembles that observed in chronic angina (see Chaps. 7 and 18), but it is usually more severe and is more likely to be referred to as "pain." The threshold of activity causing anginal discomfort is lower in unstable angina than it is in stable angina, and sometimes angina occurs at rest or awakens the patient from sleep.[1] In unstable angina, the episodes of pain occur with increased frequency, usually last longer—up to 30 minutes—and the pain generally radiates more widely. Unstable angina, like myocardial infarction, may be accompanied by dyspnea, presumably due to impaired function of a large segment of the left ventricle. Brief episodes of pain (several seconds), lancinating or darting pain, or pain that is continuous for more than 1 hour is rarely unstable angina.

ELECTROCARDIOGRAM. In the interval between episodes of ischemia, the electrocardiogram (ECG) may be normal, it may exhibit nonspecific ST segment or T-wave changes, or it may show the Q-waves of a prior myocardial infarction.[8] During ischemic pain, ST segment

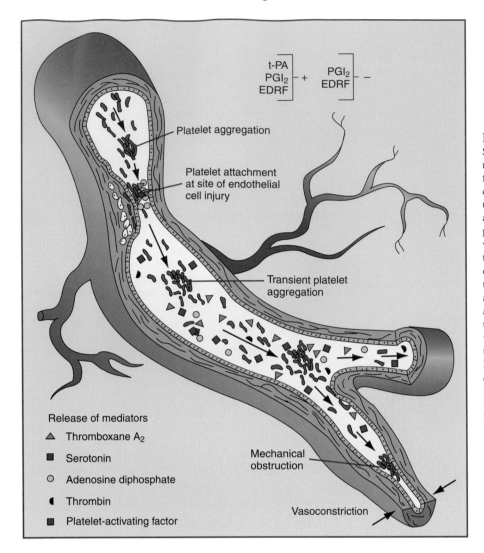

Figure 20-1
Schematic diagram suggesting probable mechanisms responsible for the conversion from chronic coronary heart disease to acute coronary artery disease syndromes, including unstable angina. Endothelial injury, usually at sites of atherosclerotic plaques with plaque ulceration or fissuring, is associated with platelet adhesion and aggregation; and the release and activation of selected mediators—including thromboxane A_2, serotonin, platelet-activating factor, thrombin, or adenosine diphosphate—promote platelet aggregation. Thromboxane A_2, serotonin, thrombin, and platelet-activating factor are vasoconstrictors at sites of endothelial injury. t-PA, tissue-type plasminogen activator; PGI_2, prostaglandin I_2; EDRF, endothelium-derived relaxing factor. (Redrawn from Willerson, J.T., and Cohn, J.N. [eds.]: Cardiovascular Medicine. New York, Churchill Livingstone, 1995, p. 335.)

deviations or T-wave changes frequently occur. The latter changes are usually transient; their persistence for more than 12 hours suggests that non–Q-wave myocardial infarction has occurred. The diagnostic significance of ST segment and T-wave changes is greater if they are not present on a tracing before or subsequent to the pain. Both are of diagnostic value, but only ST segment deviation is a marker of increased risk of an adverse clinical event (death or myocardial infarction).[9]

CORONARY ARTERIOGRAPHY. When critical coronary artery obstruction is defined as more than 70% stenosis of the luminal diameter of one or more of the three major arteries and more than 50% of the left main coronary artery, three-vessel coronary artery disease is found in approximately 40% of patients with unstable angina, two-vessel disease in 20%, one-vessel disease in 15%, left main coronary artery disease in 10%, and no critical obstruction in the remaining 15%. The culprit lesions in unstable angina are often eccentric, with scalloped or overhanging edges, reflecting a disrupted atherosclerotic plaque or partially lysed thrombus (see Fig. 20–3).[1, 4, 6]

Ventricular function, measured by contrast or radionuclide ventriculography or echocardiography, may be permanently impaired in patients with previous myocardial infarction or those who show transient impairment during and after episodes of ischemia.

EXERCISE TESTING. Exercise testing can be carried out safely after stabilization of symptoms and is of prognostic value. The prognosis is best in the approximately one-third of patients with a normal exercise ECG or myocardial perfusion scintigram. In contrast, a "high-risk" exercise stress test or perfusion scintigram (see Chap. 7) defines a group of patients in whom subsequent fatal events, myocardial infarction, or failure of medical therapy is high. Patients with positive tests that are not deemed high risk have an intermediate prognosis.

OTHER LABORATORY TESTS. The release into the circulation of biochemical markers of myocardial cell injury—such as creatine kinase (CK) and its MB isoenzyme (CK-MB), troponin T, troponin I, and myoglobin—signifies the presence of cell injury and myocyte necrosis, that is, the diagnosis of non–Q-wave myocardial infarc-

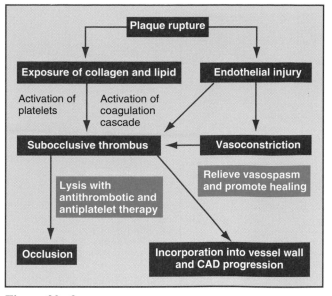

Figure 20–2

Consequences and management of rupture of an atherosclerotic plaque. CAD, coronary artery disease. (Redrawn from Langer, A., and Armstrong, P.W.: Treatment of acute ischemic syndromes in the absence of coronary occlusion: Preventing progression to acute occlusion. *In* Califf, R.M. [vol. ed.]: Acute Myocardial Infarction and Other Ischemic Syndromes. Braunwald, E. [ser. ed.]: Atlas of Heart Diseases. Vol. 8. Philadelphia, Current Medicine, 1996.)

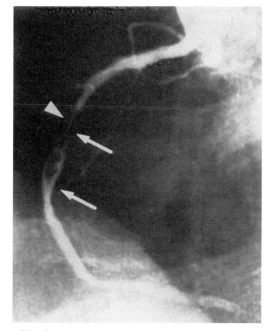

Figure 20–3

Intracoronary thrombus in unstable angina. This left anterior oblique right coronary arteriogram shows a severe stenosis in the midportion of the right coronary artery *(arrowhead)*, followed by a large filling defect surrounded by contrast medium on all sides *(arrows)*. (From Bittl, J.A., and Levin, D.C.: Coronary arteriography. *In* Braunwald, E. [ed.]: Heart Disease. 5th ed. Philadelphia, W.B. Saunders, 1997, p. 266.)

tion rather than unstable angina. Release of either troponin is associated with a higher risk of an adverse outcome.[10]

Natural History

The risk of death in unstable angina is intermediate between those of stable angina and acute myocardial infarction.[8] In one registry of patients considered to have unstable angina, approximately 20% "ruled in" for non–Q-wave myocardial infarction. Of the remainder, 2.5% died during the subsequent 6 weeks and another 3% developed a new myocardial infarction.[11] In patients with unstable angina who stabilized on medical therapy, almost 60% developed an adverse coronary event (myocardial infarction or a repeated episode of unstable angina) during an 8-month period.[1, 4] Older patients and those with significant ST segment changes on the ECG are at higher risk of an adverse outcome.

MANAGEMENT

In 1994, the Agency for Health Care Policy and Research developed practice guidelines for the treatment of unstable angina (Fig. 20–4).[8]

Initial Therapy

Patients with symptoms suggesting unstable angina should be evaluated by a physician immediately. The first step is to obtain a directed history, carry out a directed physical examination, and obtain a 12-lead ECG—if possible while the patient is experiencing pain—in order to estimate the likelihood of the presence of significant coronary artery disease (Table 20–3). A history of prior myocardial infarction, definite angina, or the presence of ST segment deviations or marked T-wave changes during pain make the likelihood of coronary artery disease high. The risk of death or nonfatal myocardial infarction should then be determined (Table 20–4). Prolonged pain at rest and the presence of unstable angina with evidence of left ventricular failure (hypotension, rales, or transient mitral regurgitation) place the patient at high risk.

In patients at high or intermediate risk of coronary artery disease, therapy should be begun wherever the patient is first encountered, that is, in the emergency department or in the physician's office.[12] Patients who have ongoing chest pain should be placed at bedrest and given supplemental oxygen. Unless there is a contraindication, they should be started on aspirin as well as anti-ischemic therapy with beta blockers and sublingual nitroglycerin tablets (Table 20–5). After initial treatment and stabilization in the emergency department, patients at high risk for adverse outcomes (see Table 20–4) should be transferred to an intensive care unit, whereas patients at intermediate risk may be in a regular bed with electrocardiographic monitoring. Patients at low risk may be managed as outpatients but should undergo detailed evaluation within 72 hours.

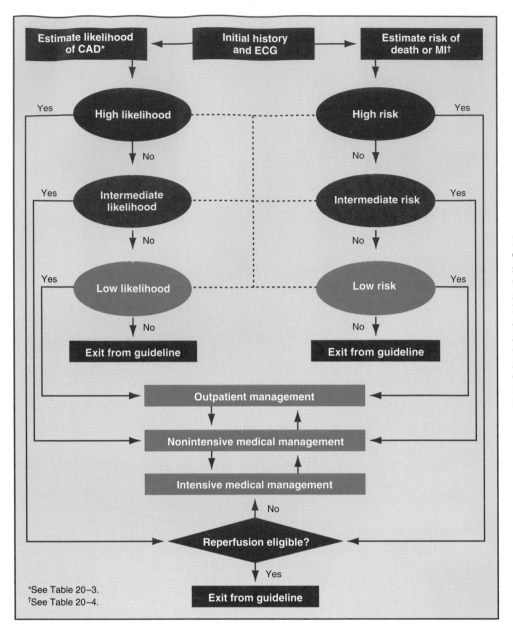

Figure 20–4

Overall strategy for diagnosis and risk stratification for patients with unstable angina according to the Agency for Health Care Policy and Research guidelines. CAD, coronary artery disease; ECG, electrocardiogram; MI, myocardial infarction. (Redrawn from Lee, T.H.: Practice guidelines in cardiovascular medicine. *In* Braunwald, E. [ed.]: Heart Disease. 5th ed. Philadelphia, W.B. Saunders, 1997, p. 1980.)

Many aspects of care of patients with unstable angina can be managed by primary care physicians. Cardiac consultation should be sought in high-risk patients, as well as in patients who fail to respond to therapy or who develop complications such as heart failure and when coronary revascularization is considered.

Intensive Medical Treatment (Fig. 20–5)

All patients with unstable angina should be evaluated for noncoronary causes of unstable angina, such as valvular heart disease or hypertrophic obstructive cardiomyopathy, and for extracardiac conditions, such as severe anemia, thyrotoxicosis, or infection, that may precipitate

unstable angina in a patient with chronic stable angina. The routine management of the hematocrit and serum thyroxine is recommended. Mild sedation or treatment with an anxiolytic drug is usually advisable. The aggressiveness of pharmacologic therapy described later depends on the severity of the ischemia and often requires multiple adjustments during hospitalization and after discharge.

NITRATES. Nonhypotensive patients at high risk (see Table 20–4) and those whose symptoms are not fully relieved with up to three sublingual nitroglycerin tablets should receive intravenous nitroglycerin. This drug should be administered by continuous infusion commencing at a dose of 5 to 10 μg/min and titrated up by 10 μg/min every 5 to 10 minutes until relief of symptoms or limiting side effects occur. Patients on intra-

Table 20–3	Likelihood of Significant CAD in Patients with Symptoms Suggesting Unstable Angina	
High Likelihood (e.g., 0.85–0.99)	**Intermediate Likelihood (e.g., 0.15–0.84)**	**Low Likelihood (e.g., 0.01–0.14)**
Any of the following features: History of prior MI or sudden death or other known history of CAD Definite angina: males ≥60 or females ≥70 Transient hemodynamic or ECG changes during pain Variant angina (pain with reversible ST segment elevation) ST segment elevation or depression ≥1 mm Marked symmetric T-wave inversion in multiple precordial leads	Absence of high-likelihood features and any of the following: Definite angina: males <60 or females <70 Probable angina: males ≥60 or females ≥70 Chest pain probably not angina in patients with diabetes Chest pain probably not angina and two or three risk factors other than diabetes Extracardiac vascular disease ST segment depression 0.05–1 mm or T-wave inversion ≥1 mm in leads with dominant R-waves	Absence of high- or intermediate-likelihood features but may have: Chest pain classified as probably not angina One risk factor other than diabetes T-wave flattening or inversion <1 mm in leads with dominant R-waves Normal ECG

From Braunwald, E., Mark, D.B., Jones, R.H., et al.: Unstable Angina: Diagnosis and Management. Clinical Practice Guideline no. 10 (amended). AHCPR Publication no. 94–0602. Rockville, MD, Agency for Health Care Policy and Research and the National Heart, Lung, and Blood Institute, Public Health Service, U.S. Department of Health and Human Services, May 1994.

Abbreviations: MI, myocardial infarction; CAD, coronary artery disease; ECG, electrocardiogram.

venous nitroglycerin should be switched to oral or topical nitrate therapy once they have been symptom-free for 24 hours.

MORPHINE SULFATE. When ischemic symptoms are not relieved by three serial sublingual nitroglycerin tablets or when symptoms recur despite adequate anti-ischemic therapy, in addition to intravenous nitroglycerin, morphine sulfate at a dose of 2 to 5 mg intravenously is recommended, unless contraindicated by hypotension or a history of intolerance. Morphine may be repeated every 5 to 10 minutes as needed to relieve symptoms and maintain patient comfort.

BETA-ADRENERGIC BLOCKERS. Patients at high risk of an adverse event and without contraindications (bradycardia, hypotension, left ventricular failure, atrioventricular block or reactive airway disease) should receive intravenous beta blockers, for example, metoprolol in up to three 5-mg increments, atenolol, or esmolol (see Table 20–5). Intravenous treatment should be followed by oral beta blockers. Intermediate- and low-risk patients do not require intravenous therapy and may be started on oral beta blockers directly. Target heart rates of 50 to 60 beats per minute at rest are appropriate.

CALCIUM ANTAGONISTS. These drugs may be used to control ongoing or recurrent ischemic symptoms or hypertension in patients already on adequate doses of nitrates and beta blockers, in those unable to tolerate adequate doses of one or both of these agents, and in those with Prinzmetal's angina (see p. 294). Calcium antagonists should be avoided in patients with pulmonary edema or evidence of left ventricular dysfunction. Short-acting nifedipine should *not* be used in the absence of concurrent beta blockage.

ANTIPLATELET AGENTS. There is substantial evidence that aspirin is useful both acutely and chronically in patients with unstable angina (Fig. 20–6).[13–15] The initial dose should be 160 mg or 324 mg; subsequently, the dose should be 80 to 324 mg/day. Patients unable to

take aspirin may be started on ticlopidine 250 mg twice a day as a substitute. Potent new antiplatelet drugs that block the platelet glycoprotein IIb/IIIa receptor appear to be promising, but at the time of this writing, these have not been approved for the treatment of unstable angina except as an adjunct for percutaneous transluminal coronary angioplasty in high-risk patients.

HEPARIN. Intravenous heparin is indicated in patients at high or intermediate risk of an adverse outcome (Fig. 20–7) and should be begun immediately and continued for 2 to 5 days or until coronary revascularization is performed.[13, 16] The initial dose is 80 units/kg by intravenous bolus followed by an infusion of 18 units/kg/min, maintaining the activated partial thromboplastin time (aPTT) at 1.5 to 2.5 times control (see Table 20–5). When a therapeutic level has been achieved, the aPTT should be remeasured every 24 hours. Some studies suggest that low-molecular-weight heparin may be superior to unfractionated heparin.[17] Hemoglobin or hematocrit and platelet count should be measured daily while the patient is on heparin.

THROMBOLYSIS. Even though thrombosis plays a significant role in the pathogenesis of unstable angina, well-controlled studies have shown no benefit from thrombolytic therapy.

EMERGENCY/URGENT CARDIAC CATHETERIZATION. If chest discomfort with objective evidence of ischemia persists for more than 1 hour after the commencement of aggressive medical therapy, and there is no obvious contraindication to coronary revascularization such as a serious concurrent disease, *emergency* cardiac catheterization should be strongly considered. Patients with continued ischemia despite therapy, especially those who are hypotensive, can benefit from stabilization by means of intra-aortic balloon counterpulsation as a bridge to cardiac catheterization and/or surgery. Intra-aortic balloon counterpulsation may also be used to stabilize patients who require interhospital transfer. *Urgent* cardiac

Table 20–4   **Short-Term Risk of Death or Nonfatal Myocardial Infarction in Patients with Unstable Angina**

High Risk	Intermediate Risk	Low Risk
At least one of the following features must be present: Prolonged ongoing (≥20 min) rest pain Pulmonary edema, most likely related to ischemia Angina at rest with dynamic ST changes ≥1 mm Angina with new or worsening mitral regurgitation murmur Angina with S₃ or new/worsening rales Angina with hypotension	No high-risk feature but must have any of the following: Prolonged (>20 min) rest angina, now resolved, with moderate or high likelihood of CAD Rest angina (>20 min or relieved with rest or sublingual nitroglycerin) Nocturnal angina Angina with dynamic T-wave changes New-onset Canadian Cardiovascular Society class III or IV angina in the past 2 weeks with moderate or high likelihood of CAD Pathologic Q-waves or resting ST depression ≤1 mm in multiple lead groups (anterior, inferior, lateral) Age >65 years	Absence of high- or intermediate-likelihood features but may have any of the following: Increased angina frequency, severity, or duration Angina provoked at a lower threshold New-onset angina with onset 2 weeks to 2 months before presentation Normal or unchanged ECG

From Braunwald, E., Mark, D.B., Jones, R.H., et al.: Unstable Angina: Diagnosis and Management. Clinical Practice Guideline no. 10 (amended). AHCPR Publication no. 94–0602. Rockville, MD, Agency for Health Care Policy and Research and the National Heart, Lung, and Blood Institute, Public Health Service, U.S. Department of Health and Human Services, May 1994.

Abbreviations: CAD, coronary artery disease; ECG, electrocardiogram.

catheterization should be considered in patients with unstable angina who have recurrent ischemic episodes despite appropriate medical therapy or who have high-risk unstable angina. This strategy may require transfer of the patient to a hospital with a cardiac catheterization laboratory.

Laboratory Testing

Total CK and CK-MB should be measured every 6 to 8 hours for the first 24 hours after admission. Troponin T, troponin I, or lactate dehydrogenase isoenzymes may be useful in patients presenting 24 to 72 hours after symptom onset if serial CK and CK-MB levels are normal; there is some evidence that the troponins are superior to CK as markers of adverse prognosis.[10] Serum lipid levels should be obtained, unless the patient has had a recent determination. Follow-up ECGs should be recorded every 8 hours for 24 hours, then every 24 hours, and whenever the patient has recurrent symptoms or a change in clinical status, and before discharge. A chest radiogram should be obtained in all patients.

Nonintensive Medical Management

When ischemia at rest in a high-risk patient has been brought under control by medical management for at least 24 hours, the patient may be transferred out of the intensive care/coronary care unit and placed on a maintenance medical regimen consisting of oral long-acting nitrates (e.g., 10 to 60 mg isosorbide dinitrate po, bid or tid), a beta blocker, aspirin, and heparin. During the following period of at least 24 hours, the patient is observed closely, if possible in a monitored bed, to identify ST segment/T-wave changes and arrhythmias. If ischemic episodes, left ventricular failure, serious tachyarrhythmias,

or hypotension develops or recurs on medical management, the patient should be returned to the intensive care unit or the cardiac catheterization laboratory or transferred to a hospital where such a facility is available (Fig. 20–8). If ischemia is controlled, activity should be increased as tolerated.

USE AND TIMING OF NONINVASIVE TESTS. Exercise or pharmacologic stress testing should be performed before discharge in patients who have responded to medical therapy and have been free of angina at rest or minor exertion and of congestive heart failure for a minimum of 24 hours. It is also an integral part of the expeditious outpatient evaluation of low-risk patients with unstable angina. The exercise treadmill test is a suitable mode of stress testing in patients with a normal resting ECG who are not taking digoxin. Patients with widespread or marked resting ST segment depression (≥1 mm), ST segment changes secondary to digoxin, left ventricular hypertrophy, left bundle branch block, intraventricular conduction defect, or ventricular preexcitation should be tested using myocardial perfusion scintigraphy. In patients unable to exercise owing to physical limitations, a pharmacologic stress should be used in combination with myocardial perfusion scintigraphy or echocardiography. Patients with unstable angina should also have an assessment of left ventricular function. Left ventriculography may be carried out at the time of cardiac catheterization; alternatively, two-dimensional echocardiography or radionuclide ventriculography may be employed.

CORONARY ARTERIOGRAPHY. Cardiac catheterization and coronary arteriography are ordinarily not indicated in patients with extensive co-morbidities contraindicating revascularization as well as in those who do not wish to undergo this therapy. Two strategies, an *early invasive* strategy and an *early conservative* strategy have been compared in patients with unstable angina who do not require emergency or urgent cardiac catheterization.[18]

Table 20–5	Drugs Commonly Used in Intensive Medical Management of Patients with Unstable Angina		
Drug Category	**Clinical Condition**	**When to Avoid***	**Dosage**
Aspirin†	Unstable angina	Hypersensitivity Active bleeding Severe bleeding risk	324 mg (160–324) daily
Heparin	Unstable angina in high-risk category	Active bleeding History of heparin-induced thrombocytopenia Severe bleeding risk Recent stroke	80 units/kg IV bolus Constant IV infusion at 18 U · kg⁻¹ · hr⁻¹ Titrated to maintain aPTT between 1.5 and 2.5 times control
Nitrates	Symptoms are not fully relieved with three sublingual nitroglycerin tablets and initiation of beta blocker therapy	Hypotension	5–10 μg/min by continuous infusion Titrated up to 75–100 μg/min until relief of symptoms or limiting side effects (headache or hypotension with a systolic blood pressure <90 mm Hg or more than 30% below starting mean arterial pressure levels if significant hypertension is present) Topical, oral, or buccal nitrates are acceptable alternatives for patients without ongoing or refractory symptoms

Beta blockers‡	Unstable angina	PR interval (ECG) >0.24 sec
		2° or 3° atrioventricular block
		Heart rate <60 beats/min
		Blood pressure <90 mm Hg
		Shock
		Left ventricular failure with congestive heart failure
		Severe reactive airway disease
			Metoprolol
			  5-mg increments by slow (over 1–2 min) IV administration
			  Repeated every 5 min for a total initial dose of 15 mg
			  Followed in 1–2 hr by 25–50 mg by mouth every 6 hr
			  If a very conservative regimen is desired, initial doses can be reduced to 1–2 mg
			Propranolol
			  0.5–1.0 mg IV dose
			  Followed in 1–2 hr by 40–80 mg by mouth every 6–8 hr
			Esmolol
			  Starting maintenance dose of 0.1 mg · kg⁻¹ · min⁻¹ IV
			  Titration in increments of 0.05 mg · kg⁻¹ · min⁻¹ every 10–15 min as tolerated by blood pressure until the desired therapeutic response has been obtained, limiting symptoms develop, or a dose of 0.20 mg · kg⁻¹ · min⁻¹ is reached
			  Optional loading dose of 0.5 mg/kg may be given by slow IV administration (2–5 min) for more rapid onset of action
			Atenolol
			  5-mg IV dose
			  Followed 5 min later by a second dose
			  5-mg IV dose and then 50–100 mg orally every day initiated 1–2 hr after the IV dose

Calcium channel blockers	Patients whose symptoms are not relieved by adequate doses of nitrates and beta blockers or in patients unable to tolerate adequate doses of one or both of these agents or in patients with variant angina	Pulmonary edema Evidence of left ventricular dysfunction	Dependent on specific agent
Morphine sulfate	Patients whose symptoms are not relieved after three serial sublingual nitroglycerin tablets or whose symptoms recur with adequate anti-ischemic therapy	Hypotension Respiratory depression Confusion Obtundation	2–5-mg IV dose May be repeated every 5–30 min as needed to relieve symptoms and maintain patient comfort

From Braunwald, E. (panel chair), Jones, R.H., Mark, D.B., et al.: Diagnosing and managing unstable angina. Circulation 90:613–622, 1994.

Abbreviations: IV, intravenous; aPTT, activated partial thromboplastin time; ECG, electrocardiogram; 2°, second-degree; 3°, third-degree.

* Allergy or prior intolerance is a contraindication for all categories of drugs listed in this chart.

† Patients unable to take aspirin because of a history of hypersensitivity or major gastrointestinal intolerance should be started on ticlopidine 250 mg twice a day as a substitute.

‡ Choice of the specific agent is not as important as ensuring that appropriate candidates receive this therapy. If there are concerns about patient intolerance owing to existing pulmonary disease, especially asthma, left ventricular dysfunction, or risk of hypotension or severe bradycardia, initial selection should favor a short-acting agent, such as propranolol or metoprolol or the ultra–short-acting agent esmolol. Mild wheezing or a history of chronic obstructive pulmonary disease should prompt a trial of a short-acting agent at a reduced dose (e.g., 2.5 mg IV metoprolol, 12.5 mg oral metoprolol, or 25 μg · kg⁻¹ · min⁻¹ esmolol as initial doses) rather than complete avoidance of beta blocker therapy.

Note: Some of the recommendations in this guide suggest the use of agents for purposes or in doses other than those specified by the U.S. Food and Drug Administration. Such recommendations are made after consideration of concerns regarding nonapproved indications. Where made, such recommendations are based on more recent clinical trials or expert consensus.

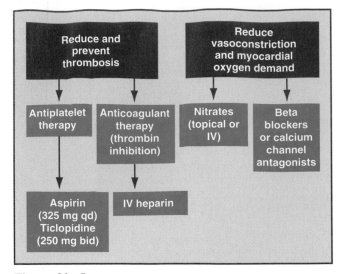

Figure 20–5

Initial management of acute ischemic syndromes in the absence of coronary occlusion. IV, intravenous. (Redrawn from Langer, A., and Armstrong, P.W.: Treatment of acute ischemic syndromes in the absence of coronary occlusion: Preventing progression to acute occlusion. *In* Califf, R.M. [vol. ed.]: Acute Myocardial Infarction and Other Ischemic Syndromes. Braunwald, E. [ser. ed.]: Atlas of Heart Diseases. Vol. 8. Philadelphia, Current Medicine, 1996.)

In the former, cardiac catheterization is performed routinely in all hospitalized patients with unstable angina without contraindications to catheterization or revascularization, usually within 48 hours of presentation. In the early conservative strategy, cardiac catheterization is performed only in patients who have persistent or recurrent pain/ischemia, congestive heart failure, left ventricular dysfunction (ejection fraction [EF] < 0.5), malignant ventricular arrhythmia, or a clearly positive, high-risk (see Table 18–6), noninvasive study. In this strategy, patients who respond to therapy with a negative exercise

or pharmacologic stress test and normal or only mildly impaired left ventricular function can be managed medically without catheterization. Patients with a positive, although not high-risk, exercise test without significantly impaired left ventricular function (EF > 0.5) should be referred for additional testing, either an exercise imaging study or a cardiac catheterization.

MYOCARDIAL REVASCULARIZATION. In the early invasive strategy, revascularization is carried out promptly on all patients without specific contraindications whose anatomy is suitable, regardless of the response to therapy or the findings on noninvasive testing. In the early conservative strategy, patients found at arteriography to have significant obstruction of the left main coronary artery (≥50%), significant (≥70%) three-vessel disease with depressed left ventricular function (EF < 0.5), two-vessel disease with proximal severe subtotal stenosis (≥95%) of the left anterior descending artery, and depressed left ventricular function should be referred promptly for coronary revascularization. Other patients with significant coronary artery disease should also be considered for prompt revascularization if they have any of the following: failure to stabilize with medical treatment; recurrent angina/ischemia at rest or with moderate-level activities; ischemia accompanied by symptoms of congestive heart failure, a third heart sound gallop, new or worsening mitral regurgitation, or if they are deemed at high risk by noninvasive testing (see Table 18–6).

These two strategies result in similar outcomes with respect to death or myocardial infarction. However, in patients in whom the early conservative strategy is applied, there are high rates of recurrence of unstable angina, more persistent and severe chronic stable angina requiring more intensive antianginal medical therapy, and a higher rate of hospital readmission. For this reason, many cardiologists prefer the invasive strategy for patients initially admitted to a tertiary center with the facilities and personnel experienced in the revascularization treatment of unstable angina. In patients admitted to hos-

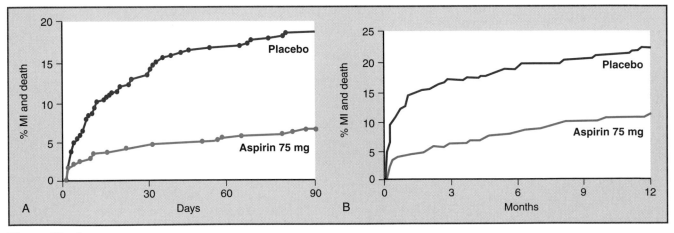

Figure 20–6

A and *B*, Risk of myocardial infarction (MI) and death during treatment with aspirin or placebo. (*A*, Redrawn from the RISC Group: Risk of myocardial infarction and death during treatment with low-dose aspirin and intravenous heparin in men with unstable coronary artery disease. Volume 336, issue 8719, pp. 827–830. © by The Lancet Ltd., 1990. *B*, Redrawn with permission from the American College of Cardiology [Journal of the American College of Cardiology, 1991, vol. 18, pp. 1587–1593].)

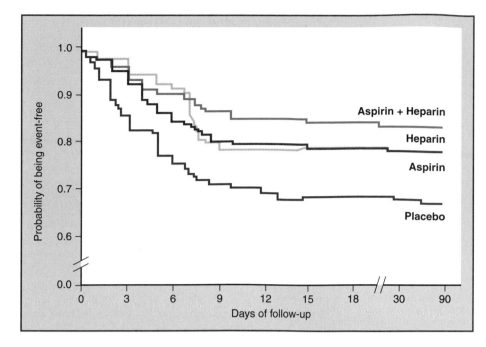

Figure 20–7

Effects of 7 days of therapy with placebo, aspirin, or the combination on clinical events. (Redrawn from Califf, R.M.: Spectrum of acute ischemic heart disease: Unstable angina to acute myocardial infarction. *In* Califf, R.M. [vol. ed.]: Acute Myocardial Infarction and Other Ischemic Syndromes. Braunwald, E. [ser. ed.]: Atlas of Heart Diseases. Vol. 8. Philadelphia, Current Medicine, 1996; data from Theroux, P., Waters, D., Lam, J., et al.: Reactivation of unstable angina after the discontinuation of heparin. N. Engl. J. Med. 327: 141–145, 1992.)

pitals without such facilities in whom transfer is required, either strategy is satisfactory. The conservative strategy requires careful follow-up of the patient with particular attention to the adjustment of anti-ischemic medication (nitrates, beta blockers, and calcium antagonists).

The choice between the two modes of revascularization—surgery or catheter-based revascularization—depends largely on the coronary anatomy, as described in Chapter 18. Patients with multiple, diffuse lesions are generally more suitable for coronary artery bypass grafting, as are those with left main coronary artery disease, three-vessel coronary artery disease, or significantly impaired left ventricular function. The immediate risk of angioplasty and other catheter-based interventions in patients with unstable angina may be reduced by the prior administration of abciximab (ReoPro), an inhibitor of platelet glycoprotein IIb/IIIa receptors;[19] there is some evidence that the monoclonal antibody may also reduce the rate of restenosis after angioplasty.

Discharge from Hospital and Postdischarge Care

Patients may be discharged after recovery from revascularization or, in those who do not undergo revascularization, 24 to 48 hours after ischemia has been controlled and noninvasive testing has been completed. Aspirin (80 to 324 mg/day) should be continued for an indefinite period, regardless of whether revascularization has been carried out. Patients who are not revascularized may be continued on beta blockers and long-acting nitrates, supplemented by sublingual nitroglycerin as needed. High-risk patients should be seen as outpatients in follow-up 1 to 2 weeks after discharge and lower-risk patients at 2 to 6 weeks. During follow-up, secondary prevention measures are undertaken—treating hypertension and hyperlipidemia, encouraging the cessation of smoking, and em-

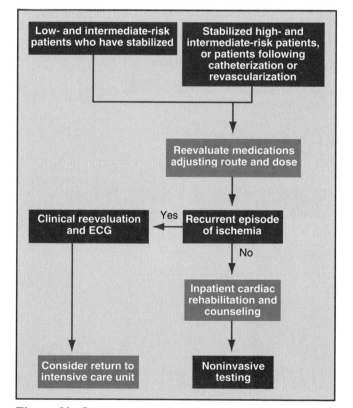

Figure 20–8

Nonintensive management of unstable angina. ECG, electrocardiogram. (Redrawn from Archibald, N.D., and Jones, R.H.: Guidelines for treatment of unstable angina. *In* Califf, R.M. [vol. ed.]: Acute Myocardial Infarction and Other Ischemic Syndromes. Braunwald, E. [ser. ed.]: Atlas of Heart Diseases. Vol. 8. Philadelphia, Current Medicine, 1996.)

barking on an exercise program. Patients should be advised to contact their primary care physician if symptoms recur or become more severe. In patients found at coronary arteriography not to have a critical obstruction in the coronary vascular bed, the unstable angina may have been caused by a subtotal thrombotic occlusion superimposed on a nonobstructive plaque with subsequent lysis of the thrombus. Alternatively, the unstable angina might have been caused by epicardial vasospasm (Prinzmetal's angina), described later, or by vasoconstriction in the coronary microcirculation. Patients with the latter condition usually respond to calcium antagonists and have an excellent prognosis.

Initial Outpatient Management

Initial management on an outpatient basis is advisable in patients with unstable angina considered to be at low

risk of adverse events at the time of the initial evaluation (Fig. 20–9; see also Table 20–4). Workup should include a search for noncardiac factors that may have caused or precipitated unstable angina or lack of compliance with a regimen previously designed for chronic stable angina. If the patient's symptoms are well controlled on the medical regimen, noninvasive stress testing and risk stratification may be undertaken on an outpatient basis.

PRINZMETAL'S VARIANT ANGINA

This uncommon form of angina also causes ischemic pain at rest. However, its pathogenesis differs from the usual form of unstable angina in that it is caused by severe focal spasm of one of the epicardial coronary arteries.[1, 20]

Patients with Prinzmetal's angina are usually in their 40s or 50s, generally one or two decades younger than those with unstable angina caused by coronary atherosclerosis. They often do not exhibit coronary risk factors, except for cigarette smoking. Prinzmetal's angina has been reported to occur in association with migraine, Raynaud's phenomenon, and aspirin-induced asthma. It may be precipitated by alcohol withdrawal, emotional distress, and the administration of 5-fluorouracil and cyclophosphamide. The attacks of pain occur most frequently in the early morning hours, may awaken the patient from sleep, are usually quite severe, and may be accompanied by tachyarrhythmias that can cause syncope. In contrast to the unstable angina caused by coronary atherosclerosis, exercise capacity may be normal (unless the patient has coexistent atherosclerotic coronary artery disease [see later]). Again, in contrast to unstable angina, the progression from exercise-induced angina to rest pain is rarely observed in Prinzmetal's angina.

The principal feature on laboratory investigation that distinguishes Prinzmetal's angina from unstable angina is the ST segment *elevation* during ischemia in the former and the ST segment *depression* in the latter. ST segment elevation is often asymptomatic and may be detected on continuous (Holter) ECG monitoring. With prolonged, severe ST segment elevation, myocardial infarction can occur and transient intraventricular and atrioventricular conduction disturbances and ventricular tachyarrhythmias may develop.

Approximately half of patients with Prinzmetal's angina also have a fixed obstructive lesion in a proximal coronary artery. The site of spasm is usually within 1 cm of the fixed obstruction. The diagnosis of Prinzmetal's angina can be confirmed in the catheterization laboratory by observing localized coronary spasm or inducing it with gradually escalating doses of intravenous ergonovine[21] or the intracoronary injection of acetylcholine or by hyperventilation.

MANAGEMENT. Episodes of Prinzmetal's angina respond to nitrates, given sublingually or intravenously. Oral calcium antagonists are usually effective in preventing recurrence,[22] but these may have to be given at doses

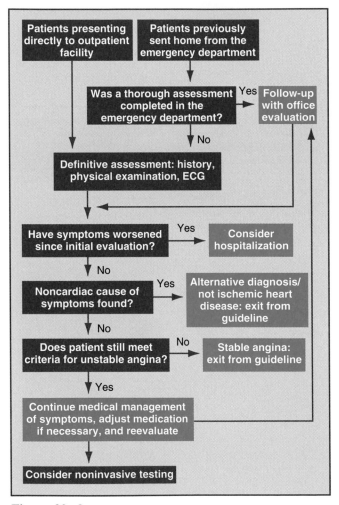

Figure 20–9

Outpatient management of unstable angina. ECG, electrocardiogram. (From Archibald, N.D., and Jones, R.H.: Guidelines for treatment of unstable angina. *In* Califf, R.M. [vol. ed.]: Acute Myocardial Infarction and Other Ischemic Syndromes. Braunwald, E. [ser. ed.]: Atlas of Heart Diseases. Vol. 8. Philadelphia, Current Medicine, 1996.)

higher than those usually employed in the management of chronic stable angina or unstable angina (see Table 18–12). The episodes of rest pain do not respond to, and cannot be prevented by, beta blockade. Surgical or catheter-based revascularization is indicated in patients with Prinzmetal's angina who have a severe, discrete *fixed* obstruction and severe exercise-induced angina that does not respond adequately to medical therapy.

Prinzmetal's angina is often cyclical, with an acute, active phase—characterized by frequent episodes of rest pain–followed by periods of inactivity. Patients who develop tachyarrhythmias during episodes of ischemia are at high risk of sudden death and require intensive therapy with calcium antagonists and nitrates. Patients who are maintained under active treatment with calcium antagonists and nitrates have an excellent prognosis with a 5-year survival rate of more than 90%.

References

1. Gersh, B.J., Braunwald, E., and Rutherford, J.D.: Chronic coronary artery disease. *In* Braunwald, E. (ed.): Heart Disease. 5th ed. Philadelphia, W.B. Saunders, 1997, pp. 1289–1365.
2. Braunwald, E.: Unstable angina: A classification. Circulation 80: 410, 1989.
3. van Miltenburg-van Zijl, A.J., Simoons, M.L., Veerhoek, R.J., and Bossuyt, P.M.: Incidence and followup of Braunwald subgroups in unstable angina pectoris. J. Am. Coll. Cardiol. 25:1286, 1995.
4. Ribiero, P.A., and Shah, P.M.: Unstable angina: New insights into pathophysiologic characteristics, prognosis, and management strategies. Curr. Probl. Cardiol. 21:669–732, 1996.
5. Merlini, P.A., Bauer, K.A., Oltrona, L., et al.: Persistent activation of coagulation mechanism in unstable angina and myocardial infarction. Circulation 90:61, 1994.
6. Freeman, M.R., Williams, A.E., Chisholm, R.J., et al.: Intracoronary thrombus and complex morphology and unstable angina: Relation to timing of angiography and in-hospital cardiac events. Circulation 80:17, 1989.
7. Sherman, C.T., Litvack, F., Grundfest, W., et al.: Coronary angioscopy in patients with unstable angina pectoris. N. Engl. J. Med. 315:913, 1986.
8. Braunwald, E., Mark, D.B., Jones, R.H., et al.: Unstable angina: Diagnosis and management. Clinical Practice Guideline no. 10. AHCPR Publication no. 94–0602. Rockville, MD, Agency for Health Care Policy and Research and the National Heart, Lung, and Blood Institute, Public Health Service, U.S. Department of Health and Human Services, May 1994, pp. 28, 92.
9. Cannon, C.P., McCabe, C.H., Stone, P.H., et al., for the TIMI III Registry ECG Ancillary Study Investigators: The electrocardiogram predicts one-year outcome of patients with unstable angina and non–Q-wave myocardial infarction: Results of the TIMI III Registry ECG Ancillary Study. J. Am. Coll. Cardiol. 30:133, 1997.
10. Antman, E.M., Tanasijevic, M.J., Thompson, B., et al.: Cardiac-specific troponin I levels to predict the risk of mortality in patients with acute coronary syndromes. N. Engl. J. Med. 335:1342–1349, 1996.
11. Stone, P.H., Thompson, B., Anderson, H.V., et al.: The influence of race, sex and age on management of unstable angina and non–Q-wave myocardial infarction: The TIMI III Registry. JAMA 275: 1104–1112, 1996.
12. Mark, D.B., and Braunwald, E.: Medical management of unstable angina. *In* Fuster, V., Ross, R., and Topol, E. (eds.): Atherosclerosis and Coronary Artery Disease. Philadelphia, Lippincott-Raven, 1996, pp. 1315–1320.
13. Theroux, P., Ouimet, J., McCans, J., et al.: Aspirin, heparin, or both to treat unstable angina. N. Engl. J. Med. 319:1105, 1988.
14. Cairns, J.A., Gent, M., Singer, J., et al.: Aspirin, sulfinpyrazone, or both in unstable angina. N. Engl. J. Med. 313:1369, 1985.
15. Selwyn, A.P., and Braunwald, E.: Ischemic heart disease. *In* Fauci, A.S., Braunwald, E., Isselbacher, K.J., et al. (eds.): Harrison's Principles of Internal Medicine. 14th ed. New York, McGraw-Hill, 1998, pp. 1365–1375.
16. Theroux, P., Waters, D., Qiu, S., et al.: Aspirin versus heparin to prevent myocardial infarction during the acute phase of unstable angina. Circulation 88:2045, 1993.
17. Gurfinkel, E.P., Manos, E.J., Mejail, R.I., et al.: Low-molecular-weight heparin versus regular heparin or aspirin in the treatment of unstable angina and silent ischemia. J. Am. Coll. Cardiol. 26:313, 1995.
18. The TIMI IIIA Investigators, Braunwald, E. (chairman): Early effects of tissue-type plasminogen activator added to conventional therapy on the culprit coronary lesion in patients presenting with ischemic cardiac pain at rest. Circulation 87:38–52, 1993.
19. The EPIC Investigators: Use of a monoclonal antibody directed against the platelet glycoprotein IIb/IIIa receptor in high-risk coronary angioplasty. N. Engl. J. Med. 330:956, 1994.
20. Gersh, B.J., Bassendine, M., Forman, R., et al.: Coronary artery spasm and myocardial infarction in the absence of angiographically demonstrable coronary artery disease. Mayo Clin. Proc. 56:700, 1981.
21. Nakamura, Y., Yamaguro, T., Inoki, I., et al.: Vasomotor response to ergonovine of epicardial and resistance coronary arteries in the nonspastic vascular bed in patients with vasospastic angina. Am. J. Cardiol. 74:1006, 1989.
22. Morikami, Y., and Yasue, H.: Efficacy of slow-release nifedipine on myocardial ischemic episodes in variant angina pectoris. Am. J. Cardiol. 68:580, 1991.

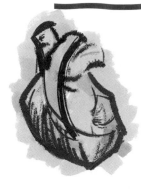

Chapter 21

Recognition and Management of Patients with

Hypertension

Michael H. Alderman

High blood pressure affects 15% to 18% of adults, more than 50 million Americans, and its management is the most common reason for physician office visits. Hypertension is a principal risk factor for myocardial infarction, stroke, renal failure, and other vascular diseases that together account for the majority of all deaths in the United States and the entire industrialized world. The enormous reduction in cardiovascular mortality and morbidity since the mid-1970s has resulted, in large part, from the wide application of effective antihypertensive therapy. The very magnitude of the problem of hypertension dictates that its management must be on a population-wide basis and that it can be achieved only through the delivery of medical care by a system in which the primary care physician plays a central role.

EPIDEMIOLOGY

An understanding of blood pressure and its relation to cardiovascular disease, as well as its treatment, depends, in large measure, on the fruits of epidemiologic investigation. The latter are especially relevant to primary care physicians, who, in the evolving system of managed health care, are responsible not only for the individual patients who seek their help but also for a defined patient panel. Indeed, the primary care physician's practice will increasingly become a population whose total health is the responsibility of that physician.

The basis of modern strategies to manage blood pressure lies in two sets of population-based studies. Observational studies of large populations, such as at Framingham, in which healthy persons have been followed prospectively after a comprehensive initial evaluation[1] and large clinical trials of antihypertensive therapy.[2] In these prospective observational studies, baseline characteristics such as blood pressure and other risk factors have been related to the subsequent occurrence of cardiovascular events. This approach has firmly established the existence of a strong, positive, and continuous relation between blood pressure and the occurrence of both heart attack and stroke. No threshold separates those patients with and those without risk for cardiovascular events. The meta-analysis shown in Figure 21–1 describes *relative,* not absolute risk. Thus, for example, in regard to stroke, for every 7.5 mm Hg increase in diastolic pressure, there is almost a 50% increase in events. The *absolute* number of events depends on a variety of risk factors in addition to blood pressure. For example, at any level of blood pressure, the event rate in older persons is higher than that in younger ones. Although relative risk increases throughout the range of blood pressure, and is highest for those with the highest pressures, paradoxically, the largest actual number of events (depicted by the size of the squares at each level of pressure in the *right panel* of Fig. 21–1), actually occurs in persons at the middle range of pressures. Indeed, most myocardial infarctions are observed in individuals with diastolic pressures in the mid- and upper 80s. This finding can be explained by the fact that only a very small percentage of the population have the highest pressures, and even though they are at high individual risk, together they contribute relatively few events. By contrast, many more persons have "high-normal" pressures, and hence, although their individual risk is small, in the aggregate they contribute most of the population's events.

There are important practical implications of these find-

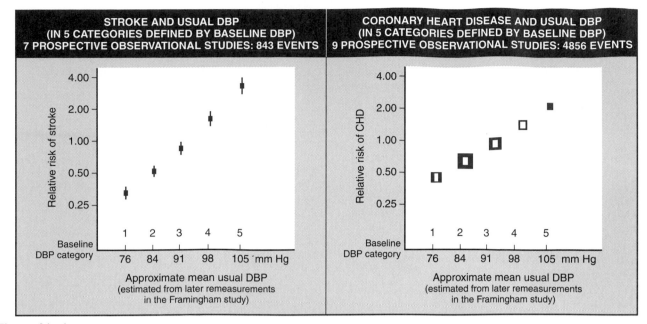

Figure 21–1

The relative risks of stroke and coronary heart disease (CHD), estimated from the combined results of the prospective observational studies, for each of five categories of diastolic blood pressure (DBP). Estimates of the usual DBP in each baseline DBP category are taken from mean DBP values 4 years after baseline in the Framingham study. The *solid squares* in the left panel represent disease risks in each category relative to risk in the whole study population; the *sizes of the squares* in the right panel are proportional to the number of events in each DBP category; and 95% confidence intervals for the estimates of relative risk are denoted by *vertical lines* in the left panel. (Redrawn from MacMahon, S., Peto, R., Cutler, J., et al.: Blood pressure, stroke, and coronary heart disease. Part I. Prolonged differences in blood pressure: Prospective observational studies corrected for the regression dilution bias. Volume 335, issue 8692, pp. 765–774, © by The Lancet Ltd, 1990.)

ings for primary care physicians. First of all, blood pressure must be recognized for what it is: a risk factor whose level strongly affects the likelihood of coronary and cerebrovascular events—but not a *cause* of disease. Not everyone with hypertension, even severe hypertension, develops a myocardial infarction or a stroke, and not everyone with a low pressure avoids these events. Thus, a strategy designed to identify and treat only those subjects with an arbitrarily defined level of pressure termed "hypertensive" may ignore the biologic message inherent in the available epidemiologic data. Instead, the message is that an effort to reduce blood pressure in the entire population would actually prevent more cardiovascular events than the current strategy, which focuses only on subjects with the highest pressures.[3]

Risks in Patients versus Populations

The clinical value of antihypertensive therapy has been demonstrated in large, population-based clinical trials.[2] However, the primary care physician should recognize that what is found in a trial might not actually apply to a particular patient with characteristics different from those of the group enrolled in the trial. Thus, although decision-making for the individual patient should be informed by the outcomes of clinical trials, it must take into account the assessment of the individual patient.[5] Whereas the reduction of blood pressure is, by definition, the *immediate* goal of antihypertensive therapy, the ultimate purpose

of treatment is the prevention of vascular complications. Particular interventions may lower arterial pressure but that, in itself, does not ensure clinical benefit.[5]

The early antihypertensive drug trials carried out by the Veterans Administration Study Group proved conclusively that it is possible to prolong life by lowering elevated blood pressure. Subsequent studies, largely based on treatment with diuretics and beta blockers, have consistently reaffirmed the clinical benefit of antihypertensive therapy. New classes of effective, well-tolerated antihypertensive drugs, such as angiotensin-converting enzyme (ACE) inhibitors, and calcium antagonists have subsequently been developed. However, their effectiveness in improving clinical outcome relative to diuretics and beta blockers has *not* been established. It must also be appreciated that all effective antihypertensive drugs can produce adverse effects. A consideration of the latter is especially important in the treatment of low-risk subjects, who are increasingly the target of antihypertensive therapy.

DIAGNOSTIC EVALUATION

The purpose of the initial evaluation of the patient in regard to blood pressure is to answer four questions:[6] What is the usual blood pressure level? Is a secondary or correctable cause of hypertension present? What is the absolute risk for the occurrence of cardiovascular disease?

Are there indications or contraindications for any particular antihypertensive drug?

The first step in the hypertensive patient is to perform the appropriate general medical evaluation with special emphasis on the cardiovascular system. This is described in Chapter 11. The next step is to determine, as accurately as possible, the usual level of blood pressure. This requires repeated measurements. Before labeling an asymptomatic person with minimally or inconsistently elevated pressure as "hypertensive," a period of observation is encouraged. In the absence of signs of target-organ damage such as enlarged heart, funduscopic changes, evidence of renal, coronary, or cerebrovascular dysfunction or accelerated hypertension, it is reasonable to follow the patient for at least 4 weeks. Whenever possible, the same observer should adhere to standardized measurement techniques under approximately the same conditions, recording the pressures at least three times in both arms, and averaging the last two pressures (assuming that no more that 5 mm Hg separates the individual readings). Spurious elevations sometimes occur owing to "white-coat" hypertension; this is seen most commonly in the elderly and particularly in older women. Home recordings, obtained with either a 24-hour recording device or a simple home instrument, may distinguish such persons. However, confirmation of office readings does not seem necessary unless, over time, it appears that the office finding is inconsistent with the clinical situation. (For further discussion, see Chap. 11.)

Several laboratory tests are appropriate on a routine basis (see Table 11–7). These include determination of hematocrit, serum creatinine, fasting blood sugar, cholesterol, including high- and low-density fractions, and potassium. Urinalysis should be performed to determine whether urinary albumin or protein is present.[7] Although the electrocardiogram is a less-sensitive guide to enlargement of the ventricular mass than is the echocardiogram, the former is generally preferred for reasons of cost and availability, and it is used to detect left ventricular hypertrophy, evidence of ischemic heart disease, or arrhythmia. In borderline situations where uncertainty about the degree of risk exists, the echocardiogram can provide helpful information regarding the presence of ventricular hypertrophy. It may also be helpful when cardiomegaly is found on the chest radiogram and when cardiac signs or symptoms are present.

Risk Assessment

Conventional practice is often guided by the use of a threshold blood pressure to distinguish those who do from those who do not merit pharmacologic reduction of blood pressure.[8] As already pointed out, this strategy is consistent with the link between blood pressure and cardiovascular events. As recent meta-analyses have shown (see Fig. 21–1), at every level of pressure, even within the usual range, a lower pressure is desirable.[1] At any level of blood pressure, treating persons at higher risk will prevent a larger number of events than will similar treatment directed at a lower-risk group. Figure 21–1 depicts the potential impact of similar reductions of systolic pressure in persons with different levels of absolute risk. The per-

centage reduction of events is the same, but the absolute numbers who benefit are quite different. Another way to describe the impact of absolute risk is by presenting treatment implications on the basis of the number of persons who need to be treated to prevent a single event during a fixed period of time, generally 1 year. Among low-risk participants in the British Medical Research Council Trial of Antihypertensive Therapy, it was necessary to treat 850 persons for 1 year to prevent one stroke. On the other hand, in high-risk patients characterized by cigarette smoking, an elevated blood sugar and cholesterol, and electrocardiographic signs of left ventricular hypertrophy, only 40 patients would have to be treated for 1 year to prevent one stroke.[9]

The implications of these findings are clear. Many persons currently receiving treatment, who are relatively young (<50 years) and female and who do not have other risk factors or evidence of cardiovascular disease, are at minimal risk of an event and therefore unlikely to benefit from antihypertensive treatment. In these circumstances, the side effects and costs of therapy become relatively more important. But, at the same time, there are many patients with pressures below an arbitrary cutoff point of 140/90 mm Hg whose combination of vascular disease and other risk factors produces a likelihood of disease so great that a fall in pressure would produce substantial benefit. Unfortunately, the firm data needed to support the policies of withholding antihypertensive treatment from low-risk persons and of intervening in high-risk individuals are not available. However, at the borderline range (140 to 160 mm Hg systolic and 85 to 90 mm Hg diastolic), where so many patients fall, it seems appropriate to apply an assessment of absolute risk to the process of determining whether or not to initiate drug therapy. To simply treat all borderline hypertensive persons would vastly increase the number of low-risk patients under treatment.

Although a variety of strategies based on epidemiologic data have been developed to precisely quantify risk, the application of this information remains an imprecise science in the individual case. Absolute risk is the sum of all factors that influence the likelihood of events. Of these, age is perhaps most powerful (Fig. 21–2), followed by the presence of target-organ disease, male gender (Fig. 21–2), and associated risk factors for vascular disease, such as the presence of diabetes, hypercholesterolemia, and cigarette smoking. Additional sensitive techniques are becoming available to measure risk. For example, the echocardiographic measurement of cardiac mass, the presence of albumin in the urine, the arm/ankle blood pressure index, as well as insulin levels and plasma renin activity all help in the assessment of risk. Together, these measure provide powerful tools for the stratification of patients, although a precise format for incorporating these new techniques in estimation of risk of individual patients has not yet been developed.

Three European societies (European Society of Cardiology, European Atherosclerosis Society, and European Society of Hypertension) have suggested that if the 10-year risk of developing symptomatic coronary artery disease exceeds 20% (or will exceed 20% if projected to age 60 years), treatment for all risk factors is required. The presence of *any* clinical vascular disease increases the 10-year

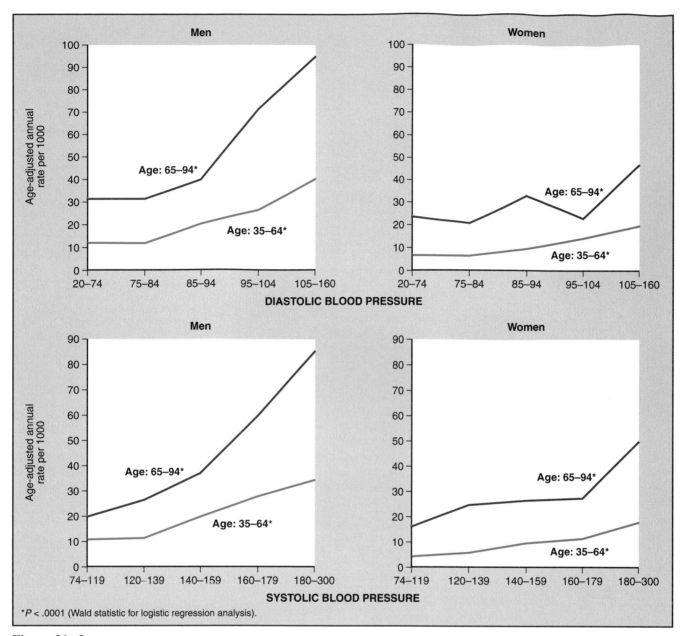

Figure 21–2

Cardiovascular risk curves. (Redrawn from J. Hypertension 6:53–59, 1988, Vokonas, P.S., Kannel, W.B., and Cupples, L.A.: Risk of hypertension in the elderly: The Framingham Study, by permission of Rapid Science Publishers Ltd.)

risk to more than 20%. The interaction between age, gender, total cholesterol, and systolic pressure, based on a risk function derived from the Framingham Study, is shown in Figure 21–3. The risk of developing CHD in a 10-year period in a 30-year-old nonsmoking woman with a systolic pressure of 180 mm Hg and a cholesterol of 300 mg/dl is less than 5%. This contrasts sharply with a risk exceeding 40% in a 70-year-old male smoker with a similarly elevated total cholesterol and a systolic pressure of only 140 mm Hg. Whereas the *relative* risk will be reduced in both of these individuals, with blood pressure lowering, the *absolute* risk will be reduced substantially more in the latter patient than in the former. As shown in Figures 21–3 and 21–4, the risk of developing clinical manifestations of coronary heart disease and stroke varies

over an eightfold range in persons of the same age and systolic pressure, depending on the presence or absence of other risk factors.

MANAGEMENT

Nonpharmacologic Interventions

In Western societies, blood pressure tends to rise with age, so that the majority of persons above the age of 65 years have pressures that exceed conventional standards for hypertension. Earlier notions that this age-related rise

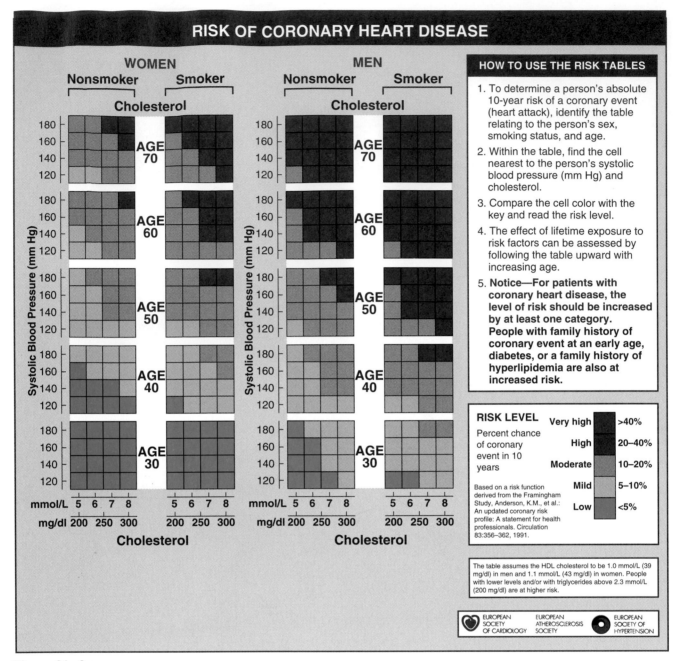

Figure 21-3

Absolute risk (percentage) of having a cardiovascular event in 10 years according to age, systolic pressure, and total serum cholesterol. (Redrawn courtesy of Bristol-Myers Squibb; adapted from Pyorala, K., De Backer, G., Graham, I., et al.: Prevention of coronary heart disease in clinical practice. Recommendations of the Task Force of the European Society of Cardiology, the European Atherosclerosis Society, and the European Society of Hypertension, published in Eur. Heart J. 15:1300–1331, 1994, and in Atherosclerosis, vol. 110, pp. 121–161, Copyright 1994, with permission from Elsevier Science.)

in pressure was either benign or even desirable have long since given way to the recognition that lower pressures are associated with improved survival. Since this rise in blood pressure generally occurs gradually over time, the possibility of arresting this progress is understandably attractive. Nonpharmacologic intervention has attracted considerable attention as a means to both prevent blood pressure elevation and reduce existing pressure slightly. The problem is whether such an approach is effective.

The nonpharmacologic methods generally believed to be effective include weight loss, sodium restriction, potassium intake increase, exercise, and moderation of alcohol consumption (Table 21–1).[10] In tightly controlled, short-term studies, each of these interventions has been shown to lower blood pressure of at least some participants, and in general, the impact of all of these interventions is proportional to the original level of the pressure. However, there is little information on the long-term effects of these interventions. Thus far, they have revealed little, if

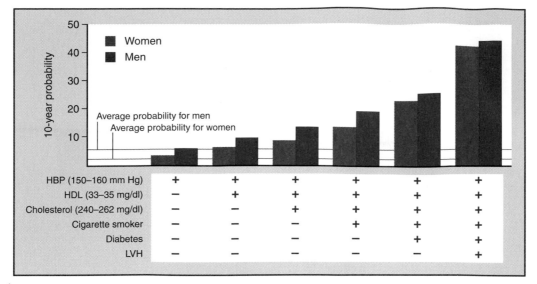

HBP (150–160 mm Hg)	+	+	+	+	+	+
HDL (33–35 mg/dl)	–	+	+	+	+	+
Cholesterol (240–262 mg/dl)	–	–	+	+	+	+
Cigarette smoker	–	–	–	+	+	+
Diabetes	–	–	–	–	+	+
LVH	–	–	–	–	–	+

Figure 21–4

Risk of coronary disease in hypertension by increasing number of risk factors in patients aged 42 to 43 years with a systolic pressure ranging from 150 to 160 mm Hg depends on the extent of associated atherogenic cardiovascular risk factors. These include low high-density lipoprotein (HDL) cholesterol, modest hypercholesterolemia, cigarette smoking, diabetes, and left ventricular hypertrophy (LVH). HBP, high blood pressure. (Redrawn from Kannel, W.B.: Natural history of cardiovascular risk. *In* Hollenberg, N.K. [vol. ed.]: Hypertension: Mechanisms and Therapy. Braunwald, E. [ser. ed.]: Atlas of Heart Diseases. Vol. 1. Philadelphia, Current Medicine, 1995, pp. 5.1–5.22; adapted from Kannel, W.B.: Potency of vascular risk factors as the basis for antihypertensive therapy. Eur. Heart J. 13:34–42, 1992.)

any, meaningful sustained effect and have not demonstrated a reduction in clinical events.

The target groups for nonpharmacologic intervention include persons with high-normal pressures, labile hypertension, white-coat hypertension (see Chap. 11), a family history of hypertension, obesity, high sodium intake, excessive alcohol consumption, and a sedentary lifestyle—characteristics that predispose them to future elevations of blood pressure. A vigorous commitment by both physician and patient is required for sustained success in these efforts.

Nonpharmacologic strategies for blood pressure reduction are not incompatible with pharmacologic approaches. Whereas antihypertensive drug therapy has been shown

not only to have a rather substantial effect on blood pressure but also to prevent stroke and myocardial infarction, thus far no nonpharmacologic intervention has been shown to produce these clinical benefits.

The Decision to Institute Drug Treatment

Many patients present to the primary care physician already receiving antihypertensive medication. It is useful to attempt to withdraw all drug therapy in subjects without severe hypertension or complicating signs or symptoms. Patients must be carefully followed after withdrawal of therapy—normal pressures are sometimes maintained for prolonged periods. These patients will be spared drug therapy for some time, although the majority will ultimately require treatment as pressure rises. Several studies of drug withdrawal under well-controlled conditions indicate the safety of this approach.[11] Presumably, a rise in pressure precedes any untoward outcomes, thus permitting reinitiation of treatment in a timely fashion, as long as the patient is carefully *monitored*.

Although most guidelines recommend drug therapy if blood pressure remains above 140 mm Hg systolic or 95 mm Hg diastolic after nonpharmacologic therapy has been applied (Fig. 21–5), a strong argument can be made for a more individualized approach that considers the patient's absolute risk based not only on blood pressure but also on other risk factors. At the extremes of pressure, above a systolic pressure of 170 mm Hg or a diastolic of 100 mm Hg, thresholds that include about 5% of the adult population, drug therapy is desirable regardless of the absolute cardiovascular risk status. By the same to-

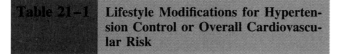

Table 21–1	Lifestyle Modifications for Hypertension Control or Overall Cardiovascular Risk

Lose weight if overweight

Limit alcohol intake to ≤1 oz/day of ethanol (24 oz of beer, 8 oz of wine, or 2 oz of 100-proof whiskey)

Exercise (aerobic) regularly

Reduce sodium intake to less than 100 mmol/day (<2.3 gm of sodium or approximately <6 gm of sodium chloride)

Maintain adequate dietary potassium, calcium, and magnesium intake

Stop smoking and reduce dietary saturated fat and cholesterol intake for overall cardiovascular health; reducing fat intake also helps reduce caloric intake—important for control of weight and type II diabetes

From Hollenberg, N.K.: Summary of the Joint National Committee (JCN)–V and WHO/International Society of Hypertension (ISH) Special Reports. *In* Hollenberg, N.K. (vol. ed.): Hypertension: Mechanisms and Therapy. Braunwald, E. (ser. ed.): Atlas of Heart Diseases. 2nd ed. Vol. 1. Philadelphia, Current Medicine, 1998, p. 13.15.

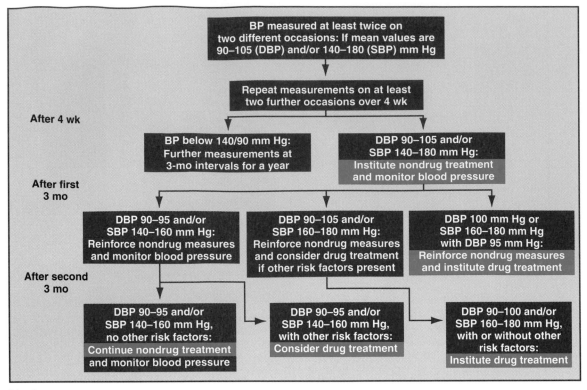

Figure 21–5

Management of mild hypertension defined as diastolic blood pressure (DBP) of 90 to 105 mm Hg or systolic blood pressure (SBP) of 140 to 180 mm Hg, or both. Drug treatment should be instituted more promptly in patients with evidence of substantial risk of cardiovascular disease. BP, blood pressure. (Redrawn from Hollenberg, N.K.: Summary of the Joint National Committee [JNC]–V and WHO/International Society of Hypertension [ISH] special reports. *In* Hollenberg, N.K. [vol. ed.]: Hypertension: Mechanisms and Therapy. Braunwald, E. [ser. ed.]: Atlas of Heart Diseases. 2nd ed. Vol. 1. Philadelphia, Current Medicine, 1998, p. 13.15.)

ken, in view of the generally low risk, patients with pressures below 140/85 mm Hg usually need not be considered for drug therapy. It is in the range between these two extremes of pressure that the absolute risk can most usefully be applied to assist decision-making about the desirability of drug therapy. No rigid guideline of risk level can be defined to separate those who should be treated from those who should not. Persons with established cardiovascular disease, manifested by a previous myocardial infarction, stroke, transient ischemic attack, or peripheral vascular disease within the broad range described previously, usually merit aggressive blood pressure reduction. Beyond that, the presence and magnitude of other risk factors such as adult-onset diabetes or glucose intolerance, hypercholesterolemia, or a family history of premature coronary artery disease tend to tip the balance toward intervention. In patients less than 55 years of age with borderline pressures—between 140/85 mm Hg and 170/100 mm Hg—and the absence of target-organ disease or other risk factors, the clinical benefit that can be achieved with pharmacotherapy is small. For such patients, probably 20% to 30% of all so-called hypertensive persons, watchful waiting while maintaining nonpharmacologic therapy is a reasonable course. By the same token, it is clear that sustained blood pressure elevation contributes to vascular disease development; if pressures do not fall after 6 to 9 months of observation, drug therapy is indicated. Moreover, if pressure rises over time, or if any suggestion of target-organ damage appears, therapy should be initiated. The safety and efficacy of low-dose (12.5 to 25 mg) chlorothiazide are well established, and its use is well justified in such patients.

Choice of Drug Therapy

The purpose of drug therapy is to prevent the occurrence of coronary artery disease and stroke. The reduction of blood pressure is the intermediate objective. Many drugs are available to reduce blood pressure, but it is not yet clear that all have equal cardiovascular protective capacity. Diuretics and beta blockers have provided the most compelling evidence of benefit in hypertensive patients. Clinical trials in *secondary* prevention have demonstrated the capacity of ACE inhibitors to prevent cardiovascular events.[12] While calcium antagonists, angiotensin II–receptor blockers, and alpha-adrenergic antagonists are all effective antihypertensive agents, there is no evidence as yet that these agents reduce the incidence of cardiovascular or cerebrovascular events.

The range of effective antihypertensive agents is enormous and growing rapidly. They can be classified as (1) diuretics, (2) ACE inhibitors, (3) calcium channel entry blockers, (4) centrally acting antiadrenergic agents,

Table 21–2 Selected Antihypertensive Drugs

Class	Generic Name	Dose Range (mg)*	Comments
		Diuretics	
Thiazide-type	Hydrochlorothiazide	12.5–25/qd or bid	Standard diuretic
	Chlorthalidone	12.5–50/bid or tid	Long-acting >24 hr, potassium depletion
Loop-acting	Furosemide	20–80/bid or tid	Potassium depletion
Potassium-sparing	Amiloride	5–10/qd	Useful with thiazide-type
	Triameterene	50–100/qd or bid	Useful with thiazide-type
	Spironolactone	25–100/bid	
Beta Blockers			
Nonselective	Propranolol	40–80/bid	Lipid-soluble
	Propranolol	40–160/qd	LA
	Nadolol	20–120/qd	Long-acting
	Pindolol	5–30/bid	With ISA
Beta, selective	Metoprolol	25–100/bid	Available in IV form
	(also once-a-day formulation)		Long-acting
	Atenolol	25–100/qd	Without ISA
	Bisoprolol	5–10/qd	Mild ISA
	Acebutolol	200–800/qd	
Angiotensin-Converting Enzyme Inhibitors			
	Captopril	12.5–75/bid	Short-acting low-dose effective with congestive heart failure
	Enalapril	2.5–40/qd	Available in intravenous form
	Lisinopril	5–40/qd	Long-acting
Angiotensin II–receptor blockers	Losartan	25–50/qd	
Calcium Channel Entry Blockers			
Nondihydropyridines	Verapamil	40–120/tid	Negative inotropic and chronotropic effects
	Verapamil, sustained release	120–480 qd	Heart block may occur
	Diltiazem	30–90/tid	
	Diltiazem CD	180–300 qid	
Dihydropyridines	Nifedipine	10–30/tid	Vasodilator
	Nifedipine XL	30–90 qd	More vasoselective than nifedipine
	Nicardipine	20–40/tid	
	Amlodipine	2.5–10/qd	Long-acting, vasoselective
Centrally Acting Antiadrenergic Agents			
	Clonidine	0.05–0.6/bid	Alpha$_2$ agonist, drowsiness, dry mouth
	Guanabenz	4–16/bid	Longer duration than clonidine
	Methyldopa	250–1000/bid	False transmitter
Peripherally Acting Antiadrenergic Agents			
	Guanethidine	10–50/qd	Long-acting adrenergic neurotransmitter depleter
	Prazosin	1–10/bid	Alpha$_2$ receptor antagonist, favorable lipid effects
	Terazosin	1–5/bid	Long-acting
	Phenoxybenzamine	10–40/qd or bid	Special for pheochromocytoma
	Labetalol	100–400/bid	Combined alpha/beta blocker
		IV 2/min	

Abbreviations: qd, every day; bid, twice a day; tid, three times a day; LA, long-acting; ISA, intrinsic sympathomimetic activity; CD, extended release; XL, extended release; IV, intravenous; qid, four times a day.

*All doses in milligrams except where noted.

and (5) peripherally acting antiadrenergic agents (Table 21–2). All are effective and well-tolerated antihypertensive agents. All have side effects, but these generally affect only a small fraction of those exposed, and thus it is usually possible to achieve blood pressure control with few side effects.

Diuretics are the antihypertensive agents with which there has been the widest and longest experience. These include the commonly used thiazides, the loop diuretics, and the potassium-sparing agents. Concerns about electrolyte imbalance and the possible risk of sudden death with large doses of thiazides have been advanced as reasons to consider potassium-sparing agents. However, no clinical trial data support the superior protective capacity of the latter. In patients without cardiac disease and, particularly, evidence of congestive heart failure, potassium-sparing agents are preferred. Otherwise, thiazides are appropriate. Beta blockers, both cardioselective and not, are available with and without intrinsic sympathomimetic activity, although, again, no clear advantage for either type has been established. Long- and short-acting ACE inhibitors are available. No important differences have been observed within the converting enzyme inhibitor class. Although the locus of action of the angiotensin II–receptor blockers differs from that of the ACE inhibitors, their interference with the renin-angiotensin system is similar, and these former agents have the advantage of not producing cough, a complication of ACE inhibitors that affects about 5% of the population.

A variety of calcium antagonists are available, including both the dihydropyridine (nifedipine, nicardipine, and amlodipine) and the nondihydropyridine types (diltiazem and verapamil). Both types are available in long- and short-acting formulations. Short-acting dihydropyridines have not been approved for antihypertensive therapy, and a growing body of data suggests that they may increase the risk of cardiovascular events, making them inappropriate for chronic antihypertension therapy.[5]

The recommendations of professional organizations and national hypertension committees for initiation of drug therapy differ.[13] Some prefer diuretics and beta blockers on the basis of their demonstrated ability to reduce cardiovascular or cerebrovascular events, whereas others resist distinguishing between effective classes. Clinical trial data suggest variations in response to the different classes based on the patient's baseline characteristics.[14] For example, a Veterans Administration trial has suggested that calcium antagonists and diuretics are more effective in African-Americans, whereas beta blockers and converting enzyme inhibitors tend to be more effective in whites.[15] Both vasoconstriction and volume expansion are important in the pathogenesis of hypertension. Diuretics and calcium antagonists are more likely to be effective in volume-expanded subjects, and ACE inhibitors and beta blockers, by interfering with the renin-angiotensin-aldosterone system, are more likely to be effective in patients whose blood pressure elevation is primarily determined by vasoconstriction.[16]

The presence of concomitant conditions often dictates therapy (Table 21–3). Thus, beta blockers are logical first-line drugs in hypertensive patients with angina or a history of myocardial infarction, but they would not be appropriate for patients with chronic obstructive pulmonary disease. Diuretics have their place in patients with congestive heart failure, and alpha blockers are effective in those with benign prostatic hypertrophy.

Although initial therapy merits careful selection because the right choice will facilitate attainment of blood pressure control and therefore encourage adherence to therapy, it is only the first step in a process that is likely to be lifelong and require periodic adjustments. Thus, if the first agent selected does not lead to optimal results (see later), neither the patient nor the physician should be discouraged—instead they should recognize that they have embarked on a process whose goal is attainable, but sometimes only after multiple midcourse corrections.

Goals of Therapy and the J-Shaped Curve

Whereas the immediate goal of antihypertensive therapy is blood pressure reduction, the long-term goal of cardiovascular protection must constantly be kept in view. Remarkably, clinical trial data do not provide a ready answer to the critical question of the level to which pressure should be reduced. In the absence of a clearly defined, absolute optimal blood pressure level, the degree of reduction sought should be based on the initial height of the pressure, the magnitude of absolute risk, and the response to therapy. The higher the initial pressure, the greater the total fall should be. Not surprisingly, higher pressures generally fall further with treatment than do those closer to average.

Concerns about the limits to blood pressure lowering reflect the repeatedly observed "J-shaped" curve, in which there appears to be a level of diastolic pressure, or an attained level of 80 mm Hg, beyond which a further fall is associated with an increase in coronary events.[17, 18] Although the J-shaped curve is consistent and highly reproducible across studies, the meaning of the observation remains uncertain. It has been suggested that patients with stiff, atherosclerotic vessels, as reflected by a wide pulse pressure, are most likely to experience increased events with marked reduction in pressure.[19] Thus, it is most likely that a J-shaped curve reflects an effect rather than a cause of disease.

For the present, it is advisable to lower pressure to at least below 140 mm Hg systolic, and to the lower 80s diastolic, when the required therapy is tolerable. However, treatment should be individualized and both the risks of the hypertension and the severity of the adverse

Table 21–3	Individualized Choices of Therapy				
Coexisting Condition	**Diuretic**	**Beta Blocker**	**Alpha Blocker**	**Calcium Blocker**	**ACEI**
Older age (>65 yr)	+ +	±	+	+	+
Black race	+ +	±	+	+	±
Angina	±	+ +	+	+ +	+
Post–myocardial infarction	+	+ +	+	±*	+ +
Congestive failure	+ +	±	+	−	+ +
Cerebrovascular disease	+	+	±	+ +	+
Renal insufficiency	+ +	±	+	+ +	+ +
Diabetes	±	−	+ +	+	+ +
Dyslipidemia	−	−	+ +	+	+
Asthma or COPD	+	−	+	+	+
Benign prostatic hypertrophy			+ +		

From Kaplan, N.M.: Systemic hypertension: Therapy. *In* Braunwald, E. (ed.): Heart Disease. 5th ed. Philadelphia, W.B. Saunders, 1997, pp. 840–862.

Abbreviations: ACEI, angiotensin-converting enzyme inhibitors; + +, preferred; +, suitable, ±, usually not preferred; −, usually contraindicated; *, dihydropyridines may be contraindicated; COPD, chronic obstructive pulmonary disease.

effects of drug therapy should be balanced. Thus, for example, subjects at low risk, even those with very high levels of blood pressure, need not be required to accept serious drug side effects to lower the pressure to some arbitrary level. By contrast, a high-risk subject, albeit with a rather modest elevation of pressure, might well be asked to accept some side effects to achieve a sizable drop in pressure, based on the expectation of substantial benefit. Clinical trials in patients with mild disease have repeatedly documented widespread tolerability of long-term hypotensive therapy with diuretics and beta blockers. More recently, it has been shown that a variety of quality-of-life measures were more favorable in pharmacologically treated, mildly hypertensive patients compared with those managed with lifestyle modification alone.[13]

In selecting a target blood pressure, it should be recalled that the systolic pressure is probably more tightly linked to cardiac and cerebrovascular events than is the diastolic pressure. Both epidemiologic and intervention trial data support this view. The notion that a rising systolic pressure associated with advancing age is a benign finding has certainly been invalidated by a number of successful clinical trials showing the clinical benefits of lowering isolated systolic hypertension. In addition, these studies have demonstrated that treatment of patients with normal diastolic pressures is both tolerable and effective in the pursuit of a lower systolic pressure. Although no specific data address the issue of systolic levels between 140 and 159 mm Hg, substantial evidence suggests that intervention is justified in individuals whose absolute risk is high.

Follow-Up and Drug Withdrawal

In the patient without accelerated hypertension or vascular signs that portend a near-term complication, a gradual fall in pressure is appropriate. The first prescription should be for the smallest effective dose of the drug. In many cases, particularly when a diuretic is administered, continued gradual blood pressure lowering on the first dose may occur over weeks. In many patients, there is an inadequate response, and this should be followed by a slow increase in drug dosage before considering the addition of another agent. However, the dose of the diuretic should be no greater (and usually less) than the equivalent of 50 mg of hydrochlorothiazide.

If the first drug does not produce the desired effect, or is intolerable, a second drug from a different class of antihypertensive agents can be substituted (or added, if some response has been achieved from the first drug). When two agents are used, one of them should be a diuretic. Almost all antihypertensive drugs are effective in about half of patients. Approximately half of patients who do not respond to the first agent will respond to the second. If control of blood pressure has been achieved by the addition of a second agent, an attempt should be made to withdraw the initial drug, but it may have to be replaced if pressure rises again.

Just as there is no recognized standard for the frequency of follow-up visits (the author's policy is a minimum of four visits per year), no schedule exists for laboratory measurements. For patients begun on diuretics, it is desirable to measure serum potassium at 3 months. An annual re-evaluation should be carried out. If the blood pressure is not controlled or any clinical manifestations of hypertension become evident, standard blood tests, as well as assessment of cardiac status by electrocardiogram or echocardiogram, should be obtained. Urinary albumin excretion (measured on a spot sample by test strip) should be obtained to monitor the course of vascular disease. Evidence of advancing renal or cardiac disease on effective hypotensive therapy merits consideration of intensifying or altering therapy.

It is not uncommon, after a long period of satisfactory treatment, for blood pressure to rise. If the change is sudden, the possibility of the development of a secondary cause, such as renal artery obstruction, should be considered (see Chap. 11). More commonly, the rise reflects a gradual increase in the severity of the essential hypertension, and an increase in the dose of the single agent previously found to be effective—or the addition of an antihypertensive in a different class—is indicated. Since the natural history of essential hypertension is unpredictable and because, in some patients, prolonged blood pressure control can be followed by sustained normotension for periods up to several years after discontinuation of medication, it makes sense to attempt, in well-controlled patients, discontinuation of therapy.[11] Several formal studies have demonstrated not only that withdrawal of therapy is possible but also that there appears to be little risk associated with this if the patients are followed carefully. The majority will require the resumption of drugs within a year or two. A reasonable practice is to slowly discontinue treatment in all patients who have maintained pressures below 140/90 mm Hg for at least 6 months; in patients with evidence of target-organ disease, the threshold might be lower, perhaps 135/85 mm Hg.

Management under Special Circumstances

The Elderly

Blood pressure, especially systolic pressure, tends to rise throughout life. Thus, the incidence and prevalence of hypertension, of both the isolated systolic and the combined types, generally exceed 50% in persons over 65 years old. Manifestations of atherosclerosis also increase in prevalence, rendering older patients with elevated pressures at greater absolute risk of cardiovascular events. Evidence of vascular disease can be found in a widening pulse pressure[19]—itself an independent risk factor for both stroke and myocardial infarction—as well as peripheral vascular disease manifested by a reduced ankle/arm index (< 0.9), left ventricular hypertrophy on the electrocardiogram or echocardiogram, and evidence of renal dysfunction reflected in microalbuminuria. With aging, the capacity of the cardiovascular system to adjust to environmental variation is also impaired. Baroreceptor function is diminished and plasma renin activity and responsiveness are also reduced, compromising the ability to maintain a stable blood pressure with changes in blood volume or position; hence, orthostatic symptoms are more common in the elderly, especially when they receive antihypertensive drugs. Associated with these changes in structure and function is an increased incidence of stroke, transient ischemic attacks, and myocardial infarction. Atherosclerotic renal artery disease, accounting for both new-onset hypertension and aggravation of the course of established hypertension, is an increasing problem of the elderly.

The reduction of elevated pressure, including isolated systolic pressure, is both feasible and desirable in elderly hypertensive patients, and its benefit, in absolute terms, is likely to exceed equally effective treatment of younger subjects who are at lower risk. The rules of management are generally similar to those applied in younger subjects. Weight control and moderation of alcohol continue to be of value in the elderly, in whom exercise is often curtailed. Diuretic-based therapy has been shown, in clinical trials, to be effective and beneficial, even among that large fraction of elderly hypertensives with concomitant adult-onset diabetes. In the Systolic Hypertension in the Elderly (SHEP) trial, isolated systolic pressure in the elderly was found to respond well to a diuretic/beta blocker–based regimen.[20] ACE inhibitors have been useful in patients with evidence of congestive failure or in cases of renal dysfunction. In contrast, beta blockers may aggravate peripheral vascular disease and contribute to serious bradycardia in the susceptible elderly. In the absence of these side effects, the cardioprotective value of these agents ensures their continuing widespread use in patients over 65 years old.

In view of the high prevalence of hypertension in the elderly and the great potential for treatment benefit in this large subgroup, management of such patients is likely to account for a large portion of the primary care physician's practice. Cautious introduction and modification of medications is essential. Depression, frequently masked in the elderly, can complicate therapy. But, in the final analysis, the yield of effective treatment will more than compensate for the time and energy that must often be invested in the care of elderly hypertensive patients.

Diabetes

A majority of insulin-dependent diabetics ultimately develop hypertension. There is universal agreement that aggressive control of blood pressure is necessary to slow the progress of vascular disease and to protect the kidneys in these patients. Clinical data support the theoretical value of ACE inhibition in the diabetic hypertensive, and these drugs are the agents of first choice in insulin-requiring diabetics. Indeed, there is evidence that ACE inhibitors are useful in nonhypertensive insulin-dependent diabetics as well. If blood pressure control is not achieved with an ACE inhibitor, the cautious addition of a small dose of a thiazide diuretic is often effective (Fig. 21–6).

Aging and obesity both increase insulin resistance, glucose intolerance, and non–insulin-dependent diabetes. The combination of hypertension and non–insulin-dependent diabetes mellitus probably exceeds 10% in the el-

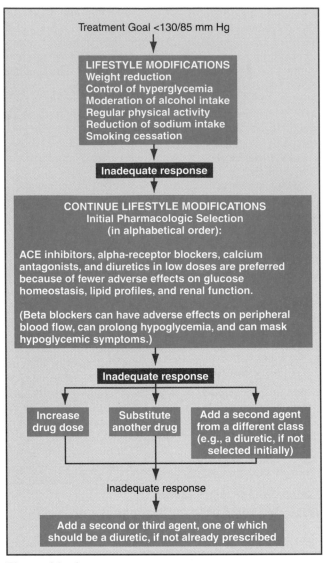

Figure 21–6

Algorithm for the treatment of hypertension in patients with diabetes. ACE, angiotensin-converting enzyme. (Redrawn from the National High Blood Pressure Education Program Working Group report on hypertension in diabetes. Hypertension 23:145, 1994. Redrawn with permission from Hypertension. Copyright 1994 American Heart Association.)

derly population, and this incidence is greater than would be expected by the independent prevalence of these two conditions. There is substantial evidence of increased cardiovascular risk not only in diabetic patients but also in those with impaired glucose tolerance without frank diabetes as well. Whether insulin resistance is an independent, reversible risk factor has yet to be demonstrated. In any event, weight reduction can often lower both pressure and insulin resistance and is to be steadfastly encouraged.

Most patients with hypertension and non–insulin-dependent diabetes mellitus require antihypertensive drug therapy. Although diuretics have consistently shown benefit in clinical antihypertensive trials in elderly diabetic patients similar to that achieved in nondiabetic hypertensives, there is some concern that these drugs may further

Table 21–4 Causes of Inadequate Response to Therapy

Pseudoresistance

"White-coat" or office elevations

Nonadherence to Therapy

Side effects of medication
Cost of medication
Lack of consistent and continuous primary care
Inconvenient and chaotic dosing schedules
Instructions not understood
Inadequate patient education
Organic brain syndrome (e.g., memory deficit)

Drug-Related Causes

Doses too low
Inappropriate combinations (e.g., two centrally acting adrenergic inhibitors)
Rapid inactivation (e.g., hydralazine)
Drug interactions

Nonsteroidal anti-inflammatory drugs	Oral contraceptives
Sympathomimetics	Adrenal steroids
Nasal decongestants	Licorice (chewing tobacco)
Appetite suppressants	Cyclosporine
Cocaine	Erythropoietin
Caffeine	Cholestyramine

Antidepressants (MAO inhibitors, tricyclics)
Excessive volume contraction with stimulation of renin-aldosterone
Hypokalemia (usually diuretic-induced)
Rebound after clonidine withdrawal

Associated Conditions

Smoking
Increasing obesity
Sleep apnea
Insulin resistance/hyperinsulinemia
Ethanol intake more than 1 oz a day (>3 portions)
Anxiety-induced hyperventilation or panic attacks
Chronic pain
Intense vasoconstriction (Raynaud's arteritis)

Secondary Hypertension

Renal insufficiency
Renovascular hypertension
Pheochromocytoma
Primary aldosteronism

Volume Overload

Excessive sodium intake
Progressive renal damage (nephrosclerosis)
Fluid retention from reduction of blood pressure
Inadequate diuretic therapy

From Kaplan, N.M.: Systemic hypertension: Therapy. *In* Braunwald, E. (ed.): Heart Disease. 5th ed. Philadelphia, W.B. Saunders, 1997, pp. 840–862; modified from Joint National Committee: Fifth report of the Joint National Committee on detection, evaluation, and treatment of high blood pressure (JNC V). Arch. Intern. Med. 153:154. 1993. Copyright 1993 American Medical Association.
Abbreviation: MAO, monoamine oxidase.

aggravate the impairment of glucose metabolism. The author believes that many patients with uncomplicated hypertensive adult-onset diabetes who are not insulin-dependent can be safely and effectively treated with low-dose thiazide diuretics. If potassium depletion becomes a problem, a potassium-sparing agent can be added or substituted. However, for patients with any evidence of renal dysfunction, including microalbuminuria, an ACE inhibitor is the agent of choice. Beta blockers or ACE inhibitors, or both, should be used in hypertensive diabetic patients with coronary artery disease.

Pregnancy

Hypertension antedating pregnancy is quite uncommon and not a contraindication to pregnancy. The hypertensive pregnant patient should be managed in close cooperation with the patient's obstetrician. In pre-eclampsia, hypertension in late pregnancy is accompanied by renal, neurologic, or hepatic involvement. When sustained elevations of pressure are present in a young woman, the possibility of a curable secondary form of hypertension should be considered, so that its correction might precede pregnancy. For women with borderline or mild elevations of arterial pressure (140 to 169 mm Hg systolic/85 to 95 mm Hg diastolic) in whom there is no evidence of target-organ disease, antihypertensive therapy might well be withheld throughout pregnancy because, for the most part, pressure tends to decline during gestation. ACE inhibitors are contraindicated in pregnant women. Alphamethyldopa and hydralazine are the drugs of choice for pregnancy-related blood pressure rise as well as for pregnant women with essential hypertension. Labetolol and calcium antagonists are sometimes useful as well. Frequently, after pregnancy, pressure declines in patients who were previously mildly hypertensive and therefore treatment needs to be re-evaluated after delivery. When hypertension is a complication of pre-eclampsia, it usually does not extend beyond the end of pregnancy.

Surgery

Hypertension itself is not a contraindication to major surgery. Effective control of blood pressure during the preoperative period reduces any potential hazard. Good communication with the anesthesiologist to ensure adequate knowledge of medications and prior cardiovascular history is necessary. Continuation of therapy up to and including the surgical procedure is appropriate. In most cases, a tablet can be taken with a small sip of water up to a few hours before the induction of anesthesia. The availability of injectable hypotensive and vasoconstrictor agents ensures that blood pressure control can always be maintained. Postoperatively, the dangers of hypotension and inadequate coronary perfusion are threats that can usually be countered by careful fluid management. Frequently, blood pressure remains low for several days after major surgery. However, most patients will require antihypertensive therapy and should be closely followed to ensure its timely reinstitution.

Resistant Hypertension

Fewer than 5% of patients with essential hypertension are nonresponders, defined as the failure of systolic blood pressure to fall by more than 10 mm Hg and diastolic pressure by more than 5 mm Hg after an adequate trial of three-drug therapy in compliant patients.[21] The most common reasons for inadequate response are, in fact, not resistant hypertension, but rather failure of compliance or inadequate therapy (Table 21–4). Occasionally, a drug interaction may prevent the hypotensive effect of the pre-scribed agent. Weight gain, nonsteroidal analgesics, oral contraceptives, cyclosporine, and glucocorticosteroids are all capable of interfering with blood pressure control. Not infrequently, with the progression of atherosclerosis, blood pressure control becomes more difficult to achieve and requires change or addition to the regimen. In some patients, the development of atherosclerotic renal artery stenosis may interfere with blood pressure control; this form of secondary hypertension (see Chap. 11) should be considered in drug-resistant cases. It is possible that the white-coat syndrome may explain an apparent failure of pressure to fall in a compliant patient. Home monitoring or 24-hour ambulatory blood pressure recording may un-cover persistent variance between office and usual pres-sures.

Renal Disease

Hypertension may be both the result and the cause of renal dysfunction. It may be secondary to renal parenchy-mal disease and to stenosis in the major renal arteries (see Chap. 11). Essential hypertension is associated with renal arteriolar nephrosclerosis and a consequent reduc-tion of the viable nephron populations. As the number of nephrons decreases, the blood volume and pressure to which the remaining glomeruli are subjected rise. This stimulates the intrarenal renin-angiotensin system, thus further compromising renal hemodynamics. The reduction of stroke and myocardial infarction demonstrated in clini-cal trials of antihypertensive therapy, and reflected in na-tional mortality and morbidity trends, has not been dem-onstrated in regard to hypertension-related renal disease. Some observations suggest that reductions in blood pres-sure more marked than those usually obtained slow the progression of renal deterioration. Since more vigorous treatment does not appear to carry additional risk, it seems appropriate to attempt to bring blood pressure down to at least 120/80 mm Hg in hypertensives with renal dysfunction. Drugs that interfere with the intrarenal renin-angiotensin system, such as ACE inhibitors, angio-tensin II–receptor blockers, and beta blockers, are reason-able first-choice agents for patients with hypertension and renal arteriolar nephrosclerosis as well as for those with hypertension secondary to unilateral renal artery stenosis. These drugs may, however, precipitate acute renal failure in patients with bilateral renal artery stenosis and can cause hyperkalemia in patients with renal failure second-ary to parenchymal renal disease.

Hypertensive Crises

(see also Chap. 17)

Malignant hypertension, or the accelerated expression of essential hypertension, is defined as markedly elevated blood pressure in association with papilledema and retinal hemorrhages, renal damage, or hypertensive encephalopa-thy. The manifestations of the last include headache, blurred vision, nausea, vomiting, seizures, and focal ab-normalities. This syndrome can be distinguished from in-tracerebral mass lesions or encephalitis by computed to-mographic scanning or examination of the cerebrospinal fluid. Cardiac manifestations and complications of malig-nant hypertension include pulmonary edema, unstable an-gina, and aortic dissection.

Widespread antihypertensive therapy has substantially reduced, but not eliminated, hypertensive crises. Although not simply a manifestation of a particular level of pres-sure, hypertensive crises generally occur when the dia-stolic pressure exceeds 130 mm Hg, usually when the rise in pressure has taken place over a short period of time. The clinical manifestations of hypertensive emergencies and their treatment are shown in Table 21–5 (see also Table 17–7). A constant intravenous infusion of nitro-prusside 0.25 to 10 μg/kg/min is most useful but requires monitoring with an intra-arterial line. The addition of intravenous furosemide 40 to 80 mg is extremely useful and reduces the dose of intravenous hypotensive agents required. In patients with hypertensive crises who are not deemed to be in immediate danger, labetalol 200 mg po may be effective.

Organizing for Successful Management

As already pointed out, high blood pressure is a mea-sure of relative risk and a contributor to absolute cardio-vascular risk. Since hypertension is not a disease, its treatment reduces but does not abolish risk. In most in-stances, lifetime treatment is required. Most patients do not have symptoms referable to blood pressure, and there-fore, neither drugs nor onerous lifestyle modifications are likely to produce any tangible benefits—beyond the hope of avoiding some later but probably unexpected complica-tion. Under these circumstances, it is not surprising that persistent compliance with therapy is difficult to achieve.

National survey data, clinical trials, and considerable research directed to this issue confirm that noncompliance is probably (at least for part of the time and for most persons) the rule rather than the exception. Failure of compliance occurs in all social classes, both genders, and all racial and ethnic groups. A single solution to this problem has not been identified. However, a combination of interventions can be helpful. Large, multicenter clinical trials, employing facilitated access to a team of therapists, have routinely produced excellent compliance. Work-site treatment and special clinics in the Veterans Administra-tion system have also been shown to keep patients in care. Through these and other experiences, three general approaches to achieving compliance have evolved.

The first approach is *cognitive*: Information about the nature of hypertension and its consequences may be use-ful, but what really seems to matter is more specific detailed information about the treatment itself. What do the medications actually do? What symptoms are to be expected? Can social drinking be continued? What effect will the medications have on sexual function? What hap-pens if a dose is skipped? What is the real value of treatment? Finally, of course, the cost of the drugs is an important issue for many patients.

The second set of compliance interventions may be considered to be *behavioral*. Physicians might alter their appointment scheduling and shorten waiting time. In cer-

Condition	Drug of Choice	Contraindicated
Hypertensive encephalopathy	Nitroprusside	Methyldopa
CNS catastrophes	Nitroprusside	Methyldopa
Subarachnoid hemorrhage	Nimodipine	
Aortic dissection	Beta blocker+nitroprusside	Hydralazine, diazoxide
Eclampsia	Hydralazine	Nitroprusside, trimethaphan
Heart failure	Nitroprusside, nitroglycerin	Labetalol
Cardiac ischemia or angina	Nitroglycerin	Hydralazine
Catecholamine-related emergencies	Phentolamine	
Clonidine withdrawal	Clonidine	
Postoperative hypertension	Nitroprusside	
Post-CABG hypertension	Nitroglycerin	

Table 21–5 Drugs for Hypertensive Emergencies

From Elliott, W.J., and Black, H.R.: Special situations in the management of hypertension. *In* Hollenberg, N.K. (vol. ed.): Hypertension: Mechanisms and Therapy. *In* Braunwald, E. (ser. ed.): Atlas of Heart Diseases. 2nd ed. Vol. 1. Philadelphia, Current Medicine, 1998, p. 12.8.
Abbreviations: CNS, central nervous system; CABG, coronary artery bypass grafting.

tain settings, adjunctive attention at a workplace or public facility such as the firehouse can enhance compliance. Sometimes cues are important in improving pill taking. Linking it to mealtime or teeth brushing can be helpful. The use of pill-organizing containers is another behavioral tool. Some physicians have found that a simple wallet card with relevant clinical and therapeutic information can be an effective reinforcing tool. Finally, there is the *social support* component of chronic care. Encouragement by the health care team, involvement of family members, and the use of group techniques can be helpful for some patients.

All of these interventions, in some combination, are useful in establishing and maintaining compliance. In the presence of a genuine partnership between the primary care physician and the hypertensive patient, the extraordinary progress in understanding the mechanism of hypertension and its treatment has made it possible to convert hypertension from an intractable threat to life and health into a marker that signals the opportunity to improve health outcome.

References

1. MacMahon, S., Peto, R., Cutler, J., et al.: Blood pressure, stroke and coronary heart disease. Part 1, Prolonged differences in blood pressure: Prospective observational studies corrected from the regression bias. Lancet 335:765–774, 1990.
2. Collins, R., Peto, R., MacMahon, S., et al.: Blood pressure, stroke and coronary heart disease. Part 2, Short-term reductions in blood pressure: Overview of randomised drug trials in their epidemiological context. Lancet 335:827–838, 1990.
3. Rose, G.: Strategy of prevention: Lessons learned from cardiovascular disease. BMJ 282:1847–1851, 1981.
4. Menard, J., Day, M., and Chatellier, G.: Individualized drug therapy: Is it time for a change from mass strategies? *In* Laragh, J.H., and Brenner, B.M. (eds.): Hypertension: Pathophysiology, Diagnosis, and Management. 2nd ed. New York, Raven Press, 1995, pp. 3035–3045.
5. Yusuf, S.: Calcium antagonists in coronary artery disease and hypertension—Time for reevaluation? Circulation 92:1079–1082, 1995.
6. Joint National Committee on Detection, Evaluation, and Treatment of High Blood Pressure: The Sixth Report of the Joint National Committee on Detection, Evaluation, and Treatment of High Blood Pressure (JNC-VI). Arch. Intern. Med. 157:2413, 1997.
7. Agewall, S., Wikstrand, J., Ljungman, S., et al.: Does microalbuminuria predict cardiovascular events in nondiabetic men with treated hypertension? Am. J. Hypertens. 8:337–342, 1995.
8. Alderman, M.H.: Blood pressure management: Individual treatment based on absolute risk and the potential of benefit. Ann. Intern. Med. 119:329–335, 1993.
9. Medical Research Council Working Party: MRC trial of treatment of mild hypertension: Principal results. BMJ 291:97–104, 1985.
10. Alderman, M.H.: Non-pharmacological treatment of hypertension. Lancet 344:307–312, 1994.
11. Alderman, M.H., Davis, T.K., Gerber, L.M., and Robb, M.: Antihypertensive drug therapy withdrawal in a general population. Arch. Intern. Med. 146:1309–1311, 1986.
12. The SOLVD Investigators: Effect of enalapril on survival in patients with reduced left ventricular ejection fractions and congestive heart failure. N. Engl. J. Med. 325:293–302, 1991.
13. Alderman, M.H., Cushman, W.C., Hill, M.N., and Krakoff, L.R.: International roundtable discussion of national guidelines for the detection, evaluation, and treatment of hypertension. Am. J. Hypertens. 6:975–981, 1993.
14. Neaton, J.D., Grimm, R.H., Jr., Prineas, R.J., et al., for the Treatment of Mild Hypertension Research Group. Treatment of Mild Hypertension Study (TOMHS): Final results. JAMA 270:713–724, 1993.
15. Materson, B.J., Reda, D.J., Cushman, W.C., et al.: Single-drug therapy for hypertension in men: A comparison of six antihypertensive agents with placebo. N. Engl. J. Med. 328:914–921, 1993.
16. Sealey, J.E., and Laragh, J.H.: The renin-angiotensin-aldosterone system for normal regulation of blood pressure and sodium and potassium homeostasis. *In* Laragh, J.H., and Brenner, B.M. (eds.): Hypertension: Pathophysiology, Diagnosis, and Management. 2nd ed. New York, Raven Press, 1995, pp. 1763–1796.
17. Hansson, L.: The J-shaped curve and how far should blood pressure be lowered? *In* Laragh, J.H., and Brenner, B.M. (eds.): Hypertension: Pathophysiology, Diagnosis, and Management. 2nd ed. New York, Raven Press, 1995, pp. 2765–2770.
18. Farnett, L., Mulroy, C.D., Linn, W.D.H., et al.: The J-curve phenomenon and the treatment of hypertension. JAMA 265:489–495, 1991.
19. Madhavan, S., Ooi, W.L., Cohen, H., and Alderman, M.H.: Relation of pulse pressure and blood pressure reduction to the incidence of myocardial infarction. Hypertension 23:395–401, 1994.
20. Fang, J., Madhavan, S., Cohen, H., Alderman, M.H.: Isolated diastolic hypertension: A favorable finding among young and middle-aged hypertensive subjects. Hypertension 26:377–382, 1995.
21. Systolic Hypertension in the Elderly Program: Prevention of stroke by antihypertensive drug treatment in older persons with isolated systolic hypertension—Final results of the Systolic Hypertension in the Elderly Program (SHEP). JAMA 265:3255–3264, 1991.
22. Bravo, E.L.: Resistant hypertension. [Review]. Nephrology 11:571–575, 1991.

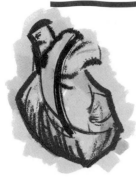

Chapter 22

Recognition and Management of Patients with

Heart Failure

LYNNE WARNER STEVENSON AND
EUGENE BRAUNWALD

Heart failure is commonly defined as the condition in which an abnormality in cardiac function is responsible for the inability of the heart to pump the quantity of blood required for ordinary activity from a normal filling pressure. Heart failure affects approximately 1% to 2% of the population. In most Western nations, heart failure accounts for 3% of the entire national health care budget, with 60% to 70% of that cost resulting from hospitalization. Now that medical therapies have been shown to improve survival and to diminish the need for hospitalization in all stages of heart failure, the identification and diligent treatment of these patients have become especially important.[1-8] The primary care physician is likely to continue to play a vital role in the recognition and in, at least, the initial care of these patients.

CLINICAL DIAGNOSIS AND ASSESSMENT

The first step is to identify the patient with heart failure (Table 22–1). Patients with a history of myocardial infarction, valvular heart disease, or severe hypertension merit particular vigilance for evidence of heart failure.

The presence of heart failure should be considered in any patient with reduced exercise tolerance, although many other causes may be responsible for this symptom. The symptoms or signs of elevated filling pressures (e.g., orthopnea, edema, or jugular venous distention) or systemic hypoperfusion (e.g., cool extremities or narrow pulse pressure) at rest are more specific but generally occur later in the disease. Many patients with chronic pulmonary disease in whom the concomitant diagnosis of heart failure is missed receive months of bronchodilator therapy for presumed exacerbation of bronchoconstriction. Patients with abdominal pain secondary to congestive hepatomegaly caused by heart failure may undergo extensive gastrointestinal evaluation before the signs of elevated right heart pressures are recognized. Occult heart failure may be diagnosed incidentally from cardiomegaly found on a routine chest radiograph, after a suspected arrhythmic or embolic event, or during an evaluation for chest pain.

History

The clinical manifestations of congestive heart failure occur not only in patients with a dilated heart and the impaired ability to eject blood (systolic failure) but also

Table 22–1	Clinical Evidence Suggesting the Diagnosis of Heart Failure	
Type of Evidence	**Highly Suggestive**	**Less Specific**
Symptoms	Orthopnea Paroxysmal nocturnal dyspnea	Decreased exercise tolerance Nocturnal cough Discomfort when bending
Signs	Jugular venous distention S$_3$ gallop Displaced left ventricular impulse Rales Narrow pulse pressure Pulsatile hepatomegaly	Tachycardia Hypotension Ascites Peripheral edema
Chest x-ray Response to diuretics	Cardiomegaly Decreased orthopnea Improved exercise tolerance Rapid weight loss > 3 lb without dizziness	Pleural effusion

Adapted from Kannel W.B., and Belander, A.J.: Epidemiology of heart failure. Am. Heart J. 1221:951, 1991.
Abbreviation: S$_3$, third heart sound.

The history should also include questions related to the cause of heart failure. For example, Is there a history of myocardial infarction? Of a heart murmur in childhood suggesting congenital heart disease? Patients with heart failure should also be questioned regarding symptoms suggestive of transient cerebral ischemic attacks or peripheral embolic events resulting from intracardiac thrombi. In addition, any history of cardiac arrest, syncope or presyncope, unexplained dizziness, or sustained palpitations should raise concern regarding cardiac dysrhythmias, which in patients with heart failure generally warrant immediate evaluation by a specialist.

Physical Examination
(Table 22–2)

In addition to the rapid clinical estimation of hemodynamic status, the cardiovascular examination should include careful assessment of the pulse for rhythm, intensity, and pulsus alternans, which when present often indicates severe left ventricular dysfunction. Postural vital signs should be measured in any patient complaining of dizziness or weakness when standing. A decline of over 10 mm Hg in systolic blood pressure with standing rarely occurs in patients with heart failure unless they have hypovolemia, excessive vasodilator effect, or autonomic neuropathy such as may be seen in amyloidosis. In addi-

in those with impaired ventricular filling (diastolic failure). The cardinal symptoms and signs of heart failure generally reflect the hemodynamic abnormalities. These occur initially during heavy exertion, then during routine activity, and ultimately at rest (see Table 3–4). When heart failure progresses slowly to the symptomatic stage, the first symptom is usually either *exertional dyspnea* or *fatigue*. At the initial evaluation and at each subsequent visit, the duration and frequency of activity responsible for these symptoms should be elicited. Specific questions could include the number of blocks the patient can walk, the tolerance for climbing stairs, which routine chores are difficult to carry out, and so on. The inability to dress without stopping to rest usually signifies the presence of severe heart failure. Patients with severe limitation of exercise but no clinical evidence of cardiac disease require a careful history to identify other causes of fatigue, such as pulmonary disease or anemia.

Orthopnea is the symptom most sensitive to baseline elevation of left ventricular filling pressure.[9] Although usually described as dyspnea in the recumbent position, orthopnea may occasionally be manifest as nocturnal cough or severely disturbed sleep. The spouse may describe *Cheyne-Stokes* respirations (cyclical hyperventilation and hypoventilation or apnea) during the patient's sleep. *Paroxysmal nocturnal dyspnea* also reflects severely elevated left ventricular filling pressures. Many patients with systemic venous congestion describe anorexia, early satiety, or abdominal discomfort. These symptoms can occur even in the absence of edema or ascites but are usually accompanied by hepatomegaly.

Table 22–2	Physical Findings to Pursue When Examining Patients with Heart Failure
Vital Signs	**Pulmonary Signs**
Pulse rate, rhythm, and quality	Rales
Determination of proportional pulse pressure	Rhonchi Friction rub
Blood pressure response to Valsalva's maneuver	Wheezes Dullness to percussion
Positional blood pressure	**Abdominal Signs**
Respiratory rate, depth, and periodicity	Ascites
Temperature	Hepatosplenomegaly
Cardiovascular Signs	Pulsatile liver
Neck vein distention	Decreased bowel sounds Ileus
Abdomino-jugular neck vein reflex	**Systemic Signs**
Cardiomegaly on palpation/percussion	Edema
Chest wall pulsatile activity	Cachexia
Gallop rhythm on auscultation	Petechiae/ecchymoses
Heart murmurs	Rash
Diminished S$_1$ or S$_2$	Arthritis
Prominent P$_2$	
Friction rub	
Peripheral pulses	
Temperature of extremities	
Neurologic Signs	
Mental status abnormalities	

Adapted from Young, J.B.: Assessment of Heart Failure. *In* Colucci, W.S. (vol. ed.): Heart Failure: Cardiac Function and Dysfunction. *In* Braunwald, E (ser. ed.) *Atlas of Heart Diseases.* vol. 4. Philadelphia, Current Medicine 1994, p 7.6.
Abbreviations: S$_1$, first heart sound; S$_2$, second heart sound; P$_2$, second pulmonic heart sound.

tion to auscultation of lungs for rales, rhonchi, wheezes, or effusion, the respiratory rate and depth and any periodic respiratory pattern should be observed.

Other components of the directed examination should focus on the potential causes of heart failure (the presence of systemic disease such as thyrotoxicosis or alcoholism), exacerbating factors such as infection, and indications of the severity of disease such as cachexia.

Clinical Assessment of Hemodynamic Profile

The severity of heart failure has traditionally been scored by the New York Heart Association (NYHA) classification and the Goldman classification (see Table 3–4). Based on both the history and the physical examination, patients can rapidly be classified according to the presence or absence of congestion or compromised perfusion (Table 22–3). Ventricular filling pressures can be normal or elevated regardless of cardiac output, whereas cardiac output can be normal or depressed regardless of filling pressure. Many patients with a low ejection fraction can still maintain normal or near-normal stroke volume with ventricular dilatation, whereas some patients with a nor-

mal ejection fraction may have a low stroke volume if the ventricular cavity is small. The four clinical profiles of heart failure are (1) no congestion with adequate resting cardiac output, (2) congestion with adequate resting cardiac output, (3) no congestion with inadequate resting cardiac output, and (4) congestion with inadequate cardiac output.[10] The last profile occurs predominantly in patients with heart failure who have received intensive diuretic therapy.

The presence of rales and peripheral edema is relatively specific but not very sensitive for elevated filling pressures in chronic heart failure, which are better identified by the presence of orthopnea and jugular venous distention.[9] Hepatic enlargement and pulsation, when present, confirm elevated right atrial pressure accompanied by tricuspid regurgitation. Rales (which may reflect alveolar edema) often develop with a pulmonary capillary wedge pressure of about 25 mm Hg. However, rales are often not present in patients with chronic heart failure, despite left ventricular filling pressures that are chronically elevated to three times normal or even higher, except when left ventricular dysfunction deteriorates suddenly. This occurs because the pulmonary lymphatic system can adapt chronically to increase alveolar fluid clearance 10- to 20-

---

Table 22–3 Initial Clinical Assessment of Resting Hemodynamic Profile for Patients with Heart Failure

	Congestion Absent	Congestion Present
Perfusion adequate	Classes I–II* Commonly underrecognized	Class III, often class IV Most common presentation of HF
Perfusion inadequate	Class III Uncommon presentation of HF before aggressive therapy	Usually class IV Common presentation of HF

Sample Profiles of Patients with Left Ventricular Ejection Fraction < 25%

No Congestion, Adequate Perfusion	*Congestion, Adequate Perfusion*	*No Congestion, Inadequate Perfusion*	*Congestion, Inadequate Perfusion*
Works parttime as store clerk	Walks ½ block, stopped by dyspnea	Walks 1 block, stopped by dyspnea or fatigue	Walks ½ block, stopped by dyspnea
Walks 1 mile daily in 20 min	Rests while dressing	Frequent inertia	Rests while dressing
No orthopnea	Three-pillow orthopnea	No orthopnea	Three-pillow orthopnea
Good appetite	Anorexia, early satiety, abdominal discomfort	Good appetite	Anorexia, early satiety, abdominal discomfort
BP 90/65	BP 90/65	BP 85/70	BP 90/80
HR 78	HR 92	HR 88	HR 98
Chest clear	Chest clear	Chest clear	Chest clear
JVP 6 cm	JVP 16 cm	JVP 6 cm	JVP 16 cm
Liver span 7 cm	Liver span 12 cm	Liver span 7 cm	Liver span 12 cm
No edema	May have edema or not	No edema	May have edema or not
Displaced LV impulse with or without S₃	Displaced LV impulse with or without S₃ Likely to have palpable RV enlargement	Same as with Adequate Perfusion, except more likely to have RV enlargement Regurgitant murmurs present but usually less prominent than in patients with congestion	Displaced LV impulse with or without S₃ Likely to have palpable RV enlargement
I–II/VI mitral regurgitation	Often II–III/VI systolic murmur may be heard at apex and base		Often II–III/VI systolic murmur may be heard at apex or base

Adapted from Stevenson, L.W.: Therapy tailored for symptomatic heart failure. Heart Failure 11:87–107, 1995.
Abbreviations: HF, heart failure; BP, blood pressure; HR, heart rate; JVP, jugular venous pressure; LV, left ventricular; S₃, third heart sound; RV, right ventricular.
* As defined by New York Heart Association.

fold.[11] Dyspnea and orthopnea occur, however, as a consequence of interstitial edema and resultant decreased lung compliance, even in the absence of rales. Elevation of left ventricular filling pressures in heart failure of recent onset can cause rales at filling pressures less than 20 mm Hg.

An inadequate cardiac output—chronic hypoperfusion—may not be apparent from the patient's general clinical appearance. However, cool extremities, altered mentation, and progressive deterioration of renal function, when present, suggest hypoperfusion at rest. Narrowing of the proportional pulse pressure ([systolic pressure − diastolic pressure]/systolic pressure) may be a helpful clue to a severely reduced cardiac output.[9] A proportional pulse pressure below 25% suggests a cardiac index below 2.2 L/min/m^2, which represents a critical level of decreased perfusion. In some older patients with a low cardiac output, the pulse pressure may be relatively preserved owing to decreased vascular elasticity.

The presence of a third heart sound (S_3) or the murmurs of mitral and tricuspid regurgitation support the diagnosis of heart failure. The new appearance of an S_3 or of mitral or tricuspid regurgitation in a patient with heart failure suggests increasing ventricular diastolic pressures. The development of a high-pitched, brief, early-diastolic murmur along the left sternal border in patients with heart failure (Graham-Steel murmur of pulmonary regurgitation) usually signifies pulmonary hypertension, often as a result of severe long-standing elevation of left atrial pressure. A right ventricular heave along the left sternal border and in the subxiphoid area indicates right ventricular distention. All these physical findings may become less prominent after successful treatment of heart failure.

Laboratory Evaluation

The electrocardiogram may provide clues to the cause and severity of the heart failure. A completely normal electrocardiogram is rare in patients with symptomatic heart failure. Patients with left ventricular dilatation often exhibit an RV_6 greater than RV_5, and a tall R in aVL. Low voltage suggests chronic constrictive pericarditis, cardiac tamponade, severe chronic obstructive pulmonary disease, or cardiac amyloidosis. A myocardial infarct pattern with deep Q- or QS-waves suggests that ischemic heart disease is the cause of heart failure. Poor R-wave progression in the precordial leads is common with both ischemic and nonischemic cardiomyopathy. Left bundle branch block or less-specific intraventricular conduction delays can result from ischemic heart disease and also occur commonly in patients with nonischemic cardiomyopathy. Sinus tachycardia (heart rate greater than 100 beats per minute) may reflect the high sympathetic tone characteristic of cardiac decompensation.

Echocardiography provides considerable information without risk or discomfort and is a key test in the evaluation of patients with established or suspected heart failure.[2,12] The echocardiogram can be used to detect both systolic and diastolic dysfunction—predominant systolic

dysfunction is a more common cause of heart failure, and it is characterized by a low ejection fraction and dilated ventricle. However, it is important to identify patients with diastolic dysfunction in whom filling is impaired but the ejection fraction is preserved (see Patients with Primary Diastolic Heart Failure), since therapy will be different[13] (see later). Echocardiography often suggests potential causes of heart failure such as ischemic heart disease, primary valvular disease, or amyloidosis.

A patient with newly diagnosed heart failure deserves specialized evaluation to determine the cause of ventricular dysfunction and guide further therapy directed toward decreasing the progression of the disease and improving clinical status.[1-3] This may involve thallium or sestamibi perfusion imaging (see Chap. 4) to identify regional hypoperfusion, as occurs in ischemic heart disease. Cardiac catheterization and coronary angiography are often indicated. Endomyocardial biopsy is not routinely indicated (Table 22-4). A chest x-ray may be the first image documenting the presence of cardiac disease (see Chap. 14) and this occasionally suggests the cause, as in left ventricular aneurysm, mitral stenosis, or congenital heart disease. Since the left ventricle often dilates in the anteroposterior direction, the cardiac silhouette may appear deceptively normal. Once heart failure is advanced, the enlarged right ventricle forms the left border of the cardiac silhouette. The presence of enlargement of vessels to the upper lobes, fluid in the fissures, peribronchial cuffing, and pulmonary interstitial and alveolar edema are all indicative of pulmonary venous hypertension (Fig. 22-1). Echocardiography is especially useful in identifying valvular abnormalities and in assessing their severity. In addition, this technique separates patients with predominant systolic heart failure (dilated ventricle, markedly depressed ejection fraction) from those with diastolic heart failure (nondilated ventricle, high, normal, or only slightly depressed ejection fraction[13,14]). Patients with heart failure secondary to ischemic heart disease often demonstrate regional wall motion disorders.

Blood tests that may be helpful include serum sodium and indices of renal and hepatic function, which often reflect disease severity. Thyroid-stimulating hormone, serum iron studies for hemochromatosis, and hematocrit may be helpful in the search for a cause (Table 22-4). Electrolyte measurements and coagulation studies are useful for management.

Precipitating Factors

A careful search should be made for reversible precipitating factors that could have caused or exacerbated heart failure (Table 22-5). In many patients, symptomatic heart failure is precipitated by an acute disturbance that places an extra hemodynamic load on the heart, such as an infection or tachyarrhythmia. Perhaps the most frequent cause of reversible cardiac decompensation is failure of compliance with the therapeutic regimen. Increase of dietary sodium intake or inappropriate discontinuation of medications can precipitate heart failure in patients with asymptomatic left ventricular dysfunction.

Table 22–4	Selected Recommendations from Guidelines for Heart Failure	
Topic	**Recommendation**	**Strength of Evidence***
Prevention in asymptomatic patients	Asymptomatic patients with moderately or severely reduced left ventricular systolic function (EF < 35%–40%) should be treated with an ACE inhibitor	A
Initial evaluation	Patients with symptoms highly suggestive of heart failure should undergo echocardiography or radionuclide ventriculography to measure left ventricular function even if physical signs of heart failure are absent	C
Diagnostic testing	Practitioners should perform a chest x-ray; ECG; CBC; serum electrolytes, serum creatinine, serum albumin, liver function tests; and urinalysis for all patients with suspected or clinically evident heart failure.	C
	A T_4 and TSH level should also be checked in all patients over age 65 years with heart failure and no obvious cause, and in patients who have atrial fibrillation or other signs or symptoms of thyroid disease	
	Routine use of myocardial biopsy is not recommended	
Screening for arrhythmias	Screening evaluation for arrhythmias such as ambulatory ECG is not routinely warranted.	A
Activity recommendations	Regular exercise should be encouraged for all patients with stable NYHA classes I–III heart failure	C
Diet	Dietary sodium should be restricted to as close to 2 gm/day as possible	C
ACE inhibitors	Patients with heart failure due to left ventricular systolic dysfunction should be given a trial of ACE inhibitors unless specific contraindications exists: (1) history of intolerance or adverse reactions to these agents, (2) serum potassium greater than 5.5 mEq/L that cannot be reduced, or (3) symptomatic hypotension	A
	Patients with systolic blood pressure less than 90 mm Hg have a higher risk of complications and should be managed by a physician experienced in utilizing ACE inhibitors in such patients	
	Caution and close monitoring are also required for patients who have a serum creatinine greater than 3.0 mg/dl or an estimated creatinine clearance of less than 30 ml/min; half the usual dose should be used in this setting	
Digoxin	Digoxin should be used routinely in patients with severe heart failure and should be added to the medical regimen of patients with mild or moderate heart failure who remain symptomatic after optimal management with ACE inhibitors and diuretics	C
Hydralazine/isosorbide dinitrate	The combination of isosorbide dinitrate and hydralazine is an appropriate alternative in patients with contraindications or intolerance to ACE inhibitors and may be added as adjunctive therapy when symptoms persist despite aggressive therapy with ACE inhibitors and diuretics	B
Anticoagulation	Anticoagulation is not routinely recommended in the absence of atrial fibrillation, mobile thrombi, or previous embolic events	C

From Lee T.H.: Practice guidelines in cardiovascular medicine. In Braunwald, E. (ed.): Heart Disease. 5th ed. Philadelphia: W.B. Saunders, 1997, pp. 1939–1996; adapted from Konstam, M., Dracup, K., Baker, D.W., et al.: Heart failure: Evaluation and care of patients with left-ventricular systolic dysfunction. Clinical Practice Guideline No. 11. AHCPR Publication no. 94–0612. Rockville, MD, Agency for Health Care Policy and Research, Public Health Service, U.S. Department of Health and Human Services, June 1994.

Abbreviations: EF, ejection fraction; ACE, angiotensin-converting enzyme; ECG, electrocardiogram; CBC, complete blood count; T_4, thyroxine; TSH, thyroid-stimulating hormone; NYHA, New York Heart Association.

* Strength of evidence: A, good evidence of treatment from randomized trials; B, fair evidence; C, expert opinion.

In patients with *ischemic heart disease* and new or worsening heart failure, the possibility of reversible ischemia causing myocardial hibernation needs to be considered.[2] Viable myocardium with impaired resting blood flow is most commonly identified by delayed thallium uptake in a region of myocardium that exhibits failure of contraction. In such patients, coronary revascularization may be very effective in improving ventricular function and diminishing heart failure (see Chap. 18).

Although *hypertension* is now an uncommon sole cause of heart failure, it may be an important contributor. Even modest elevations in arterial pressure can further compromise a ventricle impaired by another process such as previous myocardial infarction. Therefore, hypertension should be treated aggressively.

Heavy alcohol consumption has been estimated to cause approximately 10% of all cases of dilated cardiomyopathy in adults and is probably underrecognized. Even two drinks daily may be sufficient to worsen heart failure in patients with left ventricular dysfunction of other causes. Illicit drug use may also contribute to cardiomyopathy. *Cocaine use* may cause acute coronary syn-

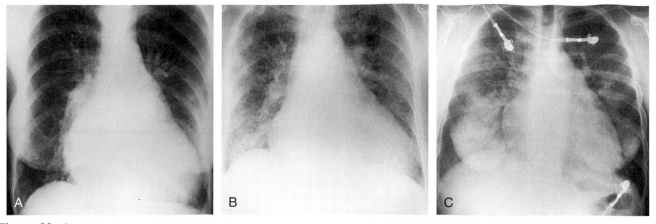

Figure 22–1

Cardiac radiograph in heart failure. *A,* Pulmonary blood flow redistribution. Enlargement of the upper lobe vessels in this patient with ischemic cardiomyopathy and elevated pulmonary venous pressure. *B,* Pulmonary interstitial edema. The vessels are indistinct and enlarged. There is peribronchial cuffing. *C,* Pulmonary alveolar edema in a patient with congestive cardiomyopathy. The central parahilar distribution of edema, termed *bat wing* edema, is typical of cardiovascular or fluid overload (uremic) pulmonary alveolar edema. (*A–C,* From Steiner, R.M., and Levin, D.C: Radiology of the heart. *In* Braunwald, E. [ed.]: Heart Disease. 5th ed. Philadelphia, W.B. Saunders, 1997, pp. 204–239.)

dromes but can also produce a chronic cardiomyopathy similar to that seen with pheochromocytoma.

Tachyarrhythmias can cause cardiomyopathy in otherwise normal hearts but more often may aggravate left ventricular dysfunction of other causes. Atrial fibrillation, present in approximately 20% of patients with heart failure, is a major target for therapy, since rates during exertion are often excessive. Conversion to sinus rhythm or at least aggressive rate control is usually associated with marked clinical improvement.

Both *hyperthyroidism* and *hypothyroidism* may compromise cardiac function. These conditions should be considered, especially in patients receiving amiodarone, since the iodine contained in this antiarrhythmic drug can cause hypothyroidism or hyperthyroidism. *Severe obesity* is the most common metabolic abnormality contributing to heart failure; weight loss often improves symptoms and sometimes the ejection fraction as well. Obesity may also be associated with sleep apnea, which can compromise cardiac function. *Pregnancy* may unmask previously asymp-

tomatic heart disease, but it can also cause a cardiomyopathy (peripartum cardiomyopathy). *Anemia,* both acute and chronic, can precipitate decompensation of patients with previously stable left ventricular dysfunction.

Patients with heart failure are at risk of developing deep venous thrombosis and *pulmonary embolism* (see Chap. 30), which in turn can exacerbate heart failure and precipitate acute decompensation.

A variety of *drugs* may exacerbate heart failure. First-generation calcium antagonists have been associated with clinical deterioration and decreased survival of patients with heart failure. Usually prescribed for hypertension, angina, or control of the ventricular response in atrial fibrillation, these agents should be replaced by other therapies in most patients with cardiac decompensation. Current trials are evaluating newer calcium antagonists, such as amlodipine, which may not have the same deleterious effects. Antiarrhythmic agents that severely depress myocardial contractility, such as disopyramide and sotalol, may aggravate systolic heart failure. Beta blockers are beneficial in some patients with heart failure (see later), but they may aggravate heart failure when they are initiated rapidly or given in high doses or in patients with severe congestive symptoms. Nonsteroidal anti-inflammatory agents can cause fluid retention and deterioration of renal function, hence worsening the symptoms and signs of heart failure.

Table 22–5	Potentially Reversible Factors in Heart Failure

Noncompliance with therapeutic regimen
Superimposed systemic infection
Pulmonary embolism
Extensive myocardial ischemia
Primary valvular disease
Tachycardias
Hypertension
Heavy alcohol consumption
Cocaine, amphetamines, or excess use of bronchodilators
Anemia
Metabolic factors (thyroid disease, hemochromatosis, obesity, electrolyte disorders)
Pregnancy
Medications

MANAGEMENT OF HEART FAILURE (Figs. 22–2 and 22–3)

The goals of therapy are to reduce the symptoms of heart failure, prevent or reverse progression of ventricular dysfunction, and prolong survival.[3] The relative importance of these goals varies according to the presence and severity of the symptoms of heart failure. In the asympto-

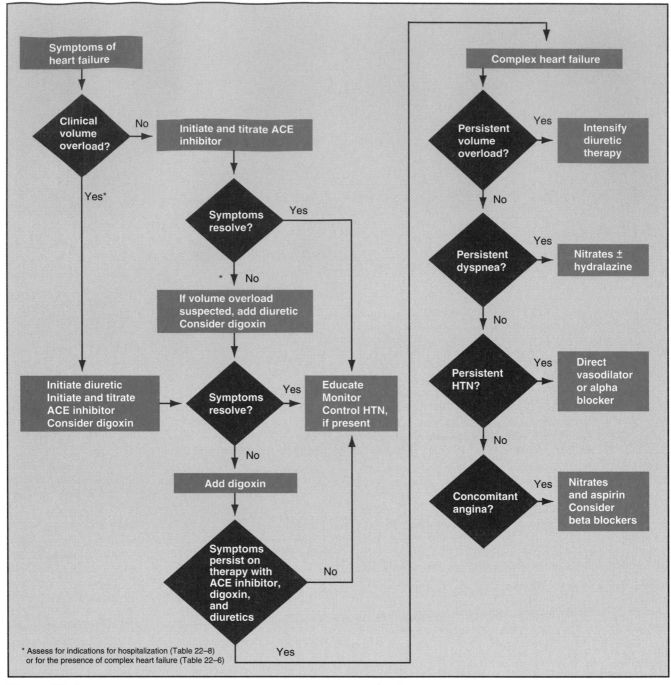

Figure 22–2

Algorithm for treating symptoms of heart failure, emphasizing the importance of determining fluid status and recognizing "complex" heart failure or other indications for hospitalization. (See Tables 22–6 and 22–8.) ACE, angiotensin-converting enzyme; HTN, hypertension. (Adapted from Konstam, M.A., Dracup, K., Baker, D.W., et al.: Heart Failure: Evaluation and care of patients with left-ventricular systolic dysfunction. Clinical Practice Guideline no. 11. AHCPR Publication no. 94–0612. Rockville, MD, Agency for Health Care Policy and Research, Public Health Service, U.S. Department of Health and Human Services, June 1994.)

matic or mild stages of heart failure, emphasis is on arresting disease progression, whereas in later stages of decompensation, it is on improving the quality as well as the length of life.

Depending on the clinical severity of decompensation, treatment of *reversible* underlying or precipitating causes should be undertaken along with the adjustment of phar-

macologic therapy. For example, alleviation of ischemia, anemia, or infection may lead to resolution of heart failure symptoms. Discontinuation of heavy alcohol consumption often improves the clinical status and ventricular function.

Asymptomatic ventricular dysfunction may be diagnosed by echocardiography or radionuclide angiography after

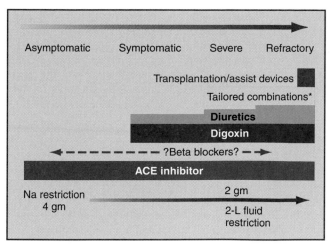

Figure 22–3

Escalation of therapy for left ventricular dysfunction in relation to the severity of symptoms and hemodynamic decompensation. Angiotensin-converting enzyme (ACE) inhibition has been demonstrated to improve prognosis for patients at all levels of heart failure. Digoxin decreases symptoms of heart failure once they have developed. It is not yet known which patients may benefit from beta-adrenergic blocking agents. Cardiac transplantation or implantable ventricular assist devices are considered only for a very small population with heart failure refractory to all other therapies. * The term *tailored combinations* refers to the use of additional vasodilators (usually in combination with an ACE inhibitor) and, when necessary, short-term hemodynamic monitoring and use of intravenous nitroprusside or dobutamine. (Redrawn from Smith, T.W., Kelly, R.A., Stevenson, L.W., and Braunwald, E.: The management of heart failure. *In* Braunwald, E. [ed.]: Heart Disease. 5th ed. Philadelphia, W.B. Saunders, 1997, pp. 492–514.)

cardiomegaly is found incidentally on a routine chest radiograph, during evaluation of a suspected arrhythmia or embolic event, or referral for atypical chest pain. A history of myocardial infarction warrants screening to detect asymptomatic left ventricular dysfunction, since such patients have been shown to benefit from intervention. Angiotensin-converting enzyme (ACE) inhibitors are the only class of drugs that have been shown to benefit asymptomatic patients with left ventricular dysfunction (see Table 22–4).

Symptomatic Heart Failure

The development of symptoms heralds a worsening prognosis for patients with left ventricular dysfunction. After confirming the diagnosis and addressing potentially reversible factors, the approach to symptoms of heart failure requires assessment of the hemodynamic profile, as discussed previously (see Table 22–3).

Some patients develop symptoms of heart failure while already on ACE inhibitors for previous hypertension or asymptomatic left ventricular dysfunction. Other patients are not diagnosed with left ventricular dysfunction until they present with symptoms of heart failure. In either case, ACE inhibitors should be titrated as tolerated to "target doses." These drugs can be expected to improve

symptoms, slow disease progression, and prolong survival.

If, despite ACE inhibitors, patients continue to have congestion, as evidenced by orthopnea or other evidence of volume overload, they should be evaluated for the presence of resting hypoperfusion or other criteria for complex heart failure (Table 22–6), which might warrant referral for specialized heart failure management. If systemic perfusion appears to be adequate, diuretic therapy can be added to ACE inhibitors, recognizing the need to avoid excessive reduction of blood pressure.

Digitalis is clearly indicated in patients with heart failure and atrial fibrillation. Although the addition of digoxin does not appear to prolong life in patients with heart failure and sinus rhythm, it does reduce the incidence of hospitalization for heart failure. Discontinuation of digitalis in patients with a history of symptomatic heart failure and sinus rhythm has been shown to result in clinical deterioration.[15]

Relief of Congestion

As a general goal in patients with systolic heart failure, filling pressures should be reduced by vasodilators and diuretics to a level at which orthopnea, edema, rales, and ascites are absent and jugular venous pressure is not elevated. In patients with diastolic heart failure, including those with acute myocardial ischemia or infarction, optimal filling pressures may be higher, but it is usually possible to achieve relief of symptomatic congestion at rest and during routine activity (Table 22–7).

Patients should be considered for hospitalization if there is evidence of decompensation despite therapy (Table 22–8). Even in the absence of acute deterioration, referral for specialist management should be considered for other evidence of complex heart failure (see Table 22–6).

Table 22–6	Complex Heart Failure

Acute Decompensation

Profile suggesting simultaneous congestion and hypoperfusion (see Table 22–2)

Heart failure in the presence of other active cardiac problems
    Examples: Angina or other evidence of active ischemia
              Hemodynamically significant aortic valve disease
              Syncope or symptomatic ventricular arrhythmias

Symptoms of heart failure in the presence of major noncardiac conditions complicating assessment/therapy
    Examples: Suspected exacerbation of pulmonary disease
              Progressive renal dysfunction
              Active systemic infection

Anticipated difficulty with initiation or adjustment of ACE inhibitors
    Systolic blood pressure < 90 mm Hg with decompensation
    Serum sodium < 134 mEq/L
    Major symptoms of heart failure and history of intolerance to ACE inhibitors

Chronic Failure despite Standard Therapy

Patients with persistent class III or IV symptoms of heart failure or an emergency room visit or hospitalization for heart failure despite ≥1 month of attempted therapy with ACE inhibitors, digoxin, and diuretics

Abbreviation: ACE, angiotensin-converting enzyme.

Table 22–7 **Systolic versus Diastolic Dysfunction in Heart Failure**

Parameters	Systolic	Diastolic
History		
Coronary heart disease	++++	+
Hypertension	++	++++
Diabetes	+	+++
Valvular heart disease	++++	–
Paroxysmal dyspnea	++	+++
Physical examination		
Narrow pulse pressure	+++	–
Cardiomegaly	+++	+
Soft heart sounds	++++	+
S₃ gallop	+++	+
S₄ gallop	+	+++
Mitral regurgitation	+++	+
Edema	++	++
Jugular venous distention	+++	++
Chest radiogram		
Cardiomegaly	+++	+
Pulmonary congestion	+++	+++
Electrocardiogram		
Low voltage	+++	–
Left ventricular hypertrophy	++	++++
Left ventricular dilatation	+++	–
Q-waves	+++	+
Echocardiogram		
Low ejection fraction	++++	–
Left ventricular dilatation	+++	–
Atrial dilatation alone	–	+++
Left ventricular hypertrophy	++	++++
Mitral regurgitation	+++	++

Adapted from Young, J.B.: Assessment of heart failure. *In* Colucci, W.S. (vol. ed.): Heart Failure: Cardiac Function and Dysfunction. Braunwald, E. (ser. ed.): Atlas of Heart Diseases. Vol. 4. Philadelphia, Current Medicine 1994, p. 7.6.

Abbreviations: S₃, third heart sound; S₄, fourth heart sound

Maintenance of Perfusion

Systemic perfusion, which is a function of cardiac output and peripheral vascular resistance, can usually be maintained even when the left ventricular ejection fraction is low. The "arithmetic of cardiac output" demonstrates that stroke volume can be preserved despite a low ejection fraction in the presence of ventricular dilatation. For example, in patients with chronic heart failure with left ventricular ejection fractions one-third of normal (20%), the left ventricular end-diastolic volumes may exceed three times normal. Stroke volume may be only marginally reduced and a slight compensatory tachycardia may contribute to a normal cardiac output at rest. However, as left ventricular dilatation progresses, functional mitral regurgitation often develops, despite an anatomically normal mitral valve. This dynamic mitral regurgitation is very sensitive to changes in loading conditions and may cause a marked reduction of forward stroke volume. As heart failure progresses, similar factors operate on the right ventricle, with tricuspid regurgitation affecting right ventricular stroke volume. Systemic perfusion may also decline when ejection fraction falls acutely before compensatory dilatation has occurred.

The majority of patients with low ejection fraction and impaired perfusion derive benefit from peripheral vasodilatation, which reduces the load on the left ventricle. Ad-

justment of doses to achieve "target" doses of ACE inhibition for patients with few or no symptoms of heart failure is usually continued until a systolic blood pressure of 90 to 100 mm Hg is reached or until dizziness or other evidence of postural hypotension develops. On the other hand, patients with more severe heart failure may tolerate systolic pressures as low as 80 mm Hg.

Preservation of Renal Function

The majority of patients with chronic congestive heart failure demonstrate a slight increase in serum creatinine and blood urea nitrogen (BUN) as therapy relieves congestion. Therapy should not be decreased or discontinued for a serum creatinine less than 2.0 mg/dl or an increase from baseline levels of less than 1.0 mg/dl. Continued increases in serum creatinine require close surveillance, but the majority of patients achieve a stable level early after therapy has been intensified and often show subsequent improvement in renal function as their hemodynamic status stabilizes. In some patients, particularly those with intrinsic renovascular disease associated with atherosclerosis, hypertension, and diabetes, a compromise must be achieved between impaired renal function and the intensive diuresis and vasodilatation required to relieve cardiac symptoms. This usually requires participation of a specialist.

Management of Complex Heart Failure

In patients with evidence of hypoperfusion at rest, even cautious initiation or increase of therapy with ACE inhibitors can precipitate severe hypotension, whereas oral loop diuretics are often ineffective in initiating diuresis.

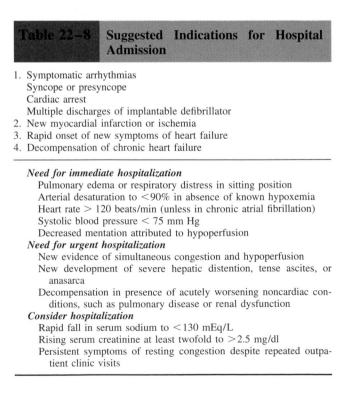

Table 22–8 **Suggested Indications for Hospital Admission**

1. Symptomatic arrhythmias
   Syncope or presyncope
   Cardiac arrest
   Multiple discharges of implantable defibrillator
2. New myocardial infarction or ischemia
3. Rapid onset of new symptoms of heart failure
4. Decompensation of chronic heart failure

Need for immediate hospitalization
   Pulmonary edema or respiratory distress in sitting position
   Arterial desaturation to <90% in absence of known hypoxemia
   Heart rate > 120 beats/min (unless in chronic atrial fibrillation)
   Systolic blood pressure < 75 mm Hg
   Decreased mentation attributed to hypoperfusion
Need for urgent hospitalization
   New evidence of simultaneous congestion and hypoperfusion
   New development of severe hepatic distention, tense ascites, or anasarca
   Decompensation in presence of acutely worsening noncardiac conditions, such as pulmonary disease or renal dysfunction
Consider hospitalization
   Rapid fall in serum sodium to <130 mEq/L
   Rising serum creatinine at least twofold to >2.5 mg/dl
   Persistent symptoms of resting congestion despite repeated outpatient clinic visits

Although adding a second diuretic such as metolazone, a drug that blocks sodium reabsorption at different sites from those targeted by the loop diuretics, may initiate dramatic diuresis, this drug may also cause dangerous hypotension and electrolyte disturbances. Often, patients with combined congestion and hypoperfusion do not respond well to any oral medications and continue in a downward spiral of deterioration. These patients are often managed best in the hospital, where diuretics, vasodilators, and if necessary, intravenous inotropic agents can be adjusted simultaneously, sometimes with the aid of a temporary pulmonary artery catheter.

Patients with evidence of simultaneous congestion and ischemia should also be considered to have complex heart failure that requires special evaluation, generally in the hospital. Angina may be aggravated by increased myocardial oxygen requirements and compromised subendocardial perfusion that accompany elevated left ventricular filling pressures, and it may improve markedly once optimal loading conditions are restored. On the other hand, the exacerbation of heart failure may arise from recent infarction or new ischemia, or both, which may require specific intervention.

Noncardiac conditions can also render heart failure complex because they either complicate hemodynamic assessment or restrict the limits within which therapy can be safely adjusted. For example, the continued use of high-dose adrenergic bronchodilators in patients with chronic pulmonary disease and left ventricular failure can cause tachycardia that can worsen left ventricular function and may precipitate arrhythmias. On the other hand, even mild fluid retention in such patients can worsen pulmonary function. Patients with chronic renal failure may be particularly dependent on circulating volume to preserve renal function. The ideal compromise between cardiac and renal function requires careful titration of diuretics and other medications, as discussed later.

HEART FAILURE IN SPECIAL PATIENT GROUPS

Patients with Primary Diastolic Heart Failure

The different features in systolic and diastolic heart failure are summarized in Table 22–7. In systolic heart failure, the primary abnormality is the inability to eject sufficient blood. This condition is associated with a marked reduction of the left ventricular ejection fraction, usually to below 35% in symptomatic patients. In diastolic heart failure, impaired ventricular relaxation leads to elevation of ventricular end-diastolic pressure with little reduction of the ejection fraction. In up to 40% of patients with clinical evidence of heart failure, the left ventricular ejection fraction exceeds 35%,[13] and they may have either isolated diastolic heart failure or coexistent systolic and diastolic failure. Diastolic heart failure may be caused by reduced ventricular diastolic capacity, as occurs in hypertrophic, restrictive, or hypertensive cardio-

myopathy, constrictive pericarditis, myocardial infiltration, or impaired ventricular relaxation. Diastolic dysfunction should be suspected in patients with heart failure and hypertension or diabetes, although these conditions can cause systolic dysfunction as well.

As discussed earlier, since the stroke volume is the product of ejection fraction and ventricular diastolic volume, any process that restricts myocardial dilatation leads to a lower stroke volume and cardiac output and thus more severe limitation of cardiac reserve. In the extreme example of hypertrophic cardiomyopathy, the left ventricular ejection fraction may be as high as 80%, but even 80% of a severely diminished left ventricular cavity volume can yield a low stroke volume.[14]

The physical examination usually reveals a fourth heart sound, sometimes an S_3. The symptoms and signs of elevated left- and right-sided filling pressures can be as severe as in systolic failure but are not often accompanied by evidence of hypoperfusion. The diagnosis is best confirmed by echocardiography, which may demonstrate abnormal ventricular filling patterns in the presence of relatively preserved systolic function and little, if any, ventricular dilatation.

Management

The tendency to retain fluid is often the most prominent feature on clinical assessment in patients with impaired diastolic function. These patients should be treated with diuretics until symptoms resolve or until further symptom reduction is prevented by postural hypotension or unacceptable reductions in renal function. Calcium antagonists may improve diastolic function in some patients, but the benefits in the absence of hypertension have not been proved. ACE inhibitors are another reasonable choice for control of hypertension in such patients. Efforts should be made to slow heart rate and thereby prolong the diastolic filling period. Digoxin is occasionally indicated to control the heart rate in atrial fibrillation, although beta blockers, amiodarone, or verapamil may be more effective for this purpose in patients with diastolic dysfunction. The atrial contribution to ventricular filling should be maintained. This may require cardioversion in patients with atrial fibrillation and sequential atrioventricular pacing in those without a properly timed atrial contraction. Vigorous afterload reduction is generally *not* indicated in patients with diastolic dysfunction and may be deleterious except in the control of hypertension.

The Elderly

Half of all patients with heart failure in the United States are over 70 years old; nearly 1 in 10 persons over 80 years old has this condition. Predominant diastolic dysfunction as a cause of heart failure is increased in the elderly.[13] Heart failure in these patients is frequently combined with diffuse coronary artery disease or aortic valve sclerosis. Vascular disease in the carotid arteries and lower extremities and noncardiac co-morbid conditions such as diabetes mellitus, pulmonary disease, and renal disease may complicate the diagnosis and management.

The options and intensity of therapy for heart failure

are limited by the aging circulation. Whereas younger patients often tolerate systolic blood pressures as low as 80 mm Hg, and this low pressure aids in the maintenance of stroke volume, patients over the age of 70 years should probably be maintained at a systolic pressure of at least 90 mm Hg; those with cerebrovascular disease may require systolic pressures of 120 mm Hg or even higher. Owing to altered autonomic regulation, unacceptable postural hypotension resulting from vasodilator therapy may be a greater problem in the elderly, who are also more prone to develop progressive renal dysfunction during diuresis. However, in most elderly patients, by careful manipulation of the therapeutic measures, an acceptable balance can be reached where jugular venous pressure, creatinine, and BUN are all slightly elevated but stable.

Affiliation of the patient and family with a physican–nurse–social services team specialized in the care of patients with heart failure (see Expectations after Hospitalization) may require particular emphasis in the elderly population, in whom other conditions often limit compliance and physical function. When compared with standard care, a team of experts in heart failure and geriatrics can improve the quality of life and reduce hospitalizations for heart failure in the elderly.[16]

Patients with Chronic Heart Failure despite Standard Therapy

According to the Agency for Health Care Policy and Research guidelines, patients on therapy with ACE inhibitors, digoxin, and diuretics who nonetheless demonstrate persistent symptoms limiting daily activity or who require repeated hospitalizations, are considered to have complex, chronic heart failure. The outcome for such patients receiving care from a multidisciplinary, specialized heart failure team has improved since the mid-1980s.[17] As for all patients with heart failure, the goals include achievement of optimal fluid balance and vasodilator regimen, but for complex heart failure, this may be facilitated by intravenous vasodilators such as nitroprusside or infusions of inotropic agents such as dobutamine or milrinone for initial stabilization, often guided by invasive hemodynamic monitoring.

The optimal blood pressure needed to reduce left ventricular workload while maintaining peripheral perfusion in these patients may be lower than that usually tolerated, with systolic blood pressures commonly 80 to 90 mm Hg. High doses and combinations of vasodilators and inotropic agents may be required. The balance between cardiac and renal compensation may be particularly delicate in these patients. Modestly elevated levels of creatinine and BUN may have to be accepted in order to maintain relief from congestive symptoms.

Frequent, routine telephone contact from a heart failure program helps to avert decompensation. In selected, highly motivated patients, instruction in home blood pressure measurement may facilitate minor adjustments in medications. Once an effective regimen has been initiated, further changes must be made very carefully. Even for symptomatic hypotension attributed to excessive vasodila-

tation or diuresis, doses of medication should in general be reduced by small amounts rather than discontinued. Any change in vasodilator or diuretic medication requires re-evaluation within 3 days. Although many patients with complex heart failure can be stabilized, continued vigilance is required to detect early signs of recurrent decompensation.

Patients Who Are Candidates for Cardiac Transplantation

This procedure provides a good quality of life and a 60% to 70% 5-year survival for carefully selected patients (Table 22–9).[18, 19] Unfortunately, this option is limited by the donor heart supply to fewer than 2500 patients yearly in the United States, where an estimated 40,000 patients could benefit from transplantation each year. Transplant recipients assume the burdens of rejection, immunosuppression, and accelerated graft coronary artery disease. More than half of the recipients continue to be restricted in their activities and fewer than half return to work. Many patients who can be stabilized on a carefully tailored medical regimen with a left ventricular ejection fraction less than 25% have quality of life and rates of survival similar to those expected after cardiac transplantation. The primary care physician should refer patients with complex heart failure to heart failure/transplant centers for consideration early in their disease if they are potentially eligible.

DRUGS IN THE MANAGEMENT OF HEART FAILURE (Table 22–10)

ACE Inhibitors

ACE inhibitors have been shown to decrease hospitalization at all stages of heart failure when the left ventricular ejection fraction is less than 40%.[4, 8] Initial therapy usually consists of 12.5 mg tid of captopril, 2.5 mg bid of enalapril, or 2.5 mg daily of lisinopril. Upward titration of oral ACE inhibitors should proceed, generally in the outpatient setting, with optimal doses established by 4 to 6 weeks. Although target doses should be sought, a dose that consistently produces symptomatic hypotension should be avoided.

Although ACE inhibitors reduce the diuretic requirements of patients with heart failure, they are rarely adequate for relieving congestion at rest without concomitant use of diuretics (see Fig. 22–2). However, it is prudent to avoid major increases in the doses of ACE inhibitors and diuretics simultaneously, except in hospitalized patients, because of the risk of hypotension.

Approximately 5% to 10% of patients cannot tolerate ACE inhibitors, primarily because of cough. There is currently no good evidence to suggest that the frequency of cough varies with different agents. In many patients with heart failure treated with ACE inhibitors, cough is actually a sign of elevated left-sided filling pressures, and will

Table 22-9	Cardiac Transplantation

Selection Criteria

I. Accepted indications
   1. Peak $VO_2 \leq 10$ ml/kg/min with achievement of anaerobic metabolism
   2. Severe ischemia consistently limiting routine activity not amenable to bypass surgery or angioplasty
   3. Recurrent symptomatic ventricular arrhythmias refractory to all accepted therapeutic modalities
II. Probable indications
   1. Peak $VO_2 < 14$ ml/kg/min and major limitation of the patient's daily activities
   2. Recurrent unstable ischemia not amenable to bypass or angioplasty
   3. Instability of fluid balance/renal function not due to patient noncompliance with regimen of weight monitoring, flexible use of diuretic drugs, and salt restriction
III. Inadequate indications
   1. Ejection fraction $\leq 20\%$
   2. History of previous functional class III or IV symptoms of heart failure
   3. Previous ventricular arrhythmias
   4. Peak $VO_2 > 15$ ml/kg/min without other indications
IV. Continuing evaluation
   1. Clinical assessment by heart failure/transplant team at least every 1–2 months
   2. Re-evaluation at 6-month intervals to include assessment of clinical stability and measurement of peak oxygen consumption

Contraindications

General
   Any noncardiac condition that would itself shorten life expectancy or increase the risk of death from rejection or from complications of immunosuppression, particularly infection
Specific
   Over the upper age limit of 55–65 years (various programs)
   Active infection
   Active ulcer disease
   Severe diabetes mellitus with end-organ damage
   Severe peripheral vascular disease
   *Pulmonary function (FEV$_1$, FVC) < 60% or history of chronic bronchitis
   *Creatinine clearance < 40–50 ml/min
   *Bilirubin > 2.5 mg/dl, transaminases > 2 times normal
   *Pulmonary artery systolic pressure > 60 mm Hg
   *Mean transpulmonary gradient > 15 mm Hg
   Active substance abuse
   High risk of noncompliance

Selection Criteria: Adapted from Mudge, G.H., Goldstein, S., Addonizio, L.J., et al.: Cardiac transplantation: Recipient guidelines/prioritization. Reprinted with permission from the American College of Cardiology. J. Am. Coll. Cardiol. 22:21, 1993.

Abbreviations: VO$_2$, volume of oxygen consumption; FEV$_1$, forced expiratory volume in 1 sec; FVC, forced vital capacity.

* May need to demonstrate reversibility after aggressive therapy to improve hemodynamic status.

diminish with treatment of heart failure. Of the remaining patients, some can tolerate low doses of these agents. Angioneurotic edema and agranulocytosis are rare complications of ACE inhibition. Angiotensin II–receptor blockers are now being studied as substitutes for the minority of patients who cannot tolerate ACE inhibitors and as an addition to ACE inhibitors in those patients who require additional therapy. These newer agents, often used in the treatment of hypertension, improve hemodynamics and exercise tolerance in a manner similar to that of ACE inhibitors. The effects on disease progression and survival are not known.

ACE inhibitors often improve renal function in patients with mild to moderate heart failure. However, in severe heart failure, inhibition of the renin-angiotensin system may reduce the glomerular filtration rate. Renal artery stenosis should be considered if renal function deteriorates markedly with ACE inhibitor therapy. When serum creatinine levels exceed 2 mg/dl or the serum BUN level exceeds 50 mg/dl, or both, the initiation or adjustment of ACE inhibitor therapy should be done only by those with extensive experience.

Symptomatic hypotension occurring repeatedly even with low doses of ACE inhibitors in a patient with persistent heart failure symptoms signifies the presence of complex heart failure, which should be evaluated by a specialist. Similarly, when moderate or severe symptoms of heart failure persist despite therapy with digoxin, diuretics, and target doses of ACE inhibitors, or when target doses are not tolerated, heart failure also should be considered to be *complex* and should be evaluated for the purpose of adding other agents. In patients hospitalized with decompensation and hypertension, the shorter-acting ACE inhibitor captopril is frequently used because it is more easily titrated and may also decrease the possibility of renal dysfunction.[8]

Diuretics (See also Chap. 9)

Diuretics should be administered for the control of congestion and fluid retention (see Figs. 22–2 and 22–3). Although thiazide diuretics are well tolerated and effective in mild heart failure, these agents are frequently inadequate for the chronic prevention of fluid retention in moderate or severe heart failure and have been associated with hyponatremia. Recurrent fluid retention often responds best to a loop diuretic such as furosemide, with initial oral daily doses of 10 or 20 mg. Patients may be begun on diuretic therapy on an outpatient basis. They should be instructed to weigh themselves daily and should be contacted by telephone within 3 days of initiating diuretics to discuss the response and possible adjustment in the dose of diuretics and of potassium replacement (see later). They should return to see their physician within the next 3 to 7 days for further clinical assessment, including repeat assessment of their serum potassium concentration. During the initiation of diuretic therapy in ambulatory patients, weight loss should not exceed 1 or 2 lb daily. If there is no response to a given initial dose, it should be increased by at least 50%. If there is no improvement after two dosage increases, the patient should be re-evaluated for evidence of other factors that render heart failure complex (see Table 22–6); hospitalization may sometimes be necessary to establish safe and effective diuresis. Intravenous administration may be required to initiate diuresis in patients who are already on high doses of oral diuretics. Early experience with the oral loop diuretic torsemide indicates that its better absorption and earlier peak effect than those of furosemide may in some cases improve diuretic responsiveness without the need for intravenous administration.

Table 22–10 Oral Medications Commonly Used in the Treatment of Heart Failure

Drug	Initial Dose (mg)	Target Dose (mg)	Recommended Maximal Dose (mg)
ACE Inhibitors			
Captopril	6.25*–12.5 tid	50 tid	100 qid
Enalapril	2.5 bid	10 bid	20 bid
Lisinopril	5 qd	20 qd	40 qd
Quinapril	5 bid	20 bid	†
Ramipril	1 bid	5 bid	†
Zofenopril	10 bid	30 bid	†
Trandolapril	1	4	†
Nitrates			
Isosorbide dinitrate	10 tid	As needed with ACE inhibitors (40 mg tid with hydralazine)	80 tid
Mononitrates		Little experience in heart failure	
Nitrate patches		Generally considered to be less effective than isosorbide dinitrate	
Hydralazine	25 tid	75 qid	150 qid
Loop Diuretics (often first-line diuretic)			
Furosemide	10–40 qd	As needed	240 bid
Bumetanide	0.5–1.0 qd	As needed	10 qd
Torsemide‡	20	As needed	200 mg daily
Thiazide Diuretics (less commonly used than loop diuretics)			
Hydrochlorothiazide	25 qd	As needed	50 qd
Chlorthalidone	25 qd	As needed	50 qd
Thiazide-Related Diuretics			
Metolazone (usually given only in conjunction with loop diuretic)	2.5* 1/2 hr before loop diuretic dose	As needed, most effective with intermittent use	10 qd
Potassium-Sparing Diuretics			
Spironolactone	25 qd	As needed	50 bid§
Triamterene	50 qd	As needed	50 bid§
Amiloride	5 qd	As needed	20 qd§

Adapted in part from Konstam, M.A., Dracup, K., Baker, D.W., et al. Heart failure: Evaluation and care of patients with left-ventricular systolic dysfunction. Clinical Practice Guideline no. 11. AHCPR Publication no. 94–0612. Rockville, MD, Agency for Health Care Policy and Research, Public Health Service, U.S. Department of Health and Human Services, June 1994.

Abbreviations: ACE, angiotensin-converting enzyme; qd, once a day; bid, twice a day; tid, three times a day, qid, four times a day.

* Given as a single test dose initially.

† Little experience with doses above target doses in heart failure.

‡ Dose of 20 mg assumes previous loop diuretic therapy with decreasing response.

§ These doses may lead to high risk of life-threatening hyperkalemia in heart failure and are rarely used.

Once optimal fluid balance has been restored, the maintenance dose of the diuretic is lower than that required to initiate diuresis. When the total daily dose of furosemide is less than 80 mg, once-daily diuretic dosing in the morning may decrease the inconvenience of nocturia.

The patient should understand that monitoring fluid status requires continued vigilance. The adjustment of diuretics for heart failure has been compared with the adjustment of insulin for diabetes: the needs change from day to day depending on many factors. Guided by daily weights, the majority of ambulatory patients can become responsible for their own flexible diuretic regimens. They are generally instructed to double their loop diuretic (not thiazides or potassium-sparing diuretics) when a weight gain of 2 lb or more occurs. Once the baseline weight has been re-established, the previous dose can be resumed. When daily doses of furosemide exceed 160 mg, evaluation of the entire regimen by a specialist may be helpful.

Intermittent use of metolazone (2.5 or 5.0 mg) for weight gain refractory to a doubling of the dose of furosemide frequently restores fluid balance and the response to the loop diuretic. Since even a 2.5-mg dose of this diuretic in conjunction with furosemide can cause a brisk diuresis, serious hypotension, or electrolyte depletion, or a combination of these, the first dose of metolazone in patients already receiving a loop diuretic may be most safely administered in the hospital setting. Chronic, regular use of metolazone is rarely indicated, since it loses much of its diuretic effect over time and causes electrolyte depletion.

The adjunctive role of potassium-sparing diuretics such as aldactone, amiloride, or triamterene remains a subject of controversy. When added to loop diuretics, the additional diuretic effect is generally small but may be significant, particularly in patients with evidence of predominantly right-sided heart failure. Some heart failure experts advocate addition of such an agent when the potassium replacement exceeds 40 to 60 mEq daily (see later). Extreme caution is necessary to avoid hyperkalemia when adding a potassium-sparing agent to a regimen that includes ACE inhibitors, particularly when diabetes or pre-existing renal disease may further compromise potassium regulation. The peak effect may not be evident for several days, during which serum potassium levels need to be checked frequently. Potassium-sparing diuretics are particularly hazardous in the setting of fluctuating fluid balance and renal function.

Electrolyte Replacement

Diuretic therapy causes urinary losses of both potassium and magnesium. ACE inhibitors reduce potassium excretion, but most patients with good renal function require potassium supplementation during daily therapy with loop diuretics such as furosemide despite ACE inhibitor therapy. Dietary supplementation is rarely adequate. Salt substitutes, most of which contain potassium, can improve compliance with sodium restriction but should be used in moderation, as excessive consumption can cause hyperkalemia.

Hypokalemia is a well-recognized complication of diuretic therapy that can aggravate arrhythmia and precipitate severe muscle cramps during rapid diuresis. The dangers of *hyperkalemia* are less well recognized but are equally important. Serum levels of potassium over 6 mEq/L, particularly when the level has risen quickly, can depress myocardial contractility and cause arrhythmias resembling ventricular tachycardia. Aggressive repletion of potassium in the presence of ACE inhibitors and potassium-sparing diuretics has led to many episodes of life-threatening hyperkalemia, one of the causes of sudden death in heart failure. Hospitalized patients with heart failure are at greater risk for cardiac arrest from hyperkalemia than from hypokalemia.

Serum potassium levels should generally be maintained between 3.8 and 4.5 mEq/L in patients with heart failure. Serum levels of potassium can fluctuate rapidly and are a relatively poor index of total body potassium stores. In addition, replacement of total body potassium from the intravascular pool occurs very slowly. Unless hypokalemia is very severe or life-threatening, potassium should be replaced by oral administration. (In the rare instances when it is required, intravenous potassium should not be administered more rapidly than 10 mEq/hr.)

Patients who require loop diuretics usually receive maintenance doses of 20 to 60 mEq of oral potassium daily. In patients in whom aggressive diuresis is attempted in the outpatient setting, extra oral potassium should be given after the patient has noted diuresis based on urine output or weight change. Aggressive diuresis in the outpatient setting must be prescribed by an experienced physician and nurse team who are in daily or almost daily contact with the patient. Electrolytes, serum urea, and creatinine should be checked at least every 3 days when a net fluid loss of more than 2 lb is anticipated. Other than hyperkalemia, the major side effect of oral potassium preparations is gastrointestinal intolerance, which can be reduced by giving divided doses with meals.

Severe *hypomagnesemia* can also occur as a consequence of diuretic therapy and can precipitate or aggravate ventricular arrhythmias. Hypomagnesemia can aggravate hypokalemia, and some patients require chronic supplementation of both minerals. Magnesium is generally replaced to levels of approximately 2 mg/dl, but there is no evidence of benefit from chronic supplementation.

Vasodilators

Nitrates

Nitrates are added to ACE inhibition to relieve symptoms of pulmonary congestion. However, other than in combination with hydralazine, they have not been shown to prolong survival in heart failure. The addition of a nitrate to ACE inhibitor therapy may improve exercise tolerance in patients with severe exertional dyspnea. The combination of hydralazine and nitrates is useful when ACE inhibitors are not tolerated.

Nitrate therapy is generally introduced with isosorbide dinitrate at a dose of 10 mg tid and the dose may be gradually increased to 40 mg tid. Although nitrate tolerance is a well-recognized problem, it is rarely evident clinically when oral nitrates are taken three times daily with a nitrate-free interval of at least 10 hours at night. The only common side effect of nitrate is headache, which frequently improves after 24 to 48 hours of therapy but may require acetaminophen. Patients with severe headaches after 48 hours generally require dose reduction. Sublingual nitroglycerin (0.3 to 0.6 mg) is very effective for rapid, temporary relief of pulmonary edema or congestion and may be used every few minutes on an emergency basis until more definitive therapy is available. In some patients, exertional dyspnea may be decreased by nitroglycerin or sublingual isosorbide dinitrate before embarking on strenuous activity.

Other Antianginal Therapy

seek other cause of angina

Since over half of all cases of heart failure are due to ischemic heart disease, many patients with heart failure also complain of angina—for them, nitrates are the first-line therapy. When angina worsens in patients with heart failure, other conditions such as anemia or elevated left ventricular filling pressures that increase myocardial oxygen demand and reduce coronary perfusion may be present. These conditions should be sought, identified, and treated. When mechanical coronary revascularization is not possible, antianginal therapy with the cautious administration of beta-adrenergic–receptor blockers may be useful (see Beta-Adrenergic Blocking Agents). Amlodipine or felodipine may be considered for therapy of uncontrollable angina when heart failure is otherwise well compensated. Amiodarone, which was used as an antianginal agent for many years in Europe before finding wider acceptance as an antiarrhythmic agent, may also be effective in these patients (see later).

amlodipine

amiodarone

Hydralazine

Hydralazine, by itself, is only a potent arterial vasodilator and does not reduce ventricular filling pressures to the same extent as is achieved with nitrates and ACE inhibitors. When used alone, it may stimulate sympathetic tone reflexly. The combination of hydralazine and isosorbide dinitrate has been shown to decrease mortality as well as to improve left ventricular ejection fraction and exercise capacity in patients with heart failure.[20] However, this combination has been found to be less beneficial than ACE inhibitors.[5, 8] The major indications for hydralazine in combination with nitrates in heart failure are intolerance of ACE inhibitors and persistent heart failure symptoms or hypertension despite ACE inhibitors.

Calcium Antagonists

ACE-I + amlodipine

Although calcium antagonists cause vasodilatation in heart failure, the overall benefit appears to be reduced by their negative inotropic effect and by the reflex activation of the sympathetic nervous system that they can induce. One report has described beneficial effects with the newer agent amlodipine when added to ACE inhibitor therapy in heart failure caused by dilated (nonischemic) cardiomyopathy[21], but another similar agent (felodipine) has shown no benefit. Although these drugs are currently not recommended as vasodilators in systolic heart failure, they may be useful as antihypertensive agents in patients with diastolic dysfunction.

Digitalis

Cardiac glycosides are the oldest drugs still currently prescribed for heart failure. Although digitalis compounds improve contractility, their clinical benefit may result in part (or even largely) from their effects on the autonomic nervous system. Digitalis is commonly used in patients with heart failure and atrial fibrillation to decrease ventricular rate, although it is often inadequate as a single agent in this regard. Digitalis is used in symptomatic patients with normal sinus rhythm and systolic heart failure to improve functional status and decrease clinical deterioration.[15] Although it reduces the need for hospitalization for heart failure, digitalis does not improve survival of patients in sinus rhythm.[22] For outpatients with mild to moderate heart failure, there is no need to "load" with high doses to achieve an early therapeutic response. For most patients with normal renal function, initiation of 0.25 mg digoxin daily is adequate to achieve a steady state after a week. In the elderly or in patients with impaired renal function, 0.125 mg or less should be used as the daily dose.

Signs of toxicity include nausea, confusion, visual disturbances, ventricular or junctional tachyarrhythmias, and atrioventricular block. When toxicity is suspected, an electrocardiogram should be obtained and serum potassium determined. Serum digoxin levels may be checked to detect toxicity when renal function declines or after institution of drugs that can reduce digoxin clearance, such as amiodarone, quinidine, and verapamil. Increased gastrointestinal absorption of digoxin may result from therapy with antibiotics or anticholinergic agents. Serum levels of 0.8 to 1.2 ng/dl may be optimal. Serum levels above 2.0 ng/dl are generally considered to be excessive, whereas levels below 0.5 ng/dl are considered ineffective. Digoxin levels are also useful to ascertain patient compliance.

Other Therapeutic Measures

BETA-ADRENERGIC BLOCKING AGENTS. There is increasing interest in the use of beta-adrenergic blocking agents to improve ventricular function and retard disease progression in selected patients with heart failure.[23, 24] If these agents are tolerated, they result in consistent improvement in left ventricular ejection fraction when added to therapy with ACE inhibitors, digoxin, and diuretics. Initiation of beta-adrenergic blocking agents for heart failure should be supervised by a specialist.

Most experience with this therapy is with metoprolol. The initial dose is usually 6.25 mg. Because the smallest tablet currently available is 50 mg, therapy for heart failure patients requires special pharmacy formulations or use of a pill cutter. Fluid retention and symptoms of congestion frequently develop during initiation of beta blockers, requiring close observation by both patient and physician, and an increase in the dose of the diuretic may be necessary. Fatigue and dizziness commonly occur during initiation. Decompensation severe enough to require hospitalization occasionally occurs even when these agents are given in very low doses by heart failure specialists. Although this therapy frequently causes symptomatic deterioration during the first few weeks, improved left ventricular function usually occurs over 2 to 3 months. Carvedilol has recently been approved for mild to moderate heart failure. The side effects in addition to those observed with metoprolol include dizziness from the peripheral vasodilation. The initial dose is 3.125 mg twice daily.[23]

AMIODARONE. This is the safest and most effective agent for preventing atrial and ventricular arrhythmias in heart failure.[25] Even patients with severe heart failure generally tolerate oral amiodarone without an exacerbation of heart failure symptoms. However, because amiodarone reduces the clearance of digoxin and warfarin, the doses of these agents must be reduced. Major side effects of amiodarone include pulmonary toxicity, liver dysfunction, hyperthyroidism, hypothyroidism, and neuropathy. The initiation and adjustment of this drug should be supervised by a physician with extensive experience in treating heart failure.

Amiodarone, similar to beta-adrenergic blocking therapy, has been shown to reduce arrhythmia-related events after myocardial infarction and has more recently been used for the treatment of tachyarrhythmias and heart failure.[26, 27] Both therapies decrease heart rate, suppress arrhythmias, lead to chronic improvement in left ventricular ejection fraction, and may reduce hospitalizations for chronic heart failure. Although amiodarone may be considered for patients with heart failure and sinus tachycardia or severe angina in the absence of severe arrhythmias, this indication is still experimental.

THERAPY TO PREVENT SUDDEN DEATH. Up to half of all deaths in patients with chronic heart failure are sudden. Although ventricular tachycardia and fibrillation can cause sudden death in heart failure, multiple other causes include myocardial infarction, pulmonary or systemic emboli, hyperkalemia, and primary bradyarrhythmias. These precipitants should be sought and corrected.[25] Cardiac arrest and syncope in heart failure merit careful evaluation for treatable causes, including ventricular tachyarrhythmias. Amiodarone is frequently helpful in these patients. However, there are no general indications for treatment of asymptomatic nonsustained ventricular tachycardia, which can be detected in over 50% of patients with NYHA classes III and IV heart failure.

ANTICOAGULANTS. The annual incidence of systemic and pulmonary embolism in patients with chronic heart failure is 2% to 5%. By comparison, the risk for severe bleeding complications from anticoagulation in the general population is 0.8% to 2.5% yearly, but this risk may be higher in patients whose warfarin requirements are unpredictably reduced by intermittent hepatic congestion. Therefore, anticoagulation is not routinely recommended in the current guidelines for the treatment of heart failure.[2] However, anticoagulation is indicated in heart failure patients with additional specific risks for embolic events, such as atrial fibrillation, a history of pulmonary or arterial embolic events, and mobile intracardiac thrombi or marked apical dyskinesis visualized on echocardiography. The risks of chronic anticoagulation with warfarin in patients with heart failure may be reduced by careful maintenance of the International Normalized Ratio (INR) at relatively low levels (2.0 to 2.5).

SUPPLEMENTAL OXYGEN. The use of supplemental oxygen is indicated when heart failure is accompanied by arterial desaturation. Some patients develop arterial desaturation during sleep, particularly with Cheyne-Stokes breathing pattern or sleep apnea. For such patients, nocturnal oxygen therapy may improve sleep, daytime symptoms, and occasionally, cardiac function.

SPECIAL MANAGEMENT ISSUES

Education of Patients with Heart Failure

(Tables 22–11 and 22–12)

Exercise/Activity

Patient education about heart failure often emphasizes the necessary restrictions in lifestyle that are imposed by this condition and leads to a mindset that reinforces the concept of the "failure" of a vital organ. Rather than referring to the heart as "failing," it is more positive to refer to it as "handicapped" and to emphasize that handicaps require special provisions but can often be overcome. Too often, all the "don'ts" are covered first, and the "dos" are relegated to the last few minutes of the counseling session. Instead, the positive features regarding permitted activity level should be outlined initially.

In order to avoid physical deconditioning, ambulatory patients with heart failure should be encouraged to participate in a regular program of specific, uninterrupted exercise at least 4 days a week (e.g., a walking program outdoors or in an enclosed mall during inclement weather). Stationary bicycles and home treadmills can be set at low workloads equivalent to walking. Rowing machines or more vigorous aerobic exercise simulating skiing or stair climbing are too strenuous for most patients. Weight-lifting and other significant isometric effort should not be part of the regimen.

An exercise program can begin by asking the patient to walk at a comfortable pace for 10 minutes, with increases first in duration and then in speed. Daily activities such as housework or shopping are encouraged but are not equivalent to specific, uninterrupted exercise. A major benefit of a specific exercise prescription may be in convincing both patient and family that the clinical condition is helped and not hurt by activity. In making recommendations regarding employment, heavy or sustained isometric work should be avoided. Patients should not routinely lift more than 20 lb.

In general, patients without evidence of congestion at rest can safely participate in sexual activity. Dyspnea is less likely if pillows are used to elevate the chest and head. Some patients take 2.5 or 5.0 mg of sublingual

Table 22–11	Education of Patients and Family regarding Heart Failure

General Information

Cause or probable cause of heart failure
Explanation of symptoms of heart failure
Patient as leader of care team
Role of family members or other caregivers
Availability of qualified local support group
Advisability of vaccinations against influenza

Outlook with Heart Failure

Potential for good function and survival
Undulating disease course
Life expectancy
Advance directives
Family recognition of risk for sudden death

Self-Monitoring

Heart failure diary
Daily weights
Home blood pressure monitoring, if appropriate
Surveillance for common symptoms
Instructions for when to contact care team (see Table 22–12)

Medications

Explanation and schedule of medications
Likely side effects and appropriate responses
Plan of diuretic adjustment for weight increase, with subsequent electro-
    lyte management
Anticoagulation management, if necessary
Availability of lower-cost medications or financial assistance

Dietary Recommendations

Sodium restriction, label reading, and meal planning
Lipid restriction for patients with known vascular disease
General fluid limit (even if liberal)
Alcohol restriction or elimination

Activity Recommendations

Recommendations for work, leisure activities
Regular aerobic activity
Sexual activity
Encouragement of midday rest period, if appropriate

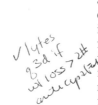

Adapted from Kostam et al.,[2] Smith et al.,[3] and Stevenson.[10]

isosorbide dinitrate before sexual activity to reduce breathlessness.

In patients with heart failure who work outside the home, extra rest on weekends is advisable and sometimes it may be necessary to curtail professional, community, and family responsibilities to allow continued employment. Intermittent rest such as a scheduled nap or afternoon rest period each day is often helpful to prevent excessive fatigue. Rest at home for several days is indicated after a bout of overt heart failure.

Sodium and Fluid Restriction

After having emphasized what patients *can* do, it is necessary to be very firm about restrictions on sodium and, in some cases, fluid intake.[2, 10] For many patients, sodium restriction is perceived as a severe penalty, and considerable education and encouragement regarding other seasoning options are required. Patients with hyper-

tension or early left ventricular dysfunction should be advised to avoid adding salt to meals and should limit their intake of salty foods, such as potato chips, cheese, and canned soups. Once the daily furosemide requirement exceeds 80 mg, patients should limit their daily sodium intake to 2 gm. This can be accomplished by emphasis on fresh foods and careful attention to labels on packaged food. If patients remain clinically stable for more than 3 months without the need for frequent adjustment of diuretics, they may *occasionally* indulge in pizza or "fast" food. However, they should be warned to watch their weight particularly closely over the next few days. Some patients even learn to take extra furosemide prophylactically when escaping their sodium restriction. Such transgressions should not be encouraged but, if carefully managed in stabilized patients, may ultimately lead to better overall compliance.

Although salt restriction is widely advised, the importance of fluid restriction has been underemphasized. Even before heart failure becomes severe, patients should understand that their ability to excrete an excess fluid load is impaired. Patients with frequent exacerbations of heart failure may require lower diuretic dosages and fewer hospitalizations when limited to 2 quarts of fluid intake daily. The only patients for whom temporary tighter restrictions might be considered are those whose serum sodium is below 125 mEq/L, and these patients ordinarily require in-hospital management. To make the most of a limited fluid allotment, patients should drink fluids other than water and may want to include ice, frozen juices, and frozen grapes as part of their daily fluid intake.

Other Dietary Restrictions

Prohibition of alcohol should be considered in all patients with a reduced left ventricular ejection fraction, since decrements in left ventricular function can be de-

Table 22–12	Specific Instructions for Patient about When to Contact Physician's Office*

Weight gain ≥ 3 lb, not responding to predesignated diuretic change
Uncertainty about how to increase diuretics
New swelling of the feet or abdomen
Worsening shortness of breath with mild exercise
Onset of inability to sleep flat in bed or awakening from sleep because
    of shortness of breath
Worsening cough
Persistent nausea/vomiting or inability to eat
Worsening dizziness or new spells of sudden dizziness not related to
    sudden changes in body position
Prolonged palpitations
If you, the patient, experience any sudden severe symptoms, you may
    need to call 911 or the equivalent emergency phone number to arrange a trip to the emergency room. (These sudden severe symptoms may include **but are not limited to** chest pain, severe shortness of breath, loss of consciousness not due to sudden standing, new cold or painful arm or foot, sudden new visual changes, or impairment of speech or strength in an extremity.)

Note: This is only a sample list and is not intended to include all potential problems for which a patient with heart failure should seek urgent medical advice.

tected after the consumption of even one alcoholic beverage. Patients with alcoholic cardiomyopathy must abstain completely.

Most patients whose heart failure is secondary to ischemic heart disease should be counseled about the need to reduce the intake of fats and cholesterol. An American Heart Association step I diet[28] is indicated in such patients, although during periods of acute decompensation and shortly thereafter, risk from fat intake assumes a lower priority.

Predicting Survival

Patients with heart failure and their families seek and deserve to know the prognosis. However, even specialists in the field are repeatedly humbled by their inability to predict how long these patients will survive. Therefore, it is a disservice to cite a specific period of time during which the patients and family unconsciously count down the days, at the end of which nothing happens. If it seems essential to provide a range, the cliché of "less than 6 months to live" should be avoided and instead the longest possible range in which outcome could be positive should be offered—"Many patients like you are alive over a year later." At the same time, it is vital to inform families that a patient with serious heart disease can die suddenly at any time.[25] Although the specter of sudden death is often frightening, it is important to inform patients and families at the outset that half of all deaths in patients with heart failure are sudden. This expectation may allow important conversations to take place in time and also prevent years of self-recrimination following a sudden death that occurred after traveling, arguing, or bringing in the groceries. It is also helpful for patients to prepare advance directives regarding their preferences for life-sustaining therapies.

Clinical status remains the strongest general predictor of survival. Among patients with NYHA class I or II heart failure, the average annual mortality is 5% to 10%, depending on the index event. Those in NYHA class III have an annual mortality approaching 20%, whereas patients with persistent class IV symptoms have an annual mortality in the range of over 50%.

In patients with mild to moderate symptoms of heart failure, left ventricular ejection fraction is a strong prognostic indicator, with a predicted 3-year mortality of almost 50% in patients with an ejection fraction less than 20% and approximately 25% with an ejection fraction between 30% and 35%.[6, 7] Although the prognosis for patients with predominantly diastolic dysfunction has not been well defined, overall mortality appears to be lower in this group than in those with systolic dysfunction.[13]

The patient's trajectory over time provides important prognostic information. Patients who appear to be improving often continue to do so, whereas those who are deteriorating despite treatment may continue to deteriorate. Even when class IV symptoms are present at the time of the initial evaluation, the potential for improvement is illustrated by the experience with ambulatory patients awaiting cardiac transplantation, up to one-third of whom may improve sufficiently to leave the transplant list for a quality of life and 2-year survival that are equivalent to that attained after transplantation.[29]

Prognosis is better in patients in whom acute decompensation has been precipitated by a specific event, such as pulmonary embolism, recurrence of which can be prevented, than in those in whom it appears related to progression of the underlying illness. The potential for spontaneous improvement in left ventricular function should also be recognized, particularly in patients with heart failure symptoms of recent onset. This is most likely for patients without ischemic heart disease in whom an unrecognized viral infection may have caused reversible dysfunction.

Continuing Care

For patients with newly diagnosed left ventricular dysfunction as reflected in cardiomegaly or an abnormally depressed ejection fraction, evaluation by a specialist to determine the underlying cause and to ascertain whether it can be corrected or ameliorated is recommended. Cardiac specialists can also work with the primary care physician in the management of acute, severe decompensation and in the establishment of a long-term treatment program. The latter may, ordinarily, be supervised by the primary care physician. The most important aspect of continuing care in heart failure is the ability to recognize early signs of clinical deterioration. Symptoms of congestion and those suggestive of arrhythmias or embolic events should be sought. Syncope in a patient with heart failure usually warrants hospital admission for specialized evaluation. Mortality among such patients approaches 30% during the next year.[25]

Physicians who are following patients with chronic heart failure often find it helpful to maintain a specific flow sheet (Table 22–13). Routine questions should include recent weight/diuretic history and activity level.

Interval Laboratory Evaluations

Electrolytes, creatinine, and BUN should be measured within 24 to 48 hours of a major diuresis, after a major change of therapy, with the development of severe decompensation, and every 3–6 months in patients who are in stable, mild heart failure on a constant target dose of an ACE inhibitor alone. Patients in whom warfarin anticoagulation is indicated (see earlier) require checking of the prothrombin time to keep the INR within a safe range (2 to 3) and not less frequently than every 4 to 6 weeks.

Once major symptoms of heart failure have developed, serum sodium is a very sensitive indicator of the patient's overall state of compensation.[30] A level below 134 mEq/L in a patient with major symptoms generally indicates that the heart failure has become complex and is not likely to respond to simple adjustments in therapy. A serum sodium of less than 125 mEq/L or a decline of 5 mEq/L to less than 130 mEq/L often warrants hospital admission. Magnesium levels should be determined initially and after major changes in the diuretic regimen. Other laboratory

Table 22–13	Clinic Flow Sheet for Chronic Heart Failure*

Vital Information

Blood pressure (sitting, standing [after 3 min])
Heart rate (sitting, standing)
Clinic weight/home weight
Recent emergency room or hospital visits
Recent need for extra diuretics

Interim History

Routine activity level
Specific exercise
Limitation while dressing
Orthopnea/paroxysmal nocturnal dyspnea
Gastrointestinal symptoms
Angina
Palpitations/syncope
Symptoms of embolic events

Cardiovascular Examination (+ Vital Signs Above)

Jugular venous pressures
Peripheral edema
Ascites
Hepatomegaly
Warmth of extremities
Right heart prominence
Change in S_3, S_4, or murmurs

Summary

Fluid overload (yes/no)
Activity level (I–IV)
Compared with last visit (worse/same/better)
Clinically stable (yes/no)

---

* To be recorded at each encounter.
Abbreviations: S_3, third heart sound; S_4, fourth heart sound.

tests may be necessary depending on the medical regimen. Digoxin levels do not need to be obtained routinely but are usually checked when there is concern regarding toxicity, a change in renal function, or noncompliance.

A white blood cell count should be obtained before and after ACE inhibitor therapy is begun to check for the rare case of agranulocytosis. Hematocrit should be determined when a stable patient deteriorates. The electrocardiogram generally does not need to be repeated at every visit, except for patients receiving antiarrhythmic therapy (to check the Q-T interval) or when recent symptoms suggest ischemia or arrhythmias. Chest radiographs are not routinely necessary during follow-up but may be useful for identifying pneumonia or other pulmonary processes that may be causing exacerbations of dyspnea.

Once the clinical assessment and routine laboratory tests are completed, it is important to synthesize the information into an overall assessment of volume status and stability. If changes in the medical regimen are required, they should be made gradually, if possible. For example, for postural hypotension in the absence of suspected hypovolemia, vasodilator doses can be decreased by 25%. For suspected volume depletion, the diuretic can be stopped for 1 or 2 days and restarted at doses that are 25% lower. Drugs for heart failure should rarely be discontinued abruptly except in the event of toxicity or allergy.

Hospital Admission

Indications for hospital admission are summarized in Table 22–8. New heart failure symptoms of *rapid onset,* even if relatively mild, should be considered grounds for admission, as deterioration can occur rapidly.

Expectations after Hospitalization

For the patient admitted primarily for therapy of heart failure, the plan for hospitalization should include the components shown in Table 22–14. These may be provided most effectively by a specialist or a team experienced in caring for such patients both in the hospital and during their transition through a high-intensity clinic early after discharge. Experience has repeatedly shown that a major factor in successful outcome after discharge is the adequacy of patient education, including specific instructions about when to contact the medical care system (see Table 22–12). These instructions should be provided in the hospital and reiterated after discharge.

There is increasing conviction that after hospitalization for heart failure, patients should move first into a special program (if it is available) that can provide specialized physician, nurse, and in some cases, nutritionist support until the outpatient course becomes stable. During this time, telephone contact should be made twice weekly and a physical assessment carried out every 1 or 2 weeks. A formal program of specialized heart failure management may decrease re-hospitalizations by up to 80%.[31] If the patient's condition remains stable for at least 4 weeks after discharge, patients may "graduate" to more standard care. Patients are then followed regularly, as described previously, and should be returned to the specialized program if there is new or recurrent evidence of complex heart failure.

Table 22–14	Expectations from Hospitalization for Heart Failure

Elucidation of cause or exacerbating factors, if necessary
Plan of treatment for reversible conditions
Achievement of optimal fluid status and definition of "dry weight" or plan for achieving dry weight at home (often unsuccessful if not achieved before discharge)
Definition of optimal vasodilator doses and associated blood pressure limits
Institution of therapy for ischemia, if needed
Institution of therapy for arrhythmias, if needed
Adequate anticoagulation regimen, if indicated
Estimation of capacity for daily activity after discharge
Decision regarding home health care
Education of patient and family (see Table 22–11)
Written information to patient, including
    Wallet card indicating diagnosis and medical regimen
    Written medication schedule
    Scheduled office evaluation in 5–10 days
    24-hr phone number of physician familiar with recent regimen
    Instructions regarding indications for urgent call (see Table 22–12)

References

1. American College of Cardiology/American Heart Association Task Force Report: Guidelines for the evaluation and management of heart failure. J. Am. Coll. Cardiol. 26:1376–1398, 1995.
2. Konstam, M.A., Dracup, K., Baker, D.W., et al.: Heart failure: Evaluation and care of patients with left-ventricular systolic dysfunction. Clinical Practice Guideline no. 11. AHCPR Publication no. 94–0612. Rockville, MD, Agency for Health Care Policy and Research, Public Health Service, U.S. Department of Health and Human Services, June 1994.
3. Smith, T.W., Kelly, R.A., Stevenson, L.W., and Braunwald, E.: The management of heart failure. In Braunwald, E. (ed.): Heart Disease. 5th ed. Philadelphia, W.B. Saunders, 1997, pp. 492–514.
4. Pfeffer, M.A., Braunwald, E., Moye, L.A., et al., on behalf of the SAVE Investigators: Effect of captopril on mortality and morbidity in patients with left ventricular dysfunction after myocardial infarction: Results of the Survival and Ventricular Enlargement trial. N. Engl. J. Med. 327:669–677, 1992.
5. Braunwald, E.: Heart failure. In Fauci, A.S., Braunwald, E., Isselbacher, K.J., et al. (eds.): Harrison's Principles of Internal Medicine. 14th ed. New York, McGraw-Hill, 1998, pp. 1286–1298.
6. The SOLVD Investigators: Effect of enalapril on mortality and the development of heart failure in asymptomatic patients with reduced left ventricular ejection fractions. N. Engl. J. Med. 327:685–691, 1992.
7. The SOLVD Investigators: Effect of enalapril on survival in patients with reduced left ventricular ejection fractions and congestive heart failure. N. Engl. J. Med. 325:293–302, 1991.
8. Fonarow, G.C., Chelimsky-Fallick, C., Stevenson, L.W., et al.: Effect of direct vasodilation with hydralazine versus angiotensin-converting enzyme inhibition with captopril on mortality in advanced heart failure: The Hy-C Trial. J. Am. Coll. Cardiol. 19:842, 1992.
9. Stevenson, L.W., and Perloff, J.K.: The limited reliability of physical signs for estimating hemodynamics in chronic heart failure. JAMA 26:884, 1989.
10. Stevenson, L.W.: Therapy tailored for symptomatic heart failure. Heart Failure 11:87–107, 1995.
11. Braunwald, E.: Normal and abnormal myocardial function. In Fauci, A.S., Braunwald, E., Isselbacher, K.J., et al. (eds.): Harrison's Principles of Internal Medicine. 14th ed. New York, McGraw-Hill, 1998, pp. 1278–1286.
12. Lee T.H.: Practice guidelines in cardiovascular medicine. In Braunwald, E. (ed.): Heart Disease. 5th ed. Philadelphia, W.B. Saunders, 1997, pp. 1939–1996.
13. Vasan, R.S., Benjamin, E.J., and Levy, D.: Prevalence, clinical features and prognosis of diastolic heart failure: An epidemiologic perspective. J. Am. Coll. Cardiol. 26:1565–1574, 1995.
14. Maron, B.J., Bonow, R.O., Cannon, R.O., et al.: Hypertrophic cardiomyopathy—Interrelations of clinical manifestations, pathophysiology and therapy. N. Engl. J. Med. 316:780–789, 1987.
15. Packer, M., Gheorgiade, M., Young, J.B., et al., for the RADIANCE Study Group: Withdrawal of digoxin from patients with chronic heart failure treated with angiotensin-converting enzyme inhibitors. N. Engl. J. Med. 329:1–7, 1993.
16. Rich, M.W., Beckham, V., Wittenberg, C., et al.: A multidisciplinary intervention to prevent the readmission of elderly patients with congestive heart failure. N. Engl. J. Med. 333:1190–1195, 1995.
17. Stevenson, W.G., Stevenson, L.W., Middlekauff, H.R., et al.: Improving survival for patients with advanced heart failure: A study of 737 consecutive patients. J. Am. Coll. Cardiol. 26:1417–1423, 1995.
18. Hunt, S. (chair.): 24th Bethesda Conference on Cardiac Transplantation. J. Am. Coll. Cardiol. 22:1–64, 1993.
19. Mudge, G.H., Goldstein, S., Addonizio, L.J., et al.: Cardiac transplantation: Recipient guidelines/prioritization. J. Am. Coll. Cardiol. 22:21–31, 1993.
20. Cohn, J.N., Archibald, D.G., Ziesche, S., et al.: Effect of vasodilator therapy on mortality in chronic congestive heart failure: Results of a Veterans Administration cooperative study. N. Engl. J. Med. 314:1547–1552, 1986.
21. Packer, M., O'Connor, C., Ghali, J.K., et al.: Effect of amlodipine on morbidity and mortality in severe chronic heart failure. N. Engl. J. Med. 335:1107–1114, 1996.
22. The Digitalis Investigation Group: The effect of digoxin on mortality and morbidity in patients with heart failure. N. Engl. J. Med. 336:525–533, 1997.
23. Waagstein, F., Bristow, M.R., Swedberg, K., et al.: Beneficial effects of metoprolol in idiopathic dilated cardiomyopathy. Lancet 342:1442–1446, 1993.
24. Packer, M., Bristow, M.R., Cohn, J.N., et al.: The effect of carvedilol on morbidity and mortality in patients with chronic heart failure. N. Engl. J. Med. 334:1349–1355, 1996.
25. Stevenson, W.G., Stevenson, L.W., Middlekauff, H.R., and Saxon, L.A.: Sudden death prevention in patients with advanced ventricular dysfunction. Circulation 88:2953–2961, 1993.
26. Doval, H.C., Nul, D.R., Grancelli, H.O., et al., for Grupo de Estudio de la Sobrevida en la Insuficiencia Cardiac en Argentina (GESICA): Randomized trial of low-dose amiodarone in severe congestive heart failure. Lancet 344:493–498, 1994.
27. Singh, S.N., Fletch, R.D., Fisher, S.G., et al., for the Survival Trial of Antiarrhythmic Therapy in Congestive Heart Failure Trial: Amiodarone in patients with congestive heart failure and asymptomatic ventricular arrhythmia. N. Engl. J. Med. 333:77–82, 1995.
28. Expert Panel on Detecting, Evaluating and Treatment of High Blood Cholesterol in Adults: Second report. Circulation 89:1329, 1994.
29. Stevenson, L.W., Steimle, A.E., Fonarow, G., et al.: Improvement in exercise capacity of candidates awaiting heart transplantation. J. Am. Coll. Cardiol. 25:163–170, 1995.
30. Lee, W.H., and Packer, M.: Prognostic importance of serum sodium concentration and its modification by converting enzyme inhibition in patients with severe chronic heart failure. Circulation 73:257–267, 1986.
31. Fonarow, G.C., Stevenson, L.W., Walden, J.A., et al.: Impact of a comprehensive heart failure management program on hospital readmission and functional status of patients with advanced heart failure. J. Am. Coll. Cardiol. 30:725–732, 1997.

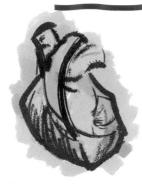

Chapter 23

Recognition and Management of Patients with

Tachyarrhythmias

MELVIN M. SCHEINMAN

In assessing patients with suspected or known tachyarrhythmias, the physician must determine the possible severity of the arrhythmia and any underlying cardiologic and noncardiologic conditions. This chapter reviews the common cardiac arrhythmias seen by primary care physicians, identifies the appropriate diagnostic procedures for different types of patients, and indicates when further specialized care is required.

OFFICE EVALUATION OF A PATIENT WITH A SUSTAINED ARRHYTHMIA

History

The office evaluation of a patient with a new sustained arrhythmia must be brief and directed to specific questions that relate to proper diagnosis and therapy. Arrhythmias are often evanescent; hence, one of the most important initial maneuvers is to record the arrhythmia on a 12-lead electrocardiogram (ECG). While the ECG is being recorded, the physician must discern several key elements in the history. For example, was the arrhythmia preceded or is it accompanied by anginal chest pain? Is there a prior history of structural heart disease? A new-onset sustained arrhythmia in a patient with established cardiac disease should suggest the presence of ventricular tachycardia (VT). In contrast, a history of abrupt-onset tachycardia in a younger, otherwise healthy individual would favor a diagnosis of supraventricular tachycardia (SVT).[1] An accurate drug history may be of paramount importance. A common cause of VT in younger patients is due to suicide attempts using tricyclic antidepressants. Intravenous cocaine use should always be considered as a cause of VT. The type and amount of drug therapy, particularly antiarrhythmic therapy, is extremely important. Has the patient been treated with digitalis preparations, quinidine-type drugs, or sotalol, and what is the time relationship of the new arrhythmia to drug initiation? It is also important to record use of diuretic agents, since severe electrolyte disorders, particularly hypokalemia, may exacerbate arrhythmias related to the use of antiarrhythmic drugs. The clinician should search out the presence of severe hypoxia or acid-base disturbances. Patients with severe lung disease will often present with atrial fibrillation, multifocal atrial tachycardia, or frequent ventricular premature depolarizations. Other important noncardiac causes of cardiac arrhythmias include hyperthyroidism and pheochromocytoma. Sinus tachycardia is common to both of these diagnoses. Atrial fibrillation is a frequent sequela of hyperthyroidism, whereas both SVT and VT may be associated with pheochromocytoma.

The Physical Examination

The physical examination is geared toward assessment of the nature of the arrhythmia as well as its hemodynamic consequences. If the physical examination shows evidence of periodic large A-waves in the jugular venous pulse, variation in the intensity of the first heart sound and in the systolic blood pressure, then the presence of atrioventricular (AV) dissociation and, hence, VT should be suspected. Findings on physical examination also guide the response to therapy. For example, signs (and symptoms) of cardiac failure or severe hypotension mandate emergency measures that should be initiated in the office (see later under Treatment).

Interpretation of the ECG

The 12-lead ECG is key to understanding arrhythmia categorization as well as mechanism. The first analysis is directed toward the division of the arrhythmia into narrow complex versus wide complex tachycardia (Table 23–1). A QRS complex of 0.12 second or more in any lead is diagnostic of a wide complex tachycardia. The wide complex tachycardias are further divided into those due to VT, to SVT with aberrant conduction (or bundle branch block), or to pre-excited tachycardias. The latter are less common but may occur in patients with accessory pathways who have arrhythmias manifest by antegrade conduction over a bypass tract. If during wide complex tachycardia one discerns evidence of AV dissociation, then a diagnosis of VT is certain. Since only 20% of patients with VT will show clear-cut evidence of AV dissociation, a stepwise approach can help to distinguish VT from SVT with aberrancy (Fig. 23–1). It is important to remember that SVT with wide QRS complexes may be seen in patients with hyperkalemia, tricyclic overdose, or various antiarrhythmic agents (i.e., flecainide). In all series of patients with wide complex tachycardias, VTs outnumber SVTs by about 3:1.

Distinctions among the narrow complex tachyarrhythmias can usually be made based on ECG criteria: the regularity of the rhythm (see Table 23–1) and the rela-

Table 23–1	Types of Tachycardias

Wide complex tachycardias QRS ≥ 0.12 sec
  Ventricular tachycardia (with or without detectable AV dissociation)
    Monomorphic (each beat looks similar)
      Polymorphous—beats vary, often with an oscillating pattern; torsades de pointes
  Supraventricular tachycardia (with or without apparently conducted or retrograde P-waves)
    With aberrant conduction in the His-Purkinje system in the ventricles
    With antegrade conduction via an accessory pathway
Narrow complex tachycardias QRS < 0.12 sec
  Irregularly irregular—atrial fibrillation (see Fig. 23–3)
  Irregular—Multifocal atrial tachycardia
      Any supraventricular rhythm with irregular AV conduction or superimposed premature beats
  Regular—Sinus tachycardia
    Atrial flutter (see Fig. 23–4)
    Paroxysmal supraventricular tachycardia (see Fig. 23–2)
      AV nodal reentry
      Accessory pathway
    Ectopic atrial tachycardia from an accelerated atrial focus (see Fig. 23–2)
    Junctional ectopic tachycardia

Abbreviation: AV, atrioventricular.

tionship of the P-wave to the QRS complex (Fig. 23–2). The physician must first distinguish sinus tachycardia from tachyarrhythmias. Sinus tachycardia is defined as a sinus rate above 100 beats per minute, and it rarely exceeds 180 beats per minute in the adult. It can often be distinguished from paroxysmal supraventricular tachycardia (PSVT) by readily discernible P-waves that are upright in the inferior leads (leads II, III, and aVF), by its gradual onset and cessation, by its occasional gradual slowing in response to carotid sinus pressure, or by its variation in response to respiration or activity.

[handwritten margin note: ST 100-180]

Sinus tachycardia may be precipitated by serious conditions such as hypovolemia, heart failure, infection, anemia, electrolyte abnormalities, and thyrotoxicosis. It may also be stimulated by adrenergic agents, coffee, tea, tobacco, alcohol, or vagolytic agents. Frequently, however, it is related to emotion or stress. The sinus tachycardia itself does not require any treatment, but it serves to call attention to associated medical problems.

In most adults, atrial fibrillation, atrial flutter, and SVTs cannot be conducted at rates exceeding about 160 to 180 beats per minute because of delay in the AV node. As patients become older, these maximal rates decline.

If conduction to the ventricle exceeds 160 to 180 beats per minute with a wide QRS complex, an accessory pathway should be suspected. Conversely, if patients have atrial fibrillation, atrial flutter, or other nonsinus rhythms with rates below 100 to 120 beats per minute in the absence of medications, intrinsic disease of the AV node should be suspected. Since an SVT itself may be a manifestation of sinus node dysfunction, these patients with slow AV conduction commonly have the so-called brady-tachy syndrome (see Chap. 24). In patients with the brady-tachy syndrome, it is often impossible to treat the tachyarrhythmia successfully with medications without simultaneously causing symptomatic bradycardia. The patient may require catheter ablation of the source of the SVT, the combination of ablation of the AV node with a pacemaker to guard against symptomatic bradycardia, or the combination of medications to prevent the tachyarrhythmia with a pacemaker.

Management (Table 23–2)

If patients present with hemodynamically unstable VT, ventricular flutter or fibrillation, or atrial fibrillation associated with very rapid response owing to accelerated conduction over an accessory pathway, then immediate direct-current cardioversion is necessary. Once the patient is stable, arrangements must be made for expeditious transfer for hospital admission. If VT is associated with stable hemodynamics, then a trial of drug therapy is in order while the clinician awaits for the emergency medical team to transport the patient to an emergency room facility. If the diagnosis of VT cannot be excluded, initial therapy includes the use of intravenous lidocaine or intravenous procainamide (Table 23–3).

For patients with a regular SVT who are hemodynamically unstable, emergency direct-current countershock may be necessary. Most often, these patients are sufficiently stable to allow for a trial of carotid sinus massage,

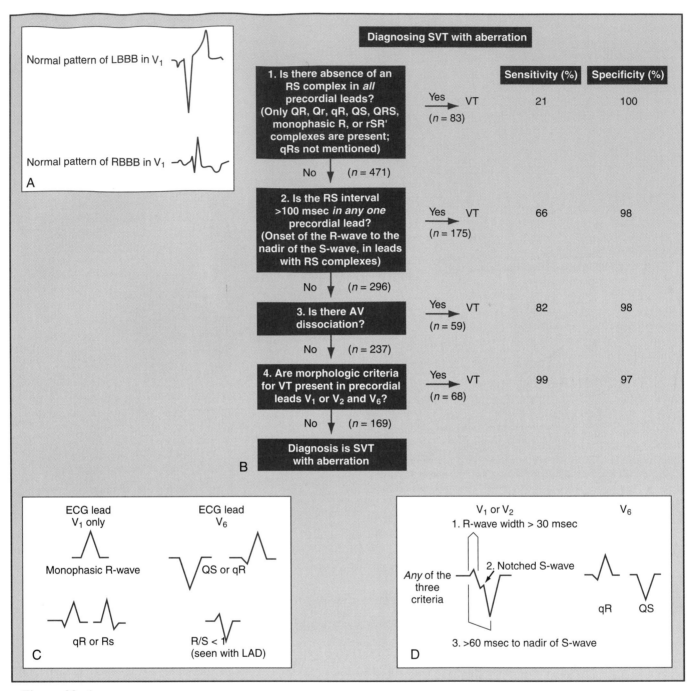

Figure 23–1

The 12-lead electrocardiogram (ECG) in the differential diagnosis of wide complex tachycardia. Brugada and colleagues analyzed 384 cases of ventricular tachycardia (VT) and 170 cases of supraventricular tachycardia (SVT) with aberrancy, representing 554 patients with tachycardia (those taking antiarrhythmic medications were excluded). They then devised a systematic approach for diagnosing wide QRS complex tachycardia with regular rhythm. *A,* The first step is to exclude sinus tachycardia or atrial tachycardia with right bundle branch block (RBBB) or left bundle branch block (LBBB). This can usually be done by finding P-waves: The ST segment and T-wave are always smooth, unless distorted by a P-wave. However, missing this diagnosis should not affect the ability to diagnose VT or SVT, unless the patient is taking QRS-lengthening drugs. *B,* Steps in the diagnosis of SVT with aberration. A "Yes" answer at any point indicates that no further steps need to be taken. When the answer is "No," proceed to the next step. The cumulative sensitivity using this method is 97% and the specificity is 99%. AV, atrioventricular. *C,* Morphologic criteria favoring diagnosis of VT in the presence of RBBB-type QRS complexes (dominant positive in V₁). LAD, left axis deviation. *D,* Morphologic criteria used to diagnose VT in the presence of LBBB-type QRS complexes (dominant *negative* in V₁). (*A–D,* Adapted from Brugada, P., Brugada, J., Mont, L., et al.: A new approach to the differential diagnosis of a regular tachycardia with a wide QRS complex. Circulation 83:1649, 1991.)

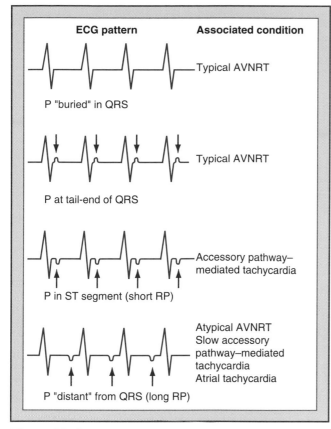

ECG pattern	Associated condition

P "buried" in QRS — Typical AVNRT

P at tail-end of QRS — Typical AVNRT

P in ST segment (short RP) — Accessory pathway–mediated tachycardia

P "distant" from QRS (long RP) — Atypical AVNRT Slow accessory pathway–mediated tachycardia Atrial tachycardia

Figure 23–2

Electrocardiogram (ECG) patterns of narrow complex tachycardias. The most important clue to the mechanism of a narrow complex tachycardia is the relationship of the P-wave to the QRS complex. No visible P-wave often means that the P-wave is buried in the QRS complex. This is usually due to typical atrioventricular (AV) nodal reentry. With typical AV nodal reentry, the P-wave may also be located just at the start or the end of the QRS complex, giving a qRs or Rsr' pattern. When the P-wave is located close to the previous QRS complex, it is identified as a short-RP tachycardia. This is often seen with accessory pathway–mediated tachycardia and is due to retrograde atrial activation over the accessory pathway. The P-wave may also be far from the previous QRS complex and classified as a long-RP tachycardia. If the P-wave is inverted, it may be the result of atypical AV node reentry, or it may be using a slowly conducting accessory pathway in the retrograde direction. AVNRT, atrioventricular nodal reentry tachycardia. (Redrawn from Grogin, H.R.: Supraventricular tachycardia. In Scheinman, M. [vol. cd.]: Arrhythmias: Electrophysiologic Principles. Braunwald, E. [ser. ed.]: Atlas of Heart Diseases. Vol. 9. Philadelphia, Current Medicine, 1996, pp. 5.1–5.17.)

which is preceded by careful auscultation of the carotid arteries. The procedure is performed by applying pressure to the carotid bifurcation with the patient in a supine position, neck extended, and head turned away from the side being stimulated. Pressure is initially applied lightly on one side only, then more firmly for about 5 seconds in a massaging or rotating manner to stimulate carotid sinus baroreceptors and cause a reflex increase in vagal tone. Care must be taken not to massage atherosclerotic carotid arteries, from which some risk of embolization may ensue. Although massage of each side individually may be

Table 23–2	Office-Based Treatment of Sustained Cardiac Arrhythmias
Arrhythmia	**Treatment**
Hemodynamically unstable ventricular tachycardia Atrial fibrillation with rapid conduction via a bypass tract Ventricular fibrillation	Emergency direct-current countershock
Hemodynamically stable monomorphic ventricular tachycardia	IV lidocaine IV procainamide
Polymorphous ventricular tachycardia	IV Mg^{2+}
Supraventricular tachycardia	IV adenosine or IV verapamil

Abbreviation: IV, intravenous.

beneficial, simultaneous bilateral massage should never be performed.

Carotid sinus massage often causes a gradual slowing of sinus tachycardia, may increase the degree of AV block in patients with atrial flutter, may somewhat slow the rate of atrial fibrillation, and may cause sudden termination of a reentrant SVT. It can rarely terminate VT.

As an alternative to carotid sinus massage, patients may use the Valsalva maneuver or may suddenly immerse the face in cold water. Application of pressure to the eyeballs should not be tried, since retinal detachment has been reported. Each of these maneuvers, which may be taught to the patient if of proven success under a physician's observation, is associated with an increase in vagal tone that may be adequate to terminate an SVT. However, patients with symptoms of more than palpitations alone, such as those with dyspnea, dizziness, or chest pain, need further medical attention urgently if simple attempts are not rapidly successful.

If carotid massage is unsuccessful in a patient with a regular PSVT, intravenous adenosine or verapamil is remarkably effective (>95%) in terminating the episode. If the SVT is readily terminated and was not associated with evidence of acute myocardial ischemia or hemodynamic instability, then hospitalization is not required but the patient should be referred to a cardiac specialist for further treatment. There are currently a wide variety of effective pharmacologic as well as nonpharmacologic treatment modalities (Table 23–4), and early referral to a specialist is recommended to help chart the most appropriate therapies.

DIAGNOSIS AND TREATMENT OF SPECIFIC TACHYARRHYTHMIAS

Atrial Fibrillation

DIAGNOSIS. Atrial fibrillation, which is the most common sustained clinical arrhythmia, is diagnosed by

Table 23-3 Common Antiarrhythmic Medications

Class	Drug	IV Loading Dose	Maintenance Dose	Major Side Effects	Excretion
1A	Quinidine sulfate	10 mg/kg	200–400 mg po q 6 hr	Diarrhea, thrombocytopenia, torsades de pointes, tinnitus, hypotension	Hepatic
	Quinidine gluconate	—	324–628 mg po q 8 hr		Hepatic
	Procainamide	10–15 mg/kg	1000 mg po q 8 hr	Nausea, lupus syndrome, torsades de pointes	Renal/hepatic
1B	Lidocaine	1 mg/kg	1–4 mg/min IV	Seizures, respiratory arrest	Hepatic
1C	Flecainide	—	100–150 mg po q 12 hr	Headache, visual disturbances, ventricular tachycardia	Hepatic/renal
	Propafenone	—	150–300 mg q 8 hr	Metallic taste, nausea, ventricular arrhythmias	Hepatic/renal
III	Amiodarone	5 mg/kg IV 1.2 gm/day × 10 days po	200–400 mg/day	Thyroid, pulmonary fibrosis, corneal deposits, hepatic fibrosis, gray-blue skin discoloration	Lacrimal ducts/hepatic
	Sotalol	—	80–160 mg q 12 hr	Bradycardia, bronchospasm, fatigue, increased congestive failure, torsades de pointes	Renal

Abbreviations: IV, intravenous; po, by mouth; q, every.

obtaining a 12-lead ECG and finding an irregularly irregular ventricular rhythm without discrete P-waves (Fig. 23–3). The QRS complex is usually narrow because of the supraventricular origin, but it may be wide if there is aberrant conduction or bundle branch block. Atrial fibrillation associated with the Wolff-Parkinson-White syndrome may occur at a very rapid rate and be life-threatening. This arrhythmia is diagnosed by its very rapid irregular rate associated with wide pre-excited QRS complexes and requires emergency treatment (see later).

EPIDEMIOLOGY. Approximately 4% of the popula-

Table 23-4 Ablation of Cardiac Arrhythmias

Arrhythmia	Approach
Atrial fibrillation	Catheter ablation of AV node and implantation of a pacemaker The maze operation (experimental)
Ectopic atrial focus	Catheter ablation of the focus
PSVT (pre-excitation)	Catheter ablation of anomalous AV connection
PSVT (AV nodal)	Catheter ablation of AV slow pathway Retronodal surgical resection, division of His bundle, implantation of pacemaker
Ventricular tachycardia (coronary heart disease)	Endocardial resection guided by mapping
Ventricular tachycardia (arrhythmogenic right ventricular dysplasia)	Simple ventriculotomy; isolation of arrhythmic site
Ventricular tachycardia (after repair of tetralogy of Fallot)	Resection of infundibulectomy scar
Multiform ventricular tachycardia (long QT syndrome)	Left stellate ganglionectomy

From Bigger J.T.: Cardiac arrhythmias. *In* Bennett, J.C., and Plum, F. (eds.): Cecil Textbook of Medicine. 20th ed. Philadelphia, W.B. Saunders, 1996, p. 252.
Abbreviations: AV, atrioventricular; PSVT, paroxysmal supraventricular tachycardia.

tion over age 60 years has sustained atrial fibrillation, with a particularly steep increase in prevalence after the seventh decade of life. The most powerful predictor for risk of this arrhythmia in the past was rheumatic heart disease, but since this diagnosis is rare in developed countries, it accounts for only a small number of cases. Other correlates include congestive heart failure, hypertensive cardiovascular disease, and coronary artery disease. Moreover, both sustained and paroxysmal atrial fibrillation have important implications for the development of cerebrovascular accident or the risk of death. It is estimated that 15% to 20% of cerebrovascular accidents in nonrheumatic patients are due to atrial fibrillation, and there is an even higher incidence for those with rheumatic mitral valve disease.

RISK AND PRECIPITATING FACTORS. When called on to manage patients with new-onset atrial fibrillation, it is important to establish the precipitating factors, since the type of associated condition determines long-term prognosis (Table 23–5). Atrial fibrillation may result from acute intercurrent ailments. For example, this arrhythmia may occur in patients with hyperthyroidism or after either cardiac or pulmonary surgery or during a bout of pneumonitis, especially in older patients. These arrhythmias may occur in patients with acute pulmonary embolism, myocarditis, or after acute myocardial infarction, particularly when complicated by either right coronary occlusion or acute congestive heart failure. When atrial fibrillation occurs in these settings, it almost always abates spontaneously if the patient recovers from the underlying problem. Hence, management usually involves administration of drugs to achieve rate control, and chronic antiarrhythmic therapy is generally not needed.

Alternatively, atrial fibrillation may occur in association with organic cardiac disease. Important associated conditions include rheumatic mitral stenosis, hypertension, hypertrophic cardiomyopathy, or chronic congestive heart failure. In contrast to patients with acute intercurrent ailments, those with structural heart disease may expect

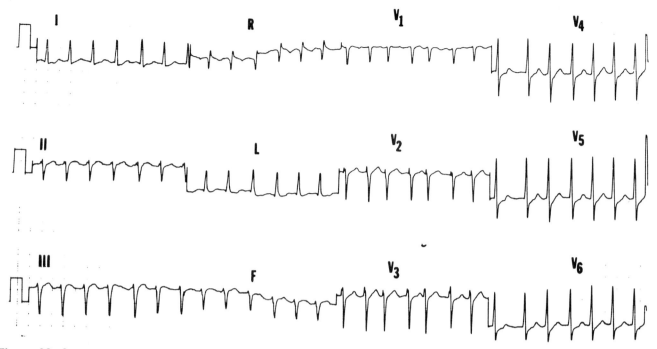

Figure 23–3

A 12-lead ECG shows atrial fibrillation with rapid ventricular response. Note that the ventricular rate is irregular and no discrete P-waves are recorded.

(even with antiarrhythmic therapy) many recurrences until chronic atrial fibrillation supervenes.

When atrial fibrillation is not associated with a precipitating cardiac or noncardiac diagnosis, patients are known as "lone fibrillators." The natural history of the atrial fibrillation in these patients is similar to that in patients with structural cardiac disease, in that atrial fibrillation is likely to recur.

Management

The objectives of therapy include (1) achieving rate control, (2) restoring sinus rhythm (where feasible), and (3) decreasing the risk of cerebrovascular accident.

INITIAL EVALUATION. The initial evaluation of patients with new-onset atrial fibrillation includes a detailed history keying on possible precipitating factors as well as the presence of organic cardiac disease. As such, the initial evaluation includes, at a minimum, a careful physical examination, 12-lead ECG, chest x-ray, echocardiogram, and tests of thyroid function. Further testing will depend on various aspects of the history or physical examination. For example, if atrial fibrillation is usually precipitated by exercise, then an exercise treadmill test is appropriate. In the patient with frequent episodes of paroxysmal atrial fibrillation, a 24- to 48-hour Holter recording may discern whether atrial fibrillation was triggered by another arrhythmia, such as when a premature atrial complex during a rapid paroxysmal atrial tachycardia may cause the immediate onset of atrial fibrillation.

RATE CONTROL. If the patient presents with atrial

fibrillation and rapid rate associated with severe heart failure or cardiogenic shock, emergency direct-current cardioversion is indicated. For patients with atrial fibrillation associated with rapid rate but with stable hemodynamics, attempts to achieve acute rate control are indicated. Drugs to slow the rate of atrial fibrillation include digitalis preparations, calcium channel blockers (verapamil or diltiazem), and beta blockers (Table 23–6). If rapid rate control is desired, then the latter two types of

Table 23–5 Precipitating Factors for Atrial Fibrillation

Associated Cardiac Abnormalities

Hypertension, congestive heart failure, coronary artery disease
Valvular heart disease (mitral or tricuspid)
Inflammatory/infiltrative disease (pericarditis, amyloid)
Congenital (atrial septal defect)
Metastatic atrial disease
Triggering arrhythmias (atrial flutter, paroxysmal supraventricular tachycardia)

Other Precipitants

Drugs or intoxicants (alcohol, carbon monoxide)
Postoperative, especially after cardiac or pulmonary surgery
Acute or chronic pulmonary disease
Enhanced vagal tone/enhanced sympathetic tone
Metabolic abnormalities: e.g., hypokalemia, hyperthyroidism, pheochromocytoma
Exertion-related

Lone Atrial Fibrillation

Table 23-6   **Drugs Used for Acute Rate Control**

Drug	Dose	Side Effects	Primary Metabolic Route
Digoxin	0.5 mg followed by 0.25 mg q 2–6 hr to total dose of 1–1.5 mg	Nausea, emesis, disturbed vision, atrial or ventricular arrhythmias, or both	Renal
Diltiazem	20 mg IV as loading dose (if necessary), followed by 5–15 mg/hr infusion	Hypotension, peripheral edema, headache, sinus node depression, AV block	Hepatic
Verapamil	0.15 mg/kg loading dose, 5–10 mg q 30 min as needed	Same as above	Hepatic
Esmolol	0.5 mg/kg/min (load) 0.05–0.2 mg/kg/min (maintenance)	Negative inotropic effects, suppression of sinoatrial and AV nodal function, bronchospasm	Hepatic

Abbreviations: q, every; IV, intravenous; AV, atrioventricular.

agents are far more effective than digitalis, which may require many hours before rate control is achieved. In addition, a common misconception is that digitalis therapy is associated with acute conversion to sinus rhythm, but carefully controlled studies have shown that conversion to sinus rhythm is no more likely with digoxin than with placebo. As emphasized later, digitalis and intravenous calcium channel blocker therapy are contraindicated for patients presenting with Wolff-Parkinson-White syndrome and atrial fibrillation. Intravenous diltiazem has been shown to be safe and effective for patients with atrial fibrillation and congestive heart failure.

CHRONIC ANTIARRHYTHMIC THERAPY AND ELECTIVE CARDIOVERSION. For patients presenting with a single, initial episode of self-limited atrial fibrillation, no specific therapy is required because recurrences may be delayed for many years. In contrast, patients who manifest frequent recurrences may be candidates for chronic antiarrhythmic therapy (Table 23–7) with class IA (quinidine, procainamide, and disopyramide), class IC (propafenone and flecainide), or class III (sotalol and amiodarone) agents, all of which are more effective than placebo in maintaining sinus rhythm.[2]

Unfortunately, these agents have important drawbacks. First, even with drug therapy, recurrence rates for atrial fibrillation approach 50% per year (as opposed to recurrences with placebo therapy of 75% per year). In addition, these agents may be associated with significant side effects. For class IA drugs, these include induction of torsades de pointes. For example, a recent meta-analysis compared quinidine with placebo for patients with atrial fibrillation and found that all cause mortality was *higher* in the groups treated with quinidine. In addition, in the Stroke Prevention in Atrial Fibrillation (SPAF) trials, substantial numbers of patients were treated with antiarrhythmic agents; in patients with congestive heart failure, those treated with class IA or IC drugs had significant excess mortality compared with those not treated with antiarrhythmic drugs. Great care must be exercised in the use of these agents, balancing the benefits against the potential for adverse effects. General rules include avoidance of all class IA drugs in the face of torsades de pointes associated with one of these agents and avoidance of class IC agents for those patients with structural heart disease. In addition, sotalol is contraindicated for patients with severe depression of the left ventricular ejection fraction.

The only drug that appears to be both effective and safe for patients with congestive heart failure and atrial fibrillation is amiodarone. This agent is associated with a

Table 23-7   **Overview of Drug Therapy of Arrhythmias**

Arrhythmia	Acute Management (IV)	Chronic Therapy	Chronic Anticoagulants
Atrial fibrillation	Digoxin, verapamil, diltiazem	Classes IA, IC, sotalol, amiodarone	Yes
Atrial fibrillation with rapid rate owing to Wolff-Parkinson-White syndrome	Procainamide; avoid IV verapamil or digoxin	Class IC, sotalol, amiodarone	No
Atrial flutter	Digoxin, verapamil, diltiazem	Classes IA, IC, sotalol, amiodarone	Yes
Paroxysmal supraventricular tachycardia	Adenosine, verapamil, propranolol, esmolol	Beta blockers, calcium channel blockers, classes IA, IC, sotalol	No
Monomorphic ventricular tachycardia	Lidocaine, procainamide, amiodarone	Sotalol, amiodarone	No
Polymorphous ventricular tachycardia (congenital)	Propranolol, cardiac pacing	Cardiac pacing, beta-blockers	No
Polymorphous ventricular tachycardia (acquired)	IV Mg^{2+}/correct electrolyte abnormalities	Avoid offending drug class	No

Abbreviation: IV, intravenous.

host of both cardiac (e.g., severe sinus bradycardia or arrest or AV block) and noncardiac (e.g., thyroid abnormalities, pulmonary fibrosis) adverse effects, but low-dose amiodarone (i.e., ≤200 mg/day) appears to be very well tolerated. Great care must be used in treatment of patients with sinus node dysfunction.

ANTICOAGULANT THERAPY. The beneficial effects of warfarin for patients with atrial fibrillation associated with mitral stenosis is well known, but until recently, the high risk of stroke in patients with nonrheumatic atrial fibrillation was not appreciated. Recent studies have documented that the risk of cerebrovascular accident in patients with nonrheumatic atrial fibrillation is 4% to 7% per year.[3] Patients at particularly high risk include those with hypertension, age over 70 years, history of congestive heart failure, increased left atrial size, or prior stroke.[4] Stroke is similar in patients with paroxysmal versus chronic atrial fibrillation. A host of studies have documented the remarkable efficacy of warfarin in decreasing the risk of embolic phenomena by 45% to 85% in patients with nonrheumatic atrial fibrillation with a low risk of significant hemorrhage, provided the International Normalized Ratio (INR) is in the range of 2.0 to 2.5.[3, 6–9] Still controversial is the need for anticoagulant therapy in younger patients with lone atrial fibrillation, since the risk for embolic phenomena is very low in this group.

The role of aspirin therapy for patients with atrial fibrillation remains controversial. In one study, 75 mg of aspirin failed to decrease the stroke risk compared with placebo (5.5% per year).[10] In contrast, the SPAF I trials showed that a higher dose of aspirin, 325 mg, appeared to be of benefit in patients under 75 years of age.[8] In a follow-up study (SPAF II), the incidence of stroke was higher with aspirin (4.8%) compared with warfarin (3.6%).[10] Recent results of the SPAF III trials demonstrated that aspirin (325 mg/day) and fixed low-dose warfarin (1, 2, or 3 mg) proved ineffective for stroke prevention.[11] Therefore, the weight of current data favors warfarin with an INR of 2.0 to 2.5 as the best strategy to prevent systemic embolization.[12]

DIRECT-CURRENT CARDIOVERSION. Direct-current cardioversion is a very effective technique for restoration of sinus rhythm. Because of the benefits of sinus rhythm in terms of improved cardiac output and decreased risk of embolic phenomena in general, at least one attempt should be made to restore sinus rhythm. Several precautions are in order. The patient must be pretreated with an antiarrhythmic agent, since reversion to atrial fibrillation after shock therapy is very high. In addition, unless urgent cardioversion is required because of hemodynamic decompensation or secondary ischemia, consideration must be given to pre- and postcardioversion anticoagulation. One approach is for the patients to be fully anticoagulated for about 2 to 3 weeks before and for about 4 weeks after attempted direct-current cardioversion to decrease the risk of an embolism after successful reversion to sinus rhythm.

An alternative is to perform transesophageal echocardiography (TEE), which provides excellent ability to detect clot in the left atrium or the left atrial appendage. Both the finding of clot and spontaneous echo contrast in the left atrium are associated with higher risks of systemic embolization. Data suggest that if the TEE shows no atrial clots or spontaneous contrast, then it is usually safe to proceed with cardioversion without prior anticoagulation, although thromboemboli may rarely occur despite a negative TEE.[13, 14] Current evidence suggests that patients with recent-onset atrial fibrillation with no evidence of atrial clots or spontaneous contrast by TEE may undergo direct-current cardioversion after initiation of anticoagulant therapy, but without a course of full anticoagulant treatment.[15, 16] It must be appreciated that atrial function is depressed after cardioversion and that anticoagulant therapy is recommended for at least 1 month after cardioversion. For those patients with clot or spontaneous echo contrast with TEE, full anticoagulant therapy is recommended for at least 2 to 3 weeks before cardioversion.

Direct-current external shock is usually performed in a monitored area under supervision of an anesthesiologist. It is wise to check the arterial oxygen saturation, serum potassium level, digoxin, or antiarrhythmic blood drug levels before the cardioversion. Direct-current shocks beginning with at least 200 joules are used in order to achieve sinus rhythm. If the patient fails to revert after maximal external shocks (360 joules), then internal cardioversion with small energy shocks delivered between the coronary sinus and the right atrium is almost always effective.

LONG-TERM APPROACH. One should be especially careful to seek those patients with atrial fibrillation in whom cure is possible. This may be true for patients with hyperthyroidism as well as for those with other cardiac arrhythmias that appear to trigger atrial fibrillation. For example, patients with atrial flutter or PSVT may experience atrial premature impulses during tachycardia, which gives rise to atrial fibrillation. It is possible in selected patients to apply catheter ablation to cure the underlying arrhythmia and, hence, prevent the trigger for atrial fibrillation. Therefore, in the evaluation of patients who present with atrial fibrillation, initial testing should include obtaining a thyroid-stimulating hormone assay, an echocardiogram, and a 48-hour ambulatory ECG recording for those with paroxysmal atrial fibrillation. In analyses of these recordings, the clinician seeks evidence for triggering arrhythmias. In addition, one looks for vagal triggers of atrial fibrillation, such as sinus bradycardia associated with sleep or heavy meals, that may be initially treated with vagolytic antiarrhythmic agents such as disopyramide. Alternatively, if atrial fibrillation appears only with enhanced sympathetic tone, such as with exercise, a trial of beta blocker therapy is appropriate. In some patients, episodes of atrial fibrillation may be initiated by caffeine, alcohol, or marijuana.

The natural history of atrial fibrillation associated with structural cardiac disease or in patients with lone atrial fibrillation is for spontaneous recurrence of the arrhythmia. Unfortunately, no drug is universally effective, and the decision of how many drugs to try before a judgment is made to terminate antiarrhythmic drugs and focus on rate control depends on how symptomatic the patient is during atrial fibrillation. If the episodes are poorly tolerated, then multiple drug trials or even various ablative procedures may be required (see later). On the other hand, if rate control can be readily achieved with drugs, such as digoxin, beta blockers, or calcium antagonists, that block the AV node and the patient has a good symptomatic outcome, then a completely acceptable alternative is to use drugs to control rate combined with chronic anticoagulant treatment.

ROLE OF CATHETER ABLATION. Various ablative techniques have been successfully applied for treatment of patients with symptomatic atrial fibrillation refractory to drug therapy. The most used technique involves application of radiofrequency energy to the region of the AV junction to produce complete AV block. In this situation, complete arrhythmia control is achieved, but chronic pacemaker therapy is required. Newer modifications of this technique involve application of radiofrequency energy to the posterior or midseptal areas to modify but not completely destroy AV nodal conduction.

A number of surgical centers are currently using the maze procedure to try to cure atrial fibrillation. This procedure involves placing transmural lesions over both atria, in such a manner that the fibrillatory impulses cannot complete a reentrant circuit. The maze procedure involves all of the risks of major open-heart surgery.

Patients with persistent tachycardia may suffer from a tachycardia cardiomyopathy with left ventricular failure superimposed on their native cardiac disease. Hence, in the management of patients with chronic atrial fibrillation, rate control is an important objective that must be achieved either via AV nodal blocking drugs or, failing these, with catheter ablative procedures.

WHEN TO CALL A CARDIOLOGIST. There are several points in the life cycle of patients with atrial fibrillation when expert consultation is strongly recommended. For those clinicians who do not use antiarrhythmic agents on a regular basis, it is useful to obtain expert consultation to sequence drug therapy, especially when newer agents such as propafenone, sotalol, and amiodarone are being considered. Similarly, if the clinician is not experienced in the performance of direct-current cardioversion, it is well to ask for expert assistance in preparing a patient for this procedure and performing it. When sinus rhythm cannot be maintained, catheter ablative procedures should be considered in patients who remain symptomatic despite attempts to control their heart rate.

Atrial Flutter

Diagnosis

The treatment of patients with atrial flutter is very similar to that of atrial fibrillation, but there are several important differences. Atrial flutter has been separated into two types. *Typical* atrial flutter is usually manifest by negative flutter waves in the inferior leads and positive waves in lead V₁ (Fig. 23–4). This has been termed *counterclockwise flutter*. Alternatively, typical flutter may show regular flutter waves that are positive in the inferior leads and negative in V₁ *(clockwise flutter)*. These mor-

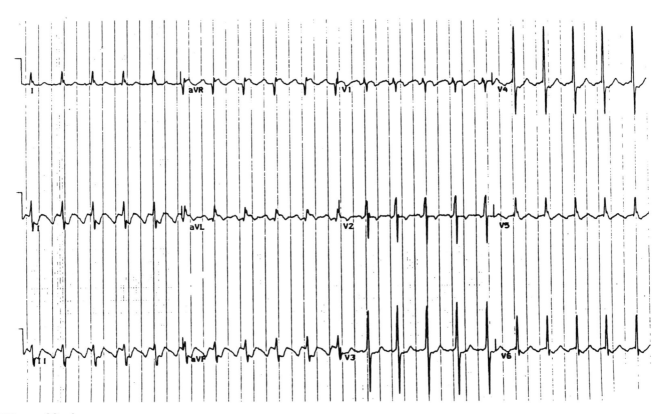

Figure 23–4

A 12-lead ECG shows the pattern of typical atrial flutter. Note the inverted flutter waves in the inferior leads and the positive flutter waves in V₁. Atrial flutter is accompanied by 2:1 atrioventricular block.

phologic features are associated with a very regular flutter rate of approximately 300 complexes per minute. *Atypical* flutter shows either positive or negative flutter waves in the inferior leads, is associated with more rapid rates (350/min) that are often irregular, and may precede the onset of atrial fibrillation.

CAUSE, RISK FACTORS, AND PATHOPHYSI-OLOGY OF ATRIAL FLUTTER. Atrial flutter may occur in patients without cardiac disease, but it most often occurs in association with mitral or tricuspid valve disease or after repair of certain congenital abnormalities. Atrial flutter commonly occurs after cardiac surgery and in approximately 5% of patients after acute myocardial infarction. In patients with atrial flutter, the rhythm may subsequently change to atrial fibrillation.

MECHANISMS. Typical atrial flutter is now known to be a reentrant arrhythmia localized to the right atrium with a critical zone of conduction at the base of the right atrium between the tricuspid annulus and the eustachian ridge. With counterclockwise rotation around the flutter isthmus, a negative flutter wave is found in leads II, III, and aVF and a positive flutter wave in V_1. Clockwise flutter produces positive waves in leads II, III, and aVF and negative deflection in V_1. In contrast, in patients with atypical flutter, the precise circuit has not been defined; these patients will often develop atrial fibrillation.

Management

INITIAL EVALUATION. Initial evaluation can proceed in an orderly fashion if the patient is hemodynamically stable with this arrhythmia. Such evaluation includes a careful history with emphasis on the presence of cardiac disease, a 12-lead ECG, and an echocardiogram.

TREATMENT. Direct-current cardioversion is very effective at even low energy, and patients with atrial flutter are often converted to sinus rhythm with 20 to 50 joules of delivered energy. In patients with hemodynamic compromise, this is the indicated therapy and it is generally recommended for all patients with atrial flutter. A less-effective alternative is application of AV nodal blocking drugs to slow the ventricular response (see Table 23–6), which is more difficult in patients with atrial flutter than with atrial fibrillation. Medications are usually not effective in converting the rhythm to sinus, and rate control may be the preferred option when reversion to sinus rhythm is not possible. Patients with typical atrial flutter are generally responsive to atrial overdrive pacing. If direct-current cardioversion is to be avoided or if the patient already has an atrial pacemaker lead in place, then rapid overdrive pacing should be attempted to terminate this arrhythmia.

Current information suggests that patients with chronic atrial flutter carry a risk for systemic embolization. Anticoagulant therapy should be seriously considered in patients with chronic or recurrent atrial flutter, particularly if the TEE shows spontaneous echo contrast or frank clot formation.

LONG-TERM TREATMENT. Patients with chronic atrial flutter can be treated in a manner very similar to that outlined for patients with atrial fibrillation. This approach involves use of antiarrhythmic agents and AV nodal blockers for rate and rhythm control. However, chronic drug therapy is often ineffective for patients with atrial flutter. In contrast, catheter ablative techniques to produce a line of block between the tricuspid annulus and the inferior vena cava can interfere with the flutter circuit and have a success rate of about 85%, suggesting that this approach should supplant drug therapy as the treatment of choice. Successful ablation obviates the need not only for antiarrhythmic therapy but also for chronic anticoagulant treatment.

WHEN TO CALL A CARDIOLOGIST. Since atrial flutter is often very resistant to drug therapy, the patient is best served by early referral to a cardiologist. The latter can aid the primary physician with cardioversion or overdrive pacing, outline drug therapy if appropriate, and recommend when to intervene with catheter ablation.

Paroxysmal Supraventricular Tachycardia

Diagnosis

The diagnosis of PSVT is suspected from a history of abrupt onset and abrupt termination of palpitations.[17] The diagnosis is confirmed by recording a narrow complex tachycardia during an episode of palpitations (Fig. 23–5). Evaluation of these patients should include obtaining data from an event recorder (which the patient activates) or a 24- to 48-hour ambulatory ECG recorder, depending on the frequency of symptoms. The recorded symptoms depend on the tachycardia rate, relationship of the P-wave to the QRS complex, and associated cardiac disease. In some patients, the overriding symptom complex may revolve around severe anxiety, and the episode may be misdiagnosed as a hysterical reaction or panic attack.

Most instances of PSVT (see Fig. 23–2) are due to reentrant arrhythmias involving the AV nodal region, an accessory extranodal pathway, or a circuit localized within the atrium. The most common mechanism is AV nodal reentry and is due to *dual AV nodal* pathways. These pathways are designated as "fast" and "slow" (Fig. 23–6). In these patients, the PSVT is usually triggered by a critically timed atrial premature complex that results in conduction block in the fast pathway and antegrade conduction over the slow pathway. If conduction in the slow pathway is sufficiently slow, the return impulse now finds the fast pathway excitable, and this sequence may give rise to a circus movement tachycardia involving the AV junctional area. Risk factors that may exacerbate the triggering of premature beats include stress, caffeine, or beta receptor agonists.

A similar mechanism is known to occur in patients with *accessory AV nodal pathways*. In some two to three per thousand live births in the United States each year, babies are born with an accessory pathway that is separate from the normal AV node–His axis. This pathway consists of microscopic muscular tissue that bridges the atrium to the ventricle over the AV groove. The pathway may be located almost anywhere on the right or left annulus or may occur in the septum. The accessory path-

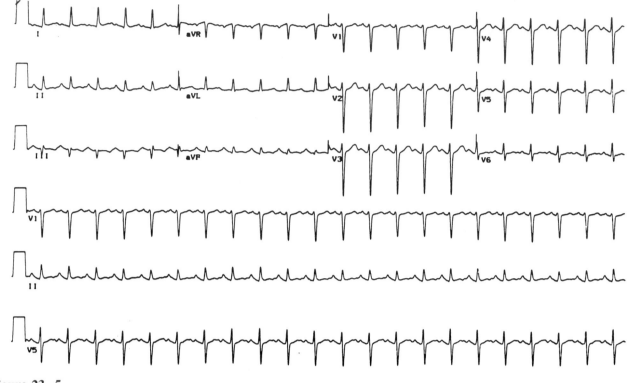

Figure 23–5
A 12-lead ECG of a patient with atrial tachycardia. Note that the P-wave usually just precedes the QRS in patients with atrial tachycardia.

way usually has a longer refractory period compared with the AV node; hence, a premature impulse will tend to block in the pathway and conduct over the AV node and His bundle to the ventricle. If the ventricular impulse finds the accessory pathway excitable, then that impulse returns to the atrium and initiates a circus movement tachycardia (see Fig. 23–6). Since antegrade conduction usually proceeds over the AV node, the QRS complex during tachycardia will either be normal or show a pattern of aberrant supraventricular conduction.

Some 90% of patients presenting with PSVT have one of the two mechanisms described previously. The bulk of the remainder have atrial tachycardia that may be due to reentry within the atrium or to abnormal automaticity of an atrial focus.

Management

INITIAL EVALUATION. Most patients with PSVT are young and without evidence of cardiac disease; hence, except in special circumstances, extensive evaluation is not required. A number of practical points bear emphasis. The ECG during and even after an episode of rapid tachycardia will often show persistent ST depression. This finding, in and of itself, does not require hospitalization and does not require coronary angiography. An echocardiogram should be obtained in selected patients with PSVT to evaluate possible occult cardiac abnormalities. For example, patients with right-sided accessory pathways may have manifest or occult Ebstein's anomaly.

TREATMENT. Since the predominant mechanisms of

PSVT involve AV nodal conduction, initial therapy for patients presenting with narrow complex tachycardia involves maneuvers or drugs that block conduction at the AV node. Carotid sinus massage, for example, is a safe and often effective maneuver for tachycardia termination. Care must be taken to exclude significant carotid stenosis (by careful auscultation over the carotids) before applying carotid massage. Children with PSVT are often treated by application of facial cold packs, which is a potent vagal maneuver. These maneuvers increase vagal tone, which delays conduction and prolongs refractoriness in the AV node. If the tachycardia fails to terminate with vagal maneuvers, then intravenous drug treatment is indicated.

Adenosine and verapamil are very rapidly acting, effective, and safe.[17, 18] Adenosine is administered in bolus infusions to adults at an initial dose of 6 mg; repeat doses of 12 and 18 mg may be attempted if the lower dose proves ineffective. The half-life of adenosine is approximately 10 seconds, so that adverse effects are quickly dissipated. Adenosine is effective in approximately 95% of patients with PSVT, and the chief adverse effect is transient dyspnea and chest tightness. Intravenous verapamil is used in a dose of 0.15 mg/kg and should not be used in patients with underlying sinus or AV node dysfunction or in those pretreated with beta blockers. The chief advantage of adenosine is its short half-life. One advantage of verapamil is its relatively low cost, but this drug may aggravate underlying sinus or nodal disease or congestive heart failure in patients with depressed left ventricular function. Short-acting beta blocking agents (esmolol) or intravenous propranolol may be used, partic-

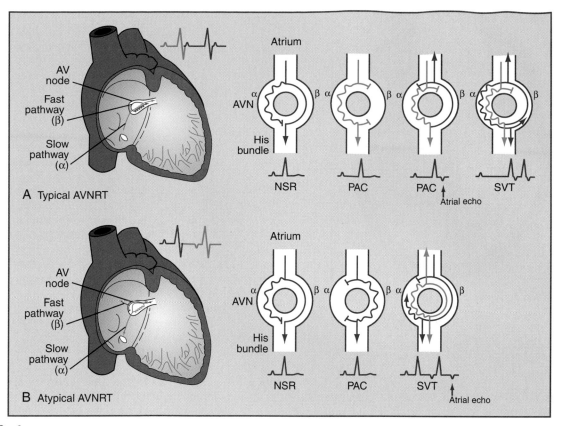

Figure 23–6

Schema for typical and atypical atrioventricular node reentrant tachycardia (AVNRT). *A,* Typical atrioventricular (AV) node [AVN] reentry. An impulse from the atrium enters the AV node and travels down both the slow (α) and the fast (β) pathways. It quickly travels down the fast pathway, resulting in activation of the ventricles with a short PR interval and in the blocking of the impulse from the slow pathway when it reaches the terminal portion of the AV node, since the tissue is still refractory. A premature atrial contraction (PAC) results in the conduction of the impulse down the slow pathway and thus a longer PR interval. It blocks in the fast pathway, since that tissue has a longer refractory period. If the tissue of the fast pathway regains conduction, the impulse after traveling down the slow pathway can return retrogradely back to the atrium via the fast pathway, resulting in an atrial echo beat. A key component of the circuit is that the retrograde impulse finds the fast pathway no longer refractory. For this to occur there must be a suitable delay in antegrade conduction over the slow pathway. The QRS complex is narrow because the ventricle is being activated via the normal His-Purkinje system (HPS). Retrograde activation over the fast pathway happens quickly, and on the surface ECG the retrograde P-wave is usually "buried" or at the tail end of the QRS complex. This can give the appearance of a "pseudo" right bundle branch pattern in lead V_1. This is a short-RP tachycardia. *B,* When the circuit is reversed, as during atypical AV node reentry, antegrade conduction occurs over the fast pathway and retrograde conduction over the slow pathway. In atypical AV node reentry, a PAC is conducted over the fast pathway. The PR interval remains short. If there is retrograde activation over the slow pathway to the atrium, then supraventricular tachycardia (SVT) may be initiated. The QRS complex remains narrow because activation of the ventricle is still via the normal HPS. Retrograde atrial activation over the slow pathway takes longer compared with conduction over the fast pathway, resulting in a long-RP interval. This is a long-RP tachycardia. NSR, normal sinus rhythm. (*A* and *B,* Redrawn from Grogin, H.R.: Supraventricular tachycardia. *In* Scheinman, M. [vol. ed.]: Arrhythmias: Electrophysiologic Principles. Braunwald, E. [ser. ed.]: Atlas of Heart Diseases. Vol. 9. Philadelphia, Current Medicine, 1996, pp. 5.1–5.17.)

ularly if the patient fails to respond to adenosine. Medications are so effective that direct-current cardioversion is seldom required, except for instances associated with hemodynamic collapse. Similarly, anticoagulant therapy is not required for patients with PSVT.

SPECIAL CASE OF THE WOLFF-PARKINSON-WHITE SYNDROME. Patients with Wolff-Parkinson-White syndrome have an accessory pathway from the atrium to the ventricle that bypasses the usual delay in the AV node. When the patient is in sinus rhythm, dual conduction down this pathway as well as through the AV node will often cause a delta wave, which is the initial slurred deflection at the beginning of the QRS complex that results from initial activation of the QRS complex by conduction over the accessory pathway (Fig. 23–7). The

presence of an alternative AV pathway in patients with Wolff-Parkinson-White syndrome makes them prone to develop PSVT, which may then cause atrial fibrillation.

These patients as well as those with variants of the Wolff-Parkinson-White syndrome, such as those with a short resting PR interval in sinus rhythm but without a delta wave (accelerated AV nodal conduction), may present with atrial fibrillation with a rapid ventricular response. Patients with Wolff-Parkinson-White syndrome or other accessory pathways are also slightly more likely to have other congenital cardiac abnormalities that are associated with higher risks of PSVT, atrial fibrillation, and atrial flutter.

In patients with short refractory periods of the abnormal pathway, rapid, life-threatening arrhythmias may oc-

WPW or other accessory pathways - may develop very fast wide complex tachycardia. Shock then procainamide. NEVER use dig or verapamil.

342 ❖ Part 3 ❖ Recognition and Management of Patients with Specific Cardiac Problems

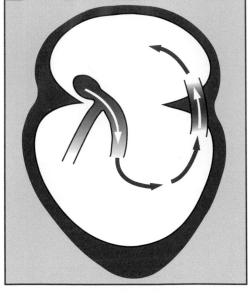

Figure 23–7

Schema showing reentrant pathway in patients with accessory pathways. The tachycardia circuit usually involves antegrade conduction over the AV node and retrograde conduction over the accessory pathway.

cur (Fig. 23–8). This situation, which is recognized by an irregular wide complex (pre-excited QRS) with very rapid rate (i.e., RR intervals less than 250 msec) on the ECG, should be considered as dangerous and requiring urgent attention. Emergency direct-current countershock followed by intravenous infusion of procainamide is the treatment of choice for atrial fibrillation or atrial flutter in patients with accessory pathways and very rapid AV conduction. These patients should generally be admitted to the hospital for further evaluation by a cardiologist and should be

recommended to undergo catheter ablation of the pathway. It is critical to remember *not* to use intravenous digoxin or verapamil in these patients. Lidocaine or intravenous beta blockers are not deleterious but are usually not effective for rate control in patients with rapid atrial fibrillation via an accessory pathway, and hence, their use delays appropriate care.

LONG-TERM TREATMENT OF PATIENTS WITH RECURRENT PSVT. Chronic drug therapy of patients with recurrent episodes of PSVT includes use of agents that block at the AV node (digoxin, calcium antagonists, or beta blockers) (see Table 23–6) or agents that act primarily on fast pathway or accessory pathway conduction (i.e., class IA agents: quinidine/procainamide/disopyramide; or class IC agents: propafenone, flecainide) (see Table 23–7). Class III antiarrhythmic agents (amiodarone, sotalol) act on both the normal and the fast or accessory pathways. Chronic digoxin therapy is contraindicated for patients with the Wolff-Parkinson-White syndrome.

In patients with recurrent SVTs of relatively short duration who are asymptomatic except for palpitations, an alternative to catheter ablation or chronic antiarrhythmic treatment may be episodic therapy for the occasional arrhythmia. In some patients, 10 to 40 mg of propranolol, or equivalent doses of other beta blockers, may be adequate to terminate a supraventricular arrhythmia; in others, a concomitant 0.25-mg dose of digoxin may provide an effective "cocktail." Use of intermittent therapy is discouraged, since patients may develop symptomatic prolonged pauses when the arrhythmia terminates. More complex arrhythmia will commonly require chronic medications or referral to a cardiologist.

The advent of radiofrequency catheter ablative procedures has completely changed the approach to the long-term management of patients with recurrent PSVT and

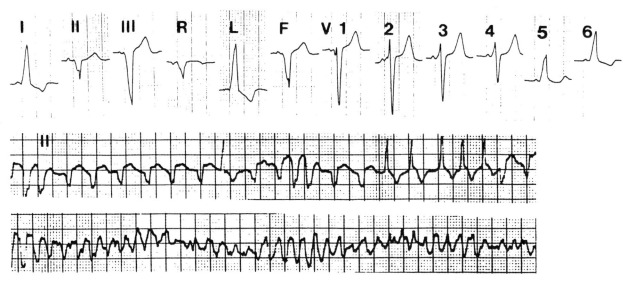

Figure 23–8

Top, a 12-lead ECG from a patient with the Wolff-Parkinson-White syndrome. Note the delta wave between the P-wave and the onset of the QRS complex in lead V_2. *Middle* and *bottom,* A lead II rhythm strip (not continuous) initially shows atrial fibrillation with rapid ventricular response, which quickly deteriorated into ventricular fibrillation *(bottom)*. Atrial fibrillation with rapid ventricular response is the most dangerous arrhythmia for patients with the Wolff-Parkinson-White syndrome.

Class I act on fast pathway
Class III (amiodarone, sotalol) act on sl + fast pathways.

other SVTs (Table 23–8).[19–22] These catheter techniques involve use of invasive electrophysiologic studies to localize the abnormal pathway(s), which are then destroyed by application of radiofrequency energy. The technique is effective in 90% to 98% of attempts and is associated with a very low incidence of adverse effects.

WHEN TO REFER TO A CARDIOLOGIST. Referral for specialist care is indicated for all patients with manifest Wolff-Parkinson-White syndrome and episodes of palpitations or syncope. Patients with Wolff-Parkinson-White syndrome carry the distinct risk of sudden cardiac death because of atrial fibrillation with rapid rate. In addition, all patients with recurrent PSVT who either fail a course of medical therapy or are disinclined to take lifelong drug therapy are candidates for catheter ablation and should be referred to a specialist who can adequately discuss the benefits and possible adverse effects of the catheter procedure. Ablative techniques have also proved to be safe and effective for patients with atrial tachycardia.

Premature Atrial Contractions

Half or more of the adult population will have premature atrial complexes, which will often be asymptomatic. Premature atrial contractions are probably the most common arrhythmic cause of palpitations (see Chap. 10) and can occasionally precipitate a sustained SVT in patients with the appropriate substrate (see Fig. 23–2). Frequent or recurrent premature atrial contractions may be an early sign of a dilated atrium in patients with mitral or tricuspid valve disease, congestive heart failure, or congenital heart disease. They may also be caused by any of the same types of stresses that precipitate sinus tachycardia.

Premature atrial contractions are preceded by a detectable P-wave that differs from the sinus P-wave with a PR interval of 0.12 second or greater. The premature contrac-

tion may or may not be associated with effective ventricular ejection and a detectable pulse, depending on whether the premature contraction is very early. For very early premature contractions, the P-wave may be difficult to find in the preceding T-wave, and some very early premature atrial contractions may be blocked because the AV node is still in its refractory period. In such situations, a blocked premature atrial contraction may be misdiagnosed as a sinus pause or sinus node dysfunction. Conducted premature atrial contractions may be associated with aberrant ventricular conduction and, hence, a wide ventricular complex. Premature atrial contractions are not commonly associated with a compensatory pause because, unlike a premature ventricular contraction, they commonly cause immediate resetting of the sinus node. In some patients, however, the premature atrial contraction may not be effectively conducted back into the sinus node; in these situations, a compensatory pause will occur.

Premature atrial contractions commonly require no treatment. Patients with symptomatic palpitations due to atrial premature contractions should be reassured as to their benign nature, and drug therapy should be discouraged. For those patients in whom premature atrial contractions trigger SVTs, treatment is as described previously.

Wandering Atrial Pacemaker and Multifocal Atrial Tachycardia

 heart

lung

When patients have more than two different P-wave morphologies, the rhythm is termed *wandering atrial pacemaker* (if the heart rate is less than 100 beats/min) or multifocal atrial tachycardia (if the heart rate is above 100 beats/min). Wandering atrial pacemaker is often a prelude to a sustained atrial tachycardia or, more commonly, atrial fibrillation in a patient with intrinsic heart

Table 23–8	Overview of Catheter Ablation		
Type of Arrhythmia	**Site of Ablation (e.g., accessory pathway, AV node)**	**Success Rate for Catheter Ablation (%)**	**Indications for Ablation**
Wolff-Parkinson-White syndrome	Accessory pathway (see Fig. 23–7)	85–95 (right-sided) 95+ (left-sided)	Episodes of PSVT* Episodes of atrial fibrillation
AV node reentry	Slow AV nodal pathway (see Fig. 23–6)	95+	Symptomatic PSVT* in patients who do not want chronic drug therapy Symptomatic PSVT* resistant to drug therapy
Atrial fibrillation	AV junction	100	Rapid ventricular response uncontrolled with medications
Typical atrial flutter	Linear lesion between inferior vena cava and tricuspid annulus	80–90	Rapid ventricular response uncontrolled with medications or first-line therapy in those who do not wish to take chronic antiarrhythmic drugs and anticoagulants
Atrial tachycardia	Atrial focus	70–80	Rapid ventricular response uncontrolled with medications Patients who wish to avoid lifelong drug therapy

* For PSVT, catheter ablation has matured to be used as first-line therapy.
Abbreviations: AV, atrioventricular; PSVT, paroxysmal supraventricular tachycardia.

disease. Multifocal atrial tachycardia most commonly is an arrhythmia found in patients with advanced pulmonary disease, sometimes associated with an exacerbation of the pulmonary disease itself and sometimes with the medications used to treat the pulmonary disease.

As with sinus tachycardia and premature atrial contractions, wandering atrial pacemaker and multifocal atrial tachycardia may be precipitated by a variety of noncardiac conditions whose successful treatment will often result in termination of the arrhythmia. If the arrhythmia itself is causing important secondary problems, verapamil is the recommended medication, provided the patient does not have severe left ventricular dysfunction.

Premature Ventricular Complexes and Nonsustained VT

Diagnosis

Ventricular arrhythmias may be separated into various categories. These include isolated *premature ventricular complexes* (PVCs) (Fig. 23–9), *nonsustained VT* (three or more successive PVCs), and *sustained monomorphic VT* (Fig. 23–10), which is defined as VT persisting for 30 seconds or requiring termination by intervention. Ventricular arrhythmias in these categories generally show a single morphology; patients with multiple types of monomorphic VT are referred to as having a *pleomorphic pattern*. A separate category of ventricular arrhythmia includes patients with *polymorphic VT*, which is defined as a rapid ventricular arrhythmia with beat-to-beat changes in the ventricular complexes.

MAKING THE DIAGNOSIS. Ventricular premature beats are recognized by premature wide complexes followed by compensatory pauses. The cause of the compensatory pause is related to the fact that the premature ventricular contraction penetrates the AV node, making it refractory to the next sinus impulse. In addition, ventricular premature beats have distinct morphologic features that distinguish them from supraventricular beats with aberrancy (see Fig. 23–1).

Management

Most patients with PVCs do not require antiarrhythmic treatment. Long-term studies have shown that individuals with PVCs or nonsustained VT and no structural heart disease have a benign long-term prognosis, and no specific therapy is indicated.[23] In patients with these arrhythmias, sudden cardiac death most often occurs in the setting of ischemic cardiac disease. Patients surviving an acute myocardial infarction who show high-density PVCs (i.e., ≥ 10 PVCs/hr) or complex forms have a higher risk of early (2-year) mortality. This finding is of limited value, since 40% of postinfarction patients will show either high-density PVCs or nonsustained VT and most will have a benign prognosis. Another factor that greatly influences prognosis is poor left ventricular ejection fraction ($< 40\%$).

The signal-averaged ECG, which is a simple noninva-

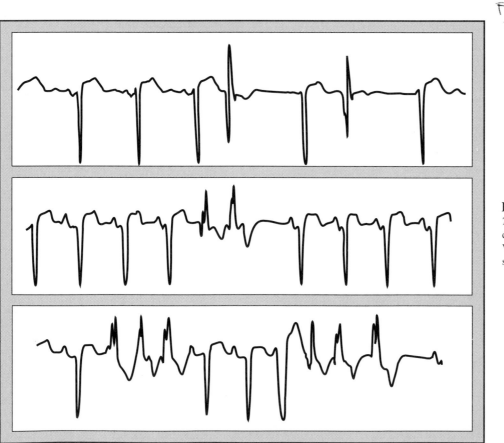

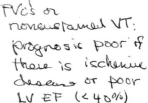

PVC's or nonsustained VT: prognosis poor if there is ischemic disease or poor LV EF (< 40%)

Figure 23–9
Top, Single premature ventricular complexes. *Middle* and *bottom,* Ventricular couplets and triplets, respectively.

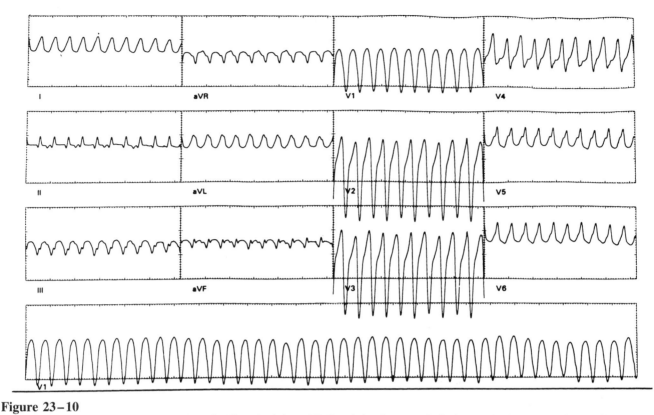

Figure 23–10

A 12-lead ECG shows wide complex tachycardia. There is obvious AV dissociation (best seen in lead II), which is most consistent with ventricular tachycardia.

sive test obtained in a fashion similar to that of an ordinary ECG, appears to help detect patients at risk for VT or sudden death. In this test, the electrical signals are processed to obtain simultaneous electrical activity from all three surface planes. The signals are processed to allow passage of high-frequency electrical events, and usually 200 complexes are averaged to exclude random noise. It has been found that late, low-amplitude, high-frequency signals correlate with the presence of intraventricular conduction delay and, hence, may represent the substrate for VT.

Recent studies have shown that postinfarction patients with high-density PVCs (or nonsustained VT), decreased ejection fraction, and a positive signal-averaged ECG have a 17-fold risk for developing either sustained VT or sudden cardiac death compared with patients without these risk factors.[24] Despite these impressive results, it should be emphasized that although a high-risk group (as defined) can be identified, the best treatment for these patients is still under debate.

The evaluation of patients with ventricular premature beats is critically dependent on the presence of organic cardiac disease. For patients with atrial or ventricular premature beats without cardiac disease, no further therapy is required. An echocardiogram, chest x-ray, and exercise stress test should be obtained if premature complexes occur with exercise. If the patient has just recovered from an acute myocardial infarction, an ejection fraction should be determined to assess prognosis. The role of the signal-averaged ECG and invasive electrophysiologic testing to

define prognosis and guide therapy is currently uncertain, but patients with ejection fractions below 40% and with episodes of sustained or nonsustained VT should be referred to a cardiologist with expertise in arrhythmias for consideration of electrophysiologic testing.

HIGH-RISK POST–MYOCARDIAL INFARCTION PATIENTS WITH HIGH-DENSITY PVCs. A number of studies have documented the salutary effect of beta blocker therapy for post–myocardial infarction patients (see Chap. 19). The benefits of such therapy appear to be greater for those with poor left ventricular function. There appears to be no role for the use of the class I antiarrhythmic agents for post–myocardial infarction patients. Large post–myocardial infarction trials of moricizine and sotalol showed no significant difference in mortality between treated and placebo groups.[26, 27] Several larger trials from Europe and Canada showed a decreased incidence of arrhythmia deaths in post–myocardial infarction patients treated with amiodarone, but no significant change in overall mortality.[28, 29] Hence, at this point in time, beta blockers should be used in all patients who can tolerate them, but no additional specific antiarrhythmic agent can be advocated. Some agents (class I) are clearly contraindicated.

Post–myocardial infarction patients with nonsustained VT who do not have inducible sustained VT during invasive electrophysiologic studies have a benign prognosis. In contrast, those with inducible sustained VT have a higher risk of developing sustained VT or sudden death.

A recent trial to assess the benefit of implantable defibrillators for patients with nonsustained VT and coronary artery disease showed a significant benefit of implantable cardioverter defibrillators (ICDs) in those patients with nonsustained VT who have inducible sustained VT that is refractory to intravenous procainamide.[30] A second study found that defibrillator therapy was significantly better than amiodarone or sotatol for patients with symptomatic VT or VF.[31]

ROLE OF THE PRIMARY CARE PHYSICIAN. PVCs are very frequent, and most patients with this problem do not require therapy, especially those who have no structural cardiac disease. Patients without structural heart disease are not at increased risk of subsequent cardiac events. Even exercise-induced nonsustained VT is not associated with an increased risk of cardiac events in subjects without apparent cardiac disease. Primary care physicians should identify patients with high-density PVCs and coronary artery disease or other underlying cardiac abnormalities who should be referred for specialty care, recognizing that treatment at this time may vary among specialists.

Sustained VT

Diagnosis

VT often occurs in the setting of high-density PVCs and should be distinguished from SVT with aberrant conduction (see Table 23–1). AV dissociation is the most definitive ECG finding in VT.

Patients presenting with sustained VT deserve careful evaluation, looking for specific causes (Table 23–9). Approximately 75% of patients with sustained VT have underlying coronary artery disease. For these patients, the extent of coronary disease, the presence of impaired left ventricular function, and evidence of myocardial ischemia are important prognostic factors. Sustained VT in patients with familial hypertrophic cardiomyopathy carries a high risk for sudden cardiac death among young individuals. Other causes of VT include acquired valvular heart disease, idiopathic cardiomyopathy, or congenital cardiac disease. It is now well appreciated that patients successfully operated on for correction of tetralogy of Fallot or ventricular septal defect are at risk for late development of VT. Another recently described but rare cause of either sustained VT or sudden cardiac death in young adults is known as *arrhythmogenic right ventricular dysplasia*.[32] The right ventricular muscle is replaced with fibrofatty tissue, a diagnosis that can be made by echocardiography. It may be confirmed by echocardiogram showing a dilated right ventricle or by cardiac magnetic resonance imaging.

VT WITHOUT STRUCTURAL CARDIAC DISEASE. In contrast to patients with structural heart disease and VT are those in whom VT occurs in the setting of no structural disease. These patients fall into two general categories, with VT emanating either from the right or left ventricular outflow tract or, less commonly, from a left septal focus. The right ventricular outflow tract VTs are often exercise induced and may respond to beta blocker therapy. Patients with idiopathic left septal VT are characterized by an unusual form of VT that usually

Table 23–9	Causes of Sustained VT or VF	
Structural Cardiac Disease	**Nonstructural Cardiac Disease**
Coronary Artery Disease	*Long QT Syndrome*
	Congenital/acquired
Cardiomyopathy	*Other*
Hypertrophic	Coronary artery spasm
Dilated	Catecholamine-induced VT
Restrictive	Right ventricular outflow VT
Valvular Heart Disease	Left septal VT
Congenital	
Corrected congenital lesions (VSD repair, tetralogy of Fallot)	
Anomalous origin of left coronary artery	
Right ventricular dysplasia	

Abbreviations: VT, ventricular tachycardia; VF, ventricular fibrillation; VSD, ventricular septal defect.

responds to intravenous verapamil therapy and may respond acutely to vagal maneuvers. Patients with either right ventricular outflow tract or idiopathic left septal VT may be excellent candidates for permanent cure of the tachycardia by catheter ablation.

Management

Patients who present with VT require careful evaluation directed at diagnosing the presence, type, and severity of any underlying cardiac disease. As such, most of these patients will require echocardiography. If coronary artery disease is known or suspected, coronary arteriography is often required to discern the extent and severity of coronary disease. VT is commonly seen in patients with large myocardial infarctions or in areas of myocardial aneurysm formation. Invasive electrophysiologic studies can guide decisions among drug, ablative, or ICD therapy.

For patients with VT without structural heart disease, attention is directed at obtaining a 12-lead ECG during VT to help localize the origin of this VT. In these patients, the VT is often induced by exercise, so a treadmill test may be required to make the diagnosis.

ACUTE MANAGEMENT. Initial therapy depends on an accurate diagnosis. For example, although intravenous verapamil may be highly effective for patients with SVT, this agent may be lethal for those with VT. Direct-current cardioversion should always be used in the face of hemodynamic instability. Initial drug therapy for patients with VT should include a bolus infusion of lidocaine followed by a lidocaine drip (see Table 23–3). If the patient fails to respond, intravenous therapy with procainamide is indicated. This drug is infused at a rate of 50 mg/min followed by an infusion of 2 to 4 mg/min. Infusion of bretylium (a class III agent) may be tried if the patient fails to respond to lidocaine and procainamide. Intravenous amiodarone, which has recently been approved for treatment of patients with hemodynamically unstable VT or ventricular fibrillation resistant to conventional therapy, may be preferable to bretylium, since the latter is seldom effective in patients with VT and is associated with hypotension. Intravenous amiodarone is infused into a central venous line in a dextrose solution. An initial loading dose of 5 mg/kg is administered over 30 to 45 minutes, followed by an infusion of 1 gm over 24 hours. After stabilization, the patient is switched to oral amiodarone in doses of 200 to 400 mg/day. Drugs such as intravenous bretylium or amiodarone must be used with great care and should be supervised by physicians well versed in their use.

ROLE OF THE PRIMARY CARE PHYSICIAN. The primary care physician should attempt to distinguish VT from SVT with aberration and should be responsible for emergency treatment of patients with sustained VT or fibrillation. After the patient is stabilized, workup is directed at establishing the cause of this arrhythmia. If there is not a reversible cause, multiple treatment options exist (Table 23–10).

DRUG THERAPY. Two modes have been suggested to assess the efficacy of drug therapy in patients with a history of sustained ventricular arrhythmia. One approach uses the reduction of ambient PVCs or nonsustained VT as assessed by 24-hour Holter recordings, whereas another makes use of serial electrophysiologic testing. The latter technique requires insertion of a temporary transvenous electrode catheter with attempted induction of VT before and after drug intervention. By either technique, patients whose arrhythmia is suppressed have a much better prognosis (in terms of arrhythmia recurrence) than those in whom drugs are ineffective. Two randomized studies[33, 34] compared the invasive with the noninvasive approaches with conflicting results, although the larger and more recent trial found Holter monitoring to be as predictive as electrophysiologic testing (Fig. 23–11). As noted earlier, empiric amiodarone therapy is superior to therapy with other antiarrhythmic drugs whether assessed by invasive or noninvasive approaches.

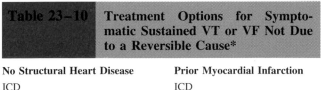

Table 23–10	**Treatment Options for Symptomatic Sustained VT or VF Not Due to a Reversible Cause***

No Structural Heart Disease	**Prior Myocardial Infarction**
ICD	ICD
Drugs	Class I or III drugs guided by EP
Beta blockers	testing or Holter monitor
Calcium channel blockers	Map-guided surgery
Class I or III agents	RF catheter ablation
RF catheter ablation	Nonpharmacologic

Idiopathic Cardiomyopathy

ICD
Drugs (especially amiodarone)
RF catheter ablation for bundle
   branch reentrant VT

Modified from Lesh, M.D.: Ventricular tachycardia: Mechanisms, diagnosis, and treatment. *In* Scheinman, M. (vol. ed.): Arrhythmias: Electrophysiologic Principles. Braunwald, E. (ser. ed.): Atlas of Heart Diseases. Vol. 9. Philadelphia, Current Medicine, 1996, pp. 6.1–6.6.

Abbreviations: VT, ventricular tachycardia; VF, ventricular fibrillation; RF, radiofrequency; EP, electrophysiologic: ICD, implantable cardioverter/defibrillator.

* Treatment options for patients with VT or VF. The therapy recommended depends on presentation and substrate.

DEVICE THERAPY. The use of the ICD has had dramatic impact on the therapy of patients with malignant ventricular arrhythmias. These devices, which now may be placed intravenously (Fig. 23–12), operate by detecting VT or ventricular fibrillation and initiating either antitachycardia pacing or a rescue shock where appropriate. ICDs are currently recommended for specific indications (Table 23–11), but these indications may broaden pending the results of ongoing randomized trials. Since this is a rapidly evolving field, such patients should be managed in consultation with a cardiologist experienced in arrhythmias. At present, ICD therapy is the preferred treatment option for patients with symptomatic sustained VT, VT poorly responsive to conventional medical therapy such as with amiodarone, or VF except when in the setting of an acute myocardial infarction. Such patients should be referred to a cardiologist experienced in treating arrhythmias.

CATHETER ABLATION. Only modest results have been reported in the use of ablative techniques for patients with ischemic heart disease, in part related to the greater complexity of VT compared with SVT and the frequent occurrence of multiple reentrant circuits.[22] Certain types of VT are, however, very effectively treated by catheter ablation. One such arrhythmia is bundle-to-bundle reentry. These patients usually present with syncope or a history of aborted sudden death. The basic mechanism is reentry involving both right and left bundle branches. Catheter ablation of the right bundle branch is curative. Catheter ablation is also effective for treatment of patients with either right ventricular outflow tract VT or left septal VT. In selected individuals with good left ventricular function who require cardiac surgery for other reasons (e.g., coronary bypass surgery, valve surgery, or correction of congenital abnormalities), other needed surgery can be combined with excision of a VT focus.

VENTRICULAR FIBRILLATION. Evaluation of patients with ventricular fibrillation is similar to that described for patients with VT. In the absence of obvious participating causes (e.g., drugs, electrolyte abnormalities, severe hypoxemia, or acidosis), these patients should be treated with an ICD. If the ventricular fibrillation occurred as the result of an acute (<48 hr) myocardial infarction, no chronic treatment may be needed. If the arrhythmia was precipitated by transient myocardial ischemia, coronary revascularization may be critical. An ICD is recommended in patients in which the cause of VF has not been diagnosed or who are at substantial risk of a recurrence. As with VT, these decisions should be made in conjunction with a cardiologist.

Polymorphous VT

Diagnosis

DIAGNOSTIC CONSIDERATIONS. Polymorphous VT is defined as a rapid ventricular arrhythmia with beat-to-beat changes in the QRS complex. A subset of polymorphous VT is an arrhythmia denoted by the term *torsades de pointes*. This arrhythmia consists of beat-to-beat changes in QRS complex polarity, so that the QRS com-

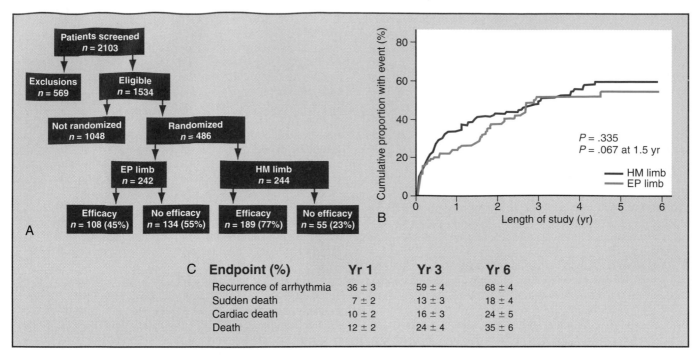

C	**Endpoint (%)**	**Yr 1**	**Yr 3**	**Yr 6**
Recurrence of arrhythmia	36 ± 3	59 ± 4	68 ± 4
Sudden death	7 ± 2	13 ± 3	18 ± 4
Cardiac death	10 ± 2	16 ± 3	24 ± 5
Death	12 ± 2	24 ± 4	35 ± 6

Figure 23–11

A, The Electrophysiologic Study Versus Electrocardiographic Monitoring (ESVEM) trial. The ESVEM trial attempted to determine whether electrophysiologic (EP) testing or Holter monitoring (HM) was best in predicting drug efficacy in patients with sustained ventricular tachycardia (VT) or those surviving cardiac arrest. Of 2103 patients screened, 486 were randomized to HM or EP testing to guide antiarrhythmic drug therapy. HM had a greater chance of predicting antiarrhythmic drug efficacy, defined as 100% suppression of runs of VT greater than 15 beats, 90% reduction of shorter runs, 80% of pairs, and 70% of ventricular ectopic beats and absence of exercise-induced VT ($P < .0001$). *B,* In 297 subjects for whom drug efficacy was predicted and who were censored on drug discontinuation, the rate of arrhythmia recurrence was the same, regardless of the method of guiding therapy. In both cases, the risk of recurrent VT was approximately 70% at 6 years. *C,* The actuarial rates for arrhythmia recurrence and sudden, cardiac, and total death are shown for those patients treated with a drug predicted to be effective by EP study or HM. Treatment with amiodarone or nonpharmacologic therapy (surgery, ablation, or implanted devices) was not an option in the ESVEM trial. (*A–C,* Redrawn from Lesh, M.D.: Ventricular tachycardia: Mechanisms, diagnosis, and treatment. *In* Scheinman, M. [vol. ed]: Arrhythmias: Electrophysiologic Principles. Braunwald, E. [ser. ed]: Atlas of Heart Diseases. Vol. 9. Philadelphia, Current Medicine, 1996, pp. 6.1–6.16.)

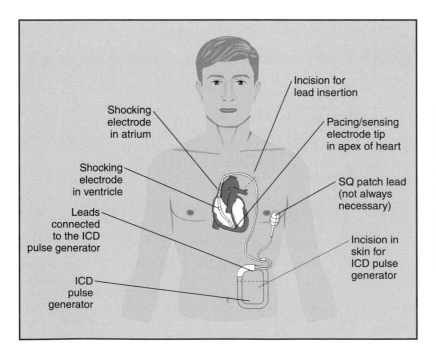

Figure 23–12

Nonthoracotomy lead system. Perhaps the single most significant advance in implantable defibrillator technology to date has been the development of transvenous lead systems that do not require thoracotomy for implantation. ICD, implantable cardioverter-defibrillator; SQ, subcutaneous. (Redrawn from Cockrell, J.L., and Siu, A.: Implantable defirilllators for the management of cardiac rhythm disorders. *In* Scheinman, M. [vol. ed]: Arrhythmias: Electrophysiologic Principles. Braunwald, E. [ser. ed]: Atlas of Heart Dieseases. Vol. 9. Philadelphia, Current Medicine, 1996, pp. 9.1–9.16; adapted from Cardiac Pacemakers, Inc., St. Paul, MN.)

Table 23–11	Devices for Ventricular Tachycardia: Indications for ICD

Failure of diagnosis
  Sudden death, noninducible, negative Holter monitor recording
Failure of therapy
  Clinical recurrence on a drug predicted effective by electrophysiologic testing
  Clinical recurrence on amiodarone
  Clinical recurrence after surgery or ablation
Predicted failure of therapy
  Still inducible on type I drug
  Amiodarone with multiple risk factors
  Inducible after surgery or ablation
  Symptomatic VT/VF as first-line therapy

Modified from Lesh, M.D.: Ventricular tachycardia: Mechanisms, diagnosis, and treatment. *In* Scheinman, M. (vol. ed.): Arrhythmias: Electrophysiologic Principles. Braunwald, E. (ser. ed.): Atlas of Heart Diseases. Vol. 9. Philadelphia, Current Medicine, 1996, pp. 6.1–6.16.
Abbreviation: ICD, implantable cardioverter/defibrillator.

plex appears to be rotating about the baseline. Another typical feature of torsades de pointes is its association with a long QT interval. It should be emphasized that patients with more than one form of monomorphic VT may show a pattern resembling polymorphous VT with change from one monomorphic configuration to another (pleomorphic VT).

The pathogenesis and treatment of polymorphous VT are very different from those for monomorphic VT. Polymorphous VT may be divided into hereditary versus acquired forms (Table 23–12).

HEREDITARY. Hereditary forms of polymorphic VT are known as the *idiopathic long QT syndrome*. This syndrome consists of patients at great risk for sudden cardiac death associated with prolonged QT intervals and may be inherited as an autosomal dominant trait without hearing loss (Romano-Ward syndrome) or an autosomal recessive trait with hearing loss (Jervell and Lange-Nielsen syndrome). The syndrome should be suspected in children or young adults presenting with seizures, syncope, or aborted sudden death. Untreated patients face a very high risk for sudden cardiac death owing to polymorphous VT that degenerates into ventricular fibrillation. A voluntary worldwide registry suggests that 75% of untreated patients will die suddenly. In contrast, those treated with beta blockers have a much improved prognosis but still face a 6% risk of sudden cardiac death. The pathogenesis of polymorphous VT appears to be related to abnormal prolongation of the membrane action potential, related to detectable genetic abnormalities that cause the long QT syndrome.

ACQUIRED. The most common cause of acquired polymorphous VT is drug related (Fig. 23–13). The chief offenders appear to be the class IA drugs (quinidine, procainamide, disopyramide) or sotalol, each of which prolongs the action potential duration. These agents are usually, but not always, associated with QT prolongation, and the polymorphous VT is almost always provoked by a preceding pause. Other drugs incriminated in the induction of polymorphous VT include the tricyclic antidepressants as well as phenothiazine derivatives. More recently,

polymorphous VT has been found associated with the use of terfenadine (Seldane) or astemizole (Hismanal). The parent compounds are associated with prolongation of the QT interval, but the metabolites are harmless. In patients with severe liver disease, or in those with normal liver function exposed to drugs that impair the metabolism of these agents, high levels of the parent compound may provoke polymorphous VT. Drugs that impair the metabolic breakdown of terfenadine include erythromycin and ketoconazole and the latter drugs should not be used in combination with terfenadine. Moreover, erythromycin has been shown independently to cause prolongation of the action potential owing to block of K$^+$ channels.

Other agents implicated in the genesis of polymorphous VT include ketanserin, probucol, organic phosphate insecticides, or high-protein liquid diets. Electrolyte abnormalities, particularly hypokalemia, hypocalcemia, and hypomagnesemia, may either cause or be associated with provoking drug-induced polymorphous VT.

Another important cause of polymorphous VT is found in patients with severe ischemia. The true incidence of this arrhythmia is not known, since many patients do not survive to reach the hospital. In these patients, episodes of polymorphous VT are usually preceded by symptoms or ECG signs of acute myocardial ischemia. Polymorphous VT is usually preceded by sinus tachycardia, and the QT interval is normal.

Management

A careful family and drug history, together with the baseline ECG as well as the ECG recorded during the arrhythmia, usually allows the clinician to separate acquired from congenital long QT syndrome. Patients with the congenital long QT syndrome usually have a family

Table 23–12	Causes of Polymorphous Ventricular Tachycardia

Congenital
  Jervell and Lange-Nielsen
  Romano-Ward (abnormalities on chromosomes 3, 4, and 7 have been described)
Acquired (drugs)
  Antiarrhythmic drugs
    Class IA (quinidine, procainamide, disopyramide)
    Class III (sotalol, amiodarone [rare])
  Psychotropic drugs
    Tricyclic antidepressants
    Phenothiazines
  Antibiotics
    Erythromycin, pentamidine, ampicillin
  Antihistamines
    Terfenadine, astemizole
  Miscellaneous drugs
    Probucol, ketanserin, cocaine, papaverine, organophosphates
Electrolyte disorders
  Hypokalemia, hypocalcemia, hypomagnesemia
Severe ischemia
  Post–myocardial infarction
  Coronary spasm
Normal hearts/no drugs
  Exercise-induced
  Short-coupled premature ventricular complexes

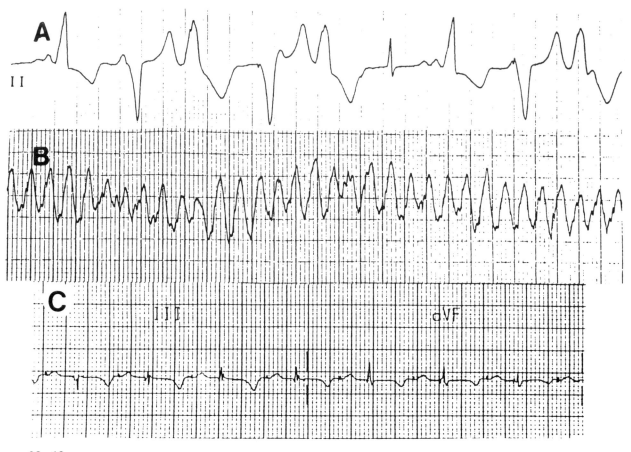

Figure 23–13

A, Strips show multiform ventricular complexes in a patient treated with quinidine. Note that the normally conducted beat (narrow QRS complex) is associated with marked prolongation of the QT interval. *B,* An episode of polymorphous VT that required emergency cardioversions. *C,* The efficacy of atrial overdrive pacing.

history of syncope or sudden cardiac death at a young age. Special evaluation may be required in patients who present with syncope and a borderline-prolonged QT interval. Since the arrhythmia (torsades de pointes) is often precipitated by startle, attempts to provoke the arrhythmia (while the patient is under ECG monitoring) by startle are appropriate, as is the use of the exercise stress test to assess whether the QT interval shortens appropriately with increases in heart rate. On rare occasions, patients with the long QT syndrome will actually show paradoxical lengthening of the QT interval with increases in heart rate.

The acquired long QT syndrome is usually due to drug or electrolyte abnormalities. The most important element in making the diagnosis is a careful drug history. The most common offenders are the class IA drugs and sotalol. Other drugs that have been implicated include psychotropic agents, antihistamines, and various antibiotics (see Table 23–12). Patients should also be evaluated for possible unstable acute ischemic heart disease.

TREATMENT OF THE IDIOPATHIC LONG QT SYNDROME. The efficacy of beta blocker therapy has been demonstrated, and these remain the drug of first choice for patient management. Failing this therapy, other available options include a left cervicosympathectomy, cardiac pacing with maximal doses of beta blockers, or

use of a defibrillator. The available data suggest that although symptoms are reduced, there is, nevertheless, a significant incidence of recurrent syncope (40%) or sudden cardiac death (8%) in patients undergoing cervicothoracic sympathectomy. The rationale for use of chronic cardiac pacing rests on the observations that in most patients with the long QT syndrome, polymorphous VT may be triggered by pauses. The recurrence rate of syncope or torsades de pointes in patients treated with combined therapy is less than 10%. There is a growing experience in the use of ICD therapy for these patients, especially with the availability of smaller generators and transvenous insertions. Even in patients undergoing ICD treatment, adjunctive therapy with beta blockers and cardiac pacing may be required to decrease the incidence of device discharges.

TREATMENT OF DRUG-INDUCED POLYMORPHOUS VT. The most important aspect of treatment depends on a proper diagnosis with prompt cessation of the offending drug. The diagnosis should be suspected if a patient treated with the previously mentioned drugs presents with syncope, seizures, or palpitations. Electrolyte abnormalities should be sought and corrected. If polymorphous VT recurs, then a bolus infusion of Mg^{2+} (1 to 2 gm over 10 minutes followed by continuous infusions) is indicated. The most effective acute therapy is insertion of a temporary transvenous cardiac pacemaker, by which method the cardiac rate is adjusted to mitigate the length of the pause that appears critical for the induction of polymorphous VT. As the arrhythmia is brought under control, the paced rate is gradually reduced and the pacemaker ultimately removed.

For patients with unstable ischemic heart disease, treatment with beta blockers, nitrates, or intravenous amiodarone may be effective, whereas traditional antiarrhythmic agents appear to be of limited value. Where feasible, prompt revascularization is the treatment of choice.

Polymorphous VT may also occur in patients with normal hearts who have not been exposed to drugs. These arrhythmias may be catecholamine (or exercise) related, may be due to coronary artery spasm, or may be of completely unknown origin. Some of these patients (especially those in the exercise-related group) may respond to beta blockers or calcium channel blockers. Since the mortality among these patients is high and drug therapy is not reliable, an ICD should be strongly considered.

The primary physician should try to distinguish between monomorphic and polymorphous VT because these arrhythmias have different mechanisms and modes of treatment. The clinician must also separate the acquired from the congenital forms of polymorphous VT. Patients with the congenital long QT syndrome are rare and are at very high risk for sudden cardiac death. Expert consultation is required for determining the role of drug/pacemaker or ICD therapy. In addition, expert advice is often needed to resolve issues relating to genetic testing of family members, treatment of asymptomatic affected family members, and proper family counseling.

The Patient Who Has Survived Sudden Cardiac Death

In patients who have survived an episode of cardiac sudden death, the precipitating arrhythmia may be a tachyarrhythmia or bradyarrhythmia. In patients with evidence for bradyarrhythmias, a permanent pacemaker implantation is commonly indicated (see Chap. 24). If a tachyarrhythmia is known to be the cause, specific evalu-

ation and treatment should be targeted for the known tachyarrhythmia.

In many patients, however, the specific arrhythmic cause of sudden cardiac death cannot be determined. In patients in whom the event occurred in conjunction with an obvious acute myocardial infarction, evaluation and subsequent treatment should proceed as guided by the presentation of the acute myocardial infarction, its complications, and it sequelae (see Chap. 19). In other patients, the sudden cardiac death may clearly be attributed to an acute episode of myocardial ischemia, even in the absence of acute myocardial infarction. In such patients, treatment of the underlying coronary artery disease, commonly with revascularization, is paramount (see Chap. 20). Occasionally, the evaluation may reveal critical aortic valvular stenosis, hypertrophic cardiomyopathy, massive pulmonary embolism, or other less-common causes of sudden cardiac collapse that have specific indicated treatments.

In many patients, however, the episode of cardiac arrest cannot be attributed to a potentially reversible coronary or noncoronary cause. In such patients, a comprehensive clinical history and examination should be accompanied by at least an ECG, echocardiogram, and stress test to define whether any underlying structural heart disease is present, even if it may not be directly remediable by surgical or medical means. Then, the evaluation and treatment should proceed with standard electrophysiologic testing to determine whether inducible ventricular arrhythmias are present and whether medications can successfully suppress any inducible arrhythmia (Fig. 23–14). Treatment is then an ICD combined with medications that can prevent the need for ICD discharge in the individual patient. The evaluation and treatment of these patients should be performed in conjunction with a cardiologist with experience in arrhythmias, who normally would also participate in the follow-up care of such patients.

References

1. Brugada, P., Brugada, J., Mont, L., et al.: A new approach to the differential diagnosis of a regular tachycardia with a wide QRS complex. Circulation 83:1649, 1991.

Figure 23–14

Diagnostic workup of patients with aborted sudden cardiac death. ECG, electrocardiogram; ECHO, echocardiogram; EP, electrophysiologic; SVT, supraventricular tachycardia; ICD, implantable cardioverter-defibrillator. (Adapted from Fitzpatrick, A.: Syncope and sudden cardiac death. *In* Scheinman, M. [vol. ed]: Arrhythmias: Electrophysiologic Principles. Braunwald, E. [ser. ed]: Atlas of Heart Diseases. Vol. 9. Philadelphia, Current Medicine, 1996, pp. 12.1–12.13.)

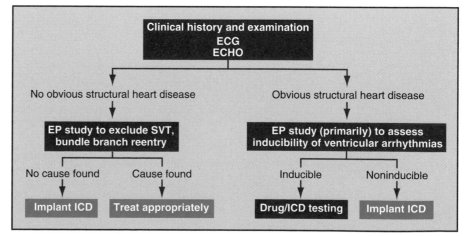

2. Golzari, H., Cebul, R.D., and Bahler, R.C.: Atrial fibrillation: Restoration and maintenance of sinus rhythm and indications for anticoagulation therapy. Ann. Intern. Med. 125:311–323, 1996.
3. The Boston Area Anticoagulation Trial for Atrial Fibrillation Investigators: The effect of low-dose warfarin on the risk of stroke in patients with non-rheumatic atrial fibrillation. N. Engl. J. Med. 323:1505–1511, 1990.
4. Stroke Prevention in Atrial Fibrillation Investigators: Predictors of thromboembolism in atrial fibrillation. I. Clinical features of patients at risk. Ann. Intern. Med. 116:1–5, 1992.
5. Stroke Prevention in Atrial Fibrillation Investigators: Predictors of thromboembolism in atrial fibrillation. II. Echocardiographic features of patients at risk. Ann. Intern. Med. 116:6–12, 1992.
6. Ezekowitz, M.D., Bridgers, S.L., James, K.E., et al.: Warfarin in the prevention of stroke associated with nonrheumatic atrial fibrillation. N. Engl. J. Med. 327:1406–1412, 1992.
7. Connolly, S.J., Laupacis, A., Gent, M., et al.: Canadian Atrial Fibrillation (CAFA) study. J. Am. Coll. Cardiol. 18:349–355, 1991.
8. Stroke Prevention in Atrial Fibrillation Investigators: Stroke Prevention in Atrial Fibrillation Study final results. Circulation 84:527–539, 1991.
9. Petersen, P., Boysen, G., Godtfredsen, J., et al.: Placebo-controlled, randomised trial of warfarin and aspirin for prevention of thromboembolic complications in chronic atrial fibrillation. The Copenhagen AFA-SAK Study. Lancet 1:175–179, 1989.
10. Stroke Prevention in Atrial Fibrillation Investigators: Warfarin versus aspirin for prevention of thromboembolism in atrial fibrillation. Stroke Prevention in Atrial Fibrillation II study. Lancet 343:687–691, 1994.
11. Stroke Prevention in Atrial Fibrillation Investigators: Adjusted-dose warfarin versus low-intensity, fixed-dose warfarin plus aspirin for high-risk patients with atrial fibrillation: Stroke Prevention in Atrial Fibrillation III randomised trial. Lancet 348:633–638, 1996.
12. The Atrial Fibrillation Investigators. The efficacy of aspirin in patients with atrial fibrillation. Analyses of pooled data from 3 randomized trials. Arch. Intern. Med. 157:1237–1240, 1997.
13. Manning, W.J., Silverman, D.I., Gordon, S.P.F., et al.: Cardioversion from atrial fibrillation without prolonged anticoagulation with use of transesophageal echocardiography to exclude the presence of atrial thrombi. N. Engl. J. Med. 328:750–756, 1993.
14. Klein, A.L., Grimm, R.A., Black, I.W., et al.: Cardioversion guided by transesophageal echocardiography: The ACUTE Pilot Study. A randomized, controlled trial. Ann. Intern. Med. 126:200–209, 1997.
15. Manning, W.J., Silverman, D.I., Keighley, C.S., et al.: T.E.E. facilitated early cardioversion of atrial fibrillation using short term anticoagulation. J. Am. Coll. Cardiol. 25:1354–1361, 1995.
16. Weigner, M.J., Caulfield, T.A., Danias, P.G., et al.: Risk for clinical thromboembolism associated with cardioversion to sinus rhythm in patients with atrial fibrillation lasting less than 48 hours. Ann. Intern. Med. 126:615–620, 1997.
17. Ganz, L.I., and Friedman, P.L.: Supraventricular tachycardia. N. Engl. J. Med. 332:162–173, 1995.
18. Madson, C.D., Pointer, J.E., and Lynch, T.G.: A comparison of adenosine and verapamil in the pre-hospital setting. Ann. Emerg. Med. 25:649–655, 1995.
19. Lesh, M.D., Van Hare, G.F., Epstein, L.M., et al.: Radiofrequency catheter ablation of atrial arrhythmias. Results and mechanisms. Circulation 89:1074–1089, 1994.
20. Deshpande, S., Jazayeri, M., Dhala, A., et al.: Catheter ablation in supraventricular tachycardia. Annu. Rev. Med. 46:413–430, 1995.
21. McIntosh-Yellin, N.L., Drew, B.J., and Scheinman, M.M.: Safety and efficacy of central intravenous bolus administration of adenosine for termination of supraventricular tachycardia. J. Am. Coll. Cardiol. 22:741–745, 1993.
22. Scheinman, M.M.: NASPE survey on catheter ablation. Pacing Clin. Electrophysiol. 18:1474–1478, 1995.
23. Kennedy, H.L., Whitlock, J.A., Sprague, M.K., et al.: Long-term follow-up of asymptomatic healthy subjects with frequent and complex ventricular ectopy. N. Engl. J. Med. 312:193–197, 1985.
24. El-Sherif, N., Denes, P., Katz, R., et al.: Definition of the best prediction criteria of the time domain signal-averaged electrocardiogram for serious arrhythmic events in the postinfarction period. The Cardiac Arrhythmia Suppression Trial/Signal-Averaged Electrocardiogram (CAST/SAECG) Substudy Investigators. J. Am. Coll. Cardiol. 25:908–914, 1995.
25. Roden, D.M.: Risks and benefits of antiarrhythmic therapy. N. Engl. J. Med. 331:785–791, 1994.
26. The Cardiac Arrhythmia Suppression Trial II Investigators: Effect of the antiarrhythmic agent moricizine on survival after myocardial infarction. N. Engl. J. Med. 327:227–233, 1992.
27. Waldo, A.L., Camm, A.J., de Ruyter, H., et al: Effect of D-sotalol on mortality in patients with left ventricular dysfunction after recent and remote myocardial infarction. Lancet 348:7–12, 1996.
28. Julian, D.G., Camm, A.J., Frangin, G., et al.: Randomised trial of effect of amiodarone on mortality in patients with left ventricular dysfunction after recent myocardial infarction: EMIAT. Lancet 349:667–674, 1997.
29. Cairns, J.A., Connolly, S.J., Roberts, R., and Gent, M., for the Canadian Amiodarone Myocardial Infarction Arrhythmia Trial Investigators: Randomised trial of outcome after myocardial infarction in patients with frequent or repetitive ventricular premature depolarisations: CAMIAT. Lancet 349:675–682, 1997.
30. Moss, A.J., Hall, W.J., Cannom, D.S., et. al.: Improved survival with an implanted defibrillator in patients with coronary disease at high risk for ventricular arrhythmia. N. Engl. J. Med. 335:1933–1940, 1996.
31. The Antiarrhythmics vs. Implantable Defibrillators (AVID) Investigators: A comparison of antiarrhythmic drug therapy with implantable defibrillators in patients resuscitated after near-fatal ventricular arrhythmias. N. Engl. J. Med. 337:1576–1583, 1997.
32. Marcus, F.I., Fontaine, G.: Arrhythmic right ventricular dysplasia cardiomyopathy. A review. Pacing Clin. Electrophysiol. 18:1298–1314, 1995.
33. Mitchell, L.B., Duff, H.J., Manyari, D.E., and Wyse, D.G.: A randomized clinical trial of the noninvasive and invasive approaches to drug therapy of ventricular tachycardia. N. Engl. J. Med. 317:1681–1687, 1987.
34. Mason, J.W.: A comparison of electrophysiologic testing with Holter monitoring to predict antiarrhythmic drug efficacy for ventricular tachyarrhythmias. N. Engl. J. Med. 329:445–451, 1993.

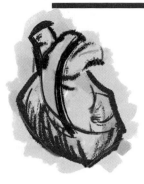

Chapter 24

Recognition and Management of Patients with

Bradyarrhythmias

NORA GOLDSCHLAGER

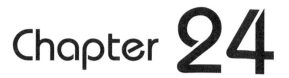
OFFICE EVALUATION OF THE PATIENT WITH BRADYCARDIA

Bradycardia may be an incidental finding or it may be present in severely symptomatic individuals, whether or not structural heart disease coexists. In many patients, the bradycardia can impact negatively on prognosis.[1-3] In all persons with bradycardia, a focused history and physical examination are necessary to define the significance of the bradycardia in order to advise the patient regarding the importance of further investigation into its nature, appropriate management, and follow-up.

When bradycardia is detected by physical examination or when symptoms consistent with cerebral hypoperfusion are reported, an electrocardiogram (ECG) is critical for diagnosis. In some patients, bradycardia or cardiac conduction system abnormalities may be detected first by the ECG in the absence of suspicious symptoms. The recommended evaluation and treatment depend on the ECG findings as well as a careful history and physical examination (Fig. 24–1).

12-Lead ECG

The ECG can provide identification of not only the rhythm but also the existence of associated conditions that need to be recognized. These latter include disorders of the atrioventricular (AV) and intraventricular conduction system (such as first-degree [1°] AV block and bundle branch block) and evidence of atrial abnormalities (suggesting atrial hypertrophy or intra-atrial conduction delay) and ventricular hypertrophy. Conduction system disease is often diffuse, with up to one-third of patients

with sinus node dysfunction having AV and intraventricular conduction disease and a similar percentage of patients with AV block having sinus node dysfunction.[4, 5] Patients with ventricular hypertrophy may be especially reliant on atrial contraction to fill a poorly compliant ventricle and may suffer from reduced stroke volume and concomitant symptoms in the absence of this atrial "kick."

Sinus rhythm normally occurs at a rate of 60 to 100 beats per minute with the patient at rest. Sinus bradycardia is considered to be present when the resting sinus rate is less than 60 beats per minute. Neither sinus tachycardia nor sinus bradycardia per se indicates sinus node dysfunction or organic heart disease. Some patients with bradycardia from sinus nodal and sinoatrial dysfunction also develop supraventricular tachyarrhythmias, including atrial fibrillation and flutter and reentrant tachycardias (but not multifocal atrial tachycardia). In this condition, known as the *bradycardia-tachycardia syndrome,* patients complain of symptoms referable to both bradycardia and tachycardia; the latter are often perceived as uncomfortable palpitations and the former as dizziness and presyncope.

Symptoms and Their Underlying Pathophysiology

The clinical presentation of patients with bradycardia, due either to intrinsic abnormalities of impulse formation or to intrinsic conduction system disease, is determined by the presence of three conditions: the slow heart rate itself, inability to increase the heart rate in response to an increase in metabolic need, and inappropriately timed atrial and ventricular depolarization and contraction sequences (Table 24–1). The symptoms of bradycardia thus reflect varying degrees of cerebral hypoperfusion, low

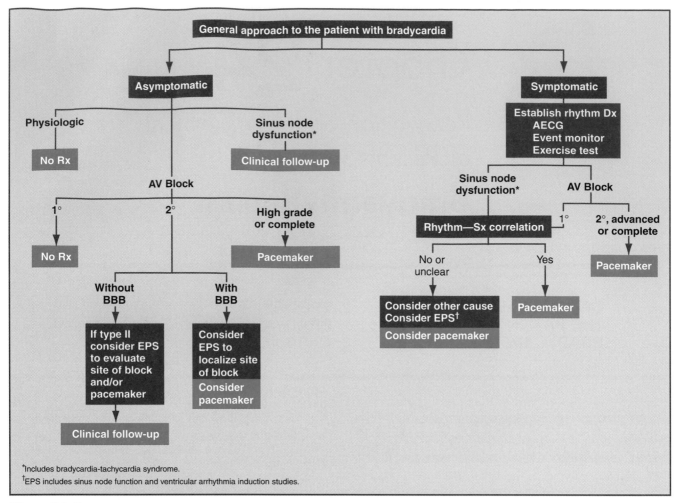

Figure 24–1

General approach to the patient with bradycardia. Rx, treatment; Dx, diagnosis; AECG, ambulatory electrocardiography; AV, atrioventricular; Sx, symptoms; 1°, first-degree; 2°, second-degree; BBB, bundle branch block; EPS, electrophysiologic study.

Table 24–1	Clinical Presentation of Patients with Bradycardia

Symptoms Due to Cerebral Hypoperfusion
Syncope and presyncope
Confusion
Memory loss
Bradycardia-dependent tachyarrhythmias (atrial fibrillation, polymorphic ventricular tachycardia)
Symptoms Due to Chronotropic Incompetence
Effort fatigue, weakness, breathlessness, hypotension
Symptoms Due to AV Dyssynchrony Resulting from Varying AV Intervals or VA Conduction
Pulmonary congestion and pulmonary edema
Hypotension
   Due to loss of atrial "kick"
   Due to atrial stretch (caused by inappropriate AV relationships)–mediated atrial baroreceptor stimulation with reflex hypotension

Abbreviations: AV, atrioventricular; VA, ventriculoatrial.

cardiac output at rest or during exercise, and an impaired hemodynamic state. Symptoms can be episodic or chronic and can change over time and with advancing age. Because patients often adapt their lifestyles to compensate for the impairment in heart rate, they may not volunteer significant symptoms unless they are closely questioned about ability and time required to perform specific activities or are actually observed during performance of these activities.

Syncope is the classic symptom of cerebral hypoperfusion resulting from severe bradycardia; however, symptoms of presyncope such as dizziness, lightheadedness, weakness, and confusion reflect the same pathophysiology and warrant the same aggressive approach to diagnosis and management. It should be emphasized that patients with cerebral hypoperfusion may have memory impairment surrounding the symptomatic episodes and may therefore be unable to provide an adequate or accurate history of the events.

Patients with sinus node dysfunction or AV block, in whom the escape focus is unresponsive to autonomic nervous system input (such as fascicular or ventricular escape foci), cannot increase their heart rates in response to increases in the oxygen demand imposed by physical stress. As a result, they are intolerant of effort and will report symptoms of exercise-related breathlessness, weakness, and fatigue. The sometimes vague and episodic nature of the symptoms may confuse the clinician unless a high index of suspicion for this rhythm disorder is maintained. The symptoms, which can be disabling, are often confused with other conditions such as underlying heart disease, medication, hypothyroidism, or simply advanced age. The impaired heart rate response to increases in metabolic need has been termed *chronotropic incompetence.*

During periods of AV block, the atria and ventricles depolarize and contract asynchronously. Right and left atrial pressure and volume increase to variable extents, depending on the degree to which the AV valves are open or closed at the onset of ventricular systole. The resulting atrial stretch and stimulation of atrial natriuretic peptide secretion produce reflex systemic hypotension and consequent cerebral hypoperfusion. In addition, the increases in left atrial and pulmonary venous pressures can cause or contribute to shortness of breath and pulmonary venous congestion, including frank pulmonary edema, sometimes leading to the mistaken diagnosis of refractory left ventricular failure.

More rarely, bradycardias can lead to a potentially lethal form of ventricular tachycardia known as *pause-dependent* or *bradycardia-dependent ventricular tachycardia.* Pause- or bradycardia-dependent ventricular tachycardia is usually polymorphous and can be associated with a bradycardia-related long QT interval; nonconducted extrasystoles, postextrasystolic pauses, or merely a slowing of heart rate can cause the bradycardia. Symptoms in these patients can include not only palpitations, syncope, and presyncope but also cardiac arrest.

Physical Examination

The physical findings in the patient with bradycardia reflect the origin of the QRS rhythm (sinus, atrial escape, junctional, fascicular, or ventricular) and the AV relationships (associated-synchronous or dissociated-dyssynchronous)—often to a greater degree than does the rate itself. Junctional or ventricular escape rhythms arising as a result of atrial bradycardia or AV block cause AV dyssynchrony, which leads to varying amounts of atrial contribution to ventricular filling and therefore varying stroke output. Thus, the systolic blood pressure may vary accordingly.

In patients with AV dissociation or 1:1 retrograde ventriculoatrial conduction, examination of the venous pulse contour in the neck reveals cannon A-waves from atrial contraction against closed mitral and tricuspid valves. Cannon A-waves should not be confused with an elevated central venous pressure, a fairly common physical finding that is independent of the venous pulse contour. Occasionally, especially if the A-wave is prominent, the diagnosis of AV block can be made from inspection of the neck vein pulse contours.

The carotid pulse may be variable in volume and upstroke velocity when AV dyssynchrony is present. Examination of the chest may disclose rales, which reflect increased pulmonary venous pressure. Since AV dyssynchrony causes changes in the positions of the mitral and tricuspid valves relative to their fully closed or open positions, the intensity of the first heart sound will vary, as will the audibility of atrial (fourth heart) gallop sounds and the presence and intensity of AV valve regurgitant murmurs. Since AV dyssynchrony results in varying stroke outputs, semilunar valve ejection murmurs can also vary in intensity.

The liver may be enlarged and may pulsate because of transmitted A- and CV-waves. Peripheral edema may also be present but is unusual.

These same physical findings can also be present in patients who have single-chamber ventricular pacemakers and an independent atrial rhythm, since AV dissociation will exist if the ventricular rhythm is paced. In these patients, the symptoms of weakness, fatigue, and congestive heart failure, together with physical findings indicating AV dyssynchrony, constitute the *pacemaker syndrome,*[6] which is treated by changing the implanted single-chamber ventricular pacing system to a dual-chambered system, in which sensing of the atrial rhythm triggers a paced ventricular response to restore AV synchrony (see later).

Further Diagnostic Testing to Detect Bradyarrythmias

AMBULATORY ECG MONITORING. Since the 12-lead ECG usually is not sufficient to make a definitive diagnosis, ambulatory ECG (Holter) monitoring is commonly the next test to document rhythm abnormalities in patients with symptoms suggesting bradycardia. These devices employ an "alarm" button that is activated by the patient on perception of symptoms; newer monitors can be programmed to retain in memory the cardiac rhythm for only a specific number of seconds before and after the alarm is activated by the patient. Wristwatch monitors are less cumbersome than Holter monitors and are preferred by many patients.

Because the patient must be able to trigger the alarm for precise correlation between the heart rhythm and symptoms, ambulatory ECG devices are best utilized in patients who have daily symptoms but who do not have frank syncope or severe presyncopal symptoms. Precise rhythm-symptom correlation is, however, difficult to obtain, in part because patients may focus on staying conscious and avoiding personal injury rather than on depressing an event marker. In patients who have recurrent symptoms of cerebral hypoperfusion but do not develop symptoms during ambulatory monitoring, further diagnostic evaluation, such as event monitoring and exercise testing, are indicated (see Fig. 24–1), especially if suggestive bradyarrhythmias were noted on continuous ambulatory monitoring.

EVENT MONITORING. In contrast to the ambulatory ECG recording device, which must be worn continuously by the patient, the event recorder is carried by the patient for weeks to months and placed on the skin and turned on only when symptoms are occurring. The device contains electrodes on its surface to record the rhythm from the skin onto a small tape.

The taped rhythm can be transmitted over telephone lines to a monitoring center for immediate interpretation or can be sent in its entirety to the center for writeout and interpretation. The event monitor is extremely useful in patients with inconstant and episodic symptoms but without frank syncope or severe presyncope, since participation by the patient in the recording of the rhythm is required.

In both ambulatory ECG monitoring and event recording, documentation of a normal rhythm and rate during symptoms can exclude an arrhythmia as the cause of the symptoms. Alternatively, the correlation of symptoms with a rhythm disturbance is diagnostic. In the absence of symptoms, the physician must decide whether to proceed to additional testing.

TREADMILL EXERCISE TESTING. Formal exercise testing is necessary to evaluate heart rate response to effort in patients suspected of having chronotropic incompetence. The importance of recognizing the condition of chronotropic incompetence has increased in recent years, in part due to the development of rate-adaptive cardiac pacemakers that, through sensor technology, can increase and decrease the pacing rate in response to activities of daily living (see later). Special exercise protocols are often used by arrhythmia specialists to determine whether the heart rate is appropriate for various activities as well as for maximal exercise capacity.

The Role of the Primary Care Physician

Depending on the particular community in which a physician practices, some or all of the aforementioned noninvasive tests for bradycardia may be available; if not, referral to a specialist is warranted for expeditious workup of the patient. The role of the primary care physician is crucial, however, in suspecting the diagnosis of bradycardia in symptomatic patients and in planning the diagnostic approach. Similarly, the primary care physician must be relied on to recognize those bradycardic rhythms that are benign and without prognostic impact, thus obviating the need for expensive and unnecessary workup.

Since most patients with symptomatic bradycardia and some with asymptomatic bradycardia require cardiac pacing, referral to a pacemaker specialist is often necessary for definitive therapy. This is true whether or not the bradycardia is due to the use of medications that must be continued to treat other medical illnesses.

SPECIFIC BRADYARRHYTHMIAS

Sinus Arrhythmia

Respiratory sinus arrhythmia, in which the sinus rate increases with inspiration and decreases with expiration by more than 0.16 second, is a normal physiologic rhythm and is most commonly found in young healthy subjects. Nonrespiratory sinus arrhythmia, in which phasic changes in sinus rate are not due to respiration, may be accentuated by the use of vagal agents such as digitalis and morphine; its mechanism is unknown. Patients with nonrespiratory sinus arrhythmia are usually older and have underlying cardiac disease; however, this arrhythmia is not a marker for structural heart disease, and its presence should not prompt a cardiac workup.

Sinus Node Dysfunction

Sinus node dysfunction is usually a degenerative process involving the sinus node and sinoatrial area (Table 24–2). Rarely, the syndrome is familial. The degenerative process and associated fibrosis often involve the AV node and intraventricular conduction system as well as the sinus node area; as many as 25% to 30% of patients with sinus node dysfunction have evidence of AV block and bundle branch block.

Sinus node dysfunction is present when profound sinus bradycardia, pauses in sinus rhythm (sinus arrest), sinoatrial block, or a combination of these exists (Fig. 24–2). Transient sinus node dysfunction can be medication-related and reversible when the offending agent is withdrawn.

Sinus Pause

Some normal individuals without structural heart disease experience marked sinus bradycardia and pauses in sinus rhythm under conditions of high vagal tone (Fig. 24–3). In some subjects, a trigger such as vomiting can be identified. Vagal stimulation is also responsible for significant sinus (and ventricular) bradyarrhythmias in patients in the intensive care setting (Tables 24–3 and 24–4; Fig. 24–4).

Sinoatrial Block

In some patients, the sinus node itself may not be dysfunctional but the impulse generated within it may be blocked before it can activate the atrium. Sinoatrial block may take the form of progressive delay in transmission of the sinus-generated impulse through the sinoatrial node to the atrium, finally resulting in a nonconducted sinus impulse and absence of a P-wave (Wenckebach, or type I second-degree [2°] exit block) or abrupt failure of transmission of the sinus impulse to the atrium (type II 2° exit

Table 24–2	Causes of Sinus Bradycardia*

Idiopathic
    Degenerative processes (e.g., Lev's disease, Lenegre's disease)
Medications
    Beta blockers
    Some calcium channel blockers (diltiazem, verapamil)
    Digoxin (when vagal tone is high)
    Class I antiarrhythmic agents (e.g., procainamide)
    Class III antiarrhythmic agents (amiodarone, sotalol)
    Clonidine
    Lithium carbonate
Acute myocardial ischemia and infarction
    Right or left circumflex coronary artery occlusion or spasm
High vagal tone

* Includes sinus arrest and sinoatrial block.

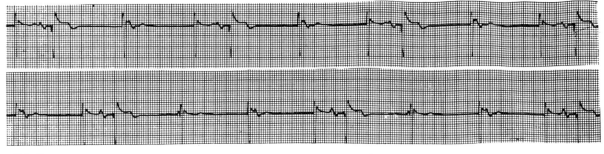

Figure 24–2

This rhythm strip was recorded in a 48-year-old healthy, active man who complained of breathlessness during moderately strenuous exercise. There was no evidence of structural heart disease on physical examination and an echocardiogram was normal. The atrial rhythm is marked sinus bradycardia at a rate of about 43 beats per minute. The narrow QRS rhythm is mostly regular at a rate of 50 beats per minute, suggesting a junctional origin. Occasionally, P-waves are associated with earlier than expected QRS complexes; these represent capture beats. The rhythm is thus sinus bradycardia, atrioventricular (AV) dissociation with intermittent capture, and junctional escape rhythm. The long PR interval of captured beats may not indicate AV nodal disease, since it may represent concealed retrograde conduction of the junctional impulse retrogradely into the AV node, delaying transmission of the subsequent sinus depolarization. Although the sinus bradycardia was atropine-sensitive, the patient declined chronic anticholinergic therapy and opted for a dual-chamber rate-adaptive pacemaker, which allowed both appropriate rate response to physical activity and restoration of AV synchrony. The patient has remained asymptomatic.

block). In type I 2° exit block, the increment in delay in impulse transmission through the sinoatrial nodal tissue is progressively less (analogous to type I 2° AV nodal block); thus, the PP intervals become progressively shorter until a P-wave fails to occur. In type II 2° sino-atrial exit block, abrupt failure of sinus impulse conduction to the atria can take the form of 2:1, 3:1, or higher degrees of block. Fixed high-grade sinoatrial block can mimic sinus bradycardia on the ECG.

Bradycardia-Tachycardia Syndrome

Bradycardia-tachycardia syndrome is characterized by episodes of both bradycardia and supraventricular tachycardia (Fig. 24–5). The bradycardia is due to sinus node dysfunction with associated junctional or ventricular escape rhythms. The supraventricular tachycardias may be atrial tachycardia, atrial flutter, atrial fibrillation, or even AV nodal reentry tachycardia; more than one type may occur in the same patient. Bradycardia-tachycardia syndrome is caused by diffuse disease of the cardiac conduction system but is not necessarily associated with structural heart disease. Owing to the paroxysmal atrial fibrillation, the incidence of systemic embolism is relatively high and these patients usually require anticoagulation as well as a permanent pacemaker unless antiarrhythmic agents can suppress the tachyarrhythmias without precipitating important bradycardia.

Approach to Office Management of Sinus Bradycardias

Outpatient evaluation of sinus bradycardia must include a review of the medications the patient is receiving (see Table 24–2). Withdrawal of offending agents, if possible, can cure the problem; if the medications are necessary to treat specific conditions, cardiac pacing will be required to provide rate support. If the bradycardia is due to acute myocardial ischemia or infarction, the patient is likely to be able to provide the history compatible with this underlying diagnosis; moreover, the acute infarction process will be clear from the 12-lead ECG. However, since up to 25% of myocardial infarctions are clinically "silent" or present with atypical symptoms, attention to this diagnosis as documented by the ECG is mandatory.

Since the sinus arrhythmias are benign, documentation of their existence is all that is required. Vagally mediated atrial bradyarrhythmias are also generally benign; however, the occasional patient can have highly symptomatic vagally mediated bradycardic episodes, especially if there is also a significant vasodepressor response resulting in cerebral hypoperfusion (the *neurocardiogenic syndromes*).

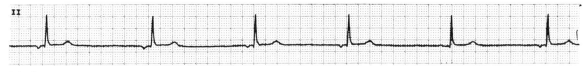

Figure 24–3

Lead II rhythm strip recorded in a 32-year-old well-conditioned, healthy man during a routine physical examination. The inverted P-waves in this lead indicate a junctional or low atrial focus of origin (the next to last P-wave is possibly of sinus origin). This rhythm is not in and of itself abnormal, since it may be an escape rhythm due to the sinus bradycardia so commonly seen in conditioned individuals. Neither workup nor treatment of the rhythm is required in cases like this. Exercise testing, with its associated vagolysis and enhancement of sympathetic tone, would be expected to demonstrate an increase in sinus rate.

Table 24–3	Conditions and Situations Associated with Vagally Mediated Bradyarrhythmias

Sleep
Urination
Defecation
Swallowing
Valsalva maneuver
Vomiting, retching
Intubation
Suctioning
Elevated intracranial pressure
Extreme hypertension
Isotonic exercise conditioning
Left ventricular mechanoreceptor stimulation (e.g., neurally mediated syncope)

Table 24–4	Features of Vagally Mediated Bradyarrhythmias

Transient, often situational
Slowing of sinus rate
Irregular sinus rhythm
AV block with changing PR intervals and irregular sinus rates
Atypical type I or II 2° block sequences, often with inconstant PP intervals
Inconstant rates of escape foci
Can be abolished by intravenous atropine or increase in sympathetic tone

Abbreviations: AV, atrioventricular; 2°, second-degree.

These individuals may require referral to a specialist for head-up tilt-table testing to confirm the diagnosis and to guide therapy (see Chap. 12). Vagally mediated sinus bradycardias respond to intravenous atropine or isoproterenol, although the latter is not routinely used owing to its effects of increasing myocardial oxygen consumption and causing ventricular ectopy. The expected normal heart rate response to 2 to 3 mg of intravenous atropine is an increase of about 15% to rates of 85 to 90 beats per minute. Walking briskly around the office or running in place produces immediate vagolysis and will also serve to increase the sinus rate in vagally mediated sinus bradycardias. Oral theophylline has also been used with some success. These maneuvers, together with the usual good health of the patients, can aid in the clinical judgment of the benignity of these rhythms.

Patients with sinus node dysfunction may or may not respond to intravenous atropine or exercise by consistently and immediately increasing their heart rates;[7] since many if not most of these patients have some underlying heart disease (most commonly, hypertension and coronary artery disease), intravenous isoproterenol is not recommended. Ambulatory ECG monitoring is the preferred approach to documenting the presence of sinus node dysfunction.

Electrophysiologic studies have both a variable sensitivity and a low specificity for detecting and excluding suspected sinus node dysfunction as the cause of a patient's symptoms and are recommended only if the symptoms suggest bradycardia but documentation cannot be achieved in a reasonable period of time using other available diagnostic techniques. Referral to a specialist will of course be required for pacemaker insertion (see later). Patients with the bradycardia-tachycardia syndrome are also usually referred to a specialist, both for pacemaker implantation and for optimal choice of therapy for tachyarrhythmias.

AV Nodal–His Block

Pathophysiology and Natural History

Like sinus node dysfunction, AV nodal–His block (and bundle branch block) in adult patients often results from sclerodegenerative processes. Acquired AV nodal block is frequently due to acute ischemia and infarction, infection, trauma, and medications (Table 24–5).

The three areas of the AV node or junction—atrionodal, central compact, and nodal-His portions—merge, without clear separation, with the His bundle. Cells in the atrionodal area have a relatively fast intrinsic depolarization rate (45 to 60 beats/min) and are responsive to auto-

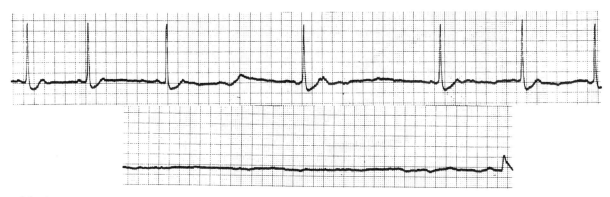

Figure 24–4
Vagal bradycardia and asystole in an intubated hospitalized patient during suctioning. Although long pauses in rhythm like this are not uncommon in the hospital setting (where they require no treatment), they can occur in healthy individuals with neurocardiogenic syncopal syndromes and can be reproduced during head-up tilt-table testing.

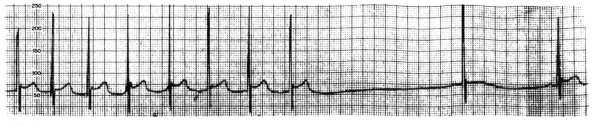

Figure 24–5
This rhythm strip illustrates the bradycardia-tachycardia syndrome. A junctional tachycardia at a rate of 81 beats per minute present in the beginning of the strip abruptly extinguishes, resulting in a pause of 3.8 seconds. The pause is terminated by sinus rhythm at 36 beats per minute. Patients with this syndrome commonly experience palpitations during the tachycardias and presyncopal symptoms during the bradycardias. Treatment is permanent cardiac pacing and antiarrhythmic drugs.

nomic nervous system input. Cells in the nodal-His region have a slower intrinsic depolarization rate (about 40 beats/min) and, because of sparse autonomic innervation, are generally unresponsive to these neural influences. The site of origin of a junctional rhythm will therefore determine its rate and responsiveness to vagal and adrenergic tone and, consequently, the presence and severity of clinical symptoms. The QRS complex duration is an unreliable guide to origin of a QRS rhythm, since rhythms originating in the longitudinally separated predivisional region of the His bundle can have a wide QRS complex.

AV block can be congenital or acquired. Patients with congenital AV block usually have escape pacemakers arising from within the AV node or His bundle. In contrast, only about 25% of patients with acquired AV block have escape pacemakers arising within the AV node; escape rhythms originate within the His bundle in about 15% to 20% and distal to the His bundle in about 70% (Fig. 24–6).[4]

The natural history of patients with AV block depends on the underlying cardiac condition; however, the site of the block and the resulting rhythm disturbances themselves undoubtedly contribute to prognosis. 1° AV block has little prognostic import.[8] Both chronic (i.e., established) 2° (types I and II) and third-degree (3°) AV block

Table 24–5	Causes of Acquired AV Nodal–His Block

Idiopathic fibrosis (Lenegre's disease)
Sclerodegenerative processes (e.g., Lev's disease with calcification of the mitral and aortic annuli)
AV node or His bundle radiofrequency ablation procedures
Medications (e.g., digitalis, beta blockers, calcium channel blockers, class III antiarrhythmic agents)
Acute inferior wall myocardial infarction
Inflammatory diseases (myocarditis)
Infections (e.g., endocarditis involving the aortic valve or valve ring, Chagas' disease, Lyme disease)
Infiltrative processes (e.g., hemochromatosis, sarcoidosis, amyloidosis, neoplasm)
Trauma (including cardiac surgical procedures)
Collagen-vascular diseases
Aortic root diseases (e.g., spondylitis)
Electrolyte abnormalities (e.g., extreme hyperkalemia)

Abbreviation: AV, atrioventricular.

can be associated with adverse outcomes, including death, unless the arrhythmias are vagally mediated or are due to other reversible causes.[8–11]

Diagnosis

His bundle electrography has provided important information regarding normal and abnormal AV conduction in humans and indicating the site of AV conduction delay. The technique involves positioning of a multipolar electrode catheter across the tricuspid valve in proximity to the AV nodal–His bundle to record electrical activity as it passes through the level of the low right atrium (A), His bundle (H), and proximal right bundle branch; ventricular electrical activity (V) is also recorded. Normally, the conduction time through the AV node is 90 to 150 msec and the conduction time through the His-Purkinje system is 22 to 55 msec. In patients with prolonged PR interval, a long AH interval signifies conduction delay within the AV node, and a long HV time represents conduction delay within the His bundle or in the bundle branches.

1° AV BLOCK (Fig. 24–7). 1° AV block is defined as a PR interval greater than 0.20 second. In 1° AV block (delay in conduction between the atria and the ventricles), all atrial impulses are conducted to the ventricles. The components of the PR interval are interatrial conduction (10 to 50 msec), AV nodal conduction (90 to 150 msec), and intra-His and His-Purkinje conduction (25 to 55 msec). The conduction delay in 1° AV block can thus represent prolonged interatrial, intra–AV nodal, or His-Purkinje conduction. Although His bundle recordings can clarify the site of conduction delay, such testing is rarely if ever indicated in persons with 1° AV block.

2° AV BLOCK. In 2° AV block, not all atrial impulses are conducted to the ventricle. Type I (Wenckebach) 2° AV block (Fig. 24–8) is present when the conduction of atrial impulses to the ventricles is progressively delayed because of AV nodal refractoriness, with eventual failure of conduction of an atrial impulse to the ventricles. The AV conduction ratio in type I 2° AV block can be 2:1, 4:3, 8:7, and so on. Because type I 2° AV block usually occurs within the AV node, the PR interval of the first conducted P-wave of the Wenckebach period is often prolonged; and because this conduction

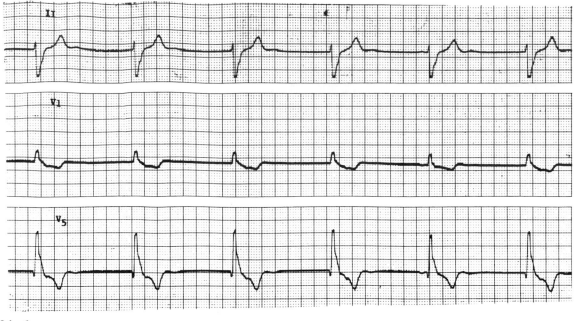

Figure 24–6

Simultaneously recorded leads II, VI, and V₅ in a 42-year-old patient presenting with syncope. The QRS rhythm shows a pattern of left and superior axis deviation and right intraventricular conduction delay, suggesting a fascicular origin; the rate is about 39 beats per minute. Deformities in the early portions of the T-waves can be seen to occur at relatively constant intervals, possibly representing retrogradely (ventriculoatrial [VA]) conducted P-waves (an exception is the next to last P-QRS complex). Patients with VA conduction can have severe symptoms of cerebral hypoperfusion and effort intolerance due to both reflex hypotension caused by the atrial stretch-mediated baroreceptor stimulation and by the inability of this cardiac pacemaker (originating in ventricular tissue) to increase its firing rate in response to increases in metabolic need.

disturbance does not involve the bundle branches, the QRS complexes are expected to be narrow and normal-appearing unless concomitant bundle branch disease is present. In a typical, or classic, Wenckebach period, the PR intervals progressively lengthen and the RR intervals progressively shorten.

In type II 2° AV block (Fig. 24–9), atrial impulses fail to be transmitted to the ventricles but there is no discernible increase in conduction delay before the failure of conduction. Because measurable prior conduction delay does not occur, the failure of antegrade conduction is abrupt and unpredictable. In contrast to type I 2° AV block, in which the conduction delay is in the AV node, the conduction delay in type II 2° AV block can be within the His bundle or, more commonly, distal to the His bundle in the bundle branches. If the block is within the His bundle, the QRS complexes are usually narrow and appear to be normal or only mildly aberrant.

If the block is distal to the His bundle, the QRS complexes will have a bundle branch block pattern. In contrast to type I 2° AV block, the PR interval of the conducted P-waves is essentially constant and often normal.

A 2:1 AV conduction ratio may represent either type I or type II 2° AV block. Since two consecutive PR intervals are not recorded, the presence or absence of progressive PR interval prolongation cannot be ascertained and the differential diagnosis may be difficult. Certain guidelines can be useful: If the PR interval of the conducted P-waves is prolonged and the QRS complexes are narrow and normal-appearing, type I 2° AV block (supra- or intra-His) is probably present. If the PR interval of the conducted P-waves is prolonged and the QRS complexes have a bundle branch block pattern, it may not be possible to distinguish between the two types. Altering the AV conduction ratio from 2:1 to 3:2 or greater by means of carotid sinus massage (to produce a slower sinus rate) or

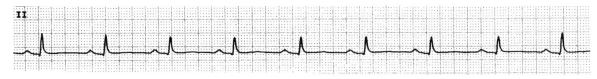

Figure 24–7

Lead II rhythm strip demonstrating first-degree (1°) AV block (PR interval >0.20 sec). The PR interval is prolonged to about 0.25 second. The PR interval contains within it interatrial conduction, AV nodal conduction, and His-Purkinje conduction; the site of conduction delay in 1° AV block is usually the AV node, especially when the QRS complexes are narrow and normal-appearing.

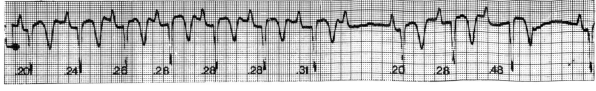

Figure 24–8

Type I second-degree (2°) AV block (Wenckebach) is illustrated in this rhythm strip by the increasing PR intervals (designated by the numbers) before failure of conduction of a P-wave. The sinus rate is constant at about 70 beats per minute. The first period has an 8:7 AV conduction ratio. Long AV conduction ratios are often atypical, as in this example, in which the three PR intervals before the last PR intervals do not progressively increase. (Other atypical features can include failure of RR intervals to shorten before the nonconducted P-wave.) The second period has a 4:3 AV conduction ratio; the nonconducted P-wave deforms the last T-wave of the period. This shorter period is typical of type I 2° AV block. The usual site of conduction delay in type I 2° AV block is the AV node, especially when the QRS complexes are narrow and normal-appearing.

intravenous atropine (to enhance AV nodal conduction) will often allow identification of the nature of the AV block and thus its probable location.

HIGH-DEGREE (INCLUDING COMPLETE) AV BLOCK. In high-grade AV block, the AV conduction ratio is 3:1 or greater. Multiple levels of block may exist (Fig. 24–10), causing irregularity in the PR intervals and ventricular rate.

When complete AV block occurs, no atrial impulses are conducted to the ventricles despite temporal opportunity for this to occur, and the atria and ventricles are depolarized by their respective pacemakers, independent of each other. Complete AV block may be paroxysmal and life-threatening. The atrial rate in complete AV block is almost always faster than the ventricular rate, but a notable exception is digitalis toxicity, which can cause

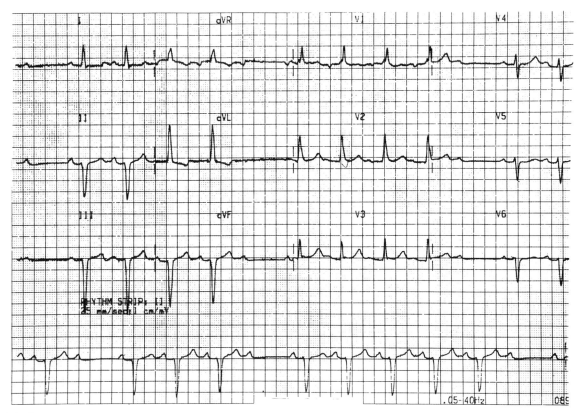

Figure 24–9

Type II 2° AV block is illustrated in this 12-lead electrocardiogram (ECG) and accompanying lead II rhythm strip. The sinus rate is constant at about 76 beats per minute. The PR intervals of conducted impulses are also constant, at about 0.23 second. The QRS complexes have a pattern of left anterior fascicular block and right-sided conduction delay, suggesting bifascicular block. Nonconducted P-waves are not preceded by progressive lengthening of the PR intervals and occur unpredictably; these are the hallmarks of type II 2° AV block. The usual site of conduction block in type II 2° AV block is below the AV node, in either the His bundle or the Purkinje network. Thus, type II 2° AV block is usually accompanied by other evidence of fascicular disease (as in this example). The long PR interval in this ECG could represent conduction delay either within the AV node or in the fascicular system; the presence of the AV block suggests the latter.

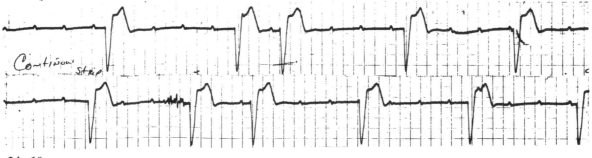

Figure 24–10

This continuously recorded rhythm strip was obtained in a 74-year-old man being treated for hypertension with beta blockers, calcium channel blockers, and long-acting nitrates, who presented to the emergency department with 2 days of dizziness and falling. The atrial rhythm is sinus and high-degree AV block is present, with ventricular rates as low as 30 beats per minute. The QRS complexes have a left bundle branch block pattern, suggesting the possibility of advanced conduction system disease; old ECGs would be helpful in ascertaining the age of the bundle branch block. Despite the absence of sinus bradycardia, which would be expected in view of the drugs the patient is receiving, this rhythm must be assumed to be due to the medications until proved otherwise, and the medications should be discontinued. Temporary cardiac pacing is often required for rate support, especially in older patients. Should these medications be necessary to treat the patient's underlying medical illness, permanent cardiac pacing will be required. If the AV block does not resolve on discontinuing the AV nodal blocking agents, the rhythm must be considered to be due to intrinsic and diffuse conduction system disease, and permanent cardiac pacing should be undertaken.

acceleration of a junctional pacemaker in addition to the AV block. In high-grade AV block, the QRS rhythm originates distal to the site of the AV block and may be in the AV junction, bundle of His, bundle branches, or distal Purkinje system, and it is an escape rhythm.

If the atrial rhythm is not sinus, the existence of advanced or complete AV block is diagnosed by the presence of a slow and regular rate. Atrial fibrillation and flutter may be associated with advanced AV block and slow ventricular rates, often because of medications that slow AV conduction. The rate of the ventricular rhythm, as well as the QRS complex morphology, will depend on the site of origin of the rhythm. Its regularity indicates that it is not being stimulated by the atrial rhythm but by an independent pacemaker originating below the level of the conduction block.

In vagotonic block, a high degree of vagal tone, such as occurs in conditioned athletes or withdrawal of sympathetic tone during sleep, may be associated with marked slowing of the sinus rate, pauses in rhythm, variable degrees of AV conduction delay manifested by (often irregular) PR interval prolongation, and failure to conduct P-waves resembling type I or II 2° AV block (see Table 24–4). It is crucial to recognize vagotonic block, since it usually occurs in normal individuals but can occur in patients with inferior or right ventricular myocardial infarction or any other clinical condition in which hypervagotonia is present (see Table 24–3).[12] Vagally mediated bradycardia can add to the effects of certain medications, such as beta-adrenergic blocking agents, some antihypertensive drugs, and digitalis. It can also be seen during swallowing (deglutition bradycardia), coughing (tussive bradycardia), yawning, and even assumption of an upright posture ("postural heart block").[13] In the critical care setting, vagally mediated bradycardia (including AV block) can occur during endotracheal suctioning or esophagogastric intubation and in patients with elevated intracranial pressure.

Approach to Office Management

INCREASED VAGAL TONE. Outpatient evaluation of AV block must begin with a recognition of the major reversible causes of AV conduction delay or block: hypervagotonia and medications. High vagal tone can cause or contribute to both atrial and ventricular bradycardia even in the absence of withdrawal of sympathetic tone. Vagally mediated bradycardias are usually transient and not accompanied by symptoms of severe presyncope or frank syncope, and no specific treatment is indicated. If necessary, intravenous atropine can be used to facilitate AV nodal conduction, thus avoiding ventricular bradycardia; however, if the atropine induces an increase in atrial rate, paradoxical slowing of ventricular rate can occur as a result of more rapid stimulation of the AV node with encroachment on the refractory period of the AV conduction system. The effects of intravenous atropine are short-lived, and its chronic use is accompanied by significant side effects. Should it be deemed necessary to treat vagally mediated bradycardia, oral theophylline and transdermal scopolamine have been used with some success;[14] chronic therapy is usually not required.

In contrast to the majority of vagally mediated bradyarrhythmias, some vasovagal episodes (hypotension with variable degrees of bradycardia) can be frequent, unpredictable, abrupt, and disabling (see Chap. 12). These highly symptomatic episodes (referred to as *neurocardiogenic, cardioneurogenic,* or *neurovascular* syndromes) can require heart rate support with oral theophylline, ephedrine, and even permanent dual-chamber cardiac pacing as well as intravascular volume support with fluids, mineralocorticoids, and support hose. Since left ventricular baroreceptor stimulation (from vigorous systolic contraction) and consequent reflex peripheral vasodilatation play a role in this syndrome, drugs that have negative inotropic effects (e.g., beta blockers, verapamil, disopyramide) are often used in management. Because of a central nervous system component, anticholinergic agents (e.g., transdermal scopolamine, serotonin reuptake inhibitors such as sertraline) can also be useful. Patients in whom these malignant vasovagal syndromes are known or suspected should be referred to a specialist to document the extent of hypotension and bradycardia during head-up tilt-table testing; tilt-table–guided therapy is more successful than empiric therapy in managing this disorder.[15]

MEDICATIONS. Commonly used medications that cause or contribute to bradycardia do so by enhancing vagal tone (e.g., digitalis), reducing sympathetically mediated enhancement of AV conduction (e.g., beta blockers, including ophthalmic preparations), or acting directly on sinoatrial and AV conduction tissue (e.g., verapamil, diltiazem, and beta blockers). Thus, a thorough review of the patient's medications is important. Withdrawal of these drugs is often associated with reversal of the AV block, and permanent cardiac pacing is not required. An exception exists if the drugs cannot be withdrawn, in which case pacemaker therapy is required. If the ventricular rhythm is slow in the absence of these agents, intrinsic AV conduction system disease is present, and referral to a cardiologist for permanent cardiac pacing is indicated. Electrical cardioversion of an atrial arrhythmia associated with slow ventricular rate in the absence of medications should be undertaken with extreme caution, if at all, since postcardioversion bradycardia or even asystole can occur owing to the diffuse underlying conduction disease.

ASYMPTOMATIC AV BLOCK. Occasionally, AV block with slow ventricular rates is discovered incidentally on a routine ECG recording. As with atrial bradycardias, it is most important to obtain a focused, thorough history seeking clues to the presence of symptoms of bradycardia, which can be vague, subtle, and nonspecific. If the patient is truly asymptomatic and the AV block is supra-His in location (deduced from the presence of narrow, normal-appearing QRS complexes), frequent careful observation may be all that is warranted. However, if the AV block is potentially infra-His (i.e., type I or II 2° block with bundle branch block), referral for electrophysiologic study is indicated, and "prophylactic" pacemaker therapy is often prudent and may improve prognosis. Many bradycardic patients without definitive symptoms will feel remarkably better after permanent pacemaker implantation, suggesting they have adapted their lifestyle and expectations to match their diminished ability to raise cardiac output.

HIGH-DEGREE (INCLUDING COMPLETE) AV BLOCK. Outpatients with high-grade or complete AV block of any cause who have symptoms (including those of acute myocardial infarction) should be considered emergencies and transferred immediately to an intensive care unit where monitoring facilities are available in case temporary or permanent transvenous pacing be required. In-office trials of intravenous atropine are time-consuming and essentially irrelevant unless delay in transfer is expected. Many patients, even elderly ones, can tolerate extremely slow heart rates (25 to 30 beats/minute) if they are supine (to maximize intravascular volume) and intravascular volume is enhanced by fluid administration. If available, transcutaneous pacing can be employed (see later), but it is unreliable and not well tolerated for prolonged periods of time. Very rarely, cardiopulmonary resuscitative procedures must be used.

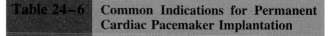

CARDIAC PACING

Temporary or permanent cardiac pacing is indicated in any situation in which bradycardia causes symptoms of cerebral hypoperfusion or hemodynamic decompensation (Table 24–6). Patients with bradycardia-dependent ventricular tachycardia may require pacing to prevent pauses in rhythm, thus eliminating the tachyarrhythmia. Although emergency pacing can be effected temporarily by transcutaneous pacing, in all but the most critical situations, temporary pacing is best accomplished by the transvenous route.[16] Permanent cardiac pacing is almost always performed through the transvenous route; in some circumstances, however, epicardial placement of electrodes via thoracotomy or a subxiphoid approach is used.

Temporary Pacing

Transcutaneous pacing, in which electrical current is delivered to the heart via large surface electrodes, is generally reserved for standby or prophylactic use in patients at high risk for bradycardia—for example, during acute inferior and large anterior wall myocardial infarctions—and in some patients with sinus node dysfunction who are undergoing elective cardioversion. Availability of transcu-

Table 24–6	**Common Indications for Permanent Cardiac Pacemaker Implantation**

Sinus node dysfunction
  With symptoms of cerebral hypoperfusion or chronotropic incompetence with or without symptoms but with escape rates less than 40 beats/min, and whether or not due to necessary medications
Acquired AV block
  Complete or high-grade
    With symptoms, whether or not the symptoms are due to necessary medication
    With asystolic pauses exceeding 3 sec
    With escape pacemaker rates less than 40 beats/min
  Second-degree
    Type I or II, with symptoms
Neurally mediated ("vasovagal") syndromes
  With recurrent syncope or presyncope and bradycardia and hypotension during head-up tilt testing
Carotid sinus hypersensitivity
  With symptoms due to bradycardia provoked by carotid sinus massage in patients with recurrent syncope or presyncope
  With asystolic pauses in rhythm exceeding 3 sec in response to carotid sinus massage in patients with recurrent syncope

Adapted from ACC/AHA Task Force Report: Guidelines for implantation of cardiac pacemakers and antiarrhythmia devices. J. Am. Coll. Cardiol. 18:1–13, 1991.
Abbreviation: AV, atrioventricular.

taneous pacemakers has heretofore been limited to hospitals and some cardiologists' offices. However, they do have a place in cardiopulmonary resuscitation, and depending on the particular practice and community, their use should become more widespread. Because of its ease of use and relative efficacy, this pacing modality has virtually eliminated the need for transmyocardial pacing in emergency situations.

The *transcutaneous pacing system* uses two large low-impedance surface electrodes placed on the anterior and posterior chest walls. A long pulse duration of 20 to 40 msec and programmable current output of up to 100 mA are often necessary to overcome the impedance of the chest wall and intrathoracic structures. The transcutaneous pacemaker paces the ventricle unless it senses spontaneous ventricular electrical activity, thus functioning in VVI (demand) mode (Table 24–7). Ventricular capture (depolarization) is best seen on the pacemaker generator's oscilloscope and strip-chart recording (Fig. 24–11). Substantial distortion of the QRS complex is present on bedside rhythm monitors or ECG recordings, and paced QRS complexes cannot be identified by these means. Ventricular capture should be verified by palpating the pulse. Skeletal muscle twitching (not to be considered a sign of myocardial stimulation) occurs at a stimulus output of 30 mA, but ventricular capture does not usually occur until 35 to 80 mA. Sedation of an awake patient is usually required to mitigate the painful muscle contractions.

Transcutaneous cardiac pacing can be effective in up to 70% of patients. Most poor outcomes result from its use in advanced stages of cardiopulmonary arrest. If cardiac arrest has been present for more than 15 minutes, successful pacing is accomplished in only 33% to 45% of patients, with little effect on outcome. Temporary transvenous and esophageal pacing are accomplished in hospital settings and in intensive care units by specialists and are indicated when reliable emergent pacing is required[16] (see Chap. 17).

Permanent Pacing

Pacing system design is complex, but all pacemaker generators can be described by a standardized code (see Table 24–7). Current pacemakers have several functions that can be changed noninvasively by a programmer.[17, 18] The programmable features of a pacing system allow for optimal benefit for the patient while conserving battery energy.

Single-Chamber Demand Pacing (VVI, AAI)

Both sensing and pacing circuits are present in these units. When a spontaneous intracardiac signal is sensed, VVI and AAI pulse generators inhibit their output and no pacemaker output occurs.

Electrical signals sensed by demand-pulse generators can originate not only from the heart but also from the environment (e.g., electrocautery, microwave ovens), from the patient (e.g., muscle potentials), or occasionally, from the pacing system itself. The sensed signals can inhibit

Table 24–7	Commonly Programmed Modes of Pacemaker Function*
AAI	Demand atrial pacing; output inhibited by sensed atrial signals.
AAIR	Demand atrial pacing; output inhibited by sensed atrial signals. Atrial pacing rates decrease and increase in response to sensor input up to the programmed sensor based upper rate.
VVI	Demand ventricular pacing; output inhibited by sensed ventricular signals.
VVIR	Demand ventricular pacing; output inhibited by sensed ventricular signals. Ventricular paced rates decrease and increase in response to sensor input up to the programmed sensor based upper rate.
VDD	Paces ventricle; senses in both atrium and ventricle; synchronizes with atrial activity and paces ventricle after a preset atrioventricular interval up to the programmed upper rate.
VDDR	Paces ventricle, senses in both atrium and ventricle; synchronizes with atrial activity and paces ventricle after a preset atrioventricular interval up to the programmed upper rate; in absence of spontaneous atrial activity, functions as VVIR.
DDD	Paces and senses in both atrium and ventricle; paces ventricle in response to sensed atrial activity up to programmed upper rate.
DDDR	Atrial and ventricular paced rates can both increase and decrease in response to sensor input up to the programmed sensor upper rate.

Abbreviations: A, atrium; V, ventricle; D, dual (both atrium and ventricle); I, inhibition; D, inhibition and triggering (pacing in response to another event); R, rate adaptation available.

* By convention, the first letter refers to the chamber(s) in which pacing occurs, the second letter to the chamber(s) in which sensing the intracardiac signal occurs, and the third letter to the mode of response to sensed signals. An R in the fourth position signifies rate responsiveness.

output and result in pauses in paced rhythm, a phenomenon termed *oversensing,* which can cause symptoms of cerebral hypoperfusion. This problem can generally be corrected by noninvasive programming to raise the sensing threshold, obviating the need for surgical revision.

P-Synchronous Pacing Systems (VDD) (Fig. 24–12)

VDD pacing systems are dual-chamber systems in which electrodes are located in both the atrium and the ventricle. Some new systems use a single lead, the tip of which is positioned in the right ventricular apex for ventricular sensing and pacing and in which the sensing-only atrial electrodes are located on the lead at the level of the atrium. When the atrial electrodes sense an electrical signal, a ventricular pacing stimulus is delivered after a programmable AV delay that corresponds roughly to the PR interval. If a spontaneous QRS complex occurs, the ventricular output is inhibited. Thus, the ventricular pacing stimulus is either triggered by a sensed atrial signal or inhibited by a native QRS event.

"Universal Pacing" (DDD)

DDD pulse generators are capable of sensing and pacing on demand in both the atrium and the ventricle. They therefore attempt to mimic the physiology of normal AV conduction in many patients who require cardiac pacing.

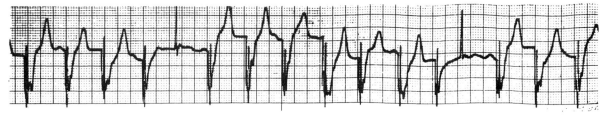

Figure 24–11

Rhythm strip illustrating transcutaneous cardiac pacing, recorded from the pacing device's ECG monitor. The pacing stimuli are delivered over a 40-msec interval and thus can obscure the onset of the paced QRS complexes. Transcutaneous pacing systems function in VVI mode (see text) and are inhibited by spontaneous ventricular depolarizations. In this rhythm strip, the 5th and 13th QRS complexes are upright and not preceded by a pacing stimulus and are therefore native in origin; they appropriately inhibit the output of the pacing device. The pacing stimuli preceding these spontaneous QRS complexes (4th and 12th stimuli) do not produce paced ventricular depolarizations, and therefore there are no associated T-waves (the presence of a T-wave is helpful in indicating ventricular depolarization when the QRS complexes are obscured). Thus, intermittent failure to capture is present. Paper speed changes account for the slight irregularity in paced rhythm.

The ability to sense retrograde atrial depolarizations can trigger ventricular pacing; if the paced ventricular depolarization conducts retrograde to the atrium, the process can become repetitive, creating a "pacemaker-mediated tachycardia."[6] Specific pulse-generator features are designed to terminate these tachycardias automatically.

Dual-chamber devices depend on a stable atrial rhythm for optimal function. Because of their potential to facilitate rapid-paced ventricular rates, these systems should not be used in patients with atrial arrhythmias such as chronic fibrillation, refractory atrial flutter, multifocal atrial tachycardia, or refractory supraventricular tachycardia. Instead, single-chamber VVI devices are commonly utilized in these patients. Alternatively, newer devices can change their mode of function automatically from DDD to single-chamber VVI(R) function on sensing an atrial arrhythmia; such devices are appropriate for patients with paroxysmal atrial arrhythmias when there is an advantage to producing AV synchrony during sinus or atrial paced rhythm yet protect against a pacemaker-facilitated tachycardia when the atrial rhythm is not sinus.

Rate-Responsiveness

Rate-adaptive pacing systems (see Table 24–7) are appropriate for patients with persistent or refractory atrial arrhythmias who are not candidates for DDD devices and for patients with sinus node dysfunction that prevents rate acceleration in response to increases in metabolic demand. Current commonly used sensors measure muscle activity or minute ventilation and then adjust the paced rate. The same option is available on many DDD pacemakers. Sensor-based pacing rates depend on the individual sensor and the programmed rate-response parameters. Patient dissatisfaction with rate-adaptive pacing almost always reflects inappropriate programmed parameters; determining optimal settings often requires considerable time and expertise.

The type of pacing system, model, and serial number are indicated on an identification card supplied to the patient by the manufacturer; patients should carry this card with them at all times. It is important to note, however, that the information provided by the card does not guarantee the current status of any programmable function.

ECG Patterns of Paced Complexes

The configuration of paced P-waves and QRS complexes reflects how myocardium is depolarized (Fig. 24–

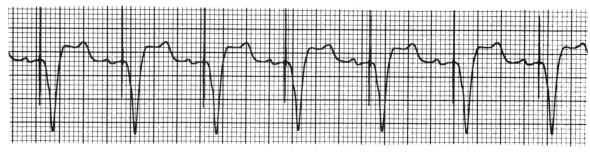

Figure 24–12

P-synchronous pacing in a 64-year-old woman with complete AV block. The atrial rhythm is sinus. All P-waves are sensed and followed at a constant AV interval by paced QRS complexes. Thus, "tracking" of the atrial rhythm is present. The parameters of intact pacing system function demonstrated in this illustration are atrial sensing and ventricular pacing; atrial pacing and ventricular sensing are not seen and are thus not verified. This pacing system could be either a DDD or a VDD system (see text). The tracking of sinus rhythm and rate allow not only AV synchrony but also rate adaptation to increase in metabolic need.

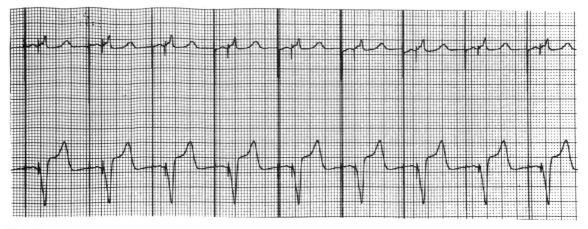

Figure 24–13

AV pacing is illustrated in these simultaneously recorded leads I and II. Since all P-waves and QRS complexes are paced and no native complexes are seen, sensing function cannot be evaluated. The large atrial pacing artifact is due to the unipolar configuration of the atrial lead; the smaller ventricular pacing artifact is due to the bipolar configuration of the ventricular lead. Note the changing amplitude and polarity of the ventricular pacing stimuli, an artifact of the recording equipment. The patient's native heart rate and rhythm are not known, since all complexes are paced.

13). Paced atrial complexes reflect the sequence of atrial activation initiated by the pacing impulse and thus also the site of the stimulating electrode(s). Since the atrial electrodes can be located in the atrial appendage or screwed into any portion of atrial tissue, paced P-waves will have variable contours. Atrial hypertrophy and conduction delay cannot be diagnosed if the P-waves are paced.

Pacing from the right ventricular endocardium or epicardium produces paced QRS complexes having a left bundle branch block configuration (reflecting right ventricular depolarization beginning before left ventricular depolarization). Occasionally, pacing from the interventricular septum can cause paced QRS complexes having an indeterminate conduction delay pattern; they can even be narrow and relatively normal-appearing, reflecting near-simultaneous activation of both the right and the left sides of the interventricular septum. Paced QRS complexes usually have a duration of 0.12 to 0.18 second; if they are substantially longer, intrinsic myocardial disease, rapid-paced rate, hyperkalemia, or antiarrhythmic drug therapy should be suspected. Spontaneous QRS complexes occurring in patients with pacemakers often show marked T-wave inversion of unknown cause.

Choice of Cardiac Pacing System and Relative Costs

State-of-the-art pacing systems can be costly. The cost of single-chamber, non–rate-adaptive devices, including pulse generator and lead, is about $6000 to 6500, and that of single-chamber, rate-adaptive devices is around $7000. Dual-chamber non–rate-adaptive devices (pulse generator and two leads) can cost up to $10,000, and rate-adaptive ones can cost $11,000 or more, depending on the availability of special algorithms to recognize paroxysmal arrhythmias and alter mode of function, retain ECG data in memory, and other sophisticated technical design features. These high up-front costs notwithstanding, studies have clearly shown the advantages of appropriate device selection, including programmable features, in many patients.[19, 20, 21] Device selection should probably always take advantage of the patient's spontaneous sinus rhythm to preserve AV synchrony and normal rate response; rate adaptation in patients with atrial bradycardia also serves to preserve the normal sequence of depolarization and contraction and thus hemodynamic function. Patients with supraventricular arrhythmias generally should be prescribed dual-chamber devices to take advantage of normal rhythm, when it is present, and to reduce the frequency of paroxysmal arrhythmias.

Numerous observational and retrospective studies have suggested an advantage for dual-chamber over single-chamber pacing systems in patients with atrial rhythm other than chronic fibrillation. In one randomized trial, the incidence of atrial arrhythmias and systemic embolism was reduced by the use of dual-chamber systems in appropriate patients,[22] but mortality was not changed. Several randomized controlled studies are currently in progress to assess whether dual-chamber pacing improves quality of life or mortality and whether it is cost effective compared with single-chamber pacing.

Pacing System "Malfunctions"

Pacing system "malfunctions" fall into four general categories, the general nature of which should be recognized by the primary care physician. These include undersensing, or failure to sense; oversensing, or sensing unwanted signals; failure to capture; and failure of output.

Failure to sense spontaneous complexes and to inhibit output appropriately results in the delivery of an earlier than expected pacing stimulus. Failure to sense can occur because of lead dislodgment, fibrous reaction at the lead site, or the end of battery life (Fig. 24–14). Occasionally,

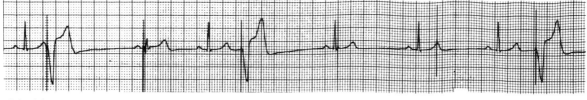

Figure 24–14

Failure to sense in a 37-year-old woman with a VVI pacing system (see text) implanted for "congenital complete AV block" 18 years earlier. Pacing function is intact. The pacing rate is about 39 beats per minute and the pulse generator is at end of life. The failure to sense intrinsic QRS complexes results in fixed-rate asynchronous stimulus delivery. The third QRS complex is a fusion complex in which the ventricles are depolarized by both the sinus-stimulated QRS complex and the paced complex. The fourth and fifth pacing stimuli do not produce a QRS complex; however, since they fall in the refractory period of ventricular muscle, failure to capture should not be diagnosed.

a delay in native conduction prevents the native depolarization from reaching the lead electrode early enough to inhibit the pacing stimulus.

Oversensing refers to sensing of unwanted electrical signals such as T-waves, myopotentials, and environmental signals (e.g., electrocautery, cell phones). Oversensing inhibits output and can produce long asystolic pauses in rhythm. Programming the pulse generator to a higher sensing threshold so as to ignore electrical signals below it will often solve the problem. When a programmer is not available or the pulse generator cannot be identified, placing a magnet over the generator will eliminate the oversensing while the patient is urgently transported for definitive care.

Failure to pace is present when pacing stimuli do not depolarize the otherwise receptive nonrefractory myocardium (Fig. 24–15). This condition may result from poor electrode position, too low a programmed output, end of battery life with resulting reduction in energy output, or an increase in myocardial stimulation threshold.

Failure to capture often can be managed by noninvasive programming to a higher energy output, but lead repositioning or implantation of a new generator, or both, may be required. Failure to pace, even if asymptomatic, requires urgent referral to a pacemaker specialist.

The difference between failure to capture when the stimulus artifact is present and absence of stimulus output should be clearly understood. Applying a magnet will aid in determining the cause for the lack of stimulus

output. If no output is present, the pulse generator must be replaced.

Monitoring the Patient with a Pacemaker and the Role of the Primary Care Physician

All patients with pacemakers should be monitored on a routine basis by a pacemaker specialist; the specialist may or may not be the implanting cardiologist and is generally not an implanting surgeon. Additional transtelephonic monitoring, set up by the pacemaker specialist, can be utilized routinely to reduce the number of visits to the specialist as well as to provide follow-up support for those patients who reside considerable distances from pacemaker centers or who are physically unable to get to the center. Rhythm strips and pacemaker rate information are routinely sent to the pacemaker specialist for inclusion in the patient's pacemaker file. It is the responsibility of the specialist routinely to interrogate the pacemaker, assess battery status, perform pacing and sensing threshold(s) to optimize programmed parameters and thus prolong pulse generator life, and assess underlying rhythm and rate and degree of pacemaker dependency. Moreover, since it is the specialist who receives advisories of real and potential pacemaker-related problems, as well as of manufacturer- or government-initiated recalls of devices

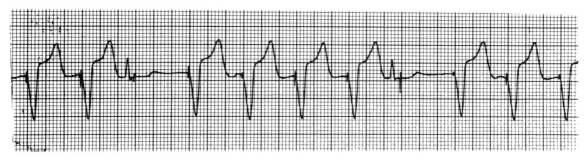

Figure 24–15

Asynchronous fixed-rate ventricular pacing illustrating episodic noncapture (third and eighth pacing stimuli) due to ventricular refractoriness produced by the preceding spontaneous QRS complexes. This should not be interpreted as failure to capture. True capture failure requires that temporal opportunity to capture exists.

found to be actually or potentially defective, the specialist is in the best position to evaluate the patient in a timely manner in light of the potential device failures, some of which can be life-threatening. In general, once a patient has stabilized after pacemaker implantation and the wound has been checked, routine office follow-up can be carried out at 3 months, then semiannually, and finally annually until battery end of life approaches, which is currently at around 5 to 7 years but which depends substantially on how the pacemaker is programmed and may change with evolving technology. Current guidelines for pacemaker follow-up by transtelephonic monitoring help to ensure continuity of evaluation of pulse generator status.[23] Depending on the particular pacing system, after about the fourth year postimplantation, monthly telephone transmissions are prescribed to ensure detection of subtle rate changes that indicate battery end of life. Telephone transmissions do not, however, substitute for office follow-up visits, during which interrogation of battery status directly through the programmer can disclose information not available from rate data alone.[18]

The primary care physician must ensure that the paced patient has formal follow-up with a cardiologist who has up-to-date, state-of-the-art knowledge of cardiac pacing. Communication among the patient's physicians is necessary, so that each knows the concerns of the others. This is particularly important if patients are receiving medications that can affect pacing and sensing thresholds, so that appropriate programming changes can be made if necessary. Wound infections, upper extremity thrombophlebitis, and pacing system infections can occur months to years after implantation, and these should be recognized because referral will be required. Intercurrent events that can affect pacemaker function, such as myocardial infarction and development of renal insufficiency, should prompt referral for additional pacemaker checks. Especially in patients with rate-adaptive pacing systems, the pacemaker specialist will want to know the perception by the primary care physician of the patient's actual effort tolerance and general sense of well-being in order to program the most appropriate rate-response settings. Patients who are undergoing surgical procedures of any kind need not have antibiotic therapy for endocarditis prophylaxis.

In patients with pacemakers, any symptoms that are new or otherwise unexplained warrant an evaluation by the pacemaker specialist (Table 24–8), since noninvasive programming may be able to correct or ameliorate those that can be identified as being caused or contributed to by the pacing system. In patients with unexplained fevers, specialized studies such as echocardiography may be necessary to exclude infection of the pacing system that would require aggressive antibiotic therapy and likely removal of the entire system. Patients who develop new pulmonary hypertension require evaluation for lead-related thromboembolism, whether septic or sterile, and appropriate treatment should be undertaken. It is crucial to bear in mind the possibility that a patient's symptoms might in fact be pacemaker-related before undertaking unnecessary diagnostic workups or prescribing nonindicated therapies.

Finally, it is the responsibility of the specialist to provide the patient and the primary care physician with a copy of the most recent programmed settings obtained by interrogation. The pacemaker specialist should counsel the patient as to which types of activities or diagnostic or therapeutic procedures might cause adverse pacemaker interactions, so that either appropriate programming changes can be made or certain activities and occupations can be avoided entirely to allow protection of both the pacing system and the patient. The primary care physician should be apprised of these conditions as well, so that continued reinforcement can occur.

Table 24–8	Symptoms in Patients with Pacing Systems
Symptom	**Possible Pacemaker-Related Cause**
Palpitations	Inappropriate rate settings or rate-adaptive parameters
	Pacemaker-mediated tachycardias
Weakness	Pacemaker syndrome
	Inappropriate rate-adaptation settings
	Failure to capture
	Oversensing leading to pauses in rhythm
	Battery end of life with slow rate or no output
Breathlessness, nocturnal dyspnea, fatigue	Pacemaker syndrome
	Inappropriate upper rate setting
	Inappropriate rate-adaptation setting
	Battery end of life with slow rate or no output
Hiccups, cough	Diaphragmatic pacing
Muscle twitching	Lead insulation failure
	Unipolar stimulation
Swelling, suffusion of upper extremity	Thrombophlebitis (subclavian vein, inferior vena cava)
Dyspnea, edema	Right heart failure due to lead-related pulmonary emboli (including septic emboli)
Fever of unknown origin	Pacing system infection

References

1. Sutton, R., and Kenny, R.A.: The natural history of sick sinus syndrome. Pacing Clin. Electrophysiol. 9:1110, 1986.
2. Tresch, D.D., and Fleg, J.L.: Unexplained sinus bradycardia: Clinical significance and long-term prognosis in apparently healthy persons older than 40 years. Am. J. Cardiol. 58:1009, 1986.
3. Wharton, J.M., and Goldschlager, N.: Temporary cardiac pacing. In Saksena, S., and Goldschlager, N. (eds.): Electrical Therapy for Cardiac Arrhythmias. Philadelphia, W.B. Saunders, 1990, p. 107.
4. Puech, P., Grolleau, R., and Guimond, C.: Incidence of different types of A-V block and their localization by His bundle recordings. In Wellens, H.J.J., Lie, K,I., and Janse, M.J. (eds.): The Conduction System of the Heart: Structure, Function, and Clinical Implications. Philadelphia, Lea & Febiger, 1976, p. 467.
5. Narula, O.S.: Atrioventricular conduction defects in patients with sinus bradycardia. Circulation 44:1096, 1971.
6. Ausubel, K., and Furman, S.: The pacemaker syndrome. Ann. Intern. Med. 103:420, 1985.
7. Cappato, R., Alboni, P., Paparella, N., et al.: Bedside evaluation of sinus bradycardia: Usefulness of atropine test in discriminating organic from autonomic involvement of sinus automaticity. Am. Heart. J. 114:1384, 1987.
8. Mymin, D., Mathewson, F.A.L., Tate, R.B., and Manfreda, J.: The

natural history of primary first-degree atrioventricular heart block. N. Engl. J. Med. 315:1183, 1986.

9. Massie, B., Scheinman, M.M., Peters, R., et al.: Clinical and electrophysiologic findings in patients with paroxysmal slowing of the sinus rate and apparent Mobitz type II atrioventricular block. Circulation 58:305, 1978.

10. Shaw, D.B., Kekwick, C.A., Veale, D., et al.: Survival in second degree atrioventricular block. Br. Heart J. 53:587, 1985.

11. Strasberg, B., Lam, W., Swiryn, S., et al.: Symptomatic spontaneous paroxysmal AV nodal block due to localized hyperresponsiveness of the AV node to vagotonic reflexes. Am. Heart J. 103:795, 1982.

12. Goldschlager, N.: Conduction disorders and cardiac pacing. *In* Crawford, M. (ed.): Current Diagnosis and Treatment in Cardiology. Norwalk, CT, Appleton & Lange, 1995, p. 246.

13. Seda, P.E., McAnulty, J.H., and Anderson, C.J.: Postural heart block. Br. Heart J. 44:221, 1980.

14. Benditt, D.G., Benson, W., Jr., Kreitt, J., et al.: Electrophysiologic effects of theophylline in young patients with recurrent symptomatic bradyarrhythmias. Am. J. Cardiol. 52:1223, 1983.

15. Natale, A., Sra, J., Dhala, A., et al.: Efficacy of different treatment strategies for neurocardiogenic syncope. Pacing Clin. Electrophysiol. 18:655, 1995.

16. Le, K., and Goldschlager, N.: Temporary cardiac pacing in the intensive care unit. J. Intensive Care Med. 11:57, 1996.

17. Kusumoto, F.M., and Goldschlager, N.: Cardiac pacing. N. Engl. J. Med. 334:89, 1996.

18. Ludmer, P.L., and Goldschlager, N.: Cardiac pacing in the 1980s. N. Engl. J. Med. 311:1671, 1984.

19. Crossley, G.H., Gayle, D.D., Simmons, T.W., et al.: Reprogramming pacemakers enhances longevity and is cost-effective. Circulation 94(Suppl II):II-245–II-247, 1996.

20. Sutton, R., and Bourgeois, I.: Cost benefit analysis of single and dual chamber pacing for sick sinus syndrome and atrioventricular block: An economic sensitivity analysis of the literature. Eur. Heart J. 17:574–582, 1996.

21. Kamalvand, K., Tan, K., Kotsakis, A., et al.: Is mode switching beneficial? A randomized study in patients with paroxysmal atrial tachyarrhythmias. J. Am. Coll. Cardiol. 30:496–504, 1997.

22. Andersen, H.R., Theusen, L., Bagger, J.P., et al.: Prospective randomised trial of atrial versus ventricular pacing in sick-sinus syndrome. Lancet 344:1523–1528, 1994.

23. Medicare, Cardiac Pacemaker Evaluation Services: Coverage Issues Manual. HCFA Publication no. 6. Health Care Financing Administration, Washington, DC, 1984, sect. 50-1.

Chapter 25

Recognition and Management of Patients with
Valvular Heart Disease
BLASE A. CARABELLO

Five million Americans have some form of valvular heart disease. In addition to its magnitude, further importance is added to the recognition and management of valve disease because, unlike coronary disease, which often progresses despite therapy, proper management of valvular heart disease usually leads to a normal life span in most instances. On the other hand, misdiagnosis or improper management may result in a shortened life span or persistent congestive heart failure.

All valvular disease imparts a hemodynamic overload on either the left or the right ventricle, or both, that may be well tolerated for years. However, eventually the overload can produce myocardial damage that may become irreversible. In some patients, medical therapy may forestall this damage; in others, surgical intervention is the only effective therapy. This chapter addresses the recognition of valvular heart disease and emphasizes the best modalities for evaluation and follow-up. It also focuses on when to refer patients for the specialized care leading to surgical intervention.

AORTIC STENOSIS

Aortic stenosis is the most common of the primary valvular heart diseases. It is estimated that up to 1% of

Americans are born with a bicuspid aortic valve, which is the most common cardiac congenital abnormality (see Chap. 26). Of this group, a substantial proportion eventually develops significant aortic valvular obstruction. Other patients develop stenosis of a previously normal tricuspid valve. In either situation, aortic stenosis is due to idiopathic degeneration and calcification of the valve. Rarely today, in industrialized societies, rheumatic heart disease may cause aortic stenosis. However, in rheumatic aortic stenosis, the mitral valve is almost always abnormal. Thus, the diagnosis of rheumatic aortic stenosis should not be made in the face of an echocardiographically normal mitral valve.

As aortic stenosis progresses, an increasingly higher left ventricular systolic pressure is required to drive blood across the obstructed valve, resulting in a pressure gradient between the left ventricle and the aorta. This extra pressure work that the left ventricle must perform results in concentric left ventricular hypertrophy. Initially, the hypertrophy is compensatory because the increased muscle mass allows the ventricle to generate the higher pressure required by the obstruction to flow. However, eventually the hypertrophied myocardium takes on pathologic characteristics, resulting in the development of symptoms, morbidity, and mortality.[1]

pressure gradient between LV + aorta >50 mmHg severe AS

Figure 25–1

The natural history of aortic stenosis. There is a long latent period during which survival is about the same as that for the normal population. However, once the symptoms of angina, syncope, or congestive heart failure develop, survival declines dramatically. Within 5 years, half the patients complaining of angina will die unless corrective surgery is performed. For patients complaining of syncope, 50% survival is only for 3 years, and for patients who complain of the symptoms of congestive heart failure, 50% survival is only 2 years without aortic valve replacement. Av, average. (Redrawn from Ross, J., Jr., and Braunwald, E.: Aortic stenosis. Circulation 38[Suppl 5]: V-61, 1968. Reproduced with permission from Circulation. Copyright 1968 American Heart Association.)

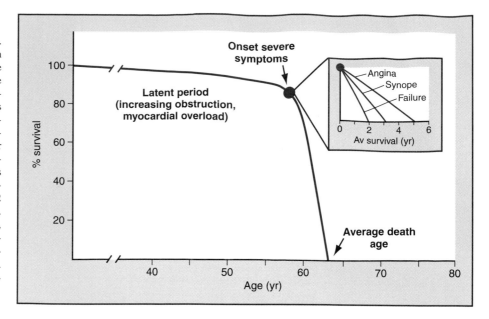

Diagnosis

may cause angina, syncope, CHF

History

Most patients with aortic stenosis are asymptomatic. As shown in Figure 25–1, survival is nearly normal during this asymptomatic phase. However, when the classic symptoms of angina, syncope, or congestive heart failure develop, there is a rapid increase in the risk of death unless aortic valve replacement is performed. Although aortic stenosis is rarely the cause of angina, syncope, or congestive heart failure in the large population of patients who complain of these common symptoms, this diagnosis should never be overlooked when those symptoms present, since aortic stenosis is lethal if uncorrected, yet it has an excellent outcome after aortic valve surgery.

Physical Examination

The physician usually discovers aortic stenosis because of the typical systolic ejection murmur that is heard best in the aortic area and radiates to the neck. The murmur has a harsh quality and initially may be quite loud. However, as the disease progresses, the murmur peaks progressively later in systole, and its intensity usually decreases as cardiac output falls. The murmur may disappear over the sternum and reappear at the apex, giving the false impression that mitral regurgitation is present (Gallivardin's phenomenon). When the severity of aortic stenosis becomes hemodynamically significant, the carotid upstroke becomes reduced in volume and delayed. This may be appreciated as the physician palpates his or her own carotid pulse with one hand while simultaneously palpating the patient's carotid pulse with the other. A graphic example of this important physical finding is demonstrated in Figure 25–2. An additional finding helpful in assessing the severity of aortic stenosis on physical examination is the quality of the second heart sound (S_2). As stenosis severity worsens, valve motion is

reduced and the aortic component of S_2 disappears. Thus, a single soft S_2 representing the closure of the pulmonic component is a typical finding in severe aortic stenosis. More rarely, S_2 may be paradoxically split.

Laboratory Studies

The *electrocardiogram* in aortic stenosis usually shows left ventricular hypertrophy. The chest x-ray may demonstrate a boot-shaped heart consistent with the development of left ventricular concentric hypertrophy. Occasionally, aortic valve calcification is seen on the lateral view. However, *echocardiography* is the principal laboratory method by which aortic stenosis is diagnosed and quantified. Two-dimensional echocardiography demonstrates thickened valve leaflets with restricted motion. It also gauges left ventricular ejection fraction and the extent of concentric left ventricular hypertrophy. Ejection fraction is the percent of the left or right ventricle's end-diastolic volume (EDV) ejected during systole, that is, $\frac{\text{stroke volume}}{\text{EDV}}$. Precise measurement of the transvalvular gradient is afforded by Doppler interrogation of the valve. For blood flow to remain constant, blood stream velocity must increase when it reaches the stenosis. The magnitude of this increase can be quantified using the Doppler technique. The transducer both emits and receives the reflected sound waves. If the blood stream moving toward the transducer accelerates, it compresses the sound waves and the frequency received by the transducer is greater than that that it emitted. This is the same principle by which the pitch of an oncoming train increases as the train approaches an observer and decreases as it moves away from the observer. Using the modified Bernoulli formula (gradient $= 4 \times V^2$, where V $=$ flow velocity in m/sec), the transvalvular gradient can be calculated (Fig. 25–3). In general, in resting subjects who are not in heart failure, gradients higher than 50 mm Hg indicate severe

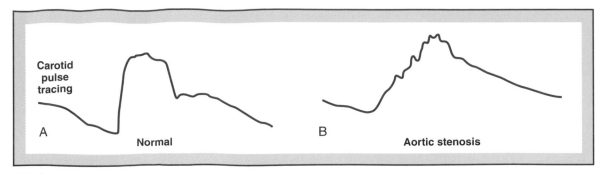

Figure 25–2

The carotid pulse tracing of a normal subject is demonstrated *(A)* and compared with the carotid pulse tracing of a patient with aortic stenosis *(B)*. The marked delay in upstroke that can be seen here can also be easily palpated during physical examination. (*A* and *B*, Redrawn from Boro, K.M., and Wynne, J.: External pulse recordings, systolic time intervals, apexcardiography, and phonocardiography. *In* Cohn, P.F., and Wynne, J. [eds.]: Diagnostic Methods in Clinical Cardiology. Boston, Little, Brown, 1982.)

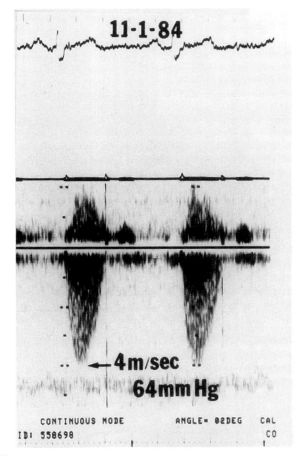

Figure 25–3

The Doppler interrogation of the aortic valve in a patient with aortic stenosis demonstrates high-velocity blood flow at 4 m/sec. Using the modified Bernoulli equation (see text), a gradient of 64 mm Hg is calculated. (From Assey, M.E., Usher, B.W., and Carabello, B.A.: The patient with valvular heart disease. *In* Pepine, C.J., Hill, J.A., and Lambert, C.R. [eds.]: Diagnostic and Therapeutic Cardiac Catheterization. 2nd ed. Baltimore, Williams & Wilkins, 1994.)

aortic stenosis, although lower gradients may also signify severe stenosis when the cardiac output is reduced.

Since most patients with aortic stenosis are in an age range where concomitant coronary artery disease is likely, adult patients with aortic stenosis should undergo cardiac catheterization before surgery. During this procedure, coronary angiography displays the coronary anatomy and the transvalvular gradient is confirmed by direct pressure measurement.

Management

Apart from prophylaxis against infective endocarditis, there is no effective medical management for aortic stenosis. If the patient is asymptomatic, no therapy is required. If the symptoms of angina, syncope, or heart failure have developed, immediate valve replacement is indicated as a lifesaving measure. Nitrates and diuretics may be employed cautiously to treat angina and heart failure, respectively, in the interim between when the diagnosis is made and when surgery is performed. Beta blockers that may precipitate cardiovascular collapse should be avoided in the treatment of angina. Angiotensin-converting enzyme (ACE) inhibitors and other vasodilators used prominently in the treatment of most forms of congestive heart failure may precipitate syncope and even death in aortic stenosis and are relatively contraindicated. However, in some individuals with concomitant systemic hypertension, cautious use of vasodilators may reduce symptoms.

In severely symptomatic patients who are not candidates for aortic valve replacement (because of other life-limiting illnesses such as terminal cancer), balloon aortic valvotomy affords temporary improvement in the transvalvular gradient and may relieve symptoms in some patients. During this procedure, a large balloon catheter is advanced percutaneously from the femoral artery and over a guide wire to the aortic valve orifice. There, balloon inflation modestly increases valve cusp mobility. Unfortunately, the stenosis returns to its original severity within 6 months in approximately half of the patients in whom this procedure is attempted. Balloon aortic valvuloplasty in adults with critical, calcific aortic stenosis does not ame-

Gradient = 4 × V²

β-blockers + ACE-I
Contraindicated

Table 25–1	Aortic Stenosis: Guidelines for Medical Therapy and for Referral for Specialized Care	
Symptoms	Doppler Gradient (Peak to Peak)	Course of Action
None	<30 mm Hg	Observe
None	>30 mm Hg	Observe
Equivocal	>30 mm Hg	Refer for further evaluation
Angina, syncope or CHF	>30 mm Hg	Refer for further evaluation
CHF	Any level	Refer for further evaluation
Angina syncope	<30 mm Hg	Consider another cause
Symptomatic but aortic valve surgery contraindicated	>30 mm Hg	Consider balloon aortic valvotomy

Abbreviation: CHF, congestive heart failure.

liorate the high mortality in these patients, although in those at high risk of operation it may serve as a "bridge" to valve replacement.

Overall Strategy

When aortic stenosis is detected on the physical examination of an *asymptomatic* patient, an echocardiogram should be performed to quantify severity. If the peak gradient is less than approximately 50 mm Hg, the patient can be followed yearly with a history and physical examination.[2] If the peak gradient exceeds approximately 50 mm Hg, follow-up should be performed every 6 months. In patients who are physically active, repeat echocardiography is indicated if the patient reports the onset of one or more of the triad—angina, syncope, or heart failure. At that time, an echocardiogram can be repeated to determine whether there has been a change in the severity of the stenosis and whether left ventricular dysfunction has developed. At that point, the patient should be referred promptly for final workup before aortic valve replacement. In sedentary patients, more frequent echocardiograms may detect the onset of left ventricular dysfunction before the onset of symptoms. In the rare circumstance where there has been a clear decrement in left ventricular performance in the still-asymptomatic patient, aortic valve replacement is probably advisable.[3] On occasion, the patient may complain of vague symptoms not typical of the classic triad of symptoms. In such cases, stress testing may be useful in assessing symptomatic status. However, exercise testing in patients with aortic stenosis is controversial, must be performed with extreme caution, and probably should be left in the hands of the cardiologist.

At the other end of the spectrum, even patients who present with advanced heart failure and severe left ventricular dysfunction may still benefit from aortic valve replacement, especially if the mean transvalvular gradient exceeds 30 mm Hg. In this case, surgery affords an acute reduction in left ventricular afterload, permitting immedi-

ate improvement in left ventricular performance. Thus, many such patients are still surgical candidates and should be referred for evaluation.

Table 25–1 summarizes the clinical and echocardiographic markers that guide the primary care physician's timing for referral of aortic stenosis patients for specialized care.

MITRAL STENOSIS

Almost all cases of acquired mitral stenosis result from rheumatic heart disease. Although the attack rate of rheumatic fever is slightly higher in men than in women, mitral stenosis develops far more frequently in women than men, with a 4:1 female-to-male ratio.[3,4] Typically, symptoms of mitral stenosis develop in the fourth and fifth decades of life. In many cases, the woman with mitral stenosis is asymptomatic until her first pregnancy, when increased hemodynamic demand results in cardiac decompensation. Although it has been debated for decades, it appears that in most cases of mitral stenosis occurring in Western countries, the rheumatic disease spares the myocardium and muscle function is normal. Thus, the symptoms of mitral stenosis usually do not accrue from contractile dysfunction but rather are due to the obstruction to blood flow across the mitral valve itself.

Opening of the normal mitral valve in early diastole creates a common chamber between the left atrium and the left ventricle, allowing for equalization of left atrial and left ventricular pressures early in diastole. However, as shown in Figures 25–4 and 25–5, mitral stenosis obstructs blood flow and causes a persistent pressure gradient between the left atrium and the left ventricle. This obstruction to flow reduces filling of the left ventricle, raises left atrial pressure, and causes pulmonary congestion and reduced cardiac output. Thus, the classic features of left-sided congestive heart failure are manifested without overt left ventricular muscle dysfunction. Since it is the right ventricle that has the responsibility for generating the force that drives blood across the mitral valve, the stenosis places a progressive pressure overload on the right ventricle. Secondary, reversible pulmonary vasoconstriction and pulmonary vascular thickening often develop along with the mitral stenosis, further adding to the burden on the right ventricle. As pulmonary pressure increases, right ventricular performance is reduced and symptoms of right heart failure may develop together with those of left heart failure.

[margin note: pressure grad. between LA + LV]

Diagnosis

History

In industrialized nations, the history that the patient with mitral stenosis suffered from acute rheumatic fever many years in the past is frequently unreliable. Thus, many patients who contend they have suffered from rheumatic fever have no evidence of valvular heart disease,

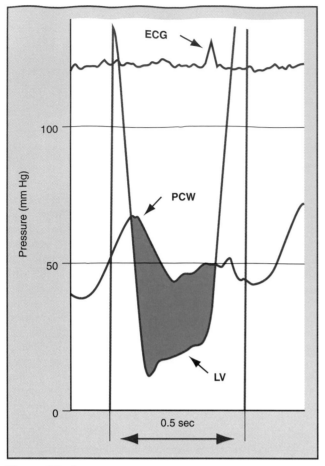

Figure 25-4

Pressure tracings taken from a patient with mitral stenosis demonstrate a large diastolic pressure gradient *(shaded area)* between the pulmonary capillary wedge pressure (PCW) representing left atrial pressure and the left ventricular pressure (LV). ECG, electrocardiogram. (Redrawn from Carabello, B.A., and Grossman, W. Calculation of stenotic valve orifice area. *In* Baim, D.S., and Grossman, W. [eds.]: Cardiac Catheterization, Angiography, and Intervention. 5th ed. Baltimore, Williams & Wilkins, 1996.)

whereas the majority of patients who clearly have rheumatic valvular deformities deny ever contracting acute rheumatic fever.

The typical symptoms of mitral stenosis are dyspnea on

Figure 25-5

Diagram of simultaneous pressure curves, auscultatory findings at the apex, and blood flow in mitral stenosis. When left ventricular (LV) pressure exceeds left atrial (LA) pressure, the mitral valve closes (M_1). When LV pressure falls below aortic (Ao) diastolic pressure, the aortic valve closes (A_2). When LV pressure falls below LA pressure, the mitral valve opens and an opening snap (OS) is heard as the valve is abnormal. Blood flow through the abnormal mitral valve is turbulent, generating a mid-diastolic murmur (MDM) and a presystolic murmur (PSM). (From Sutton, G.C.: Examination of the cardiovascular system. *In* Julian, D.G., et al. [eds.]: Diseases of the Heart. 2nd ed. London, W.B. Saunders, 1996, p. 150.)

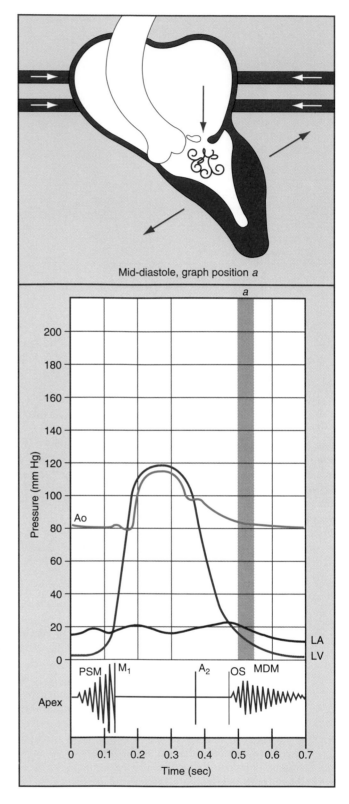

Mid-diastole, graph position *a*

exertion, orthopnea, and paroxysmal nocturnal dyspnea, which resemble the symptoms produced by left ventricular failure. As right-sided failure develops, ascites and edema are frequent complaints. Symptoms more specific for mitral stenosis (although less common) include hemoptysis, hoarseness, sudden decompensation when rapid atrial fibrillation develops, and systemic embolism. Hemoptysis occurs when high left atrial pressure ruptures small bronchial veins. Hoarseness develops as the enlarged left atrium impinges on the left recurrent laryngeal nerve (Ortner's syndrome). Atrial fibrillation with a rapid ventricular response—which is a common arrhythmia in mitral stenosis—reduces diastolic filling, thereby increasing left atrial pressure while simultaneously reducing left ventricular stroke volume, leading to abrupt cardiac decompensation. Atrial fibrillation together with mitral stenosis causes left atrial blood stasis and thrombus formation with potential for systemic embolization. Occasionally, otherwise asymptomatic patients present with a systemic embolism as the first manifestation of the condition. In some patients with vague symptoms, exercise testing is useful to objectively evaluate exercise tolerance.

Physical Examination

The typical murmur of mitral stenosis is a soft, low-pitched diastolic rumble best heard at the apex with the patient in the left lateral decubitus position. It is often missed if the patient is lying quietly. Hand-grip exercise or a few sit-ups may help to accentuate the murmur. The murmur is preceded by the sound of the stenotic mitral valve opening (opening snap) (see Fig. 25–5). High left atrial pressure in severe disease opens the mitral valve early in diastole, causing the interval between S_2 and the opening snap to be short (60 to 80 msec). In less-severe cases of mitral stenosis, lower left atrial pressure delays opening of the mitral valve and the S_2–opening snap interval is longer (>100 msec).

Another important clue to the presence of mitral stenosis is a loud first heart sound (S_1). In some cases where neither an opening snap nor a mitral rumble is audible, a loud S_1 may be the only clue on physical examination that mitral stenosis is present. The S_1 is typically loud in mitral stenosis because the transmitral gradient holds the valve open until it is closed by the force of ventricular systole. This varies from the normal condition where the mitral valve leaflets drift closed toward the end of diastole and thus move less and produce a softer S_1 when ventricular systole causes valve closure.

If pulmonary hypertension has developed, a loud second pulmonic heart sound and a right ventricular lift are noted. If pulmonary hypertension has led to right-sided heart failure, distended neck veins, ascites, and edema are usually found.

Laboratory Studies

The electrocardiogram frequently shows atrial fibrillation. If the patient is in sinus rhythm, a large notched P-wave is present in standard lead II and in lead V_1 (P

mitrale). In cases of pulmonary hypertension, a large R-wave in lead V_1 and a large S-wave in lead V_6 indicate right ventricular hypertrophy. The chest x-ray demonstrates several features typical of mitral stenosis. These include straightening of the left heart border due to left atrial enlargement, a double density along the right heart border as the left atrial shadow is seen inside the right atrial shadow, enlargement of the pulmonary arteries if pulmonary hypertension has developed, and the presence of Kerley B lines in the lung fields indicative of lymphatic hypertrophy secondary to increased pulmonary venous pressure.

However, despite the utility of the physical examination, electrocardiogram, and chest x-ray in diagnosing mitral stenosis, echocardiography is the best technique for evaluating the patient with this disorder (Fig. 25–6). Doppler interrogation can derive the transvalvular gradient and estimate the flow rate and mitral valve orifice area. In addition, the echocardiographic appearance of the valve is an excellent guide as to whether balloon mitral valvotomy, a nonsurgical procedure for relief of the stenosis, is applicable. Those patients with relatively pliant valve leaflets, little involvement of the subvalvular apparatus, limited mitral valve calcification, and no or mild mitral regurgitation are excellent candidates for balloon mitral valvotomy. Left ventricular ejection fraction and pulmonary artery pressure can also be estimated. If even mild tricuspid regurgitation exists, Doppler interrogation of the tricuspid valve can assess the reverse gradient between the right ventricle and the right atrium during systole. This in turn can be used to calculate pulmonary artery systolic pressure. If, for instance, the echocardiographically estimated systolic gradient across the tricuspid valve were 36 mm Hg and the right atrial pressure were judged to be 10 mm Hg by physical examination, then the peak right ventricular systolic pressure would be estimated at 46 mm Hg, which, in the absence of pulmonary stenosis, would also be the pulmonary artery systolic pressure.

Cardiac catheterization is usually not necessary to define the severity of mitral stenosis. However, catheterization is performed in older patients to identify coronary disease or as a precursor to balloon valvotomy.

Management

No therapy is required in asymptomatic patients in normal sinus rhythm. Symptoms of mild pulmonary congestion usually can be controlled with diuretics alone. For patients in sinus rhythm, digitalis is of little benefit, since contractile function is usually normal and the symptoms of congestive heart failure are due primarily to valve obstruction rather than to a contractile deficit. However, if the patient develops atrial fibrillation, prompt slowing of the heart rate is necessary, since, as noted previously, a rapid heart rate reduces mitral inflow, thereby increasing left atrial pressure and reducing cardiac output. Although digoxin is usually the drug of choice for chronically maintaining control of the ventricular response, intravenous diltiazem or esmolol may be preferable in the acute

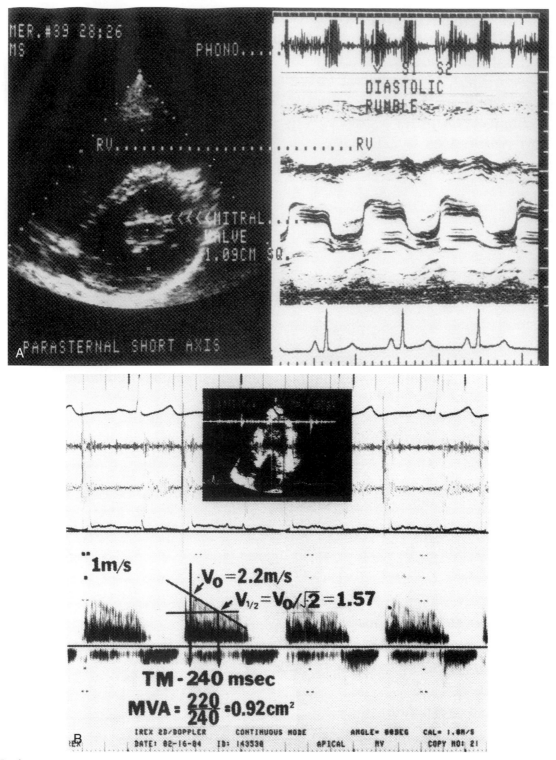

Figure 25–6

A, Cross-sectional image of the mitral valve used to planimeter its area. M-mode echocardiogram is at the *right*. This very stenotic valve has an orifice area of 1.09 cm². RV, right ventricle. *B,* The Doppler flow pattern for a patient with mitral stenosis. It demonstrates delay in decay of flow velocity that is maintained by the transmitral gradient. This principle, in turn, is used to calculate the pressure half-time that is divided into the empirical constant of 220 to calculate a mitral valve area (MVA). V_o, velocity at valve opening; TM, time from T_o to $T_{1/2}$. (*A* and *B,* from Assey, M.E., Usher, B.W., and Carabello, B.A.: The patient with valvular heart disease. *In* Pepine, C.J., Hill, J.A., and Lambert, C.R. [eds.]: Diagnostic and Therapeutic Cardiac Catheterization. 2nd ed. Baltimore, Williams & Wilkins, 1994.)

Figure 25–7

The steps of a balloon mitral valvotomy. *Top left,* Puncture of the interatrial septum with a guide wire *(curved arrow)* advanced across the septum through the mitral valve. *Bottom left,* A large sheath has been advanced over the guide wire *(curved arrow). Top right,* (1) An Inoue balloon catheter has been advanced across the mitral valve and the distal portion has been inflated and retracted snugly against the mitral valve. *Middle right,* (2) The proximal portion of the balloon has been partially inflated, leaving a waist at the site of the mitral valve stenosis. *Bottom right,* (3) The balloon has now been fully inflated and the waist has nearly disappeared, indicating successful separation in at least one of the commissures. (From Berman, A.D., McKay, R.G., and Grossman, W.: Balloon valvuloplasty. *In* Baim, D.S., and Grossman, W. [eds.]: Cardiac Catheterization, Angiography, and Intervention. 5th ed. Baltimore, Williams & Wilkins, 1996.)

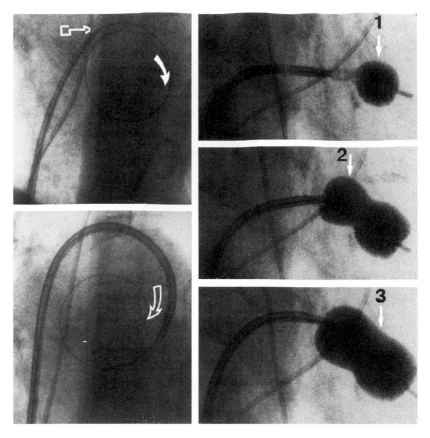

setting when a more rapid reduction in heart rate is required. Once heart rate has been reduced, restoration of sinus rhythm with quinidine or procainamide is usually achieved. If this therapy fails to restore sinus rhythm, electrical cardioversion is indicated.

If atrial fibrillation cannot easily and consistently be reverted to sinus rhythm, if sinus rhythm cannot be maintained, or if symptoms increase to greater than New York Heart Association classification II, that is, if patients develop symptoms on mild or moderate exertion, or if there is evidence that pulmonary hypertension is developing, mechanical correction of mitral stenosis is usually warranted because further delay worsens the prognosis. Unlike in aortic stenosis, in mitral stenosis, in most cases an excellent durable commissurotomy can be performed by balloon mitral valvotomy[5] (Fig. 25–7). In this procedure, transseptal catheterization is performed by advancing a sheathed catheter and needle from the right femoral vein to the right atrial side of the intra-atrial septum. The needle is advanced to puncture the septum, and the sheath is passed over the needle into the left atrium. A guide wire is passed through the sheath into the left ventricle. A balloon dilatation catheter is placed over the guide wire across the mitral orifice where it is inflated, producing a separation of the valve leaflets at the commissures. Typically, this results in doubling of the mitral valve area and reduces the transmitral valve gradient to 6 mm Hg or less, in turn improving symptomatic status. If the valve anatomy is unfavorable for balloon valvotomy, as can be determined by echocardiography (see earlier), open surgical commissurotomy or mitral valve replacement should be performed.

In patients with mitral stenosis and chronic atrial fibrillation who are not candidates for operation or balloon valvotomy because of coexisting disease or refusal to undergo the procedure, anticoagulation is desirable because the combination of atrial fibrillation and mitral stenosis produces an incidence of stroke of 5% to 10% per year in the absence of anticoagulation.

Table 25–2	**Mitral Stenosis: Guidelines for Medical Therapy and for Referral for Specialized Care**		
Symptoms (Including Atrial Fibrillation)	Valve Area (cm²)	Evidence of Pulmonary Hypertension (Clinical or Doppler)	Course of Action
None	>1.0	No	Observe
None	<1.0	No	Exercise to evaluate symptoms objectively; refer if exercise is severely limited
Mild	>1.0 <1.5	No	Observe
None	<1.5	Yes	Refer for further evaluation
Atrial fibrillation	<1.5	No or yes	Refer for further evaluation
Moderate	<1.5	No or yes	Refer for further evaluation

[handwritten annotation at top: MR Compensates c̄ dilatation of LV which somewhat ↓ the pulm HTN which would otherwise develop]

In summary, patients with mitral stenosis should undergo echocardiography when the disease is suspected or first detected. Patients are then followed by repeated clinical examination and echocardiography until symptoms limit lifestyle, atrial fibrillation occurs, or pulmonary hypertension (systolic pressure ≥ 50 mm Hg) develops. At this time, the patient should be referred for definitive mechanical correction of the stenosis.

In patients who present with far-advanced disease with severe pulmonary hypertension, surgical risk is increased. However, it is important to note that after successful operation, pulmonary artery pressure usually returns to or toward normal. Thus, pulmonary hypertension by itself is not a contraindication to referral for surgery or valvotomy.

Table 25–2 contains clinical and echocardiographic markers that guide the primary care physician in timing referral of mitral stenosis patients for specialized care.

MITRAL REGURGITATION

The mitral valve apparatus is composed of the mitral annulus, the mitral leaflets, the chordae tendineae, and the papillary muscles. When abnormalities of any of these four components cause mitral regurgitation, the regurgitation is classified as *primary*. In disease states where ventricular dilatation and changes in ventricular geometry cause malalignment of the papillary muscles, the regurgitation is considered to be *secondary*. Common causes of primary mitral regurgitation include endocarditis, spontaneous rupture of chordae tendineae, rheumatic heart disease, myocardial ischemia, the mitral valve prolapse syndrome, and collagen vascular disease.

Mitral regurgitation places a volume overload on the left ventricle. Normally, all of the blood that the left ventricle ejects enters the aorta and constitutes the effective forward cardiac output. In mitral regurgitation, a portion of the left ventricular end-diastolic volume is ejected into the left atrium; this regurgitation may be considered to be wasted or ineffective cardiac output.[6] Additionally, the regurgitant volume increases left atrial pressure, which is referred to the lungs where it causes pulmonary congestion. As shown in Figure 25–8, in acute mitral regurgitation when left ventricular hypertrophy has not yet had time to develop, there is a modest increase in end-diastolic volume as sarcomeres are stretched by the volume overload. This use of the Frank-Starling mechanism allows a modest increase in total stroke volume and also increases the work-generating capability of the ventricle. As the disease becomes more chronic, eccentric hypertrophy develops, allowing forward stroke volume to be returned toward normal. Additionally, the increased volume of both the left atrium and the left ventricle that develops with time allows the regurgitant volume to be accommodated at a lower diastolic pressure, reducing the symptoms of pulmonary congestion. This compensated stage may persist for several years but, if uncorrected, eventually leads to left ventricular muscle dysfunction.[7] A major goal of the management of mitral regurgitation is early recognition of left ventricular dysfunction, so that surgery can be performed to correct the mitral regurgitation before left ventricular dysfunction becomes permanent. It should be emphasized that the increased preload that results from the volume overload and the tendency for the regurgitant orifice to unload the ventricle during systole (reduced afterload) augment ventricular performance and cause ejection fraction to be higher than normal. In patients with mitral regurgitation, a fall of ejection fraction into the mid-normal range usually indicates the presence of muscle dysfunction.

Diagnosis

History

The patient with mitral regurgitation in the compensated phase of the disease is usually asymptomatic. Even fairly strenuous exercise is relatively well tolerated. However, in the acute phase before compensation has developed or later in the disease when decompensation is beginning to develop, symptoms typical of left-sided congestive heart failure (dyspnea on exertion, orthopnea, and paroxysmal nocturnal dyspnea) occur or the new onset of atrial fibrillation in the absence of other symptoms may presage the onset of left ventricular dysfunction.

Figure 25–8

The pathophysiologic stages of mitral regurgitation (MR). *A,* Normal physiology (N) is contrasted with that of acute mitral regurgitation (AMR). In AMR, the volume overload of MR increases sarcomere length (SL), augmenting preload. Increased SL is reflected by an increase in end-diastolic volume (EDV). The new pathologic pathway for ejection into the left atrium (LA) reduces afterload as quantified by end-systolic stress (ESS), allowing the left ventricle to eject more completely. Enhanced ejection is reflected by a fall in end-systolic volume (ESV). As a result, the total stroke volume increases to 140 cc, but because 50% is regurgitated into the LA (regurgitant fraction [RF] 0.50), forward stroke volume (FSV) falls. Ejection fraction (EF) increases, although contractile function (CF) is normal but not increased. *B,* AMR is contrasted with chronic compensated mitral regurgitation (CCMR). In CCMR, eccentric cardiac hypertrophy produces a further increase in EDV. This allows for a large increase in total stroke volume (190 cc) so that FSV returns to nearly normal. The now-enlarged LA can accommodate the regurgitant volume at a lower pressure, so that left atrial pressure declines. CF remains normal, and EF remains increased. *C,* CCMR is contrasted with chronic decompensated mitral regurgitation (CDMR). In this phase, CF has been reduced from muscle damage caused by prolonged severe volume overload. Reduced CF reduces the effectiveness of left ventricular ejection and ESV increases. There is a further increase in diastolic volume, which is not compensatory for the increase in ESV, resulting in a fall in total and forward stroke volume. Concomitantly, increased EDV worsens the MR by annular dilatation and papillary muscle malalignment and regurgitant fraction increases. EF is reduced from the CCMR state but often remains within the normal range. (*A–C,* Redrawn from Carabello, B.A.: Mitral regurgitation. Part 1: Basic pathophysiological principles. Mod. Concepts Cardiovasc. Dis. 57:53–58, 1988.)

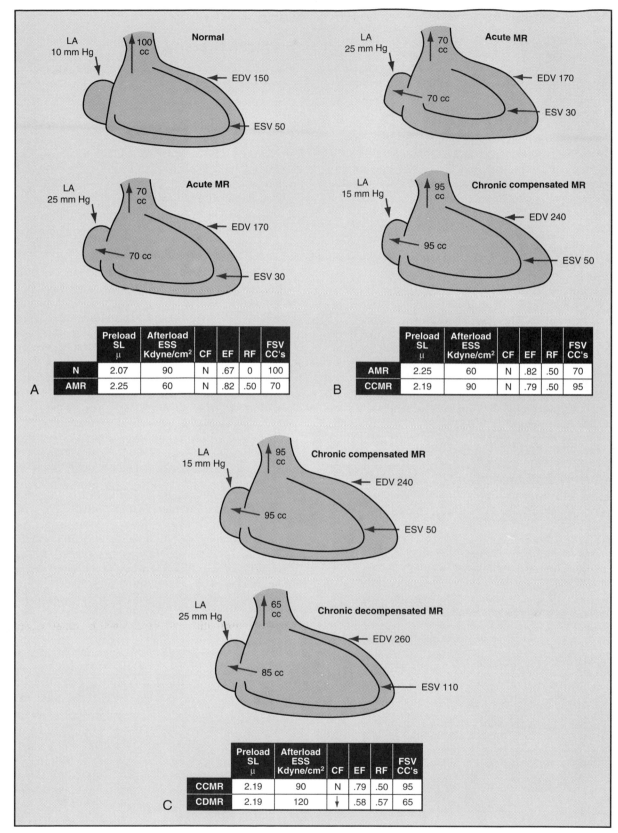

Figure 25–8 *See legend on opposite page*

[handwritten: MR should be corrected before EF falls <60% or ESD > 45 mm. (minor axis)]

Physical Examination

[handwritten: S₃ may not mean CHF]

Mitral regurgitation is most commonly recognized by the presence of a holosystolic murmur heard best at the apex, often radiating to the axilla. It is often accompanied by a systolic thrill. The enlarged volume-overloaded left ventricle causes a hyperactive precordium while displacing the point of maximal impulse downward and to the left. The rapid filling of the left ventricle in diastole by the large volume of blood stored in the left atrium during systole usually creates a third heart sound (S_3). As such, an S_3 in mitral regurgitation may simply be an indicator of the severity of the regurgitation and does not necessarily mean that the patient is in congestive heart failure. If secondary pulmonary hypertension has developed, findings of right-sided failure may also be present.

Laboratory Studies

The electrocardiogram shows left atrial abnormality and left ventricular hypertrophy. The chest x-ray shows an enlarged left ventricle and pulmonary congestion if the patient is in heart failure. The finding of a normal-sized heart on chest x-ray suggests either that the mitral regurgitation is relatively mild or that it is acute and eccentric hypertrophy has not yet had time to develop.

As in other valvular disorders, echocardiography is key in the assessment of mitral regurgitation (Fig. 25–9). During echocardiography, left ventricular dimensions and performance are gauged.[4, 7, 8] Color-flow Doppler provides an estimate of the severity of the mitral regurgitation. Often, the pathoanatomy that has produced the mitral regurgitation is discernible during transthoracic echocardiography. If not, transesophageal echocardiography that achieves superb imaging of the mitral valve is usually capable of diagnosing the cause of the mitral regurgitation.

Because the echocardiographic assessment of the severity of mitral regurgitation is occasionally inaccurate, cardiac catheterization usually is performed before surgery to assess hemodynamics, the ventriculographic severity of mitral regurgitation, and the coronary anatomy.

Management

Surgical Therapy

The only definitive treatment for mitral regurgitation is mitral valve surgery.[4] Surgery should be timed to occur before irreversible left ventricular dysfunction has developed. As noted earlier, the favorable loading conditions of mitral regurgitation augment ejection performance. Thus, a supernormal ejection fraction is "normal" in mitral regurgitation. In order to achieve a surgical outcome that allows for a normal postoperative life span, relief of symptoms, and normal postoperative ejection performance, mitral regurgitation should be corrected before left ventricular ejection fraction falls below 60% or before echocardiographic end-systolic minor-axis diameter exceeds 45 mm. Further delay in operation, even in *asymptomatic* patients, may result in persistent postoperative left ventricular dysfunction or reduced life span.

Currently, three types of operation are performed for the correction of mitral regurgitation—mitral valve replacement with removal of the mitral valve apparatus, mitral valve replacement with preservation of at least part of the mitral valve apparatus, and mitral valve repair in which a prosthetic valve is avoided and the native valve is reconstructed so that it becomes competent. Recently, the importance of the mitral valve apparatus in maintaining left ventricular function has been recognized. The mitral valve apparatus not only prevents mitral regurgitation but also acts as an internal skeleton integrating left ventricular contraction. Destruction of the apparatus reduces ejection performance and worsens postoperative outcome. Thus, every attempt should be made to conserve the continuity between the valve leaflet and the papillary muscle of at least a part of the mitral apparatus, even when a prosthetic valve is inserted. Mitral valve repair is the most desirable operation, since the mitral valve apparatus is conserved, retaining its function of augmenting left ventricular performance while at the same time avoiding the risks of a prosthesis, which include prosthetic valve failure, endocarditis, and thromboembolism.[9]

[handwritten: importance of mitral valve apparatus]

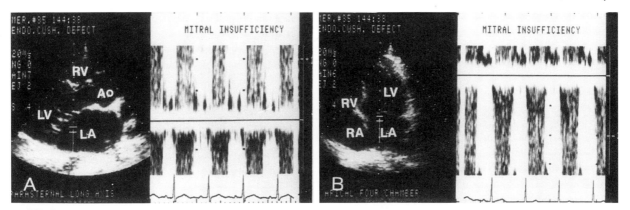

Figure 25–9

Parasternal long axis *(A)* and apical four-chamber *(B)* views of the heart of a patient with mitral regurgitation. Both left ventricular and left atrial enlargement are seen. Continuous-wave Doppler interrogation demonstrates mitral regurgitant flow. RV, right ventricle; Ao, aorta; LV, left ventricle; LA, left atrium; RA, right atrium. *(A and B,* From Assey, M.E., Usher, B.W., and Carabello, B.A.: The patient with valvular heart disease. *In* Pepine, C.J., Hill, J.A., and Lambert, C.R. [eds.]: Diagnostic and Therapeutic Cardiac Catheterization. 2nd ed. Baltimore, Williams & Wilkins, 1994.)

Medical Therapy

Medical therapy in mitral regurgitation is reserved for acute symptomatic mitral regurgitation and for patients with chronic symptomatic mitral regurgitation deemed not to be surgical candidates. In *acute* mitral regurgitation, the use of vasodilators such as ACE inhibitors or nitroprusside guided by Swan-Ganz catheterization is the mainstay of therapy. By reducing afterload, vasodilators increase aortic flow preferentially, at once increasing forward flow while reducing regurgitant volume and left atrial pressure. Concomitantly, vasodilator-mediated reduction in preload helps to relieve the symptoms of pulmonary congestion and also reduces left ventricular volume, which in part restores mitral valve competence. If acute mitral regurgitation has resulted in hypotension, intra-aortic balloon pumping, which reduces afterload while maintaining blood pressure, is substituted for vasodilators. In asymptomatic patients, no medical therapy is indicated.

Unlike in aortic regurgitation, where the use of vasodilators may forestall surgery in patients with asymptomatic chronic disease (see later), there is no convincing evidence that vasodilator therapy is of benefit in *chronic asymptomatic* mitral regurgitation. In patients with symptomatic chronic mitral regurgitation, digoxin diuretics and vasodilators form the mainstay of medical therapy.

In summary, asymptomatic patients with mitral regurgitation should be followed yearly with history, physical examination, and echocardiography. If symptoms develop or if ejection fraction declines to or approaches 60% or left ventricular end-systolic minor-axis diameter approaches 45 mm, the patient should be referred for preoperative evaluation. When possible, patients should be referred to surgeons known for excellence in mitral valve repair.

In patients with far-advanced disease, referral also is indicated for assessment for surgery. Such patients may still improve, provided the mitral valve apparatus can be preserved at the time of operation. If surgery is not deemed feasible, therapy with digoxin, diuretics, and an ACE inhibitor is indicated.

In severe acute mitral regurgitation, patients are usually unstable and require specialized therapy with intravenous vasodilators or intra-aortic balloon counterpulsation.

Table 25–3 presents markers that guide the primary care physician in the timing of referral of patients with mitral regurgitation for specialized care.

Table 25–3	Guidelines for Referral for Valve Surgery in Patients with Severe Mitral Regurgitation		
Symptoms	**ESD (mm)**	**EF**	**Course of Action**
None	<45	>0.60	Observe
Mild	<45	>0.60	Observe
>Mild	<45	>0.60	Refer for further evaluation
None	>45	or <0.60	Refer for further evaluation
Yes	>45	or <0.60	Refer for further evaluation

Abbreviations: ESD, end-systolic left ventricular diameter; EF, ejection fraction.

Pts c̄ MR should be referred for eval if more than mild sy, ESD >45 or EEF <60

MITRAL VALVE PROLAPSE

Mitral valve prolapse refers to a group of conditions in which one or both mitral valve leaflets become superior to the plane of the mitral annulus (prolapse into the left atrium) during systole.[4] The causes of mitral valve prolapse range from variations of normal physiology to severe anatomic deformity of the mitral valve. The former include normal subjects during the Valsalva maneuver as well as patients with atrial septal defect, in whom the left ventricle is reduced in volume; this reduces tension on the mitral apparatus, allowing the mitral valve to prolapse into the left atrium during systole. On release of the Valsalva maneuver or after repair of the atrial septal defect, left ventricular volume returns to normal and the mitral valve prolapse disappears. This variety of mitral valve prolapse is probably completely benign.

The most common pathologic cause of mitral valve prolapse is myxomatous degeneration of the valve. Other causes of pathologic prolapse include the Marfan syndrome, collagen vascular disease, and coronary artery disease. The term *mitral valve prolapse syndrome* refers to a degenerative condition of the mitral valve in which thickened and redundant leaflets are associated with atypical chest pain, autonomic dysfunction, and a modest risk of complications, including progression to severe mitral regurgitation, stroke, and infective endocarditis.

Diagnosis

HISTORY. Most patients with mitral valve prolapse are asymptomatic. A minority complain of atypical chest pain, palpitations, fatigue, and orthostatic lightheadedness. When mitral regurgitation is severe, the symptoms described previously in the section on Mitral Regurgitation may be present.

Physical Examination

Another name for the mitral valve prolapse syndrome is the *click-murmur syndrome,* derived from the findings during physical examination of patients with the disease. Classically, mitral valve prolapse produces a mid-systolic click and a late-systolic murmur (see Chap. 13). The click occurs as the elongated mitral valve apparatus reaches the end of its tether in mid systole. At this point, the valve leaflets pass the point of coaptation, causing mitral valve incompetence, and the murmur of mitral regurgitation commences. In some patients, only the click or only the murmur is present. In others, neither physical finding is present despite mitral valve prolapse proved by echocardiography.

The presence of the click and murmur and their position in the systolic portion of the cardiac cycle vary with maneuvers that alter left ventricular volume (see Chap. 13). Maneuvers that decrease volume, such as assuming the upright position or the Valsalva maneuver, cause the valve to prolapse earlier, so that the click is heard earlier in systole and the murmur becomes more holosystolic in nature. Maneuvers that increase left ventricular volume,

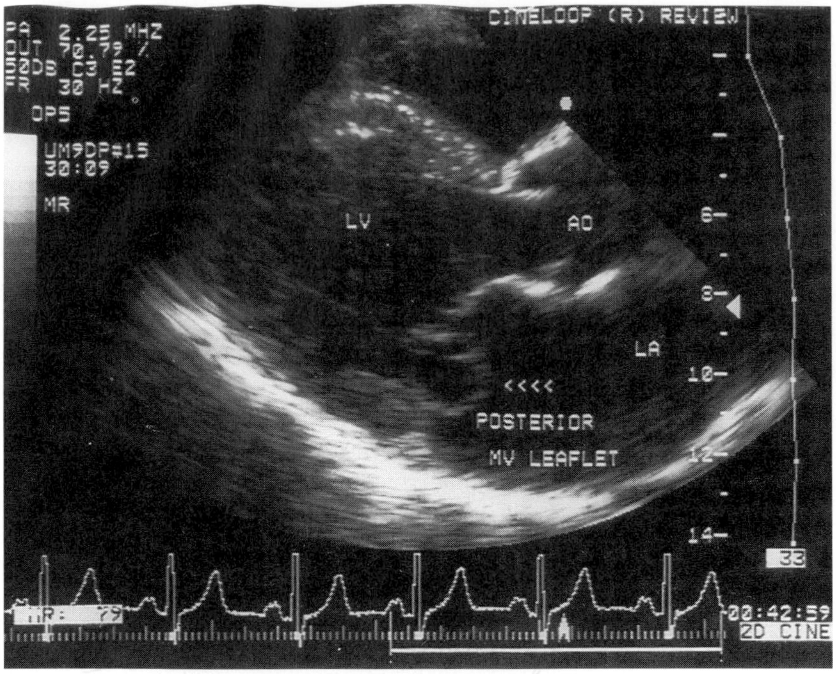

Figure 25–10
Two-dimensional echocardiogram shows severe prolapse of a thickened posterior mitral valve (MV) leaflet. LV, left ventricle; Ao, aorta; LA, left atrium. (From Carabello, B.A., Ballard, W.L., and Gazes, P.C.: Cardiology Pearls. Sahn, S.A., and Heffner, J.E. [ser. eds.]. Philadelphia, Hanley & Belfus, Inc., 1994.)

such as assuming recumbency or squatting, reduce the amount of prolapse and may cause the click and murmur to disappear entirely. With time, in some patients, degeneration of the valve worsens, so that the murmur becomes progressively more holosystolic as the degree of mitral regurgitation increases.

Laboratory Studies

The electrocardiogram in mitral valve prolapse is often normal, but it may demonstrate nonspecific ST and T-wave abnormalities, especially in the inferior leads.

Echocardiography is the diagnostic modality of choice to confirm this condition. The diagnosis of mitral valve prolapse is based on the appearance of one or both leaflets of the mitral valve superior to the annular plane in systole. However, the plane of the mitral annulus is not flat but rather has the configuration of a saddle (hyperbolic paraboloid). This configuration may cause the mitral valve to appear to be prolapsing in the echocardiographic apical four-chamber view when, in fact, prolapse is absent. Thus, the diagnosis of mitral valve prolapse seen in the apical four-chamber view must be confirmed in the parasternal long-axis view to avoid overdiagnosis of this condition. Diagnoses of mitral valve prolapse made before general recognition of this principle in 1987 may therefore have been made in error. Perhaps more important than diagnosing the prolapse itself (which can usually be detected on physical examination), echocardiography displays the morphology of the mitral valve (Fig. 25–10). As noted earlier, it is those patients whose valves are clearly anatomically abnormal (misshapen, redundant, and thickened) who are at risk for most of the complications of the disease. Doppler interrogation of the valve also allows estimation of the degree of mitral regurgitation that might be present.

Management

The majority of patients with mitral valve prolapse are asymptomatic and require no therapy. Those patients who have clearly abnormal valvular anatomy and who also have the murmur of mitral regurgitation should undergo endocarditis prophylaxis for those procedures that cause a bacteremia (see Chap. 16). In patients who complain of chest pain or palpitations, beta blockers, diltiazem or verapamil may be effective therapy. Some patients with mitral valve prolapse are at risk for stroke. These appear to be those patients who have anatomically misshapen valves and the murmur of mitral regurgitation. It has been speculated that this combination results in valve damage or perhaps denudation of the endothelium in the left atrium, providing a nidus for clot formation, which in turn, might embolize. In patients with thickened and redundant mitral valves, daily low-dose aspirin therapy is probably indicated, although no trials have been performed to substantiate this recommendation. When mitral valve prolapse has led to severe mitral regurgitation, the regurgitation is treated using the same principles detailed previously for the treatment of mitral regurgitation from any cause.

CHRONIC AORTIC REGURGITATION

The aortic valve may become incompetent due to pathology of either the aortic valve leaflets or the aortic root. Endocarditis and rheumatic heart disease are common valvular causes of aortic regurgitation. Idiopathic aortic root dilatation (annuloaortic ectasia) associated with hypertension and aging, Marfan's syndrome, aortic dis-

valve
endocarditis
rheumatic

root HTN, aging, Marfan's, dissection, syphilis, collagen vasc disease

section, syphilis, and collagen vascular disease affect the aortic root, leading to aortic regurgitation (see Chap. 27). A more complete list of the causes of aortic regurgitation is provided in Table 25–4.

As in mitral regurgitation, aortic regurgitation exerts a volume overload on the left ventricle. However, unlike mitral regurgitation, the excess stroke volume is ejected into a high-pressure chamber, the aorta, where it increases pulse pressure. Thus, systolic hypertension frequently accompanies aortic regurgitation, making it a combined pressure and volume overload. Appropriately, the ventricular hypertrophy that occurs differs from that of mitral regurgitation. In aortic regurgitation, there are both eccentric hypertrophy to accommodate the volume overload and modest concentric hypertrophy to compensate for the pressure overload. As with severe mitral regurgitation, severe aortic regurgitation may be tolerated for a prolonged period of time. Eventually, however, left ventricular function declines. Thus, as with mitral regurgitation, aortic regurgitation should be corrected before left ventricular dysfunction becomes severe and irreversible.

Diagnosis

History

Patients with severe aortic regurgitation and normal left ventricular function may be remarkably asymptomatic, even during strenuous exertion. When symptoms do develop, they are usually those of left-sided congestive heart failure. Occasionally, angina occurs in patients with aortic regurgitation, although much less frequently than in patients with aortic stenosis. Angina probably develops in part due to the relative diastolic hypotension that develops due to the valve incompetence. Since the coronary arteries fill in diastole, a lowered diastolic blood pressure reduces the driving force filling the coronary arteries and reduces coronary blood flow. When angina does occur in aortic regurgitation, it is frequently associated with vasodilatation and flushing. Less common complaints in patients with aortic regurgitation include syncope, an unpleasant awareness of the heartbeat, or carotid artery pain.

Physical Examination

The typical murmur of aortic regurgitation is a high-pitched, early-decrescendo blowing diastolic murmur heard best along the left sternal border when the patient is sitting upright. As the regurgitant jet impinges on the mitral valve, it may cause partial valve closure and a low-pitched rumble of physiologic mitral stenosis (Austin Flint murmur). In chronic aortic regurgitation, the precordium is extremely active and the point of maximal impulse is displaced downward and to the left. The high total stroke volume and wide pulse pressure produce a myriad of signs. These include Corrigan's pulse (a brisk carotid upstroke with a rapid decline), de Musset's sign (bobbing of the head), Duroziez's sign (a systolic and diastolic bruit when the femoral artery is compressed by

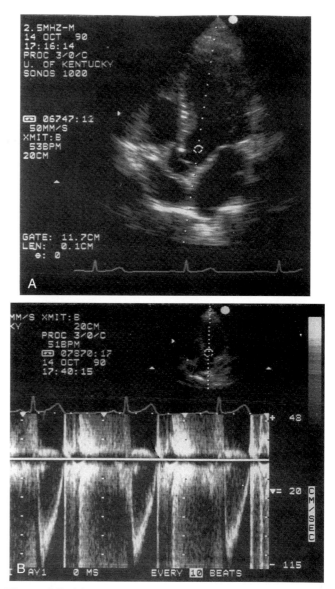

Figure 25–11

Pulsed-wave mapping technique for quantitating aortic regurgitation. Two-dimensional echocardiogram still frames were taken from the apical four-chamber view and show the location of the pulsed-wave sample volume (*A*) and spectral recordings from each site (*B*). Sample volume located just below the aortic valve and pulsed-wave recording demonstrate holodiastolic, high-velocity, and broad-banded signal indicative of turbulent regurgitant flow. (*A* and *B*, From Smith, M.D.: Evaluation of valvular regurgitation by Doppler echocardiography. *In* Carabello, B.A., [guest ed.]: Valvular Heart Disease. Cardiol. Clin. Vol. 9, May 1991.)

Table 25–4	Causes of Aortic Regurgitation	
Aortic Root Cause	**Valve Leaflet Cause**
Aortic dissection	Infective endocarditis
Marfan's syndrome	Rheumatic heart disease
Annuloaortic ectasia	
Syphilis	
Ehlers-Danlos syndrome	
Ankylosing spondylitis	
Aortitis of any cause	
Pseudoxanthoma elasticum	
Systemic lupus erythematosus	

the bell of the stethoscope), Hill's sign (augmentation of the systolic femoral blood pressure of greater than 30 mm over brachial systolic pressure), and Quincke's pulse (systolic plethora and diastolic blanching of the nail bed when gentle pressure is placed on the nail).

Laboratory Studies

In severe aortic regurgitation, the electrocardiogram usually shows left ventricular hypertrophy. The chest x-ray demonstrates an enlarged heart, often with dilatation of the proximal aorta. The echocardiogram demonstrates an enlarged left ventricle (Fig. 25–11). The valvular or aortic root anatomy responsible for aortic regurgitation may be detected. Color-flow Doppler interrogation of the aortic valve demonstrates the aortic regurgitation and helps quantify its severity (Fig. 25–12).

When surgery is contemplated, cardiac catheterization is usually performed to confirm the echocardiographic estimate of regurgitant severity by aortography. Coronary arteriography is also performed to assess the presence of coronary artery disease.

Management *usually replacement is necessary.*

TIMING OF OPERATION. As with mitral regurgitation, correction of aortic insufficiency must be performed before the development of irreversible left ventricular dysfunction, if the symptoms of heart failure (if present) are to be relieved and the patient is to attain a normal postoperative life span. Unlike in mitral regurgitation, however, in most cases of aortic regurgitation, valve replacement instead of repair is necessary. Thus, in deciding when to operate, the risks of a prosthesis must be weighed against the risk of delaying surgery.[10] The "55 rule" has been extremely useful in making this decision. Sound studies demonstrate that a good outcome can be

ECHO q2yrs if ESD < 40
refer for surgical eval
if ESD > 55 mm
or EF < 55%
or > mild sympt

asymptomatic — vasodilators

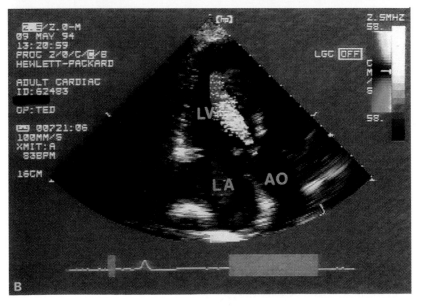

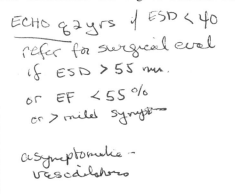

Figure 25–12

A, Apical five-chamber view of the heart with color-flow Doppler shows aortic regurgitation with a jet extending from the aortic valve leaflets almost to the apex of the left ventricle consistent with moderately severe aortic regurgitation. RV, right ventricle; RA, right atrium; LA, left atrium; AO, aorta; *B,* Apical long-axis view of the left ventricle (LV) in the same patient shows a regurgitant aortic jet extending from the aortic valve leaflets to the apex of the ventricle consistent with moderately severe aortic regurgitation. (*A* and *B,* From Young, G.D., and St. John Sutton, M.: Echocardiography and Doppler ultrasound. *In* Julian, D.G., Camm, A.J., Fox, K.M., et al. [eds.]: Diseases of the Heart. 2nd ed. London, W.B. Saunders, 1996, Plate 16.1.)

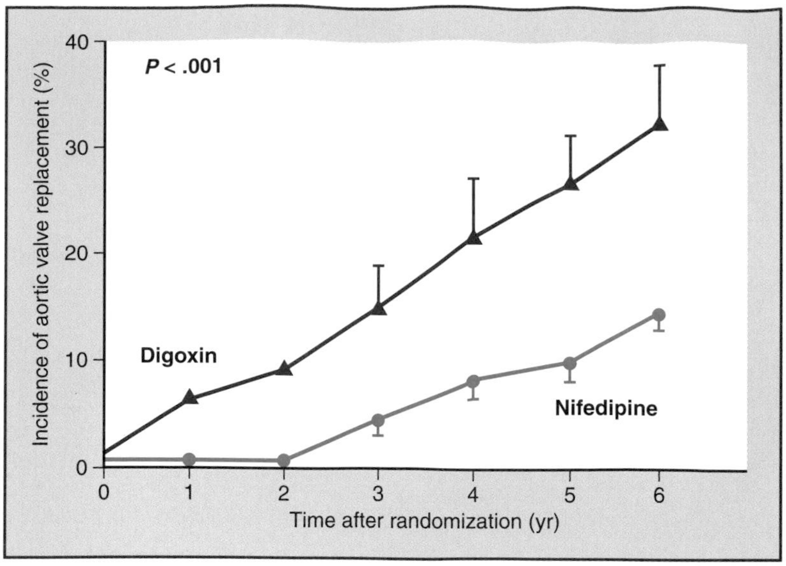

Figure 25–13

The need for aortic valve replacement for asymptomatic patients with aortic regurgitation is compared for a group of such patients treated with digoxin versus a group treated with nifedipine. Nifedipine delayed the onset of symptoms and reduced the need for aortic valve replacement. (Redrawn from Scognamiglio, R., Rahimtoola, S.H., Fasoli, G., et al.: Nifedipine in asymptomatic patients with severe aortic regurgitation and normal left ventricular function. N. Engl. J. Med. 331:689–694, 1994. Copyright 1994 Massachusetts Medical Society. All rights reserved.)

expected, provided that the left ventricular echocardiographic end-systolic minor-axis diameter does not exceed 55 mm and that the left ventricular ejection fraction is not lower than 55%. Thus, for asymptomatic patients, operation can be delayed until either symptoms develop or the aforementioned thresholds are approached. If end-systolic diameter is less than 40 mm, it is unlikely that ventricular dysfunction will develop within 2 years, and thus, echocardiography can safely be performed at 2-year intervals. For end-systolic diameters between 40 and 50 mm, yearly echocardiographic follow-up is recommended, and if end-systolic diameter is greater than 50 mm but less than 55 mm, echocardiographic follow-up should be performed every 6 months. When symptoms of heart failure develop in a patient with severe aortic regurgitation, surgery should be performed regardless of the echocardiographic findings because the new onset of heart failure indicates cardiac decompensation.

There is increasing evidence that vasodilator therapy in asymptomatic patients with normal left ventricular function can delay both the onset of left ventricular dysfunction and the need for surgery (Fig. 25–13).[11] The best documentation for this effect exists for nifedipine, although it is likely that other dihydropyridine calcium channel blockers and possibly ACE inhibitors may provide the same benefit.

OVERALL STRATEGY. Asymptomatic patients with moderate to severe chronic aortic insufficiency should receive long-acting nifedipine, 30 to 60 mg per day. In the future, other vasodilators may be shown to be equally effective to nifedipine. Thus, it is probably reasonable to substitute other dihydropyridine calcium blockers such as amlodipine or an ACE inhibitor if nifedipine is poorly tolerated. Clinical and echocardiographic follow-up should be performed at intervals determined by left ventricular end-systolic dimension. When either symptoms develop or ejection fraction approaches 0.55 or end-systolic diameter approaches 55 mm, patients should be referred for preoperative workup including cardiac catheterization, aortography, and coronary arteriography. Table 25–5 provides markers that guide the primary care physician in timing of referral of the patient with aortic regurgitation for specialized care.

ACUTE AORTIC REGURGITATION

Acute aortic regurgitation often constitutes a medical emergency, but unfortunately, this condition may be difficult to recognize. In acute aortic regurgitation, there is a sudden fall in cardiac output, resulting in hypotension, and a sudden rise in left ventricular diastolic pressure, both events acting in concert to reduce coronary blood flow.[12] Perhaps because of this coronary pathophysiology, the mortality of acute aortic regurgitation treated medically approaches 75% if even mild heart failure develops. On the other hand, surgical treatment has a mortality of less than 25%. Most cases of severe acute aortic regurgitation are caused by infective endocarditis. Although there is a persistent fear that a prosthetic valve might become reinfected if it is implanted early in the patient's course of antibiotic therapy, reinfection is relatively rare, occurring in only 10% of prosthetic valves even when they are implanted within 48 hours of the last positive blood culture (see Chap. 16).

Table 25–5	Guidelines for Referral for Patients with Severe Chronic Aortic Regurgitation			
Symptoms	**ESD (mm)**		**EF**	**Course of Action**
None	<55		>0.55	Begin vasodilators, observe
>Mild	<55		>0.55	Refer for further evaluation
None	≥55	or	<0.55	Refer for further evaluation
Yes	≥55	or	<0.55	Refer for further evaluation

Abbreviations: ESD, left ventricular end systolic diameter; EF, ejection fraction.

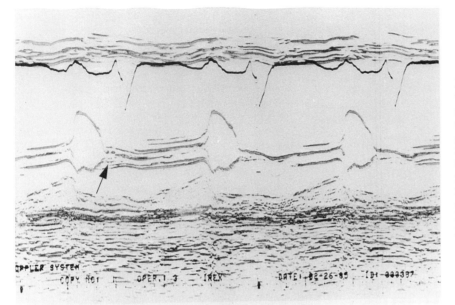

Figure 25–14

The M-mode echocardiogram in a patient with acute severe aortic regurgitation. The mitral valve tracings are shown just below the electrocardiogram. The mitral valve is seen to close well before the QRS (mitral valve preclosure, *arrow*), indicating very high left ventricular end-diastolic pressure and the need for urgent aortic valve replacement. (From Carabello, B.A., Usher, B.W., and Gwinn, N.S.: Cardiology. *In* Sahn, S.A., and Heffner, J.E. [eds.]: Critical Care Pearls. Philadelphia, Hanley & Belfus, 1989.)

[Handwritten margin notes:] in acute MR most physical signs are absent short, blowing diastolic murmur ↓ S₁ (MV preclosure) Seen on M-mode

As noted previously, a large total stroke volume and wide pulse pressure and the resultant eccentric hypertrophy cause most of the signs of chronic aortic regurgitation. In acute aortic regurgitation, eccentric hypertrophy has not yet developed and both the wide pulse pressure and the large stroke volume are absent, as are most of the signs of aortic regurgitation. In fact, a short, blowing diastolic murmur may be the only clue of this condition on physical examination.

Diagnosis

Because it is the onset of heart failure that makes the outcome of medical therapy poor, the signs of even mild heart failure should be carefully elicited on physical examination. Besides listening for the typical murmur, close attention should be directed to S₁. In severe acute aortic regurgitation, left ventricular filling from the aorta closes the mitral valve before ventricular systole (mitral valve preclosure), decreasing the intensity of S₁. Mitral valve preclosure suspected on physical examination and confirmed echocardiographically is an ominous sign indicating the need for urgent aortic valve replacement.

ECHOCARDIOGRAPHY. Once acute aortic regurgitation is suspected, prompt echocardiography is mandatory. An M-mode echocardiogram is used to search for premature mitral valve closure (demonstrated in Fig. 25–14), an important indicator regarding the timing of operation. In addition, aortic valve vegetations confirming the diagnosis of endocarditis and Doppler flow interrogation of the aortic valve to assess the severity of aortic regurgitation can be obtained.

In most cases of acute aortic regurgitation, cardiac catheterization is not necessary. Most cases affect younger patients in whom there is no reason to suspect coronary artery disease. Thus, the data needed to judge whether operation is necessary usually can be obtained during physical examination and echocardiography.

Management

In patients who are entirely asymptomatic, conservative management is possible. If infective endocarditis is the cause of the acute aortic regurgitation, appropriate antibiotic therapy is employed (see Chap. 16). Such patients should be followed carefully clinically for signs of heart failure. If these occur, referral for preoperative workup is indicated. In some cases, preoperative improvement is afforded by using hemodynamic monitoring and vasodilators. However, this strategy should not be used to delay surgery but rather as an attempt to improve the patient's condition preoperatively.

TRICUSPID REGURGITATION

The most important cause of primary tricuspid regurgitation is infective endocarditis (see Chap. 16). Tricuspid valve involvement occurs in only 10% of the general population who develop endocarditis but increases to 50% among users of illicit intravenous drugs who develop endocarditis. Most tricuspid regurgitation is secondary to right ventricular dilatation and failure, which in turn may be caused by left heart failure, primary lung disease, primary pulmonary hypertension, or an intracardiac shunt. Although the volume overload imposed on the right ventricle by tricuspid regurgitation may worsen the patient's overall condition, the right ventricle tolerates tricuspid regurgitation remarkably well. Therefore, treatment is usually aimed at improving the diseases responsible for the tricuspid regurgitation rather than at surgical correction.

Diagnosis

HISTORY. There are no features in the patient's history specific for tricuspid regurgitation. Its presence worsens the symptoms of right ventricular failure, including fatigue, edema, and ascites.

PHYSICAL EXAMINATION. The murmur typical of tricuspid regurgitation is a holosystolic murmur heard along the left sternal border. The murmur increases with inspiration as negative intrathoracic pressure increases right ventricular inflow and outflow. However, in end-stage right ventricular failure, inspiration fails to augment right ventricular filling, and the inspiratory increase in the murmur does not occur. On physical examination, there are also signs of right ventricular enlargement, most commonly manifest as a parasternal lift. Examination of the neck veins reveals large V-waves. This corresponds to systolic expansion of the liver, which may be palpated in the right upper quadrant. The liver may be tender if right ventricular failure has been rapid in onset.

LABORATORY STUDIES. The electrocardiogram shows right-axis deviation and evidence of right ventricular hypertrophy. Right ventricular enlargement is seen on the chest x-ray as obliteration of the retrosternal air space.

The echocardiogram demonstrates both right atrial and right ventricular enlargement. Doppler interrogation of the tricuspid valve demonstrates retrograde systolic tricuspid flow (Fig. 25–15). Pulmonary artery pressure can be esti-

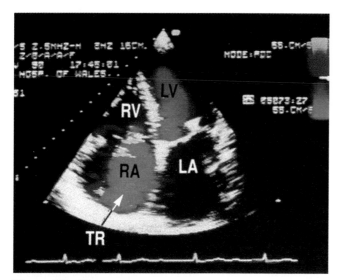

Figure 25–15

Apical four-chamber view with color-flow Doppler of a patient with severe tricuspid regurgitation (TR). Most of the right atrium (RA) is filled with blue, which represents the TR. RV, right ventricle; LV, left ventricle; LA, left atrium. (From Hall, R.J.C., and Nitter-Hauge, S.: Other valve disorders; a] tricuspid-pulmonary and mixed lesions; b] prosthetic valves. *In* Julian, D.G., Camm, A.J., Fox, K.M., et al. [eds.]: Diseases of the Heart. 2nd ed. London, W.B. Saunders, 1996, Plate 42.1.)

mated and is used to identify pulmonary hypertension as the cause of right ventricular decompensation. If endocarditis is the primary cause of tricuspid regurgitation, vegetations are often imaged.

Cardiac catheterization is rarely indicated in the diagnosis of tricuspid regurgitation. Right ventriculography to demonstrate tricuspid regurgitation is not commonly practiced because introduction of a catheter across the tricuspid valve to perform the study can by itself cause tricuspid regurgitation, introducing the possibility of artifact into the study. If cardiac catheterization is performed, right atrial pressure tracings show a large V-wave; as the tricuspid regurgitation worsens, the right atrial pressure tracing progressively resembles more that of a right ventricular pressure tracing.

Management

The management of tricuspid regurgitation is usually aimed at treating the disease responsible for right ventricular decompensation. Thus, if left heart failure caused right heart failure, the focus is on improving left ventricular performance. In chronic secondary tricuspid regurgitation, diuretics are the mainstay of therapy in reducing right ventricular volume overload. Vasodilators, which have such an important role in the treatment of left ventricular failure, have little effect on the pulmonary vascular bed and, thus, usually do little to help reduce primary tricuspid regurgitation. Since most cases of primary tricuspid regurgitation stem from infective endocarditis secondary to illicit drug use, there is usually little enthusiasm for tricuspid valve replacement, for fear that the valve prosthesis will become infected during subsequent drug use. However, in some cases, especially those in which infected emboli have produced pulmonary hypertension, tricuspid valve replacement may be necessary. Although there is only modest experience with tricuspid valve repair, this strategy is attractive because it avoids a prosthesis and may be appropriate therapy for some patients.

VALVE PROSTHESES

All valvular prostheses have their own inherent drawbacks.[13,14] Although insertion of the prosthesis improves the condition for which it was inserted and, when operation is timed properly, can offer the patient a normal life span, thromboembolism, endocarditis, and primary valve failure all complicate the use of prosthetic valves. Further, all prostheses are inherently stenotic compared with normal native valve. For this reason, emphasis on valve repair is increasing, and it is agreed that, whenever possible, the patient's native valve should be repaired rather than replaced with a prosthesis. Repair is now possible in most cases of nonrheumatic mitral regurgitation and in about 10% to 15% of cases of aortic regurgitation. Balloon valvotomy is successful in the long-term treatment of pulmonic stenosis and in many cases of mitral stenosis, permitting correction of these conditions without the use of a prosthesis. However, in acquired calcific aortic

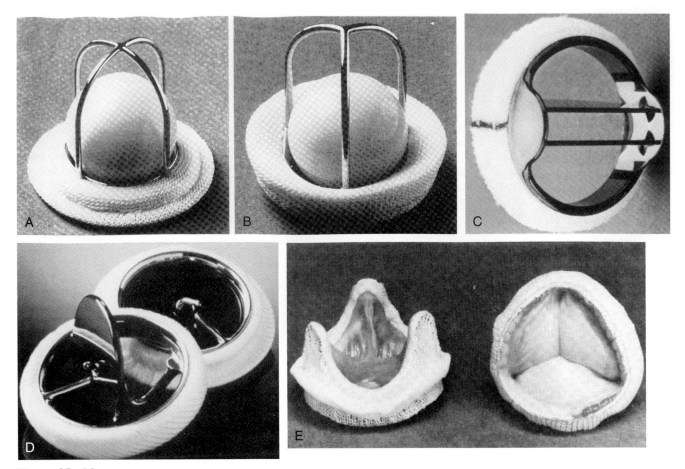

Figure 25-16
Several types of valve prostheses. *A,* Starr-Edwards caged-ball mitral prosthesis. *B,* Starr-Edwards caged-ball aortic prosthesis. *C,* St. Jude Medical bileaflet valve. *D,* Medtronic-Hall tilting disk valve. *E,* The Carpentier-Edwards bioprosthesis. (*A–E,* From Wernley, J.A., and Crawford, M.H. Choosing a prosthetic heart valve. *In* Carabello, B.A. [guest ed.]: Valvular Heart Disease. Cardiol. Clin. Vol. 9, May 1991.)

stenosis, valve degeneration is so extensive that repair is virtually impossible and a prosthesis must be inserted. Options for prosthetic valves include bioprosthetic heterografts, bioprosthetic homografts, and mechanical valves. Transplantation of the patient's pulmonary valve into the aortic position, with use of a homograft in the pulmonary position (the Ross procedure), is attractive in young patients because the pulmonary autograft can grow with the patient. Some of the commonly used prosthetic valves are demonstrated in Figure 25-16.

Bioprosthetic Heterografts

Bioprosthetic heterografts are typically made from porcine aortic valves that can be inserted in any position. Their advantage is a low incidence of thromboembolism, and therefore, anticoagulation is not required. Their major drawback is primary valve failure. The younger the patient, the sooner deterioration occurs, and the older the patient, the more delayed deterioration is. For example, in a 30-year-old patient, deterioration often occurs within 5 years of implantation, whereas in the 70-year-old patient, valvular function is likely to remain normal for at least

10 years. Thus, these valves are particularly appropriate for use in older patients. They also are used in young women who wish to become pregnant, since warfarin anticoagulation, which has a high risk for causing fetal damage, is not required. However, in such cases, the need for eventual valve rereplacement is almost certain. Stent-free human homograft valves are sewn into the aortic position and, occasionally, can be modified for use in the mitral position. They do not require anticoagulation and seem especially resistant to endocarditis. They appear durable, although long-term follow-up is limited.

Mechanical Valves

Mechanical valves are extremely durable, and some have an excellent hemodynamic profile with low transvalvular gradients even in small-sized valves. However, all require lifetime anticoagulation to avoid the high risk of thromboembolism. Mechanical valves are particularly useful in patients with a small aortic annulus and in young patients with a long life expectancy. They should be avoided in patients who are unwilling to take warfarin faithfully or who are at high risk for bleeding.

In choosing a valve prosthesis, the need for durability,

Table 25–6		Characteristics of Commonly Used Prosthetic Valves		
Name	**Type**	**Anticoagulant**	**Durability**
Carpentier-Edwards	B	No, unless large LA and AF	5–15 yr
Hancock	B	Same	5–15 yr
St. Jude	M, L$_2$	Yes	Unlimited
Medtronic-Hall	M, TD	Yes	Unlimited
Starr-Edwards	M, CB	Yes	Unlimited

Abbreviations: B, bioprosthesis; LA, left atrium; AF, atrial fibrillation; M, mechanical; L$_2$, bileaflet; TD, tilting disk; CB, caged ball.

the risk of anticoagulation, the hemodynamics of the prosthesis, and patient preference must all be considered. The ultimate decision is often not made until the native valve has been examined at operation, at which time the surgeon chooses a valve that maximizes benefit and minimizes risk.

Table 25–6 lists some of the characteristics of commonly used prosthetic valves.

References

1. Ross, J., Jr., and Braunwald, E.: Aortic stenosis. Circulation 38(Suppl V):V-61, 1968.
2. Pellikka, P.A., Nishimura, R.A., Bailey, K.R., et al.: The natural history of adults with asymptomatic, hemodynamically significant aortic stenosis. J. Am. Coll. Cardiol. 15:1012, 1990.
3. Roy, S.B., and Gopinath, N.: Mitral stenosis. Circulation 38(Suppl V):V-68, 1968.
4. Braunwald, E.: Valvular heart disease. *In* Fauci, A.S., Braunwald, E., Isselbacher, K.J., et al. (eds.): Harrison's Principles of Internal Medicine. 14th ed. New York, McGraw-Hill, 1998, pp. 1311–1324.
5. Reyes, V.P., Raju, B.S., Wynne, J., et al.: Percutaneous balloon valvuloplasty compared with open surgical commissurotomy for mitral stenosis. N. Engl. J. Med. 331:961, 1994.
6. Carabello, B.A.: Mitral regurgitation. Part 1: Basic pathophysiologic principles. Mod. Concepts Cardiovasc. Dis. 57:53, 1988.
7. Zile, M.R., Gaasch, W.H., Carroll, J.D., et al.: Chronic mitral regurgitation: Predictive value of preoperative echocardiographic indexes of left ventricular function and wall stress. J. Am. Coll. Cardiol. 3:235, 1984.
8. Enriquez-Sarano, M., Tajik, A.J., Schaff, H.V., et al.: Echocardiographic prediction of survival after surgical correction of organic mitral regurgitation. Circulation 90:830, 1994.
9. Goldman, M.E., Mora, F., Guarino, T., et al.: Mitral valvuloplasty is superior to valve replacement for preservation of left ventricular function: An intraoperative two-dimensional echocardiographic study. J. Am. Coll. Cardiol. 10:568, 1987.
10. Bonow, R.O., Lakatos, E., Maron, B.J., et al.: Serial long-term assessment of the natural history of asymptomatic patients with chronic aortic regurgitation and normal left ventricular systolic function. Circulation 84:1625, 1991.
11. Scognamiglio, R., Rahimtoola, S.H., Fasoli, G., et al.: Nifedipine in asymptomatic patients with severe aortic regurgitation and normal left ventricular function. N. Engl. J. Med. 331:689, 1994.
12. Mann, T., McLaurin, L., Grossman, W., et al.: Assessing the hemodynamic severity of acute aortic regurgitation due to infective endocarditis. N. Engl. J. Med. 293:108, 1975.
13. Lindblom, D., Lindblom, U., Qvist, J., et al.: Long-term relative survival rates after heart valve replacement. J. Am. Coll. Cardiol. 15:566, 1990.

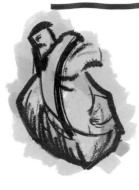

Chapter 26

Recognition and Management of Adults with

Congenital Heart Disease

ELYSE FOSTER AND MELVIN D. CHEITLIN

Congenital heart disease occurs in 0.3% of all live births. Most patients with congenital heart disease are recognized in infancy or childhood and appropriately treated. Since cardiopulmonary bypass capabilities were developed in the early 1950s, amazing advances in surgical treatment for infants and children with major congenital heart lesions have permitted survival into adulthood. Most patients with major congenital heart disease who have been surgically corrected or palliated will reach adulthood and child-bearing age. Even lesions such as transposition of the great arteries, which invariably was fatal in the first year of life, are now surgically ameliorated. Thus, it is estimated that the number of patients with congenital heart disease reaching adulthood is 20,000 per year in the United States alone.[1] Since patients with congenital heart disease have an increased risk of bearing offspring with congenital heart disease, the prevalence of congenital heart disease in newborns may also be rising.

Because the embryology of the formation of the heart and cardiovascular system is complex, there are many stages at which abnormalities can occur, leading to a wide variety of congenital heart abnormalities. All congenital heart lesions will fall into one or more of the following anatomic-pathophysiologic categories listed in Table 26–1: (1) predominant left-to-right shunts, (2) predominant right-to-left shunts, (3) stenotic or atretic valves and hypoplastic ventricles, (4) great vessel abnormalities, (5) positional abnormalities, and (6) other congenital syndromes. Examples of specific lesions falling into each of these categories are listed in Table 26–1.

Therefore, the aims of this chapter are:

1. To describe the clinical presentation, recommended diagnostic evaluation, and indications for surgery of the most common unoperated congenital lesions encountered in the adult patient (Tables 26–2 and 26–3).
2. To describe the most common complications that arise after palliative surgery for congenital heart disease.[2]
3. To describe the interaction between congenital heart disease and systemic illnesses.

Prospective clinical trials comparing treatments for the various types of congenital heart disease have not been performed. Recommendations for treatment are based on experience and the well-documented natural history of the disease.[3] It is not reasonable to expect a primary care physician to manage patients with complicated congenital heart disease without the aid of a cardiologist experienced in the care of these patients.

The primary care physician will see the adult patient with congenital heart disease in the following ways:

1. *Minor congenital abnormalities.* Examples include single anomalous pulmonary vein, bicuspid aortic valve, and mild coarctation of the aorta. In these conditions, the problem for the primary care physician is, first, to recognize the abnormality and, second, to understand the natural history of these lesions. For instance, a patient with a bicuspid aortic valve may do well until age 40 or 50 years when progressive valve calcification leads to severe aortic stenosis.
2. *Major untreated congenital heart disease.* At times, significant congenital heart disease can be overlooked during childhood. The most common lesion is an atrial septal defect, but occasionally, a ventricular septal defect or even a patent ductus arteriosus is missed. A second type of patient has untreated congenital heart disease because there was previously or is at present no adequate palliative surgical procedure. Such conditions include pulmonary vascular disease and pulmonary hypertension, as well as lesions that markedly restrict pulmonary blood flow because of small pulmonary arteries that can be neither grafted nor shunted successfully. These patients can be very difficult to treat, and usually, their only option is lung transplantation with or without heart transplantation or intracardiac repair. Rarely, previously untreated patients will have "single-ventricle" lesions, usually associated

Table 26–1	**Anatomic-Pathophysiologic Classification of Congenital Heart Disease**		
	Definition	**Level**	**Example (e.g., Lesion)**
I. Left-right shunt	Pulmonary venous return shunted to right heart (PBF > SBF)	At venous level	Pulmonary vein draining into superior vena cava
		At atrial level	Atrial septal defect
		At ventricular level	Interventricular septal defect
		At arterial level	Patent ductus arteriosus
II. Right-left shunt	Systemic venous return shunted to left heart* (SBF > PBF) "cyanotic heart disease"	At venous level	Superior vena cava into left atrium
		At atrial level	Tricuspid atresia
		At ventricular level	Tetralogy of Fallot
		At arterial level	Transposition of the great vessels
			Truncus arteriosus
III. Stenotic and hypoplastic valves or ventricles			Congenital aortic stenosis
			Congenital pulmonic stenosis
			Pulmonary atresia
			Left heart hypoplasia
IV. Great vessel abnormalities		Arterial	Coarctation of the aorta
		Venous	Total anomalous pulmonary venous drainage
V. Positional abnormalities			Corrected transposition (L-TGV)
			Dextrocardia dextraposition
			Transposition of the great vessels
VI. Other congenital syndromes with aortic involvement			Marfan's syndrome
			Muscular dystrophy

Abbreviations: PBF, pulmonary blood flow; SBF, systemic blood flow; L-TGV, L-transposition of the great vessels.
* Also reversal of left-to-right shunt at atrial, ventricular, or arterial level in a patient with Eisenmenger's physiology.

with pulmonary stenosis in those surviving to adulthood.

3. *Significantly palliated lesions.* This category includes the most frequently seen patients with significant congenital heart disease. Here, the palliation can be partial, for instance, patients with Blalock-Taussig or a Potts shunt, or those with total correction of tetralogy of Fallot, or Mustard procedure for transposition of the great arteries. All of these patients have potential late postrepair complications and none can be considered completely cured[2, 4] (see Tables 26–2 through 26–4).

4. *Patients who have been "cured."* These are the least common patients with congenital heart disease,

Table 26–2	Findings in Selected Uncomplicated Congenital Cardiac Defects*		
Type	**Physical Findings**	**ECG**	**Chest Radiograph**
Atrial septal defect	Ejection murmur across pulmonic valve Widely and fixed split S$_2$ Diastolic flow murmur across tricuspid valve Parasternal (RV) impulse	rSr' or rSr's'; left axis with ostium primum defect	Large pulmonary artery and increased pulmonary vascular markings (pulmonary plethora)
Ventricular septal defect	Holosystolic left parasternal murmur ± thrill Normal or moderately split S$_2$ Diastolic flow murmur and S$_3$ Apical impulse prominent and displaced laterally; also parasternal impulse	Biventricular or left ventricular hypertrophy	Cardiomegaly Prominent pulmonary artery and pulmonary plethora
Patent ductus arteriosus	Widened arterial pulse pressure Hyperdynamic apical impulse Continuous "machinery" murmur	LV hypertrophy	Prominent pulmonary artery and pulmonary plethora; enlarged LA, LV; occasionally calcified ductus
Congenital valvular aortic stenosis	Decreased pulse pressure and carotid upstroke Sustained apical impulse S$_4$; systolic ejection murmur ± thrill Single or paradoxical splitting of S$_2$ Concomitant aortic regurgitation common	LV hypertrophy	Poststenotic aortic dilatation Prominent LV
Valvular pulmonic stenosis	Large jugular A-wave RV parasternal impulse Pulmonic ejection sound Systolic ejection murmur ± thrill at second left intercostal space Widely split S$_2$ with soft (or inaudible) P$_2$ Right ventricular S$_4$	RV hypertrophy RA abnormality	Pulmonary blood flow normal or reduced Poststenotic dilatation of main or left pulmonary artery RA and RV enlargement
Coarctation of aorta	Reduced lower extremity blood pressure; delayed, diminished femoral pulses Mid-systolic coarctation murmur at left sternal border or posterior left intrascapular area Continuous murmur from collaterals Sustained apical impulse; S$_4$ Evidence of associated bicuspid aortic valve common	LV hypertrophy	Prominent ascending aorta; LV enlargement Poststenotic aortic dilatation Notching of inferior rib surfaces from collateral flow in intercostal arteries
Ebstein's anomaly	Acyanotic or cyanotic (right-to-left shunt owing to increased RA pressure) Increased jugular pressure and regurgitant wave Systolic murmur of tricuspid regurgitation increased with inspiration Wide splitting of S$_2$; S$_4$ and S$_3$	RA abnormality Right bundle branch block PR prolongation Ventricular preexcitation	Enlarged RA Pulmonary vascularity normal or decreased
Tetralogy of Fallot	Usually cyanotic Clubbing may be present Prominent ejection murmur at left sternal border Soft or absent P$_2$	RV hypertrophy RA abnormality	"Boot"-shaped heart owing to RV hypertrophy, small pulmonary artery, and small LV Pulmonary vascularity normal or reduced

From Andreoli, T.E., Bennett, J.C., Carpenter, C.C.J., and Plum, F. Congenital heart disease. *In* Cecil Essentials of Medicine. 4th ed. Philadelphia, W.B. Saunders, 1977, p. 41.

Abbreviations: ECG, electrocardiogram; S$_2$, second heart sound; RV, right ventricle; S$_3$, third heart sound; LV, left ventricle; LA, left atrium; S$_4$, fourth heart sound; RA, right atrium; P$_2$, second pulmonic heart sound.

* Findings vary depending on severity of lesions and associated abnormalities (see text).

Table 26–3 Indications for Primary Surgery, Common Postoperative Complications, and Indications for Reoperation in Congenital Heart Disease

Lesion	Indication for Primary Repair	Postrepair Complications	Indication for Reoperation
Atrial septal defect	Qp:Qs ≥ 1.8 : 1	Atrial fibrillation* CVA*	Secundum: large residual shunt Primum: MR
Ventricular septal defect	Qp:Qs ≥ 1.5 : 1	Patch leak Endocarditis† Progressive PHTN	Patch leak when Qp:Qs ≥ 1.5 : 1
Patent ductus arteriosus	Qp:Qs > 1.5 : 1	Persistent shunt Endoarteritis† Progressive PHTN	Persistent shunt
Atrioventricular canal defect	Qp:Qs > 1.5 : 1	Patch leak Endocarditis Progressive MR Atrial fibrillation Atrioventricular block	MR Patch leak
Anomalous pulmonary venous drainage	Qp:Qs > 1.5 : 1	Obstruction of the pulmonary veins	Significant obstruction
Tetralogy of Fallot	No previous repair	Patch leak Pulmonary insufficiency Residual PS Heart block Ventricular and atrial arrhythmias Sudden death Endocarditis	Hemodynamically significant PI or PS
Transposition of great vessel	N/A	**Postatrial Switch:** RV failure TR Baffle obstruction Atrial arrhythmias Heart block Endocarditis **Postarterial Switch:** Supravalvar aortic stenosis Coronary artery stenosis	Significant baffle obstruction Progressive RV failure TR
Ebstein's anomaly	Severe TR RV failure	Atrial arrhythmias Progressive TR	Severe TR
Tricuspid atresia	N/A	**Post-Fontan's** Atrial arrhythmias Protein-losing enteropathy Ascites	Conduit obstruction
AS	AVA < 0.8 cm² in the presence of symptoms	**Postvalvotomy** Progressive AI or restenosis Ventricular arrhythmias Sudden death Endocarditis	Severe AS or AI in the presence of symptoms or LV dysfunction
Subaortic stenosis	Gradient > 30 mm Hg or development of AI at a lower gradient	Progressive AI Restenosis Endocarditis	Severe AI or recurrent stenosis in the presence of symptoms
Pulmonary stenosis	Transpulmonary gradient > 50 mm Hg Transpulmonary gradient < 50 mm Hg with RV hypertrophy or symptoms	Restenosis Pulmonic valve insufficiency Endocarditis rare	Severe PS or PI in the presence of symptoms
Coarctation of aorta	Upper extremity HTN Transcoarctation gradient > 25 mm Hg	Residual HTN Saccular aneurysm Dissecting aneurysm Circle of Willis aneurysm—CVA Premature CAD AS/AI Endocarditis or endarteritis	Recurrent coarctation AS/AI (see above) CAD Saccular or dissecting aneurysm

Abbreviations: Qp:Qs, pulmonary–to–systemic flow ratio; CVA, cerebrovascular accident; MR, mitral regurgitation; PHTN, pulmonary hypertension; PI, pulmonic valve insufficiency; PS, pulmonary stenosis; RV, right ventricle; TR, tricuspid regurgitation; AS, aortic stenosis; AVA, aortic valve area; AI, aortic insufficiency; LV, left ventricle; HTN, hypertension; CAD, coronary artery disease.

* These complications are most common when repair is performed at age >40 yr.

† Endocarditis and endarteritis likely only in the presence of persistent shunt.

Table 26–4	Primer of Palliative Surgery	
Procedure	**Anatomy**	**Comment**
Systemic Arterial–Pulmonary Arterial		
Classic Blalock-Taussig	Subclavian artery directly to PA	Absent ipsilateral radial pulse; continuous murmur
Modified Blalock-Taussig	Subclavian to PA conduit	Preserved pulse; continuous murmur
Central shunt	Aorta to PA conduit	Continuous murmur
Waterston	Ascending aorta to RPA	Continuous murmur*
Potts	Descending aorta to LPA	Continuous murmur*
Systemic Venous to PA		
Glenn	Superior vena cava to PA	No murmur 2° to shunt; arrhythmias uncommon
Fontan	Total cavopulmonary shunt	No murmur; atrial arrhythmias common
Other		
Mustard and Senning	Atrial baffle for TGV	No murmur
		Obstruction and atrial arrhythmias common
Jatene	Arterial switch for TGV	Possible murmur owing to aortic insufficiency or supravalvar stenosis
Rastelli	Right ventricle–pulmonary artery	Valve degeneration may lead to pulmonary insufficiency murmur

Adapted from Foster, E., and Cheitlin, M.: Hemodynamically unstable presentations of congenital heart disease in adults. *In* David L. Brown (ed.): Cardiac Intensive Care. Philadelphia, W.B. Saunders, 1997.

Abbreviations: PA, pulmonary artery; RPA, right pulmonary artery; LPA, left pulmonary artery; 2°, secondary; TGV, transposition of the great vessels.

* Continuous murmur may disappear in the presence of pulmonary hypertension.

consisting of some patients with closure of atrial or ventricular septal defect and ligation and division of patent ductus arteriosus.[4, 5]

Finally, the primary care physician will likely see only the commonest of the congenital heart lesions. McNamara and Latson[2] estimated from the prevalence of various congenital heart diseases at birth that patients with the following conditions will constitute 60% of those with congenital heart disease seen as adults: atrial septal defect, ventricular septal defect, patent ductus arteriosus, tetralogy of Fallot, coarctation of the aorta, and congenital aortic stenosis.

Differential diagnosis of congenital heart disease in the adult requires a thorough history and physical examination, chest x-ray, and electrocardiogram (ECG). A definitive diagnosis, together with an extensive amount of information concerning pathophysiology, is often obtainable with a complete echocardiographic examination. Additional information can be obtained by magnetic resonance imaging (MRI); for example, the size of the pulmonary arterial branches may be better seen with this noninvasive technique. Cardiac catheterization and angiography are indicated after a noninvasive evaluation when there is a need to measure pulmonary vascular resistance or to examine the pulmonary and coronary arteries.

LESIONS CHARACTERIZED BY A LEFT-TO-RIGHT SHUNT

Interatrial Septal Defect

Pathophysiology

In this group of lesions, a defect in the interatrial septum allows pulmonary venous return to pass from the left to the right atrium. Because this left-to-right shunt increases the venous return to the right ventricle, the right ventricular stroke volume and pulmonary blood flow are increased compared with the systemic blood flow.

There are three types of atrial septal defects: (1) ostium secundum defect in the center of the atrial septum, (2) ostium primum defect in the lower part of the septum and frequently associated with abnormalities of the mitral or tricuspid valves, resulting in valvular regurgitation, and (3) sinus venosus defect that is usually superior and posterior in relation to the superior vena cava and frequently associated with an anomalous drainage of one or more pulmonary veins into the right atrium.

Recognition and Diagnosis

HISTORY AND PHYSICAL EXAMINATION. Young patients with atrial septal defect are frequently asymptomatic and are identified only because of a murmur, an abnormal chest x-ray, or an abnormal ECG. With increased diastolic filling of the right ventricle and increased right ventricular stroke volume, the patient often has a right ventricular precordial lift. The most significant abnormality on physical examination is the widely split and fixed second heart sound (S_2), which is caused by a consistent increase in right ventricular diastolic filling unaltered by the respiratory cycle. A grade II or III/VI, rarely grade IV, systolic ejection murmur is heard in the second interspace to the left of the sternum because of the increased pulmonary flow across a normal pulmonic outflow tract and valve. There may also be a rumbling mid-diastolic murmur along the left sternal border caused by increased diastolic flow across a normal tricuspid valve. With an ostium primum defect, the associated cleft mitral valve may cause an apical pansystolic murmur of mitral regurgitation. The murmur may be well heard along the left sternal border because the jet may be directed into the right atrium through the low atrial septal defect.

LABORATORY

CHEST X-RAY. With a significant left-to-right shunt, the cardiac silhouette is enlarged mainly because of the right ventricular dilatation. The pulmonary vascular markings are increased (Fig. 26–1).

ECG. The ECG shows signs of right ventricular enlargement with an rsR′ in V_1. Patients with an ostium primum defect atrial septal defect have characteristic severe left axis deviation, owing to the abnormal course of the conduction system, in addition to the rsR′ in V_1.

OTHER DIAGNOSTIC PROCEDURES AND REFERRAL FOR CARDIOLOGY CONSULTATION.

Transthoracic echocardiography (TTE) with a contrast study should be the initial investigation in patients with suspected atrial septal defect. Although the defect is rarely visualized directly in the adult, indirect evidence of an atrial septal defect includes right-sided chamber enlargement and appearance of saline contrast in the left heart chambers. Doppler echocardiography can demonstrate flow across the atrial septum. The next step in the evaluation would be referral to a cardiologist for transesophageal echocardiography (TEE) or catheterization and for coronary angiography in patients over age 40 years to detect coronary artery disease (Fig. 26–2). These studies should determine the need for surgical referral.

Course and Complications

Most patients are asymptomatic or minimally symptomatic into early adulthood. Young women tolerate pregnancy well as long as they have not developed significant pulmonary hypertension. However, if the left-to-right shunt is large, most patients will eventually become symptomatic with congestive heart failure and frequently

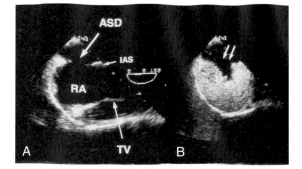

Figure 26–2

Transesophageal echocardiogram of a 24-year-old man with an ostium secundum atrial septal defect (ASD). *A,* The defect in the midportion of the interatrial septum (IAS) is demonstrated. RA, right atrium; TV, tricuspid valve. *B,* The negative contrast effect of intravenously injected saline solution when unopacified left atrial blood enters the right atrium *(double arrow)* is shown.

atrial fibrillation. In older patients without pulmonary vascular disease, the magnitude of the left-to-right shunt can increase as left ventricular compliance falls owing to diastolic dysfunction. Whereas aging alone may reduce diastolic compliance, hypertension and coronary artery disease may make it even worse. Pulmonary vascular disease with pulmonary hypertension, reversal of the shunt, and development of cyanosis occurs in approximately 10% to 15% of patients. Even in the absence of pulmonary hypertension, patients with unoperated atrial septal defect do not have a normal life expectancy. Early natural history studies demonstrate only about 50% survival beyond the age of 40 years.[3] If atrioventricular (AV) valvular regur-

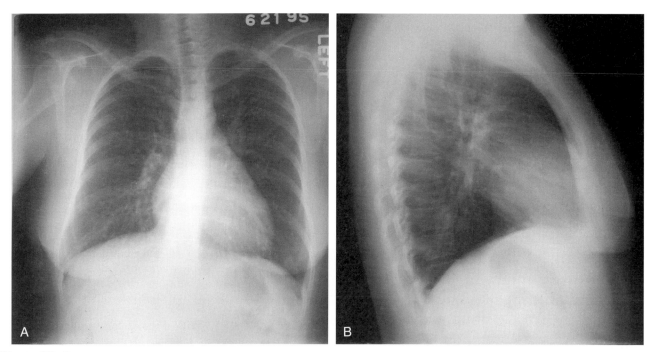

Figure 26–1

A, Chest x-ray, posteroanterior (PA) view, of a 32-year-old woman with ostium secundum atrial septal defect. Note the prominent pulmonary vascular markings and increased cardiothoracic ratio. *B,* Chest x-ray, lateral view. Note the right ventricular enlargement.

gitation is present in the patient with an ostium primum defect, congestive heart failure may occur at an earlier age. Because of the abnormal interatrial communication, occasionally paradoxical embolization may result in systemic embolization, even in the absence of pulmonary hypertension.

Primary or patch closure of an atrial septal defect in childhood provides excellent operative results and nearly normal long-term survival in adults.[4, 5] Additionally, a recent retrospective study suggested improved 10-year survival in patients over the age of 40 years treated surgically (95%) compared with those treated medically (84%).[6] However, late repair does not appear to reduce the incidence of arrhythmias, which are generally related to atrial dilatation.

Treatment

Operative patch closure is generally recommended if the shunt is large with a pulmonary blood flow–to–systemic blood flow ratio of 1.8 : 1 or higher and right ventricular enlargement. Percutaneous closure with a variety of devices is currently experimental and rarely would be considered in adults at this time. Patients with smaller shunts have a lower incidence of congestive heart failure, pulmonary hypertension, and arrhythmias but are at risk for paradoxical embolization. Even in elderly patients with large shunts, operative closure can be done at low risk and with good results in reducing symptoms. If the patient has severe pulmonary vascular disease and a reversed shunt with arterial oxygen saturations at rest below 90% and little or no residual left-to-right shunt, operative closure is contraindicated.

In patients with ostium primum defects, surgical valve repair with or without annuloplasty may reduce the severity of the mitral and tricuspid regurgitation. If severe mitral regurgitation persists, valve re-repair or replacement is necessary. In sinus venosus defects, it is frequently necessary to patch the atrial septal defect in such a way as to ensure that the anomalous pulmonary venous drainage is diverted into the left atrium.

MANAGEMENT OF THE POSTOPERATIVE PATIENT. The patient with atrial septal defect closure in childhood can lead a completely normal life without the need to impose exercise restrictions, unless the patient has persistent or progressive pulmonary hypertension. Likewise, in the absence of pulmonary hypertension, pregnancy is safe. Atrial fibrillation is common; anticoagulation is indicated in postoperative patients with this arrhythmia because of the high risk of stroke. However, the risk for endocarditis is extremely low and prophylactic antibiotics are recommended only for the first 6 months after surgery, unless other lesions such as mitral regurgitation are present.

Interventricular Septal Defect

Pathophysiology

Patients with unoperated ventricular septal defect are encountered less frequently than those with atrial septal defect because large defects are usually closed surgically in childhood when there is evidence of congestive heart failure or pulmonary hypertension, and small defects have a high rate of spontaneous closure. The ventricular septal defect permits a left-to-right shunt to occur at the ventricular level. When the increased pulmonary blood flow returns to the left ventricle, left ventricular diastolic volume and stroke volume increase.

Ventricular septal defects can be classified by anatomic location: perimembranous ventricular septal defects, the AV canal ventricular septal defect, multiple muscular ventricular septal defects, and the so-called supracristal ventricular septal defect.

Recognition and Diagnosis

HISTORY AND PHYSICAL EXAMINATION. A murmur is frequently detected shortly after birth. The young adult with an uncorrected ventricular septal defect and normal pulmonary artery pressures is usually asymptomatic but may have suffered an episode of endocarditis. When the shunt ratio exceeds 2 to 3 : 1, exertional dyspnea may develop after the age of 30 years; symptoms are rare in patients with smaller shunts. The most disabled group with pulmonary hypertension and cyanosis (i.e., Eisenmenger's physiology) is discussed separately.

If the ventricular septal defect is small (restrictive), there is a large pressure difference between the left and the right ventricles in systole. The resulting high-velocity jet across the defect causes the loud, frequently grade IV/VI, pansystolic murmur heard along the left sternal border in the third or fourth intercostal space characteristic of this lesion.

If the ventricular septal defect is large (nonrestrictive), there is no pressure difference between the left and the right ventricles; then, the magnitude of the shunt depends on the ratio of pulmonary vascular resistance to systemic vascular resistance. If the pulmonary vascular resistance is lower than the systemic vascular resistance, the left-to-right shunt can be large and the pansystolic murmur may be loud. As the pulmonary vascular resistance approaches the systemic vascular resistance, the left-to-right shunt diminishes and the systolic murmur becomes softer and finally disappears.

With large left-to-right shunts, the left ventricle dilates and becomes hypertrophied, causing a hyperdynamic, displaced left ventricular apex. There may be a diastolic rumbling murmur at the apex because of increased blood flow in diastole across the mitral valve. If the pulmonary pressures are high, the pulmonic component of S_2 becomes loud and a right ventricular lift may develop.

Patients with a supracristal ventricular septal defect may develop a diastolic blowing murmur of aortic regurgitation. The pansystolic murmur followed immediately by a blowing diastolic murmur may simulate a continuous murmur.

LABORATORY

CHEST X-RAY. With a small left-to-right shunt, the chest x-ray may be normal. With a large left-to-right shunt, cardiomegaly may be caused by left ventricular dilatation, left atrial dilatation, and possibly, right ventricular dilatation. The main pulmonary artery is prominent, and the pulmonary vascular markings are increased. When pulmonary vascular resistance is increased, the chest x-ray will show evidence of right ventricular prominence, dilatation of the main pulmonary artery, and peripheral "pruning" of pulmonary vessels.

ECG. This may be within normal limits, or it may show left ventricular hypertrophy or biventricular hypertrophy, depending on the size of the shunt and the pulmonary artery pressure.

OTHER DIAGNOSTIC PROCEDURES AND REFERRAL FOR CARDIOLOGY CONSULTATION. TTE with color-flow Doppler imaging usually defines the location and size of a ventricular septal defect. TEE is particularly helpful when transthoracic imaging is limited. If the left-to-right shunt is large, the left atrium and left ventricle are dilated. Right ventricular dimension is normal unless there is pulmonary hypertension. The pulmonary artery systolic pressure can usually be estimated by Doppler. The presence of associated defects (e.g., pulmonary stenosis) or expected complications (e.g., aortic insufficiency with a supracristal ventricular septal defect) can be confirmed.

Once a clinically significant ventricular septal defect is diagnosed, referral to a cardiologist is indicated to assist in the decision as to whether cardiac catheterization or surgical closure is indicated.

Course and Complications

With a small perimembranous or muscular ventricular septal defect, the only danger is that of infective endocarditis. The patient should repeatedly be informed of the importance of receiving appropriate antibiotics at the time of dental work or other procedures causing bacteremia (see Chap. 16).

By the time the patient has reached adolescence or early adulthood, there is virtually no chance that the ventricular septal defect will close spontaneously. If the left-to-right shunt is large, congestive heart failure is possible. If a large ventricular septal defect is associated with pulmonary hypertension, the chance of the development of pulmonary vascular disease is high. In adults diagnosed with ventricular septal defect, the overall 10-year survival after initial presentation is approximately 75%. Functional class greater than 1, cardiomegaly, and elevated pulmonary artery pressure (>50 mm Hg) are clinical predictors of an adverse prognosis.[7]

Treatment

With a small ventricular septal defect, prophylaxis against infective endocarditis should be recommended. With a large ventricular septal defect in the adolescent or adult, closure of the defect should be performed as long as there is a dominant left-to-right shunt. Once the pulmonary vascular resistance exceeds 60% to 70% of systemic vascular resistance and the left-to-right shunt diminishes, closure of ventricular septal defect is no longer indicated. If aortic regurgitation develops in the presence of a supracristal ventricular septal defect, closure of the ventricular septal defect will help prevent progression of the aortic regurgitation and is therefore indicated.

Management of the Postoperative Patient

The patient with ventricular septal defect closure in childhood usually leads a normal life. There is no need to impose restrictions on exercise or pregnancy unless there is progressive pulmonary hypertension. Prophylactic antibiotics are indicated only for the first six postoperative months unless there is a residual defect.

Patent Ductus Arteriosus

Pathophysiology

The patent ductus arteriosus connects the proximal descending aorta with the pulmonary artery at its bifurcation. The magnitude of the left-to-right shunt depends on the size of the patent ductus and the pulmonary vascular resistance–to–systemic vascular resistance ratio in a manner similar to that of the ventricular septal defect. In the absence of pulmonary vascular disease, aortic pressures exceed pulmonary artery pressures throughout the cardiac cycle, resulting in continuous left-to-right shunting of blood and a "continuous murmur" or "machinery murmur."

When the patent ductus arteriosus is large and the pulmonary vascular resistance is low compared with the systemic vascular resistance, a large left-to-right shunt causes a loud, continuous, so-called machinery, murmur. The marked increase in pulmonary blood flow results in left-sided volume overload with an increase in the size of the left atrium, left ventricle, ascending aorta, and aortic arch. The left ventricular volume overload can result in congestive heart failure.

Recognition and Diagnosis

HISTORY AND PHYSICAL EXAMINATION. If the patent ductus arteriosus is small, the heart will be normal and the only finding will be the continuous murmur, usually loudest under the left clavicle or in the second interspace along the left sternal border. With a large patent ductus arteriosus and relatively low pulmonary vascular resistance, the continuous murmur will be louder, the left ventricular apex will be displaced and hyperactive, and a low-pitched diastolic murmur may be heard at the apex because of increased diastolic flow across a normal mitral valve.

With a large patent ductus arteriosus and high pulmonary vascular resistance, the murmur is no longer continuous; it may be heard only in systole or may even be absent. The pulmonic component of S_2 is increased, and the only audible murmur might be the high-pitched, decrescendo murmur of pulmonic valve regurgitation along the left sternal border—a murmur that may be indistinguishable from the murmur of aortic regurgitation. In patients with patent ductus arteriosus and pulmonary vascular disease with reversed shunting, the key to the diagnosis is the presence of "differential cyanosis and clubbing" in the lower extremities (i.e., toes) and absence of these findings in the fingers (see Former Left-to-Right

Shunts with Pulmonary Vascular Disease [Eisenmenger's Physiology]).

LABORATORY

CHEST X-RAY. With a small patent ductus arteriosus, the chest x-ray may be normal. With a large patent ductus arteriosus with a large left-to-right shunt, the left ventricle and the left atrium may be enlarged. The main pulmonary artery and major branches of the pulmonary artery are increased, and the pulmonary vascular markings are increased. The pulmonary arteries are pruned in the presence of pulmonary hypertension.

ECG. With a large patent ductus arteriosus, there may be left ventricular hypertrophy and left atrial enlargement. With increased pulmonary vascular resistance, right ventricular hypertrophy often appears.

OTHER DIAGNOSTIC PROCEDURES AND REFERRAL FOR CARDIOLOGY CONSULTATION. On two-dimensional echocardiography, the ductus itself is rarely seen, but visualization of abnormal, continuous, high-velocity "aliased" flow within the main pulmonary artery near the left branch is seen on color-flow Doppler imaging (Fig. 26–3). Pulmonary artery systolic pressures can also be accurately estimated.

If a hemodynamically significant patent ductus arteriosus is suspected, referral to a cardiologist is indicated to assist in the decision as to whether closure is needed.

Course and Complications

With a small patent ductus arteriosus, the only danger is that of infective endocarditis; prophylactic antibiotics should be given at the time of dental work or other procedures causing bacteremia. With a large left-to-right shunt, especially with high pulmonary artery pressures, the danger of congestive heart failure and development of pulmonary vascular disease and Eisenmenger's syndrome must be considered.

Treatment

With a small patent ductus arteriosus in a young or middle-aged person, ligation preferably with division of the patent ductus is indicated because of the long-term

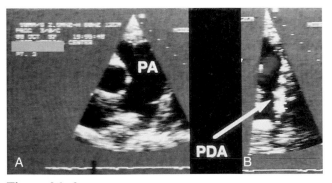

Figure 26–3

Transthoracic echocardiogram of an adult patient with a patent ductus arteriosus (PDA). *A,* The basal short-axis view demonstrates the dilated pulmonary artery (PA) with the adjacent circular ascending aorta. *B,* In the same view, the color-flow jet through the PDA is seen entering the PA. The flow was continuous on real-time imaging.

danger of infective endarteritis. Currently, some centers are closing smaller patent ductuses percutaneously using intravascular devices with an approximately 95% success rate at intermediate follow-up; long-term follow-up is not yet available. With a large left-to-right shunt, especially with elevated pulmonary artery pressures, ligation of the patent ductus arteriosus, preferably with division, is indicated at any age.

In a patient over the age of 60 to 65 years with a small patent ductus arteriosus, the danger of developing infective endarteritis must be balanced against the dangers of the surgery. In an older, asymptomatic patient, antibiotic prophylaxis is indicated but surgical correction is generally not recommended.

Occasionally, a small "silent" patent ductus arteriosus is detected serendipitously on Doppler echocardiography performed for another indication. Closure is not usually recommended in patients with inaudible shunts, but antibiotic prophylaxis is prudent.

MANAGEMENT OF THE POSTOPERATIVE PATIENT. The patient with closure of a patent ductus arteriosus early in childhood before the development of pulmonary hypertension usually leads a normal life.[4] Prophylactic antibiotics are recommended only when a murmur persists postoperatively, and their use is controversial when the shunt is detected only by color-flow Doppler imaging.

Complete AV Septal Defect (AV Canal Defect)

Pathophysiology

In this lesion, there is failure of the endocardial cushions to complete their task of closing the atrial septum, the ventricular septum, and the formation of the mitral and tricuspid valve. As a result, patients have a ventricular septal defect, an atrial septal defect, and varying degrees of AV valve regurgitation. AV septal defects, formerly known as endocardial cushion defects, are commonly encountered in children with trisomy 21 (Down's syndrome). With large left-to-right shunts at the atrial and ventricular levels and systemic pressures in the right ventricle because of the ventricular septal defect, pulmonary vascular disease occurs very early.

Recognition and Diagnosis

HISTORY AND PHYSICAL EXAMINATION. Most adults with uncorrected complete AV septal defects are cyanotic with Eisenmenger's syndrome and are not candidates for correction. When the repair has been performed in childhood, residual mitral or tricuspid regurgitation often remains.

LABORATORY

CHEST X-RAY. Depending on the severity of the left-to-right shunt and of the AV valve regurgitation, the right and left ventricles are dilated, as are the left and right atria. Pulmonary vascularity is increased when a left-to-right shunt persists; the pulmonary arteries show "pruning" in the presence of pulmonary vascular disease.

ECG. The characteristic ECG shows severe left axis deviation suggestive of a left anterior hemiblock.

OTHER DIAGNOSTIC PROCEDURES AND REFERRAL FOR CARDIOLOGY CONSULTATION. The two-dimensional echocardiogram of a complete AV defect demonstrates complete absence of the crux of the heart, with both low atrial and high ventricular septal defects. In the adult, color-flow imaging and Doppler studies show regurgitation of both AV valves and evidence of pulmonary artery hypertension.

Adults with this lesion should be referred to a cardiologist experienced in congenital heart disease to determine operability for a primary repair or to evaluate and treat residual disease.

Course, Complications, and Treatment

Because most untreated patients with complete AV septal defects will not survive the first year, these children are usually corrected in infancy. The surgery consists of patch closure of the atrial and ventricular septal defects and repair of the AV valves. The unoperated adult with a complete AV septal defect is rarely a candidate for a complete repair because of the frequent and early development of pulmonary vascular disease, but she or he may be a candidate for heart-lung transplantation or lung transplantation with intracardiac repair.

MANAGEMENT OF THE POSTOPERATIVE PATIENT. The most common postoperative sequela is progressive mitral valve regurgitation owing to an inadequate repair. Tolerance for pregnancy depends on the presence of pulmonary hypertension and the severity of valvular dysfunction. Mitral valve regurgitation places the patient at continued risk for endocarditis, and prophylactic antibiotics are indicated. Complete heart block is relatively common after surgical repair, may appear late in the postoperative course, and requires a pacemaker.

Anomalous Pulmonary Venous Drainage

Pathophysiology

One, more than one, or all pulmonary veins can drain anomalously into the right heart and create a left-to-right shunt, which increases venous return to the right ventricle and increases right ventricular stroke volume as in an atrial septal defect. When all of the pulmonary veins drain anomalously into the systemic venous system, an atrial septal defect must be present to return oxygenated blood to the left side of the heart.

Recognition and Diagnosis

HISTORY AND PHYSICAL EXAMINATION. The patient is usually asymptomatic with a normal physical examination in the presence of a single anomalous vein. When the anomalous pulmonary vein is associated with a sinus venosus atrial septal defect, the patient will have the findings of the atrial septal defect.

LABORATORY

CHEST X-RAY. Anomalous veins may be visible on the x-ray. With multiple anomalous pulmonary veins, the pulmonary vascular markings will be increased and the right ventricle enlarged.

ECG. The ECG may be normal unless the left-to-right shunt is large; then, an rsR′ or RV hypertrophy will be present.

OTHER DIAGNOSTIC PROCEDURES AND REFERRAL FOR CARDIOLOGY CONSULTATION. Color-flow Doppler imaging may reveal a flow disturbance when the vein drains into the inferior vena cava. TEE can be used to identify the entrance of the pulmonary veins. Referral to a cardiologist experienced in congenital heart disease is indicated to determine the need for surgery.

Course, Complications, and Treatment

The benign course of patients with a single anomalous pulmonary vein supports the recommendation that surgical correction is not indicated in the absence of an associated sinus venosus atrial septal defect. If there are multiple veins draining anomalously, then the course and complications are similar to those of an interatrial septal defect. When the pulmonary blood flow is increased to 1.8 to 2 times systemic blood flow, surgical repair with redirection of the pulmonary veins into the left atrium should be performed. The rare adult presenting de novo with total anomalous pulmonary venous drainage usually remains a surgical candidate.

PREDOMINANT RIGHT-TO-LEFT SHUNTS (CYANOTIC HEART DISEASE)

Former Left-to-Right Shunts with Pulmonary Vascular Disease (Eisenmenger's Physiology)

Pathophysiology

In the adult with cyanotic congenital heart disease, Eisenmenger's physiology is the commonest cause. In patients with an interatrial septal defect, interventricular septal defect, or patent ductus arteriosus, the development of pulmonary vascular disease occurs only in the presence of a large left-to-right shunt. With a large ventricular septal defect or patent ductus arteriosus, the pulmonary hypertension may be present from birth. The excessive pulmonary blood flow and high pulmonary artery pressure inevitably results in intimal hyperplasia, medial arterial smooth muscle hypertrophy, and a relative paucity of small pulmonary arteries as the lung grows. Once the pulmonary vascular resistance reaches 60% to 70% of systemic vascular resistance, the process is irreversible and may progress even if the shunt is closed. In patients with atrial septal defects, the pulmonary vascular resistance and pressure fall after birth. The development of pulmonary hypertension is more insidious but is usually established by adolescence if it is going to occur.

Because of the development of pulmonary vascular disease, there is a marked increase in pulmonary vascular resistance. The magnitude of the left-to-right shunt, therefore, is decreased or even absent. The severe pulmonary hypertension presents an afterload burden to the right ventricle, causing right ventricular hypertrophy and, finally, right heart failure. The shunt then becomes balanced or predominantly right-to-left.

Recognition and Diagnosis

HISTORY AND PHYSICAL EXAMINATION. Patients are symptomatic with a limitation of physical activity owing to dyspnea and fatigue. Other symptoms include syncope, chest pain, and hemoptysis. There may be a history of endocarditis or septic embolization. Headaches and fatigability may be due to polycythemia.

On physical examination, there is cyanosis of the lips, fingers, and toes and clubbing of the fingers and toes (Table 26–5). The murmurs of the respective shunt lesions are no longer typical and may be entirely absent. The physical findings may confirm right heart failure with an increased central venous pressure, tricuspid regurgitation, pulmonic regurgitation, and right-sided fourth heart sound and third heart sound gallops. All three anatomic lesions have a similar clinical presentation when pulmonary vascular disease is present, and they may be difficult to distinguish from one another.

However, with a patent ductus arteriosus, the desaturated blood passes through the ductus and down the aorta, causing the toes to be cyanotic while the fingers of the right hand or both hands are pink, depending on whether the desaturated blood goes into the left subclavian artery.

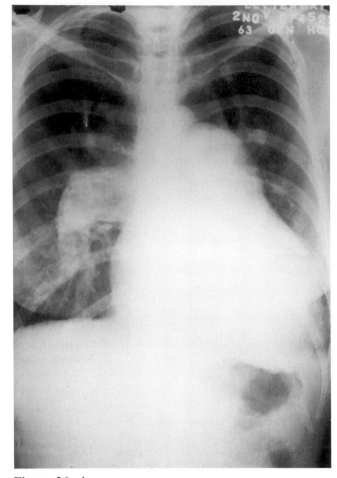

Figure 26–4

Chest x-ray, PA view. The patient is a 40-year-old woman with Eisenmenger's syndrome due to a ventricular septal defect. Note the enlarged heart and monstrous enlargement of the pulmonary artery and proximal branches of the right pulmonary artery. There is a calcification due to atherosclerosis in the right pulmonary artery. Note the clear lateral lung fields ("pruning").

Table 26–5	Findings of Eisenmenger's Physiology*

Signs of pulmonary arterial hypertension
    Prominent jugular A-wave (decreased ventricular compliance owing to RV hypertrophy)
    Jugular regurgitant wave (if functional tricuspid regurgitation present)
    Left parasternal (right ventricular) lift
    Palpable pulmonary artery pulsation (second left intercostal space)
    Pulmonic ejection murmur
    Loud P_2
    Diastolic decrescendo murmur of pulmonic insufficiency (Graham Steell's murmur)
    Holosystolic murmur of tricuspid regurgitation
Cyanosis
Clubbing of fingers
Erythrocytosis

From Andreoli, T.E., Bennett, J.C., Carpenter, C.C.J., and Plum, F. Congenital heart disease. *In* Cecil Essentials of Medicine. 4th ed. Philadelphia, W.B. Saunders, 1977, p. 42.
    Abbreviations: RV, right ventricle; P_2, second pulmonic heart sound.
    * Not all findings are present in each case.

LABORATORY. The oxygen saturation is low, and there is evidence of secondary polycythemia with an increased hematocrit. The bleeding time may be prolonged owing to an associated bleeding diathesis. Uric acid levels may be elevated.

CHEST X-RAY. The chest x-ray shows evidence of right ventricular enlargement, prominent proximal pulmonary arteries with peripheral oligemia, and "pruning" (Fig. 26–4) of the peripheral pulmonary vessels.

ECG. The ECG shows evidence of right atrial enlargement and right ventricular hypertrophy, usually with a rightward axis. A superior axis suggests an ostium primum atrial septal defect or an AV septal defect as the underlying cause (Fig. 26–5).

OTHER DIAGNOSTIC PROCEDURES AND REFERRAL FOR CARDIOLOGY CONSULTATION. TTE demonstrates right atrial enlargement and severe right ventricular hypertrophy with varying degrees of right ventricular dilatation and dysfunction. The level of shunt can usually be discerned by two-dimensional imag-

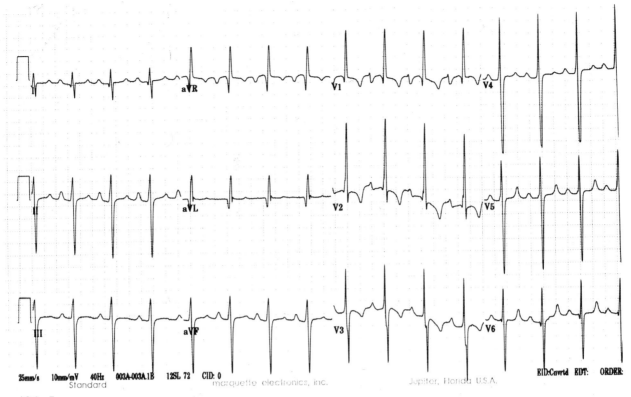

Figure 26–5

Electrocardiogram from a 36-year-old patient with Eisenmenger's syndrome due to an atrioventricular septal (canal) defect. Note the evidence of right ventricular and biatrial enlargement with a superior and leftward QRS axis.

ing, in conjunction with color-flow Doppler and saline contrast injection. The pulmonary artery systolic pressure can be estimated from the peak velocity of the tricuspid regurgitant jet. The peak right ventricular systolic pressure is equal to four times the velocity squared (by a modified Bernoulli equation) added to an estimated right atrial pressure (jugular venous pressure).

Referral to a cardiologist is indicated to confirm the diagnosis and to determine whether the pulmonary vascular disease is reversible or not. The latter determination may require cardiac catheterization.

Course and Complications

Death occurs from the mid-third decade to as late as the sixth decade of life. Although life expectancy is shortened in patients with Eisenmenger's physiology, careful medical management may reduce mortality. The most common causes of death include pulmonary infarction and hemoptysis, arrhythmias with sudden death, progressive right ventricular failure, and brain abscess. Pregnancy carries an extremely high fetal and maternal mortality (approximately 50%) and should be avoided.[8]

Treatment

When pulmonary vascular resistance is high enough to cause a predominant right-to-left shunt, surgical closure of the defect is contraindicated. When the patient is sufficiently symptomatic, right ventricular failure has oc-

curred, or the patient has developed ventricular arrhythmias causing syncope, heart and lung transplant or lung transplant with intracardiac repair should be considered.

Tetralogy of Fallot

Pathophysiology

Tetralogy of Fallot refers to a combination of lesions consisting of an interventricular septal defect, infundibular stenosis with or without valvular pulmonic stenosis, and an aorta overriding the ventricular septal defect. The fourth lesion inferred by the word *tetralogy* is right ventricular hypertrophy, which is a compensatory response to the other lesions. The right ventricular obstruction and large ventricular septal defect result in a high right ventricular pressure that is similar to left ventricular pressure. When the resistance due to the right ventricular outflow obstruction is greater than systemic vascular resistance, there is a right-to-left shunt, arterial desaturation, and if severe, cyanosis. If the right ventricular outflow obstruction is not severe, there may be little or no right-to-left shunt. The shunt may even be left-to-right, and the pulmonary valve and arteries may be normal or large. This lesion is sometimes referred to as "pink" or "acyanotic" tetralogy of Fallot.

In tetralogy of Fallot, the aortic arch is right-sided in about 10% of patients. In pulmonary atresia, a right-sided aortic arch is present in 20% to 30% of patients.

Recognition and Diagnosis

HISTORY AND PHYSICAL EXAMINATION. Patients are frequently diagnosed in infancy when cyanosis appears at the usual time of ductal closure. The rare adult encountered with untreated tetralogy of Fallot usually has severe exercise intolerance.

The patient has a systolic ejection murmur, usually grade III or IV/VI, in the second to third intercostal space at the left sternal border caused by the infundibular pulmonic stenosis. S_2 is single. Later, the patient develops clubbing and cyanosis of the upper and lower extremities. There may be a precordial lift owing to right ventricular hypertrophy. After a primary total repair, there is usually a systolic murmur owing to residual stenosis and a murmur of pulmonary insufficiency. When the patient has had a palliative systemic to pulmonary shunt (see later), there is a continuous murmur.

LABORATORY

CHEST X-RAY. The heart size is normal. The apex is rounded and lifted off the left hemidiaphragm. These findings give the appearance of the boot-shaped heart, so-called coeur en sabot (Fig. 26–6). The pulmonary arteries are normal or small, and the lung fields are clear. A right-sided aortic arch may be present.

ECG. Invariably, there is right ventricular hypertrophy. After primary repair, there is frequently a right bundle branch block and, occasionally, varying degrees of AV block.

OTHER DIAGNOSTIC PROCEDURES AND REFERRAL FOR CARDIOLOGY CONSULTATION. In patients with unrepaired tetralogy of Fallot, transthoracic echocardiography demonstrates severe right ventricular hypertrophy including the infundibulum usually with a thickened, malformed pulmonary valve. There is a large ventricular septal defect in the vicinity of the membranous septum (i.e., perimembranous) with evidence of right-to-left shunting and a dilated overriding aorta. The gradient across the right ventricular outflow tract can be measured. In the patient with total primary repair, there is usually some degree of residual stenosis and nearly always pulmonary insufficiency. Referral to a cardiologist is indicated to determine eligibility for surgery in unrepaired patients and to determine the severity of residual lesions in repaired patients.

When TTE is nondiagnostic, biplane or multiplane transesophageal echocardiography may supplement the information. In patients considered for surgery, catheterization is indicated to measure pulmonary vascular resistance and to define anomalous coronary arteries and the size of the pulmonary arteries.

Course and Complications

Most patients with tetralogy of Fallot have had palliative operations or corrective surgery by the time they are teenagers. Occasionally, a patient reaches the third decade of life without surgery. Sometimes patients present with only palliative systemic to pulmonary arterial shunts such as Blalock-Taussig shunt (subclavian to pulmonary artery), Potts' shunt (descending aorta to left pulmonary

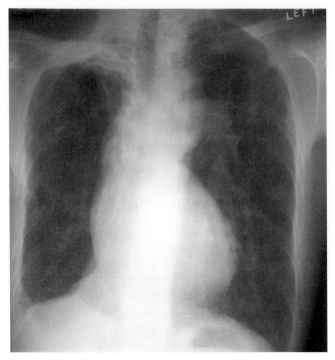

Figure 26–6

Chest x-ray, PA view. The patient is a 52-year-old man with tetralogy of Fallot and a left-sided aortic arch. Note the "elevated" left ventricular apex. Interstitial lung markings are increased in this patient owing to chronic pulmonary disease.

artery), or Waterston's shunts (ascending aorta to right pulmonary artery). Before surgical correction was possible, most patients died in the second decade of life.

Although it is an extremely successful operation, total intracardiac repair (see later) for tetralogy of Fallot has several potential significant postoperative residua, including residual right ventricular outflow tract obstruction, pulmonary valve regurgitation, and arrhythmias. In the early and intermediate follow-up period, important residual right ventricular outflow tract obstruction appears to be the major source of morbidity and mortality. However, in the late follow-up period, pulmonary insufficiency with eventual right ventricular failure owing to volume overload and ventricular arrhythmias may lead to disability and even death. Survival in postoperative tetralogy of Fallot is about 90% at about 30 years after surgery.[9]

Treatment

All patients who are unoperated should have an attempted surgical correction. Patients with only palliative shunts should have these taken down and surgical repair performed unless pulmonary vascular resistance has become severely elevated. The operation consists of patching the ventricular septal defect and relieving the right ventricular outflow tract obstruction.

MANAGEMENT OF THE POSTOPERATIVE PATIENT. After palliative procedures or total intracardiac repair, patients are at risk for endocarditis and should receive antibiotic prophylaxis during procedures associated with bacteremia. Those patients with intracardiac repair are at risk for tachyarrhythmias (atrial and ventricular) and complete heart block. Premature ventricular contractions are also common and may predict sudden death but should not be treated empirically. Patients with nonsustained ventricular tachycardia or syncope should be referred to an electrophysiologist with experience in congenital heart disease.

The hemodynamic residua after a total intracardiac repair may include residual right ventricular outflow tract obstruction, pulmonary valve insufficiency, peripheral pulmonary artery stenosis of one or both pulmonary arteries, and ventricular septal patch leaks. The presence and severity of residual lesions can usually be determined noninvasively, and patients should be followed by an experienced cardiologist to decide whether and when repeat surgery is indicated. Pregnancy is generally well tolerated unless the residual right ventricular outflow obstruction is severe. Unless right ventricular failure is present, pulmonic valvular insufficiency is not a contraindication to pregnancy.

Transposition of the Great Arteries

These infants are born with the great arteries arising from the wrong ventricle. The aortic valve arises anteriorly from the right ventricle and the pulmonic valve posteriorly from the left ventricle. Without cross-connections, such as a patent foramen ovale, atrial septal defect, ventricular septal defect, or patent ductus arteriosus, this lesion is incompatible with life.

Infants with this condition rarely survive without intervention; thus, with only rare exceptions, adults have had palliative procedures (such as the Mustard or Senning procedures), after which the right ventricle usually continues to serve the systemic circulation. More recently, an arterial switch operation, the Jatene procedure, was developed to reconnect the great arteries to their proper ventricle, reconnect the coronary arteries to the new aortic location, and restore a "normal" circulation. Postoperative patients should be followed by a cardiologist as well as a primary care physician. Medical therapy to treat failure of the systemic right ventricle includes afterload reduction with vasodilators, digoxin, and diuretics. Noninvasive and invasive studies may demonstrate the need for further surgical palliative procedures.

Ebstein's Anomaly

Pathophysiology

In Ebstein's anomaly, the septal and posterior leaflets of the tricuspid valve are dysplastic and displaced from the tricuspid annulus apically into the body of the right ventricle. Thus, a portion of the right ventricle is above the tricuspid valve (the atrialized right ventricle) and enlarges the true right atrium. The valve may be regurgitant, and if a patent foramen ovale or an atrial septal defect is present, there can be a large right-to-left shunt. These patients are cyanotic, are likely to present in infancy, and

may have had palliative procedures with atrial septal defect closure. The presentation in adolescents or adults is more likely related to progressive tricuspid regurgitation and heart failure or arrhythmias than to cyanosis.

Recognition and Diagnosis

HISTORY AND PHYSICAL EXAMINATION. There may be a history of dyspnea and intermittent cyanosis leading to exercise intolerance, atypical chest pain, and palpitations or syncope. On physical examination, these patients frequently have widely split first heart sound and S_2. After one or more loud systolic clicks owing to prolapse of the redundant leaflets, a systolic murmur of tricuspid regurgitation with accentuation on inspiration may be present. Since the regurgitant jet may be eccentric owing to the displaced leaflet, it is not unusual to hear the tricuspid regurgitation murmur best at the apex—thus, resembling the murmur of mitral regurgitation.

LABORATORY

CHEST X-RAY. Classically, the chest x-ray shows a globular heart with a long sweep of right atrium. The lung fields are usually normal but may show diminished pulmonary blood flow. The normal prominent bulge of the main pulmonary artery segment may be absent.

ECG. The classic ECG reveals a low-voltage right bundle branch block, often a first degree AV block, and right atrial abnormality. Wolff-Parkinson-White syndrome may be present, and the patient may have runs of paroxysmal atrial tachycardia.

OTHER DIAGNOSTIC PROCEDURES AND REFERRAL FOR CARDIOLOGY CONSULTATION. The echocardiogram is diagnostic, demonstrating the morphology of the abnormal tricuspid valve with a tricuspid regurgitant jet arising apically within the right ventricle.

Referral to a cardiologist is indicated for evaluation of the symptomatic patient. Catheterization is rarely necessary but may be indicated preoperatively when surgical treatment is necessary. Electrophysiology studies should be performed in a center where radiofrequency ablation is available to treat bypass tract–related arrhythmias.

Course and Complications

Once the patient has survived childhood, the prognosis is favorable, even with severe displacement of the tricuspid valve. If the tricuspid regurgitation is severe, then the ability to increase cardiac output may be diminished and the patient may have progressive limitation of activity with fatigability.

Treatment and Management Issues

If an unoperated patient is symptomatic, closure of an atrial septal defect and reconstruction of the tricuspid valve with an annuloplasty or even replacement has been done with success. If atrial tachycardia is present with an anomalous muscle connection, radiofrequency ablation of the AV pathway can successfully treat the paroxysmal atrial tachycardia. Patients with persistent tricuspid regurgitation after valve repair and those who have had tricuspid valve replacement require antibiotic prophylaxis.

Other Cyanotic Lesions

Tricuspid atresia, single ventricle, and truncus arteriosis are uncommon lesions that are almost uniformly fatal in childhood without surgical palliative procedures. When possible, they should be managed in conjunction with a service specializing in adult congenital heart disease.

STENOTIC AND ATRETIC VALVES AND HYPOPLASTIC VENTRICLES

Congenital Aortic Stenosis (see Chap. 25)

Pathophysiology

The pathophysiology of congenital aortic stenosis is similar to that of acquired aortic stenosis. However, in congenital aortic stenosis, the anatomic level of obstruction is more likely to be supravalvular or subvalvular than in acquired aortic stenosis, which is almost always valvular. Valvular aortic stenosis is due to a malformed valve that is usually functionally bicuspid. Patients with the most severely malformed and stenotic valves may require intervention in childhood. Even with a less-restricted orifice, the disturbed flow through the valve causes progressive thickening and calcification and may eventually result in severe stenosis and varying degrees of valvular insufficiency that become manifest later in life. Intervening endocarditis may hasten valve destruction and cause predominant valvular insufficiency.

In supravalvular aortic stenosis, the narrowing is usually above the level of the sinuses of Valsalva. Therefore, the coronary arteries arise from the aorta proximal to the obstruction and are subjected to an elevated systolic pressure equal to that of the left ventricle. The high pressures cause coronary artery dilatation and may accelerate atherosclerosis.

In the most common form of subaortic stenosis, there is a discrete membrane immediately below the aortic valve, resulting in a systolic jet that traumatizes the valve tissue, causing aortic regurgitation. There is frequent association of left ventricular outflow tract obstruction with coarctation of the aorta and also mitral valve abnormalities. Obstructive hypertrophic cardiomyopathy and the tunnel types of left ventricular outflow tract subvalvular aortic stenosis are not discussed in this chapter.

Recognition and Diagnosis

HISTORY AND PHYSICAL EXAMINATION. Congenital valvular aortic stenosis has a similar presentation to that of acquired disease and is covered in Chapter 25. In congenital aortic stenosis, an ejection click is usually heard as long as the leaflets remain flexible. This click disappears as calcification and immobility of the valve progress. Other aspects of the physical examination are similar to that of acquired disease.

With supravalvular aortic stenosis, the obstruction is above the aortic valve and, thus, there is no ejection click and no aortic regurgitation. The systolic jet arises in the ascending aorta, directing the percussion wave into the innominate artery. This mechanism raises systolic blood pressure in the right arm by 10 to 20 mm Hg compared with that in the left arm.

In patients with discrete membranous subaortic stenosis, there is no ejection click. Eighty percent of patients have a murmur of aortic regurgitation.

LABORATORY

CHEST X-RAY. The chest x-ray is similar to that in patients with acquired aortic stenosis with poststenotic dilatation of the aorta and calcification of the valve. The findings in supravalvular aortic stenosis are similar with one important distinction—there is no poststenotic dilatation of the ascending aorta. Calcification can be seen in the atherosclerotic dilated coronary arteries in some patients. Similarly, in patients with discrete membranous subvalvular aortic stenosis, the chest x-ray shows no poststenotic dilatation.

ECG. In young patients with severe aortic stenosis, the ECG may be normal, and thus, the absence of left ventricular hypertrophy on the ECG does not exclude the diagnosis in this population.

OTHER DIAGNOSTIC PROCEDURES AND REFERRAL FOR CARDIOLOGY CONSULTATION. TTE is diagnostic in valvular aortic stenosis with direct visualization of the valve leaflets by two-dimensional imaging and measurement of the pressure gradient across the left ventricular outflow tract by Doppler interrogation. The valve area can be accurately derived. However, surface imaging is limited in its ability to visualize a subaortic membrane or supravalvar stenosis; in these cases, TEE may be indicated.

Referral to a cardiologist is indicated for symptomatic patients or those with moderate or severe asymptomatic stenosis or to clarify the severity of the stenosis when a discrepancy exists between the clinical findings and the noninvasive data.

Course and Complications

The complications of congenital aortic stenosis in the adult are similar to those of acquired aortic stenosis. As soon as symptoms begin, there is a rapid increase in mortality, with one-quarter to one-third of deaths occurring suddenly. With discrete membranous subvalvular aortic stenosis, progressive aortic regurgitation can occur.

After aortic valvotomy for severe stenosis during childhood, approximately one-fourth of patients will need repeat surgery for recurrent stenosis or progressive aortic insufficiency in the next 25 years.[10] With medical treatment, approximately one-third of children with systolic gradients below 50 mm Hg and about 80% of those with gradient 50 to 79 mm Hg will need surgery within 25 years.[10]

Treatment

With symptomatic, hemodynamically significant valvular aortic stenosis (i.e., an aortic valve area less than 0.8 cm^2) and a flexible noncalcified valve, balloon valvotomy may have therapeutic success similar to that of operative valvotomy even in young adults. However, when there is calcification or associated aortic insufficiency, valve replacement is required. The Ross procedure, which places a homograft in the pulmonary valve position and uses the patient's own pulmonary valve in the aortic position, has had promising early results. The advantages of this innovative, although technically challenging, approach are that it obviates the need for anticoagulation without using bioprosthetic valves with their excess rate of degeneration.[11]

The indications for repair in supravalvular aortic stenosis are a significant gradient or coronary artery dilatation, or both. In patients with discrete membranous subvalvular aortic stenosis and any associated aortic regurgitation, operative repair with adequate resection of the membrane and underlying myocardium should be performed in an attempt to prevent progressive aortic regurgitation or regrowth of the membrane.[12]

MANAGEMENT OF THE POSTOPERATIVE PATIENT. Patients treated surgically for valvular, supravalvar, and subvalvar aortic stenosis in childhood are at risk for endocarditis, regardless of the type of surgery performed. Those who underwent surgical valvotomy as well as those with prior resection of a subaortic membrane must be followed for progressive aortic insufficiency.

Pulmonic Valvular Stenosis

Pathophysiology

Although pulmonic valve stenosis may be progressive, it is congenital in origin. The obstruction to outflow puts an afterload burden on the right ventricle, resulting in concentric right ventricular hypertrophy. With severe right ventricular hypertrophy, increased systolic compression of the right ventricle may compromise the intramural coronary arteries, causing subendocardial ischemia.

Recognition and Diagnosis

Symptoms vary with the severity of obstruction. In patients with severe obstruction (peak right ventricular–pulmonary artery pressure gradient >80 mm Hg), dyspnea, fatigue, symptoms of right ventricular failure, and syncope may be present. On physical examination, the sound of pulmonary closure is inaudible or soft. The fourth heart sound and prominent A-waves in the jugular venous pulse are often present. Typical findings include a right ventricular heave, a right parasternal systolic thrill, and an early systolic ejection sound, followed by a loud (≥ 3/6) systolic ejection murmur at the upper left sternal border.

LABORATORY

CHEST X-RAY. The chest x-ray usually shows a normal overall heart size but with right ventricular prominence, normal pulmonary vascularity, and poststenotic dilatation of the main and left pulmonary arteries.

ECG. The ECG typically shows right axis deviation and exhibits right ventricular hypertrophy and right atrial enlargement.

ECHOCARDIOGRAPHY. Two-dimensional echocardiography shows the stenotic pulmonary valve and thickening of the free wall of the right ventricle. Accurate measurements of the pressure gradient across the right ventricular outflow tract are possible with Doppler interrogation. Referral to a cardiologist is indicated for catheterization and pulmonary arteriography when needed and to assist in the decision to intervene.

Course and Complications

It is unusual to see an adult with severe valvular pulmonary stenosis. Adult patients with valvular pulmonary stenosis in general do well; however, eventually, right ventricular failure can occur. In children followed medically for pulmonary stenosis without surgical intervention, the likelihood of developing symptomatic stenosis requiring surgery depends on the initial gradient—less than 25 mm Hg: 5%; 25 to 49 mm Hg: 20%; and 50 to 79 mm Hg: 76%. Symptoms may occur during pregnancy in patients with moderately severe or severe pulmonary stenosis.

Surgical valvotomy has been an extremely successful operation for relieving pulmonary valve obstruction long term. A recent natural history study of surgically treated severe (gradient ≥ 80 mm Hg) pulmonic stenosis demonstrated an excellent 25-year survival of 95%, equivalent to the normal population. Approximately 50% of patients did have mild to moderate regurgitation, but reoperation was rarely necessary (5%) at 25 years.[13]

Treatment

In the adult, severe pulmonary valve stenosis requiring intervention is defined as a peak systolic gradient in excess of 60 mm Hg. The decision to treat moderate stenosis (gradient between 40 and 60 mm Hg) is based on the presence of symptoms, the age of the patient, and the degree of right ventricular hypertrophy.

In patients with severe valvular pulmonary stenosis, percutaneous balloon valvuloplasty is the current treatment of choice and has replaced surgical valvotomy in patients with flexible valves (see Chap. 25). In patients with mild to moderate pulmonary stenosis, especially if there is no right ventricular hypertrophy, observation with recommendation for prophylactic antibiotics to prevent infective endocarditis is indicated without surgical or nonsurgical intervention.

MANAGEMENT OF THE POSTOPERATIVE PATIENT. Recurrent valvular pulmonary stenosis is uncommon and routine serial echocardiography is not indicated, although a baseline study is indicated when an adult patient is first encountered. Thereafter, additional studies need be performed only when a change in clinical status is suggested by the development of symptoms or a change in the physical examination. Patients treated either surgically or by balloon valvuloplasty for valvular pulmonary stenosis in childhood have a low risk for endocarditis. Thus, antibiotic prophylaxis is recommended only in those with a murmur of residual stenosis or insufficiency.

The endocarditis risk is probably higher in those treated for infundibular or supravalvar stenosis, if only because the repair is more likely to have hemodynamic residua. Arrhythmias are less common than in patients with repaired aortic valve stenosis.

GREAT VESSEL AND CORONARY ARTERIAL ABNORMALITIES

Coarctation of the Aorta

Pathophysiology

In the most common form of aortic coarctation, there is narrowing at the level of the ligamentum arteriosus. The constriction may take the form of a localized hourglass narrowing or a hypoplastic segment of the distal arch proximal to the ligamentum. On occasion, the aorta can be completely interrupted at that level.

Proximal to the aortic obstruction, arterial hypertension is usually present. Since there is a lower pressure in the aorta distal to the obstruction, the brachiocephalic vessels form collateral arterial channels with the intercostal arteries and superior and inferior recurrent epigastric arteries, which carry blood around the coarctation to the distal aorta. The key physical findings are femoral pulses that are either absent or delayed and diminished compared with the right brachial pulse. The blood pressure differential between the upper and the lower extremities reflects the pressure drop across the coarctation.

As many as 80% of patients with coarctation of the aorta have an associated bicuspid aortic valve. Aortic aneurysms can occur around the area of the coarctation or elsewhere in the aorta and in the branches of the circle of Willis (so-called berry aneurysms).

Recognition and Diagnosis

HISTORY AND PHYSICAL EXAMINATION. The adult with uncorrected coarctation is usually asymptomatic. Nonspecific symptoms may develop, including exertional dyspnea, headache, epistaxis, and leg fatigue, as well as the symptoms of congestive heart failure. Unfortunately, the presentation of untreated coarctation may be catastrophic, most commonly between the ages of 15 and 40 years, owing to aortic rupture or dissection, infective endocarditis or endarteritis, and cerebral hemorrhage.

Hypertension is present in the right arm or both arms. Usually, in the adult with coarctation, the hypertension is not severe and is predominantly systolic. On palpation, the femoral pulses are diminished and delayed compared with the brachial pulses and may even be absent. Systolic blood pressure is usually 10 to 20 mm Hg higher in the legs; in coarctation, blood pressure in the thighs is lower than in the arms, especially after exercise. With the patient leaning forward, arterial pulsation may be felt posteriorly in the intercostal spaces owing to the pulsations of the enlarged collateral periscapular and intercostal vessels.

Coarctation of the thoracic aorta causes a late-systolic ejection murmur that is usually audible in the second and third interspaces at the left sternal border but also posteriorly to the left of the spine in the interscapular area. At times, the murmur is best heard in the back. If a bicuspid aortic valve is present, there may also be a systolic murmur, a faint aortic regurgitation murmur, and a systolic ejection click.

LABORATORY

CHEST X-RAY. The aortic knob may be enlarged because of lateral displacement of the left subclavian artery. On barium swallow, the esophagus can be seen to have a double indentation, the so-called reversed-3 sign, due to the aortic knob superiorly and a second indentation due to the poststenotic dilatation of the descending aorta distal to the coarctation. Frequently, in the adult, notching of the inferior surfaces of the ribs posteriorly can be seen due to erosion of the ribs by the collateral arteries (Fig. 26–7).

ECG. The ECG frequently is normal or shows left ventricular hypertrophy.

OTHER DIAGNOSTIC PROCEDURES AND REFERRAL FOR CARDIOLOGY CONSULTATION. It is difficult to visualize the actual site of the coarctation in the adult patient with transthoracic two-dimensional echocardiography. However, Doppler studies of the descending aorta, which are not part of routine echocardiography, in the suprasternal notch view may identify and measure the degree of obstruction, even when images are suboptimal. An associated bicuspid aortic valve can also be identified by surface two-dimensional imaging. Angiography or MRI is usually needed to define the site and extent of narrowing.

Referral to a cardiologist is advised to assist with the

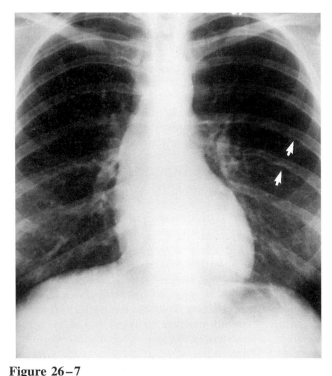

Figure 26–7

Chest x-ray, PA view, of a 25-year-old patient with coarctation of the aorta and a bicuspid aortic valve. Note the prominence of the ascending aorta due to poststenotic dilatation owing to the bicuspid aortic valve and rib notching, especially in the left posterior ribs *(arrows)*.

often-difficult decision of when to operate on patients, especially those with milder degrees of coarctation. Coronary angiography should be performed preoperatively in most adults over the age of 30 years because of the high incidence of premature coronary artery disease.

Course and Complications

The patient may be asymptomatic. However, coarctation and hypertension can lead to the complications of hypertension—stroke, congestive heart failure, and premature coronary artery disease and its complications. In one necropsy series of unrepaired coarctation, 50% of patients died by about age 30 years and 90% by age 60 years.[14] Before the age of 30 years, proximal aortic rupture, aortic dissection, and cerebral hemorrhage due to rupture of a berry aneurysm may occur, and after the age of 40 years, the incidence of congestive heart failure increases. Infective endarteritis (at the site of coarctation) or endocarditis (on a bicuspid aortic valve) is a danger.[15]

Treatment

If the coarctation is severe enough to cause proximal hypertension with a gradient of greater than 25 to 30 mm Hg across the coarctation, repair should be undertaken. Most of these patients will have multiple collateral vessels seen on aortography and atheromatous changes at the site of the coarctation, which can complicate surgery. If the gradient is less than 20 mm Hg and no collaterals are present, repair is not indicated. In some patients, primary balloon dilatation has been used successfully.

MANAGEMENT AND TREATMENT OF THE POSTOPERATIVE PATIENT. Patients with repaired coarctation require continued close clinical follow-up. Hypertension, requiring medical therapy, is likely to persist in those patients repaired after the first 10 years of life. Postoperative patients require antibiotic prophylaxis because of the persistent danger of endocarditis on the bicuspid aortic valve and at the site of repair. A preexistant aneurysm of the circle of Willis may cause a cerebrovascular accident even after coarctation repair.

MRI should be performed as a baseline examination in all postoperative adults with coarctation repair for detection of potential complications including recoarctation, focal saccular aneurysms, and dissecting aneurysms. The incidence of recurrent coarction requiring surgery at 20-year follow-up is about 3%.[16] Focal saccular aortic aneurysms may develop at the site of the repair.[17] Rupture of these aneurysms, more likely in women and during pregnancy, is heralded by the occurrence of paraspinal pain and hemoptysis. Thus, a woman with an aneurysm who is contemplating pregnancy should probably undergo prophylactic reoperation before conception. There is also an ongoing risk of aortic dissection even in the absence of an aneurysm.

The mortality at 20-year follow-up after successful repair is approximately 5%, mostly owing to cardiovascular disease and cerebrovascular accidents.[4] Approximately 10% of patients require subsequent cardiovascular surgery, the majority for aortic valve replacement.[16]

Coronary Artery Anomalies

Although coronary artery anomalies are rare, they should be considered a potential cause in young patients (usually in the second or third decade of life) presenting with symptoms suggestive of ischemia, including exertional syncope or chest pain. The suspicion for a coronary anomaly should be highest when there are no risk factors for premature atherosclerotic disease and there is no evidence of valvular heart disease or cardiomyopathy. The most common coronary anomalies seen in adults are anomalous origin of the left circumflex coronary artery from the right sinus of Valsalva, coronary to pulmonary artery fistulas, coronary cameral fistulas (fistulous connection between the coronary artery and the coronary chamber, usually right atrium or right ventricle), and abnormal origin of the left coronary artery from the anterior sinus of Valsalva or the right coronary artery from the left posterior sinus of Valsalva. Hypoplasia of the coronary arteries with small underdeveloped distal epicardial vessels is a rare condition.

As with other forms of ischemia, the ECG may be normal at rest; exercise testing may be required to detect an abnormality. However, in patients with anomalous origin of a coronary artery, ischemia may not be precipitated by stress, even in patients who have had a previous serious ischemic episode.[18] TTE is rarely diagnostic, although on rare occasions, an anomalous coronary artery may be detected serendipitously when an echocardiogram is obtained for another purpose.

Referral to a cardiologist is indicated for diagnosis and treatment. In some cases, TEE can accurately identify an anomalous origin of the proximal coronary arteries.[19] However, coronary angiography is mandatory in patients requiring surgery and is usually the best next test after an exercise test. When ischemia is definitively demonstrated or the patient has had a syncopal episode during exertion, surgical intervention is the only treatment, given the mechanical origin of the ischemia. The management of asymptomatic anomalies is less certain and depends on their anticipated potential for ischemic complications. With coronary arteriovenous fistulas or coronary cameral fistulas, surgical closure is indicated when the left-to-right shunt exceeds 1.5 : 1.

POSITIONAL ABNORMALITIES

Physiologically "Corrected" Transposition (L-Transposition)

Pathophysiology

This lesion is characterized by malposition of the great vessels and ventricular inversion, with the left ventricle connected to the right atrium and pulmonary artery and the right ventricle connected to the left atrium and aorta.

Blood flow is physiologically correct, but an anatomic right ventricle serves as the systemic ventricle. Most previously undiagnosed adults with this lesion have no other abnormalities.

Recognition and Diagnosis

HISTORY AND PHYSICAL EXAMINATION. With no other abnormalities, this lesion may remain undetected until the patient presents with syncope owing to complete heart block. Since the aortic valve is leftward and anterior in the position of the normal pulmonic valve, S_2 may be very loud and similar to that in a patient with pulmonary hypertension.

LABORATORY

CHEST X-RAY. The radiographic findings depend on whether accompanying defects are present.

ECG. Reversal of the conduction system leads to abnormal septal depolarization with no R-wave in V1 and no Q-waves in V5 and V6. There may be varying degrees of AV block.

Treatment, Course, and Complications

Without additional lesions, patients with corrected transposition may live to old age. The development of complete heart block is common and occurs at a rate of approximately 5% per year in adults. In the presence of severe accompanying lesions, surgical correction may be possible. However, even without additional lesions, the systemic ventricle, an anatomic right ventricle, may show progressive failure requiring medical treatment. Cardiac consultation is indicated to evaluate any accompanying defects and coordinate follow-up.

Dextrocardia and Dextroposition

Pathophysiology

With dextrocardia and situs inversus, the vena cava, atria, ventricles, and great vessels are all reversed and, thus, connected appropriately. Frequently, there are associated congenital heart lesions and the right lung may be hypoplastic.

Recognition and Diagnosis

HISTORY AND PHYSICAL EXAMINATION. The patient is asymptomatic in the absence of other lesions. The abnormality is suspected by palpitating the cardiac activity over the right chest instead of the left. The position of the left ventricular point of maximal impulse can be extremely helpful in making a diagnosis, with it being either in the right mid-clavicular line or at the right sternal border or epigastrium.

LABORATORY

CHEST X-RAY. The definitive diagnosis is made by the radiographic appearance of dextrocardia.

Cardiac consultation is indicated to evaluate whether any associated cardiopulmonary defects are present.

CONGENITAL SYNDROMES ASSOCIATED WITH CARDIAC ANOMALIES

Marfan's Syndrome

Marfan's syndrome, a genetic disorder of connective tissue, is by far the most common syndrome likely to be encountered in the adult patient. It is transmitted as an autosomal dominant trait but has a 30% rate of spontaneous mutation.[20] The most important cardiac manifestations are aortic root dilatation and mitral valve prolapse with mitral regurgitation. The aortic root dilatation is progressive and may be complicated by aortic valve insufficiency, aortic dissection, and rupture. These patients should be followed by serial echocardiography, and prophylactic aortic root repair should be considered when the aortic diameter exceeds 5.0 cm, although other authors have suggested intervention at an earlier stage.[21] Aortic dissection may occur even before the aorta enlarges to that degree, and pregnant women are at particularly high risk. Prophylactic therapy with beta blockers significantly reduces the rate of aortic dilatation and the incidence of aortic insufficiency and dissection.[22] In addition to the aortic complications, progressive mitral regurgitation may occur, especially due to endocarditis and chordal rupture.

A related connective tissue disorder is Ehlers-Danlos syndrome, which is associated with similar cardiac features.

Muscular Dystrophies

Many forms of muscular dystrophy have associated involvement of the myocardium or cardiac conduction system, and these cardiac abnormalities also may be present in some heterozygotic carriers who may not have obvious abnormalities of skeletal muscle function. A baseline ECG and chest x-ray should be obtained, and patients with cardiac symptoms or abnormalities in these screening tests should be referred for cardiac consultation.

SYSTEMIC MANIFESTATIONS OF CONGENITAL HEART DISEASE AND OTHER LIFE ISSUES

Hematology

Patients with significant cyanosis due to congenital heart disease develop secondary erythrocytosis. When these patients are in the "compensated" state, they are asymptomatic with stable hematocrits (usually <65%) and no evidence of iron deficiency.[23] The absolute value for the hematocrit does not determine the clinical state, and occasional patients may even tolerate a hematocrit of 70%. "Decompensated" patients have increasing hematocrits (>65%) and symptoms of hyperviscosity (headache, fatigability, and coagulation abnormalities).[23] Phlebotomy should be performed for headache, fatigability, and hematocrits greater 65% in the presence of symptoms. Moreover, iron deficiency should be excluded as a cause of symptoms and treated if present. A mild bleeding diathesis is also associated with cyanotic heart disease, necessitating preoperative phlebotomy to a hematocrit just below 65% before elective surgery.[23]

Hyperuricemia

The mechanism for hyperuricemia in cyanotic congenital heart disease is poorly understood but does not seem to be based on red cell turnover alone and is likely related to decreased urate clearance by the kidneys. Gout is fairly common and can be treated with conventional therapy; nephrolithiasis is uncommon.[23]

Pulmonary Disease

Hemoptysis most commonly occurs in cyanotic heart disease due to Eisenmenger's syndrome. There are multiple causes including pulmonary edema, pulmonary infection, pulmonary infarction, and pulmonary arteriolar rupture.[24] Moreover, multiple thoracic surgeries, hypoplastic lungs, and a predisposition to frequent pulmonary infections may lead to chronic lung disease. It is important to consider the confounding role of pulmonary disease in the patient with symptomatic dyspnea. In the patient with obstructive lung disease, bronchodilator therapy must be used with caution, so as not to exacerbate underlying arrhythmias. Conversely, in those requiring treatment of arrhythmias with amiodarone, it is important to follow their pulmonary status with serial pulmonary function tests.

Infectious Disease and Endocarditis Prophylaxis

The major risk of infection for patients with congenital heart disease is that due to endocarditis or endarteritis (see Chap. 16). The indications for prophylactic antibiotics are summarized in Table 26–6.[25] Persistent fevers in any patient with congenital heart disease warrant a careful examination for the stigmata of endocarditis. Blood cultures should be obtained if there is any suspicion of endocarditis, but the decision to treat while waiting for results depends on the clinical status of the patient. Careful attention to dental hygiene, skin infections, and other potential sources of bacteremia (e.g., genitourinary tract, especially in sexually active women) is an important adjunctive part of the preventive medical regimen.

Table 26–6	Risk of Endocarditis in Congenital Heart Disease according to Defect		
Defect	**Associated Defects**	**Risk of Endocarditis**	**Prophylaxis Indicated**
Acyanotic			
Bicuspid AV	Coarctation	High	Yes
Valvular PS	VSD (see TOF), Noonan's syndrome	Low (mild PS)	Yes
		Intermediate (severe PS)	Yes
ASD secundum	Mitral valve prolapse	Low	No‡
ASD primum, AV canal	Bridging AV valve leaflets, trisomy 21	Intermediate (with MR)	Yes
VSD	PS (see TOF), AI	Intermediate-high (unoperated or w/AI)	Yes
		Low (operated w/o AI)	No*
PDA	Coexists with many complex syndromes	Low (ligated)	No
		Intermediate (patent)	Yes
Coarctation	Bicuspid AV	Low (operated†)	Yes
		Intermediate (unRx)	Yes
L-TGV	VSD, infundibular PS	Low (isolated L-TGV)	No‡
Ebstein's anomaly	ASD	Low-intermediate	Yes
	PFO		
Cyanotic			
TOF	RAA, ASD	Intermediate	Yes
Eisenmenger's syndrome	VSD, ASD, PDA	Intermediate	Yes
Tricuspid atresia	Pulmonary atresia, ASD, VSD	?	Yes
Pulmonary atresia/intact septum		?	Yes
Postoperative			
Fontan		Low	Yes
Glenn		Low	Yes
Blalock-Taussig		High	Yes
Prosthetic valve		High	Yes
RV-PA conduit		High	Yes

Adapted from Foster, E.: Congenital heart disease in adults. *In* Crawford, M. (ed.): Clinical Diagnosis and Treatment in Cardiology. Norwalk, CT, Appleton & Lange, 1994.

Abbreviations: AV, aortic valve; PS, pulmonic stenosis; VSD, ventricular septal defect; TOF, tetralogy of Fallot; ASD, atrial septal defect; MR, mitral regurgitation; AI, aortic insufficiency; w/, with; w/o, without; PDA, patent ductus arteriosus; unRx, untreated; L-TGV, congenitally corrected transposition of the great vessels; PFO, patent foramen ovale; RAA, right-sided aortic arch; RV, right ventricle; PA, pulmonary artery.

* Indicated for first 6 months postoperative.
† Unless there is associated bicuspid AV.
‡ Indicated in the presence of other lesions.

Reproductive Issues

As patients with congenital heart disease reach reproductive age, birth control and pregnancy need to be specifically addressed. The method of contraception should be individualized and chosen with respect to a number of important issues, including (1) the risk of pregnancy and childbirth for the patient; thus, surgical sterilization might be considered for those at highest risk (i.e., patients with Eisenmenger's syndrome and Marfan's syndrome); (2) the social situation, including the number of partners and the frequency of sexual intercourse; (3) the risk of thrombotic disorders; and (4) the presence of hypertension (e.g., in a patient with unrepaired coarctation). For example, barrier methods (e.g., diaphragm, condom, vaginal sponge) may be employed when there is infrequent sexual intercourse and minimal or low risk of pregnancy. Current hormonal methods—including low-dose estrogen pills, progesterone-only pills, and implanted progesterone—appear to be associated with a low risk of thromboembolic disease and hypertension. Intrauterine devices are relatively contraindicated because of the risk of salpingitis, especially in patients with multiple partners and those at highest risk for endocarditis. The relative advantages and disadvantages of each of these methods should be addressed in conjunction with an experienced gynecologist to help the patient make the most suitable choice.

In the patient who wishes to become pregnant, advance planning is desirable. The patient will then be able to weigh the risks of pregnancy, determined on the basis on her functional class and specific lesion, against her desire to conceive and proceed with pregnancy. Because of the risk of transmission of congenital heart disease (approximately 10% for both the mother and the father), fetal echocardiography is strongly recommended.[26] Nevertheless, with careful management, more and more women with congenital anomalies are able to have successful pregnancies. Both maternal and fetal mortality depend on the maternal functional class; in mothers in New York

Heart Association (NYHA) class I, the risk is 0% and 0.4%, respectively, compared with NYHA class IV with a risk of 30% and 6.8%, respectively.[8] In Eisenmenger's syndrome, maternal mortality is extremely high (50%), but it is much lower with other cyanotic lesions.[27] However, these patients should be aware that the rate of fetal demise may be as high as 50%.

Thus, patients—regardless of the nature of their congenital heart disease—who are in functional class III or IV as well as those with pulmonary vascular disease and Marfan's syndrome should be strongly advised against pregnancy. For all but the lowest-risk patients (functional class I), prenatal care should generally include a high-risk obstetrics service in consultation with a cardiologist. Other issues to consider for maternal and fetal welfare include the presence of ventricular dysfunction, arrhythmias, and their therapy, and the need for antibiotic prophylaxis and anticoagulation. The safest management of anticoagulation during pregnancy for patients with prosthetic valves is an unresolved issue and, therefore, should be planned on an individual basis in consultation with a high-risk obstetrics service and a cardiologist.

Exercise Guidelines

Adult patients with congenital heart disease frequently request guidelines for physical exercise and participation in sports. In a recent conference, general guidelines for exercise were outlined and some of these recommendations are summarized in Table 26–7.[28] However, exercise prescriptions must be individualized with an emphasis on the severity of the lesion and the patient's clinical status. The clinical features that seriously limit exercise tolerance and increase the risk of exercise include cyanosis, pulmonary hypertension, ventricular dysfunction, and arrhythmias. The specific lesions considered to place the patient at highest risk during exercise are severe aortic stenosis, anomalous origin of the left coronary artery, Marfan's syndrome, and severe mitral valve prolapse. Exercise test-

Table 26–7	Exercise Guidelines for Patients with Congenital Heart Disease	
Unrestricted	**Low-Intensity Sports***	**No Competitive Sports**
ASD, VSD—operated† or small	ASD, VSD—moderate	ASD, VSD with CHF or Eisenmenger's
PDA—operated† or small	PDA—moderate	PDA with CHF or Eisenmenger's
PV stenosis (<50 mm Hg)	PV Stenosis (>50 mm Hg)	Severe PV stenosis with symptoms
AV stenosis (<25 mm Hg‡)	AV stenosis (25–49 mm Hg‡)	AV stenosis (>50 mm Hg‡)
Coarctation—treated§	Coarctation (<20 mm Hg differential)	Coarctation (>20 mm Hg differential)
	Unoperated or palliated cyanotic heart disease	
Repaired TOF w/o residua	Repaired TOF with mild RV pressure or volume overload	Repaired TOF with severe residua
TGV s/p arterial switch	TGV status post atrial switch	
	Anomalous left coronary artery	
	Marfan's syndrome¶	

Adapted from Graham, T.P., Bricker, J.T., James, F.W., and Strong, W.B.: 26th Bethesda Conference: Recommendations for determining eligibility for competition in athletes with cardiovascular abnormalities. Task Force 1: Congenital heart disease. Reprinted with permission from the American College of Cardiology (J. Am. Coll. Cardiol. 24:867–873, 1994).

Abbreviations: ASD, atrial septal defect; VSD, ventricular septal defect; CHF, congestive heart failure; PDA, patent ductus arteriosus; PV, pulmonary valve; AV, aortic valve; TOF, tetralogy of Fallot; w/o, without; RV, right ventricular; TGV, transposition of the great vessels.

* Low-intensity sports include those with low static and dynamic activity: billiards, bowling, cricket, curling, golf, and riflery.

† Operated, without residual pulmonary hypertension.

‡ Peak gradient.

§ Treated without residual BP difference and without significant hypertension.

¶ No body-contact sports.

ing to detect ischemia, arrhythmias, and hemodynamic instability may be helpful in evaluating the safety of exercise in an individual patient. As isometric (i.e., static) exercise raises blood pressure to high levels in a short period of time, patients with lesions potentially exacerbated by increased afterload (e.g., those with aortic insufficiency or systemically functioning right ventricle) should avoid weightlifting and similar activities.

Occasionally, physicians are consulted as to the safety of scuba diving in cardiac patients. During decompression, gas bubbles are found in the venous circulation. In the presence of an abnormal intracardiac communication, such as an uncorrected ventricular septal defect or atrial septal defect, there may be paradoxical embolization of these gas bubbles.[29] Patients with uncorrected atrial or ventricular septal defects should therefore refrain from recreational or professional diving. There also appears to be a greater than normal incidence of patent foramen ovale in divers who suffer decompression sickness, but screening for patent foramen ovale, found normally in up to 25% of the population, is generally not recommended.[30]

Work, Travel, and Insurance

Many people with congenital heart disease have been successful in school and are gainfully employed. The work must be tailored to any physical limitations (see earlier). The ability to maintain employment is critical to the patient's overall well-being, and efforts should be made to help the patient continue working.

The safety of airplane travel was recently addressed in a study of cyanotic patients in both simulated and actual commercial flights.[31] The fall in arterial oxygen saturation was similar to that in normal patients and was well tolerated. Thus, as long as the stress of travel is not excessive on the basis of other medical considerations (e.g., heart failure or arrhythmias), air travel is probably safe without the need for supplemental oxygen.

Medical insurance and life insurance are frequently unavailable to many patients with congenital heart disease. Thus, in the current medical environment, the high-cost medical care that these patients require may be difficult to deliver, posing important ethical and economic issues.

CONCLUSIONS

The primary care physician will not see many patients with significant congenital heart disease compared with all the other problems in his or her practice. However, with the increasing probability that these patients will survive to adulthood, they will occasionally be encountered in a primary care practice. Their medical problems are varied, at times complicated and challenging. It is imperative that the primary care doctor be able to recognize these patients and be aware of their ongoing problems. The interaction between their congenital heart disease and other medical illnesses must be appreciated. In this way, these patients can receive proper and appropriate care.

References

1. Congenital heart disease after childhood: An expanding patient population. 22nd Bethesda Conference, Bethesda, MD, October 18–19, 1990. J. Am. Coll. Cardiol. 18:311–342, 1991.
2. McNamara, D.G., and Latson, L.A.: Long-term follow-up of patients with malformations for which definitive surgical repair has been available for 25 years or more. Am. J. Cardiol. 50:560–568, 1982.
3. Perloff, J., and Child, J.: Natural survival patterns. In Perloff, J., and Child, J. (eds.): Congenital Heart Disease in Adults. Philadelphia, W.B. Saunders, 1991.
4. Morris, C., and Menashe, V.: 25-year mortality after surgical repair of congenital heart defect in childhood. A population-based cohort study. JAMA 266:3447–3452, 1991.
5. Murphy, J.G., Gersh, B.J., McGoon, M.D., et al.: Long-term outcome after surgical repair of isolated atrial septal defect. Follow-up at 27 to 32 years. N. Engl. J. Med. 323:1645–1650, 1990.
6. Konstantinides, S., Geibel, A., Olschewski, M., et al.: A comparison of surgical and medical therapy for atrial septal defect in adults. N. Engl. J. Med. 333:469–473, 1995.
7. Ellis, J.R., Moodie, D.S., Sterba, R., and Gill, C.C.: Ventricular septal defect in the adult: Natural and unnatural history. Am. Heart J. 114:115–120, 1987.
8. Perloff, J.K.: Pregnancy and congenital heart disease. J. Am. Coll. Cardiol. 18:340–342, 1991.
9. Murphy, J.G., Gersh, B.J., Mair, D.D., et al.: Long-term outcome in patients undergoing surgical repair of tetralogy of Fallot. N. Engl. J. Med. 329:593–599, 1993.
10. Keane, J.F., Driscoll, D.J., Gersony, W.M., et al.: Second natural history study of congenital heart defects. Results of treatment of patients with aortic valvar stenosis. Circulation 87:I-16–I-27, 1993.
11. Ross, D., Jackson, M., and Davies, J.: Pulmonary autograft aortic valve replacement: Long-term results. J. Am. Coll. Cardiol. 23:69–75, 1994.
12. van Son, J.A., Schaff, H.V., Danielson, G.K., et al.: Surgical treatment of discrete and tunnel subaortic stenosis. Late survival and risk of reoperation. Circulation 88:II-159–I-169, 1993.
13. Hayes, C.J., Gersony, W.M., Driscoll, D.J., et al.: Second natural history study of congenital heart defects. Results of treatment of patients with pulmonary valvar stenosis. Circulation 87:I-28–I-37, 1993.
14. Campbell, M.: Natural history of coarctation of the aorta. Br. Heart J. 32:633–640, 1970.
15. Liberthson, R., Pennington, D., Jacobs, M., and Daggett, W.: Coarctation of the aorta: Review of 234 patients and clarification of management problems. Am. J. Cardiol. 43:835–840, 1979.
16. Cohen, M., Fuster, V., Steele, P.M., et al.:. Coarctation of the aorta. Long-term follow-up and prediction of outcome after surgical correction [see comments]. Circulation 80:40–45, 1989.
17. Parks, W.J., Ngo, T.D., Plaurth, W.H., et al.: Incidence of aneurysm formation after Dacron patch aortoplasty repair for coarctation of the aorta: Long-term results and assessment utilizing magnetic resonance angiography with three-dimensional surface rendering. J. Am. Coll. Cardiol. 26:266–271, 1995.
18. Hoffman, J.E.: Congenital anomalies of the coronary vessels and the aortic root, In Emmanouilides, G.C., Riemenschneider, T.A., Allen, H.D., and Gutgesell, H.P. (eds.): Heart Disease in Infants, Children and Adolescents: Including the Fetus and Young Adult. Baltimore, Williams & Wilkins, 1995, pp. 769–791.
19. Fernandes, F., Alam, M., Smith, S., and Khaja F.: The role of transesophageal echocardiography in identifying anomalous coronary arteries. Circulation 88:2532–2540, 1993.
20. Pyeritz, R., and Murphy, E.: Genetics and congenital heart disease: Perspectives and prospects. J. Am. Coll. Cardiol. 13:1458–1468, 1989.
21. Francke, U., and Furthmayr, H.: Marfan's syndrome and other disorders of fibrillin. N. Engl. J. Med. 330:1384–1385, 1994.
22. Shores, J., Berger, K.R., Murphy, E.A., and Pyeritz, R.E.: Progression of aortic dilatation and the benefit of long-term beta-adrenergic blockade in Marfan's syndrome [see comments]. N. Engl. J. Med. 330:1335–1341, 1994.
23. Territo, M.C., and Rosove, M.H.: Cyanotic congenital heart disease: Hematologic management. J. Am. Coll. Cardiol. 18:320–322, 1991.

24. Graham, T.: The Eisenmenger syndrome. *In* Roberts, W.C. (ed.): Adult Congenital Heart Disease. Philadelphia, F.A. Davis, 1987, pp. 567–581.

25. Dajani, A.S., Taubert, K.A., Wilson, W., et al.: Prevention of bacterial endocarditis. Recommendations by the American Heart Association [see comments]. Circulation 96:358–366, 1997.

26. Whittemore, R., Wells, J.A., and Castellsague, X.: A second-generation study of 427 probands with congenital heart defects and their 837 children. J. Am. Coll. Cardiol. 23:1459–1467, 1994.

27. Presbitero, P., Somerville, J., Stone, S., et al.: Pregnancy in cyanotic congenital heart disease. Outcome of mother and fetus. Circulation 89:2673–2676, 1994.

28. Graham, T.P., Bricker, J.T., James, F.W., and Strong, W.B.: 26th Bethesda Conference: Recommendations for determining eligibility for competition in athletes with cardiovascular abnormalities. Task Force 1: Congenital heart disease. J. Am. Coll. Cardiol. 24:867–873, 1994.

29. Bove, A.A.: Cardiovascular disorders and diving. *In* Bove, A.A., and Davis, J.C. (eds.): Diving and Medicine. Philadelphia, W.B. Saunders, 1990, pp. 239–248.

30. Moon, R.E., Camporesi, E.M., and Kisslo, J.A.: Patent foramen ovale and decompression sickness in divers. Lancet 1:513–514, 1989.

31. Harnick, E., Hutter, P.A., Hoorntje, T.M., et al.: Air travel and adults with cyanotic congenital heart disease. Circulation 93:272–276, 1996.

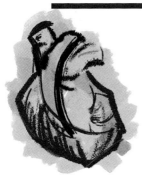

Chapter 27

Recognition and Management
of Patients with

Diseases of the Aorta: Aneurysms and Dissection

PATRICK T. O'GARA

The Normal Aorta

The aorta is the primary conduit through which the cardiac output is delivered to the systemic arterial bed. It is divided at the level of the diaphragm into thoracic and abdominal segments. The thoracic aorta can be further subdivided into the ascending, arch, and descending portions. The ascending aorta arises from the base of the left ventricle and courses superiorly and rightward. The aortic arch gives rise to the brachiocephalic vessels. The descending thoracic aorta is a posterior mediastinal structure with attachments to the thoracic cage and comprises the segment between the left subclavian artery and the diaphragm. The abdominal aorta extends from the diaphragmatic hiatus to its bifurcation into the common iliac arteries and is divided into suprarenal and infrarenal segments.

The wall of the aorta, like that of other arteries, is composed of three layers: intima, media, and adventitia. Its tensile strength derives primarily from the elastic lamellar units of the media and secondarily from smooth muscle cells, collagen, and ground substances. With age, the elastic fibers of the media degenerate, a process accelerated by hypertension or inflammation—conditions that predispose the aorta to aneurysmal enlargement or dissection. The terms *aneurysm* and *dissection* are not synonymous. The former implies pathologic enlargement or expansion, whereas the latter refers to the process by which a cleavage plane is created between the inner and the outer portions of the wall by the surging column of blood as it is propelled forward during each cardiac contraction. An aortic dissection can occur in a previously aneurysmal segment. Alternatively, the dissection process may lead to aneurysm formation if the false lumen continues to expand.

AORTIC ANEURYSM

Classification

Ectasia and *aneurysm* are descriptive terms indicative of vessel enlargement. The former refers to mild dilatation and usually some degree of uncoiling or tortuosity, whereas the latter implies luminal expansion beyond 1.5 to 2.0 times the normal aortic diameter. Aneurysms are generally of three types: fusiform (diffuse) (Fig. 27–1), saccular (asymmetric and protruding) (Fig. 27–2), and false. Fusiform and saccular aneurysms are "true" aneurysms in that their walls are composed of all three aortic layers. "False" aneurysms are contained ruptures whose outer walls are composed of periadventitial hematoma (Table 27–1).

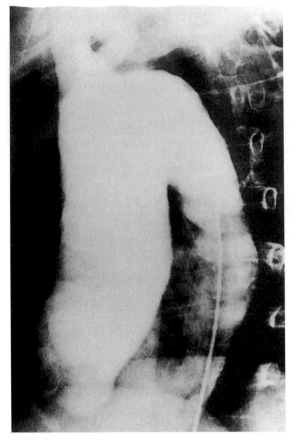

Figure 27–1

Contrast aortogram in the left posterior oblique projection demonstrates diffuse aneurysmal enlargement of the entire ascending and arch portions of the thoracic aorta. (From Creager, M.A., Halperin, J.L., and Whittemore, A.D.: Aneurysmal disease of the aorta and its branches. *In* Loscalzo, J., Creager, M.A., and Dzau, V.J. [eds.]: Vascular Medicine: A Textbook of Vascular Biology and Diseases. Boston, Little, Brown, 1992, pp. 903–930.)

Thoracic Aortic Aneurysm

Ascending Aortic Aneurysms

Aneurysms of the ascending aorta are asymptomatic in the majority of patients and are usually first detected on a chest x-ray obtained for other indications (Fig. 27–3). In some patients, enlargement of the aortic root, especially when it exceeds 5 cm in diameter, is accompanied by a murmur of aortic regurgitation due to malcoaptation of the leaflets. Radiation of the murmur predominantly to the right, rather than to the left, of the sternum suggests that the regurgitation is secondary to disease of the aortic root rather than of primary valvular origin. Rarely, a right superior parasternal pulsation can be appreciated.

CAUSE. The majority of ascending aortic aneurysms are fusiform. The most common cause is *cystic medial necrosis*, a noninflammatory degenerative process of the aortic media with fragmentation of elastic fibers, drop-out of smooth muscle cells, and pooling of mucoid-like ground substances. This process weakens the wall of the aortic root and predisposes to aneurysm formation or dissection, or both. Specific diseases associated with cystic medial necrosis include Marfan's syndrome and, less commonly, other inherited disorders of connective tissue, such as Ehlers-Danlos syndrome, osteogenesis imperfecta, and the mucopolysaccharidoses (Hunter's and Hurler's syndromes).

Marfan's syndrome is caused by a mutation in the gene for *fibrillin*, a protein that is critical to the structural integrity of the aortic media. Common clinical manifestations of the syndrome include an abnormally long arm span, arachnodactyly, ectopia lentis, high-arched palate, scoliosis, pectus excavatum, and aortic and mitral regurgitation.[1] Not all patients with cystic medial necrosis on pathologic examination of an aortic aneurysm specimen have a recognizable connective tissue disorder, but certain clinical clues are commonly present, such as a history of spontaneous pneumothoraces or inguinal hernias. The term *annuloaortic ectasia* is a clinical and pathoanatomic descriptor that is applied to the condition affecting a sub-

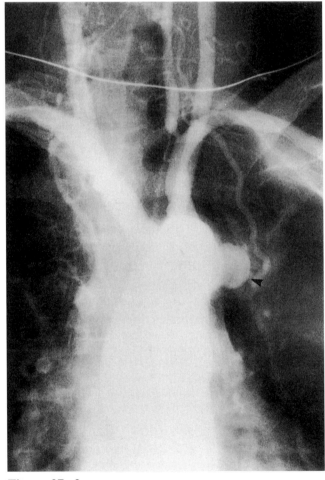

Figure 27–2

Contrast aortogram in an anteroposterior (AP) projection demonstrates a saccular aneurysm *(arrowhead)* that protrudes from the distal arch. (From Creager, M.A., Halperin, J.L., and Whittemore, A.D.: Aneurysmal disease of the aorta and its branches. *In* Loscalzo, J., Creager, M.A., and Dzau, V.J. [eds.]: Vascular Medicine: A Textbook of Vascular Biology and Diseases. Boston, Little, Brown, 1992, pp. 903–930.)

Table 27–1.	Classification of Aortic Aneurysms

Type
Fusiform
Saccular
False (pseudo-)

Location

Thoracic
   Ascending
   Arch
   Descending
Thoracoabdominal
Abdominal
   Suprarenal
   Infrarenal

set of patients with aneurysms involving the aortic root, associated with aortic regurgitation, but not accompanied by other evidence of connective tissue abnormalities.[2]

Atherosclerosis is a distinctly *uncommon* cause of ascending aortic aneurysm. When atherosclerotic changes are present in this portion of the aorta, evidence of the disease in other segments of the aorta and systemic vascular beds is usually quite obvious. In contrast to aneurysms that result from cystic medial necrosis, which are confined to the ascending aorta, atherosclerotic changes extend into and, often, beyond the arch.

In recent years, there has been an increasing appreciation for the importance of inflammatory conditions that affect the aorta and predispose to its aneurysmal enlargement.[3] These include *giant cell arteritis,* which predominantly affects the large and medium-sized muscular arteries, often including the temporal arteries, and occurs most commonly in elderly women. Associated symptoms such as low-grade fever, fatigue, headache, and proximal girdle stiffness (polymyalgia rheumatica) are common. The involvement of the aorta typically occurs in the ascending portion but spares the root and annulus. Both the arch and the descending thoracic aorta can be involved as well. Aortic dissection has also been described.

Takayasu's arteritis, on the other hand, affects a younger population (mean age at diagnosis = 29 years), 90% of whom are women.[4] Although traditionally described as "pulseless disease" owing to proximal obliteration of the major arch vessels, there are both aneurysmal and stenotic variants, even in the same patient. The granulomatous inflammation within the adventitial and medial layers causes systemic inflammation, with fever and weight loss, and pain and tenderness over affected arteries, with hypertension and symptoms of vascular insufficiency of the upper extremities.

A *congenital sinus of Valsalva aneurysm* is a pathologic enlargement of the aorta confined to one of the three sinuses. This condition does not usually become clinically evident until the aneurysm ruptures spontaneously, typically into a right heart chamber, causing chest pain, dyspnea, and a loud, continuous, or to-and-fro murmur.

Aortic Arch Aneurysms

Isolated aneurysms of the aortic arch are uncommon. Pathologic conditions affecting this portion of the aorta typically involve either or both the ascending and descending segments as well. Cystic medial necrosis, inflammation, and atherosclerosis are the most common causes. Since the major vessels originate from the arch, the surgical approach to this portion of the aorta is complex.

Descending Thoracic Aortic Aneurysms

Atherosclerosis is by far the most common cause of descending thoracic aortic aneurysm. Aneurysms of the descending thoracic aorta are usually asymptomatic and are most often detected on chest x-rays performed for the evaluation of other problems. When symptoms do occur, they range from a nondescript, dull ache in the left posterior chest to dysphagia secondary to extrinsic compression of the esophagus, to hoarseness because of impingement of the left recurrent laryngeal nerve, or to dyspnea/cough/wheezing or stridor owing to compression of the left main stem bronchus or its major branches. When aneurysms of the descending aorta cross the diaphragm, they are termed *thoracoabdominal aneurysms,* which may present with symptoms or signs related chiefly to the abdominal component, such as a prominent epigastric pulsation.[5]

Trauma due to a rapid deceleration injury, such as a motor vehicle accident, may result in transection of the descending thoracic aorta and false aneurysm formation. Because of the threat of rupture, prompt surgical repair of posttraumatic aneurysms is mandated.

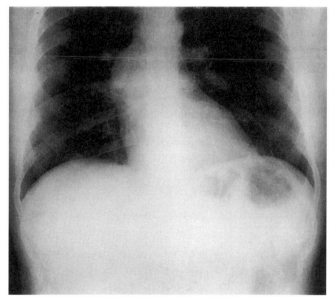

Figure 27–3
Chest x-ray of a 43-year-old man with an asymptomatic ascending aortic aneurysm. (From Creager, M.A., and Halperin, J.L.: Aortic and arterial aneurysms. *In* Creager, M.A. [vol. ed.]: Vascular Disease. Braunwald, E. [ser. ed.]: Atlas of Heart Diseases. Philadelphia, Current Medicine, 1996, pp. 1.1–1.19.)

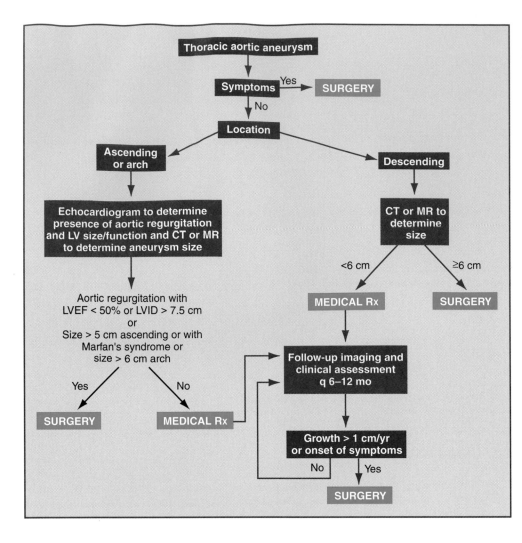

Figure 27–4

Approach to the patient with a thoracic aortic aneurysm. The first branch point is to ascertain whether symptoms suggestive of growth (pain, compression of adjacent structures) are present. If so, prompt surgical referral should be made. The location, extent, and size of the aneurysm should otherwise be documented. For any patient with Marfan's syndrome, referral to a cardiovascular specialist should be made. An additional concern in the patient with an ascending aortic aneurysm is the possible coexistence of aortic valve regurgitation, the presence of which may pose another set of criteria for surgical repair independent of the aneurysm's size. Isolated arch aneurysms are rare and are usually addressed in concert with either the ascending or the descending aortic component. A schedule of clinical and radiographic surveillance must be established to ensure continued aggressive medical therapy (as, e.g., against hypertension) and to measure the size and rate of growth of the aneurysm. SURG, surgery; AR, aortic regurgitation; CT, contrast chest computed tomography scan; MR, magnetic resonance scan; ECHO, transthoracic echocardiogram; MED Rx, medical therapy; LVEF, left ventricular ejection fraction; LVID, left ventricular internal diastolic dimension; F/U, follow-up; q, every.

Approach to the Patient

(Fig. 27–4)

The history should include special reference to those symptoms that suggest aortic expansion or threatened rupture—that is, pain or features such as dysphagia or hoarseness that suggest encroachment on adjacent structures. In the presence of aortic valve involvement by an aneurysm leading to aortic regurgitation, left ventricular failure may be a warning sign of aneurysmal expansion. Questions should also be posed regarding familial involvement (suggesting Marfan's syndrome, osteogenesis imperfecta, or other inheritable disorders of connective tissue), associated problems that suggest a connective tissue or inflammatory condition, prior trauma, infections, and a history of the risk factors for atherosclerotic vascular disease, such as hypercholesterolemia, hypertension, cigarette smoking, or diabetes.

Physical Examination

The physical examination should note body size and habitus. The blood pressure should be measured in all four extremities, and careful notation should be made of all major arterial pulses. The presence of a bruit over the carotid, subclavian, and femoral arteries, as well as the abdominal aorta, should be sought. The cardiac examination should ascertain heart size and the presence of heart murmurs, especially aortic regurgitation. The skin, eyes, skeletal system, and joints should be examined for any clues as to the presence of an underlying connective tissue or systemic inflammatory condition; the latter may occur in giant cell arteritis and Takayasu's arteritis.

Diagnostic Tests

The location, extent, size, shape, and when possible, the rate of growth of the aneurysm should then be defined. A chest x-ray is a very useful starting point, and every effort should be made to obtain previous chest x-rays for comparison. Simple visual comparison of radiographs often allows an appreciation of the rate of growth of the aneurysm.

Every patient with an aneurysm of the ascending aorta and an aortic diastolic murmur should have transthoracic echocardiography (TTE) to define the severity of the regurgitation, to measure left ventricular chamber size, and to assess left ventricular systolic function. Because the ascending aorta is an anterior structure within the mediastinum, TTE can also provide clear images for several centimeters above the level of the aortic valve in most patients. TTE, however, is much *less* useful for the evaluation of aneurysms of the aortic arch and descending thoracic aorta. Transesophageal echocardiography (TEE) is more valuable for the latter,[6] but noninvasive cross-sectional imaging, as can be accomplished with contrast computed tomography (CT) (Fig. 27–5) or magnetic resonance imaging (MRI) (Fig. 27–6), is more appropriate for an elective examination in a patient in whom an acute dissection is not suspected. Both of the latter modalities offer a relatively wider field of view and greater resolution. In the assessment of the patient with an ascending aortic aneurysm with or without aortic regurgitation, if the TTE windows prove technically inadequate or if concern is raised that the aneurysm extends beyond the field of view, then either a contrast CT scan or MRI should be obtained to provide better clarification and definition. The choice of which modality to pursue depends primarily on the local availability of equipment and radiologic expertise. Invasive contrast aortography is usually not necessary for screening, diagnosis, or assessment of the growth of the aneurysm, but it is often useful in planning surgical repair.

Patients with suspected Marfan's syndrome should undergo TTE even in the absence of findings that suggest the presence of aortic root involvement, since this portion of the aorta may be hidden within the cardiomediastinal silhouette on chest x-rays. Because the prognosis in these patients is dependent on the size of the aortic root, it is important to measure this dimension accurately and to follow it closely on serial measurements. The echocardiogram is also a useful means for assessing the mitral valve apparatus that is often involved in patients with Marfan's syndrome.

The need for and type of laboratory testing depend on the suspected cause and associated complications. There is no specific laboratory testing that is routine. A rapid plasma reagin test for syphilis should be obtained in appropriate patients with a calcified aneurysm of the ascending aorta. An erythrocyte sedimentation rate may be a helpful guide to immunosuppressive therapy in patients with an inflammatory aortitis (giant cell, Takayasu's). Blood cultures should be obtained in patients with suspected infection of an aortic aneurysm.

Management

The natural history of thoracic aortic aneurysms is variable and depends on the underlying cause, size, and associated features that promote continued expansion. Aneurysmal size and rates of enlargement are the strongest predictors for rupture. Aneurysms greater than 5 cm in maximal diameter or that grow rapidly (a diameter increase greater than 0.5 cm/yr) are at high risk for rupture, as are those associated with pain, which also suggests expansion. The incidence of rupture does *not* seem to be related to the anatomic segment of the thoracic aorta involved. Surveillance imaging should be done on an annual basis, or every 6 months should there be concern about rapid growth. Such imaging may be accomplished with simple posteroanterior and lateral chest films for many patients with a descending thoracic aortic aneurysm, but it usually must involve contrast CT scanning or MRI studies in patients with ascending or arch involvement.

As extrapolated from the clinical experience with the medical management of patients with acute aortic dissection as well as from a randomized controlled trial in patients with Marfan's syndrome,[7] treatment with a beta blocker to control blood pressure and its rate of rise appears to be useful in slowing expansion and decreasing the associated risk of rupture. The corrective surgery for a thoracic aortic aneurysm is difficult, usually requires cardiopulmonary bypass, and should be undertaken only in

Figure 27–5
Contrast chest computed tomography (CT) scan of the same patient as in Figure 27–3. This image is obtained at the level of the right ventricular outflow tract and confirms the presence of an ascending aortic aneurysm. (From Creager, M.A., and Halperin, J.L.: Aortic and arterial aneurysms. *In* Creager, M.A. [vol. ed.]: Vascular Disease. Braunwald, E. [ser. ed.]: Atlas of Heart Diseases. Philadelphia, Current Medicine, 1996, pp. 1.1–1.19.)

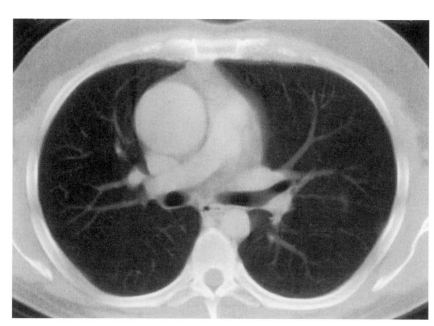

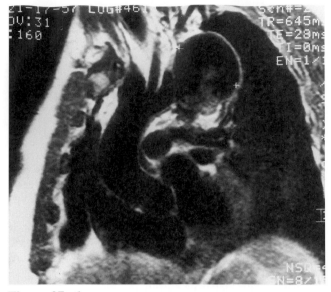

Figure 27–6

Magnetic resonance imaging (MRI) scan through the long axis of the aorta of a 28-year-old man with a large saccular aneurysm. This man had undergone repair of an aortic coarctation 10 years previously and developed a false aneurysm at the proximal suture line that incorporated the origin of the left subclavian artery.

centers with a skilled and experienced surgical team. Because aneurysms in patients with Marfan's syndrome have a higher risk of rupture than atherosclerotic aneurysms, these patients must be managed more aggressively.

Referral to a Cardiovascular Specialist

Patients with an aneurysm of the thoracic aorta should be referred to a cardiovascular specialist with the presence of any of the following:

1. Symptoms, especially pain
2. Marfan's syndrome
3. Maximal aortic diameter greater than 5.0 cm
4. Rate of growth greater than 0.5 cm/yr
5. Hypertension that is difficult to control
6. Suspected false aneurysm, regardless of size
7. Associated coronary or peripheral vascular disease that would potentially complicate surgical management

The optimal timing of surgery for thoracic aortic aneurysms remains a subject of controversy, given the variable natural history as a function of cause, the high prevalence of associated cardiovascular disorders that independently affect long-term outcome, and the inherent risks of such technically demanding surgery. Surgical repair is recommended as shown in Table 27–2.[8, 9]

Aneurysms that involve the root of the aorta and that are accompanied by severe aortic regurgitation usually require combined replacement of the ascending aorta and aortic valve, which adds to the risk of operation. Aneurysms that extend from the ascending aorta into the arch

are also more difficult to repair, and such surgery entails a higher risk of cerebrovascular complications, with stroke or neuropsychiatric changes occurring in as many as 10% to 15% of patients.[9] The most feared complication of surgery on the descending aorta is postoperative paraplegia from ischemic spinal cord damage, which occurs in approximately 5% of patients despite the adoption of a variety of techniques to perfuse the distal circulation during the period of cross-clamping.[9]

Postoperative Management

After the patient's recovery from operation, it is critical for the primary care physician to (1) continue aggressive efforts at blood pressure control, using a beta blocker whenever possible; (2) aggressively modify other cardiovascular risk factors; (3) establish a schedule of periodic imaging studies to screen for complications related to the operation (such as late false aneurysm formation) and to ensure that aneurysmal disease does not appear or progress in other segments of the aorta, especially in susceptible persons, such as those with Marfan's syndrome or those previously identified as having involvement of multiple aortic segments; and (4) supervise appropriate anticoagulation in patients with mechanical prosthetic valves.

Thoracoabdominal Aortic Aneurysms

Classification

Thoracoabdominal aneurysms are classified into four anatomic groups: Type I involve most of the descending thoracic and suprarenal abdominal aorta; type II extend from just beyond the origin of the left subclavian artery to the aortic bifurcation with involvement of visceral and renal arteries; type III commence in the mid- to distal portion of the descending thoracic aorta and extend to the bifurcation of the abdominal aorta; type IV begin at or

Table 27–2	Indications for Surgery of Aortic Aneurysms		
Ascending Thoracic	**Descending Thoracic**	**Thoracoabdominal**	**Abdominal Aorta**
Pain	Pain	As for descending thoracic or abdominal aorta	Pain, tenderness
Severe AR	Compression of adjacent structures		Atheroemboli
Size ≥ 6 cm Marfan's ≥5 cm	Size ≥ 6 cm		Size ≥ 5 cm
Growth ≥ 1 cm/yr	Growth ≥ 1 cm/yr		Growth ≥ 1 cm/yr

Adapted from Creager, M.A., and Halperin, J.L.: Aortic and arterial aneurysms. *In* Creager, M.A. (vol. ed.): Vascular Disease. Braunwald, E. (ser. ed.): Atlas of Heart Diseases. Philadelphia, Current Medicine, 1996, pp. 1.1–1.19.

Abbreviation: AR, aortic regurgitation.

just superior to the diaphragmatic hiatus and extend beyond the origin of the renal arteries, usually to the bifurcation.[5] Type IV aneurysms are essentially synonymous with abdominal aortic aneurysms, which are discussed later. Atherosclerosis is by far the most common cause of thoracoabdominal aneurysms, which occur more commonly in men than in women.

Imaging

Attention is usually drawn to the presence of a thoracoabdominal aneurysm when the thoracic component is identified on a routine chest x-ray or when an abdominal aortic aneurysm is first appreciated by physical examination. The extent of thoracoabdominal aortic involvement and the degree of luminal enlargement can be assessed with either contrast CT scanning or MRI. Adjunctive abdominal ultrasound examinations to assess the size or rate of growth of the abdominal aortic component should not be necessary, provided that the CT or MRI studies are obtained with the appropriate windows that should extend to the pelvis. Surgical planning, however, usually requires contrast aortography for precise delineation of the relationship between the aneurysm and the major aortic branch vessels.

Management

Medical management of patients with thoracoabdominal aortic aneurysm should follow the general principles outlined previously for the thoracic aneurysms. Namely, the blood pressure must be strictly controlled, using a beta blocker whenever possible, and efforts at smoking cessation and lipid management should be intensified. Concomitant renal disease should be identified, since this may be an indicator of the presence of renal artery stenosis, which may also need to be addressed at the time of surgical repair. The indications for surgery, as for thoracic aneurysms, can be reduced to the following three: (1) symptoms of expansion, especially pain; (2) thoracic diameter greater than 6 cm or abdominal diameter greater than 5 cm; and (3) rate of growth (>1 cm/yr).

The major postoperative complications include paraplegia (in thoracic aneurysm), renal failure (which occurs in as many as 5% to 10% of patients), and myocardial infarction. Longer-term, postoperative medical management is similar to that for patients with thoracic aortic aneurysms.

Abdominal Aortic Aneurysms

Aneurysms of the abdominal aorta, which are most commonly caused by atherosclerosis, are subdivided into two major classes: suprarenal (or pararenal) and infrarenal. Nearly 90% are in the latter category. Genetic factors may play a causative role, since there is a distinct familial incidence of abdominal aortic aneurysm in families with decreased type III collagen and elastin or increased collagenase activity within the aortic wall. As many as 25% of patients with an abdominal aortic aneurysm have an affected first-degree relative.[10] There is also a 10% to 15% incidence of coexistent popliteal artery aneurysms. Infrarenal abdominal aortic aneurysms occur in men two to five times as frequently as in women. Their prevalence increases with age and is higher among patients with evidence of coexistent atherosclerotic peripheral vascular disease.

Rupture

Spontaneous rupture is the most feared complication of abdominal aortic aneurysm. Risk factors for rupture include large size, rapid rate of enlargement, and pain. In an autopsy review of 591 cases of abdominal aortic aneurysm, 118 of which had ruptured, Darling and colleagues reported that rupture occurred in 10% of aneurysms smaller than 4.0 cm in maximal diameter, 25% of those 4.0 to 7.0 cm, 45% of those 7.0 to 10.0 cm, and 60% of aneurysms greater than 10.0 cm.[11] Several other large series support the contention that the risk of rupture becomes unacceptably high once the aneurysm reaches a maximal diameter of 5.0 cm.[12] Rapid expansion, defined as an increase in diameter of more than 1.0 cm over the course of 1 year, similarly is an indicator of high risk. Likewise, pain in the flank, low back, or abdomen or tenderness localized to the epigastric pulsation may herald rupture. Aneurysmal rupture is an extremely hazardous condition; approximately 60% of patients die before reaching the operating room, and of those operated on, the mortality is 50%.[12]

Approach to the Patient

(Fig. 27–7)

In asymptomatic persons, the examiner should be able to detect an abdominal aortic aneurysm 4.0 cm or larger in diameter on palpation, except perhaps in obese individuals or those with an unusual body habitus. Suspicion of the presence of an aneurysm should be raised if the common femoral or popliteal arteries feel unusually large. It is not uncommon for the diagnosis to be established only after an abdominal or lumbar spine imaging study obtained for other clinical reasons.

Abdominal ultrasonography can detect aortic aneurysms with nearly 100% sensitivity and provide an assessment of size in the transverse and anteroposterior dimensions to within 3 mm.[9] This technique defines the longitudinal extent of the aneurysm less well, but it is otherwise extremely useful for screening and follow-up. It is safe, reproducible, and noninvasive and does not entail exposure to contrast media or ionizing radiation. Ultrasonography can also provide an assessment of mural thrombus in aneurysms. This technique, however, does not suffice for surgical planning, since it does not allow for an appreciation of the relationship between the aneurysm and the branch vessels.

Both contrast CT scanning (Fig. 27–8) and MRI offer wider fields of view and better resolution than does ultrasonography in the accurate depiction of the size, shape, and extent of abdominal aortic aneurysms.[9] Newer, computer-generated reconstruction techniques can define the relationship between the major visceral vessels and the aneurysm. In obese patients or those with an unusual

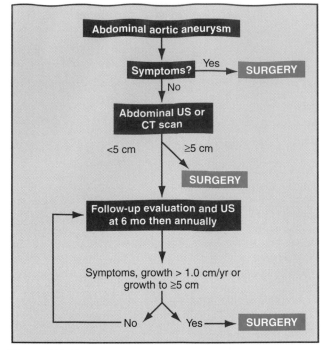

Figure 27-7

Approach to the patient with an abdominal aortic aneurysm. Symptoms referable to the aneurysm (pain) are an indication for surgical repair. In the vast majority of patients, the aneurysm can be sized accurately with abdominal ultrasonography. A maximal diameter greater than 5.0 cm, a growth rate in excess of 1.0 cm/year, or the development of symptoms during follow-up should also prompt surgical referral. The presence of significant co-morbid conditions, however, may militate against this recommendation. Alternatively, consideration may be given to endoluminal stenting, if available. Medical therapy should focus on the control of hypertension and on the reduction of associated risk factors for atherosclerotic disease. SURG, surgery; US, ultrasound; CT, contrast computed tomography.

The majority of patients with abdominal aortic aneurysms have concomitant coronary artery disease. Since perioperative myocardial ischemia/infarction is the most frequent complication of such surgery, patients with risk factors for or symptoms to suggest coronary artery disease should undergo careful evaluation before surgery[14, 15] (see Chap. 15). Clinical markers of increased perioperative risk include previous myocardial infarction, ongoing poorly controlled angina pectoris, heart failure, diabetes, and advanced age. A "high-risk" stress test with exercise-induced ischemia at a low workload or involving multiple myocardial segments on myocardial perfusion scintigraphy (see Chap. 4) is an additional and independent predictor of increased risk.

Management

Aggressive efforts at blood pressure control, risk factor modification, and lifestyle changes are appropriate. Because the risk of rupture appears to increase substantially once the aneurysm reaches a diameter of 5.0 cm, it is this size that should prompt referral for surgical repair (see Table 22-2). Patients with *symptomatic* aneurysms of smaller dimensions should also be referred. The risks of operation, however, are substantial, and the perioperative mortality rates are still in the range of 2% to 4%.[12] Surgical referral of the asymptomatic patient with a 5-cm aneurysm and significant co-morbid conditions that would independently pose a significant risk of mortality or major morbidity over the course of the next 2 years may not be appropriate. One- and 5-year survival rates after abdominal aortic aneurysm repair are in the range of 95% and 65%, respectively.[9]

Referral to a cardiologist is appropriate whenever doubt

body habitus, these cross-sectional techniques are more accurate than is ultrasonography in assessing the rate of growth. In many surgical centers, operative planning can proceed on the basis of these noninvasive imaging modalities, although contrast aortography is still preferred by many surgeons. The presence on clinical examination of important, coexistent peripheral arterial occlusive disease, especially when it affects the iliofemoral systems, should trigger angiography.

SURVEILLANCE IMAGING. Given the known propensity for aneurysms to enlarge (usually by 0.2 to 0.4 cm/yr), a schedule of surveillance imaging studies must be established on the initial detection of an asymptomatic abdominal aortic aneurysm (luminal diameter > 3.0 cm).[13] However, much variability in the rate of enlargement exists. Annual ultrasonographic examinations should suffice for asymptomatic individuals whose maximal aortic diameter is less than 4.0 cm. Once aneurysm size reaches 4.0 cm, however, repeat examinations every 6 months are advised. More frequent follow-up examinations are also recommended in patients whose aneurysm's diameter has increased more than 0.5 cm within the past 12 months.

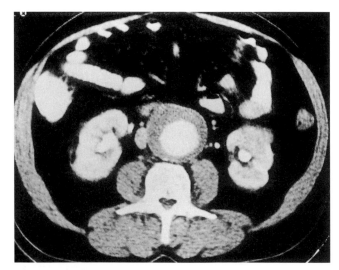

Figure 27-8

Contrast abdominal CT scan demonstrates an abdominal aortic aneurysm just anterior to the vertebral body. Extensive mural thrombus is present within the aneurysm. (From Creager, M.A., Halperin, J.L., and Whittemore, A.D.: Aneurysmal disease of the aorta and its branches. *In* Loscalzo, J., Creager, M.A., and Dzau, V.J. [eds.]: Vascular Medicine. 2nd ed. Boston, Little, Brown, 1996, pp. 901-926.)

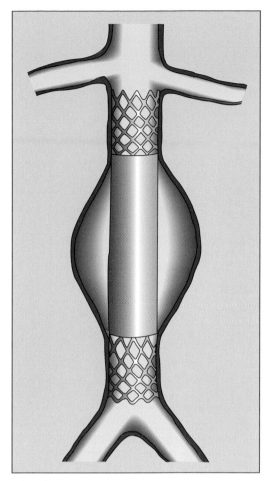

Figure 27–9

Diagram showing an intraluminal stent graft within an infrarenal abdominal aortic aneurysm. (From Parodi, C., Palmaz, J.C., and Barone, H.D.: Transformed intraluminal graft implantation for abdominal aortic aneurysms. Ann. Vasc. Surg. 5:491, 1991.)

persists regarding the relative safety of proceeding with surgery on the aneurysm.

ENDOVASCULAR STENTING. Early reports of the use of endovascular stenting for the treatment of abdominal (and thoracic) aortic aneurysms are quite promising.[16] Stenting has been widely applied in the treatment of coronary, renal, and distal peripheral vascular disease. With this technique, arterial access is gained via a direct cutdown on the femoral artery and the stent is delivered to the site of the aneurysm over a balloon catheter. Using a combination of angiographic and fluoroscopic techniques, the operator deploys the stent so that its edges protrude just beyond the margins of the aneurysm itself (Fig. 27–9). This technique essentially "excludes" the aneurysm from the circulation. Blood flow is maintained through the stent, and the circumferential arterial lumen gradually thromboses. Stenting may become the procedure of choice in patients who are considered to be at high surgical risk. It is anticipated that the technique will continue to improve and that extension to a lower-risk population will then become appropriate.

AORTIC DISSECTION

Acute dissection of the aorta is an uncommon clinical event, yet one that is fraught with catastrophic consequences. There is an annual U.S. incidence of approximately 2000 cases, which accounts for 3% to 4% of all sudden cardiovascular deaths. Untreated, mortality during the first day occurs at a rate of 1%/hr, is 75% at 2 weeks, and exceeds 90% by 1 year.[9]

Pathogenesis

Most commonly, a tear or rent in the intima allows luminal blood to gain access to the aortic media and, driven by the force of the systolic pressure, to separate the inner two-thirds from the outer one-third of the aortic wall. The dissection propagates in an anterograde direction for a variable length and then typically reenters at a more distal location. Less commonly, propagation proceeds in a retrograde fashion or even bidirectionally. In a large majority of patients with dissection who undergo postmortem examination, an intimal tear can be identified with one or more reentry sites.

The use of cross-sectional imaging techniques has spawned a greater appreciation for two other mechanisms by which medial hematoma formation can occur in the wall of the aorta.[17] Spontaneous intramural hemorrhage represents a continued leakage of blood into the aortic media from ruptured branches of the vasa vasorum. CT scanning or MRI is useful in diagnosis. The clinical presentation and natural history also are similar to that of classic aortic dissection, with a higher mortality in patients with intramural hematomas of the ascending than of the descending aorta.

In patients with advanced atherosclerotic involvement of the aorta, luminal blood may burrow under a deep atherosclerotic plaque and erode through the internal elastic lamina and gain access to the medial layer. This may result in formation of a localized ulcer, that is, a penetrating aortic ulcer,[18] false aneurysm, or frank rupture. Penetrating aortic ulcers are found almost exclusively in the mid- to distal portion of the descending thoracic aorta in older patients with hypertension and a heavy atherosclerotic burden. Aortography is useful for detecting false aneurysms resulting from penetrating atherosclerotic ulcers. Because of the risk of rupture, such aneurysms constitute an indication for operation.

Any process that leads to the weakening and degeneration of the components of the aortic media (elastic fibers, smooth muscle) can predispose to aortic dissection. Aging is accompanied by medial degeneration, a process that is further accelerated by hypertension. Aortic dissection is most common among patients in the sixth and seventh decades of life, 80% of whom are hypertensive.[19] It is seen earlier in patients with the inheritable disorders of connective tissue such as Marfan's and Ehlers-Danlos syndromes. Cystic medial necrosis is the pathologic expression of these syndromes and has been described as well in patients with bicuspid aortic valve disease or aortic coarctation, disorders that have also been associated with a higher than expected increase in the incidence of aortic dissection. A long list of other diseases has been associated with aortic dissection, including Turner's syndrome, Noonan's syndrome, polycystic kidney disease, and the inflammatory aortitides. About half of the reported aortic dissections in young women occur during the third trimester of pregnancy or in the early postpartum period. Many of these women may have previously unrecognized disorders of connective tissue. Because of the very high risk of spontaneous dissection or rupture, recognition of an aneurysm of the ascending aorta in a pregnant woman with Marfan's syndrome should be an indication for consideration of the termination of the pregnancy and urgent aortic repair.

Traumatic dissection can occur as a complication of catheterization or cannulation of the aorta during the performance of cardiovascular procedures requiring aortic cross-clamping, after incision of the aorta for aortic valve replacement, or even with the excision of small buttons of aorta for the construction of proximal vein graft anastomoses. The presence of an aortic transection with the formation of a false aneurysm must be excluded in any motor vehicle accident victim with widening of the mediastinum on chest x-ray. This can be accomplished by any of the imaging techniques useful in assessing the thoracic aorta—TEE, noninvasive cross-sectional imaging (CT or MRI), or contrast aortography.

Classification

Aortic dissections are classified both temporally and anatomically. A dissection is considered to be *acute* if the patient is observed within 2 weeks of its clinical recognition. Chronic dissections are of greater than 2 weeks' duration. The most widely used anatomic schema is the Stanford classification,[5, 9] which divides aortic dissections simply into two types (Fig. 27–10). Type A dissections involve the ascending aorta (regardless of the site of entry or origin), whereas type B dissections do not involve the ascending aorta. The importance of this distinction lies in the recognition of the natural history. Type A dissections are associated with a relatively higher incidence of early fatal complications (rupture with tamponade, severe aortic regurgitation, stroke) compared with Type B dissections. This simple distinction also underlies the treatment strategies that have evolved since the mid-1960s.

Nearly two-thirds of aortic dissections arise within the ascending aorta, just a few centimeters above the level of the aortic valve, where the hydrodynamic and torsional forces are greatest. About one-fifth occur just beyond the origin of the left subclavian artery where the relatively mobile arch becomes fixed to the posterior thoracic cage. A minority of dissections arise either in the arch itself or in the abdominal aorta.

Clinical Examination

History

Chest pain is the most common presenting feature of aortic dissection.[19, 20] Adjectives such as "ripping" and "tearing" have often been used to describe the pain of dissection, which usually begins abruptly and is often very severe. Patients can often recall the exact time at which the pain arose. Type A dissections usually are accompanied by anterior chest pain, but a posterior component may also occur. Patients with type B dissections, on the other hand, typically describe pain in the interscapular or midback region almost exclusively.

Physical Examination

Helpful findings on physical examination include asymmetry of pulse or blood pressure, a new murmur of aortic

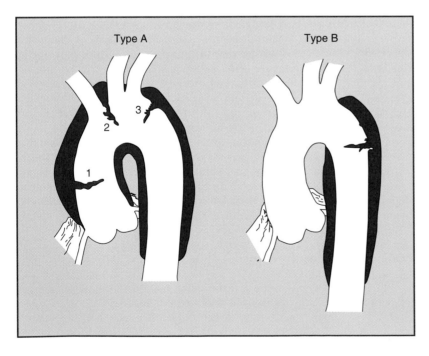

Figure 27–10

The Stanford classification system for aortic dissection. Type A refers to any dissection that involves the ascending aorta, regardless of its site of origin. In the example shown, entry site 1 is in the proximal ascending aorta, site 2 is in the arch after the take-off of the innominate artery, and site 3 is in the proximal descending thoracic aorta just beyond the origin of the left subclavian artery. Type B dissections are those that do not involve the ascending aorta. (Redrawn from Miller, D.C., Stinson, E.B., Oyer, P.E., et al.: Operative treatment of aortic dissections: Experience with 125 patients over a 16-year period. J. Thorac. Cardiovasc. Surg. 78:365, 1979.)

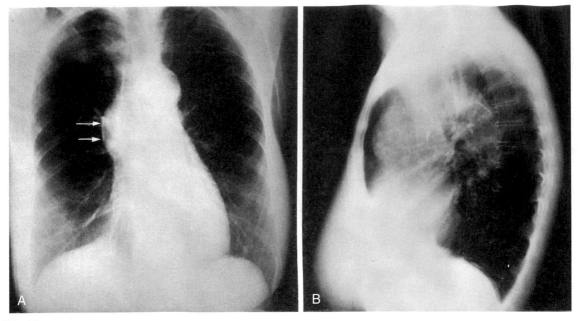

Figure 27-11

Posteroanterior *(A)* and lateral *(B)* chest x-rays of a 42-year-old woman with Marfan's syndrome and an acute type A dissection. There is an obvious bulge in the ascending aorta, which can be appreciated on both radiographic projections. The dissection originated at this point and extended into the descending thoracic aorta. (*A* and *B*, From O'Gara, P.T., and DeSanctis, R.W.: Aortic dissection. *In* Loscalzo, J., Creager, M.A., and Dzau, V.J. [eds.]: Vascular Medicine. 2nd ed. Boston, Little, Brown, 1996, p. 901.)

regurgitation, evidence of pericardial involvement, stroke, or signs of limb ischemia. Pericardial involvement is suggested by the presence of a friction rub, jugular venous distention, or pulsus paradoxus (see Chap. 28), and it implies contained rupture of a type A dissection into the pericardial space. The left pleural space is the second most common site of rupture and may be associated with both type A and type B dissections.

Diagnostic Tests

The absence of acute ischemic electrocardiographic changes is notable and helps to distinguish the severe pain of dissection from that associated with acute myocardial infarction. The chest x-ray is abnormal in about 90% of patients with aortic dissection (Fig. 27-11). When possible, the film on presentation should be compared with a previous study. The most common finding is mediastinal widening owing to aortic expansion. On occasion, an asymmetric bulge along the edge of the aorta that corresponds to the site of origin of the dissection can be identified. The "calcium sign" refers to a 1 cm or greater displacement of intimal calcium from the soft tissue border of the aorta, typically noted in the region of the aortic knob. Cardiac enlargement may signify the presence of a pericardial effusion. A left pleural effusion of variable magnitude may also be present. Effusions do not indicate rupture per se but rather are usually the expression of a sympathetic reaction to the intense aortic mural inflammation caused by the dissecting hematoma.

The diagnosis of aortic dissection can be made after careful integration of the information obtained from the history, physical examination, and chest radiograph in only about 60% of patients. Because time is of the essence, more definitive diagnostic testing should proceed promptly and efficiently.

Imaging

Four diagnostic imaging modalities for the detection and characterization of aortic dissection can be pursued, each with its own relative advantages and disadvantages.[21] The choice of technique should be based largely on local expertise. Collaboration among the primary care physician, cardiovascular specialist, radiologist, and surgeon is of paramount importance to deal successfully with this cardiovascular emergency.

In most institutions, TEE has become the procedure of choice (Fig. 27-12). It can be performed within 15 to 20 minutes by an expert operator with adjunctive sedation and the usual precautions necessary for the prevention of aspiration. The blood pressure must be monitored carefully during the performance of the procedure and the passage of the probe. Information regarding the presence or absence of involvement of the ascending aorta, concomitant aortic valve regurgitation, the status of left ventricular function, and the pericardial space can be quickly and accurately ascertained. On occasion, a TTE study might suffice, but precious minutes should not be wasted before moving promptly to a TEE investigation.

The sensitivity of TEE for the detection of aortic dissection exceeds 95%.[21] The early experience in which the specificity of this technique was less than optimal (75%) has been rectified by the introduction of multiplane probes that allow image acquisition across a 180-degree spectrum. In addition to providing information regarding

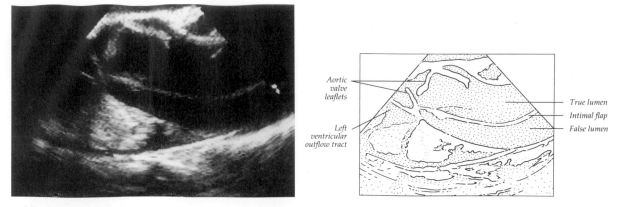

Figure 27–12

Transesophageal echocardiogram in a long-axis projection demonstrates a type A dissection with an intimal flap within the root and proximal ascending aorta. (From Cigarroa, J.E., Isselbacher, E.M., DeSanctis, R.W., and Eagle, K.A.: Diagnostic imaging in the evaluation of suspected aortic dissection: Old standards and new directions. N. Engl. J. Med. 328:35, 1993. Copyright 1993 Massachusetts Medical Society. All rights reserved.)

cardiac structure and function, TEE may allow visualization of the coronary ostia to determine their possible involvement by the dissection. This information has obviated the need for selective coronary angiography, a procedure that was performed far more frequently in the past. One of the possible disadvantages of TEE is that it can-

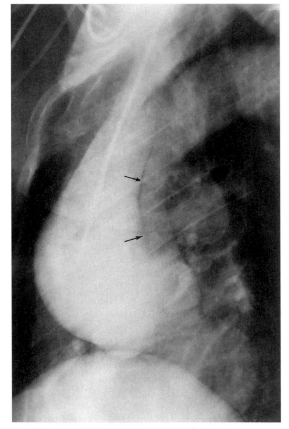

Figure 27–13

Contrast aortogram in the left posterior oblique projection demonstrates a type A dissection complicating a fusiform aneurysm of the ascending aorta. The intimal flap (*arrows*) separates the true and the false lumens.

not provide information regarding the extent of the dissection into the abdomen and beyond. Such information is infrequently necessary for the planning and performance of emergency surgery, however, and it can be obtained later via other imaging modalities.

In hospitals where there is limited or no access to TEE, contrast CT scanning is the initial procedure of choice. The sensitivity of this technique approaches 95%, albeit with a somewhat lower specificity of approximately 85%. It can be performed quickly, efficiently, and noninvasively, but it involves exposure to contrast media and ionizing radiation. Also, in current practice, the contrast CT scan does not allow an appreciation of aortic valve function nor of the involvement of major branches.

Although the sensitivity and specificity of MRI for the detection of aortic dissection both exceed 95%, this modality is constrained by issues of limited access, cost, and the problems inherent in studying acutely ill patients on intravenous medications within a magnet that is usually housed at a distance from the emergency room or operating theater.

Contrast aortography was the gold standard for the diagnostic evaluation of patients with suspected aortic dissection for many years (Fig. 27–13). More recent studies have suggested, however, that its sensitivity (88%) is actually slightly lower than that that can be achieved with TEE, contrast CT scanning, and MRI.[9] Contrast arteriography may require more than 30 to 60 minutes to accomplish and exposes the patient to contrast media and ionizing radiation. In addition, contrast aortography may actually be least sensitive for the detection of spontaneous intramural hemorrhage, as the absence of an intimal flap may create the false impression that the aorta is not pathologically involved. On the other hand, its potential advantages include its familiarity to generations of clinicians, its ability to demonstrate involvement of the aortic valve and major aortic branches, and the provision of information relative to the proximal portions of the coronary arteries. In current practice, though, contrast aortography has been relegated to no higher than third place among widely available imaging modalities for the detec-

Table 27-3	Approach to the Patient with Acute Aortic Dissection

Perform directed history and physical examination
Obtain chest x-ray
Obtain ECG to exclude myocardial ischemia
"Quick-look" TTE
TEE
   Contrast chest CT scan if TEE unavailable
Institute intravenous drug therapy (beta blockade, nitroprusside) to lower blood pressure and heart rate
Obtain surgical consultation

Abbreviations: ECG, electrocardiogram; TTE, transthoracic echocardiogram; TEE, transesophageal echocardiogram; CT, computed tomography.

tion of aortic dissection, behind both TEE and contrast CT scanning.

Management

Patients with suspected acute aortic dissection should be referred to the emergency room for prompt evaluation by a physician team including medical and surgical cardiovascular specialists (Table 27–3). Emergency medical measures to control the blood pressure and its rate of rise should be instituted without delay, even as the diagnostic workup is proceeding. Intravenous beta blockade (metoprolol 5 mg intravenously every 5 min for three doses) should be started unless specific contraindications (see Chap. 18) exist. A continuous intravenous infusion of sodium nitroprusside is the antihypertensive agent of choice (0.25 to 10 μg/kg/min) should the blood pressure remain elevated after institution of beta blockade. Monitoring of the heart rate and blood pressure is essential, but especially during transport and the performance of diagnostic testing.

Surgical Treatment

Recognition of involvement of the ascending aorta mandates emergency surgical repair unless substantial comorbidities exist, such as a dense, severe stroke, oligoanuric renal failure, and advanced age (Table 27–4). The ascending aorta should be approached primarily even if the entry tear is in a more distal segment of the aorta and the dissection has propagated in retrograde fashion.[22] Such surgery is performed through a median sternotomy, and cardiopulmonary bypass is instituted via the femoral vessels. When concomitant aortic valve replacement surgery is necessary, a valve-graft conduit is constructed and the coronary arteries are reimplanted into the conduit. Perioperative surgical mortality for type A dissections remains in the range of 10% to 15%, even in experienced centers.[20]

Medical Management

Medical therapy is initially preferred for the management of type B dissections. This preference is based on the observation that patients with acute type B dissections are at relatively lower risk for early death compared with patients with type A dissections. Patients with type B

dissections also tend to be older and have a higher prevalence of associated cardiovascular morbidity, which increases their perioperative risk. For patients with uncomplicated type B dissections, outcomes with medical and surgical therapy are comparable.[23] There are specific situations, however, in which acute surgical intervention is advised, including rupture, rapid expansion with or without formation of a localized saccular aneurysm, uncontrolled pain, and ischemia of a vital organ. In addition, acute surgical intervention is strongly recommended for patients with type B dissections and Marfan's syndrome.

Medical therapy is also advised for the management of *chronic* dissection of either the type A or the type B variety. Patients who present 2 or more weeks after the acute event are a "self-selected" group of survivors for whom surgical therapy has not been shown to offer any benefit over that that can be achieved with tight medical management alone. Surgery may be necessary for complications of the dissection, such as aneurysm formation or the development of significant aortic regurgitation with heart failure.

The management of patients with a spontaneous intramural hemorrhage in whom no intimal flap can be identified mirrors that for patients with classic dissection. Patients with penetrating aortic ulcers, on the other hand, are usually managed similarly to those with type B dissections. However, given the propensity for rupture, the re-emergence of pain after a period of quiescence should prompt surgery.

Five-year survival for the entire cohort of hospital survivors of acute aortic dissection is in the range of 80% and does not appear to differ significantly according to the type of dissection (A versus B or acute versus chronic) or the definitive therapy rendered (surgical versus medical).[24] The important long-term complications include the development of aortic regurgitation, recurrent dissection, or aneurysm formation (true or false).

Long-Term Care

The primary care physician should coordinate a program of strict antihypertensive control and surveillance noninvasive imaging with the cardiovascular specialist for all patients with aortic dissection, that is, those treated surgically and those treated medically. A chest x-ray should be obtained every 3 months for the first year, and either a contrast CT scan or an MRI study should be performed every 6 months for the first 2 years and annually thereafter. A beta blocker or, when that is contraindicated, a calcium channel antagonist with negative ino-

Table 27-4	Indications for Surgery of Aortic Dissection

Acute type A dissection
Chronic type A dissection with severe aortic regurgitation, localized aneurysm, or symptoms related to compression
Acute type B dissection with rupture, rapid expansion, refractory pain, extension, or vital organ ischemia
Chronic type B dissection with aneurysmal enlargement (>6 cm)
Marfan's syndrome

tropic properties (verapamil or diltiazem) should form the mainstay of antihypertensive therapy. Additional agents may be necessary to control blood pressure.

Late complications occur not infrequently in survivors of surgical treatment. The incidence of subsequent aneurysm formation at sites remote from the initial surgical repair is approximately 20% over 18 months of follow-up. Aneurysm formation is attributable to continued expansion of the false lumen, the walls of which are thin and inherently weak. Approximately one-third of late deaths after successful surgery can be attributed to rupture of the false lumen.[20]

References

1. Pyeritz, R.E., and McKusick, V.A.: The Marfan syndrome: Diagnosis and management. N. Engl. J. Med 300:772, 1979.
2. Lemon, D.K., and White, C.W.: Annuloaortic ectasia with aortic valve insufficiency. Am. J. Cardiol. 41:482, 1978.
3. Evans, J.M., O'Fallon, W.M., and Hunder, G.G.: Increased incidence of aortic aneurysm and dissection of giant cell (temporal) arteritis. A population-based study. Ann. Intern. Med. 122:502, 1995.
4. Kerr, G.S., Hallahan, C.W., Giordano, J., et al.: Takayasu's arteritis. Ann. Intern. Med. 120:919, 1994.
5. Creager, M.A., Halperin, J.L., and Whittemore, A.D.: Aneurysmal disease of the aorta and its variants. *In* Loscalzo, J., Creager, M.A., and Dzau, V.J. (eds.): Vascular Medicine. 2nd ed. Boston, Little, Brown, 1996, p. 901.
6. Blanchard, D.G., Kimura, B.J., Dittrich, H.C. and DeMaria, A.N.: Transesophageal echocardiography of the aorta. JAMA 272:546, 1994.
7. Shores, J., Berger, K.R., Murphy, E.A., and Pyeritz, R.E.: Progression of aortic dilatation and the benefit of long-term beta adrenergic blockade in Marfan's syndrome. N. Engl. J. Med. 330:1335, 1994.
8. Dzau, V.J., and Creager, M.A.: Diseases of the aorta. *In* Fauci, A.S., Braunwald, E., Isselbacher, K.J., et al. (eds.): Harrison's Principles of Internal Medicine. 14th ed. New York, McGraw-Hill, 1998, pp. 1394–1398.
9. Isselbacher, E.M., Eagle, K.A., and DeSanctis, R.W.: Diseases of the aorta. *In* Braunwald, E. (ed.): Heart Disease. 5th ed. Philadelphia, W.B. Saunders, 1997.
10. Webster, M.W., Ferrell, R.E., St. Jean, P.L., et al.: Ultrasound screening of first-degree relatives of patients with an abdominal aortic aneurysm. J. Vasc. Surg. 13:9, 1991.
11. Darling, R.C., Messina, C.R., Brewster, D.C., and Ottinger, L.W.: Autopsy study of unoperative abdominal aortic aneurysms: The case for early resection. Circulation 56(Suppl II):II-161, 1977.
12. Ernst, C.B.: Abdominal aortic aneurysm. N. Engl. J. Med. 328:1167, 1993.
13. Limit, E.R., Sakalihassan, N., and Albert, A.: Determination of the expansion rate and incidence of rupture of abdominal aortic aneurysm. J. Vasc. Surg. 14:540, 1991.
14. Hallett, J.W., Bower, T.C., Cherry, K.J., et al.: Selection and preparation of high-risk patients for repair of abdominal aortic aneurysms. Mayo Clin. Proc. 69:763, 1994.
15. Eagle, K.A., Brundage, B.H., Chaitman, B.R., et al.: Guidelines for perioperative cardiovascular evaluation for non-cardiac surgery. Report of the American College of Cardiology/American Heart Association Task Force on Practice Guidelines. Committee on Perioperative Cardiovascular Evaluation for Non-Cardiac Surgery. Circulation 93:1278, 1996.
16. Blum, U., Voshage, G., Lammer, J., et al.: Endoluminal stent-grafts for infra-renal abdominal aortic aneurysms. N. Engl. J. Med. 336:13, 1997.
17. Nienaber, C.A., Von Kodolitsch, Y., Petersen, B., et al.: Intramural hemorrhage of the thoracic aorta. Circulation 92:1465, 1995.
18. Stanson, A.W., Kazmier, F.J., Hollier, L.H., et al.: Penetrating atherosclerotic ulcers of the thoracic aorta: Natural history and clinical pathological correlations. Ann. Vasc. Surg. 1:15, 1986.
19. Slater, E.E., and DeSanctis, R.W.: The clinical recognition of dissecting aortic aneurysm. Am. J. Med. 60:625, 1976.
20. O'Gara, P.T., and DeSanctis, R.W.: Aortic dissection. *In* Loscalzo, J., Creager, M.A., and Dzau, V.J. (eds.): Vascular Medicine. 2nd ed. Boston, Little, Brown, 1996, p. 927.
21. Nienaber, C.A., Von Kodolitsch, Y., Nicholas, V., et al.: Definitive diagnosis of thoracic aortic dissection: The emerging role of non-invasive imaging modalities. N. Engl. J. Med. 328:1, 1993.
22. Haverich, A., Miller, D.C., Scott, W.C., et al.: Acute and chronic aortic dissections: Determinants of long-term outcome for operative survivors. Circulation 72(Suppl II):II-22, 1985.
23. Glower, D.D., Fann, J.I., Speier, R.H., et al.: Comparison of medical and surgical therapy for uncomplicated descending aortic dissection. Circulation 82(Suppl IV):IV-39, 1990.
24. Doroghazi, R.M., Slater, E.E., DeSanctis, R.W., et al.: Long-term survival of patients with treated aortic dissection. J. Am. Coll. Cardiol. 3:1026, 1984.

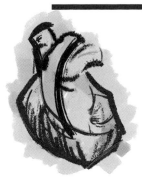

Chapter 28

Recognition and Management of Patients with

Pericardial Disease

BEVERLY H. LORELL

Functions of the Normal Pericardium

The normal human pericardium is composed of the visceral pericardium, which is a serous layer attached to the surface of the heart, and the outer parietal pericardium, which is rich in collagen and elastic fibers. The normal intrapericardial pressure is zero or negative and tracks closely with respiratory changes in intrathoracic pressure. The normal pericardium provides a physical barrier against infection between the heart and the adjacent organs. The pericardium also limits acute distention of the heart and enhances the effect that distention of one ventricle has on the pressure in the contralateral ventricle, that is, on ventricular interdependence. This effect of the pericardium on ventricular interdependence is most prominent when the heart is distended with high ventricular filling pressures. In the absence of the pericardium, intracardiac volume is larger and the pressures within the right and left ventricles are lower.

CLINICAL SYNDROMES

Acute Pericarditis

Acute pericarditis is a clinical syndrome caused by inflammation of the pericardial membrane (Table 28–1). Idiopathic or presumed viral pericarditis is most common in the outpatient setting in young healthy adults. In middle-aged and elderly patients, as well as in those referred to tertiary care centers, common causes of pericarditis include trauma, neoplasm, and uremia.

Clinical Presentation

Chest pain is the most common symptom and can usually be distinguished from the chest pain of myocardial ischemia (Table 28–2) (see Chap. 7). It is usually localized to the retrosternal region and may radiate to the neck or the trapezius ridge. Pericardial pain is often aggravated by deep inspiration, coughing, or lying supine and is eased by sitting up and leaning forward. Pericardial pain can be extremely severe and unrelenting, and it can be confused with pain of angina pectoris or acute myocardial infarction. The pleuritic nature of the pain and failure of the pain to be relieved by sublingual nitroglycerin help to discriminate acute pericarditis from angina pectoris.

Acute pericarditis is often associated with dyspnea. Dyspnea may also develop when a large pericardial effusion compresses adjacent lung tissue and bronchi. Symptoms such as a cough, prolonged fever, weight loss, and sputum production suggest the presence of underlying systemic disease that requires specific treatment, such as tuberculosis or acquired immunodeficiency syndrome (AIDS). The classic clinical features of acute pericarditis may be blunted and easily confused with other causes of chest pain in elderly patients.

Physical Examination

The pericardial friction rub is a pathognomonic physical finding. It is a high-pitched noise with a squeaking or scratching quality. In the absence of tachycardia, it has up to three distinct components that are related to cardiac motion during atrial contraction (presystole), ventricular systole, and rapid ventricular filling in early diastole. The pericardial friction rub can be notoriously evanescent and

pain

&

dyspnea

Table 28–1	Causes of Pericarditis

Idiopathic (nonspecific)
Viral infections: Coxsackie A virus, Coxsackie B virus, echovirus, adenovirus, mumps virus, infectious mononucleosis, varicella, hepatitis B, acquired immunodeficiency syndrome (AIDS)
Tuberculosis
Acute bacterial infections: pneumococcus, staphylococcus, streptococcus, gram-negative septicemia, *Neisseria meningitidis, Neisseria gonorrhoeae*
Fungal infections: histoplasmosis, coccidioidomycosis, *Candida,* blastomycosis
Other infections: toxoplasmosis, amebiasis, mycoplasma, *Nocardia,* actinomycosis, echinococcosis, Lyme disease
Acute myocardial infarction
Uremia: untreated uremia; in association with hemodialysis
Neoplastic disease: lung cancer, breast cancer, leukemia, Hodgkin's disease, lymphoma
Radiation: cardiac injury
Autoimmune disorders: systemic lupus erythematosus, rheumatoid arthritis, scleroderma, mixed connective tissue disease, Wegener's granulomatosis, polyarteritis nodosa, acute rheumatic fever
Other inflammatory disorders: sarcoidosis, amyloidosis, inflammatory bowel disease, Whipple's disease, temporal arteritis, Behçet's disease
Drugs: hydralazine, procainamide, phenytoin, isoniazid, phenylbutazone, dantrolene, doxorubicin, methysergide, penicillin (with hypereosinophilia)
Trauma: including chest trauma; hemopericardium after thoracic surgery pacemaker insertion or cardiac diagnostic procedures; esophageal rupture; pancreatic-pericardial fistula
Delayed postmyocardial-pericardial injury syndromes: postmyocardial infarction (Dressler's) syndrome; postpericardiotomy syndrome
Dissecting aortic aneurysm
Myxedema
Chylopericardium

Table 28–2	Pericardial versus Ischemic Pain

	Ischemia	Pericarditis
Location	Retrosternal; left shoulder, arm	Precordium; left trapezius ridge
Quality	Pressure, burning, buildup	Sharp, pleuritic; or dull, oppressive
Thoracic motion	No effect	Increased by breathing, rotating thorax
Duration	Stable angina: 1–15 min Unstable angina: ½ hr to hours	Hours or days
Relation to effort	Stable angina: usually Unstable angina or infarction: usually not	No relation
Posture	No effect; may sit, belch, use Valsalva's or knee-chest position for relief	Leaning forward for relief; aggravated by recumbency

From Fowler, N. O.: Acute pericarditis. *In* Fowler, N.O. (ed.): The Pericardium in Health and Disease. Mt. Kisco, NY, Futura Publishing, 1985, p. 158.

can change in quality from one examination to the next. It can be detected most easily by listening with the diaphragm of the stethoscope applied firmly to the chest at the lower left sternal border during slow inspiration and full expiration with the patient sitting up and leaning forward.

Electrocardiogram

There are four stages in the evolution of the electrocardiogram (ECG) during acute pericarditis (Table 28–3). Stage I ECG changes (Fig. 28–1) of ST segment eleva-

tion accompany the early onset of the chest pain syndrome and are virtually diagnostic of pericardial inflammation. Unlike the pattern of ST segment elevation during acute myocardial infarction, ST elevation in acute pericarditis is concave upward and usually present in all leads except V_1 and aVR. During stage I, the T-waves are upright in the leads with ST segment elevation. These ECG abnormalities occur in about 90% of patients with early pericarditis, and depression of the PR segment develops in about 80%. Stage II usually occurs hours or a few days later and is characterized by the return of the ST segments to baseline with flattening of the T-waves. In contrast, the T-waves in acute transmural myocardial infarction usually become inverted before the ST segments return completely to baseline. Stage III changes of acute pericarditis include the inversion of T-waves in most leads. In contrast to the evolution of the ECG in acute myocardial infarction, T-wave inversion during stage III of acute pericarditis is not associated with loss of R-wave voltage or the appearance of pathologic Q-waves. Stage IV of acute pericarditis includes the return of T-wave changes to baseline and may occur days to weeks later. The documentation of typical stage I changes can be diagnostic of acute pericarditis even when other

Table 28–3	Four-Stage ("Typical") ECG Evolution of Acute Pericarditis

Sequence	Leads of "Epicardial" Derivation (I, II, aVL, aVF, V_{3-6})			Leads Reflecting "Endocardial" Potential (aVR, often V_1, sometimes V_2)		
Stage	*J-ST*	*T-Waves*	*PR Segment*	*ST Segment*	*T-Waves*	*PR Segment*
I	Elevated	Upright	Depressed or isoelectric	Depressed	Inverted	Elevated or isoelectric
II early	Isoelectric	Upright	Isoelectric or depressed	Isoelectric	Inverted	Isoelectric or elevated
II late	Isoelectric	Low to flat to inverted	Isoelectric or depressed	Isoelectric	Shallow to flat to upright	Isoelectric or elevated
III	Isoelectric	Inverted	Isoelectric	Isoelectric	Upright	Isoelectric
IV	Isoelectric	Upright	Isoelectric	Isoelectric	Inverted	Isoelectric

From Lorell, B.H.: Pericardial diseases. *In* Braunwald, E. (ed.): Heart Disease. 5th ed. Philadelphia, W.B. Saunders, 1997, pp. 1478–1534; adapted from American Journal of Cardiology, vol 33, Spodick, D.H.: Electrocardiographic changes in acute pericarditis, p 470, Copyright 1974, with permission from Excerpta Medica Inc. *Abbreviations:* ECG, electrocardiogram; J-ST, junction of S- (or T-) wave with the end of the QRS complex.

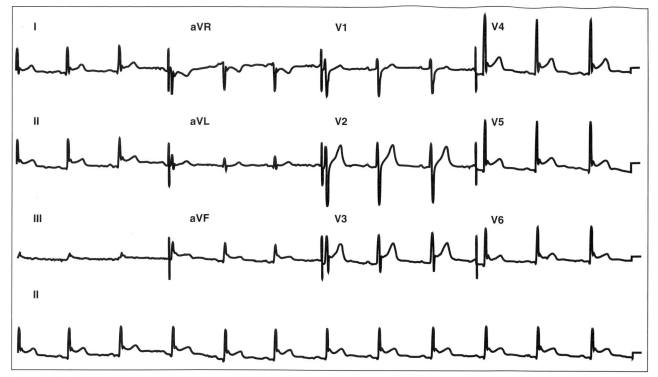

Figure 28–1

This electrocardiogram (ECG) from a 36-year-old man with pleuritic chest pain illustrates classic stage I ECG changes of acute pericarditis: ST elevation with upright T-waves in all leads except aVR and V$_1$. Note that PR segment depression is also present in multiple leads.

clinical features are misleading. Variations of this pattern are present in fewer than 50% of patients and include isolated depression of the PR segment, persistent T-wave inversion, and regional ST segment changes. The stage I changes of acute ST elevation must be differentiated from the variant of normal early repolarization.

Sinus tachycardia is a common feature of acute pericarditis, particularly in patients with fever and pain. Other atrial arrhythmias are infrequent in uncomplicated acute pericarditis and suggest the presence of underlying heart disease. Ventricular tachycardia, atrioventricular (AV) nodal block and bundle branch block are *not* features of acute pericarditis. These ECG abnormalities suggest the presence of coexisting myocarditis or myocardial ischemia.

Chest Radiograph and Echocardiogram

The chest radiograph is of limited diagnostic value in acute pericarditis, but it occasionally reveals an enlarged globular cardiac silhouette typical of pericardial effusion (Fig. 28–2). Transient pleural effusions occur in about one-fourth of patients with pericarditis and are usually left-sided (Fig. 28–3).

Transthoracic echocardiography is the most sensitive and accurate tool for the detection and quantification of pericardial fluid (Fig. 28–4). Echocardiography should be part of the initial evaluation to be sure that a currently stable patient is not at risk for acute hemodynamic decompensation, and it is a mandatory diagnostic test in

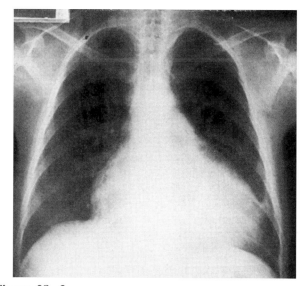

Figure 28–2

Pericardial effusion. The heart assumes a globular, rounded shape after development of a pericardial effusion. The normal indentations along the heart borders are effaced, so that the cardiac silhouette is smooth and featureless. (From Steiner, R.M., and Levin, D.C.: Radiology of the heart. *In* Braunwald, E. [ed.]: Heart Disease. 5th ed. Philadelphia, W.B. Saunders, 1997, pp. 204–239.)

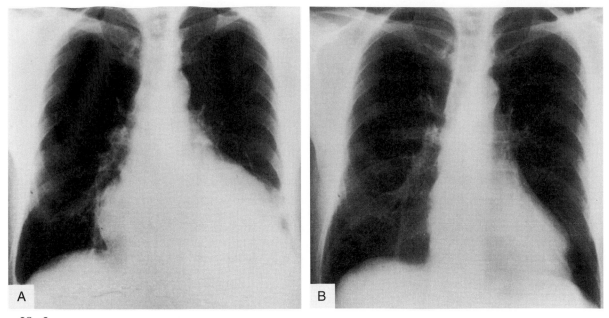

Figure 28–3

Chest radiographs of a patient with relapsing idiopathic pericarditis. *A,* An enlarged cardiopericardial silhouette with a left pleural effusion. *B,* An essentially normal radiograph was obtained during a remission after prednisone therapy. Pleural effusions occur commonly in idiopathic pericarditis and usually are either on the left side or bilateral. (*A* and *B,* From Fowler, N.O.: Pericardial disease. *In* Abelmann, W.H. [ed.]: Atlas of Heart Diseases. Vol. 2. Braunwald, E. [ser. ed.] Philadelphia, Current Medicine, 1995, pp. 13.1–13.16.)

those with suspected compression of the heart by cardiac tamponade. However, many patients with acute pericarditis do not have a detectable increase in pericardial fluid, and serial echocardiography is not required for the management of those with totally uncomplicated acute pericarditis.

Acute pericarditis is usually associated with nonspecific indicators of inflammation, including elevation of the sedimentation rate and leukocytosis. Mild elevation of the cardiac isozyme of creatine kinase (CK-MB) is common and can occur as a result of underlying epicardial inflam-

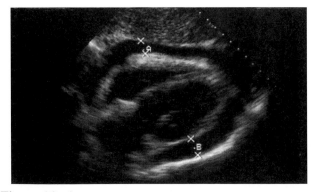

Figure 28–4

Echocardiogram shows large circumferential pericardial effusion. A indicates the anterior effusion in front of the right ventricle. B indicates the posterior effusion behind the left ventricle. X X marks the pericardial and epicardial boundaries of the effusion. (From Shabetai, R.: Diseases of the pericardium. *In* Bennett, J.C., and Plum, F. [eds.]: Cecil Textbook of Medicine. 20th ed. Vol. 1. Philadelphia, W.B. Saunders, 1996, pp. 336–342.)

mation. All patients should be evaluated for possible renal failure and tuberculosis; additional diagnostic tests may be indicated in some individuals (Table 28–4).

Management

The initial step in the management of acute pericarditis consists of determining whether the inflammation is related to underlying illness that requires specific therapy. Initial observation in the hospital, or daily examination by an experienced examiner, is warranted for all patients with acute pericarditis to exclude the development of frank cardiac tamponade, which occurs in about 15% of those with acute pericarditis.[1] Pericardial pain can be severe and should be treated with limitation of activity and nonsteroidal anti-inflammatory drugs (NSAIDs) such as aspirin (650 mg orally every 4 hours) or indomethacin (25 to 50 mg orally four times daily) for about 2 weeks. When the pain is severe and does not respond to this NSAID therapy within 5 days, corticosteroids may be carefully used. If prednisone is used, 60 to 80 mg daily in divided doses should be given. Patients should be warned of the risk of aseptic necrosis of the femoral head. After about 2 weeks, NSAIDs should be tapered. Oral warfarin anticoagulation should usually not be administered during the acute phase of pericarditis of any cause. If warfarin must be administered owing to the presence of a mechanical prosthetic heart valve, the drug should be stopped temporarily and replaced with intravenous heparin, the action of which can be promptly reversed with protamine.

Diagnostic pericardiocentesis or biopsy has very low yield in the patient with acute pericarditis and pericardial effusion who does not have tamponade, and these proce-

In All Patients

Tuberculin skin test (and control skin test to exclude anergy)
BUN and creatinine to exclude uremia

In Selected Patients

ANA and rheumatoid factor to exclude systemic lupus erythematosus or rheumatoid arthritis in patients with acute arthritis or pleural effusion

TSH and T$_4$ to exclude hypothyroidism in patients with clinical findings suggestive of hypothyroidism and in asymptomatic patients with unexplained pericardial effusion

HIV test to exclude the possibility of AIDS in patients with risk factors for HIV disease or a compatible clinical syndrome

Blood cultures in febrile patients to exclude associated possible infective endocarditis and bacteremia

Fungal serologic tests in patients from endemic areas or in immunocompromised patients

ASO titer in children or teenagers with suspected rheumatic fever

Heterophil antibody test to exclude mononucleosis in young or middle-aged patients with a compatible clinical syndrome of acute fever, weakness, and lymphadenopathy

Abbreviations: BUN, blood urea nitrogen; ANA, antinuclear antibody; TSH, thyroid-stimulating hormone; T$_4$, thyroxine; HIV, human immunodeficiency virus; AIDS, acquired immunodeficiency syndrome; ASO, antistreptolysin O.

dures are not indicated in uncomplicated pericarditis. Pericardiocentesis should be performed for diagnostic reasons in the absence of cardiac tamponade only in patients in whom there is (1) an immediate need to confirm the diagnosis of suspected purulent pericarditis based on the clinical presentation, (2) a progressive illness and enlarging effusion despite 1 week of NSAIDs, or (3) an acute illness in the context of an immunosuppressed state.

Natural History

Pericarditis of idiopathic or presumed viral cause is usually self-limited. With NSAID therapy, severe pain and dyspnea usually abate within the first few days. More subtle clinical and ECG signs of inflammation tend to abate within 2 to 4 weeks. About 1 out of every 10 patients with acute idiopathic pericarditis and associated asymptomatic pericardial effusion develops transient signs of mild cardiac constriction within the first 30 days after the signs of acute pericarditis have disappeared.

Recurrent pericarditis occurs in about 20% or less of patients and can usually be managed by reinstitution of high-dose NSAIDs that are very gradually tapered over several weeks. In one report, chronic colchicine therapy at a dose of 1 mg daily prevented further recurrence in three-fourths of patients with recurrent pericarditis over a 37-month period.[2] Pericarditis can also be complicated by the development of pericardial tamponade, pericardial effusion with or without cardiac tamponade, chronic pericardial constriction, or a combination of both effusive and constrictive pericardial disease.

Cardiac Tamponade

A pericardial effusion can be clinically silent or can elevate intrapericardial pressure and cause cardiac tam-

ponade. The normal pericardial space can accommodate between 15 and 50 ml of fluid with little increase in intrapericardial pressure. If pericardial fluid accumulates rapidly to a volume exceeding about 150 to 200 ml, a severe rise of intrapericardial pressure causes cardiac tamponade. If pericardial fluid accumulates slowly and the pericardium is able to stretch, the pericardial space can sometimes accommodate up to 2 L of fluid with minimal elevation of intrapericardial pressure. Small amounts of fluid can cause tamponade if the pericardium itself is rigid and stiff because of fibrosis or infiltration with tumor or amyloid.

Cardiac tamponade develops when fluid accumulation within the pericardial space causes the elevation and equilibration of intracardiac filling pressures, progressive limitation of ventricular diastolic filling, and the reduction of stroke volume and cardiac output. When intrapericardial pressure rises to the level of right atrial and right ventricular diastolic pressures, the transmural pressure that distends these thin-walled chambers declines to close to zero, diastolic filling falls, and cardiac tamponade occurs. If left ventricular diastolic pressure is markedly elevated at baseline owing to preexisting left ventricular disease from hypertrophy or myopathy, cardiac tamponade can occur when right atrial, right ventricular diastolic, and pericardial pressures equalize but at a much lower level than left ventricular diastolic pressure. The equalization of intrapericardial and ventricular filling pressures results in impaired diastolic filling of ventricles and a fall in stroke volume. The reduction in stroke volume is initially compensated by reflex increases in ejection fraction and tachycardia, which help to maintain forward cardiac output and to sustain the blood pressure. With severe cardiac tamponade, the stroke volume declines further, and compensatory adjustments are no longer sufficient to sustain the cardiac output and blood pressure. The suppression of tachycardia with beta-adrenergic blocker or calcium channel blocker therapy is very dangerous during the development of cardiac tamponade and can cause acute decompensation and cardiovascular collapse.

Clinical Manifestations

When cardiac tamponade occurs suddenly from intrapericardial hemorrhage owing to trauma or aortic dissection, the physical findings include (1) a precipitous fall in systemic arterial pressure, (2) marked elevation of jugular venous pressure, and (3) a small quiet heart. When cardiac tamponade develops more slowly, the major complaint is usually dyspnea related to the accumulation of interstitial lung fluid without the development of frank alveolar edema or hypoxemia. Chest pain may also be present. Additional nonspecific systemic symptoms may include weakness, weight loss, anorexia, and fatigue.

Physical Examination

Tachycardia occurs in more than 75% of patients. Pulsus paradoxus, which is an inspiratory fall in systolic arterial blood pressure of more than 15 mm Hg, is present in more than 75% of patients. Pulsus paradoxus depends on exaggerated inspiratory filling of the right heart in the presence of reduced pulmonary venous flow and filling of the left atrium and ventricle, which causes an inspiratory fall of left ventricular stroke volume and systemic arterial pressure (Fig. 28–5). Pulsus paradoxus is rarely a clinical feature of constrictive pericarditis, in which inspiratory changes of intrathoracic pressure are not communicated to the stiff, thick-walled pericardium.

Pulsus paradoxus, which can be difficult to detect in the presence of atrial fibrillation or severe hypotension, also can be present in other disorders that cause exaggerated inspiratory impairment of left heart filling, such as tension pneumothorax and severe respiratory distress due to asthma (Table 28–5). Pulsus paradoxus may be absent in the presence of cardiac tamponade in patients with atrial septal defect, severe pulmonary hypertension, or severe aortic insufficiency.

Jugular venous distention is also a common physical finding in cardiac tamponade. In medical patients with cardiac tamponade, systolic arterial hypotension (systolic arterial pressure less than 100 mm Hg) is present in only about one-third of patients and the majority of patients are alert with warm extremities and preservation of urine output owing to the presence of the compensatory mechanisms described previously.[3] Hypertension may be present in patients with developing cardiac tamponade who have preexisting hypertension owing to the increase in sympathetic tone. About one-third of patients have a pericardial friction rub.

Chest Radiograph and ECG

The heart may appear normal in size in the presence of cardiac tamponade if a small volume of fluid accumulates rapidly, but the cardiac silhouette is usually enlarged.

The ECG abnormalities of cardiac tamponade include those of acute pericarditis, as described previously, and

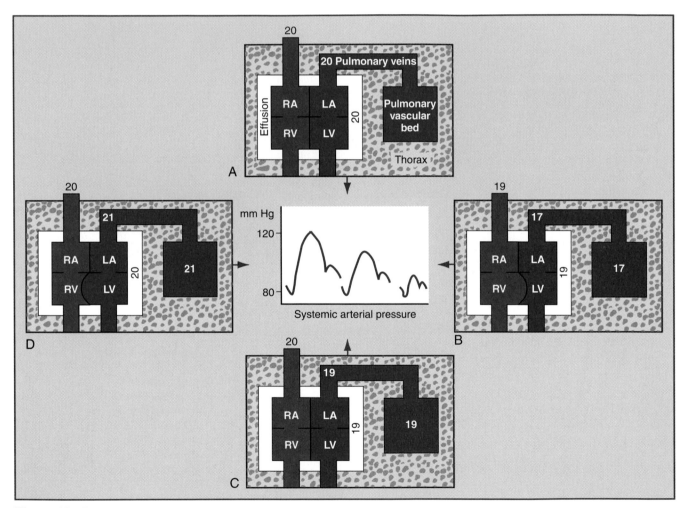

Figure 28–5

Mechanism of pulsus paradoxus at mid expiration (A), early inspiration (B), mid inspiration (C), and early expiration (D). Note that the left atrial (LA) pressure of 21 mm Hg exceeds the intrapericardial pressure of 20 mm Hg during early expiration, facilitating left ventricular (LV) filling. In early inspiration, LA pressure is 17 mm Hg, falling below the intrapericardial pressure of 19 mm Hg. This impairs LV filling, leading to decreased stroke volume and a fall in systolic arterial pressure. All values are in millimeters of mercury. RA, right atrial; RV, right ventricular. (A–D, From Fowler, N.O.: Pericardial disease. In Abelmann, W.H. [ed.]: Atlas of Heart Diseases. Vol. 2. Braunwald, E. [ser. ed.] Philadelphia, Current Medicine, 1995, pp. 13.1–13.16; adapted from Reddy, P.S.: Hemodynamics of cardiac tamponade in man. In Reddy, P.S., Leon, D.F., and Shaver, J.A. [eds.]: Pericardial Disease. New York, Raven Press, 1982, pp. 161–177.)

Table 28-5	Causes of Pulsus Paradoxus*
Cardiac tamponade	Pulmonary embolism
Acute or chronic airway disease	Right ventricular infarction
Constrictive pericarditis (rare)	Circulatory shock
Restrictive cardiomyopathy (rare)	Tension pneumothorax

Adapted from Fowler, N.O.: Pericardial disease. *In* Abelmann, W.H. (ed.): Atlas of Heart Diseases. Vol. 2. Braunwald, E. (ser. ed.) Philadelphia, Current Medicine, 1995, pp. 13.1–13.16; adapted from Fowler, N.O. (ed.): The Pericardium in Health and Disease. Mt. Kisco, NY, Futura Publishing, 1985.

*Pulsus paradoxus may be absent in cardiac tamponade with left ventricular dysfunction, regional tamponade, pulmonary arterial obstruction, hypovolemia, positive pressure breathing, atrial septal defect, or aortic insufficiency.

those of pericardial effusion including the loss of R-wave voltage and nonspecific T-wave flattening (Fig. 28–6). The development of electrical alternans (periodic beat-to-beat variations in the amplitude of the R-waves) is a much more specific indicator of tamponade and indicates pendular swinging of the heart within the pericardial space.

Echocardiogram

In patients with suspected cardiac tamponade, a transthoracic two-dimensional echocardiogram should always be performed before consideration of pericardiocentesis, except if the patient is in extremis and undergoing cardiac resuscitative efforts. The absence of echocardiographic evidence of pericardial effusion virtually excludes the diagnosis of tamponade, with the important exception of the postoperative cardiac surgery patient in whom regional loculated fluid or thrombus can cause cardiac compression. Second, the two-dimensional echocardiogram can rapidly differentiate cardiac tamponade from other causes of jugular venous pressure elevation and arterial hypotension, including constrictive pericarditis, underlying cardiomyopathy, unsuspected valvular regurgitation, and right ventricular infarction. The appearance of dense echoes or fronds within the pericardial space suggests the presence of material such as thrombus, fibrous stranding, or tumor.

Pulsus paradoxus is usually associated with exaggerated leftward motion of the interventricular septum during inspiration and an exaggerated increase in right ventricular filling. Doppler flow velocity recordings show exaggerated tricuspid and pulmonic flow velocities and reduced transmitral flow velocity with the onset of inspiration, and the opposite changes after the onset of expiration. The echocardiogram may also show the inward collapse of the right atrial or the right ventricular wall during diastole (Fig. 28–7). Right atrial and right ventricular diastolic collapse are the echocardiographic markers of the elevation and equilibration of intrapericardial pressure and right ventricular diastolic pressures. This echocardiographic finding occurs early during the development of cardiac tamponade and can be present when the patient is still well compensated. Right ventricular diastolic collapse is highly predictive but not diagnostic of the severity of cardiac tamponade, particularly during hypovolemia, and these echocardiographic signs can be reversed by volume expansion.

Management

Consultation with a cardiologist is indicated for any patient in whom the diagnosis of early cardiac tamponade is questioned, and for any in whom pericardiocentesis is considered for therapeutic or diagnostic reasons. The recognition of possible cardiac tamponade by echocardiography and the decision to proceed to cardiac catheterization and pericardiocentesis require complementary clinical and hemodynamic evaluation to distinguish those patients with mild degrees of cardiac compression from those with hemodynamic embarrassment who require the immediate drainage of pericardial fluid. Many patients with idiopathic (viral) pericarditis and echocardiographic findings of pericardial effusion and mild right heart compression can be observed very closely in the hospital if they do not have clinical findings of elevation of jugular venous pressure, tachycardia, or pulsus paradoxus. In contrast, in patients with borderline hypotension and in those with suspected cardiac perforation or rupture who have echocardiographic signs of pericardial effusion and right heart compression, immediate pericardial drainage by pericardiocentesis or surgery is mandatory. Cardiac tamponade is a *clinical* diagnosis that is definitively established by the documentation of elevation and equilibration of intrapericardial and right atrial pressure and the reversal of the finding by the evacuation of pericardial fluid. Except in an extreme emergency (see Chap. 17) in the moribund patient undergoing resuscitative efforts, pericardiocentesis

Figure 28–6

Pericardial effusion. Low-voltage QRS complexes are present throughout. Note the presence of the calibration signal indicating normal calibration on the vertical scale. (From Reynolds, G.W.: The resting electrocardiogram. *In* Julian, D.G., Camm, A.J., Fox, K.M., et al. [eds.]: Diseases of the Heart. 2nd ed. London, W.B. Saunders, 1996, p. 180.)

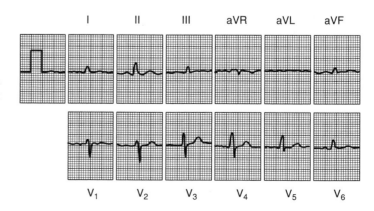

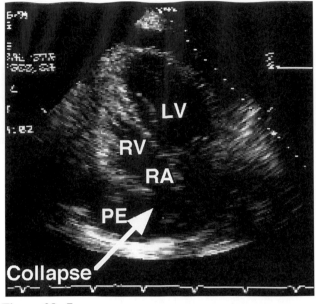

Figure 28–7

Two-dimensional echocardiogram showing a pericardial effusion (PE) as an echo-free space within the pericardial sac and partial collapse of the right atrium (RA) *(arrow),* which indicates an elevation of intrapericardial pressure and its equilibration with right heart filling pressures and strongly suggests developing cardiac tamponade. RV, right ventricle; LV, left ventricle.

should be performed by a cardiologist in conjunction with catheterization of the right heart and using the subxiphoid catheter–guide wire technique[3] (Fig. 28–8).

The presence of cardiac tamponade is confirmed by the elevation and equalization of right atrial and intrapericardial pressures. Complete drainage of the pericardial space should be attempted with the intrapericardial catheter (not needle). The successful relief of cardiac tamponade is documented by the fall of intrapericardial pressure to levels below 0 mm Hg varying with inspiration, the fall of elevated right atrial pressure and the separation between right and left heart filling pressures, the augmentation of cardiac output and stroke volume, the disappearance of pulsus paradoxus, and the restoration of normal systemic arterial pressure if hypotension was present at baseline.

Persistent jugular venous distention despite a fall of pericardial pressure should raise the question of coexisting superior vena cava obstruction, particularly in a patient with suspected malignant pericardial disease. At the completion of the pericardiocentesis, the intrapericardial catheter may be left in place to a closed drainage system. The majority of patients should be observed for about 24 hours in an intensive care setting for the recurrence of cardiac tamponade. If cardiac tamponade recurs after complete catheter pericardial drainage following this technique, percutaneous balloon pericardiotomy or surgical subxiphoid limited pericardiotomy should be considered.[4] Surgical subxiphoid pericardiotomy is usually preferred in patients with tamponade caused by purulent pericarditis and in those with the strong suspicion of tuberculous pericarditis.

Constrictive Pericarditis

Constrictive pericarditis develops when a thick, fibrotic pericardium restricts diastolic filling of the heart. This condition usually begins with an episode of acute pericarditis that may be silent clinically but progresses to chronic inflammation, fibrous scarring and thickening of the pericardium with obliteration of the free pericardial space, and the adherence of the pericardium to the surface of the heart. Pericardial constriction is usually a symmetric process that produces compression of all cardiac chambers.

Although both cardiac tamponade and constrictive pericarditis compress the heart, the pathophysiology differs and so do the clinical findings (Table 28–6). In classic constrictive pericarditis, the fibrotic thick pericardial shell limits diastolic filling of all chambers of the heart and determines the diastolic volume to which the heart may expand. This symmetric constriction results in the elevation and equilibration of diastolic pressures in all four cardiac chambers. In early diastole, when intracardiac vol-

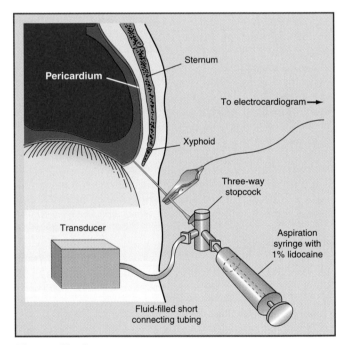

Figure 28–8

Pericardiocentesis using the subxiphoid approach, which avoids the major epicardial vessels. A hollow needle, which is attached via a stopcock to an aspiration syringe and to a short length of connecting tubing leading to a transducer, is used to enter the pericardial space. When fluid is aspirated initially, the pressure waveform at the needle tip should be examined briefly to confirm that the needle tip is in the pericardial space. A floppy-tipped guide wire is then passed through the hollow needle, and the needle is exchanged for a soft flexible catheter with end and side holes to facilitate safe and thorough drainage of the pericardial sac. (Adapted from Lorell, B.H., and Grossman, W.: Profiles in constrictive pericarditis, restrictive cardiomyopathy, and cardiac tamponade. *In* Grossman, W., and Baim, D.S. [eds.]: Cardiac Catheterization, Angiography, and Intervention. Philadelphia, Lea & Febiger, 1991, p. 643.)

Table 28–6	Clinical and Hemodynamic Compressive Pericardial Disease		
	Cardiac Tamponade	**Subacute "Elastic" Constriction**	**Chronic "Rigid" Constriction**
Duration of symptoms	Hours to days	Weeks to months	Months to years
Chest pain, friction rub	Usual	Recent past	Remote
Pulsus paradoxus	Prominent	Usually prominent	Slight or absent
Kussmaul's sign	Absent	Usually absent	Often present
Early diastolic knock	Absent	Usually absent	Often present
Heart size on chest radiograph	Usually enlarged	Usually enlarged	Usually normal, sometimes enlarged
Pericardial calcification	Absent	Rare	Often present
Abnormal P-waves or atrial fibrillation	Absent	Absent	Often present
Venous (right atrial) waveform	X or Xy	Xy or XY	XY or xY
Pericardial effusion	Always present	Often present	Absent

Abbreviations: X and Y, prominent X and Y descents, respectively; x and y, inconspicuous X and Y descents.
From Lorell, B.H.: Pericardial diseases. *In* Braunwald, E. (ed.): Heart Disease. 5th ed. Philadelphia, W.B. Saunders, 1997, pp. 1478–1534; adapted from Hancock, E.W.: On the elastic and rigid forms of constrictive pericarditis. Am. Heart J. 100:917, 1980.

ume is less than the volume that is defined by the stiff pericardial shell, atrial emptying and ventricular diastolic filling are rapid and unimpeded. Rapid early-diastolic filling of the ventricles is abruptly halted when intracardiac volume reaches the limit set by the surrounding stiff pericardium.

Tuberculosis was previously the major cause of constrictive pericarditis, but in Western nations, the largest number of cases of constrictive pericarditis today are of unknown cause (about 40%) and are probably due to previous inapparent viral pericarditis. Other contemporary causes of constrictive pericarditis include postsurgical pericarditis, prior mediastinal radiation, connective tissue disorders such as rheumatoid arthritis and systemic lupus erythematosus, and neoplastic pericardial infiltration.

Clinical Presentation

The symptoms associated with constrictive pericarditis are often mistakenly attributed to other diagnoses because the diagnosis of pericardial constriction is not considered. In patients in whom systemic venous and right atrial pressure are modestly elevated (about 15 mm Hg), symptoms related to systemic venous congestion, such as edema, abdominal swelling, and discomfort from ascites, may predominate. Vague abdominal symptoms, such as dyspepsia and anorexia with protein-losing enteropathy, may also be present. When right and left heart filling pressures are elevated to a level of 20 to 30 mm Hg, exertional dyspnea and orthopnea appear. Pleural effusion may also develop. When the cardiac output becomes fixed or reduced, severe fatigue, weight loss, and muscle wasting may develop. Chest pain that can be confused with angina pectoris is common and may be related to subendocardial hypoperfusion or chronic pericardial inflammation.

Physical Examination

The single most important finding in raising the suspicion of constrictive pericarditis is documentation of the *elevation of jugular venous pressure.* Kussmaul's sign (an inspiratory increase in the systemic venous pressure) can be detected as a rise in an already elevated jugular ve-

nous pressure during inspiration, whereas a fall in intrathoracic pressure would normally reduce jugular venous pressure. Pulsus paradoxus is uncommon and rarely exceeds 10 mm Hg unless pericardial fluid under pressure is also present. In severe cases, the most impressive physical finding during auscultation is the *early-diastolic pericardial knock* heard along the left sternal border about 0.09 to 0.12 second after the second aortic sound. It precisely corresponds in timing to the sudden cessation of ventricular filling during diastole, at the same time as a typical third heart sound gallop, and after a mitral opening snap (Fig. 28–9). Hepatomegaly is often present with prominent hepatic pulsations. Edema of the scrotum, thighs, and calves is more common in older patients. Severe muscle wasting and cachexia may lead to the incorrect diagnosis of underlying malignancy.

Chest Radiograph

The size of the cardiac silhouette may be small, normal, or large. Calcification of the pericardium, especially on the lateral chest film, is present in about half of patients and should raise the possibility of chronic tubercular pericarditis (Fig. 28–10). Pleural effusion occurs in about 60% of patients, and unexplained persistent pleural effusion can be the initial manifestation. Pulmonary redistribution of flow is common, but frank infiltrates and alveolar edema are rare.

ECG

The ECG findings of chronic constrictive pericarditis are nonspecific but include low QRS voltage, generalized T-wave flattening or inversion, and left atrial abnormalities suggestive of left atrial enlargement. Atrial fibrillation occurs in less than half of patients and may be related in part to elevation of atrial pressure and chronic atrial distention.

Echocardiogram

It is important to emphasize that severe constrictive physiology can occur in the presence of diseased but minimally thickened pericardium; conversely, pericardial

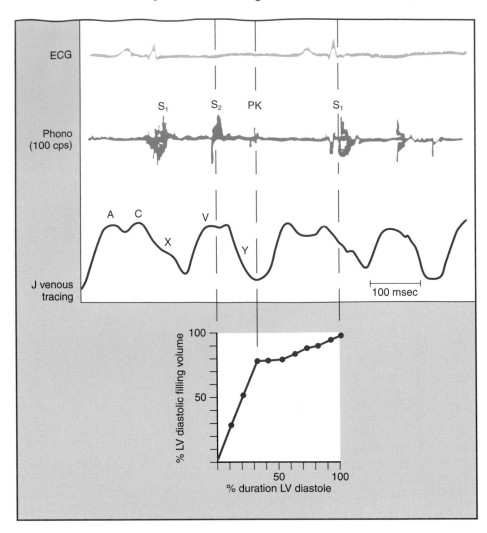

Figure 28–9

Electrocardiogram (ECG), phonocardiogram (Phono), jugular (J) venous pulse tracing, and left ventricular (LV) diastolic filling curve in a patient with constrictive pericarditis and pericardial knock (PK). The PK occurs simultaneously with the nadir of the diastolic Y descent and sudden plateau of the LV filling curve. S_1, first heart sound; S_2, second heart sound. (Redrawn from American Journal of Cardiology, Vol. 46, Tyberg, T.I., Goodyer, A.V., and Langou, R.A., Genesis of pericardial knock in constrictive pericarditis, pp. 570–575, Copyright 1980, with permission from Excerpta Medica Inc.)

thickening or calcification alone is *not* diagnostic of hemodynamically significant cardiac compression from constrictive pericarditis. The echocardiogram may show evidence of pericardial thickening and the appearance of multiple "sandwiched" parallel lines (Fig. 28–11). Two-dimensional echocardiography frequently shows an immobile, dense appearance of pericardium, abrupt displacement of the intraventricular septum during early-diastolic filling (septal bounce), dilatation of the hepatic veins and inferior vena cava, and blunted respiratory fluctuation of

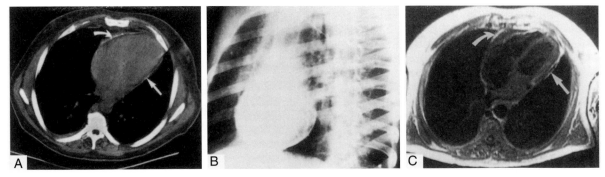

Figure 28–10

A, Computed tomography of the chest showing thickened pericardium and calcification *(arrows)* in a patient with constrictive pericarditis. *B,* Lateral chest radiograph showing pericardial calcification. *C,* Magnetic resonance imaging from a patient with constrictive pericarditis. Note a dark area of thickened pericardium over the left ventricle *(straight arrow)* and a light area of pericardial fat over the right ventricle *(curved arrow).* (*A,* From Fowler, N.O.: Pericardial disease. *In* Abelmann, W.H. [ed.]: Atlas of Heart Diseases. Vol. 2. Braunwald, E. [ser. ed.] Philadelphia, Current Medicine, 1995, pp. 13.1–13.16; adapted from Fowler, N.O.: Pericardial disease. Heart Dis. Stroke 1:85–94, 1992. *B* and *C,* Fowler, N.O.: Pericardial disease. *In* Abelmann, W.H. [ed.]: Atlas of Heart Diseases. Vol. 2. Braunwald, E. [ser. ed.]. Philadelphia, Current Medicine, 1995, pp. 13.1–13.16.)

Figure 28-11

M-mode echocardiogram shows thickening of the pericardium (TH. PERI) and abrupt displacement of the intraventricular septum during early-diastolic filling (septal bounce, *arrow*). In this patient, dilatation of the hepatic veins and venae cavae were also present. These findings are suggestive of constrictive pericarditis, which should be confirmed by cardiac catheterization.

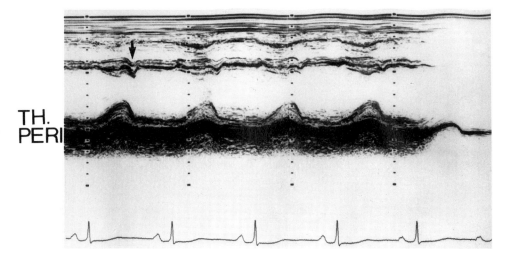

vena cava diameter (plethora). Doppler flow patterns that are strongly suggestive of constriction[5] can also occur in chronic lung disease and pulmonary hypertension.

Differential Diagnosis

Constrictive pericarditis is a great "pretender" that can be easily confused with other disorders that cause fatigue, edema, and jugular venous distention (Table 28–7). Hepatic congestion can be accompanied by low serum albumin, elevated conjugated and unconjugated serum bilirubin, and abnormal hepatocellular function tests. Elevated systemic venous pressure can also cause protein-losing enteropathy, as well as albuminuria and the nephrotic syndrome.

It can be particularly challenging to distinguish patients with constrictive pericarditis from those with restrictive cardiomyopathy (see Table 28–7). The differentiation between these two disorders is complicated by the fact that many infiltrative processes can involve the myocardium as well as the pericardium. Both constrictive pericarditis and restrictive cardiomyopathy may show nonspecific ECG abnormalities of reduced QRS voltage, nonspecific T-wave flattening, and atrial fibrillation. The development of atrioventricular block or conduction disturbances favors the diagnosis of restrictive cardiomyopathy. In patients with amyloid infiltration of the heart, echocardiography is often useful in demonstrating the presence of thickening of the ventricular myocardium with a distinctive "spark-

ling" appearance of the myocardium. Amyloidosis should also be suspected when a thick-walled heart by echocardiography is detected in the presence of diffuse low QRS voltage.

The diagnosis of restrictive cardiomyopathy is more likely when the pericardium appears normal or when marked elevation of right ventricular systolic and pulmonary artery pressures is present. Further, in classic restrictive cardiomyopathy, right ventricular diastolic pressure is usually clearly elevated but lower than left ventricular diastolic pressure. Ventricular diastolic filling in constrictive pericarditis tends to occur predominantly in early diastole, whereas it is usually more sluggish in restrictive cardiomyopathy. Magnetic resonance imaging (MRI) is probably the most sensitive imaging modality currently available for delineating the regional pericardial thickness and the relationship between extracardiac masses to the pericardium and the surface of the heart. MRI may be helpful in detecting the presence of myocardial atrophy or fibrosis, particularly in those with a remote history of radiation. In some patients, right ventricular endomyocardial biopsy may be needed to search for extensive fibrosis or infiltration with substances such as amyloid.

The definitive diagnosis of constrictive pericarditis is made by cardiac catheterization. The right and left ventricular waveforms show a characteristic "dip and plateau" in early diastole (Fig. 28–12). The early-diastolic dip corresponds to the period of rapid early-diastolic filling, whereas the plateau phase corresponds to the period of mid- and late diastole when there is no further volume expansion. The right and left atrial waveforms differ from cardiac tamponade and show a prominent and deep diastolic Y descent that is the marker of rapid atrial emptying in early diastole.

Management

Surgical pericardiectomy should be considered in patients with progressive edema or exercise limitation owing to fatigue in whom the diagnosis has been confirmed at cardiac catherization. Definitive treatment is complete surgical resection of the pericardium. In over 800 cases reported in multiple surgical series since 1981, the in-hospital operative mortality ranged from 5% to 19%,[6]

Table 28-7	Disorders Confused with Constrictive Pericarditis

Superior vena caval obstruction (usually malignant)
Primary nephrotic syndrome
Primary hepatic disease
Restrictive cardiomyopathy
    Amyloidosis
    Sarcoidosis
    Chronic radiation injury
    Hemochromatosis
    Hypereosinophilic syndrome
Tricuspid regurgitation with right ventricular dysfunction

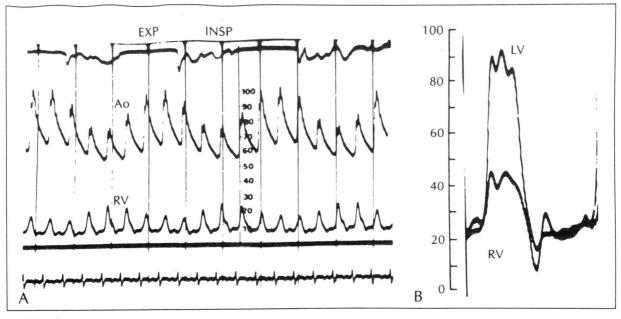

Figure 28–12

Contrasting pattern of a ventricular pressure pulse recording in cardiac tamponade *(A)* and constrictive pericarditis *(B)*. In constrictive pericarditis, there is a dip-and-plateau pattern (square-root sign) in both ventricular pressure pulse tracings with equalization of right ventricular (RV) and left ventricular (LV) end-diastolic pressures. In cardiac tamponade, there is no pronounced diastolic dip in the RV pressure pulse. The patient with cardiac tamponade demonstrates a pronounced inspiratory decline of aortic pressure (Ao) typical of pulsus paradoxus. Pressure scale is in millimeters of mercury. EXP, expiration; INSP, inspiration. *(A and B,* From Fowler, N.O.: Pericardial disease. *In* Abelmann, W.H. [ed.]: Atlas of Heart Diseases. Vol. 2. Braunwald, E. [ser. ed.] Philadelphia, Current Medicine, 1995, pp. 13.1–13.16; adapted from American Journal of Cardiology, vol 26, Shabetai, R., Fowler, N.O., and Guntheroth, W.G.: The hemodynamics of cardiac tamponade and constrictive pericarditis, pp 480–489, Copyright 1970, with permission from Excerpta Medica Inc.)

with 5-year survival of about 75% to 85%. Overall outcome is unfavorably influenced by the presence of preoperative renal insufficiency, severe preoperative functional disability (New York Heart Association class IV), the presence of extensive nonresectable calcification or incomplete pericardial resection, and the presence of prior radiation-induced cardiac injury, with fibrosis and damage of the pericardium and the myocardium. Thus, pericardiectomy should be performed *early* in the course of constrictive pericarditis in symptomatic patients because the development of severe clinical disability is associated with poor in-hospital and long-term surgical outcome. Pericardiectomy is often not warranted in very elderly patients with cachexia or baseline renal dysfunction, or in patients with limited life expectancy from other underlying disorders. Patients with known or suspected tuberculous pericarditis are usually treated with multidrug antituberculosis therapy for 2 to 4 weeks before the operation; if the diagnosis of tuberculous pericarditis is confirmed, antituberculosis therapy is usually continued for 6 months to 1 year after pericardiectomy.

Effusive Constrictive Pericarditis

Effusive constrictive pericarditis is characterized by the presence of both pericardial fluid under pressure (tamponade) and visceral pericardial constriction. The symptoms are similar to those of both chronic tamponade and con-

strictive pericarditis and include dyspnea, atypical chest pain, fatigue, and loss of exercise tolerance. The physical findings usually are those of cardiac tamponade. If the pericardial effusion under pressure is large, the chest x-ray may show cardiac enlargement. The ECG is usually abnormal with nonspecific findings of ST–T-wave abnormalities or diffuse low voltage. The two-dimensional echocardiogram may show a pericardial effusion sandwiched between thickened pericardial membranes. Cardiac catheterization is mandatory when this diagnosis is suspected in the symptomatic patient. The hallmark is continued elevation of right atrial pressure after aspiration of pericardial fluid and the restoration of the pressure within the pericardial sac to zero. Persistent elevation of right atrial pressure occurs after the relief of pericardial tamponade because of the presence of a constricting visceral pericardium. This entity is probably a stage in the development of classic constrictive pericarditis, and it is most commonly seen in patients with previous severe idiopathic or presumed viral pericarditis, neoplastic pericarditis, or mediastinal irradiation. When the diagnosis of effusive constrictive pericarditis is made at catheterization after pericardiocentesis is performed, further intervention is necessary. Pericardiocentesis can be valuable by transiently relieving symptoms and improving blood pressure as well as cardiac output. However, the unmasking of hemodynamic findings of constriction after successful pericardiocentesis indicates that surgery with total parietal and visceral pericardiectomy is needed.

Asymptomatic Pericardial Effusion

Patients who develop a pericardial effusion without the elevation of intrapericardial pressure may be completely asymptomatic and come to attention solely because of the unsuspected finding of an enlarged globular cardiac silhouette on a chest radiograph or an unexpected finding on an echocardiogram. The incidence of small pericardial effusion detected by echocardiography in asymptomatic healthy subjects ranges between 8% and 15%. In normal pregnant women, about 40% have asymptomatic small pericardial effusion evident by echocardiography that resolves within the first few weeks after delivery. Large asymptomatic pericardial effusions are extremely uncommon in healthy young and middle-aged adults. In the elderly patient with a large pericardial effusion without cardiac compression, hypothyroidism should be definitively excluded by appropriate laboratory tests.

Clinical Findings

A large asymptomatic pericardial effusion may be accompanied by muffling of the heart sounds owing to the presence of fluid between the chest wall and the cardiac chambers. Compression of the left lung base by pericardial fluid can produce Ewart's sign, which is a patch of dullness at the angle of the left scapula during auscultation. On the chest radiograph, the cardiac silhouette may be enlarged with a globular water-bottle shape when at least 250 ml of fluid accumulates. Occasionally, chronic pericardial effusion may cause loculated cystlike protuberances on the cardiac silhouette.

Transthoracic echocardiography is probably the most cost-effective and efficient tool to distinguish between cardiac enlargement from underlying cardiomyopathy versus a large pericardial effusion. If an inadequate image is obtained using echocardiography, computed tomography or MRI can be utilized to define the pericardium and the cardiac chambers. These specialized imaging tests can also be helpful in unusual situations to differentiate pericardial fluid from thick epicardial fat and to delineate other suspected pathology, including pericardial thickening and pericardial masses related to tumor.

Management

The first step is performing a rigorous history and physical examination to determine whether the patient is at clinical risk for infectious pericarditis or malignant pericardial effusion. The next management steps are outlined in Figure 28–13.

SPECIFIC CAUSES OF PERICARDIAL DISEASE

Tuberculous Pericarditis

Tuberculosis now accounts for less than 5% of patients who develop cardiac tamponade and for about 6% of those who require pericardiectomy for chronic pericardial constriction. Early tuberculous infection of the pericardium is characterized by the presence of acid-fast bacilli, deposition of fibrin, and granuloma formation. Pericardial effusion that may initially be serous or frankly hemorrhagic may then develop. As the effusion organizes, the pericardium thickens, granulomas develop, and living acid-fast bacilli may no longer be present. Constrictive pericarditis develops in almost all patients with untreated tuberculous pericarditis and in about half or less of those who receive antituberculous chemotherapy during acute tuberculous pericarditis.[7, 8]

Clinical Findings

Marked sputum production, cough, and hemoptysis, which are clinical markers of the presence of cavitary pulmonary tuberculosis, are usually absent. In the late stage of chronic tuberculous constrictive pericarditis, systemic venous congestion and low output predominate, and large pleural effusions are often present.

Diagnosis

Tuberculous pericarditis should be suspected in patients with persistent fever and unexplained pericardial effusion, especially those who are in population groups with an increased risk for tuberculosis, including severely impoverished patients, those who are immunosuppressed or at high risk for human immunodeficiency virus (HIV) infection, and those with active HIV infection. The probability of obtaining a definitive diagnosis is greatest if *both* pericardial fluid and a pericardial biopsy specimen are examined early in the effusive stage. It is important, however, to emphasize that a "negative" small pericardial biopsy specimen does not exclude tuberculous pericarditis because in some individuals examination of the entire pericardium at pericardiectomy or autopsy is needed to demonstrate histologic evidence of tuberculous pericarditis. Furthermore, the finding of isolated granulomas or caseous material without bacilli is also not absolutely diagnostic, since these findings can be present in other chronic pericardial diseases, such as sarcoidosis. Thus, it is sometimes necessary to make a presumptive clinical diagnosis of tuberculous pericarditis in severely ill patients with persistent fever, large hemorrhagic pericardial effusion, and systemic symptoms such as weight loss, even when examination of pericardial fluid and pericardial biopsy do not reveal tuberculosis. In such patients, the tuberculin skin test may not be helpful because of anergy. Infectious disease consultation is often important before embarking on a long course of multidrug antituberculosis therapy in patients at high risk for HIV infection or with known HIV disease, since atypical strains of tuberculosis may be present.

Management

Initial chemotherapy should be under the supervision of an infectious disease specialist. Constrictive pericarditis can develop even when multidrug chemotherapy is successfully initiated. In a series of 294 consecutive patients with acute pericarditis, 13 were shown to have tubercu-

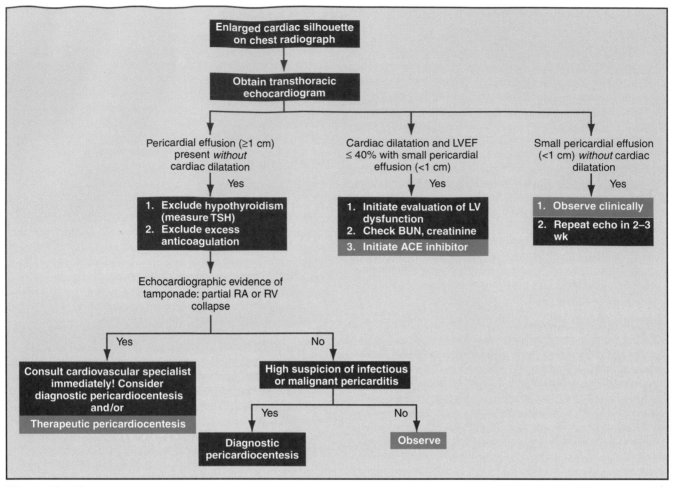

Figure 28–13

Management of asymptomatic pericardial effusion in patients with a normal physical examination. LV, left ventricular; EF, ejection fraction; TSH, thyroid-stimulating hormone; BUN, blood urea nitrogen; ACE, angiotensin-converting enzyme; RA, right atrial; RV, right ventricular.

lous pericarditis, and 54% of these developed constrictive pericarditis, requiring surgical pericardiectomy.[7] The outcome after surgical pericardiectomy for constrictive tuberculous pericarditis is favorable. In a South African study of 113 patients with constrictive tuberculous pericarditis who underwent pericardiectomy, 97% were discharged from the hospital with subsequent resolution of hepatomegaly, edema, and systemic symptoms.[8]

Purulent Bacterial Pericarditis

Despite the introduction of antibiotics, purulent pericarditis continues to occur primarily as a complication of pneumonia or empyema owing to staphylococci, pneumococci, and streptococci.[9] It can also occur with a wide spectrum of organisms as a complication of bacterial endocarditis and after thoracic surgery. Bacterial pericarditis continues to be a life-threatening complication that is detected antemortem in only about 20% of patients.

Clinical Features

Purulent bacterial pericarditis is usually an acute and fulminant illness. High fevers, night sweats, shaking chills, and dyspnea are common symptoms. The physical examination reveals tachycardia in almost all patients, whereas the presence of a pericardial friction rub occurs in less than half. The appearance of new jugular distention and pulsus paradoxus are ominous signs that suggest development of rapidly accumulating purulent fluid under pressure (cardiac tamponade). In one series, cardiac tamponade developed acutely in 38% of patients with previously unsuspected purulent bacterial pericarditis and caused death in the majority.[10]

The laboratory findings usually include a leukocytosis with a marked leftward shift. The chest film should be closely examined for evidence of underlying pneumonia and empyema or mediastinitis. The presence of a prolonged PR interval, bundle branch block, or atrioventricular dissociation suggests underlying endocarditis. A pericardial effusion, when present, usually shows polymorphonuclear leukocytosis and occasional frank thick pus. Pericardial fluid glucose level is usually depressed, whereas the protein content and lactate dehydrogenase values are increased.

Despite the lower incidence of purulent pericarditis in the present era, overall survival is poor, averaging about 30%. In the absence of randomized clinical trials, there is a general consensus that the high mortality from purulent pericarditis can be reduced substantially through the institution of appropriate intravenous antibiotic therapy as well as early surgical drainage of the pericardium. For example, in a surgical series of pericardiectomy plus intravenous antibiotic therapy, the surgical mortality was 8% with a 5-year survival of 91%, with no cases of pericardial constriction.[11] The instillation of antibiotics into the pericardial space is not warranted because of ready access of antibiotics to the pericardium during intravenous administration.

Fungal Pericarditis

Histoplasmosis

Histoplasmosis is the most common cause of fungal pericarditis[12] and should be considered in young and otherwise healthy patients suspected of having acute viral or tuberculous pericarditis and living in endemic areas. Most patients give a history of a preceding respiratory illness and have findings of pericardial chest pain and typical ECG changes of acute pericarditis. An enlarged cardiac silhouette is present in more than 90% of patients, and pleural effusion with intrathoracic adenopathy are present in about 67% of patients. In young and otherwise healthy adults with evidence of effusive pericarditis, a presumptive clinical diagnosis of histoplasmosis pericarditis can by made based on (1) residence or travel in endemic areas, (2) elevated complement fixation titer of at least 1 : 32, and (3) a positive immunodiffusion test.

Histoplasmosis pericarditis is usually a benign illness that resolves in 2 weeks and can be treated with NSAIDs to minimize and shorten the duration of chest pain and fever. However, because of the risk of rapid development of massive effusion and acute tamponade in those with histoplasmosis pericarditis, these patients should initially be hospitalized. Antibiotic therapy with amphotericin is required for only those rare patients with disseminated infectious histoplasmosis pericarditis and severe coexisting systemic disease.

Other Fungal Agents

Coccidioidomycosis pericarditis develops in patients who have inhaled fungal spores from soil or dust in endemic areas including the American Southwest, San Joaquin Valley, and Argentina.[13] Other fungal infections responsible for pericarditis include aspergillosis, blastomycosis, and those caused by *Candida* species. Fungal pericarditis from these agents usually occurs as a complication of disseminated infection in drug addicts with endocarditis, immunosuppressed patients who have received broad-spectrum antibiotics, and those recovering from complex open-heart surgery. The clinical course of pericarditis due to fungal agents other than histoplasmosis is usually characterized by fever, weight loss, and clinical findings related to the development of pericardial effusion under pressure (pericardial tamponade).

A presumptive diagnosis of coccidioidomycosis pericarditis is made in the patient with systemic illness and pericarditis who has (1) a history of dust exposure in endemic areas in the American Southwest or South America, (2) a characteristic clinical picture of disseminated coccidioidomycosis involving the lung and multiple other organs, (3) a positive serum precipitin test early in the infection followed by rising complement fixation antibody titer, and (4) microscopic evidence of the characteristic spherule in biopsy material. If pericarditis due to other fungal organisms is suspected in high-risk patients, appropriate complement fixation antibody titers should be measured and vigorous attempts should be made to obtain biopsy specimens from the pericardium and other clinically involved sites.

Drug therapy for pericarditis is essential for pericarditis associated with disseminated coccidioidomycosis, aspergillosis, and blastomycosis and usually consists of a prolonged intravenous therapy with amphotericin B. For fungal pericarditis from organisms other than histoplasmosis, surgical drainage of the pericardial space should also be considered to treat the active pericardial infection and reduce the risk of later development of constrictive pericarditis.

Pericarditis after Acute Myocardial Infarction

Pericarditis is common during the first few days after acute transmural infarction (see Chap. 19) and is present in as many as 40% of fatal transmural infarctions studied at autopsy, but thrombolytic therapy has probably lowered its incidence. It tends to occur as a regional response to inflammation and necrosis of the underlying infarcted myocardial tissue. Acute pericarditis after myocardial infarction is usually recognized clinically by the development of a pericardial friction rub or onset of severe pleuritic and positional chest pain within a few hours or on the first, second, or third day after infarction, often with a low-grade fever.[14] Acute pericarditis after infarction differs from the rare Dressler syndrome, which occurs 10 days or later after acute myocardial infarction and represents an immunologic response to the myocardial or pericardial injury. The recognition of acute postinfarction pericarditis is extremely important because it can be confused with angina pectoris. Postinfarction pericarditis is a marker of extensive infarction and worse outcomes, but its presence per se does not appear to be an independent risk factor for hospital mortality.

The typical four stages of ECG changes of acute pericarditis are rare during acute postinfarction pericarditis. The finding of a small pericardial effusion, which can be detected in about one-fourth of patients early after acute infarction, in the absence of hemodynamic compromise is not diagnostic of postinfarction pericarditis.

The development of cardiac tamponade early after an

infarction may be related to postinfarction pericarditis or to myocardial rupture into the pericardial sac. Massive cardiac hemorrhage due to cardiac rupture is usually followed by the immediate development of electrical-mechanical dissociation, although occasional patients may develop a contained false aneurysm within the pericardial space and survive after surgical repair.

Management

If pain is severe, high-dose aspirin usually provides relief in about 48 hours. The early use of drugs such as ibuprofen, indomethacin, and large doses of corticosteroids can interfere with the conversion of the myocardial infarction into a firm scar. Intravenous heparin itself does not appear to be associated with increased risk of intrapericardial hemorrhage in patients with postinfarction pericarditis, but warfarin anticoagulation should usually be avoided.

Uremic Pericarditis

Clinical uremic pericarditis now occurs in less than 20% of patients who require chronic dialysis, whereas asymptomatic pericardial effusions of small to moderate size occur in up to 60% of uremic patients who require dialysis and these are probably related to volume overload and clinical congestive heart failure. Uremic pericarditis is usually hemorrhagic and associated with the development of shaggy fibrinous exudates on the pericardial surfaces. Uremic pericarditis may present as an acute pericarditis, asymptomatic pericardial effusion, constrictive pericarditis, or pericardial tamponade.[15] Patients with effusive uremic pericarditis on dialysis usually come to attention because of the development of either hypotension during rapid fluid shifts while undergoing a routine dialysis or chest pain.

Management

Patients with uremic pericarditis should be seen in consultation by both a nephrologist and a cardiologist. Uremic patients who develop severe symptomatic pericarditis before the initiation of dialysis almost always respond to the initiation of vigorous dialysis within a period of 10 days to 3 weeks. Patients who develop symptomatic uremic pericarditis during chronic dialysis may respond to an intensification of dialysis and the initiation of therapy with NSAIDs. Percutaneous catheter pericardiocentesis with continued catheter drainage of the pericardial space for up to 48 to 72 hours is the next option, if dialysis and medications are unsuccessful. Subxiphoid pericardiotomy, balloon pericardiotomy, and surgical pericardiectomy are reserved for effusions that recur or persist despite drainage attempts.

Neoplastic Pericarditis

In a prospective series of patients with acute pericarditis of unknown cause, an unsuspected malignant origin was found in 5%.[1] Breast cancer, lung cancer, leukemia, Hodgkin's disease, and non-Hodgkin's lymphoma account for about 80% of malignant pericarditis. Less-common neoplasms that lead to pericardial involvement include ovarian and cervical cancer, gastrointestinal cancer, sarcoma, multiple myeloma, teratoma, and melanoma. Primary malignant neoplasms of the pericardium are extremely rare. In patients with AIDS, sarcoma and lymphoma can involve the pericardium.

Neoplastic pericarditis can be caused by nodular tumor deposits from hematogenous or lymphatic spread, extension to the pericardium of an adjacent malignant mediastinal tumor, diffuse pericardial thickening and infiltration with tumor, and local infiltration of the pericardium. The underlying epicardium and heart muscle are rarely involved. Asymptomatic pericardial effusions are relatively common in patients with mediastinal lymphoma and Hodgkin's disease, presumably as a consequence of compromised lymphatic drainage, and improve when therapy of mediastinal lymphoma is initiated with radiation or chemotherapy. Small, clinically unsuspected pericardial effusions detected by echocardiography may also occur in up to 50% of women with metastatic breast cancer.[16]

Clinical Presentation

In the majority of patients, neoplastic pericarditis is not suspected until symptoms and signs of severe cardiac compression (cardiac tamponade) appear. Dyspnea is the most frequent symptom, whereas chest discomfort, cough, orthopnea, and hepatomegaly are also common. Conversely, a pericardial friction rub is uncommon. The chest radiograph is abnormal in more than 90% of patients and may show pleural effusion, cardiac enlargement, mediastinal widening, or uncommonly, a nodular contour of the cardiac silhouette. The ECG is often abnormal but nonspecific.

Differential Diagnosis

Neoplastic pericarditis producing cardiac tamponade must be differentiated from other causes of jugular venous distention, edema, and hepatomegaly in cancer patients, including underlying left ventricular dysfunction and heart failure secondary to prior cardiac disease or anthracycline cardiac toxicity, superior vena caval obstruction, malignant hepatic involvement with portal hypertension, and microvascular pulmonary tumor spread with secondary pulmonary hypertension and right heart failure. The echocardiogram provides critical information regarding the presence of a pericardial effusion and the thickness and nodularity of the pericardium, and it may provide evidence of an abnormal Doppler velocity profile that supports the diagnosis of tamponade or constriction. In some instances, an MRI study may provide additional information regarding the presence and location of masses within the pericardium and the relationship to adjacent mediastinum and lungs. In about half of patients with symptomatic pericarditis and known neoplasm, the pericarditis is nonmalignant, most commonly from prior radiation or idiopathic causes.

Management

Pericardiocentesis is the cornerstone of management. Cytologic examination is diagnostic in about 85% of patients, with most false-negative results occurring in lymphoma or mesothelioma. Optically guided percutaneous pericardioscopy with biopsy is a new supplementary approach for the diagnosis of suspected neoplastic pericardial involvement.

The presence of cyanosis, hypoxemia, and the elevation of pulmonary artery pressure should raise a very strong suspicion of pulmonary microvascular tumor (lymphangitic tumor). Support for this diagnosis can be obtained at the same setting as pericardiocentesis and right heart catheterization by obtaining a sample of blood from the pulmonary capillary wedge position for cytologic analysis using the right heart catheter.

The instillation of tetracycline or other chemotherapeutic agents into the pericardial space does not appear to have a short-term or long-term advantage compared with complete catheter drainage of the pericardial space. To date, there has not been a prospective trial comparing the outcome of catheter pericardiocentesis, balloon pericardiectomy under local anesthesia, or subxiphoid pericardiectomy in the management of large malignant effusion.[4]

The subsequent management strategy and natural history strongly depend on the underlying malignancy. About 25% of patients with cardiac tamponade due to malignant pericarditis who are managed surgically or with pericardiocentesis will survive for at least 1 year, whereas the 1-year survival rate is as high as 90% in patients with cancer but nonmalignant effusion. The survival in patients with malignant pericarditis due to breast cancer is strikingly better than that of patients with malignant pericarditis and tamponade due to lung cancer or other metastatic carcinomas.[3]

Radiation Pericarditis

Factors that appear to influence the development of acute and late radiation-induced heart disease include the cumulative radiation dose, the fractionation of the dose, the volume of the heart included in the radiation field, the use of cobalt source with nonhomogeneous dose distribution versus a linear accelerator, and anterior weighting of the radiation dose. In patients who receive mantle radiation as initial treatment of Hodgkin's disease, about 2.2% develop radiation pericarditis. In breast cancer radiation therapy, in which the volume of heart included in the field is usually much less than 30%, the incidence of radiation-induced pericarditis is between 0.4% and 5%. Radiation-induced pericardial injury may become apparent during the course of treatment or, more commonly, may come to attention months or even 10 or more years later.[17] Radiation-induced pericardial injury can be associated with acute pericardial inflammation and development of pericardial effusion. The inflammation and initial effusion may resolve spontaneously or progress to constrictive pericarditis. Myocardial degeneration and coronary artery intimal proliferation and stenosis can occur.

Many patients may present with insidious and progressive development of fatigue, dyspnea, edema, and jugular venous distention due to effusive constriction or classic constrictive pericarditis. When symptoms of pericarditis with pericardial effusion or constriction occur years after apparent successful treatment of Hodgkin's disease and lymphoma, pericarditis is much more likely to be related to radiation injury than to recurrent malignant disease.

Management

Patients with asymptomatic small pericardial effusions after radiation therapy should be followed clinically without the institution of specific therapy. Percutaneous pericardiocentesis should be performed only in patients who have history, physical findings, and echocardiographic markers of probable cardiac tamponade, or when drainage of very large pericardial effusion and cytologic examination is required for management. Radiation-induced hypothyroidism occurs in about one-fourth of patients who undergo mantle irradiation, and hypothyroidism must always be excluded as a cause of delayed effusive pericarditis after radiation therapy. Pericardiectomy should be considered in symptomatic patients with large recurrent pericardial effusions refractory to management with pericardiocentesis and in those with constrictive pericarditis. The operative mortality for pericardiectomy in patients with radiation-induced constrictive pericarditis is about 21% compared with a mortality of less than 10% in those with idiopathic constrictive pericarditis.[17]

Pericarditis Related to Autoimmune Disorders

Pericarditis is detected clinically in 20% to 45% of patients with systemic lupus erythematosus (SLE) during the course of their disease, and echocardiographic abnormalities can be detected in an even higher percentage. Pericarditis tends to occur during flares of disease activity in patients with SLE, and it is the most common cardiovascular manifestation.[18] Cardiac tamponade develops in less than 10% of patients with SLE and clinically recognized pericarditis, and constrictive pericarditis is very rare. Pericarditis should be suspected when patients with SLE develop severe pleuritic chest pain, pericardial rub, or enlargement of the cardiac silhouette, suggestive of a pericardial effusion, on the chest radiograph. In patients with SLE who are treated with corticosteroids, cytotoxic agents, or immunosuppressive drugs, a meticulous physical examination, blood cultures, and a tuberculin skin test should be obtained to evaluate possible purulent, fungal, or tuberculous pericarditis. Except when purulent pericarditis is strongly suspected based on the clinical presentation, it is usually not necessary to confirm the diagnosis of SLE pericarditis by performing pericardiocentesis. In the majority of patients, pericarditis subsides when other disease manifestations become clinically inactive.

Rheumatoid Arthritis

The incidence of symptomatic pericarditis in patients with rheumatoid arthritis is about 25%.[19] Clinical features of acute pericarditis coexist with active joint inflammation, and pleural effusions on the chest radiograph are present in about two-thirds of patients. Although rheumatoid pericarditis is usually self-limited and benign, cardiac tamponade can develop abruptly.

Rheumatoid pericarditis symptoms usually subside in association with anti-inflammatory therapy administered for other manifestations of the disease, including pleuritis and acute arthritis. Suppression of recurrent effusive rheumatoid pericarditis has been reported in response to chronic colchicine treatment, but experience with this therapy is very limited. Pericardiocentesis should be performed to relieve large effusions causing cardiac tamponade. There is no clear evidence that intrapericardial steroid instillation alters the natural history of the effusion or prevents the development of constrictive pericarditis. In patients with documented effusive constrictive or constrictive rheumatoid pericarditis, pericardiectomy can provide dramatic hemodynamic and symptomatic improvement.

Pericarditis, pericardial effusion, and constrictive pericarditis can occur as a complication of other inflammatory disorders, including progressive systemic sclerosis, mixed connective tissue disease, and Sjögren's syndrome. Sarcoidosis is a rare cause of pericarditis, cardiac tamponade, and constrictive pericarditis, but the finding of thick pericardium with noncaseating granulomas may cause confusion with tuberculosis or fungal pericarditis.

Drug-Related Pericarditis

Pericarditis is reported to occur in 2% to 25% of patients with procainamide-related and hydralazine-related SLE syndrome.[20] Other drugs that can cause pericarditis in association with SLE syndrome include isoniazid and phenytoin. Pericarditis as a complication of hypersensitivity with eosinophilia has been reported after administration of penicillin, tryptophan, and cromolyn sodium. Pericarditis has also been reported in association with polymer fume fever, a syndrome of noncardiogenic pulmonary edema and pericarditis that follows inhalation of fumes from the burning of Teflon materials. Pericarditis and late pericardial constriction can also occur as a foreign body reaction in response to silicon and talc within the pericardial space.

Postpericardiotomy Syndrome

The postpericardiotomy syndrome occurs in 10% to 40% of patients after cardiac operations, usually appearing about 7 days to 2 months after surgery. Clinical features include fever, chest pain, increased sedimentation rate, pericardial effusion, and sometimes, plural effusion. Up to 50% of patients will have typical ECG findings of acute pericarditis, and many will have positive antiviral antibody titers to agents such as cytomegalovirus. The pericardial fluid is usually serosanguineous. The late development of tamponade or constriction is unusual.

Some patients develop late pericardial constriction after cardiac surgery without acute pericarditis. In these patients, blood in the tissues surrounding the opened pericardium may cause scarring and fibrosis that limits cardiac motion and results in constrictive physiology.

References

1. Permanyer-Miralda, G., Sagrista-Sauleda, J., and Soler-Soler, J.: Primary acute pericardial disease: A prospective series of 231 consecutive patients. Am. J. Cardiol. 56:623, 1985.
2. Guindo, J., Rodriguez de la Serna, A., Ramio, J., et al.: Recurrent pericarditis. Relief with colchicine. Circulation 82:1117, 1990.
3. Levine, M.J., Lorell, B.H., Diver, D.J., and Come, P.C.: Implications of echocardiographically-assisted diagnosis of pericardial tamponade in contemporary medical patients: Detection prior to hemodynamic embarrassment. J. Am. Coll. Cardiol. 17:59, 1991.
4. Ziskind, A.A., Pearce, A.C., Lemmon, C.C., et al.: Percutaneous balloon pericardiotomy for the treatment of cardiac tamponade and large pericardial effusions: Descriptions of technique and report of the first 50 cases. J. Am. Coll. Cardiol. 21:1, 1993.
5. Oh, J.K., Hatle, L.K., Seward, J.B., et al.: Diagnostic role of Doppler echocardiography in constrictive pericarditis. J. Am. Coll. Cardiol. 23:154, 1994.
6. Lorell, B.H.: Pericardial diseases. In Braunwald, E. (ed.): Heart Disease. 5th ed. Philadelphia, W.B. Saunders, 1997, p. 1478.
7. Sagrista-Sauleda, J., Permanyer-Miralda, G., and Soler-Soler, J.: Tuberculous pericarditis. Ten-year experience with a prospective protocol for diagnosis and treatment. J. Am. Coll. Cardiol. 11:724, 1988.
8. Fennell, W.M.P.: Surgical treatment of constrictive tuberculous pericarditis. S. Afr. Med. J. 62:353, 1982.
9. Sagrista-Sauleda, J., Barrabes, J.A., Permanyer-Miralda, G., and Soler-Soler, J.: Purulent pericarditis: Review of a 20-year experience in a general hospital. J. Am. Coll. Cardiol. 22:1661, 1993.
10. Rubin, R.H., and Moellering, R.C., Jr.: Clinical, microbiologic, and therapeutic aspects of purulent pericarditis. Am. J. Med. 59:68, 1975.
11. Niederhauser, U., Vogt, M., von Segesser, L.K., et al.: Pericardiectomy and acute infectious pericarditis. Schweiz. Med. Wochenschr. 122:158, 1992.
12. Wheat, L.J., Stein, L., Corya, B.C., et al.: Pericarditis as a manifestation of histoplasmosis during two large urban outbreaks. Medicine 62:111, 1983.
13. Amundson, D.E.: Perplexing pericarditis caused by coccidioidomycosis. South Med. J. 86:694, 1993.
14. Oliva, P.B., Hammill, S.C., and Talano, J.V.: Effect of definition on incidence of postinfarction pericarditis. Is it time to redefine postinfarction pericarditis? Circulation 90:1537, 1994.
15. Rutsky, E.A., and Rostand, S.G.: Treatment of uremic pericarditis and pericardial effusion. Am J. Kidney Dis. 10:2, 1987.
16. Buck, M., Ingle, J.N., Giuliani, E.R., et al.: Pericardial effusion in women with breast cancer. Cancer 60:263, 1987.
17. Cameron, J., Oesterle, S.N., Baldwin, J.C., and Hancock, E.W.: The etiologic spectrum of constrictive pericarditis. Am. Heart J. 113:354, 1987.
18. Ansari, A., Larson, P.H., and Bates, H.D.: Cardiovascular manifestations of systemic lupus erythematosus: Current perspective. Prog. Cardiovasc. Dis. 27:421, 1985.
19. Langley, R.L., and Treadwell, E. L.: Cardiac tamponade and pericardial disorders in connective tissue diseases: Case report and literature review. J. Natl. Med. Assoc. 86:149, 1994.
20. Alarcon-Segovia, D.: Drug-induced lupus syndromes. Mayo Clin. Proc. 44:664, 1969.

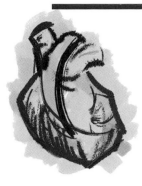

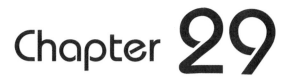

Chapter 29

Recognition and Management of Patients with

Lipoprotein Disorders

Ernst J. Schaefer

A primary contributing factor to coronary heart disease (CHD) is an elevated blood cholesterol level due to an increased level of low-density lipoprotein (LDL) cholesterol.[1] About 50% of all U.S. adults (95 million people) have cholesterol levels over 200 mg/dl, and approximately 60 million are candidates for medical advice and intervention, according to current consensus recommendations.[1]

PLASMA LIPOPROTEINS

Cholesterol and triglycerides, which are insoluble in water, are transported in blood within lipoproteins. Lipoproteins are generally spherical particles, with a surface layer composed of phospholipids with fatty acids (two fatty acids per phospholipid molecule) oriented toward the center of the particle and the polar head groups of the phospholipid on the surface of the particle (Figs. 29–1 through 29–9). Embedded within this surface phospholipid layer are molecules of proteins known as *apolipoproteins* and *free cholesterol*. Serum lipoproteins are classified on the basis of their density, electrophoretic mobility, and relative lipid and protein content.

Chylomicrons

Chylomicrons, secreted by the intestine, are large triglyceride-rich lipoproteins with more than 90% triglyceride (by weight) and 1% protein (step 1, Fig. 29–10). The protein constituents of newly formed or nascent chylomicrons include apolipoprotein (apo) B-48, apoA-I, and apoA-IV. These particles are usually not present in the serum of fasting subjects. Elevated chylomicrons in the fasting state cause markedly elevated serum triglycerides (> 1000 mg/dl or 11.3 mmol/L) and are associated with an increased risk of pancreatitis. Chylomicrons are metabolized in the blood stream by the action of lipoprotein lipase and hepatic lipase, which removes much of their triglyceride and phospholipid. During this process, chylomicrons pick up cholesterol ester and apoE from other lipoproteins and lose triglyceride and phospholipid, as well as apoA-I, apoA-IV, and the C apolipoproteins. Chylomicrons then become cholesterol ester–enriched chylomicron remnants that contain apoB-48 and apoE and are considered to be atherogenic particles.

Chylomicron remnants are taken up by the liver by specific remnant receptors (step 5, Fig. 29–10). The binding protein or ligand for this receptor is apoE. This protein may be present in plasma in three forms: apoE-3, apoE-4, and apoE-2. About 60% of the population have

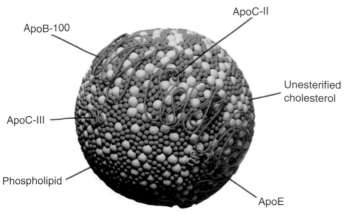

ApoB-100

ApoC-II

ApoC-III

Phospholipid

Unesterified cholesterol

ApoE

Figure 29–1

Very low density lipoprotein (VLDL). Surface view. Apo, apolipoprotein. (Redrawn from Schaefer, E.J.: Overview of the Diagnosis and Treatment of Lipid Disorders. Cambridge, MA, Copyright Genzyme Corporation, 1995, p. 4.)

the apoE-3/3 genotype, about 20% have apoE-4/3, about 15% have apoE-3/2, about 3% have apoE-4/4, about 1% have apoE-4/2, and about 1% have apoE-2/2.[2] ApoE-2-containing lipoprotein remnants are taken up more slowly by the liver than those containing apoE-3, which are taken up more slowly than those containing apoE-4. Therefore, having the apoE-2 allele, especially as apoE-2/2, results in increased levels of chylomicron and very low density lipoprotein (VLDL) remnants, upregulation of the liver LDL receptor, and decreased LDL cholesterol. Having the apoE-4 allele results in enhanced remnant uptake levels, downregulation of the liver LDL receptor, and higher LDL cholesterol levels. An elevated level of chylomicron remnants is thought to be a CHD risk factor.

Very Low Density Lipoproteins

VLDL (see Figs. 29–1 through 29–3) is synthesized in the liver and is the major vehicle for plasma triglyceride transport in the fasting state (step 2, Fig. 29–10). VLDLs are triglyceride-rich and have pre-beta mobility on lipoprotein electrophoresis. They contain about 10% of total plasma cholesterol and are precursors for LDL. The protein constituents of VLDL are apoB-100 and apoE.

They pick up the C apolipoproteins in plasma. Like chylomicrons, VLDLs are metabolized by the action of lipoprotein lipase and hepatic lipase (step 6, Fig. 29–10). During this process, much of the triglyceride and phospholipid is removed, and cholesterol ester is picked up from other lipoproteins by the action of cholesterol ester transfer protein (CETP). VLDL remnants are then formed and may be taken up by the liver by the same mechanism as chylomicron remnants (step 7, Fig. 29–10), or VLDL can be converted to form LDL by further lipolysis (step 6, Fig. 29–10). An elevated level of VLDL remnants is a probable CHD risk factor.

Low-Density Lipoproteins

LDL is the cholesterol-enriched, triglyceride-depleted product of VLDL catabolism (step 6, Fig. 29–10). LDL has beta mobility on lipoprotein electrophoresis. LDL contains and transports about 60% of total plasma cholesterol and functions to deliver cholesterol to peripheral tissues in the body, where it is used for the synthesis of cell membranes and steroid hormones. ApoB-100 is the major protein constituent of LDL. An LDL receptor that recognizes apoB-100 and apoE, but not apoB-48, allows the liver and other tissues to catabolize LDL (step 8, Fig.

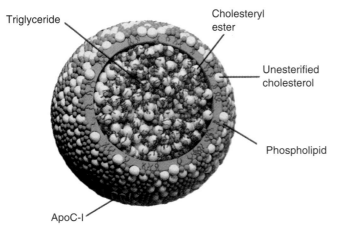

Triglyceride

Cholesteryl ester

Unesterified cholesterol

Phospholipid

ApoC-I

Figure 29–2

VLDL. Core view. Apo, apolipoprotein. (Redrawn from Schaefer, E.J.: Overview of the Diagnosis and Treatment of Lipid Disorders. Cambridge, MA, Copyright Genzyme Corporation, 1995, p. 4.)

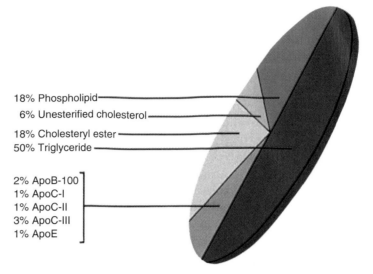

Figure 29–3

VLDL. Apo, apolipoprotein. (Redrawn from Schaefer, E.J.: Overview of the Diagnosis and Treatment of Lipid Disorders. Cambridge, MA, Copyright Genzyme Corporation, 1995, p. 4.)

18% Phospholipid
6% Unesterified cholesterol
18% Cholesteryl ester
50% Triglyceride

2% ApoB-100
1% ApoC-I
1% ApoC-II
3% ApoC-III
1% ApoE

29–10). Modified or oxidized LDL can also be taken up by a scavenger receptor on macrophages in various tissues including within the arterial wall (step 10, Fig. 29–10).

When there is an excess level of LDL in the blood, it is deposited in the blood vessel walls and becomes a major component of atherosclerotic plaque lesions. Increased LDL cholesterol levels in plasma are a cause of coronary atherosclerosis and produce an increased risk of CHD. Plasma LDL cholesterol levels are increased by diets high in saturated fat and cholesterol, mainly owing to decreased LDL receptor–mediated catabolism.[1] According to the recommendations of the National Cholesterol Education Program's (NCEP) Adult Treatment Panel (ATP), LDL cholesterol levels should be used as the basis for initiating and monitoring treatment of patients with elevated blood cholesterol.[1]

Lipoprotein(a)

Lipoprotein(a) (Lp[a]) is an LDL-like particle with an additional apolipoprotein known as apo(a) attached to it. Lp(a) may be deposited in the artery wall like LDL and may interfere with clot lysis because of its structural similarity to plasminogen. Elevated Lp(a) levels (>30 mg/dl for total particle) have been associated with premature CHD and stroke in most studies.[3] Lp(a) can be reduced with niacin or estrogen replacement therapy.

High-Density Lipoproteins

High-density lipoprotein (HDL) is synthesized in the liver and intestine (step 3, Fig. 29–10) and is responsible for transporting about 30% of the total plasma cholesterol. HDL is rich in protein and phospholipid, has a density of 1.063 to 1.21 gm/ml in plasma, and has mainly alpha mobility on lipoprotein electrophoresis. HDL acts as a vehicle for reverse cholesterol transport from tissue to the liver (proposed cardioprotective mechanism). Levels of HDL cholesterol are inversely correlated with the risk for CHD, and HDL is commonly referred to as "good" cholesterol. ApoA-I and apoA-II are the major proteins of HDL and are present in a 3:1 molar ratio. ApoA-I, but not apoA-II, is thought to be crucial for reverse cholesterol transport.

HDL picks up lipids (phospholipids, triglyceride) and proteins (A-I, E, and C apolipoproteins) from triglyceride-rich lipoproteins (chylomicrons and VLDL) as these particles undergo lipolysis. When HDL picks up free cholesterol from peripheral tissues (step 9, Fig. 29–10), the

Figure 29–4

Low-density lipoprotein (LDL). Surface view. Apo, apolipoprotein. (Redrawn from Schaefer, E.J.: Overview of the Diagnosis and Treatment of Lipid Disorders. Cambridge, MA, Copyright Genzyme Corporation, 1995, p. 6.)

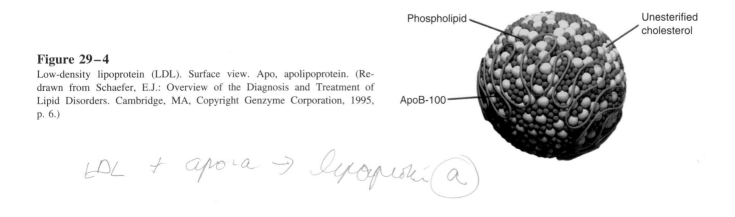

Phospholipid

Unesterified cholesterol

ApoB-100

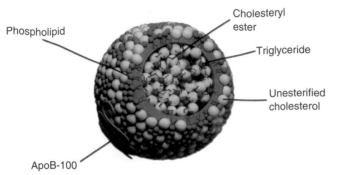

Figure 29–5

LDL. Core view. Apo, apolipoprotein. (Redrawn from Schaefer, E.J.: Overview of the Diagnosis and Treatment of Lipid Disorders. Cambridge, MA, Copyright Genzyme Corporation, 1995, p. 6.)

cholesterol is esterified by the enzyme lecithin cholesterol acyltransferase (LCAT), which transfers a fatty acid from lecithin, the major phospholipid in plasma, to cholesterol to form cholesterol ester; the cholesterol is either delivered to the liver (step 12, Fig. 29–10) or transferred to other lipoproteins (such as chylomicron or VLDL remnants), which are also taken up by the liver. Very small HDLs, which have pre-beta mobility, become somewhat larger (alpha HDL or HDL3) when they pick up cholesterol and esterify it. When this cholesterol ester is transferred to chylomicron and VLDL remnants, HDL picks up phospholipid and some triglyceride and becomes even larger (alpha HDL or HDL2). HDL2 is converted back to HDL3 by the action of hepatic lipase. There also appear to be specific HDL receptors that allow HDL to mobilize free cholesterol from tissues. HDL appears to be a major source of liver cholesterol.

RATIONALE FOR TREATMENT OF LIPID DISORDERS

Epidemiologic Evidence

A large body of epidemiologic evidence supports a direct relationship between the level of serum total and LDL cholesterol and CHD risk. This association is continuous throughout the range of cholesterol levels in the population and is curvilinear (Fig. 29–11).[1,4] The data indicate that the greatest benefit in risk reduction would be obtained in those patients with the highest cholesterol values. According to results from the third National Health and Nutrition Examination Survey (NHANES), the average LDL cholesterol level of U.S. adults is about 130 mg/dl.[1] At higher levels of total and LDL cholesterol, the direct relationship between CHD risk and cholesterol levels becomes particularly strong. For persons with cholesterol values in the top 10% of the population distribution (Fig. 29–11), the risk of CHD mortality is four times as high as the risk in the bottom 10% of the population.[1,5]

Serum LDL cholesterol levels are increased by diets high in saturated fat and cholesterol mainly because of decreased LDL receptor–mediated catabolism. Human populations on high–saturated fat/high-cholesterol diets have elevated LDL cholesterol levels and a significantly increased rate of CHD due to atherosclerosis compared with populations on low–saturated fat/low-cholesterol diets.[1] Decreased HDL cholesterol levels are also an independent risk factor for premature CHD[1,4] (Fig. 29–12). Women have higher HDL cholesterol levels than men owing to increased production of HDL constituents and, hence, a lower age-adjusted risk of CHD.

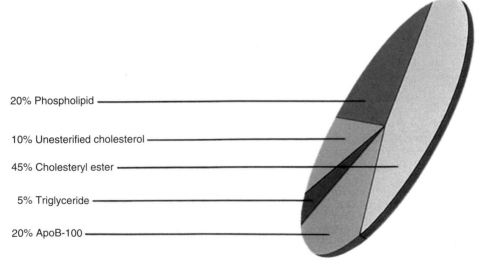

20% Phospholipid

10% Unesterified cholesterol

45% Cholesteryl ester

5% Triglyceride

20% ApoB-100

Figure 29–6

LDL. Apo, apolipoprotein. (Redrawn from Schaefer, E.J.: Overview of the Diagnosis and Treatment of Lipid Disorders. Cambridge, MA, Copyright Genzyme Corporation, 1995, p. 6.)

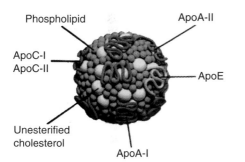

Figure 29-7

High-density lipoprotein (HDL). Surface view. Apo, apolipoprotein. (Redrawn from Schaefer, E.J.: Overview of the Diagnosis and Treatment of Lipid Disorders. Cambridge, MA, Copyright Genzyme Corporation, 1995, p. 8.)

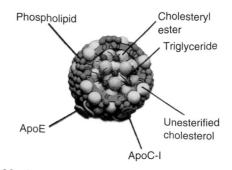

Figure 29-8

HDL. Core view. Apo, apolipoprotein. (Redrawn from Schaefer, E.J.: Overview of the Diagnosis and Treatment of Lipid Disorders. Cambridge, MA, Copyright Genzyme Corporation, 1995, p. 8.)

Genetic and Physiologic Evidence

Premature CHD can result from high LDL cholesterol levels even in the absence of other risk factors. This is most clearly demonstrated in children with the rare homozygous familial hypercholesterolemia, characterized by the absence of normal specific cell-surface receptors that remove LDL cholesterol from the circulatory system. LDL cholesterol levels can be as high as 1000 mg/dl (26 mmol/L), and severe atherosclerosis and CHD often develop before age 20 years. Patients with the more common heterozygous form of familial hypercholesterolemia and partial deficiencies of LDL-receptor function generally develop premature CHD in the middle decades of life.

Clinical Trial Evidence

Prospective studies indicate that diet treatment or diet and drug therapy that lowers LDL cholesterol can reduce subsequent CHD morbidity and mortality.[6-32] Studies in-

dicate a benefit in CHD risk reduction from both lowering LDL cholesterol and increasing HDL cholesterol. Moreover, aggressive lipid modification can result in stabilization of existing coronary atherosclerosis as well as some regression of this process.[18-28] The Coronary Primary Prevention Trial, which compared the cholesterol-lowering drug cholestyramine with a placebo, produced statistically significant reductions in LDL cholesterol levels and in the incidence of CHD.[13-15] Large prospective primary and secondary intervention studies using 3-hydroxy-3-methylglutaryl coenzyme A (HMG CoA) reductase inhibitors—specifically simvastatin and pravastatin in the Scandinavian Simvastatin Survival Study (4S),[29] the West of Scotland Study (WOSCOPS),[31] and the Cholesterol and Recurrent Events Trial (CARE)[32]—have documented significant reductions in total mortality, CHD mortality, CHD morbidity, need for coronary artery bypass surgery and angioplasty, and hospitalizations for CHD (Figs. 29-13 and 29-14).

The greatest benefit has been observed in patients with established CHD and hypercholesterolemia, in reduction not only in CHD risk but also in stroke risk.[28, 29] No benefit was noted in CHD patients with baseline LDL

Figure 29-9

HDL. Apo, apolipoprotein. (Redrawn from Schaefer, E.J.: Overview of the Diagnosis and Treatment of Lipid Disorders. Cambridge, MA, Copyright Genzyme Corporation, 1995, p. 8.)

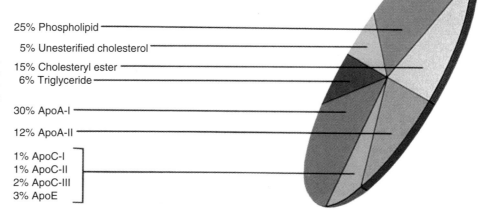

25% Phospholipid
5% Unesterified cholesterol
15% Cholesteryl ester
6% Triglyceride
30% ApoA-I
12% ApoA-II
1% ApoC-I
1% ApoC-II
2% ApoC-III
3% ApoE

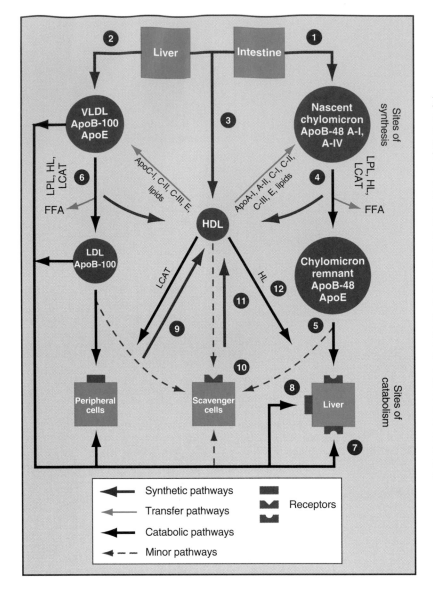

Figure 29–10

A conceptual overview of lipoprotein metabolism. Fats absorbed in the intestine are packaged into large, triglyceride-rich particles known as *chylomicrons* (step 1). These lipoproteins undergo lipolysis (removal of triglyceride) to form chylomicron remnants (step 4), which are taken up by the liver via an apoliprotein (Apo) E receptor (step 5). The liver can also secrete triglyceride-rich lipoproteins known as *very low density lipoproteins* (VLDLs) (step 2). After lipolysis, these particles can be converted to *low-density lipoproteins* (LDLs) (step 6) or taken up by the liver via an apoE receptor (step 7). The LDL formed is catabolized mainly by the liver (step 8) or other tissues via an LDL receptor that recognizes both ApoB-100 and apoE but not ApoB-48. If LDL is modified or oxidized, it can also be taken up by a scavenger receptor on macrophages or by scavenger cells (step 10). *High-density lipoprotein* (HDL) is synthesized by both the liver and the intestine (step 3). HDL picks up lipid and protein constituents from chylomicrons and VLDL as these particles undergo lipolysis (steps 4 and 6). HDL picks up free cholesterol from peripheral tissues (step 9) and macrophages (step 11) and is catabolized mainly in the liver (step 12). LPL, lipoprotein lipase; HL, hepatic lipase; LCAT, lecithin:cholesterol acyltransferase; FFA, free fatty acid. (Redrawn from Schaefer, E.J.: Overview of the Diagnosis and Treatment of Lipid Disorders. Cambridge, MA, Copyright Genzyme Corporation, 1995, p. 9.)

cholesterol values lower than 125 mg/dl in the CARE trial.[32] The efficacy, tolerability, and significant benefit noted in large placebo-controlled randomized and blinded clinical trials with HMG CoA reductase inhibitors now make these agents the drugs of choice for cholesterol lowering in asymptomatic subjects as well as those with CHD.

The combined findings of these studies support the concept that lowering total and LDL cholesterol levels will reduce the incidence of CHD events and the death rate owing to myocardial infarction.[1] Moreover, the pooled analysis of clinical trial findings suggests that intervention is as effective in preventing recurrent myocardial infarction and mortality in patients who have already had a coronary event as it is in primary prevention. The complete set of evidence strongly supports the concept that reducing elevated total and LDL cholesterol levels will reduce CHD risk in men and women, and in asymptomatic subjects, as well as in those with established CHD.[1]

It is important to recognize the magnitude of CHD reduction associated with lowering serum cholesterol levels. For individuals with serum cholesterol initially in the 250 to 300 mg/dl (6.5 to 7.8 mmol/L) range, each 1% reduction in serum cholesterol level yields approximately a 2% reduction in CHD rates.[5] Thus, it is reasonable to estimate that a 30% reduction in serum cholesterol level would reduce CHD risk by as much as 60% in this group. More modest reduction in risk could be expected in those with lower values.

APPROACH TO EVALUATION AND TREATMENT

The NCEP Guidelines— Primary Prevention

Total Cholesterol and HDL Cholesterol

The classification system of the NCEP guidelines for individuals without known CHD begins with the measure-

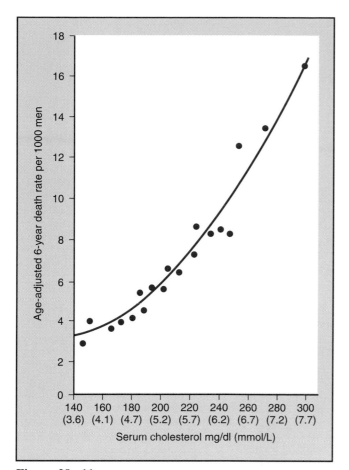

Figure 29–11

Relationship of serum cholesterol to coronary heart disease death in 356,222 men aged 35 to 57 years during an average follow-up of 6 years. Each point represents the median value for 5% of the population. Key points: (1) The risk increases steadily, particularly above 200 mg/dl (5.2 mmol/L); and (2) the magnitude of the increased risk is large—fourfold in the top 10% as compared with the bottom 10%. (Data from Stamler J, Wentworth D, Neaton JD: Is the relationship between serum cholesterol and risk of premature death from coronary heart disease continuous and graded? Findings in 356,222 primary screenees of the Multiple Risk Factor Intervention Trial [MRFIT]. JAMA 256:2823–2828, 1986; redrawn from Schaefer, E.J.: Overview of the Diagnosis and Treatment of Lipid Disorders. Cambridge, MA, Copyright Genzyme Corporation, 1995, p. 11.)

Approximately 25% of the entire adult population (more than 40 million people) in the United States (20 years of age and above) falls into the high-risk blood cholesterol classification, whereas another 54 million people have borderline-high blood cholesterol levels of 200 mg/dl or above.[1] About 20% of males and 5% of females have low HDL cholesterol levels.[4]

All patients who are screened should receive information about a step I diet (Table 29–1) and CHD risk factors (Table 29–2). According to the NCEP ATP guidelines, patients who have desirable total cholesterol and normal HDL cholesterol values should have their values checked again within 5 years. If the patient has a borderline-high value, information about other CHD risk factors should be obtained (Table 29–2).[1]

If the patient has a cholesterol value in the borderline risk category (200 to 239 mg/dl) and a normal HDL cholesterol level 35 mg/dl or higher in the absence of CHD (prior myocardial infarction, angina) or two or more CHD risk factors, dietary intervention (see later) should be advised and the cholesterol value checked within the next year.

However, if the patient has a borderline-high value (200 to 239 mg/dl) with a history of CHD or two or more CHD risk factors, or has a high-risk total cholesterol value (≥240 mg/dl) or a low HDL cholesterol value (<35 mg/dl), LDL cholesterol levels need to be assessed so an appropriate treatment regimen can be determined (Table 29–3).[1]

Another issue is whether apoA-I, apoB, LDL size, or Lp(a), should be measured for CHD risk assessment. None of these parameters has been shown to be an inde-

ment of total cholesterol and HDL cholesterol levels as a screen for the general population in the fasting or nonfasting state (Fig. 29–15). Accurate fingerstick methodology is available for both cholesterol and HDL cholesterol for screening purposes in the office setting. More recently, an accurate home cholesterol test that can be self-administered has become available.[33] Total cholesterol levels below 200 mg/dl (5.2 mmol/L) have been classified as "desirable," those between 200 and 239 mg/dl (5.2 to 6.2 mmol/L) have been classified as "borderline-high," and those of 240 mg/dl (≥6.2 mmol/L) or higher as "high risk." Levels of HDL cholesterol below 35 mg/dl (0.9 mmol/L) have been classified as "low," whereas those of 60 mg/dl (≥1.55 mmol/L) or higher have been classified as "high" and protective for CHD.

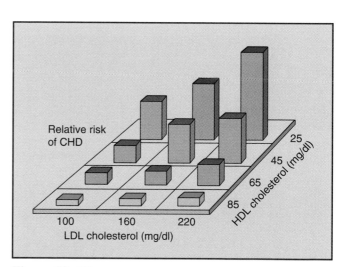

Figure 29–12

The Framingham Heart Study: Risk of coronary heart disease (CHD) by high-density lipoprotein (HDL) and low-density lipoprotein (LDL) cholesterol. Epidemiologic studies have definitely established that total and LDL cholesterol concentrations are directly correlated with clinical coronary atherosclerosis. The inverse association of HDL cholesterol concentrations with CHD endpoints have also been established in both cross-sectional and prospective epidemiologic studies. (Redrawn from Brown, W.V.: Atherosclerosis: Risk factors and treatment. In Braunwald, E. [ed.-in-chief]: Essential Atlas of Heart Diseases. Philadelphia, Current Medicine, 1997, p. 1.13.)

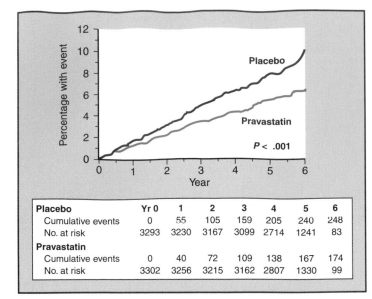

Placebo	Yr 0	1	2	3	4	5	6
Cumulative events	0	55	105	159	205	240	248
No. at risk	3293	3230	3167	3099	2714	1241	83
Pravastatin							
Cumulative events	0	40	72	109	138	167	174
No. at risk	3302	3256	3215	3162	2807	1330	99

Figure 29–13

Kaplan-Meier analysis of the time to a definite nonfatal myocardial infarction or death from coronary heart disease, according to treatment group. (Redrawn from Shepherd, J., Cobbe, S.M., Ford, I., et al.: Prevention of coronary heart disease with pravastatin in men with hypercholesterolemia. N. Engl. J. Med. 333:1301–1307. Copyright 1995 Massachusetts Medical Society. All rights reserved.)

pendent risk factor after smoking, blood pressure, diabetes, LDL cholesterol, and HDL cholesterol have been taken into account in prospective studies, except probably Lp(a).[3] Currently, some recommend that Lp(a) or Lp(a) cholesterol be measured as part of CHD risk assessment, but there is no consensus on this issue.

LDL Cholesterol

The NCEP ATP has developed guidelines for the diagnosis and treatment of individuals over age 20 years without a history of CHD but with elevated blood cholesterol levels associated with an increase in LDL cholesterol levels (Fig. 29–16).[2–4] Levels of LDL cholesterol requiring the initiation of diet and drug therapy, as well as the goals of therapy, are dependent on the presence or absence of two or more CHD risk factors (see Table 29–2). The presence of secondary causes of elevated LDL cholesterol levels (≥ 160 mg/dl or 4.1 mmol/L) must be ruled out (Table 29–4).

For patients without CHD, the cost-effectiveness of medications for cholesterol reduction varies widely depending on the patient's age and other risk factors (Figs. 29–17 and 29–18). Treatment with medications should

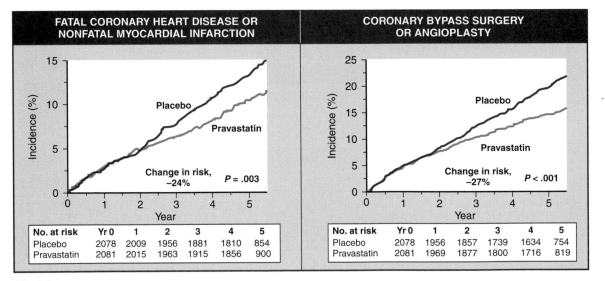

No. at risk	Yr 0	1	2	3	4	5
Placebo	2078	2009	1956	1881	1810	854
Pravastatin	2081	2015	1963	1915	1856	900

No. at risk	Yr 0	1	2	3	4	5
Placebo	2078	1956	1857	1739	1634	754
Pravastatin	2081	1969	1877	1800	1716	819

Figure 29–14

Kaplan-Meier estimates of the incidence of coronary events in the pravastatin and placebo groups. The *left-hand panel* shows data for the primary endpoint—fatal coronary heart disease or nonfatal myocardial infarction. The *right-hand panel* shows data for coronary bypass surgery or angioplasty. Changes in risk are those attributable to pravastatin. *P* values and changes in risk are based on Cox proportional-hazards analysis. (Redrawn from Sacks, F.M., Pfeffer, M.A., Moye, L.A., et al., for the Cholesterol and Recurrent Events Trial Investigators: The effect of pravastatin on coronary events after myocardial infarction in patients with average cholesterol levels. N. Engl. J. Med. 335:1001–1009. Copyright 1996 Massachusetts Medical Society. All rights reserved.)

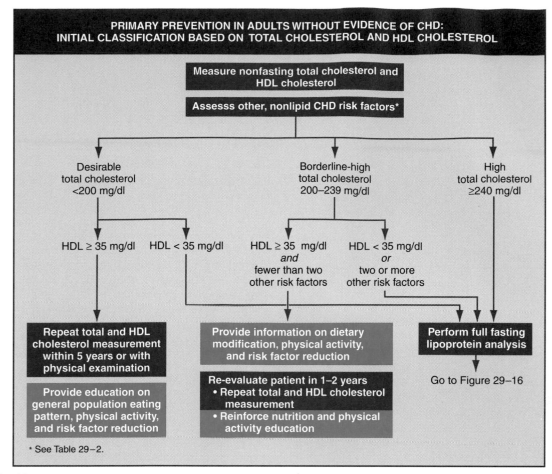

Figure 29–15

Primary prevention classification by total cholesterol. In patients without coronary heart disease (CHD), initial assessment for dyslipidemia is by total cholesterol and high-density lipoprotein (HDL) cholesterol levels (minimal approach). The physician may choose the full fasting lipoprotein analysis as the first assessment. (Redrawn from Farmer, J.A., and Gotto, A.M., Jr.: Dyslipidemia and other risk factors for coronary artery disease. *In* Braunwald, E. [ed.]: Heart Disease. 5th ed. Philadelphia, W.B. Saunders, 1997, pp. 1126–1160; from Expert Panel on Detection, Evaluation, and Treatment of High Blood Cholesterol in Adults: Summary of the second report of the National Cholesterol Education Program [NCEP] Expert Panel on Detection, Evaluation, and Treatment of High Blood Cholesterol in Adults [Adult Treatment Panel II]. JAMA 269:3015, 1993; and National Cholesterol Education Program: Second report of the Expert Panel on Detection, Evaluation, and Treatment of High Blood Cholesterol in Adults [Adult Treatment Panel II]. Circulation 89:1329, 1994.)

Table 29–1   **Dietary Therapy of High Blood Cholesterol**

Nutrient*	Recommended Intake		
	Step I Diet		*Step II Diet*
Total fat		30% or less of total calories	
Saturated fatty acids	8–10% of total calories		Less than 7% of total calories
Polyunsaturated fatty acids		Up to 10% of total calories	
Monounsaturated fatty acids		Up to 15% of total calories	
Carbohydrates		55% or more of total calories	
Protein		Approximately 15% of total calories	
Cholesterol	Less than 300 mg/day		Less than 200 mg/day
Total calories		To achieve and maintain desirable weight	

From Schaefer, E.J.: Overview of the Diagnosis and Treatment of Lipid Disorders. Cambridge, MA, Copyright Genzyme Corporation, 1995, p. 27.

* Calories from alcohol not included; approximately 50% of saturated fat and 70% of cholesterol in the U.S. diet comes from the following foods: hamburgers, cheeseburgers, meat loaf, whole milk, cheese, beef steaks, roasts, hot dogs, ham, lunch meat, cake, and eggs.

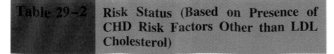

Table 29–2 Risk Status (Based on Presence of CHD Risk Factors Other than LDL Cholesterol)

Positive Risk Factors

Age
  Male: ≥45 yr
  Female: ≥55 yr or premature menopause without estrogen
           replacement therapy
Family history of premature CHD (definite myocardial infarction or
  sudden death before 55 yr of age in father or other male first-degree
  relative, or before 65 yr of age in mother or other female first-degree
  relative)
Current cigarette smoking
Hypertension (≥140/90 mmHg,* or on antihypertensive medication)
Low HDL cholesterol (<35 mg/dl* or 0.9 mmol/L)
Diabetes mellitus

Negative Risk Factor†

High HDL cholesterol (≥60 mg/dl or 1.6 mmol/L)

From Schaefer, E.J.: Overview of the Diagnosis and Treatment of Lipid Disorders. Cambridge, MA, Copyright Genzyme Corporation, 1995, p. 14.
  Abbreviations: CHD, coronary heart disease; LDL, low-density lipoprotein; HDL, high-density lipoprotein.
  * Confirmed by measurement on several occasions.
  † If the HDL cholesterol level is ≥60 mg/dl, subtract one risk factor (because high HDL cholesterol levels decrease CHD risk).

be targeted to individuals based not only on their LDL or total cholesterol level but also on their overall risk factor profile.[34, 35]

Current NCEP guidelines do not recommend specific treatment of elevated triglycerides to reduce coronary risk. Markedly elevated triglyceride levels (>1000 mg/dl in fasting state), however, warrant treatment to prevent episodes of pancreatitis.

The NCEP Guidelines— Secondary Prevention

Because of the high risk of recurrent CHD events or progressive CHD in patients with known CHD, the guidelines for initiating treatment suggest a lower threshold for secondary prevention than for primary prevention (Fig. 29–19). Data currently document the benefit of cholesterol reduction for secondary prevention for LDL levels above 125 mg/dl;[32] the NCEP guidelines are based on the logical but unproven assumption that further reduction to below 100 mg/dl will be beneficial.

For secondary prevention, cholesterol reduction with medications is not only effective but also worth the cost in nearly all situations (Figs. 29–20 and 29–21). In some

Table 29–3 LDL Cholesterol (mg/dl) for Persons 20 Years of age and Older by Race/Ethnicity, Sex, and Age: United States, 1988–1991 (NHANES III)

Race/Ethnicity, Sex, and Age	Number of Examined Persons	Mean	Selected Percentile								
			5th	10th	15th	25th	50th	75th	85th	90th	95th
Men											
20 yr and older	1669	131	75	87	95	106	129	154	167	179	194
20–34 yr	487	120	67	78	86	97	121	139	152	165	186
35–44 yr	274	134	85	92	98	111	131	156	166	176	192
45–54 yr	224	138	78	91	100	118	136	163	174	187	195
55–64 yr	228	142	78	90	104	117	143	165	175	194	205
65–74 yr	259	141	93	104	109	119	134	163	177	185	199
75 yr and older	197	132	83	88	93	106	130	154	170	186	196
Women											
20 yr and older	1673	126	69	81	88	99	122	150	165	175	191
20–34 yr	525	110	59	70	75	88	108	129	142	155	173
35–44 yr	316	117	67	85	88	97	116	138	146	155	165
45–54 yr	214	132	70	87	93	107	130	157	173	182	198
55–64 yr	213	145	79	90	101	122	145	170	184	189	209
65–74 yr	202	147	92	97	109	119	148	169	185	192	206
75 yr and older	203	147	90	102	109	121	143	168	189	197	209
Mexican Americans											
Men	448	124	70	77	85	96	120	148	161	172	188
Women	471	122	67	80	86	95	118	144	158	166	189
Non-Hispanic Black											
Men	393	126	69	76	82	96	123	146	168	186	206
Women	422	126	67	76	86	100	124	147	162	174	192
Non-Hispanic White											
Men	773	132	76	88	97	108	129	154	168	179	194
Women	729	126	69	82	89	99	122	151	166	176	192

From Schaefer, E.J.: Overview of the Diagnosis and Treatment of Lipid Disorders. Cambridge, MA, Copyright Genzyme Corporation, 1995, p. 19.
Abbreviations: LDL, low-density lipoprotein; NHANES, National Health and Nutrition Examination Survey.

patients, medications may actually save more in health care expenses than they cost.[34, 35, 35a]

NCEP Recommendations Summary

LDL cholesterol decision points for initiating diet and drug therapy and the goals of therapy are given in Table 29–5. The guidelines for secondary prevention are also strongly supported by a variety of cost analyses. For primary prevention, however, cost-effectiveness calculations suggest caution in the widespread use of expensive medications in patients who do not have risk factors other than an isolated mild to moderate elevation of LDL cholesterol.

Table 29–4	Secondary Causes	
Increased LDL Cholesterol	**Increased Triglyceride**	**Decreased HDL Cholesterol**
Hypothyroidism	Obesity	Hypertriglyceridemia
Diabetes mellitus	Diabetes mellitus	Obesity
Obesity	Lack of exercise	Diabetes mellitus
Nephrotic syndrome	Alcohol intake	Cigarette smoking
Obstructive liver disease	Renal insufficiency	Lack of exercise
Progestins	Estrogens	Beta blockers
Anabolic steroids	Beta blockers	Progestins
		Anabolic steroids

From Schaefer, E.J.: Overview of the Diagnosis and Treatment of Lipid Disorders. Cambridge, MA, Copyright Genzyme Corporation, 1995, p. 17.
Abbreviations: LDL, low-density lipoprotein; HDL, high-density lipoprotein.

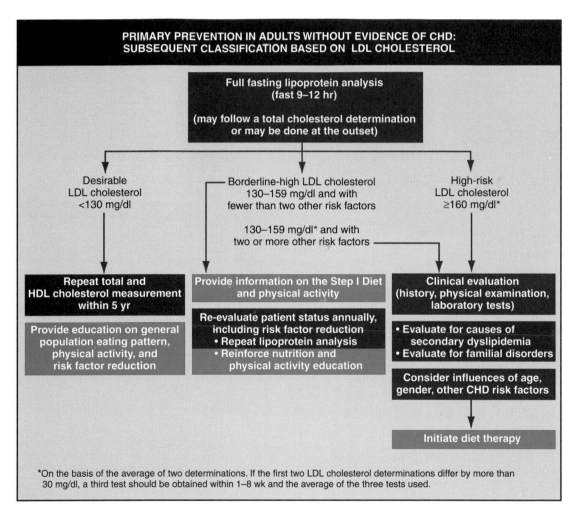

Figure 29–16

Primary prevention classification by low-density lipoprotein (LDL) cholesterol. In patients without coronary heart disease (CHD) or other atherosclerotic disease who have low high-density lipoprotein (HDL) cholesterol, borderline-high total cholesterol in the presence of two or more other risk factors, or high total cholesterol, full fasting lipoprotein analysis is required to determine LDL cholesterol level. (Redrawn from Farmer, J.A., and Gotto, A.M., Jr.: Dyslipidemia and other risk factors for coronary artery disease. *In* Braunwald, E. [ed.]: Heart Disease. 5th ed. Philadelphia, W.B. Saunders, 1997, pp. 1126–1160; from Expert Panel on Detection, Evaluation, and Treatment of High Blood Cholesterol in Adults: Summary of the second report of the National Cholesterol Education Program [NCEP] Expert Panel on Detection, Evaluation, and Treatment of High Blood Cholesterol in Adults [Adult Treatment Panel II]. JAMA 269:3015, 1993; and National Cholesterol Education Program: Second report of the Expert Panel on Detection, Evaluation, and Treatment of High Blood Cholesterol in Adults [Adult Treatment Panel II]. Circulation 89:1329, 1994.)

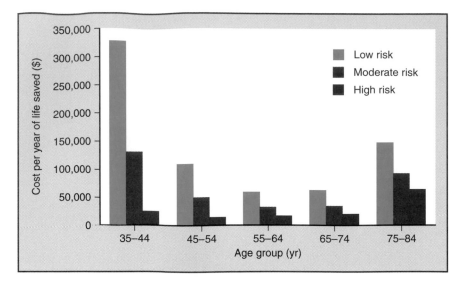

Figure 29–17

The cost-effectiveness of lovastatin (20 mg/day) for the treatment of hypercholesterolemia as primary prevention in men with a pretreatment cholesterol level exceeding 300 mg/dl, as reported by Goldman et al.[34] The ratios were derived from a computer simulation using the Coronary Heart Disease (CHD) Policy Model.[34] Estimates of CHD incidence and all-cause mortality were based on data from the Framingham Heart Study 30-year follow-up. The analysis showed that the results were sensitive to the patient's age and risk factors. Middle-age and high-risk individuals had the most favorable ratios. *High-risk patients* were defined as having a diastolic blood pressure above 105 mm Hg, being a smoker, and weighing more than 130% of ideal body weight. *Moderate-risk patients* were defined as having a diastolic blood pressure between 95 and 104 mm Hg, being a nonsmoker, and weighing 110% to 129% of ideal body weight. *Low-risk patients* were defined as having a diastolic blood pressure below 95 mm Hg, being a nonsmoker, and weighing less than 110% of ideal body weight. The authors estimated that 20 mg/day of lovastatin reduced the serum cholesterol level by 19%. The high-risk group had a cost-effectiveness ratio of less than $30,000 per year of life saved until age 75 years. The moderate-risk group had a cost-effectiveness ratio of approximately $30,000 per year of life saved from age 55 to 74 years. (Redrawn from Krumholz, H.M., and Goldman, L.: Cost-effectiveness of risk factors. *In* Brown, W.V. [vol. ed.]: Atherosclerosis: Risk Factors and Treatment. Vol. 10. Braunwald, E. [ser. ed.] Philadelphia, Current Medicine, 1996, pp. 13.1–13.12.)

LDL Cholesterol Measurement

If a patient has an LDL cholesterol level of 160 mg/dl (4.1 mmol/L), it represents approximately the 75th percentile for middle-aged Americans (see Table 29–3). It is important to confirm the presence of abnormalities by repeat determinations. Hospitalization for acute illness, including myocardial infarction, can markedly lower lipid values; therefore, lipid determinations are best carried out in stable, ambulatory persons. An elevated or borderline-high triglyceride level (≥ 200 mg/dl or ≥ 2.3 mmol/L) has not clearly been shown to be an independent risk factor for premature heart disease. However, an elevated triglyceride level is inversely associated with a low level of HDL cholesterol, which has been shown to be a significant risk factor for CHD. Common secondary causes of elevated LDL cholesterol and triglyceride values and decreased HDL cholesterol levels are shown in Table 29–3.[1] If possible, these factors should be screened for and treated before initiating diet or drug therapy for lipid disorders. Screening should include an evaluation of glucose, albumin, liver transaminases, alkaline phosphatase, creatinine, thyroid-stimulating hormone, and urinalysis, as well as asking about alcohol intake and use of beta blockers, estrogens, glucocorticoids, anabolic steroids, thiazides, and hormone preparations.

Unlike total cholesterol quantitation, currently there is no consensus-approved and -validated reference method

for the direct measurement of LDL cholesterol. Accurate measurement of LDL cholesterol first depends on the separation of LDL particles in serum from other lipoproteins, namely, chylomicrons, VLDL, and HDL.

Traditionally, LDL has been defined as all lipoproteins within the density range 1.019 to 1.063 gm/ml. However, in common practice, the definition has been broadened to include intermediate-density lipoprotein (IDL; density 1.006 to 1.019 gm/ml) or VLDL remnants (some of which are precursors of LDL) and Lp(a). Using this definition, LDL is made up of the following particles: LDL + IDL + Lp(a). This definition serves as the basis for cut-points defined by the NCEP ATP.

Currently, most clinical laboratories utilize the equation known as the Friedewald formula to estimate a patient's LDL cholesterol concentration.[36] The formula uses the following calculation: LDL cholesterol = Total cholesterol − HDL cholesterol − Triglyceride/5.

The drawbacks of using the Friedewald formula for determining levels of LDL cholesterol are (1) it is estimated by calculation; (2) it requires multiple assays and multiple steps, each adding a potential source of error, and it requires that patients fast for 12 to 14 hours before specimen collection to avoid a triglyceride bias; and (3) it is not standardized. Moreover, LDL cholesterol concentrations cannot be reported in individuals with elevated triglyceride levels (>400 mg/dl [4.5 mmol/L]).

A new, direct immunoseparation method for the measurement of serum or plasma LDL cholesterol concentra-

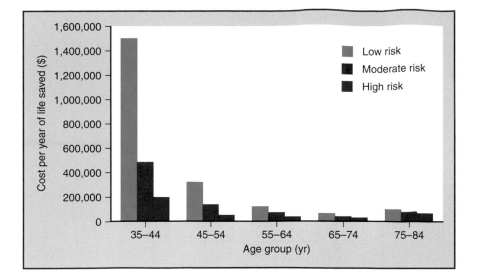

Figure 29–18

The cost-effectiveness of lovastatin (20 mg/day) for the treatment of hypercholesterolemia as primary prevention in women with a pretreatment cholesterol level exceeding 300 mg/dl. The cost-effectiveness ratios are derived from a computer simulation using the Coronary Heart Disease Policy Model.[34] Women were stratified by age and risk group. *High-risk patients* were defined as having a diastolic blood pressure above 105 mm Hg, being a smoker, and weighing more than 130% of ideal body weight. *Moderate-risk patients* were defined as having a diastolic blood pressure between 95 and 104 mm Hg, being a nonsmoker, and weighing 110% to 129% of ideal body weight. *Low-risk patients* were defined as having a diastolic blood pressure below 95 mm Hg, being a nonsmoker, and weighing less than 110% of body weight. For each age group, the cost-effectiveness ratio is most favorable for the high-risk group (i.e., lowest ratio of cost per year of life saved). In comparison with men (see Fig. 29–17), the ratios for women are less favorable at every age and for every risk level. Nevertheless, women at high risk who were between 55 and 74 years of age and those at moderate risk who were between 65 and 74 years of age had a cost-effectiveness ratio of less than $50,000 per year of life save. (Redrawn from Krumholz, H.M., and Goldman, L.: Cost-effectiveness of risk factors. *In* Brown, W.V. [vol. ed.]: Atherosclerosis: Risk Factors and Treatment. Vol. 10. Braunwald, E. [ser. ed.] Philadelphia, Current Medicine, 1996, pp. 13.1–13.12.)

tion suitable for routine use is now available.[37] This assay is especially useful for the physician who sees patients in the afternoon.

MANAGEMENT OF HYPERLIPIDEMIA

Diet Therapy

LDL cholesterol levels requiring dietary intervention are shown in Table 29–5. The cornerstone of the treatment of lipid disorders is diet therapy.[1] Approximately 50% of saturated fat and 70% of cholesterol in the U.S. diet comes from hamburgers, cheeseburgers, meat loaf, whole milk, cheese, other dairy products including ice cream, beef steaks, roasts, hot dogs, ham, lunch meat, doughnuts, cookies, cake, and eggs. These foods should be restricted. Instead, it is recommended that poultry (white meat) without skin, fish, skimmed or low-fat milk, nonfat or low-fat yogurt, and low-fat cheeses be eaten. The use of fruits, vegetables, and grains is encouraged. Oils that can be used are unsaturated vegetable oils containing polyunsaturated fat and monounsaturated fatty acids, such as canola, soybean, olive, or corn oil. However, such oils should be used only in moderation because they are rich in calories. Consumption of hydrogenated vegetable oils rich in *trans* fatty acids such as stick margarine

should be kept to a minimum as well. Soft margarine is a better alternative than stick margarine or butter. Alternatively, vegetable oil can be placed directly on bread.

Excellent patient dietary pamphlets are available from the American Heart Association. The step I diet (see Table 29–1) is recommended for the entire U.S. population. For patients with elevated LDL cholesterol, the step II diet (see Table 29–2) is recommended if lipid goals are not achieved (see Table 29–5). When pamphlets and counseling by the physician and office nurse do not achieve these goals, the patient should be referred to a registered dietitian for instruction and reinforcement of the step II diet. In most cases, diet therapy, a regular exercise program, and control of other risk factors should be tried for at least 6 months before initiating drug therapy. Dietary fat restriction to approximately 20% of calories, along with exercise, appears to be very important to prevent the age-related weight gain and obesity that so often are associated with dyslipidemia, hypertension, and diabetes in our society. Treatment with dietary fiber supplements can further reduce cholesterol levels in patients who are already on a low-fat diet (Table 29–6). Thirty minutes per day of exercise is also strongly recommended, using both aerobic and strength-building exercises.

Step II diets can be effective in significantly lowering LDL cholesterol and reducing CHD risk.[6–12] Moreover, such diets with sufficient fat restriction may promote weight loss.[12] Benefit has been noted with fish oil and vitamin E supplementation, as well as a diet rich in al-

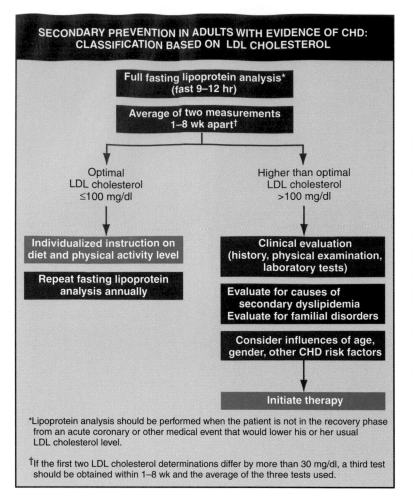

Figure 29–19

Secondary prevention classification by low-density lipoprotein (LDL) cholesterol. In patients with coronary heart disease (CHD) or other atherosclerotic disease, initial assessment for dyslipidemia is by full fasting lipoprotein analysis to determine LDL cholesterol level. (Redrawn from Farmer, J.A., and Gotto, A.M., Jr.: Dyslipidemia and other risk factors for coronary artery disease. In Braunwald, E. [ed.]: Heart Disease. 5th ed. Philadelphia, W.B. Saunders, 1997, pp. 1126–1160; from Expert Panel on Detection, Evaluation, and Treatment of High Blood Cholesterol in Adults: Summary of the second report of the National Cholesterol Education Program [NCEP] Expert Panel on Detection, Evaluation, and Treatment of High Blood Cholesterol in Adults [Adult Treatment Panel II]. JAMA 269:3015, 1993; and National Cholesterol Education Program: Second report of the Expert Panel on Detection, Evaluation, and Treatment of High Blood Cholesterol in Adults [Adult Treatment Panel II]. Circulation 89:1329, 1994.)

pha-linolenic acid.[8–10] Responsiveness to dietary therapy is related to compliance and specific genetic factors (apoE and apoA-IV phenotype) and should be monitored using LDL cholesterol levels.[1, 38]

No benefit has been noted with beta carotene supplementation.[39] Vitamin E supplementation in one study significantly reduced recurrent CHD events but led to a nonsignificant increase in total mortality,[40] and in another recent large randomized trial it showed no benefit.[40a]

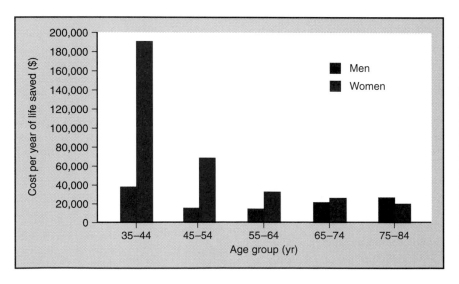

Figure 29–20

The cost-effectiveness ratios for the use of lovastatin (20 mg/day) as cholesterol-lowering therapy for secondary prevention in subjects with a pretreatment cholesterol level of less than 250 mg/dl. These estimates were derived from the Coronary Heart Disease Policy Model.[34] The therapy is more cost-effective for men than for women and for older subjects than for younger subjects. (Redrawn from Krumholz, H.M., and Goldman, L.: Cost-effectiveness of risk factors. In Brown, W.V. [vol. ed.]: Atherosclerosis: Risk Factors and Treatment. Vol. 10. Braunwald, E. [ser. ed.] Philadelphia, Current Medicine, 1996, pp. 13.1–13.12.)

Figure 29–21

The cost-effectiveness ratios for the use of lovastatin (20 mg/day) as cholesterol-lowering therapy for secondary prevention in subjects with a pretreatment cholesterol level of 250 mg/dl or more. These estimates were derived from the Coronary Heart Disease Policy Model.[34] In these subjects, the therapy is very cost-effective for men and women at all ages. For men between 35 and 54 years of age, the therapy saves both lives and money. The cost-effectiveness ratio does not exceed $30,000 per year of life saved for any group. (Redrawn from Krumholz, H.M., and Goldman, L.: Cost-effectiveness of risk factors. *In* Brown, W.V. [vol. ed.]: Atherosclerosis: Risk Factors and Treatment. Vol. 10. Braunwald, E. [ser. ed.] Philadelphia, Current Medicine, 1996, pp. 13.1–13.12.)

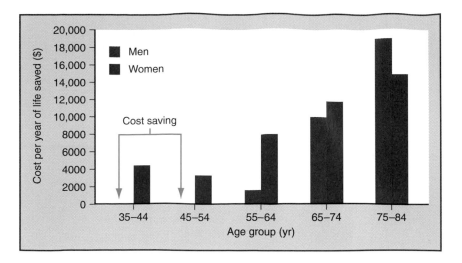

Drug Therapy

Levels of LDL cholesterol requiring drug therapy after diet treatment are shown in Table 29–5. An overview of available lipid-lowering drugs is provided in Table 29–7. Lipid-lowering medications can be divided into two general classes: drugs effective in lowering LDL cholesterol (>15% reduction), and drugs effective in lowering triglyceride levels (>15% reduction). There are currently three classes of agents that meet the LDL cholesterol-lowering criteria: (1) HMG CoA reductase inhibitors (lovastatin, pravastatin, simvastatin, fluvastatin, and atorvastatin), (2) anion-exchange resins (cholestyramine and colestipol), and (3) niacin. Of these three types of drugs, patient compliance with resins and niacin is often poor, whereas with the HMG CoA reductase inhibitors, it is generally excellent.

Safety and efficacy in CHD risk reduction in large-scale, long-term, placebo-controlled, randomized and blinded trials with HMG CoA reductase inhibitors have been documented in both primary and secondary CHD prevention studies.[29–32] Angiographic studies also indicate significant benefit with HMG CoA reductase inhibitors in preventing progression of coronary atherosclerosis and CHD risk reduction.[23–25, 27, 28] Therefore, HMG CoA reductase inhibitors are now the drugs of choice for lowering LDL cholesterol in all subjects because of efficacy, safety, and tolerability.

There are currently four agents that lower triglyceride levels by more than 15%: niacin, gemfibrozil, HMG CoA

Table 29–5	**Treatment Decisions Based on LDL Cholesterol**	

	Dietary Therapy	
	Initiation Level	*LDL Goal*
Without CHD and with fewer than two risk factors	≥160 mg/dl (4.1 mmol/L)	<160 mg/dl
Without CHD and with two or more risk factors	≥130 mg/dl (3.4 mmol/L)	<130 mg/dl
With CHD*	>100 mg/dl (2.6 mmol/L)	≤100 mg/dl

	Drug Treatment	
	Consideration Level	*LDL Goal*
Without CHD and with fewer than two risk factors	≥190 mg/dl† (4.9 mmol/L)	<160 mg/dl
Without CHD and with two or more risk factors	≥160 mg/dl (4.1 mmol/L)	<130 mg/dl
With CHD	≥130 mg/dl (3.4 mmol/L)	≤100 mg/dl

From Schaefer, E.J.: Overview of the Diagnosis and Treatment of Lipid Disorders. Cambridge, MA, Copyright Genzyme Corporation, 1995, p. 17.
Abbreviations: LDL, low-density lipoprotein; CHD, coronary heart disease.
* In CHD patients with LDL cholesterol levels 100–129 mg/dl (2.6–3.3 mmol/L), the physician should exercise clinical judgment in deciding whether to initiate drug treatment.
† In men under 35 yr of age and premenopausal women with LDL cholesterol levels 190–219 mg/dl (4.9–5.7 mmol/L), drug therapy should be delayed except in high-risk patients such as those with diabetes.

Table 29–6	Additional Effects of Dietary Fiber on Plasma Cholesterol in Individuals Consuming a Low-Fat Diet			
Fiber Type	**Test Population**	**Duration (wk)**	**Effects on Plasma Cholesterol (%)**	
Oat bran*	Normal	12	↓ 2.7	
Oatmeal*	Normal	12	↓ 3.3	
Psyllium†	Hyperlipidemic	8	↓ 7.7	
Mixed fiber‡				
Soluble	Hyperlipidemic	4–16	↓ 14	
Insoluble	Hyperlipidemic	4–16	↓ 8	

From Chait, A., and Rosenfeld, M.E.: Dietary effects on cardiovascular risk factors. *In* Brown, W.V. (vol. ed.): Atherosclerosis: Risk Factors and Treatment. Vol. 10. Braunwald, E. (ser. ed.) Philadelphia, Current Medicine, 1996, pp. 8.1–8.25.

* Data from Van Horn, L.V., Liu, K., Parker, D, et al.: Serum lipid response to oat product intake with a fat-modified diet. J. Am. Diet. Assoc. 86:759–764, 1986.

† Data from Bell, L.P., Hectorne, K., Reynolds, H., et al.: Cholesterol-lowering effects of psyllium hydrophilic mucilloid. Adjunct therapy to a prudent diet for patients with mild to moderate hypercholesterolemia. JAMA 261:3419–3423, 1989.

‡ Data from Jenkins, D.J., Wolever, T.M., Rao, A.V., et al.: Effect on blood lipids of very high intakes of fiber in diets low in saturated fat and cholesterol. N Engl J Med 329:21–26, 1993.

reductase inhibitors, and fish oil capsules. Niacin and HMG CoA reductase inhibitors also significantly lower LDL cholesterol levels, and all agents raise HDL cholesterol levels modestly. Niacin, gemfibrozil, and fish oil have also been shown to lower CHD risk prospectively.[8, 16, 17] In patients with severe (> 1000 mg/dl) fasting hypertriglyceridemia, gemfibrozil is the drug of choice because of efficacy and tolerability and because such patients often have diabetes that can be exacerbated by niacin.

Patients with Elevated LDL Cholesterol Only

For all patients with increased LDL cholesterol only, the drugs of choice are HMG CoA reductase inhibitors. If patients cannot tolerate these agents, resins, even at low doses, then niacin, or a combination of resins and niacin, should be used. The combination of an HMG CoA reductase inhibitor with an anion-exchange resin is very effective.[41] It should be noted that in postmenopausal

Table 29–7	Medications				
	Resins*	**Niacin***	**Gemfibrozil**	**HMG CoA Reductase Inhibitors**	**Probucol**
Patient Acceptance and Compliance	Often poor	Often poor	Generally excellent	Generally excellent	Generally excellent
Side Effect	Constipation Bloating Decreased absorption of certain medicines	Flushing Itching Gastritis Hepatotoxicity Hyperuricemia Hyperglycemia	Myositis Hepatotoxicity GI side effects Warfarin interaction	Hepatotoxicity Myositis GI side effects	GI side effects
Usual Dose	8–10 gm po bid	1 gm po bid with food	600 mg po bid	10–40 mg po qd	500 mg po bid
LDL Reduction	10%–20%	10%–20%	0%–15%	20%–40%	10%–15%
Triglyceride Reduction	†	40%	35%	20%	0%
HDL Increase	5%	15%–20%	5%–15%	5%–10%	‡
CHD Risk Reduction Documented	Yes 19% 7 yr	Yes 20% 5 yr	Yes 34% 5 yr	Yes	No
Long-Term Safety Documented	Yes	Yes	Yes	Yes	No

From Schaefer, E.J.: Overview of the Diagnosis and Treatment of Lipid Disorders. Cambridge, MA, Copyright Genzyme Corporation, 1995, p. 28.

Abbreviations: HMG CoA, 3-hydroxy-3-methylglutaryl coenzyme A: GI, gastrointestinal; po, by mouth; bid, twice daily; qd, every day; LDL, low-density lipoprotein; HDL, high-density lipoprotein; CHD, coronary heart disease.

* Both resins and niacin should be started at low doses and gradually increased.

† May increase triglycerides.

‡ Lowers HDL cholesterol 15%–25%.

women, estrogen replacement is quite effective in lowering LDL cholesterol and raising HDL cholesterol, but estrogens should not be used for cholesterol reduction in patients with hypertriglyceridemia because they raise triglyceride levels. Estrogen use has been associated with a significant reduction in CHD mortality in postmenopausal women.[42] In postmenopausal women with an intact uterus, estrogen is commonly combined with progesterone.[42a] A dose of either 0.625 mg or 0.3 mg of conjugated equine estrogen and 2.5 mg or 5 mg of progesterone given continuously is generally well tolerated.

Patients with Elevated LDL Cholesterol and Elevated Triglycerides

For patients with elevations in both LDL cholesterol and triglycerides (>200 mg/dl or 2.3 mmol/L), the drugs of choice are HMG CoA reductase inhibitors. For patients who cannot tolerate these agents, niacin and gemfibrozil are the next choices.

Patients with Hypertriglyceridemia and Normal LDL Cholesterol

For patients with hypertriglyceridemia only (>200 mg/dl or 2.3 mm/L) and normal LDL cholesterol levels, there are as yet no clear medication guidelines.[1] However, diet and exercise, as well as elimination of secondary causes of elevated triglycerides, are encouraged. If the patient has fasting triglycerides in excess of 1000 mg/dl (11.3 mmol/L) while on a low-fat, 2000-calorie diet, medication to reduce the risk of pancreatitis is recommended. However, before taking this step, the physician should make sure that these patients are not taking oral estrogens, thiazides, or beta blockers, are not using alcohol, or do not have uncontrolled diabetes mellitus. The drug of choice in such patients is generally gemfibrozil because most of them have glucose intolerance. In the absence of glucose intolerance, niacin can be tried. In patients in whom these agents are not effective, or if additional triglyceride reduction is needed, fish oil capsules (1 gm) at a dose of 3 to 5 capsules twice daily are effective in lowering triglycerides.

Patients with Moderate Hypertriglyceridemia or Low HDL Cholesterol, or Both

In patients with moderate fasting hypertriglyceridemia (400 to 1000 mg/dl), especially in those with HDL cholesterol deficiency, lifestyle changes, including weight reduction and an exercise program, are very helpful. If patients have established CHD, the use of either niacin, gemfibrozil, or HMG CoA reductase inhibitors should be considered to normalize their lipid levels. The goal of therapy in CHD patients is to get their LDL cholesterol below 100 mg/dl (2.6 mmol/L).[1] Some experts also recommend reduction of triglycerides to less than 200 mg/dl (2.3 mmol/L), increasing HDL cholesterol to

over 40 mg/dl (1.0 mmol/L) if possible, and decreasing the total cholesterol–to–HDL cholesterol ratio to less than 5.0. In the absence of heart disease, only lifestyle modification (diet and exercise) can currently be recommended in patients with hypertriglyceridemia or HDL cholesterol deficiency.

HMG CoA Reductase Inhibitors

These drugs inhibit HMG CoA reductase, the rate-limiting enzyme in cholesterol biosynthesis, causing upregulation of LDL receptors, and enhancing LDL catabolism (Fig. 29–22; see also step 8, Fig. 29–10). These agents decrease VLDL and LDL cholesterol production (steps 2 and 6, Fig. 29–10) and decrease plasma LDL cholesterol by 25% to 60% at maximal doses.[22–32, 43] These agents are now the drugs of choice of lipid management because of efficacy, safety, and tolerability (Table 29–8; see also Table 29–7).

The key with these agents is to start at a low dose and to gradually titrate the dose upward, since the effect may be maximized at 20 mg of any of these agents, instead of 40 mg. These drugs are generally well tolerated, but they may occasionally cause liver enzyme elevation (1% to 2%), significant creatine kinase elevation with myalgias and myositis (0.1%), and gastrointestinal side effects. Carefully controlled studies indicate that these agents do not cause cataracts, sleep problems, or daytime performance disturbances. Pravastatin use may be associated with less myositis and should be considered in patients who have developed this problem with other statins. Fluvastatin is the least expensive of these compounds, but only 25% reductions in LDL cholesterol have been reported at a dose of 40 mg/day. Atorvastatin appears to be the most potent, with a 60% reduction being noted at 80 mg/day.

Lovastatin is usually started at 20 mg po daily at suppertime and can be increased to 40 mg po qd, 20 mg po twice daily or even 40 mg po twice daily. CHD risk reduction of 25% was documented in the Monitored Atherosclerosis Regression Study (MARS) and the Canadian Coronary Atherosclerosis Intervention Trial (CCAIT).[19, 27]

Pravastatin is usually started at 10 or 20 mg po daily at bedtime, and can be increased to 40 mg po daily at bedtime. Its structure is similar to that of lovastatin, but it has greater liver selectivity. It has been successfully given in combination with gemfibrozil.

Pravastatin at 40 mg/day has been reported to lower LDL 28%, total mortality 46%, fatal and nonfatal CHD 62%, and stroke 62% in over 1800 patients with atherosclerosis.[30] Pravastatin at 40 mg/day reduced LDL 26%, total mortality 22%, fatal and nonfatal myocardial infarction (MI) 31%, and need for angioplasty or bypass surgery 37% in healthy middle-aged men with moderate hypercholesterolemia in the large prospective West of Scotland Study.[31] Pravastatin at 40 mg/day lowered LDL cholesterol 26%, fatal and nonfatal MI 24%, bypass 26%, angioplasty 23%, fatal MI 37%, and stroke 31% in post-MI patients with LDL cholesterol values in the range of 115 to 174 mg/dl (mean 137 mg/dl), in the CARE trial.[32]

Simvastatin is usually started at 10 mg po daily at suppertime, and can be increased to 20 or 40 mg po

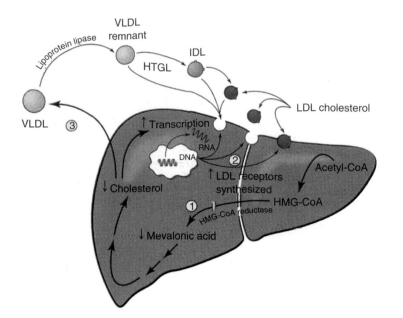

Figure 29–22

Mechanism of action of statins. The statins inhibit the rate-limiting enzyme, hydroxymethyl glutaryl–coenzyme A (HMG-CoA) reductase, in cholesterol biosynthesis (1). The associated decrease in hepatic and cellular cholesterol concentration stimulates the production of low-density lipoprotein (LDL) receptors, which increase the rate of removal of LDL from the plasma (2). There is also increased removal of very low-density lipoprotein (VLDL) remnants and intermediate-density lipoprotein (IDL), which are precursors to LDL formation. In some patients, there may also be a decrease in lipoprotein synthesis (3). The enhanced removal of VLDL remnants and IDL and the inhibition of lipoprotein synthesis may contribute to the modest triglyceride-lowering effect of the statins. Acetyl-CoA, acetyl–coenzyme A; VLDL, very low density lipoprotein; HTGL, hepatic triglyceride lipase; IDL, intermediate-density lipoprotein. (Redrawn from Brown, W.V.: Atherosclerosis: Risk factors and treatment. *In* Braunwald, E. [ed.-in-chief]: Essential Atlas of Heart Diseases. Philadelphia, Current Medicine, 1997, p. 1.30.)

daily. Its structure is similar to that of lovastatin, except that it has an additional methyl group. Simvastatin has been shown to decrease LDL 35%, total mortality 30%, nonfatal and fatal CHD 34%, stroke 37%, and angioplasty or bypass 37% in CHD patients with moderate hypercholesterolemia in the large prospective Scandinavian Simvastatin Survival Study.[29]

Fluvastatin is structurally different from the other agents, and is the first synthetic HMG CoA reductase inhibitor. It is usually started at 20 mg po daily and can be increased to 40 mg po daily. Fluvastatin lowers LDL by 22% at 20 mg/day and 25% in familial hypercholesterolemia patients at 40 mg/day. The starting dose is

20 mg/day, it is supplied as 20- and 40-mg capsules, and the maximal dose is 40 mg/day. Fluvastatin was evaluated in the recent Lipoprotein and Coronary Atherosclerosis Study (LCAS) in which 429 men and women were placed on placebo or 20 mg po twice daily of fluvastatin. LDL was reduced by 27%, triglyceride by 10%, and HDL was increased by 6%, as compared with baseline. There was significantly less angiographic progression in coronary arteries in the fluvastatin group than in the control group.[28]

Atorvastatin is a new synthetic HMG CoA reductase inhibitor, available in 10, 20, and 40 mg, with reductions in LDL of 39%, 43%, and 50%, respectively. The starting dose is 10 mg po daily, and the maximal dose is 80 mg, with LDL reduction of 60% and triglyceride reductions of 40%.[43] This new agent appears to be quite effective in lowering lipid levels in hypertriglyceridemic patients as well.

Anion-Exchange Resins

Cholestyramine and colestipol are anion-exchange resins that bind bile acids, increase conversion of liver cholesterol to bile acids, and upregulate LDL receptors in the liver.[1] This results in an increase in LDL catabolism (step 8, Fig. 29–10) and a decrease in plasma LDL by about 20%. Side effects include bloating and constipation, elevation of triglycerides, and interference with the absorption of digoxin, tetracycline, D-thyroxine, phenylbutazone, and warfarin (give drugs 1 hour earlier or 4 hours after resin). Cholestyramine (4-gm packets or scoops) or colestipol (5-gm scoops) can be started at 1 scoop or packet twice daily and gradually increased to 2 scoops twice daily (the scoops are half the price of the packets), or 2

Table 29–8	Administration of Statins

Time

Single-dose administration is always more effective in the evening.
Lovastatin is administered with the evening meal; all others are usually administered at bedtime.

Frequency

Generally administered as a single dose.
At higher doses, twice-daily administration can be considered for slightly greater efficacy, although the cost is also greater.

Usual Daily Dose Range (mg)

Lovastatin	20–80
Simvastatin	10–40
Pravastatin	10–40
Fluvastatin	20–40
Atorvastatin	10–80

Adapted from Hunninghake, D.B.: Lipid-lowering drugs. *In* Brown, W.V. (vol. ed.): Atherosclerosis: Risk Factors and Treatment. Vol. 10. Braunwald, E. (ser. ed.) Philadelphia, Current Medicine, 1996, pp. 9.1–9.19.

scoops three times daily. Colestipol is available in 1-gm tablet form as well, and a standard dose is 4 to 8 tablets twice daily. Constipation may require treatment. Cholestyramine (6 scoops/day) has been shown to lower LDL by 12.5% and reduce CHD risk prospectively by 19% over 7 years in middle-aged, asymptomatic, hypercholesterolemic men in the large, prospective, randomized, placebo-controlled Lipid Research Clinics Coronary Primary Prevention Trial (LRC-CPPT).[13, 14] Total mortality was reduced by 6%, angina by 20%, and need for bypass by 21%.[14] Most subjects on active medication took far less than the dose prescribed.

Niacin   *Not in hepatic dis on   DM NOT on insulin*

Niacin decreases VLDL by 40% (step 2, Fig. 29–10) and LDL production by 20% (Fig. 29–23; see also step 6, Fig. 29–10) and raises HDL values by 20% (Table 29–9). Niacin should be started at 100 mg po twice daily with meals and gradually increased to 1 gm po twice or three times daily with meals. Side effects include flushing, gastric irritation, and elevations of uric acid, glucose and liver enzymes in some patients. Niacin should not be used in patients with liver disease or in diabetic patients not on insulin. Long-acting niacin causes less flushing and can be used initially, but it causes excess gastrointestinal toxicity. Niacin should be discontinued if liver enzymes increase to over twice the upper normal limit.

Niacin has been shown to lower total cholesterol levels by 10% and to reduce the recurrence of MI by 20% after a 5-year period of administration in men with CHD in the Coronary Drug Project involving 8341 subjects randomized to placebo, niacin, clofibrate, D-thyroxine, and estrogen. The use of niacin was also associated with an 11% reduction in all-cause mortality 10 years after cessation of niacin.[17] No significant benefit, and in some cases, excess mortality was associated with the other therapies. Niacin in combination with clofibrate has been shown to reduce total mortality by 26% and CHD mortality by 36% in

CHD patients as compared with usual care in the Stockholm Ischemic Heart Disease Study over a 5-year period.[44]

Gemfibrozil   *NOT in CRI*

Gemfibrozil is given at a dose of 600 mg po twice daily and is generally well tolerated. The drug is very effective in lowering triglycerides and VLDL by 35% by decreasing production and enhancing breakdown of VLDL (steps 2 and 6, Fig. 29–10). The drug increases HDL by 5% to 15% and usually lowers LDL by 5% to 15%. Rarely, patients may get gastrointestinal symptoms, muscle cramps, or intermittent indigestion. The drug should not be used in patients with renal insufficiency. It also potentiates the action of warfarin.

Gemfibrozil has been found to reduce CHD risk (fatal and nonfatal MI) prospectively by 34% over 5 years in middle-aged, asymptomatic, hypercholesterolemic men as determined in the large, prospective, randomized, placebo-controlled Helsinki Heart Study.[16] CHD risk reduction was associated with HDL raising and LDL lowering,

Overview of Niacin

Commonly considered for its cost advantage or to increase HDL levels.

Favorably affects all lipid and lipoprotein levels to decrease risk for coronary heart disease; moderately lowers levels of lipoprotein(a)

Available without a prescription and can be cheaper than other lipid-lowering drugs; FDA-approved preparations are more costly.

Acceptance by both patients and health care professionals is limited because of the high frequency of side effects, especially at higher doses.

Most difficult drug to administer and to achieve compliance.

Adapted from Hunninghake, D.B.: Lipid-lowering drugs. *In* Brown, W.V. (vol. ed.): Atherosclerosis: Risk Factors and Treatment. Vol. 10. Braunwald, E. (ser. ed.) Philadelphia, Current Medicine, 1996, pp. 9.1–9.19.

Abbreviations: HDL, high-density lipoprotein; FDA, U.S. Food and Drug Administration.

Figure 29–23

Mechanisms of action of nicotinic acid. Inhibition of lipoprotein synthesis is generally considered to be the major effect of nicotinic acid (1). Inhibition of lipolysis of the stored fat in adipose tissue (2) with the resultant decrease in free fatty acids delivered to the liver could also indirectly decrease lipoprotein synthesis. Inhibition of lipoprotein synthesis decreases very low density lipoprotein (VLDL) secretion or synthesis (3), and all subsequent lipoproteins in this pathway (VLDL remnants, intermediate-density lipoproteins [IDLs] and low-density lipoproteins [LDLs]) are also decreased (4). HTGL, hepatic triglyceride lipase. (Redrawn from Brown, W.V.: Atherosclerosis: Risk factors and treatment. *In* Braunwald, E. [ed.-in-chief]: Essential Atlas of Heart Diseases. Philadelphia, Current Medicine, 1997, p. 1.32.)

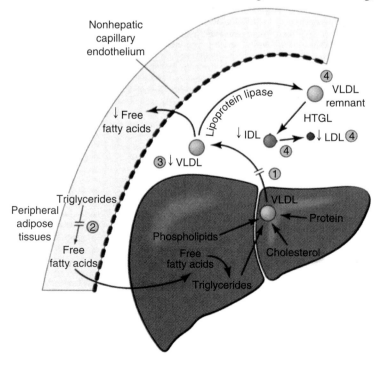

but not with triglyceride lowering.[16] No reduction in total mortality was noted, and there were nonsignificant increases in deaths from hemorrhagic stroke, accidents, and violence (homicide and suicide).[16]

Probucol

Probucol is an antioxidant given at a dose of 500 mg po twice daily and is at best a second-line drug that lowers LDL 10% to 15%. It can be used in familial hypercholesterolemia for increasing nonreceptor LDL catabolism. It may cause gastrointestinal side effects. The drug also lowers HDL by 15% to 25% by decreasing its production (step 3, Fig. 29–10). Long-term safety and efficacy in CHD risk reduction have not been established. A prospective angiographic study did not demonstrate significant benefit with probucol.[45]

Combination Therapies

HMG CoA reductase inhibitors and resins together are very effective, as are niacin and resins together, in lowering LDL cholesterol (50% to 60% reduction).[41] The combination of gemfibrozil and reductase inhibitors is not recommended because myositis incidence is quite high with the lovastatin-gemfibrozil combination. If this combination is used, it should be used with caution, and creatine kinase levels should be monitored. However, pravastatin and gemfibrozil in combination have been found to be efficacious in lipid lowering and to be well tolerated. Niacin and reductase inhibitors are also effective, but the incidence of significant liver enzyme elevation is about 10%, so this combination should be used with caution. Gemfibrozil with either fish oil capsules or niacin can be used to lower triglycerides. The new HMG CoA reductase inhibitor atorvastatin may obviate the need for combination therapy for additional LDL lowering or triglyceride lowering because of its striking efficacy.[43] Re-

sponse to drug therapy should be monitored using LDL levels.

FAMILIAL LIPOPROTEIN DISORDERS

An overview of familial hypercholesterolemic states is provided in Table 29–10.

Familial Combined Hyperlipidemia

By far the most common of these disorders is familial combined hyperlipidemia, in which affected kindred members may have elevated LDL alone (>190 mg/dl or 4.9 mmol/L), elevated triglycerides alone (>200 mg/dl or 2.3 mmol/L), or elevations of both parameters. Both abnormalities must be present in the family to make the diagnosis. These patients have been shown to have overproduction of VLDL apoB-100, but not triglyceride. They also often have decreased HDL values owing to enhanced degradation of HDL. Approximately 15% of patients with premature CHD have this disorder. Treatment consists of diet and, if necessary, use of reductase inhibitors, niacin, gemfibrozil, or combinations of these medications with anion-exchange resins. Sporadic or polygenic hypercholesterolemia is also quite common.

Familial Hypercholesterolemia

Isolated elevations of LDL are found in patients with a disorder known as *familial hypercholesterolemia* often associated with tuberous or tendinous xanthomas (Figs. 29–

Table 29–10 Familial Hypercholesterolemic States

	Familial Combined Hyperlipidemia	Familial Hypercholesterolemia	Familial Dysbetalipoproteinemia
Physical Findings	Arcus senilis	Arcus senilis Tendinous xanthomas	Arcus senilis Tuboeruptive and planar xanthomas
Associated Findings	Obesity Glucose intolerance Hyperuricemia HDL deficiency	—	Obesity Glucose intolerance Hyperuricemia
Mode of Inheritance	Autosomal dominant	Autosomal co-dominant	Autosomal recessive
Defect	Overproduction of hepatic VLDL apoB-100	Defective LDL receptor or defective apoB-100	Defective apoE
Estimated Population Frequency	1:100	1:500	1:5000
CHD Risk	+ +	+ + +	+
Treatment	Diet Niacin Resin Reductase inhibitors Gemfibrozil	Diet Niacin and resin Reductase inhibitors and resin Probucol and resin	Diet Niacin Gemfibrozil

From Schaefer, E.J.: Overview of the Diagnosis and Treatment of Lipid Disorders. Cambridge, MA, Copyright Genzyme Corporation, 1995, p. 35.

Abbreviations: HDL, high-density lipoprotein; VLDL, very low density lipoprotein; apoB-100, apolipoprotein B-100; LDL, low-density lipoprotein; apoE, apolipoprotein E; CHD, coronary heart disease.

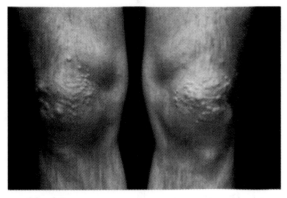

Figure 29–24
Tuberous xanthomas are yellowish nodules of varying size and occur on the elbows, buttocks, and knees. (From Mir, M.A.: Atlas of Clinical Diagnosis. London, W.B. Saunders, 1995, p. 252.)

24 and 29–25). These patients generally have marked hypercholesterolemia (>350 mg/dl or 9.1 mmol/L) with normal triglyceride values and may have defects at the LDL receptor locus or abnormalities of the apoB protein. The major metabolic abnormality in these individuals is an impaired ability to catabolize LDL (step 8, Fig. 29–10). Approximately 3% of patients with premature CHD have this disorder. Treatment generally consists of diet and a combination of medications (reductase inhibitors, resins, and niacin).[22]

Familial Dysbetalipoproteinemia (Type III Hyperlipoproteinemia)

A much rarer form of combined elevations of cholesterol and triglyceride is known as *familial dysbetalipoproteinemia* (type III hyperlipoproteinemia), in which affected subjects have accumulations of chylomicron remnants and VLDL in the fasting state. These patients usually are homozygous for a mutation in the apoE protein (apoE-2/2 phenotype) or rarely have apoE deficiency, resulting in defective hepatic clearance of chylomicron and VLDL remnants, as well as increased VLDL production (steps 2, 5, and 6, Fig. 29–10). They may also have tuboeruptive and planar xanthomas. Precise diagnosis requires quantitation of lipoprotein cholesterol values after ultracentrifugation and apoE genotyping. Treatment consists of diet, niacin, gemfibrozil, or an HMG CoA reductase inhibitor. These patients are also very responsive to gemfibrozil or niacin. Patients with both familial combined hyperlipidemia and familial dysbetalipoproteinemia often have obesity, glucose intolerance, and hyperuricemia.

Familial Hypertriglyceridemic States

An overview is provided in Table 29–11. By far the most common of these disorders is familial hypertriglyc-

eridemia (triglycerides >200 mg/dl or 2.3 mmol/L), an autosomal dominant disorder in which obesity, glucose intolerance, hyperuricemia, and HDL deficiency are often present. The disorder is associated with overproduction of hepatic VLDL triglyceride but not VLDL apoB-100 (step 2, Fig. 29–10). Some patients may have defects in VLDL clearance as well (steps 6 and 7, Fig. 29–10). CHD risk appears to be increased in those kindreds in whom HDL deficiency is also present. Approximately 15% of patients with premature CHD appear to have this disorder. HDL levels are usually low in these subjects because of enhanced degradation. Treatment with diet, exercise, and abstinence from alcohol and estrogens is recommended. In patients with CHD, niacin, gemfibrozil, or reductase inhibitors can be used to optimize lipid values.

Severe Hypertriglyceridemia

Severe hypertriglyceridemia (triglyceride values >1000 mg/dl or 11.3 mmol/L) is occasionally observed in middle-aged or elderly individuals who are obese and have glucose intolerance and hyperuricemia. These subjects usually have familial hypertriglyceridemia or familial combined hyperlipidemia that is exacerbated by other factors, such as obesity and diabetes mellitus. These patients generally also have HDL deficiency and may develop lipemia retinalis and eruptive xanthomas. They are at increased risk for developing pancreatitis owing to triglyceride deposition in the pancreas and may have paresthesias and emotional lability. These patients often have delayed chylomicron and VLDL clearance and excess VLDL production (steps 2, 4, 6, and 7, Fig. 29–10). Treatment consists of a calorie-restricted Step II diet. In patients with diabetes mellitus, it is crucial to control the blood glucose as well as possible. Medications that are effective in lowering the triglycerides to less than 1000 mg/dl (11.3 mmol/L) in these patients to reduce their risk of pancreatitis include gemfibrozil or fish oil capsules (6 to 10 capsules/day).

Patients who have severe hypertriglyceridemia in childhood or early adulthood and who are not obese often

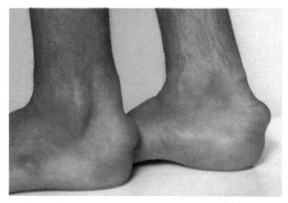

Figure 29–25
Tendinous xanthomas, from diffuse infiltration of the tendons with cholesterol, occur mainly on the extensor tendons. These lesions are strongly suggestive of familial hypercholesterolemia. (From Mir, M.A.: Atlas of Clinical Diagnosis. London, W.B. Saunders, 1995, p. 252.)

Table 29–11 **Familial Hypertriglyceridemic States**

	Familial Hypertriglyceridemia	Severe Hypertriglyceridemia	
		Early Onset	*Adult Onset*
Physical Findings	None	Lipemia retinalis Eruptive xanthomas	Lipemia retinalis Eruptive xanthomas
Associated Findings	Obesity Glucose intolerance Hyperuricemia HDL deficiency	HDL deficiency Pancreatitis	Obesity Glucose intolerance Hyperuricemia HDL deficiency Pancreatitis Paresthesias Emotional lability
Mode of Inheritance	Autosomal dominant	Autosomal recessive	Autosomal recessive

Defect	Overproduction of hepatic
	   VLDL triglyceride
		Lipoprotein lipase deficiency
		apoC-III deficiency
			Overproduction of VLDL
			   triglyceride
			Delayed catabolism of
			   chylomicrons and VLDL

Estimated Population Frequency	1 : 100	1 : 10,000	1 : 1000
CHD Risk	+	−	+
Treatment	Diet Niacin Gemfibrozil	Diet	Diet Gemfibrozil Fish oil

From Schaefer, E.J.: Overview of the Diagnosis and Treatment of Lipid Disorders. Cambridge, MA, Copyright Genzyme Corporation, 1995, p. 36.
Abbreviations: HDL, high-density lipoprotein; VLDL, very low density lipoprotein; apoC-III, apolipoprotein C-III; CHD, coronary heart disease.

have a deficiency of the enzyme lipoprotein lipase or its activator protein (apoC-II), resulting in markedly impaired removal of triglyceride. Therefore, they have a defect in chylomicron and VLDL catabolism (steps 4, 6, and 7, Fig. 29–10). These patients are at increased risk for recurrent pancreatitis; it is important to restrict their dietary fat to less than 20% of calories. Niacin or gemfibrozil, or both, are generally ineffective in these patients. However, fish oil capsules (6/day) may occasionally be helpful in certain patients to keep their triglyceride levels below 1000 mg/dl (11.3 mmol/L) and minimize the risk of pancreatitis.

Lp(a) Excess

[handwritten: only responds to niacin or hormonal therapy]

Elevated Lp(a) levels (>30 mg/dl for total mass or >10 mg/dl for cholesterol) have been associated with premature CHD in most studies. Lp(a) is a highly heritable trait, not lowered by diet or standard cholesterol-lowering medications except niacin or hormonal replacement therapy. Familial Lp(a) excess is common in patients with premature CHD. In such patients, treatment with niacin or hormonal replacement is warranted, since treatment with niacin or estrogens has been shown to reduce CHD morbidity and mortality.[17, 42] Routine screening in the general population cannot be recommended at this time.

Familial Hypoalphalipoproteinemia

Isolated deficiency of HDL (below the 10th percentile of normal) can be genetic in nature and is then known as

familial hypoalphalipoproteinemia. This disorder is found in approximately 4% of patients with premature CHD. Treatment consists of diet, weight reduction if indicated, and an exercise program. In patients with CHD, management with HMG CoA reductase inhibitors to optimize LDL cholesterol levels is the current treatment of choice.

References

1. The Expert Panel: Second report of the Expert Panel on Detection, Evaluation, and Treatment of High Blood Cholesterol in Adults (Adult Treatment Panel II). Circulation 89:1329–1445, 1994.
2. Schaefer, E.J., Lamon-Fava, S., Johnson, S., et al.: Effects of gender and menopausal status on the association of apolipoprotein E phenotype with plasma lipoprotein levels. Results from the Framingham Offspring Study. Arterioscler Thromb 14:1105–1113, 1994.
3. Bostom, A.G., Cupples, L.A., Jenner, J.L., et al.: Elevated lipoprotein (a) and coronary heart disease in men aged 55 years and younger. JAMA 276:544–548, 1996.
4. Anderson, K.M., Wilson, P.W.F., Odell, P.M., and Kannel, W.B.: An updated coronary risk profile. A statement for health professionals. AHA Medical/Scientific Statement Science Advisory. Circulation 83:356–362, 1991.
5. Stamler, J., Wentworth, D., and Neaton, J.D.: Is the relationship between serum cholesterol and risk of premature death from coronary heart disease continuous and graded? Findings in 356,222 primary screenees of the Multiple Risk Factor Intervention Trial (MRFIT). JAMA 256:2823–2828, 1986.
6. Turpeinen, O.: Effect of cholesterol-lowering diet on mortality from coronary heart disease and other causes. Circulation 59:1–7, 1979.
7. Rose, G., Tunstall, H.D., and Heller, R.F.: UK Heart Disease Prevention Project: Incidence and mortality results. Lancet 1:1062, 1983.
8. Burr, M.L., Fehily, A.M., Gilbert, J.F., et al.: Effects of changes in fat, fish, and fibre intakes on death and myocardial infarction. Diet and Reinfarction Trial (DART). Lancet 2:757–761, 1989.
9. deLorgeril, M., Salen, P., Martin, J.L., et al.: Effect of a Mediterranean type of diet on the rate of cardiovascular complications in

patients with coronary artery disease. J. Am. Coll. Cardiol. 28: 1103–1108, 1996.

10. deLorgeril, M., Renaud, S., Mamelle, N., et al.: Mediterranean alpha-linolenic acid–rich diet in secondary prevention of coronary heart disease. Lancet 343:1454–1459, 1994.

11. Watts, G.F., Lewis, B., Brunt, J.N.H., et al.: Effects on coronary artery disease of lipid lowering diet, a diet plus cholestyramine in the St. Thomas Atherosclerosis Regression Study (STARS). Lancet 339:563–569, 1992.

12. Ornish, D., Brown, S.K., Scherwitz, L.W., et al.: Can life-style changes reverse coronary heart disease? Lancet 326:129–133, 1990.

13. The Lipid Research Clinics Program: The Lipid Research Clinics Coronary Primary Prevention Trial. I. Reduction in incidence of coronary heart disease. JAMA 251:351–364, 1984.

14. The Lipid Research Clinics Program: The Lipid Research Clinics Coronary Primary Prevention Trial. II. The relationship of reduction in incidence of coronary heart disease to cholesterol lowering. JAMA 251:365–374, 1984.

15. Gordon, D.J., Knoke, J., Probstfeld, J.L., et al.: High density lipoprotein cholesterol and coronary heart disease in hypercholesterolemic men. The Lipid Research Clinics Coronary Primary Prevention Trial. Circulation 74:1217–1225, 1986.

16. Frick, M.H., Elo, O., Haapa, K., et al.: Helsinki Heart Study: Primary prevention trial with gemfibrozil in middle-aged men with dyslipidemia. N. Engl. J. Med. 317:1237–1245, 1987.

17. Canner, P.L., Berge, K.G., Wenger, N.K., et al.: Fifteen-year mortality in Coronary Drug Project patients: Long-term benefit with niacin. J. Am. Coll. Cardiol. 8:1245–1255, 1986.

18. Blankenhorn, D.H., Nessim, S.A., Johnson, R.L., et al.: Beneficial effects of combined colestipol-niacin therapy on coronary atherosclerosis and coronary venous bypass grafts. JAMA 257:3233–3240, 1987.

19. Blankenhorn, D.H., Azen, S.P., Kramsch, D.M., et al.: Coronary angiographic changes with lovastatin therapy. The Monitored Atherosclerosis Regression Study (MARS). Ann. Intern. Med. 1119: 969–976, 1993.

20. Brown, B.G., Albers, J.J., Fisher, L.D., et al.: Regression of coronary artery disease as a result of intensive lipid-lowering therapy in men with high levels of apolipoprotein B. N. Engl. J. Med. 323: 1289–1298, 1990.

21. Buchwald, H., Varco, R.L., Matts, J.P., et al.: Effect of partial ileal bypass on mortality and morbidity from coronary heart disease in patients with hypercholesterolemia. Report of the Program on Surgical Control of the Hyperlipidemias (POSCH). N. Engl. J. Med. 323:946–955, 1990.

22. Kane, J.P., Malloy, M.J., Ports, T.A., et al.: Regression of coronary atherosclerosis during treatment of familial hypercholesterolemia with combined drug regimens. JAMA 264:3007–3012, 1990.

23. Jukema, J.W., Bruschke, A.V.G., van Boven, A.J., et al., on behalf of the REGRESS Study Group: Effects of lipid lowering by pravastatin on progression and regression of coronary artery disease in symptomatic men with normal to moderately elevated serum cholesterol levels: The Regression Growth Evaluation Statin Study (REGRESS). Circulation 91:2528–2540, 1995.

24. MAAS Investigators: Effect of simvastatin on coronary atheroma: The Multicentre Anti-Atheroma Study (MAAS). Lancet 344:633–638, 1994.

25. Pitt, B., Mancini, G.B.J., Ellis, S.G., et al., for the PLAC I Investigators: Pravastatin Limitation of Atherosclerosis in the Coronary Arteries (PLAC I): Reduction in atherosclerosis progression and clinical events. J. Am. Coll. Cardiol. 26:1133–1139, 1995.

26. Sacks, E.M., Pasternak, R.C., Gibson, C.M., et al., for the Harvard Atherosclerosis Reversibility Project (HARP) Group: Effect on coronary atherosclerosis of decrease in plasma cholesterol concentrations in normocholesterolaemic patients. Lancet 344:1182–1186, 1994.

27. Waters, D., Higginson, L., Gladstone, P., et al.: Effects of monotherapy with an HMG Co-A reductase inhibitor on the progression of coronary atherosclerosis as assessed by serial quantitative arteriography: The Canadian Coronary Atherosclerosis Intervention Trial. Circulation 89:959–968, 1994.

28. The Post Coronary Artery Bypass Graft Trial Investigators: The effect of aggressive lowering of low-density lipoprotein cholesterol levels and low-dose anticoagulation on obstructive changes in sa-

phenous-vein coronary artery bypass grafts. N. Engl. J. Med. 336: 153–162, 1997.

29. Scandinavian Simvastatin Survival Study Group: Randomized trial of cholesterol lowering in 4444 patients with coronary heart disease: The Scandinavian Simvastatin Survival Study (4S). Lancet 344:1383–1389, 1994.

30. Byington, R.P., Jukema, J.W., Salonen, J.T., et al.: Reduction in cardiovascular events during pravastatin therapy: Pooled analysis of clinical events of the Pravastatin Atherosclerosis Intervention Program. Circulation 92:2419–2425, 1995.

31. Shepherd, J., Cobbe, S.M., Ford, I., et al.: Prevention of coronary heart disease with pravastatin in men with hypercholesterolemia. N. Engl. J. Med. 333:1301–1307, 1995.

32. Sacks, F.M., Pfeffer, M.A., Moye, L.A., et al., for the Cholesterol and Recurrent Events (CARE) Trial Investigators: The effect of pravastatin on coronary events after myocardial infarction in patients with average cholesterol levels. N. Engl. J. Med. 335:1001–1009, 1996.

33. McNamara, J.R., Warnick, G.R., Leary, E.T., et al.: A multi-center evaluation of a patient-administered test for blood cholesterol measurement. Preventive Med 25:583–592, 1996.

34. Goldman, L., Weinstein, M.C., Goldman, P.A., and Williams, L.W.: Cost-effectiveness of HMG-CoA reductase inhibition for primary and secondary prevention of coronary heart disease. JAMA 265:1145–1151, 1991.

35. Goldman, L., Gordon, D., Rifkind, B., et al.: Cost and health implications of cholesterol lowering. Circulation 85:1960–1968, 1992.

35a. Johannesson, M., Jönsson, B., Kjekshus, J., et al.: Cost effectiveness of simvastatin treatment to lower cholesterol levels in patients with coronary heart disease. N. Engl. J. Med. 336:332–336, 1997.

36. Friedewald, W.T., Levy, R.I., and Fredrickson, D.S.: Estimation of the concentration of low density lipoproteins separated by three different methods. Clin. Chem. 18:499–502, 1972.

37. McNamara, J.R., Cole, T.G., Contois, J.H., et al.: Evaluation of an immunoseparation method for measuring LDL cholesterol directly from serum. Clin. Chem. 41:232–240, 1995.

38. Hunninghake, D.B., Stein, F.A., Dujorne, C.A., et al.: The efficacy of intensive dietary therapy alone or combined with lovastatin in outpatients with hypercholesterolemia. N. Engl. J. Med. 328:1213–1219, 1993.

39. Hennekens, C.H., Buring, J.E., Manson, J.E., et al.: Lack of effect of long-term supplementation with beta carotene on the incidence of malignant neoplasms and cardiovascular disease. N. Engl. J. Med. 334:1189–1190, 1996.

40. Stephens, N.F., Parsons, A., Schofield, P.M., et al.: Randomized controlled trial of vitamin E in patients with coronary disease: Cambridge Heart Antioxidant Study (CHAOS). Lancet 347:781–786, 1996.

40a. Rapola, J.M., Virtamo, J., Ripatti, S., et al.: Randomized trial of α-tocopherol and β-carotene supplements on incidence of major coronary events in men with previous myocardial infarction. Lancet 349:1715–1720, 1997.

41. Mabuchi, H., Sakai, T., and Sakai, Y.: Reduction of serum cholesterol in heterozygous patients with familial hypercholesterolemia. Additive effects of compactin and cholestyramine. N. Engl. J. Med. 308:609–619, 1983.

42. Stampfer, M.J., Colditz, G.A., Willett, W.C., et al.: Postmenopausal estrogen therapy and cardiovascular disease. N. Engl. J. Med. 325: 756–762, 1991.

42a. Darling, G.M., Johns, J.A., McCloud, P.I., and Davis, S.R.: Estrogen and progestin compared with simvastatin for hypercholesterolemia in postmenopausal women. N. Engl. J. Med. 337:595–601, 1997.

43. Bakker-Arkema, R.G., Davidson, M.H., Goldstein, R.J., et al.: Efficacy and safety of a new HMG CoA reductase inhibitor in patients with hypertriglyceridemia. JAMA 275:128–133, 1996.

44. Carlson, L.A., and Rosenhamer, G.: Reduction of mortality in the Stockholm Ischemic Heart Disease Study by combined treatment with clofibrate and nicotinic acid. Acta Med. Scand. 223:405–418, 1988.

45. Walldius, G., Erikson, U., Olsson, A.G., et al.: The effect of probucol on femoral atherosclerosis: The Probucol Quantitative Regression Swedish Trial. Am. J. Cardiol. 74:875–883, 1994.

Chapter 30

Recognition and Management of Patients with

Pulmonary Embolism, Deep Venous Thrombosis, and Cor Pulmonale

SAMUEL Z. GOLDHABER

Pulmonary embolism (PE), deep venous thrombosis (DVT), and cor pulmonale are common disorders that occasionally cause death but more often confront the patient with day-to-day disability and impaired quality of life. Optimal management requires practical knowledge of epidemiology, differential diagnosis, treatment options, and preventive strategies. The evaluation of venous thromboembolism and cor pulmonale is particularly appropriate for primary care providers because of the interdisciplinary nature of these illnesses.

DIAGNOSIS OF DVT AND PE

There are two to three times as many DVTs as PEs. Most patients who are ultimately diagnosed with DVT or PE will present initially to a primary care physician. Pa-

tients with right heart failure (cor pulmonale) or systemic arterial hypotension who have suspected or proven PE are at particularly high risk of imminent demise and will usually require subspecialty consultation.

Clinical Manifestations

The first manifestation of *DVT* is often an increasingly annoying "pulling sensation" at the insertion of the lower calf muscle into the posterior portion of the lower leg. This insidious feeling can then become more pronounced and accompanied by warmth, swelling, and erythema. Tenderness may be present along the course of the involved veins, and a cord may be palpable. Additional signs include increased tissue turgor, distention of superficial veins, and the appearance of prominent venous collaterals. Homans' sign, defined as increased resistance or pain during dorsiflexion of the foot, is unreliable and nonspecific. Major considerations for differential diagno-

Table 30–1 Major Clinical Manifestations of DVT

Symptoms and Signs

Pulling sensation in lower calf (common)
Warmth, swelling, tenderness (common)
Palpable cord (occasional)
Superficial venous collateral vessels (occasional)

Differential Diagnosis

Venous insufficiency (acute or chronic)
Cellulitis or septic phlebitis
Hematoma
Ruptured Baker's cyst

Abbreviation: DVT, deep venous thrombosis.

Table 30–3 DVT Anatomic Location

Anatomic Location	All Patients (n = 150)	Symptomatic Patients (n = 120)	Asymptomatic Patients (n = 30)
Proximal	62 (41%)	49 (41%)	13 (43%)
Isolated calf	38 (25%)	30 (25%)	8 (27%)
Bilateral proximal	15 (10%)	12 (10%)	3 (10%)
Calf + proximal	14 (9%)	11 (9%)	3 (10%)
Upper extremities only	10 (7%)	10 (8%)	0 (0%)
Pelvis	5 (3%)	5 (4%)	0 (0%)
Bilateral calf	4 (3%)	1 (1%)	3 (10%)
Calf + proximal + upper	1 (1%)	1 (1%)	0 (0%)
Proximal + upper	1 (1%)	1 (1%)	0 (0%)

From Piccioli, A., Prandoni, P., and Goldhaber, S.Z.: Epidemiologic characteristics, management, and outcome of deep venous thrombosis in a tertiary-care hospital: The Brigham and Women's Hospital DVT Registry. Am. Heart J. 132: 1010–1014, 1996.
Abbreviation: DVT, deep venous thrombosis.

sis include venous insufficiency without thrombosis, cellulitis, hematoma, and ruptured Baker's cyst (Table 30–1). A clinical model for predicting pretest probability for DVT has been developed (Table 30–2). The anatomic location of DVT in a consecutive series of 150 patients is listed in Table 30–3.

Dyspnea is the most frequent symptom and tachypnea is the most frequent sign of *PE*. Whereas dyspnea, syncope, or cyanosis usually indicate a massive PE, pleuritic

Table 30–2 Clinical Model for Predicting Pretest Probability for DVT

Checklist

Major Points

Active cancer (treatment ongoing or within previous 6 mo or palliative)
Paralysis, paresis, or recent plaster immobilization of the lower extremities
Recently bedridden >3 days or major surgery within 4 wk
Localized tenderness along the distribution of the deep venous system
Thigh and calf swollen (should be measured)
Calf swelling with overall calf circumference ≥3 cm compared with the symptomless side (measured 10 cm below the tibial tuberosity)
Strong family history of DVT (≥2 first-degree relatives with history of DVT)

Minor Points

History of recent trauma (≤60 days) to the symptomatic leg
Pitting edema; symptomatic leg only
Dilated superficial veins (nonvaricose) in the symptomatic leg only
Hospitalization within previous 6 mo
Erythema

Clinical Probability

High

≥3 major points and no alternative diagnosis
≥2 major points and ≥2 minor points + no alternative diagnosis

Low

1 major point + ≥2 minor points + has alternative diagnosis
1 major point + ≥1 minor point + no alternative diagnosis
0 major points + ≥3 minor points + has alternative diagnosis
0 major points + ≥2 minor points + no alternative diagnosis

Moderate

All other combinations

From Wells, P.S., Hirsh, J., Anderson, D.R., et al.: Accuracy of clinical assessment of deep-vein thrombosis. Lancet 345:1326–1330, 1995.
Abbreviation: DVT, deep venous thrombosis.

pain, cough, or hemoptysis often suggest a small embolism located distally near the pleura.

On physical examination, young and previously healthy individuals may simply appear anxious but otherwise seem deceptively well, even with an anatomically large PE. They need not have "classic" signs such as tachycardia, low-grade fever, neck vein distention, or an accentuated pulmonic component of the second heart sound. Sometimes, a paradoxical bradycardia occurs.

In older patients who complain of vague chest discomfort, the diagnosis of PE may not be apparent unless signs of right heart failure are present. Unfortunately, because acute coronary ischemic syndromes are so common, one may overlook the possibility of life-threatening PE and may inadvertently discharge these patients from the hospital after the exclusion of myocardial infarction with serial cardiac enzymes and electrocardiograms.

The differential diagnosis of PE is broad (Table 30–4). Although PE is known as "the great masquerader," quite often another illness will simulate PE. For example, occasionally, the proposed diagnosis of PE is supposedly confirmed with a combination of dyspnea, chest pain, and an abnormal lung scan. Perhaps 12 hours later, the correct

Table 30–4 Differential Diagnosis of PE

Myocardial infarction
Pneumonia
Congestive heart failure (left-sided)
Cardiomyopathy (global)
Primary pulmonary hypertension
Asthma
Pericarditis
Intrathoracic cancer
Rib fracture
Pneumothorax
Costochondritis
"Musculoskeletal pain"
Anxiety

Abbreviation: PE, pulmonary embolism.

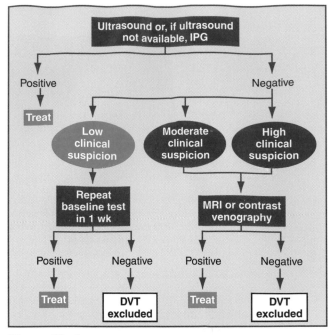

Figure 30–1

Algorithm for workup of initial deep venous thrombosis (DVT). IPG, impedance plethysmography; MRI, magnetic resonance imaging.

diagnosis of pneumonia might become apparent when an infiltrate blossoms on chest x-ray, productive purulent sputum is first produced, and high fever and shaking chills develop.

Some patients have PE and coexisting illness, such as pneumonia or heart failure. In such circumstances, a clue to the possible coexistence of PE is when clinical improvement does not occur despite standard medical treatment of the concomitant illness.

DVT: Imaging Tests

When DVT is suspected, *venous ultrasonography* should ordinarily be the first test ordered (Fig. 30–1). Sometimes referred to as a lower extremity noninvasive examination, this imaging test is usually excellent for diagnosing or excluding an initial episode of DVT in symptomatic patients. For reasons that are unclear, it is quite insensitive for detection of asymptomatic DVT, particularly after orthopedic surgery[1] or neurosurgical procedures.[2]

Venous ultrasonography routinely entails a combination (called *duplex*) of vein compression (B-mode imaging) and pulsed Doppler spectrum analysis with or without color. Normally, manual pressure of the transducer applied to the surface of the skin will cause the vein walls to collapse (Fig. 30–2*A*). Failure to compress a vein is the cardinal sign of DVT on ultrasound examination (Fig. 30–2*B* and *C*). Isolated calf vein thrombosis may be accurately detected on ultrasound examination, but this will depend on the skill of the examiners at individual institutions.[3] Impedance plethysmography (IPG) is less sensitive than ultrasonography and may occasionally fail

to detect proximal leg DVT. Therefore, IPG should not be considered a first-line diagnostic test for DVT (Table 30–5).

The venous ultrasound examination is inadequate for diagnosis of pelvic vein thrombosis; when ovarian or other pelvic vein thrombosis is suspected, magnetic resonance imaging (MRI) or contrast computed tomography (CT) are the preferred imaging tests.[4] Ultrasonography may suffice for detection of an extensive upper extremity DVT. However, because the clavicle may hinder the identification of small and medium-sized thromboses, alternative imaging tests should be considered (Table 30–6).

If the clinical suspicion of DVT is high even though the ultrasound is normal, this discrepancy should be pursued by obtaining another imaging test rather than by relying on the ultrasound examination as the final arbiter. The choice usually lies between *contrast venography* and *MRI*. The biggest disadvantage of contrast venography is that with massive DVT, none of the deep veins of the leg can be filled with contrast agent, and therefore, the diagnosis of DVT must be inferred merely by failure to fill the deep venous system. The results from a properly obtained MRI are usually more definitive than those of contrast venography. MRI can also help determine whether a visualized thrombus is acute, subacute, or chronic. Unlike venography, MRI is noninvasive and, therefore, has greater patient and physician acceptability. No contrast agent is needed, so the risks of anaphylaxis and renal failure are averted.

The diagnoses of *recurrent DVT* and *acute venous insufficiency* can mimic each other, yet their management differs drastically. Recurrent DVT requires immediate and intensive anticoagulation, whereas venous insufficiency can be managed by prescribing vascular compression stockings, without hospitalization. Therefore, distinguishing between these two conditions is crucial (Fig. 30–3). Duplex scanning may identify acute superimposed on chronic thrombus. However, if ultrasound examination is inadequate, MRI or contrast venography is usually recommended when confronted with this diagnostic dilemma.

PE: Nonimaging Tests

Arterial blood gases, which have been used for a generation in the diagnostic evaluation and triage of patients with suspected PE, are, in fact, quite often misleading

Table 30–5	Sensitivity and Specificity of Noninvasive Diagnostic Tests for DVT	
	Symptomatic Sensitivity/Specificity	Asymptomatic Sensitivity/Specificity
Ultrasound	Excellent/excellent	Fair/excellent
IPG	Fair/good	Poor/fair
MRI	Excellent/excellent	Excellent/excellent

Abbreviations: DVT, deep venous thrombosis; IPG, impedance plethysmography; MRI, magnetic resonance imaging.

and should generally not be done as part of the workup for PE. The room-air partial pressure of oxygen and the alveolar-arterial oxygen gradient do not differ between those patients who have PE at angiography and those suspected of PE who have normal pulmonary angiograms.[5]

The quantitative plasma D-dimer enzyme-linked immunosorbent assay (*ELISA*) level is elevated (>500 ng/ml) in more than 90% of patients with PE, reflecting plasmin's breakdown of fibrin and indicating endogenous (although clinically ineffective) thrombolysis.[6] A qualitative latex agglutination D-dimer, which is more readily available and less expensive than an ELISA, can be obtained initially; if elevated, the ELISA will also be elevated. However, if the latex agglutination is normal, an ELISA D-dimer should always be obtained because the ELISA is much more sensitive than the latex agglutination D-dimer, which cannot be used to exclude PE.

The plasma D-dimer ELISA has a high sensitivity (97%) and a high negative predictive value (94%) and can be used to help exclude PE. However, D-dimer levels have a low specificity of 45% and a low positive predictive value of only 50%.[6] The D-dimer will be elevated in postoperative patients as well as in those with myocardial infarction, sepsis, or almost any systemic illness.

Unfortunately, most hospital laboratories do not have assay kits for the plasma D-dimer ELISA and are able to perform only the latex agglutination D-dimer. Even when ELISA assay kits are available, they ordinarily require skilled technologic handling, with new standards run daily and many hours of turnaround time. However, a new, rapid, and technically simplified plasma D-dimer ELISA assay is available.[7] In addition, a novel whole-blood assay (SimpliRED) for D-dimer can be performed and interpreted at the bedside within 5 minutes.[8] The utility of these more rapid assays remains to be proved.

The *electrocardiogram* is most useful for helping to exclude acute myocardial infarction. Some patients with PE will manifest right ventricular strain, with new right bundle branch block, right axis deviation, S-wave in lead I plus Q-wave in lead III plus T-wave inversion in lead III, or new T-wave inversions in leads V_1 through V_3. PE can cause inferior ischemia (Fig. 30–4A and B), probably from extrinsic compression of the right coronary artery owing to increased right ventricular afterload.

PE: Imaging Tests

CHEST RADIOGRAPHY. A normal or near-normal chest x-ray in a dyspneic patient suggests PE. Well-established abnormalities include focal oligemia (Westermark's sign), a peripheral wedge-shaped density above the diaphragm (Hampton's hump), and an enlarged right descending pulmonary artery.

VENOUS ULTRASONOGRAPHY. About one-third of patients with PE have no imaging evidence of DVT. In these situations, perhaps the clot has already embolized to the lung or is in the pelvic veins, where ultrasonography is usually inadequate. Therefore, the workup for PE should continue if there is high clinical suspicion despite a normal ultrasound examination.

Table 30–6	Imaging Tests for DVT Diagnosis	
Location	**Modality**
Pelvic veins	MRI, contrast CT
Femoropopliteal veins	Ulrasound
Infrapopliteal veins	Ultrasound, MRI, or venogram
Upper extremity veins	Ultrasound, MRI, or venogram

Abbreviations: DVT, deep venous thrombosis; MRI, magnetic resonance imaging; CT, computed tomography.

LUNG SCANNING. The *lung scan* is the principal imaging test in the diagnostic workup of PE. The Prospective Investigation of Pulmonary Embolism Diagnosis (PIOPED)[9] found that high-probability lung scans identify only about half of hospitalized patients with PE (Table 30–7). Combining clinical suspicion with lung scan results is helpful (Table 30–8).

A perfusion scan defect indicates absent or decreased blood flow, possibly due to PE. Small particulate aggregates of albumin or microspheres labeled with a gamma-emitting radionuclide are injected intravenously and are trapped in the pulmonary capillary bed. Ventilation scans, obtained with radiolabeled inhaled gases, such as xenon or krypton, improve the specificity of the perfusion scan. Abnormal ventilation scans indicate abnormal nonventilated lung, thereby providing possible explanations for perfusion defects other than acute PE.

Lung scanning is particularly useful if the results are high probability (Fig. 30–5A), normal, or near-normal (Fig. 30–5B) for PE. A high-probability scan for PE is defined as having two or more segmental perfusion defects in the presence of normal ventilation. The diagnosis of PE is very unlikely in patients with normal and near-normal scans and, in contrast, is about 90% certain in those with high-probability scans. Interpretation of moderate- or indeterminate-probability scans is especially difficult (Fig. 30–5C and D) and may require subspecialty consultation to place the imaging results in proper context.

ECHOCARDIOGRAPHY. Echocardiography is useful for rapid triage of acutely ill patients who may have PE. It is most useful in patients who have more than one-third of the lung not perfused on lung scanning. Echocardiographic findings are often more specific than sensitive (Table 30–9). Bedside echocardiography can usually reliably differentiate among illnesses that have radically different treatments, including acute myocardial infarction, pericardial tamponade, dissection of the aorta, and PE complicated by right heart failure. Detection of right ventricular dysfunction due to PE helps risk-stratify, prognosticate, and plan optimal management.[10]

It appears that patients with PE and right ventricular dysfunction on echocardiogram have a special type of abnormality in which the right ventricular apex is spared and only the right ventricular free wall is hypokinetic. The border between the two zones is called the "hinge point." In situations when PE is not suspected, this distinct echocardiographic abnormality can be the first clue to the presence of PE.[11]

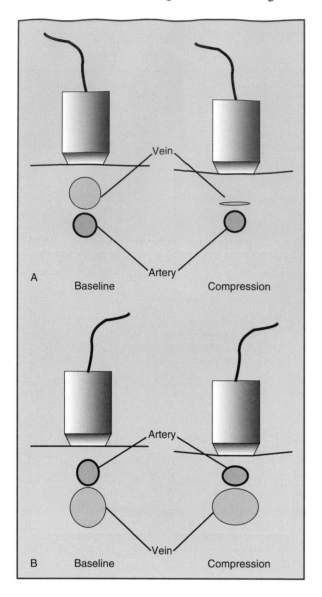

Figure 30–2

Compression venous ultrasonography. *A,* The compression maneuver is performed with the transducer held transverse to the vein. Pressure is applied to the surface of the skin through the transducer. This is transmitted to the deeper structures and causes the vein walls to collapse. Normally, as in this panel, the vein collapses easily. *B,* An abnormal compression ultrasound is defined as a failure to appose the walls of the deep vein while pressure is applied to the skin through the transducer. Sufficient pressure is applied to deform the artery wall slightly. An ancillary finding is distention of the vein. Finding echogenic material in the vein lumen reinforces the diagnosis of deep venous thrombosis (DVT). *C,* Loss of compressibility in a venous segment involved with DVT. V, common femoral vein; A, common femoral artery. *Left,* Transverse sonogram at the level of the common femoral vein and artery reveals a distended vein *(straight arrows)* lying medial to the artery *(curved arrow). Right,* Transducer has been pressed more vigorously against the skin. Vein *(straight short arrows)* now has a distorted shape and has failed to collapse completely. Sufficient pressure has been transmitted to this level of the soft tissues, causing the artery *(curved arrow)* to deform. This confirms that the common femoral vein is involved by acute DVT. (*A* and *B,* Redrawn from Polak, J.F.: Peripheral Vascular Sonography. A Practical Guide. Baltimore, Williams & Wilkins, 1992, pp. 176–177. *C,* From Polak, J.F.: Doppler ultrasound of the deep leg veins. A revolution in the diagnosis of deep vein thrombosis and monitoring of thrombolysis. Chest 99:165S–172S, 1991.)

An Integrated Approach to Diagnosis

Optimal diagnostic strategy for PE necessitates an approach that integrates clinical findings, nonimaging tests (such as the electrocardiogram, chest x-ray, or D-dimer), and radiologic imaging tests (such as ultrasonography of leg veins, lung scanning, or pulmonary angiography). Pulmonary angiography should ordinarily be pursued in the presence of moderate or high clinical suspicion for PE coupled with a nondiagnostic lung scan and negative leg ultrasound examination. When leg vein ultrasonography is undertaken as a surrogate for investigating PE, a normal result should not deter further workup because about one-third of patients with PE have normal leg ultrasound examinations.

The most widespread integrated diagnostic approach incorporates data from PIOPED and other large studies[12]

(Fig. 30–6). An alternative approach that incorporates the plasma D-dimer ELISA[13] has been tested in a series of 308 consecutive patients suspected of PE (Fig. 30–7). Neither algorithm incorporates echocardiography, which may demonstrate right ventricular dysfunction in as many as 40% of all patients with PE.

WORKUP FOR HYPERCOAGULABILITY

Once PE or DVT is diagnosed, the primary care provider must decide whether to investigate specific causes of hypercoagulability. Risk factors for venous thromboembolism formerly were divided into the two broad categories of "inherited" and "acquired." Recently, however, the theory has emerged that many PEs and DVTs occur

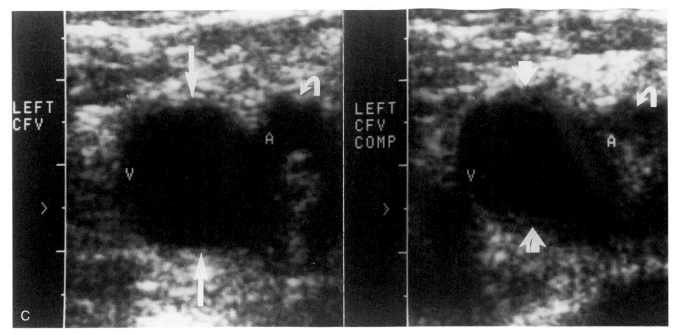

Figure 30–2
Continued

when an underlying genetic predisposition is exacerbated by a specific stress such as immobilization or pregnancy. In the Nurses' Health Study, the most important predisposing risk factors for PE were obesity, heavy cigarette smoking, and hypertension.[14] Marked obesity conferred a threefold increased risk of PE.

The classically described coagulation protein deficiencies, such as antithrombin III, protein C, and protein S, can be found in about 5% of patients with venous thrombosis. In most circumstances, determining whether these are present will be low yield and not cost-effective. However, *resistance to activated protein C* is due to a single amino acid missense mutation in Factor V (known as

Factor V Leiden) and is found more commonly in PE and DVT patients than are all of the classic coagulation protein deficiencies combined.

Patients with Factor V Leiden are at increased risk of both initial and recurrent idiopathic venous thrombosis compared with healthy controls.[15] Therefore, if a workup for hypercoagulability is pursued, assessing resistance to activated protein C is the single most cost-effective test. The next most cost-effective test is probably the plasma homocysteine level. Mild hyperhomocysteinemia is a risk factor for venous thrombosis, especially in women.[16] Finally, the most important acquired risk factor for venous thrombosis is the lupus anticoagulant (Table 30–10).

Occasionally, the diagnosis of *previously unsuspected cancer* will be established in patients with newly diagnosed venous thrombosis. For example, in a study from Malmö, Sweden, of 4399 patients undergoing venography for suspected DVT, 604 were known to have cancer at the time of venography and were excluded from further analysis. During the first 6 months after venography, 66 of 1383 patients (4.8%) with DVT were diagnosed with cancer, compared with 37 of 2412 (1.5%) who had normal venograms.[17]

Continued controversy surrounds the issue of defining the optimal cost-effective workup for occult malignancy among patients with newly diagnosed DVT. Available evidence indicates that a comprehensive medical history, physical examination—with emphasis on testicular and pelvic examinations—and routine laboratory tests such as chest x-ray, urinalysis, complete blood count, chemistries, and stool for occult blood should suffice, along with mammography.[18] Ordinarily, chest, abdominal, and pelvic CT or MRI does not appear justified. If cancer is identi-

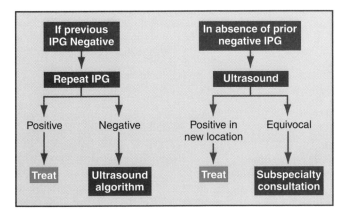

Figure 30–3
Algorithm for workup of suspected recurrent DVT. IPG, impedance plethysmography.

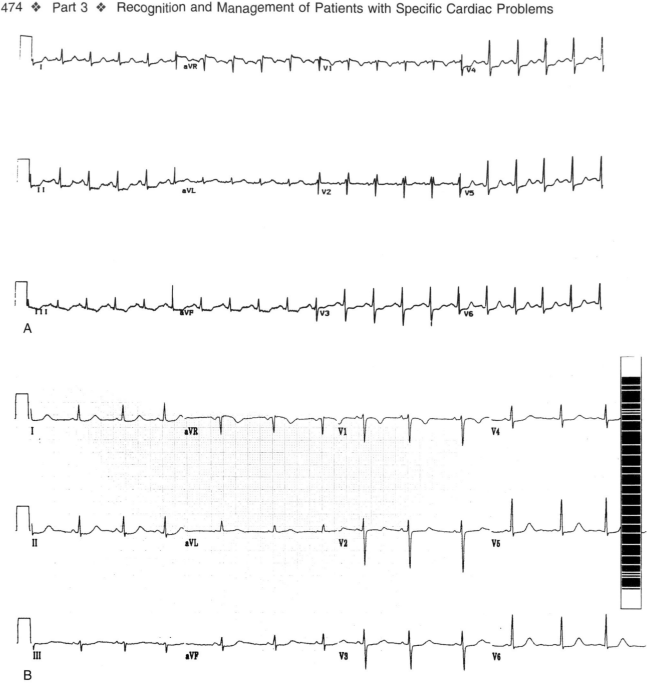

Figure 30–4

A, Electrocardiogram (ECG) of a 68-year-old woman with acute PE. Findings include sinus tachycardia, axis of 45 degrees, incomplete right bundle branch block, and inferolateral ST segment depression consistent with ischemia. *B,* After thrombolysis with recombinant tissue-type plasminogen activator (rt-PA), the patient's ECG normalized.

fied with the whole-body imaging approach, it is usually adenocarcinoma that is virtually refractory to treatment.

MANAGEMENT

Secondary Prevention

Heparin anticoagulation is the foundation for immediate management of acute PE or DVT. Heparin helps prevent new thrombus from forming and "buys time" for endogenous fibrinolytic mechanisms to lyse clot. If PE or DVT is strongly suspected, heparin should be initiated immediately, even before lung scanning or venous ultrasonography are undertaken.

Heparin can cause bleeding, thrombocytopenia,[19] and with chronic use, osteopenia. Before initiating heparin, patients should be screened for clinical evidence of active bleeding, especially with a stool analysis for occult blood. If anticoagulation is urgent, the baseline laboratory evaluation—which should include a complete blood

Table 30–7	Comparison of Scan Category with Angiogram Findings				
Scan Category	Pulmonary Embolism Present	Pulmonary Embolism Absent	Pulmonary Embolism Uncertain	No Angiogram	Total No.
High probability	102	14	1	7	124
Intermediate probability	105	217	9	33	364
Low probability	39	199	12	62	312
Near-normal/normal	5	50	2	74	131
Total	251	480	24	176	931

From PIOPED Investigators: Value of the ventilation/perfusion scan in acute pulmonary embolism. Results of the Prospective Investigation of Pulmonary Embolism Diagnosis (PIOPED). JAMA 263:2753–2759, 1990.

count, platelets, partial thromboplastin time, prothrombin time (PT) and urine dipstick for hematuria—can then be completed after heparin has been started.

For patients with PE or DVT, a traditional order for 5000 U of heparin followed by an infusion of 1000 U per hour often results in inadequate anticoagulation. An average-sized patient who is otherwise in good health should probably receive an initial bolus of 5000 to 10,000 U of heparin, followed by an infusion of approximately 1250 U per hour. Raschke and colleagues have published a particularly useful weight-based heparin nomogram (Table 30–11) that may help to achieve rapidly effective and safe levels of anticoagulation.[20]

RATIONALE FOR HEPARIN. In this era of cost-containment, it might be tempting to omit heparin altogether and begin with oral anticoagulation when patients are initially diagnosed with uncomplicated PE or DVT. Dutch investigators tested this strategy in a clinical trial of DVT patients. Unfortunately, the recurrence rate of symptomatic thrombosis was three times higher in the group that received oral anticoagulation alone.[21] Initiation of oral anticoagulants in the presence of active venous thrombosis might cause paradoxical thrombosis because of the creation of unopposed depletion of proteins C and S. Whatever the mechanism, patients with acute venous thrombosis should receive intravenous or subcutaneous heparin until oral anticoagulants have become fully effective, a process that usually takes about 5 days.

LOW-MOLECULAR-WEIGHT HEPARINS. Low-molecular-weight heparins (LMWHs) inhibit activated coagulation Factor X (FXa)—via conformational change of the antithrombin III molecule—more efficiently than they inhibit thrombin.[22] Because FXa acts earlier in the coagulation cascade than thrombin, it was hypothesized that LMWHs would produce fewer bleeding complications for a given antithrombotic efficacy. This was subsequently observed in meta-analyses of clinical trials.[23] LMWHs also react less with platelets than unfractionated heparin does and, therefore, are associated less frequently with heparin-induced thrombocytopenia.

In practice, the most relevant advantages of LMWHs are improved bioavailability and a prolonged half-life. The development of weight-adjusted dose regimens for therapeutic indications (such as DVT treatment) avoids cumbersome and costly laboratory monitoring. In contrast to unfractionated heparin, which is mainly cleared by the liver, the elimination of LMWHs occurs mostly via the kidneys.

OUTPATIENT TREATMENT OF DVT. Two separate studies reported that among low-risk patients with DVT, subcutaneously administered LMWHs could be used instead of continuous intravenous unfractionated heparin. Furthermore, almost half of LMWH patients were managed as outpatients; the others required an average of 2 to 3 days of hospitalization.[24, 25] The excellent results obtained in these two studies (Table 30–12) may

Table 30–8	PIOPED: Positive Predictive Value of PE at Angiography Based on Lung Scan Category and Clinical Likelihood of PE			
	Clinical Probability			
Lung Scan Category	*80%–100%* No. of PEs/No. of Pts. (%)	*20%–79%* No. of PEs/No. of Pts. (%)	*0%–19%* No. of PEs/No. of Pts. (%)	*0%–100%* No. of PEs/No. of Pts. (%)
High	28/29 (96)	70/80 (88)	5/9 (56)	103/118 (87)
Intermediate	27/41 (66)	66/236 (28)	11/68 (16)	104/345 (30)
Low	6/16 (40)	30/191 (16)	4/90 (4)	40/296 (14)
Very low	0/5 (0)	4/62 (6)	1/61 (2)	5/128 (4)
Total	61/90 (68)	170/569 (30)	21/228 (9)	252/887 (28)

Adapted from PIOPED Investigators: Value of the ventilation/perfusion scan in acute pulmonary embolism. Results of the Prospective Investigation of Pulmonary Embolism Diagnosis (PIOPED). JAMA 263:2757, 1990.
Abbreviations: PIOPED, Prospective Investigation of Pulmonary Embolism Diagnosis; PE, pulmonary embolism; Pts. patients.

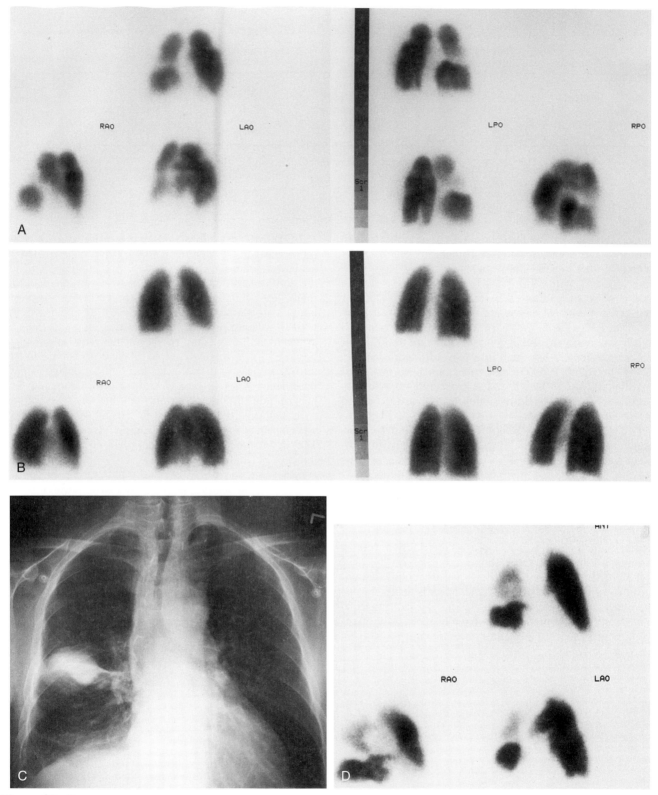

Figure 30–5

Lung scans. ANT, anterior; RAO, right anterior oblique; LAO, left anterior oblique; POST, posterior; LPO, left posterior oblique; RPO, right posterior oblique. *A,* High-probability perfusion lung scan of the same patient as in Figure 30–4, before thrombolysis. Her scan is notable for multiple bilateral segmental perfusion defects. The ventilation scan (not shown) and chest x-ray (not shown) were nearly normal. The discrepancy between near-normal ventilation ($\dot{V}$) and very abnormal perfusion ($\dot{Q}$) is called a $\dot{V}/\dot{Q}$ *mismatch. B,* Near-normal lung scan (after thrombolysis). *C,* Chest x-ray of a 54-year-old man with suspected pulmonary embolism (PE). There is a large opacity in the right middle lung zone. *D,* Perfusion scan of the same man whose chest x-ray is shown in *C.* The perfusion scan has a large defect that includes the area of the chest x-ray abnormality. The ventilation scan (not shown) is also abnormal and "matches" the chest x-ray and perfusion scan abnormalities. This perfusion scan was of "intermediate" (often called "moderate" or "indeterminate") probability of PE. (Subsequent angiography of the right middle lobe vessels revealed embolism with infarction.)

Table 30-9	Echocardiographic Signs of PE

Direct visualization of thrombus (rare)
Right ventricular dilatation
Right ventricular hypokinesis (with sparing of the apex)
Abnormal interventricular septal motion (with septum impinging on an intrinsically normal left ventricle)
Tricuspid valve regurgitation
Pulmonary artery dilatation
Lack or decreased inspiratory collapse of inferior vena cava

Abbreviation: PE, pulmonary embolism.

have been due, in part, to the vast expertise of the investigators, who worked together in "physician-nurse DVT teams" to care for these patients. Subsequently, two additional trials have confirmed the efficacy and safety of LMWH without specifically testing outpatient treatment.[25a, 25b]

Candidates for outpatient treatment must be reliable and have excellent family or community support services to enable twice-daily injections of LMWH that are based on the patient's weight. Periodic blood drawing will be needed during the first week in order to regulate the dose of warfarin. Daily telephone contact with the patient and family is also required to communicate changes in warfarin dosing and to ensure that there are no problems at home with the injection of LMWH. Often, the primary care provider will be the most knowledgeable individual about the feasibility of outpatient treatment or an abbrevi-

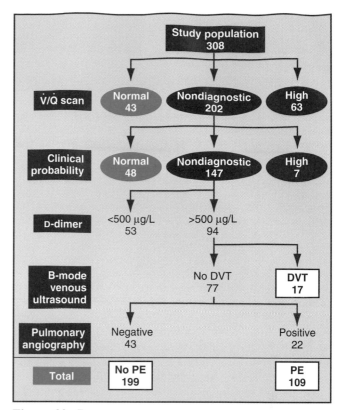

Figure 30-7

Flow chart summarizing the diagnostic workup using an integrated approach (popularized by Bounamcaux[6] in Geneva) that combines clinical probability, D-dimer enzyme-linked, immunosorbent assay (ELISA), and venous ultrasonography (US), in addition to pulmonary angiography. After 6 months of follow-up, the rate of false-negative results in the 199 patients labeled as "no PE" was 1%. V̇/Q̇, ventilation-perfusion; DVT, deep venous thrombosis; PE pulmonary embolism. (Redrawn from Perrier, A., Bounameaux, H., Morabia, A., et al.: Diagnosis of pulmonary embolism by a decision analysis–based strategy including clinical probability, D-dimer levels, and ultrasonography: A management study. Arch. Intern. Med. 156:531–536, 1996. Copyright 1996, American Medical Association.)

ated hospital stay. Either the primary care provider or a specialized "DVT team" needs to assume principal responsibility for outpatient management, especially during the first few crucial weeks when the likelihood of recurrent thrombosis or hemorrhage is greatest.

Warfarin

Warfarin is a vitamin K antagonist that prevents gamma carboxylation activation of coagulation Factors II, VII, IX, and X. The full anticoagulant effect of warfarin may not be apparent for 5 days, even if the PT, used to monitor warfarin's effect, becomes elevated more rapidly. The major toxic effect of warfarin is bleeding. Rare complications of warfarin include alopecia (that develops slowly over months), rash, and skin necrosis.

The PT, utilized to adjust the dose of warfarin, should be reported according to the International Normalized Ratio (INR), not the PT ratio or the PT expressed in seconds. The INR is essentially a "corrected" PT that adjusts

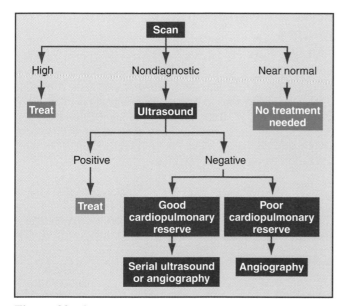

Figure 30-6

Prospective Investigation of Pulmonary Embolism Diagnosis (PIOPED)–Calgary strategy for the workup of suspected acute PE. (Redrawn from Stein, P.D., Hull, R.D., and Pineo, G.: Strategy that includes serial noninvasive leg tests for diagnostic of thromboembolic disease in patients with suspected acute pulmonary embolism based on data from PIOPED. Arch. Intern. Med. 155:2101–2104, 1995. Copyright 1995, American Medical Association.)

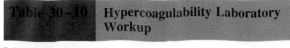 Table 30–10	Hypercoagulability Laboratory Workup

Initial PE or DVT

1. Activated protein C resistance (functional) or Factor V Leiden (DNA marker)
2. Plasma homocysteine level (treatable with B vitamins if elevated)
3. Lupus anticoagulant (may require more intensive than usual anticoagulation)

Recurrent PE or DVT (If Initial Hypercoagulability Workup Was Negative)

1. Antithrombin III deficiency
2. Protein C deficiency
3. Protein S deficiency

Abbreviations: PE, pulmonary embolism; DVT, deep venous thrombosis.

Table 30–11	The Raschke Weight-Based Heparin Nomogram
Variable	**Heparin Dose**
Initial heparin dose	80 U/kg bolus, then 18 U/kg/hr
aPTT < 35 sec (<1.2 × control)	80 U/kg bolus, then increase infusion by 4 U/kg/hr
aPTT 35–45 sec (1.2–1.5 × control)	40 U/kg bolus, then increase infusion by 2 U/kg/hr
aPTT 46–70 sec (1.5–2.3 × control)	No change
aPTT 71–90 sec (2.3–3.0 × control)	Decrease infusion by 4 U/kg/hr
aPTT > 90 sec (>3.0 × control)	Hold infusion 1 hr; then decrease infusion rate by 3 U/kg/hr

From Raschke, R.A., Reilly, B.M., Guidry, J.R., et al.: The weight-based heparin dosing nomogram compared with a "standard care" nomogram. A randomized controlled trial. Ann. Intern. Med. 119:874–881, 1993.

Abbreviation: aPTT, activated partial thromboplastin time.

for the several dozen assays used in North America and Europe. For example, within North America, a PT of 18 seconds and a PT ratio of 1.5 at one laboratory could be equivalent to a PT of 22 seconds and a PT ratio of 1.8 at another laboratory. The same blood specimen in some European laboratories might yield a PT of 30 seconds and a PT ratio of 2.5. Nevertheless, the INR for this same blood sample would be 3.0 at *all* laboratories, despite the three markedly different PT ratios and PTs given in this example.

The risk of bleeding increases as the INR increases. When the INR is used to guide anticoagulant therapy, there are fewer bleeding events compared with use of the PT ratio.[26]

CRITICAL PATHWAYS. Even within a single hospital, there can be wide variations in the management of venous thrombosis with respect to timing of the initial warfarin dose and duration of overlap of heparin and warfarin.[27] This observation provides a rationale for developing a critical pathway (Table 30–13) for the management of otherwise uncomplicated venous thrombosis.[28] Warfarin should be started, usually with a dose of 5 mg[28a] or 7.5 mg, as soon as the target partial thromboplastin time of 60 to 80 seconds has been achieved for heparin. Before heparin is in range, warfarin administration may cause paradoxical thrombosis

because of its inhibition of the natural anticoagulant protein C.

OUTPATIENT FOLLOW-UP. The efforts put into prompt diagnosis and initial therapy of venous thrombosis in hospitalized patients will be negated unless a reliable system is established to maintain effective and safe levels of outpatient anticoagulation. Although outpatient management of anticoagulation may be monotonous, repetitive, and time-intensive, expeditious and efficient outpatient monitoring and follow-up are obligatory (Table 30–14).

Special Management Issues

ISOLATED CALF VEIN THROMBOSIS. Another temptation might be to withhold anticoagulation or to use aspirin alone in patients with isolated calf vein thrombosis because such thrombi rarely embolize. However, more than one-fourth of these thrombi propagate[29] to the knee or thigh, sometimes rapidly; they may cause paradoxical embolism[30] and even fatal PE.[31] Therefore, patients with

Table 30–12	Subcutaneous LMWH versus Continuous Infusion UFH for DVT Management						
		3-Mo Follow-Up					
		Death (%)		***Recurrence (%)***		***Major Hemorrhage (%)***	
Study	**LMWH Regimen**	*LMWH*	*UFH*	*LMWH*	*UFH*	*LMWH*	*UFH*
Levine et al.[24]	Enoxaparin 1 mg/kg bid; 49% not hospitalized	4.5	6.7	5.3	6.7	2.0	1.2
Koopman et al.[25]	Nadroparin 8200 to 18,400 U bid, according to weight; 36% not hospitalized	6.9	8.1	6.9	8.6	0.5	2.0

Abbreviations: LMWH, low-molecular-weight heparin; UFH, unfractionated heparin; DVT, deep venous thrombosis; bid, twice daily.

Table 30–13	Critical Pathway for Proximal Leg DVT			
Day 1	**Day 2**	**Day 3**	**Day 4**	**Day 5**

Tests

Standard admitting labs Screen for cancer: physical examination, CXR, urinalysis, and stool for occult blood Defer testing for hypercoagulable state to outpatient setting PTT q 4–6 hr until two consecutive results within 60–80 sec PT/INR q day with target INR of 2.0–3.0	CBC, platelets qod PTT q day if stable at 60–80 sec	Arrange for inpatient or outpatient mammogram if woman >40 yr without recent mammogram		

Activity

Bed or chair, depending on pain and need to control edema	Ambulate when pain allows after 24 hr of therapeutic heparin			

Treatment

Local heat	Fit for graduated compression stockings			

Medications

In Emergency Department

Heparin bolus and drip: use weight-based nomogram Alternately, give 7500 U bolus and 1250 U/hr drip Call research nurse re: DVT trial eligibility	Heparin Adjust per nomogram Warfarin Stool softener prn	Heparin Adjust per nomogram Warfarin Stool softener prn	Heparin Adjust per nomogram Warfarin Stool softener prn	Consider discharge for uncomplicated patients after 5 days of heparin and when INR = 2–3 Warfarin Stool softener prn

On Floor

Adjust heparin by nomogram Pain relief medications prn Begin warfarin q A.M. or q P.M. as soon as PTT ≥ 60 sec Initial dosage: 5 mg or 7.5 mg q day × 2 days Stool softener				

Education

1. Risks and complications of DVT (including symptoms of pulmonary embolism) 2. Risks and complications of heparin treatment 3. Need for regulation of heparin 4. Explain activity level	1. Rationale for warfarin 2. Need for daily labs 3. Explain INR target range 4. Explain INR versus PT 5. Teach how to use stockings	1. Provide written instructions (e.g., warfarin teaching book) 2. Warfarin video 3. Review risk factor reduction strategies (e.g., smoking cessation)	Reinforce warning symptoms and signs of DVT complications	1. Arrange for next INR within 1–3 days 2. Identify the primary care physician who will be responsible for follow-up care 3. Specify how patient will communicate with the primary care physician 4. Phone or fax inpatient PT/INRs and warfarin dosages to primary care physician

Adapted from American Journal of Medicine, vol 100, Pearson, S.D., Lee, T.H., McCabe-Hassan, S., et al.: A critical pathway to treat proximal lower-extremity deep vein thrombosis, pp 283–289, Copyright 1996, with permission from Excerpta Medica Inc.

Abbreviations: DVT, deep venous thrombosis; labs, laboratory tests; CXR, chest x-ray; PTT, partial thromboplastin time; q, every; PT, prothrombin time; INR, International Normalized Ratio; CBC, complete blood count; qod, every other day; prn, as needed.

Table 30–14	Suggestions for Outpatient Anticoagulation Monitoring

Communicate explicitly and in detail among physicians and nurses from different disciplines (e.g., internal medicine and obstetrics and gynecology). **Make no assumptions** about who will regulate anticoagulation.

Explain to the patient and the family the rationale for anticoagulation and the major risks from too-intensive therapy (i.e., hemorrhage) and too-little therapy (i.e., thromboembolism). The patient and the family should understand the relationship between the PT, the INR, and dosing adjustments of anticoagulant.

Consider fingerstick testing of PT/PTT.

Use a software-supported electronic surveillance system rather than a paper notebook–based system, whenever possible. This system should flag patients in whom an expected laboratory value has not yet been reported.

Arrange for laboratory values to be reported as the INR rather than as the PT in seconds or as the PT ratio.

Consider establishment of "anticoagulation clinics."

Abbreviations: PT, prothrombin time; INR, International Normalized Ratio; PTT, partial thromboplastin time.

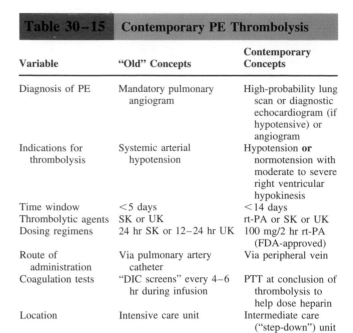

Table 30–15	Contemporary PE Thrombolysis	
Variable	**"Old" Concepts**	**Contemporary Concepts**
Diagnosis of PE	Mandatory pulmonary angiogram	High-probability lung scan or diagnostic echocardiogram (if hypotensive) or angiogram
Indications for thrombolysis	Systemic arterial hypotension	Hypotension **or** normotension with moderate to severe right ventricular hypokinesis
Time window	<5 days	<14 days
Thrombolytic agents	SK or UK	rt-PA or SK or UK
Dosing regimens	24 hr SK or 12–24 hr UK	100 mg/2 hr rt-PA (FDA-approved)
Route of administration	Via pulmonary artery catheter	Via peripheral vein
Coagulation tests	"DIC screens" every 4–6 hr during infusion	PTT at conclusion of thrombolysis to help dose heparin
Location	Intensive care unit	Intermediate care ("step-down") unit

Abbreviations: PE, pulmonary embolism; SK, streptokinase; UK, urokinase; rt-PA, recombinant tissue-plasminogen activator; FDA, U.S. Food and Drug Administration; DIC, disseminated intravascular coagulation; PTT, partial thromboplastin time.

documented calf vein thrombosis should receive routine treatment with anticoagulation.

CANCER PATIENTS. There is controversy over whether cancer patients with DVT or PE should be treated initially with heparin alone or with heparin followed by warfarin. If thrombosis occurs in more than one extremity (particularly superficial thrombosis in one limb and DVT in a different extremity), these patients have Trousseau's syndrome and may require a lifelong course of heparin in order to avoid recurrent thrombosis. Although no data are available, one generally recommended approach is to initiate a trial of warfarin, with a target INR of at least 3.0, and to reserve heparin for those patients who fail warfarin.

A prospective cohort study compared the efficacy and safety of oral anticoagulation in patients with and without cancer. The rates of bleeding and recurrent thrombosis were not statistically significantly different in the two groups of patients. However, target INRs were more difficult to maintain in the cancer patients. Therefore, cancer patients with venous thrombosis probably require more frequent monitoring of their prothrombin times than noncancer patients.[32]

ANTIPHOSPHOLIPID SYNDROME. The risk of recurrent thrombosis is high in this patient population. Therefore, whenever possible, patients with DVT or PE who also have the antiphospholipid-antibody syndrome should be maintained, often indefinitely, with a target INR of at least 3.0.[33] Chronic heparin is rarely needed.

Overall DVT Management Plan

Anticoagulation is the foundation of DVT treatment (Fig. 30–8). Patients with active and major bleeding will need placement of an inferior vena caval filter if they have pelvic or proximal leg DVT. Although the filter will not prevent continued venous thrombosis, it is usually effective in preventing fatal PE arising from the pelvic or

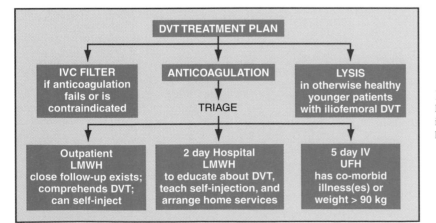

Figure 30–8
Deep venous thrombosis (DVT) treatment plan. IVC, inferior vena caval; LMWH, low-molecular-weight heparin; IV, intravenous.

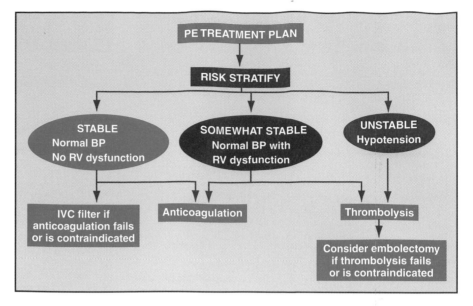

Figure 30–9
Pulmonary embolism (PE) treatment plan.
BP, blood pressure; RV, right ventricular;
IVC, inferior vena caval.

deep leg veins. The occasional patient with massive ilio-femoral venous thrombosis should be considered for thrombolytic therapy if there are no contraindications. However, only about 1 in 20 patients with DVT is an appropriate candidate for thrombolysis.

The major challenge in DVT management is triage of the vast majority of patients who will require long-term anticoagulation. Their medical, socioeconomic, and community health network environment should be factored into a decision regarding possible outpatient treatment of DVT or shortened hospitalization with LMWH.

Management: Secondary Prevention Versus Primary Therapy of PE

Anticoagulation, the cornerstone of PE management, is called "treatment" but also constitutes *secondary prevention* of recurrent PE. PEs differ markedly in size and

physiologic effect. Therefore, *risk stratification* is crucial to determine which patients will do well with anticoagulation alone and which should be considered candidates for primary treatment with thrombolysis or embolectomy (Fig. 30–9).

Echocardiography in patients with large PEs has a major role in assessing prognosis and in helping to determine whether anticoagulation alone will be effective. Patients with normal systemic arterial pressure and normal right ventricular function generally have a good prognosis after PE. For such individuals, secondary prevention is usually adequate with anticoagulation alone or placement of an inferior vena caval filter if major bleeding from anticoagulation is likely.

Systemic arterial hypotension, often a manifestation of cardiogenic shock in PE patients, confers an ominous prognosis. However, presentation with frank hemodynamic collapse is quite unusual. Much more commonly, PE patients present with normal systemic arterial pressure combined with occult right ventricular dysfunction. The

Thromboembolism Event	Low Risk*	Moderate Risk†	High Risk‡	Very High Risk§
Calf vein thrombosis (%)	2	10–20	20–40	40–80
Proximal vein thrombosis (%)	0.4	2–4	4–8	10–20
Clinical PE (%)	0.2	1–2	2–4	4–10
Fatal PE (%)	0.002	0.1–0.4	0.4–1.0	1–5
Successful preventive strategies	No specific measures	ES, LDUH (q 12 hr), and IPC	LDUH (q 8 hr), LMWH, and IPC	LMWH, oral anticoagulants, IPC (+ LDUH or LMWH), and ADH

Table 30–16   Classification of Level of Risk (Based on Published Data)

From Clagett, G.P., Anderson, F.A., Heit, J., et al.: Prevention of venous thromboembolism. Chest 108:312S–334S, 1995.
Abbreviations: MI, myocardial infarction; PE, pulmonary embolism; ES, elastic stockings; LDUH, low-dose unfractionated heparin; q, every; IPC, intermittent pneumatic compression; LMWH, low-molecular-weight heparin; ADH, adjusted-dose heparin.
  * Uncomplicated minor surgery in patients younger than 40 yr with no clinical risk factors.
  † Major surgery in patients older than 40 yr with no other clinical risk factors.
  ‡ Major surgery in patients older than 40 yr who have additional risk factors or MI.
  § Major surgery in patients older than 40 yr plus previous venous thromboembolic or malignant disease or orthopedic surgery or hip fracture or stroke or spinal cord injury.

Table 30–17	Strategies for Prevention of PE and DVT
Condition	**Strategy**
Orthopedic surgery	Warfarin (INR 2.0–2.5) × 4–6 wk IPC ± warfarin Enoxaparin 30 mg SC twice daily × 5–14 days for THR or TKR (and possibly for 1 mo[43]) Ardeparin 50 anti-Xa U/kg SC twice daily for TKR Danaparoid 750 anti-Xa U SC twice daily for THR
Gynecologic cancer surgery	Warfarin (target INR 2.0–2.5) ± IPC Standard heparin 5000 U q 8 hr ± IPC Dalteparin 2500 or 5000 U SC once daily Enoxaparin 40 mg SC once daily
Urologic surgery	Warfarin (target INR 2.0–2.5) ± IPC
Thoracic surgery	IPC plus standard heparin 5000 U q 8 hr
High-risk general surgery (e.g., prior VTE, current cancer, or obesity)	IPC *or* graded-compression stockings plus standard heparin 5000 U q 8 hr Dalteparin 2500 or 5000 U SC once daily Enoxaparin 40 mg SC once daily
General, gynecologic, or urologic surgery (without prior VTE) for benign conditions	Graded-compression stockings plus standard heparin 5000 U q 12 hr IPC alone
Neurosurgery, eye surgery, or whenever pharmacologic prophylaxis is contraindicated	Graded-compression stockings ± IPC
Pregnancy (with prior VTE)	
Antepartum	Graded compression stockings plus daily exercise program plus serial leg examinations Subcutaneous standard or LMWH
Peripartum	IPC ± SC standard or LMWH
Postpartum	Warfarin (target INR 2.0–3.0) with SC standard or LMWH continued until target INR attained
Medical conditions	Graded-compression stockings ± heparin 5000 U q 8–12 hr IPC alone

Abbreviations: PE, pulmonary embolism; DVT, deep venous thrombosis; INR, International Normalized Ratio; IPC, intermittent pneumatic compression; SC, subcutaneous; THR, total-hip replacement; TKR, total-knee replacement; q, every; VTE, venous thromboembolism; LMWH, low-molecular-weight heparin.

presence of right ventricular hypokinesis, even in the absence of systemic arterial hypotension, suggests the possibility that primary therapy of PE with thrombolysis or embolectomy will be beneficial.

Thrombolysis appears to be lifesaving in patients with massive PE.[34] Thrombolysis may also reduce the rate of recurrent PE in patients with preserved blood pressure but worsening right ventricular dysfunction,[35, 36] which may often be detected only on echocardiogram.

In our current paradigm, we consider patients potentially "hemodynamically unstable" if they have right ventricular dysfunction, even in the presence of normal systemic arterial pressure. Since the mid-1980s, the ad-

Table 30–18	Clinical Manifestations of Cor Pulmonale

Symptoms

Dyspnea on exertion
Weight gain (from fluid retention)
Abdominal distention
Syncope

General Physical Examination

Peripheral cyanosis and acrocyanosis
Digital clubbing
Distended neck veins
Abdominal ascites and peripheral edema
Hepatic congestion with right upper quadrant tenderness
Hepatojugular reflux

Cardiac Examination

Right ventricular lift
Palpable P_2; widely split S_2 with increased P_2 intensity
Right-sided S_3
Murmurs of tricuspid regurgitation and pulmonic insufficiency

Abbreviations: P_2, second pulmonic heart sound; S_2, second heart sound; S_3, third heart sound.

ministration of thrombolysis to PE patients has been streamlined so that it is safer, less expensive, and less time-consuming (Table 30–15). If thrombolysis is contraindicated or fails, suction catheter embolectomy or open surgical embolectomy may be considered for hemodynamically unstable patients.[36]

The likelihood of success can be optimized by proceeding with these primary therapeutic interventions as quickly as possible. Waiting for the development of pressor-dependent cardiogenic shock leads to an unfavorable metabolic state and poor prognosis, with increased catecholamine release and decreased perfusion of vital organs.

Prevention

Prevention strategies are of paramount importance and should be based on a patient's level of risk (Table 30–16). Virtually all hospitalized patients whose anticipated

Table 30–19	Common Causes of Cor Pulmonale	
Type	**Mechanism**	**Examples**
Obstructive vascular	Impedance to flow through large pulmonary arteries	Pulmonary thromboembolism
Obliterative vascular	Impedance to flow through small pulmonary blood vessels	Primary pulmonary hypertension, pulmonary veno-occlusive disease, collagen vascular disease
Vasoconstrictive	Impedance to flow from hypoxia-induced vasoconstriction	Chronic mountain sickness, sleep apnea syndrome
Nonvascular	Pulmonary parenchymal disease	Chronic obstructive pulmonary disease

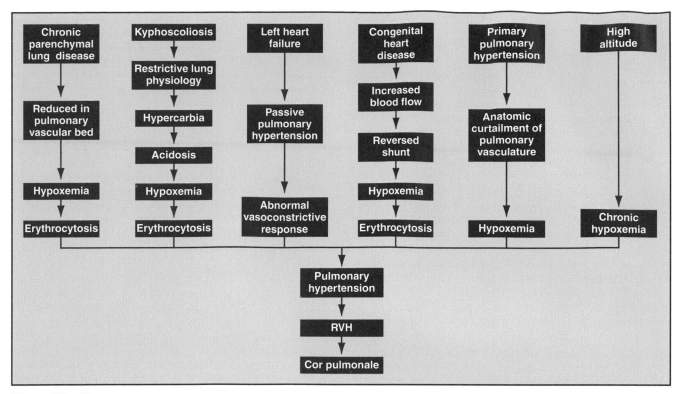

Figure 30–10

Flow diagram demonstrating the cause and pathophysiology of cor pulmonale. The final common pathway for the group of diseases that make up cor pulmonale is advanced, long-standing pulmonary hypertension. RVH, right ventricular hypertrophy. (Redrawn from Goldhaber, S.Z.: Cor pulmonale, primary pulmonary hypertension, and cardiac tumors. *In* Braunwald, E. [ed.-in-chief]: Essential Atlas of Heart Diseases. Philadelphia, Current Medicine, 1997, p. 10.2.)

Figure 30–11

Therapy for patients with advanced cor pulmonale. CPAP, continuous positive airway pressure. (Adapted from Goldhaber, S.Z.: Cor pulmonale, primary pulmonary hypertension, and cardiac tumors. *In* Braunwald, E. [ed.-in-chief]: Essential Atlas of Heart Diseases. Philadelphia, Current Medicine, 1997, p. 10.6.)

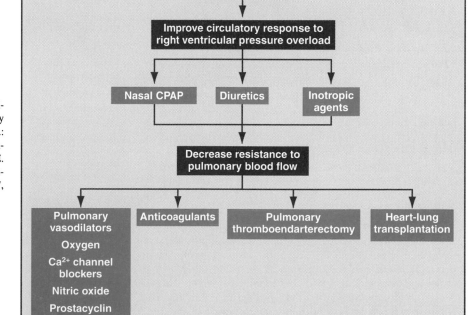

length of stay exceeds 2 days should receive mechanical, pharmacologic, or combined mechanical plus pharmacologic prophylaxis against venous thromboembolism (Table 30–17). This approach is cost-effective and medicolegally correct. *Mechanical (nonpharmacologic) measures* include graded-compression stockings, intermittent pneumatic compression of the legs or feet, and placement of an inferior venal caval filter. *Pharmacologic measures* include heparin and warfarin.

Three LMWH and one heparinoid, danaparoid, have been approved for prophylaxis. Enoxaparin is authorized by the U.S. Food and Drug Administration as a fixed dose of 30 mg subcutaneously twice daily for 7 to 10 days among patients undergoing elective total hip or knee replacement and as a fixed once daily dose of 40 mg for patients undergoing high risk general surgery. Dalteparin, another LMWH, is approved for high-risk general and pelvic surgery, in a dose of 2500 or 5000 U subcutaneously once daily. Ardeparin is the only LMWH approved for weight-adjusted dosing (50 anti-Xa units/kg twice daily) and is used to prevent venous thrombosis after total-knee replacement.[36a] Danaparoid is approved for prophylaxis of total-hip replacement but it currently is much more costly compared with the three LMWHs.

Despite available strategies for prevention of venous thrombosis, several groups of patients remain at high risk. For example, about one-third of patients in a medical intensive care unit had DVT in one survey.[37] Surprisingly, standard prophylaxis measures often appeared to fail; the overall DVT rate in patients who received any heparin or pneumatic compression prophylaxis was 34% compared with 32% in those who did not receive any prophylaxis.

DVT is a common complication in patients with major trauma and, in one major center, occurred in 58% of patients.[38] Enoxaparin 30 mg subcutaneously twice daily was compared with heparin 5000 U twice daily in a randomized controlled trial. With enoxaparin, the overall DVT rate was reduced from 44% to 31%, and the proximal DVT rate was reduced from 15% to 6%.[39]

COR PULMONALE

Cor pulmonale is usually manifested by right heart failure associated with pulmonary hypertension (Table 30–18) and can be caused by a wide spectrum of respiratory and pulmonary vascular diseases (Table 30–19 and Fig. 30–10). Undoubtedly, chronic obstructive pulmonary disease is the most common cause of cor pulmonale. Restrictive lung diseases due to intrinsic pathology (e.g., interstitial fibrosis) or extrinsic causes (e.g., obesity or kyphoscoliosis) can also precipitate pulmonary hypertension owing to alveolar hypoxia.

PE is probably the most common pulmonary vascular cause of cor pulmonale. Patients with acute PE and cor pulmonale should be considered for primary therapy with thrombolysis or embolectomy.

Patients with chronic PE and cor pulmonale should receive lifelong anticoagulation and, in addition, may be candidates for lifelong continuous oxygen therapy. However, pulmonary thromboendarterectomy is necessary if one wishes to correct the underlying problem. After institution of cardiopulmonary bypass and deep hypothermia, incisions are made in both pulmonary arteries and continued into the lower lobe branches in order to remove organized thrombus.[40] When successful, pulmonary hypertension will abate over the first few postoperative months, and quality of life will improve.

Among properly selected patients at experienced centers, the mortality rate for thromboendarterectomy is between 5% and 10%. The two major causes of mortality are: (1) inability to remove sufficient thrombotic material at surgery, resulting in persistent postoperative pulmonary hypertension and right ventricular dysfunction, and (2) severe reperfusion lung injury. Thus, at designated centers, pulmonary thromboendarterectomy can be performed with good results and at an acceptable risk among patients debilitated from cor pulmonale owing to PE.

Primary pulmonary hypertension, a diagnosis of exclusion, must be differentiated from cor pulmonale owing to chronic PE.[41] Pulmonary angiography or spiral CT scanning can rule out central pulmonary artery thrombosis. Patients with primary pulmonary hypertension should receive lifelong anticoagulation. As pulmonary artery pressures increase, these individuals should be counseled to accept continuous oxygen therapy. The most drastic intervention to improve the natural history of this illness is single-lung transplantation. Another advance in management includes the use of high doses of

Table 30–20	Indications for Subspecialty Referral

Diagnostic Dilemmas

Discordance between ultrasound and clinical suspicion
MRI not readily available or results indeterminate
Suspected recurrent DVT with equivocal ultrasound
Allergy to contrast agent or renal insufficiency

Therapeutic Dilemmas

Pregnancy
Iliofemoral venous thrombosis (massive DVT)
Massive PE
PE with normal systemic arterial pressure but right ventricular dysfunction on echocardiogram
Consideration of thrombolysis

Complications of Therapy

Hemorrhage
Heparin-induced thrombocytopenia

Mechanical Intervention

Angioplasty
Stenting
Suction thrombectomy or embolectomy
Surgery

Difficult Management Issues

Uncertainty whether outpatient or shortened hospitalization strategies should be used to treat DVT
Duration of anticoagulation
Current pregnancy
Genetic counseling and future pregnancies
Recurrent PE or DVT
Cor pulmonale due to pulmonary vascular disease

Abbreviations: MRI, magnetic resonance imaging; DVT, deep venous thrombosis; PE, pulmonary embolism.

calcium channel blockers,[42] which are effective in about one-fifth of these patients. This therapy is often guided by the pulmonary vascular response to acute drug testing performed in the cardiac catheterization laboratory. If calcium channel blockers are ineffective, lifelong continuous-infusion prostacyclin (which requires a permanent indwelling central venous catheter) or nitric oxide can be administered. Controversy exists as to whether prostacyclin can actually cause "healing" of the endothelium or whether its use merely serves as a bridge to lung transplantation.

SUBSPECIALTY REFERRAL

Despite the variety of algorithms available to help diagnose and manage PE and DVT, these conditions often pose difficult dilemmas for the primary care provider. Many patients will have individual problems outside the realm of standard critical pathways. Under these circumstances, subspecialty referral is probably appropriate (Table 30–20).

Although management of cor pulmonale owing to pulmonary vascular disease almost always requires subspecialty consultation (Fig. 30–11) the primary care provider will have a crucial role in helping the patient to choose or decline heroic interventions such as surgical bullectomy, lung transplantation, or pulmonary thromboendarterectomy. Many patients will require warfarin anticoagulation, which the primary care physician can regulate. Mobile patients with cor pulmonale, particularly those without a significant other, will often be reluctant to utilize continuous oxygen therapy. The primary care provider in this case can serve to encourage the patient to comply with this life-prolonging measure. Finally, for those patients who undertake lifelong continuous-infusion prostacyclin, the primary care physician can coordinate care of vascular access sites and prostacyclin dose adjustment. Most important, the primary care physician will be able to play a central role in giving both moral support and educational updates that the patient and family will need to cope with this ominous illness.

References

1. Wells, P.S., Lensing, A.W.A., Davidson, B.L., et al.: Accuracy of ultrasound for the diagnosis of deep venous thrombosis in asymptomatic patients after orthopedic surgery. A meta-analysis. Ann. Intern. Med. 122:47–53, 1995.
2. Jongbloets, L.M.M., Lensing, A.W.A., Koopman, M.M.W., et al.: Limitations of compression ultrasound for the detection of symptomless postoperative deep vein thrombosis. Lancet 343:1142–1144, 1994.
3. Simons, G.R., Skibo, L.K., Polak, J.F., et al.: Utility of leg ultrasonography in suspected symptomatic isolated calf deep venous thrombosis. Am. J. Med. 99:43–47, 1995.
4. Simons, G.R., Piwnica-Worms, D.R., and Goldhaber, S.Z.: Ovarian vein thrombosis. Am. Heart J. 126:641–647, 1993.
5. Stein, P.D., Goldhaber, S.Z., Henry, J.W., and Miller, A.C.: Arterial blood gas analysis in the assessment of suspected acute pulmonary embolism. Chest 109:78–81, 1996.
6. Bounameaux, H., de Moerloose, P., Perrier, A., and Reber, G.: Plasma measurement of D-dimer as diagnostic aid in suspected venous thromboembolism: An overview. Thromb. Haemost. 71:1–6, 1994.
7. de Moerloose, P., Desmarais, S., Bounameaux, H., et al.: Contribution of a new, rapid, individual and quantitative automated D-dimer ELISA to exclude pulmonary embolism. Thromb. Haemost. 75:11–13, 1996.
8. Wells, P.S., Brill-Edwards, P., Stevens, P., et al.: A novel and rapid whole-blood assay for D-dimer in patients with clinically suspected deep vein thrombosis. Circulation 91:2184–2187, 1995.
9. PIOPED Investigators: Value of the ventilation perfusion scan in acute pulmonary embolism. Results of the Prospective Investigation of Pulmonary Embolism Diagnosis (PIOPED). JAMA 263:2753–2759, 1990.
10. Wolfe, M.W., Lee, R.T., Feldstein, M.L., et al.: Prognostic significance of right ventricular hypokinesis and perfusion lung scan defects in pulmonary embolism. Am. Heart J. 127:1371–1375, 1994.
11. McConnell, M.V., Solomon, S.D., Rayan, M.E., et al.: Regional right ventricular dysfunction detected by echocardiography in acute pulmonary embolism. Am. J. Cardiol. 78:469–473, 1996.
12. Stein, P.D., Hull, R.D., and Pineo, G.: Strategy that includes serial noninvasive leg tests for diagnosis of thromboembolic disease in patients with suspected acute pulmonary embolism based on data from PIOPED. Arch. Intern. Med. 155:2101–2104, 1995.
13. Perrier, A., Bounameaux, H., Morabia, A., et al.: Diagnosis of pulmonary embolism by a decision analysis based strategy including clinical probability, D-dimer levels, and ultrasonography: A management study. Arch. Intern. Med. 156:531–536, 1996.
14. Goldhaber, S.Z., Grodstein, F., Stampfer, M.J., et al.: A prospective study of risk factors for pulmonary embolism in women. JAMA, 277:642–645, 1997.
15. Ridker, P.M., Miletich, J.P., Stampfer, M.J., et al.: Factor V Leiden and risks of recurrent idiopathic venous thromboembolism. Circulation 92:2800–2802, 1995.
16. den Heijer, M., Koster, T., Blom, H.J., et al.: Hyperhomocysteinemia as a risk factor for deep-vein thrombosis. N. Engl. J. Med. 334:759–762, 1996.
17. Nordström, M., Lindbad, B., Anderson, H., et al.: Deep venous thrombosis and occult malignancy: An epidemiological study. BMJ 308:891–894, 1994.
18. Cornuz, J., Pearson, S.D., Creager, M.A., et al.: Initial evaluation for cancer in patients with symptomatic idiopathic deep-vein thrombosis. Ann. Intern. Med. 125:785–793, 1996.
19. Warkentin, T.E.: Heparin-induced thrombocytopenia: IgG-mediated platelet activation, platelet microparticle generation, and altered procoagulant/anticoagulant balance in the pathogenesis of thrombosis and venous limb gangrene complicating heparin-induced thrombocytopenia. Transfus. Med. Rev. 4:249–258, 1996.
20. Raschke, R.A., Reilly, B.M., Guidry, J.R., et al.: The weight-based heparin dosing nomogram compared with a "standard care" nomogram. A randomized controlled trial. Ann. Intern. Med. 119:874–881, 1993.
21. Brandjes, D.P.M., Heijboer, H., Buller, H.R., et al.: Acenocoumarol and heparin compared with acenocoumarol alone in the initial treatment of proximal-vein thrombosis. N. Engl. J. Med. 327:1485–1489, 1992.
22. Weitz, JI.: Low-molecular-weight heparins. N. Engl. J. Med. 337:688–698, 1997.
23. Bounameaux, H., and Goldhaber, S.Z.: Uses of low-molecular-weight heparin. Blood Rev. 9:213–219, 1995.
24. Levine, M., Gent, M., Hirsh, J., et al.: A comparison of low-molecular-weight heparin administered primarily at home with unfractionated heparin administered in the hospital for proximal deep-vein thrombosis. N. Engl. J. Med. 334:677–681, 1996.
25. Koopman, M.M.W., Prandoni, P., Piovella, F., et al.: Treatment of venous thrombosis with intravenous unfractionated heparin administered in the hospital as compared with subcutaneous low-molecular-weight heparin administered at home. N. Engl. J. Med. 334:682–687, 1996.
25a. The COLUMBUS Investigators: Low-molecular-weight heparin in the treatment of patients with venous thromboembolism. N. Engl. J. Med. 337:657–662, 1997.
25b. Simonneau, G., Sors, H., Charbonnier, B., et al., THÉSÉE Study Group: A comparison of low-molecular-weight heparin with unfractionated heparin for acute pulmonary embolism. N. Engl. J. Med. 337:663–669, 1997.
26. Andrews, T.C., Peterson, D.W., Doeppenschmidt, D., et al.: Com-

plications of warfarin therapy monitored by the International Normalized Ratio versus the prothrombin time ratio. Clin. Cardiol. 18: 80–82, 1995.

27. Schoeneberger, R.A., Pearson, S.D., Goldhaber, S.Z., and Lee, T.H.: Variation in the management of deep vein thrombosis: Implications for the potential impact of a critical pathway. Am. J. Med. 100:278–282, 1996.

28. Pearson, S.D., Lee, T.H., McCabe-Hassan, S., et al.: A critical pathway to treat proximal lower-extremity deep vein thrombosis. Am. J. Med. 10:283–289, 1996.

28a. Harrison, L., Johnston, M., Massicotte, M.P., et al.: Comparison of 5-mg and 10-mg loading doses in initiation of warfarin therapy. Ann. Intern. Med. 126:133–136, 1997.

29. Lagerstedt, C.J., Olsson, C.G., Fagher, B.O., et al.: Need for long-term anticoagulant treatment in symptomatic calf-vein thrombosis. Lancet 2:515–518, 1985.

30. Stöllberger, C., Slany, J., Schuster, I., et al.: The prevalence of deep venous thrombosis in patients with suspected paradoxical embolism. Ann. Intern. Med. 119:461–465, 1993.

31. Pellegrini, V.D., Jr., Langhans, M.J., Totterman, S., et al.: Embolic complications of calf thrombosis following total hip arthroplasty. J. Arthroplasty 8:449–457, 1993.

32. Bona, R.D., Sivjee, K.Y., Hickey, A.D., et al.: The efficacy and safety of oral anticoagulation in patients with cancer. Thromb. Haemost. 74:1055–1058, 1995.

33. Khamashta, M.A., Cuadrado, M.J., Mujic, F., et al.: The management of thrombosis in the antiphospholipid-antibody syndrome. N. Engl. J. Med. 332:993–997, 1995.

34. Jerjes-Sanchez, C., Ramirez-Rivera, A., Garcia, M. de L., et al.: Streptokinase and heparin versus heparin alone in massive pulmonary embolism: A randomized controlled trial. J. Thromb. Thrombolysis 2:227–229, 1995.

35. Goldhaber, S.Z., Haire, W.D., Feldstein, M.L., et al.: Alteplase versus heparin in acute pulmonary embolism: Randomised trial assessing right ventricular function and pulmonary perfusion. Lancet 341:507–511, 1993.

36. Konstantinides, S., Geibel, A., Olschewski, M., et al.: Impact of thrombolytic treatment on the prognosis of hemodynamically stable patients with major pulmonary embolism: Results of a Multicenter Registry. Circulation 96:882–888, 1997.

36a. Heit, J.A., Berkowitz, S.D., Bona, R., et al.: Efficacy and safety of low molecular weight heparin (ardeparin sodium) compared to warfarin for the prevention of venous thromboembolism after total knee replacement surgery: A double-blind, dose-ranging study. Thromb. Haemost. 77:32–38, 1997.

37. Hirsch, D.R., Ingenito, E.P., and Goldhaber, S.Z.: Prevalence of deep venous thrombosis among patients in medical intensive care. JAMA 274:335–337, 1995.

38. Geerts, W.H., Code, K.I., Jay, R.M., et al.: A prospective study of venous thromboembolism after major trauma. N. Engl. J. Med. 331:1601–1606, 1994.

39. Geerts, W.H., Jay, R.M., Code, K.I., et al.: A comparison of low-dose heparin with low-molecular-weight heparin as prophylaxis against venous thromboembolism after major trauma. N. Engl. J. Med. 335:701–707, 1996.

40. Fedullo, P.F., Auger, W.R., Channick, R.N., et al.: A multidisciplinary approach to chronic thromboembolic pulmonary hypertension. In Goldhaber, S.Z. (ed.): Cardiopulmonary Diseases and Cardiac Tumors. Braunwald, E. (ser. ed.): Atlas of Heart Diseases. Vol. 3. Philadelphia, Current Medicine, 1995, pp. 7.1–7.25.

41. Rich, S., Kaufmann, E., and Levy, P.S.: The effect of high doses of calcium-channel blockers on survival in primary pulmonary hypertension. N. Engl. J. Med. 327:76–81, 1992.

42. Rubin, L.J.: Primary pulmonary hypertension. N. Engl. J. Med. 336:111–117, 1997.

43. Bergqvist, D., Benoni, G., Björgell, O., et al.: Low-molecular-weight heparin (enoxaparin) as prophylaxis against venous thromboembolism after total hip replacement. N. Engl. J. Med. 335:696–700, 1996.

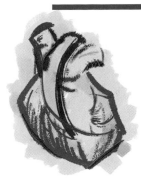

Chapter 31

Recognition and Management of Patients with

Cardiomyopathies

G. William Dec

The cardiomyopathies are a diverse group of cardiac disorders characterized by primary involvement of the ventricular myocardium. The myocardial dysfunction is not related to coronary atherosclerosis or to valvular, congenital, or hypertensive heart disease. The World Health Organization has recommended that the cardiomyopathies be classified by their anatomic appearance and abnormal physiology into dilated, hypertrophic, and restrictive types.[1] The dilated cardiomyopathies are characterized by biventricular dilatation and impaired systolic function; the hypertrophic cardiomyopathies by abnormal wall thickening, myocardial hypercontractility, and impaired diastolic function; and the restrictive cardiomyopathies by an abnormally stiff myocardium with impaired ventricular relaxation but well-preserved contractile function[2] (Table 31–1).

DILATED CARDIOMYOPATHIES

Pathology

Cardiac enlargement is the hallmark of dilated cardiomyopathy. Dilatation of all four cardiac chambers is typical (Fig. 31–1), although sometimes the disease involves only one side of the heart. Although the thickness of the ventricular wall may be mildly increased, the increase is insufficient to match the degree of ventricular dilatation. Histopathologically, there is evidence for varying degrees of myocyte degeneration, eccentric hypertrophy, and atro-

phy of the myofibrils. Interstitial and replacement fibrosis may be extensive.

A wide variety of diseases may directly affect the myocardium and result in either permanent or transient systolic dysfunction. Dilated cardiomyopathy probably represents a common expression of myocardial damage that has resulted from one or more yet to be defined myocardial insults. All potentially reversible causes of dilated cardiomyopathy should be considered, particularly excessive alcohol consumption, toxins such as cocaine or drug hypersensitivity myocarditis, ischemic heart disease, and endocrine disorders[3, 4] (Table 31–2).

Alcoholic Cardiomyopathy

Excessive alcohol consumption is one of the most common identifiable causes of dilated cardiomyopathy.[3, 5] There is substantial evidence that chronic alcohol use depresses cardiac function.[5] The typical patient with alcoholic cardiomyopathy is a middle-aged man who has consumed at least 80 gm of alcohol daily for at least a decade. As alcohol use has increased in adolescents, it is no longer rare to see young adults with this disorder. Alcoholic liver disease is rare in such patients. Cardiac failure is reversible in the majority of patients with recently diagnosed cardiomyopathy if total abstinence from alcohol is achieved.

Toxic Cardiomyopathy

Dilated cardiomyopathy can result from chronic exposure to drugs or toxins—the most common being cocaine

Table 31–1	Hemodynamic and Morphometric Features of the Cardiomyopathies		
Feature	Dilated	Hypertrophic	Restrictive
LV ejection fraction	<45%	65%–90%	50–70% <40% (late)
LV cavity size	Increased	Normal or decreased	Normal Increased (late)
Stroke volume	Markedly decreased	Normal or increased	Normal or increased
Volume : mass ratio	Increased	Decreased	Markedly decreased
Diastolic compliance	Normal to decreased	Markedly decreased	Markedly decreased
Other features	Mild/moderate MR/TR are common	Dynamic obstruction MR may be present	Often mimics constrictive pericarditis

Adapted with permission from DeSanctis, R.W., and Dec, G.W.: The cardiomyopathies. Section 1, Subsection XIV, in *Scientific American Medicine,* Dale, D.C., and Federman, D. (eds.). Copyright 1995, Scientific American Inc. All rights reserved.
Abbreviations: LV, left ventricular; MR, mitral regurgitation; TR, tricuspid regurgitation.

or antineoplastic chemotherapeutic agents, especially the anthracycline drugs. *Anthracycline cardiotoxicity* is directly related to cumulative doses of the drug and increases dramatically in patients who receive more than $400–450$ mg/m^2. Patients with preexisting left ventricular dysfunction or those who receive either concomitant mediastinal radiation or other antineoplastic drugs, such as dactinomycin, cyclophosphamide, mitomycin, or dacarbazine, are at increased risk of developing anthracycline cardiotoxicity. Although congestive heart failure may develop acutely during drug administration or within 2 months of completing the chemotherapeutic cycle, a latent period of many months or even years is more commonly observed. Mortality can exceed 60% once overt heart failure has developed.

Human Immunodeficiency Virus Cardiomyopathy

Cardiomyopathy is also common among patients with the acquired immunodeficiency syndrome (AIDS) (Table 31–3). Evidence of ventricular dysfunction has been reported in up to 20% of patients with AIDS. Fluctuations in ejection fraction are not uncommon in such patients. Myocarditis is evident at autopsy in approximately 50% of patients who die of active human immunodeficiency virus (HIV) infection. Myocardial dysfunction in patients

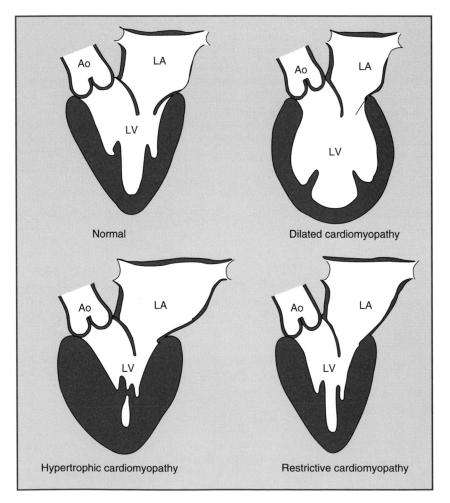

Figure 31–1
Schematic representation of the three morphometric types of cardiomyopathy—dilated, hypertrophic, and restrictive. Ao, aorta; LA, left atrium; LV, left ventricle. (Redrawn from Waller, B.F.: Pathology of the cardiomyopathies. J. Am. Soc. Echocardiog. 1:4–19, 1988.)

Table 31–2 Causes of Potentially Reversible Dilated Cardiomyopathy

Toxins

Ethanol
Cobalt
Antiretroviral agents (AZT, ddI, ddC)
Phenothiazines
Cocaine
Mercury

Metabolic Abnormalities

Nutritional (thiamine, selenium, carnitine, and taurine deficiencies)
Endocrinologic (hypothyroidism, acromegaly, thyrotoxicosis, pheno-chromocytoma)
Electrolyte disturbances (hypocalcemia, hypophosphatemia)
Hemochromatosis

Inflammatory/Infectious/Infiltrative

Infectious
    Viral (coxsackievirus, adenovirus, cytomegalovirus)
    Rickettsial (Rocky Mountain spotted fever, Q fever)
    Bacterial (diphtheria)
    Parasitic (toxoplasmosis, trichinosis)
    Spirochetal (leptospirosis, Lyme disease)
Inflammatory/infiltrative
Collagen vascular disorders (sarcoidosis)
Hypersensitivity myocarditis
Hemochromatosis
Peripartum
Sarcoidosis

Miscellaneous

Tachycardia-induced
Idiopathic

Abbreviations: AZT, zidovudine (azidothymidine); ddI, didanosine (dideoxyinosine); ddC, zalcitabine (dideoxycytidine).

with AIDS may result from active intracellular HIV replication (HIV myocarditis) or opportunistic infections such as toxoplasmosis or cytomegalovirus affecting the heart. More importantly, reversible cardiac toxicity has been described for commonly used drugs such as zidovudine (also known as AZT [azidothymidine]) and interferon alfa, agents commonly used to treat HIV and its complications. As HIV-infected patients live longer, it can be anticipated that more of them will demonstrate cardiac involvement.

Peripartum Cardiomyopathy

This is a specific dilated cardiomyopathy that usually develops during the last 6 weeks of pregnancy or in the first 3 months after parturition. A minority of cases have been shown by endomyocardial biopsy to result from active myocarditis, and these may respond to immunosuppressive therapy. Peripartum cardiomyopathy is more commonly observed in women with pre-eclampsia or multiple births. Although the majority of cases resolve with restoration of normal ventricular function, a sizable minority of patients may be left with chronic left ventricular dysfunction or require transplantation for rapidly progressive disease. Subsequent pregnancies should be avoided if residual cardiomegaly or impaired contractile function persists. Recurrence is rare if ventricular function has normalized.

Inflammatory Heart Disease

Viral myocarditis is a frequent cause of acute dilated cardiomyopathy, particularly in children and adolescents. It has long been hypothesized that subclinical viral myocarditis can initiate an autoimmune reaction that culminates in the development of an unequivocal dilated cardiomyopathy. While coxsackievirus and echoviruses frequently cause myopericarditis, these forms of myocarditis are usually mild and self-limited. Although enteroviral RNA can be recovered from endomyocardial biopsy fragments in 25% to 50% of patients with dilated cardiomyopathy, biopsy evidence of both an inflammatory infiltrate and myocyte necrosis is required to establish a histologic diagnosis of acute myocarditis. When rigorous histologic criteria are employed, only about 5% to 10% of patients with dilated cardiomyopathy have unequivocal evidence of myocarditis. The percentage is even lower when symptoms have been present for more than 1 year. Myocarditis should be considered in patients who present with acute biventricular dysfunction, unexplained life-threatening ventricular arrhythmias, or widespread T-wave inversions that occur during or immediately after an acute viral illness. The natural history of acute myocarditis is variable and ranges from early death through chronic dilated cardiomyopathy to complete recovery (Fig. 31–2).

Familial Cardiomyopathy

Cases of familial dilated cardiomyopathy are more frequent than had previously been recognized. Indeed, 20% of patients with idiopathic dilated cardiomyopathy have at least one first-degree relative with impaired ventricular function. Except for family history, no clinical or histopathologic characteristics distinguish familial from nonfamilial forms of the disease. The mode of inheritance is generally autosomal dominant, but it can be genetically heterogenous, and there are reports of autosomal recessive, X-linked recessive, and mitochondrial inheritance. Carnitine deficiency is a familial metabolic deficiency producing dilated cardiomyopathy that improves with carnitine repletion. Genotypic identification of specific mutations in dilated cardiomyopathy patients may ultimately lead to the identification and treatment of asymptomatic carriers who are at risk for development of symptomatic disease.

Table 31–3 Cardiac Lesions in AIDS

Myocarditis
Endocarditis
Pericarditis
Dilated cardiomyopathy
Kaposi's sarcoma
Malignant lymphoma
Arteriopathy
Myocardial infarction

From Glazier, J.J.: Specific heart muscle disease. *In* Abelmann, W.H. (vol. ed.): Cardiomyopathies, Myocarditis and Pericardial Disease. Braunwald, E. (ser. ed.) *Atlas of Heart Diseases.* Vol. 2. Philadelphia, Current Medicine, 1994, p. 4.2.
Abbreviation: AIDS, acquired immunodeficiency syndrome.

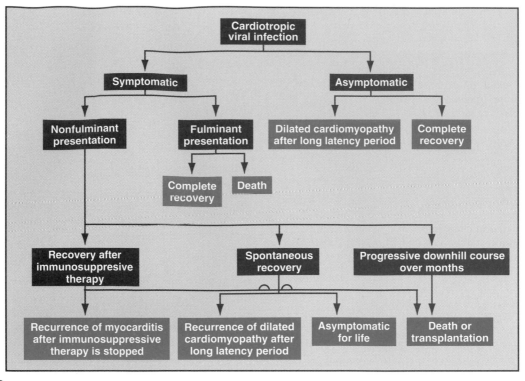

Figure 31–2

The natural history of human myocarditis. Most patients with mild symptoms of acute myocarditis are not seen by cardiologists, and most of these patients appear to recover fully. Of the patients with symptomatic heart disease typically seen by cardiologists, a small number have fulminant presentations and either die in the acute stage or appear to recover fully. Of the remaining patients with myocarditis, a few are characterized by a progressive downhill course over a period of months to years that ends in death from heart failure or intractable arrhythmias. Some spontaneously recover and remain asymptomatic for life, and others have an asymptomatic period followed by development of dilated cardiomyopathy. (Redrawn from Herskowitz, A., and Ansari, A.A.: Myocarditis. *In* Abelmann, W.H. [vol. ed.]: Cardiomyopathies, Myocarditis, and Pericardial Disease. Braunwald, E. [ser. ed.]: Atlas of Heart Diseases. Vol. 2. Philadelphia, Current Medicine, 1995, pp. 9.1–9.24.)

Idiopathic Dilated Cardiomyopathy

More than 75 specific heart muscle diseases can produce dilated cardiomyopathy.[3] However, in a sizable minority of cases, a cause is not evident despite extensive evaluation, and these patients are labeled as having idiopathic dilated cardiomyopathy.[6] This condition probably represents a final common pathway of a variety of toxic, metabolic, or infectious processes that result in acute or ongoing myocardial damage. The clinical presentation and prognosis of idiopathic dilated cardiomyopathy do not differ substantially from most secondary forms of dilated cardiomyopathy.

Ischemic Cardiomyopathy

It is uncertain whether intermittent bouts of myocardial ischemia can produce dilated cardiomyopathy in patients with *normal* epicardial coronary vessels. Although abnormal microvascular reactivity, possibly consequent to coronary vasospasm, could lead to myocardial necrosis and scarring, little direct evidence supports this theory. Small vessel disease or microvascular dysfunction is more common in patients with dilated cardiomyopathy who present

with angina-like chest pain than with symptoms of congestive heart failure.

Recurrent or extensive myocardial infarction can lead to a cardiomyopathic picture with ventricular dilatation, impaired contractility, and heart failure symptoms. Chronically ischemic but viable (so-called hibernating) myocardium can contribute to left ventricular dysfunction and ischemic cardiomyopathy. Not uncommonly, patients, particularly those with long-standing diabetes mellitus, may lack a history of angina pectoris or prior myocardial infarction despite extensive coronary artery disease, and such individuals may be clinically indistinguishable from those with idiopathic dilated cardiomyopathy. Given the high prevalence of ischemic heart disease, the possibility that impaired ventricular function may be improved through coronary revascularization should always be considered. The potential of coronary revascularization (through either coronary bypass surgery or angioplasty) is directly proportional to the extent of ischemic but noninfarcted myocardium that can be adequately revascularized.

Clinical Presentations

Patients with acute myocarditis generally have an acute presentation characterized by sudden onset of heart failure, palpitations, pleuritic or anginal-like chest pain, or even cardiogenic shock. The development and progression of symptoms is usually more gradual in patients with dilated cardiomyopathy. A minority of patients may have asymptomatic left ventricular dysfunction for months or years. The most common features are those related to left ventricular failure, particularly fatigue and dyspnea. Diminished cardiac output results in fatigue and generalized weakness. Exercise intolerance is also common and relates to both impaired cardiac output and reduced skeletal muscle performance. Right heart failure is a late and ominous feature and is associated with a particularly poor prognosis. Exertional or rest dyspnea due to chronic pulmonary congestion is a frequent symptom. Acute pulmonary edema frequently occurs in acute myocarditis but is uncommon in chronic dilated cardiomyopathy. It often occurs in response to a precipitating event such as a respiratory infection or alteration in cardiac rhythm.

Palpitations are common and reflect the occurrence of either atrial or ventricular ectopic beats. Syncope is a rare initial manifestation. When it occurs, it portends a poor prognosis. Ischemic chest discomfort occurs in 25% to 50% of patients despite angiographically normal coronary arteries and is believed to be due to a reduction in dilator reserve of the coronary vasculature. Nonanginal chest pain secondary to pulmonary emboli or abdominal pain secondary to hepatic congestion is commonly observed in the late stages of disease.

Physical Findings

The physical findings reflect the underlying severity of the left ventricular dysfunction and range from subtle signs such as unexplained premature ventricular beats or cardiomegaly on chest film to overt, decompensated biventricular heart failure. Although pulmonary rales may be heard in patients with acute dilated cardiomyopathy, clear lung fields are most common. The jugular venous pulse is often elevated, and a prominent V-wave and brisk Y descent indicative of tricuspid regurgitation are often evident. Precordial palpation typically reveals a diffuse, laterally displaced, and heaving apical impulse; often, the right ventricle is palpable as well. The most prevalent auscultatory findings are gallop sounds. A fourth heart sound (S_4 or atrial) gallop is almost universally heard when sinus rhythm is present. A third heart sound (S_3 or ventricular) gallop is typically audible in more advanced disease or during periods of decompensation. An S_3 gallop can often be elicited by stressing the heart with gentle exercise. Systolic murmurs are generally not related to primary valvular disease; the most common is mitral regurgitation consequent to progressive left ventricular dilatation. The murmurs are usually pansystolic and of grade I–II/VI. They are related to left or right ventricular cavity size and may wax and wane with worsening or improvement in heart failure. The presence of a systolic murmur louder than grade II/VI should suggest the presence of primary valvular disease.

Signs of right heart failure are initially present in fewer than 50% of patients, but they commonly develop as left ventricular dysfunction worsens and the patient enters a chronic phase of heart failure (see Chap. 22).

Diagnostic Evaluation

Noninvasive Studies

Patients presenting with unexplained dilated cardiomyopathy (see Chap. 14) should undergo a diagnostic evaluation limited initially to those studies necessary to determine the type of cardiac abnormality, uncover correctable causative factors, evaluate prognosis, and guide treatment. The American College of Cardiology and American Heart Association Task Force on Heart Failure has issued guidelines on the diagnostic approach to patients with heart failure (and cardiomyopathy) that are summarized in Table 31–4. Any evaluation should begin with a careful search for reversible secondary causes of dilated cardiomyopathy. Screening blood studies should include serum phosphorus, calcium, creatinine, urea nitrogen, and serum iron (to rule out hemochromatosis).

The chest film may suggest sarcoid or have infiltrates indicating an eosinophilic syndrome. It typically reveals

---

Table 31–4   **Diagnostic Evaluation of New-Onset Dilated Cardiomyopathy**

Class I Studies (Usually Indicated, Always Acceptable)

CBC and urinalysis
Electrolytes, renal function, glucose, phosphorus, calcium, albumin, TSH level
Chest film, electrocardiogram
Transthoracic Doppler echocardiogram
Noninvasive stress testing in patients who lack angina but who have a high probability of underlying ischemic heart disease, a known prior myocardial infarction, or extensive areas of hibernating myocardium (*Note:* Patients should be suitable candidates for revascularization if extensive ischemia is detected)

Class II Studies (Acceptable but of Uncertain Efficacy; Controversial)

Serum iron/ferritin
Noninvasive stress testing in all patients with unexplained dilated cardiomyopathy
Coronary angiography in all patients with unexplained dilated cardiomyopathy
Endomyocardial biopsy in patients with:
  Cardiomyopathy of recent onset (generally <6 mo) and rapid deterioration in ventricular function
  Clinically suspected myocarditis
  Cardiomyopathy and a systemic disease known to involve the myocardium (e.g., sarcoidosis, hemochromatosis)

Class III Studies (Generally Not Indicated)

Routine 24-hr ambulatory ECG monitoring
Serial echocardiography in clinically stable patients
Routine right heart catheterization to guide medical therapy
Endomyocardial biopsy in chronic dilated cardiomyopathy
Cardiac catheterization in patients who are not candidates for revascularization, valve replacement, or cardiac transplantation

Adapted from American College of Cardiology/American Heart Association Task Force Report: Guidelines for the evaluation and management of heart failure. J. Am. Coll. Cardiol. 26:1384–1385, 1995.
Abbreviation: CBC, complete blood count; TSH, thyroid-stimulating hormone; ECG, electrocardiogram.

cardiomegaly, often with four-chamber enlargement. Pulmonary venous redistribution is a frequent finding, whereas interstitial or alveolar edema is uncommon.

The electrocardiogram (ECG) is usually abnormal but initially may show only nonspecific repolarization abnormalities, atrial or ventricular enlargement, or sinus tachycardia. A wide variety of arrhythmias (most importantly, atrial fibrillation or ventricular tachycardia) may occur consequent to patchy interstitial fibrosis. Conduction system abnormalities are noted in more than 80% of patients and may include first-degree atrioventricular (AV) block, left anterior hemiblock, nonspecific conduction delays, and most commonly, left bundle branch block. Interestingly, right bundle branch block is quite rare. Conduction abnormalities are more common in patients with long-standing disease, progress over time, and are markers of increasing interstitial fibrosis or myocyte hypertrophy. Left ventricular hypertrophy and poor R-wave progression are also frequent ECG findings. Localized QS waves, resembling the typical pattern of myocardial infarction in the anterior leads, may be present when there is extensive left ventricular fibrosis, even without a discrete myocardial scar, or when present in multiple leads. QS waves more often reflect previous myocardial infarction and, in patients with cardiomyopathy, reflect an ischemic origin.

Transthoracic Doppler echocardiography is the most useful initial noninvasive diagnostic procedure, since it can rapidly assess systolic and diastolic function, chamber dimensions, and ventricular wall thickness and exclude clinically significant valvular heart disease. Left ventricular ejection fraction is usually less than 40%. Although global hypokinesis is often found, segmental wall motion abnormalities may occur in up to 60% of patients because of altered regional wall stress and cannot reliably be used to differentiate ischemic from nonischemic causes. Doppler interrogation often detects clinically inaudible mild to moderate mitral and tricuspid regurgitation.

Patients with a prior myocardial infarction and congestive heart failure, but without angina pectoris, are commonly evaluated with stress testing to detect ischemic or hibernating myocardium (see Chap. 18). Quantitative stress thallium scintigraphy generally provides the most clinically relevant information regarding viable myocardium in patients with left ventricular dysfunction. Radionuclide ventriculography with technetium-99m allows quantitative assessment of systolic and diastolic function but should be reserved for patients in whom echocardiography proves unsatisfactory.

Invasive Studies

Cardiac catheterization is not necessary in all patients with dilated cardiomyopathy and is not indicated for serial assessment. Right heart catheterization is most useful for tailoring medical therapy in patients with severe symptoms despite optimal treatment. Baseline hemodynamic assessment before initiation of conventional medical therapy is seldom indicated. Coronary angiography is indicated for patients with symptomatic angina pectoris, significant areas of ischemic myocardium on noninvasive stress imaging, and with unexplained cardiomyopathy and a high probability of coronary artery disease (e.g., those

with multiple coronary risk factors, segmental left ventricular dysfunction on echocardiography, or QS waves on ECGs) who are potential candidates for coronary revascularization).

Right ventricular endomyocardial biopsy has generally been used to differentiate patients with myocarditis from those with idiopathic dilated cardiomyopathy. The low diagnostic yield (< 10%) combined with the lack of an effective treatment for myocarditis has led to re-evaluation of its clinical relevance. Biopsy should be reserved for patients with rapidly progressive ventricular dysfunction and clinically suspected myocarditis (based on a preceding viral prodrome, associated pericarditis, or elevation of creatine kinase) or those in whom an active systemic disease and possible cardiac involvement (e.g., sarcoidosis, hemochromatosis, or Loeffler's eosinophilic myocarditis) is suspected.

Differential Diagnosis

Dilated cardiomyopathy must be distinguished from valvular heart disease, coronary artery disease, and hypertensive heart disease. Features that aid in differentiating dilated cardiomyopathy with accompanying functional mitral regurgitation from that due to primary mitral valve disease include the absence of a history of mitral valve prolapse, the absence of significant mitral valve calcification, the relative infrequency of atrial fibrillation, the severe depression of ventricular function, and the presence of left atrial enlargement that is proportional to the degree of left ventricular dilatation.

The clinical manifestations of end-stage aortic valve disease, either stenosis or regurgitation, may also resemble dilated cardiomyopathy. The murmur of severe aortic stenosis may be faint, but it is rarely absent. Severe elevation in left ventricular end-diastolic pressure may mask signs of aortic regurgitation and cause the diastolic murmur to disappear. Suspicion of aortic valve disease should be confirmed by noninvasive or invasive cardiac evaluation. Hypertensive heart disease is usually the result of severe, long-standing systolic and diastolic hypertension. Diastolic heart failure (see Chap. 22) rather than systolic contractile dysfunction is the more common finding in this disorder.

Natural History

Asymptomatic cardiomegaly, the first stage of dilated cardiomyopathy, may go undetected for months or years. Although the rate of progression from asymptomatic cardiomegaly to overt symptomatic disease is unknown, symptomatic patients generally have a poor prognosis. The most common complication of dilated cardiomyopathy is progressive heart failure, which is the cause of death in 75% of patients. Sudden cardiac death caused by ventricular arrhythmias or electromechanical dissociation is also frequent, especially in patients with episodes of ventricular tachycardia and severe left ventricular dysfunction. Evidence of systemic embolism or pulmonary embolism, or both, may be found at autopsy in up to 50% of patients with chronic dilated cardiomyopathy.

Emboli can also cause catastrophic complications, including embolic myocardial infarction, but they are an infrequent (<5%) cause of death.

The prognosis varies considerably, with some patients experiencing a fulminant course resulting in death or transplantation within weeks or months of presentation. Conversely, many patients do remarkably well for years. Survival data from tertiary referral centers report mortality rates of 25% to 30% at 1 year and approximately 50% at 5 years. The poor survival in early retrospective series may have reflected a substantial referral bias, since patients with more advanced disease or treatment failures are more likely to be referred to tertiary centers. More recent observations suggest substantially better survival, with an average 5-year mortality of 20% (Fig. 31–3). This reduction in mortality probably reflects earlier disease detection, a shift to population-based studies, and better treatment. A minority of patients may demonstrate a remarkably long period of clinical stability. Spontaneous improvement in ventricular function (an ejection fraction rise >10%) occurs in 20% to 40% of cases and occurs most frequently within 6 months of the initial presentation. Improvement in ventricular function is independent of the initial ejection fraction but is more likely to occur in patients with acute, rather than chronic, dilated cardiomyopathy. Active myocardial inflammation on biopsy or by radionuclide imaging techniques and lesser degrees of myocardial damage on endomyocardial biopsy correlate weakly with the likelihood of spontaneous improvement in ventricular function.

The most reliable indicator of prognosis is the severity of left ventricular dysfunction (Table 31–5). Although the relationship is certainly not linear, the lower the ejection fraction or the greater the degree of left ventricular

enlargement, the poorer the long-term prognosis. Other morphologic features that are associated with a poor prognosis include lesser degrees of left ventricular hypertrophy, a more spherical ventricular cavity, and right ventricular dysfunction.

Clinical features that portend a more favorable prognosis include female gender, age under 55 years, and New York Heart Association class less than IV. Syncope, a persistent S_3, or right-sided heart failure on physical examination all predict a poor prognosis. Although elevated serum concentrations of norepinephrine, atrial natriuretic factor, and renin have been shown to have prognostic value, they are seldom used in clinical practice. Cardiopulmonary exercise testing can provide important prognostic information and quantify a patient's extent of functional limitation. Maximal systemic oxygen uptake below 10 ml/kg/min predicts a 1-year mortality rate as high as 50% and is frequently used to identify patients in need of cardiac transplantation. Careful subjective assessment of daily functional capacity provides similar, albeit less quantitative, prognostic information and is the preferred method for following most patients, except those with advanced symptoms being considered for investigational therapies or transplantation.

Treatment

Medical Therapy

In addition to the general management of heart failure described in Chapter 22,[7] disease-specific therapies should also be considered. Abstinence from alcohol should be prescribed whenever an alcoholic cardiomyopathy is suspected. Phlebotomy is useful in treating hemochromatosis but is most effective when instituted before the development of significant left ventricular dysfunction. Correction of metabolic or endocrinologic abnormalities, such as hyperthyroidism, hypothyroidism, acromegaly, or pheochromocytoma, typically results in restoration of normal ventricular function. Adequate rate control of rapid atrial fibrillation can also lead to resolution of the cardiomyopathy.

ANTICOAGULATION. Patients with dilated cardiomyopathy are at increased risk for systemic or pulmonary embolism owing to blood stasis in the hypocontractile ventricle. The risk is greatest in patients with severe left ventricular dysfunction, established or paroxysmal atrial fibrillation, a history of thromboembolism, or echocardiographic evidence of intracardiac thrombus. Controlled trials have not evaluated the efficacy of systemic anticoagulation for dilated cardiomyopathy patients in normal sinus rhythm. Chronic warfarin therapy for such patients should be reserved for those at high risk for thromboembolism (severe heart failure, mural ventricular thrombus, history of systemic or pulmonary embolization, recent thrombophlebitis), and the International Normalized Ratio should be adjusted to achieve a value of 2 to 3.

ANTIARRHYTHMIC THERAPY. A variety of ventricular arrhythmias, including nonsustained asymptomatic ventricular tachycardia, are present during 24-hour ambulatory monitoring in the majority of patients with dilated cardiomyopathy. Sudden cardiac death accounts for 20%

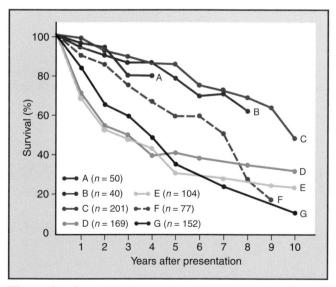

Figure 31–3

Survival among patients with dilated cardiomyopathy in seven published series reported from 1965 to 1989. The numbers in parentheses are the number of patients in each study. (Redrawn with permission from Dec, G.W., and Fuster, V.: Idiopathic dilated cardiomyopathy. N. Engl. J. Med. 331:1565, 1994. Copyright 1994 Massachusetts Medical Society. All rights reserved.)

Table 31–5	Predictors of Poor Outcome in Dilated Cardiomyopathy

Clinical Features

NYHA class IV symptoms
Older age (> 55 yr) at presentation
Male gender
Ischemic cause
History of syncope
Persistent S_3 gallop
Right-sided heart failure signs
Inability to tolerate ACE inhibitors

Hemodynamic and Ventriculographic Findings

Left ventricular ejection fraction < 20%
Right ventricular dysfunction
Pulmonary hypertension
Right atrial pressure > 8 mm Hg
Pulmonary capillary wedge pressure > 16–18 mm Hg
Cardiac index < 2.2 U/min/m²

Neurohormonal Abnormalities

Hyponatremia (serum sodium < 137 mmol/L)
Enhanced sympathetic tone (elevated plasma norepinephrine or resting sinus tachycardia)
Increased plasma atrial natriuretic factor or renin

Functional Limitations

Maximal oxygen uptake < 12 ml/kg/min

Arrhythmia Pattern

History of prior cardiac arrest
Symptomatic or asymptomatic nonsustained runs of ventricular tachycardia
Second- or third-degree AV block

Abbreviations: NYHA, New York Heart Association; S_3, third heart sound; ACE, angiotensin-converting enzyme; AV, atrioventricular.

to 40% of the mortality in this population. Unfortunately, Holter monitoring, signal-averaged ECG, and even electrophysiologic testing have not proved useful for risk stratification of patients with dilated cardiomyopathy and asymptomatic nonsustained ventricular tachycardia. Antiarrhythmic drugs have not been shown to decrease mortality, and many of these drugs actually increase risk through proarrhythmic actions. Thus, the empirical use of antiarrhythmic medications in patients with asymptomatic dilated cardiomyopathy cannot be supported at this time.

However, patients with dilated cardiomyopathy and aborted sudden cardiac death, cardiac syncope, or symptomatic ventricular tachyarrhythmias do benefit from suppression of arrhythmia. Although many respond to empirical amiodarone, the low rates of long-term success, high incidence of drug toxicity, and the increased proarrhythmic risk suggest that an implantable cardioverter-defibrillator, rather than chronic antiarrhythmic therapy, should now be considered to be the preferred treatment for such patients. Its effect on long-term survival among patients with advanced disease is less clear, since many patients will be spared an arrhythmic death only to die of progressive heart failure within 2 to 3 years.

Surgical Therapy

Given the high prevalence of ischemic heart disease and its role as the principal cause of heart failure in North America, the possibility that ventricular function may be improved through coronary revascularization should always be considered in patients with symptomatic ischemic dilated cardiomyopathy.[8] Systolic dysfunction may reflect not only fixed scar but also partially reversible effects of intermittent or prolonged ischemia (i.e., hibernating myocardium) (see Chap. 18). For patients with ischemic cardiomyopathy without angina pectoris, the potential benefit of coronary bypass surgery or multivessel angioplasty is directly proportional to the extent of ischemic, but noninfarcted, myocardium that can be adequately revascularized. The presence of reversible ischemia can often be surmised from a history of angina pectoris or demonstration of ischemic ECG changes. Favorable surgical outcome is more likely if reversible defects in two or more myocardial regions can be demonstrated by thallium scintigraphy or positron emission tomography during exercise or pharmacologic stress testing. There is growing evidence that surgical revascularization, even in the absence of angina pectoris, can improve symptoms of heart failure, exercise capacity, and long-term prognosis in carefully selected patients with extensive multivessel coronary artery disease and significantly impaired ventricular function. Patients most likely to benefit have three-vessel coronary artery disease, good distal vessels, a left ventricular ejection fraction exceeding 20%, mild or absent mitral regurgitation, and a left ventricular end-diastolic dimension less than 70 mm.

Cardiac transplantation is an effective treatment for dilated cardiomyopathy patients with advanced heart failure, but its use is limited to a small percentage of these because of an inadequate number of cardiac donors (see Chap. 22). Electrically driven, totally implantable left ventricular assist devices, particularly the Novacor and Heartmate models, may ultimately represent a better long-term solution for severe, intractable heart failure.

Referral to Cardiologists

The majority of patients with dilated cardiomyopathy do not require referral to a cardiologist for subspecialty consultation. In general, patients who may benefit from

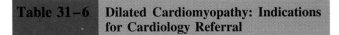

Table 31–6	Dilated Cardiomyopathy: Indications for Cardiology Referral

Progressive left ventricular dilatation, deterioration in ejection fraction, or worsening symptoms despite medical therapy
Active myocarditis
Rapidly progressive cardiac symptoms in a systemic disease known to affect the myocardium for consideration of endomyocardial biopsy
Syncope
Symptomatic or asymptomatic nonsustained ventricular tachycardia on ambulatory or in-hospital ECG monitoring
Patients with NYHA class III/IV heart failure symptoms for consideration of cardiac transplantation or participation in a heart failure clinical trial
Known ischemic cardiomyopathy with anginal symptoms or a positive stress imaging study for consideration of coronary angiography or coronary revascularization.

Abbreviations: ECG, electrocardiogram; NYHA, New York Heart Association.

specialized cardiovascular consultation include individuals who have failed conventional therapy and have progressive heart failure symptoms (Table 31–6). Patients with acute myocarditis, as well as those being considered for transplantation or enrollment in an investigational heart failure trial, should also be referred. Likewise, those who may require an invasive procedure, either an endomyocardial biopsy or coronary angiography, should be considered for referral. Finally, patients with known or suspected ischemic cardiomyopathy and poor ventricular function who are being considered for revascularization should undergo cardiac evaluation.

HYPERTROPHIC CARDIOMYOPATHIES

Hypertrophic cardiomyopathies are characterized by inappropriate myocardial hypertrophy, often predominantly involving the interventricular septum, and a hyperdynamic left ventricle.[9, 10] The myocardial hypertrophy is disproportionate to the accompanying hemodynamic load. The most prominent pathophysiologic abnormality in hypertrophic cardiomyopathy is diastolic dysfunction owing to abnormal left ventricular stiffness. A distinctive clinical feature of the disease in some patients with hypertrophic cardiomyopathy is a dynamic pressure gradient in the subaortic outflow region of the left ventricle (see Table 31–1).

Cause

Although hypertrophic cardiomyopathy may appear to develop sporadically, this condition is usually genetic. A hereditary pattern is evident on family history in more than 50% of patients, and it is transmitted as an autosomal dominant trait.[11, 12] Genetic linkage techniques reveal that the majority of familial cases are due to an abnormality on chromosome 14, which contains the gene responsible for encoding the beta heavy chain of cardiac myosin. However, a number of different genotypic abnormalities may be responsible for the development of cardiac hypertrophy. There is now convincing evidence that the specific genetic defect strongly predicts prognosis. Specific mutations have been identified that have been associated with an increased risk of sudden death and a dramatic reduction in life expectancy. It is anticipated that in the near future screening for genotypic abnormalities will be widely available and may permit a more aggressive treatment of asymptomatic patients in the hope of preventing sudden cardiac death or altering disease progression.

Hypertrophic cardiomyopathy must be differentiated from hypertensive concentric left ventricular hypertrophy. A characteristic form of hypertensive cardiomyopathy has increasingly been recognized in elderly patients. Typical features include excessive concentric left ventricular hypertrophy that is disproportionate to the severity of the hypertension, vigorous systolic contractility, and impaired diastolic function. Women and African-Americans are more commonly affected, and beta blockers often improve symptomatic pulmonary congestion.

Pathology/ Pathophysiology

The hallmark of hypertrophic cardiomyopathy is unexplained hypertrophy, predominantly of the left ventricle, and usually with thickening of the interventricular septum that is often disproportionately greater than that of the ventricular free wall. In its severest forms, the left ventricular hypertrophy may reach such massive dimensions that the walls encroach on the left ventricular cavity, which becomes small, elongated, and slitlike.[13] The left ventricular papillary muscles are greatly hypertrophied, and the anterior papillary muscle is displaced medially and anteriorly. Movement of the septal leaflet of the mitral valve may be restricted by the hypertrophied septum. The opposition of the anterior mitral leaflet to the hypertrophied septum often causes left ventricular outflow obstruction (Fig. 31–4).

Unlike the ventricular hypertrophy observed in hypertension, in which myocytes enlarge uniformly and remain in an orderly pattern, the histopathology of hypertrophic cardiomyopathy is unusual, with myofibrils demonstrating an extensive pattern of disarray. Typically they are enlarged, vary in size and shape, and show strikingly heterogenous morphology. This disarray may, in part, explain the abnormal diastolic stiffness and arrhythmias that characterize hypertrophic cardiomyopathy.

Hypertrophic cardiomyopathy may have either an obstructive or a nonobstructive form, depending on the presence or absence of a dynamic subaortic outflow pressure gradient (Fig. 31–5). The opposition of the anterior mitral leaflet and the hypertrophied septum results in dynamic outflow obstructions. Conditions that reduce left ventricular cavity size (e.g., reduced venous return) bring the mitral leaflet and septum into closer proximity and promote obstruction. Conditions that enlarge the left ventricle (e.g., increased venous return) separate them and reduce the obstruction. Interventions that increase myocardial contractility also increase outflow tract obstruction, whereas negative inotropic agents (such as beta blockers and calcium channel blockers) have the opposite effect. In addition to the presence or absence of outflow obstruction, concomitant mitral regurgitation may also contribute to symptoms. Although the dynamic systolic outflow tract obstruction may create impressive murmurs and receives significant attention in most patients, the symptoms of hypertrophic cardiomyopathy are primarily related to the increased left ventricular stiffness, which produces elevated left ventricular filling pressures and dyspnea.

Clinical Features

The majority of patients with hypertrophic cardiomyopathy are either asymptomatic or only mildly symptomatic and are identified during screening of relatives of a patient with the disease. The most common symptoms include dyspnea, exertional angina pectoris, palpitations, syncope, and near-syncope. The disease is identified most

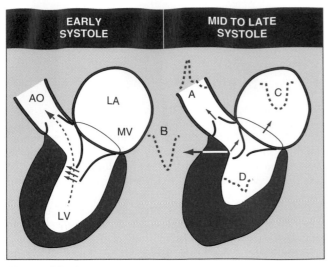

Figure 31-4

Left, Proposed mechanism of mitral valve leaflet (MV) systolic anterior motion (SAM) in early systole in hypertrophic cardiomyopathy (HCM). Ventricular septal hypertrophy causes a narrowed outflow tract, as a result of which ejection velocity is rapid and the path of ejection *(dashed line)* is closer to the MVs than is normal. This results in Venturi's forces *(three short oblique arrows* in the outflow tract) drawing anterior or posterior MVs, or both, toward the septum. Subsequent MV-septal contact results in obstruction to left ventricular outflow and concomitant mitral regurgitation, as seen on *right panel.* By midsystole, SAM-septal contact is well established, causing marked narrowing of the left ventricular outflow tract with obstruction to outflow. AO, aorta; LA, left atrium; LV, left ventricle. *Right,* Proximal to the level of SAM-septal contact, *converging lines* indicate acceleration of the jet just proximal to the obstruction and narrowing of the jet width that occurs. Distal to the obstruction, *arrows* and *diverging lines* indicate the high-velocity flow that emanates from the site of SAM-septal contact, directed posterolaterally at a considerable angle from the normal path of the aortic outflow. In late systole, although forward flow continues into the outflow tract and AO, the volume of flow is much less than in early nonobstructed systole. Typical Doppler flow patterns are shown. A, integrated Doppler flow signal in the ascending AO; B, high outflow tract velocity recorded by continuous-wave (CW) Doppler at the site of SAM-septal contact; C, presence of mitral regurgitation recorded by CW Doppler; D, late-systolic velocity peak that can be recorded in the apical region of the LV. (Redrawn from Wigle, E.D.: Hypertrophic cardiomyopathy: A 1987 viewpoint. Circulation 75:312, 1987. Copyright 1987, American Heart Association.)

often in adults during their third or fourth decades of life. Unfortunately, the first clinical manifestation of disease may be sudden cardiac death. The extent of hypertrophy and the severity of symptoms bear a general relationship but it is not absolute, since some patients have severe symptoms with only mild hypertrophy whereas others have marked hypertrophy and are virtually asymptomatic. The most common symptom is dyspnea, which is due to elevated left ventricular diastolic filling pressures secondary to impaired diastolic function. Angina pectoris occurs in 20% to 25% of symptomatic patients and may result from the markedly increased oxygen requirement of the hypertrophied myocardium and the increased pressure work resulting from outflow tract obstruction, from abnormalities of small intramyocardial arterioles, and from decreased myocardial blood flow owing to elevated left ven-

tricular diastolic filling pressures. Angina that is relieved by the patient's assuming the recumbent position is a hallmark of hypertrophic disease but is rarely encountered. Myocardial infarction may occur in older patients who develop concomitant atherosclerotic coronary disease.

Syncope or near-syncope typically occurs during or shortly after completing physical exercise. Exertional syncope may result from excessive peripheral vasodilatation, inadequate cardiac output owing to either outflow tract obstruction or impaired diastolic filling, or cardiac arrhythmias. Peripheral vasodilatation is poorly tolerated in the obstructive form of hypertrophic cardiomyopathy, since it worsens outflow tract obstruction. Syncope may also occur in the nonobstructive form of disease secondary to inadequate diastolic filling or arrhythmias ranging from atrial or ventricular tachycardias, asystole, or complete heart block. Although these symptoms in children or adolescents identify patients at increased risk of sudden death, many adult patients may have a history of near-syncope or frank syncope dating back many years.

Atrial fibrillation is a late consequence of hypertrophic cardiomyopathy and is poorly tolerated because of the loss of the presystolic atrial contribution to cardiac output and the rapid ventricular response rate, which impairs diastolic filling. Systemic embolism is a common complication of atrial fibrillation in hypertrophic cardiomyopathy, and long-term anticoagulation is necessary.

Physical Findings

The findings on physical examination depend on the presence or absence of left ventricular outflow tract obstruction, the severity of this obstruction, and the presence or absence of concomitant mitral regurgitation. In asymptomatic patients, examination typically reveals a left ventricular lift and a loud S_4 (Fig. 31-6). The initial carotid upstroke is very rapid and forceful. If obstruction to left ventricular outflow is present, a bisferiens character with a rapid initial upstroke followed by a second slower carotid impulse may be palpable (see Chap. 3). A single brisk upstroke may be converted to a double impulse if maneuvers are undertaken that elicit outflow tract obstruction.

Precordial palpation typically reveals a hyperdynamic systolic impulse and an apical impulse that is displaced laterally and inferiorly. A presystolic impulse generated by vigorous atrial contraction is often palpable.

Auscultation almost always reveals a prominent S_4 if normal sinus rhythm is maintained; an S_3 is less frequently encountered. There may be fluctuation in the spitting of the second heart sound, depending on the degree of outflow tract obstruction at any instant. The murmurs of hypertrophic cardiomyopathy may be caused by outflow tract obstruction or mitral regurgitation or both lesions. The systolic murmur characteristic of hypertrophic cardiomyopathy is harsh in character, with a crescendo-decrescendo pattern. It is most easily audible between the left sternal border and the cardiac apex and often radiates to the axilla. A holosystolic murmur, loudest at the cardiac apex, should suggest accompanying mitral regurgita-

Figure 31–5

Pathophysiologic classification of the various types of HCM. Key features include the type, location, and extent of hypertrophy; the presence or absence of a left ventricular (LV) outflow tract gradient; and the severity of accompanying mitral regurgitation, if any. (Redrawn from Yamada, G.M., and Alpert, J.S.: Hypertrophic cardiomyopathy. *In* Alpert, J.S. [ed.]: Cardiology for the Primary Care Physician. Philadelphia, Current Medicine, 1994, p. 192.)

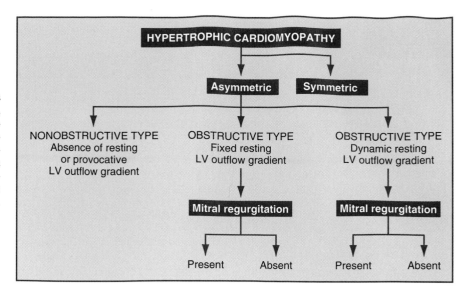

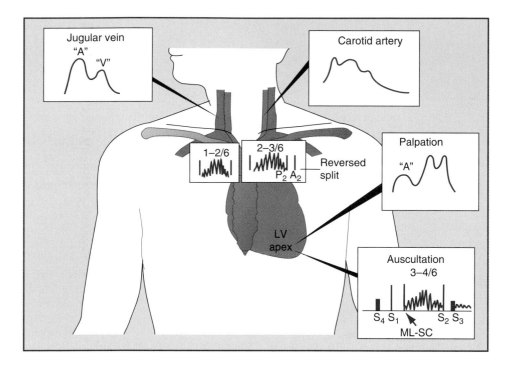

Figure 31–6

Physical examination in subaortic obstructive HCM. Seven physical signs in subaortic obstructive HCM are not found in nonobstructive HCM. On palpation, a spike-and-dome arterial pulse can often be felt in the carotid artery or in a peripheral pulse. On palpation of the left ventricular (LV) apex, there may be a triple apex beat caused by a palpable left atrial gallop and a double systolic impulse—one impulse comes before the onset of obstruction and the other after. On auscultation, at or just medial to the LV apex, there is a late-onset, diamond-shaped systolic murmur of grade 3 to 4/6 in intensity. This murmur is produced by both the subaortic obstruction and the concomitant mitral regurgitation, causing the murmur to radiate to both the left sternal border and the axilla. Because of the mitral regurgitation, there is often a short diastolic inflow murmur after the third heart sound (S_3). Rarely, a mitral leaflet–septal contact (ML-SC) sound may be heard preceding the systolic murmur at the apex. If the fourth heart sound (S_4) is palpable, there will be a double apex beat, which is quite different in timing and significance from the double systolic apex beat that occurs in subaortic obstructive HCM. In nonobstructive HCM, there is either no apical systolic murmur or, at most, a grade 1 to 2/6 murmur of mitral regurgitation. In any type of HCM, a grade 1 to 3/6 systolic ejection murmur at or below the pulmonary area may be heard. This murmur may reflect obstruction to right ventricular (RV) outflow. Examining the jugular venous pulse frequently reveals a prominent A-wave that rises on inspiration, reflecting RV diastolic dysfunction. Rarely, this is accompanied by an RV S_4. P_2, second pulmonic heart sound; A_2, aortic second sound; S_1, first heart sound; S_2, second heart sound. (Redrawn from Wigle, E.D., Kitching, A.D., and Rakowski, H.: Hypertrophic cardiomyopathy. *In* Abelmann, W.H.: Cardiomyopathies, Myocarditis, and Pericardial Disease. Braunwald, E. [ser. ed.]: Atlas of Heart Diseases. Vol. 2. Philadelphia, Current Medicine, 1995, pp. 2.1–2.22.)

Table 31–7 Bedside Maneuvers to Differentiate the Murmur of Obstructive Hypertrophic Cardiomyopathy from That of Valvular Heart Disease

Maneuver	Response of Murmur		
	Hypertrophic Cardiomyopathy	*Aortic Stenosis*	*Mitral Regurgitation*
Valsalva, hypervolemia tachycardia, standing *(decreased LV cavity)*	Increased	Decreased	Decreased
Squatting, passive leg elevation, isometric hand grip *(increased cavity size)*	Decreased	No change or slight increase	No change or slight increase

Abbreviation: LV, left ventricular.

tion. The murmur of hypertrophic cardiomyopathy demonstrates marked variability during different maneuvers. The Valsalva maneuver or abrupt standing accentuates the outflow murmur by decreasing left ventricular chamber size, whereas squatting or isometric hand grip diminishes the murmur by increasing left ventricular cavity size. Bedside maneuvers to differentiate the murmur of hypertrophic disease from aortic stenosis or mitral regurgitation are summarized in Table 31–7 and Figure 13–5.

Diagnostic Evaluation

Noninvasive Studies

The ECG typically shows left ventricular hypertrophy, nonspecific repolarization abnormalities or a strain pattern, and left atrial enlargement. Unexplained left ventricular hypertrophy or repolarization abnormalities may be the only sign of any abnormality in asymptomatic patients. Abnormal QS waves mimicking a prior myocardial infarction, often evident in the anterolateral or inferior leads (creating a pseudoinfarct pattern), are due to the massive septal hypertrophy (Fig. 31–7). Deeply inverted apical T-waves help identify patients with a variant of hypertrophic cardiomyopathy, primarily involving the apex. ECG abnormalities often precede other clinical evidence of disease, and the diagnosis of hypertrophic cardiomyopathy should be considered in any young patient whose ECG suggests a prior silent myocardial infarction or unexplained left ventricular hypertrophy.

The chest film is usually not helpful. Varying degrees of left ventricular or left atrial enlargement may be evident.

Echocardiography is the most useful initial study for confirming the diagnosis of hypertrophic cardiomyopathy. The cardinal echocardiographic feature is unexplained left ventricular hypertrophy. Asymmetric hypertrophy of the interventricular septum with a septal–to–left ventricular free-wall thickness greater than 1.3:1 is highly suggestive of the disease, although not pathognomonic (Fig. 31–8). Considerable variability in the degree and pattern of hypertrophy may be evident with concentric hypertrophy, asymmetric hypertrophy, apical hypertrophy, or hypertrophied posterior free wall.

Echocardiography also reveals the presence and severity of left ventricular outflow tract obstruction and may document whether it is fixed or labile in nature. Systolic

motion of the anterior (septal) mitral valve leaflet often accompanies hypertrophic cardiomyopathy when outflow tract obstruction exists (see Fig. 31–4). Although systolic anterior motion has rarely been described in other conditions, it is highly specific (97%) for obstructive hypertrophic cardiomyopathy. In addition to quantifying the degree of outflow tract obstruction, Doppler echocardiography is useful in assessing the severity of concomitant mitral regurgitation. Echocardiography is also extremely useful in following disease progression, particularly in children and young adults with familial disease. Provocative maneuvers such as Valsalva's or pharmacologic vasodilatation with amyl nitrite are a useful adjunct to resting echocardiographic interrogation, since they produce or intensify obstruction.

Invasive Studies

Catheterization typically reveals elevated left ventricular end-diastolic filling pressures and a prominent A-wave. The gradient in the outflow tract of the left ventricle (Fig. 31–9), if present, may be fixed or labile and range over 150 mm Hg. Left ventriculography characteristically shows a small hyperdynamic chamber. The papillary muscles are thickened, mild mitral regurgitation is common, and the apex of the ventricle is often obliterated in systole. Cardiac catheterization is usually reserved for patients in whom the diagnosis remains uncertain despite echocardiography or if surgery or dual-chamber pacing is being considered for relief of progressive symptoms. As the diagnostic accuracy of echocardiographic studies has increased, the need for invasive evaluation of hypertrophic cardiomyopathy has declined.

Electrophysiologic studies are indicated in high-risk patients, particularly those with a history of previous cardiac syncope, documented cardiac arrest, or symptomatic ventricular tachycardia. Its role in other subsets of patients, such as asymptomatic individuals with a family history of sudden cardiac death, remains unclear.

Differential Diagnosis

Hypertrophic cardiomyopathy may be confused with the left ventricular hypertrophy associated with chronic, severe, untreated hypertension. A pattern of asymmetric septal hypertrophy will differentiate the two entities, as will the history of prior blood pressure readings. The

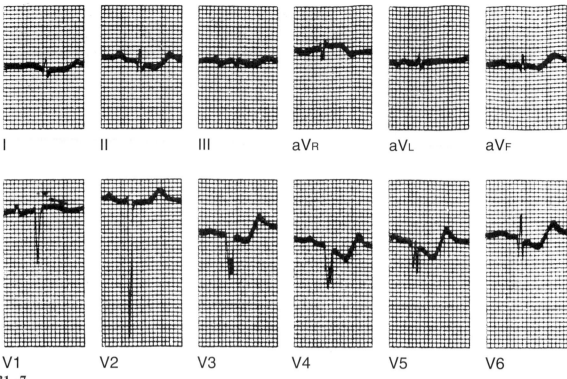

I   II   III   aV_R   aV_L   aV_F

V1   V2   V3   V4   V5   V6

Figure 31–7

Abnormal electrocardiogram from a 45-year-old woman with documented HCM. Q-waves suggestive of a prior anterior myocardial infarction (MI) are seen in leads V_3 to V_6 (a pseudo-MI pattern). (With permission from DeSanctis, R.W., and Dec, G.W.: The cardiomyopathies. Section 1, Subsection XIV, in *Scientific American Medicine,* Dale, D.C., and Federman, D. [eds.]. Copyright 1995, Scientific American Inc. All rights reserved.)

concentric form of hypertrophic cardiomyopathy has many similarities to hypertensive hypertrophic disease of the elderly. The latter entity is typically seen in older women with a prior history of hypertension and diabetes mellitus. Occasionally, restrictive or infiltrative diseases such as amyloidosis may produce marked concentric hypertrophy. Hypertrophic cardiomyopathy is occasionally confused with valvular or subvalvular aortic stenosis, chronic mitral regurgitation, infundibular pulmonic stenosis, or a small ventricular septal defect. The brisk carotid upstrokes and the variable systolic murmur with maneuvers are useful in identifying hypertrophic cardiomyopathy.

Long-term athletic training may produce an increase in left ventricular end-diastolic cavity dimension, wall thickness, and contractility that is commonly referred to as "the athlete's heart." This is a physiologic form of hypertrophy in which the left ventricular wall thickness is usually mildly increased, and overlap may exist between mild morphologic expression of hypertrophic cardiomyopathy and a more pronounced degree of physiologic hypertrophy such as that observed in rowers or weight lifters. Hypertrophic cardiomyopathy is more likely than physiologic hypertrophy when there is (1) documentation of hypertrophic cardiomyopathy in a relative of the athlete, (2) evidence of impaired left ventricular filling by transmural Doppler echocardiography, usually demonstrated as a diminished peak early-diastolic filling rate, (3) left ventricular wall thickness greater than 15 mm, and (4) left ventricular cavity size less than 45 mm.[9]

Natural History

The clinical course of hypertrophic cardiomyopathy is highly variable, although the rate of progression is generally more rapid in children and adolescents (particularly during the teenage growth years). The extent of left ventricular hypertrophy usually remains stable over time in adults; however, hypertrophy may develop during adolescence despite an initial normal echocardiogram. Progression of hypertrophic cardiomyopathy to left ventricular dilatation and systolic dysfunction (i.e., development of a dilated cardiomyopathy) occurs in up to 10% of adult patients with long-standing symptomatic disease. The best predictor of long-term outcome appears to be the specific mutation responsible for the genetic defect. Death is most often sudden in hypertrophic cardiomyopathy and may occur in previously asymptomatic individuals or in those with a stable clinical course. Those clinical features that best predict sudden death are a young age (< 30 years) at diagnosis and a family history of hypertrophic cardiomyopathy with sudden death. A history of syncope is ominous in children but less so in adults. Ventricular tachycardia on ambulatory monitoring is also associated with increased risk, particularly in patients with a history of alterations in consciousness. The presence or severity of an outflow tract gradient, the extent of left ventricular hypertrophy, and the degree of functional limitation do not correlate with the risk of sudden death.

In patients seen at major referral centers, the annual mortality averages 5% to 6% for children and 3% for

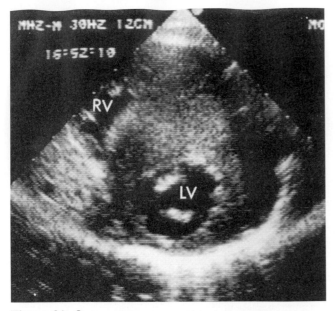

Figure 31–8

Short-axis echocardiographic image at the mitral valve level illustrates marked asymmetric ventricular hypertrophy. RV, right ventricle; LV, left ventricle. (From Levine, R.A.: Echocardiographic assessment of the cardiomyopathies. *In* Weyman, A.E. [ed.]: Principles and Practice of Echocardiography. 2nd ed. Philadelphia, Lea & Febiger, 1994, p. 784.)

adults. However, community-based studies have indicated an annual mortality of only 1%.

Treatment

Medical Therapy

Management of hypertrophic cardiomyopathy patients should be aimed at alleviating symptoms, preventing complications, and reducing the risk of sudden cardiac death (Fig. 31–10).[13] Whether asymptomatic or minimally symptomatic patients should be treated remains controversial. Some clinicians favor the use of beta-adrenergic blocking drugs or calcium channel blockers to delay progression of disease or the occurrence of sudden death. Low-dose amiodarone has also been advocated for asymptomatic patients with runs of nonsustained ventricular tachycardia. None of these treatments can be currently recommended for asymptomatic patients, since evidence concerning their efficacy is lacking.

Beta blockers have traditionally been the mainstay of medical therapy for patients with mild to moderate symptoms. They provide effective relief of angina, dyspnea, and syncope and improve exercise capacity in one-third to one-half of all patients. Although the level of ventricular ectopy often decreases, beta-adrenergic blockade has not been convincingly shown to decrease the risk of sudden death or, indeed, to alter survival in patients with hypertrophic cardiomyopathy.

Calcium channel blockers (particularly verapamil) are often useful for patients who fail to respond to beta blockers, and they have been shown to improve symptoms in up to 60% of patients unresponsive to beta blocker therapy. Although their negative inotropic properties usually lessen outflow obstruction, rarely, their peripheral vasodilating properties may actually increase obstruction and worsen symptoms. Verapamil has also been shown to prevent silent myocardial ischemia during exercise. The addition of a low-dose diuretic, such as a thiazide, may provide symptomatic improvement in patients with persistent dyspnea. For those with refractory symptoms on a single agent, the combination of a beta blocker and a calcium channel blocker may provide substantial clinical improvement. Disopyramide is a type I antiarrhythmic agent that possesses potent negative inotropic

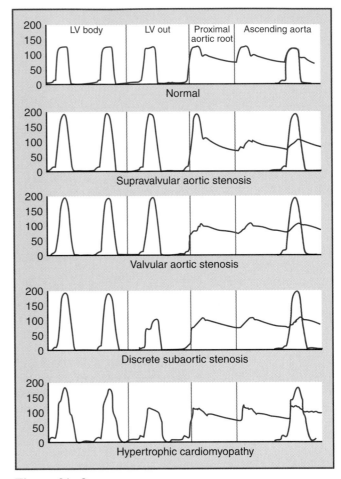

Figure 31–9

Left heart pressures in various conditions. In each *horizontal panel,* there is an idealized depiction of the pressure tracing that would be obtained as a catheter is withdrawn from the left ventricular (LV) body through the LV outflow (LV out) tract into the proximal aortic root. On the far right is a superimposition of the pressures in the LV body and in the aorta. The *vertical lines* define the boundary of the regional catheter position within the heart during withdrawal. All forms of discrete stenosis (supravalvular, valvular, and subvalvular) have delayed aortic upstroke rates downstream from the stenosis. Only in HCM is the aortic upstroke rate rapid and parallel to the LV pressure. (Redrawn from Criley, J.M., and Siegel, R.J.: Subaortic stenosis revisited: The importance of the dynamic pressure gradient. Medicine [Baltimore] 72:412, 1993.)

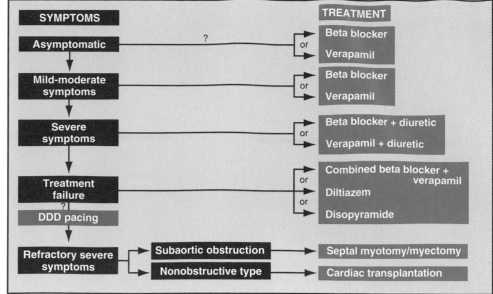

Figure 31–10
Treatment algorithm for the management of patients with HCM. *Question marks* indicate treatment recommendations that remain controversial or unproved. DDD pacing, dual-chamber pacing. (Adapted from Maron, B.J.: Hypertrophic cardiomyopathy. Curr. Probl. Cardiol. 18:686, 1993.)

properties. It has been shown to reduce obstruction and to improve symptoms in patients with the obstructive form of disease. Dosages typically range from 150 to 200 mg orally four times daily. The drug has significant disadvantages, including its anticholinergic effects and a decline in its hemodynamic benefits over time.

Management of asymptomatic, nonsustained, ventricular tachycardia remains difficult. Low-dose amiodarone (200 to 300 mg daily orally) has been suggested to diminish the risk for sudden death compared with historical controls. However, no controlled trials of this approach have been undertaken. Amiodarone may be useful in patients with a history of sudden cardiac death or symptomatic ventricular arrhythmias. The decision to use antiarrhythmic drug suppression versus an implantable defibrillator must be individualized (see Chap. 23).

EXERCISE. Strenuous exercise should be prohibited because it increases the risk of sudden death. Many persons with subclinical hypertrophic cardiomyopathy actively exercise daily. However, the risk of sudden death is real and competitive sports should be prohibited for patients with marked hypertrophy, evidence of a significant outflow tract gradient at rest, or a family history of sudden cardiac death.[14] Whether asymptomatic individuals with mild hypertrophy should have the same rigorous restraints on physical activity requires additional study. Task force recommendations on exercise in hypertrophic disease remain quite conservative.[15] Individuals with unequivocal hypertrophic cardiomyopathy should not participate in most competitive sports except those of low intensity (e.g., bowling, golf). This recommendation currently applies to individuals with or without symptoms of left ventricular outflow obstruction and is not altered by medical or surgical treatment. As sudden death risk is lower in older populations (>30 years) with hypertrophic disease, more vigorous athletic activity may be considered in individuals who lack ventricular tachyarrhythmias, a family history of sudden cardiac death, syncope, severe hemodynamic abnormalities, paroxysmal atrial fibrillation, or evidence of abnormal myocardial perfusion.[14]

Pacemaker Therapy

Growing experience with AV sequential pacing confirms its usefulness in the treatment of drug-resistant, symptomatic patients with documented outflow tract obstruction.[16] The mechanism by which the outflow gradient is reduced is uncertain, but it is probably related to decreased or paradoxical septal motion, late activation of the basal septum, or decreased left ventricular contractility. For AV sequential pacing to be successful in reducing outflow tract obstruction, there must be complete ventricular capture, which requires careful optimization of the AV delay. Dual-chamber pacing in obstructive hypertrophic cardiomyopathy represents a low-risk alternative to surgical treatment. Its effect on long-term prognosis is unknown. However, cardiac pacing is ineffective treatment for the nonobstructive form of the disease.

Surgical Therapy

Surgical myotomy/myectomy is recommended for persistently symptomatic patients with outflow tract obstruction that does not respond to medical therapy or synchronized pacing.[17] Fewer than 10% of patients with hypertrophic cardiomyopathy require surgery. Myotomy/myectomy provides more hemodynamic and symptomatic benefit for severely limited patients than any available form of medical therapy. Intraoperative transesophageal echocardiography is routinely used to guide the location and amount of upper septal muscle that is surgically resected. Mitral valve replacement is infrequently required for associated mitral regurgitation. Operative mortality rates below 5% are now routine, and over 70% of surgically treated patients report marked improvement in symptoms, functional capacity, and quality of life. Ten-

Table 31–8	Hypertrophic Cardiomyopathy: Indications for Cardiology Referral

NYHA class III/IV angina or heart failure symptoms despite conventional therapy

Children/adolescents/young adults with asymptomatic hypertrophic disease and family history of sudden death

Syncopal spells

Nonsustained ventricular tachycardia on ambulatory monitoring

Competitive athletes with a heart murmur or ECG evidence of substantial hypertrophy

Refractory heart failure or anginal symptoms leading to consideration of myectomy or dual-chamber pacing

Refractory symptoms or deterioration in left ventricular function leading to consideration of cardiac transplantation

---

Abbreviations: NYHA, New York Heart Association; ECG, electrocardiogram.

year survival rates are usually above 85%, and few patients require a second operation.[17] Unfortunately, myectomy does not prevent sudden cardiac death.

Rarely, cardiac transplantation may be required for the nonobstructive form of hypertrophic cardiomyopathy that fails to respond to maximized medical or surgical therapy. A small number of patients who develop progressive left ventricular systolic dysfunction may also benefit from transplantation.

Referral to Cardiologists

Similar to patients with dilated cardiomyopathy, most patients with hypertrophic disease do not require subspecialty consultation. Patients who may benefit from consultation include those with persistent symptoms despite beta blocker therapy in whom calcium blockers, pacemaker placement, or myectomy is being considered (Table 31–8). Likewise, patients at high risk for sudden cardiac death require consultation. Finally, patients who fail medical or surgical treatment or those with progressive left ventricular systolic dysfunction and who are in need of transplantation should undergo timely referral.

RESTRICTIVE CARDIOMYOPATHIES

The restrictive cardiomyopathies are the least commonly encountered form of heart muscle disease in Western countries. The hallmark of these disorders is abnormal diastolic function—the ventricular walls are excessively stiff and impair normal ventricular filling. Systolic function usually remains unimpaired until late in the disease.[18] Varying degrees of myocardial fibrosis, hypertrophy, endocardial thickening, or secondary infiltration are usually responsible for the disorder. Although cardiac amyloidosis and idiopathic primary restrictive cardiomyopathy are the most commonly diagnosed causes, restrictive cardiomyopathy can result from a variety of other conditions (Table 31–9). Unlike dilated and hypertrophic disease, there is rarely a familial component to restrictive cardiomyopathy.

Pathophysiology

The ventricular myocardium is rigid and noncompliant, impeding ventricular diastolic filling and producing elevation in cardiac filling pressures.[19] Systemic and venous congestion and decreased stroke volume and cardiac output are the consequences of this abnormal diastolic filling. The clinical and hemodynamic picture of restrictive cardiomyopathy mimics that of constrictive pericarditis.

Clinical Features

Congestive heart failure is the most common clinical manifestation.[20] Exertional dyspnea is a prominent feature. Exercise intolerance is also frequently encountered because of the inability of the patient to increase cardiac output by tachycardia without further compromising diastolic ventricular filling. As in constrictive pericarditis, clinical evidence of right-sided heart failure without evidence for underlying pulmonary disease of sufficient severity to serve as an explanation is a frequent initial presentation.

Physical Findings

Careful examination of the jugular venous pulse is essential for establishing the correct diagnosis. The elevated diastolic filling pressures result in chronic venous hypertension manifested by an increase in jugular venous pressure. An inspiratory increase in venous pressure (Kussmaul's sign) is commonly seen. The most prominent waveform is the Y descent. Precordial examination is generally unremarkable. The apex beat is usually in its normal position within the midclavicular line in the fifth left intercostal space. It is more likely to be palpable than in constrictive pericarditis where the pericardium is usu-

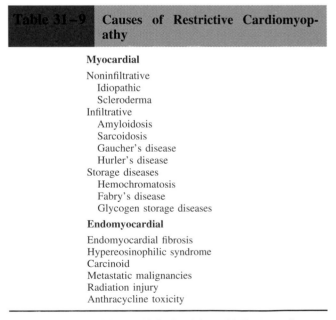

Table 31–9	Causes of Restrictive Cardiomyopathy

Myocardial

Noninfiltrative
  Idiopathic
  Scleroderma
Infiltrative
  Amyloidosis
  Sarcoidosis
  Gaucher's disease
  Hurler's disease
Storage diseases
  Hemochromatosis
  Fabry's disease
  Glycogen storage diseases

Endomyocardial

Endomyocardial fibrosis
Hypereosinophilic syndrome
Carcinoid
Metastatic malignances
Radiation injury
Anthracycline toxicity

From Wynne, J., and Braunwald, E.: Restrictive and infiltrative cardiomyopathies. *In* Braunwald, E. (ed.): Heart Disease. 5th ed. Philadelphia, W. B. Saunders, 1997, p. 1427.

ally quiet. An S_3 or S_4, or both, is usually present. Mitral and tricuspid regurgitation are frequently observed in restrictive cardiomyopathy but are quite uncommon in constrictive pericarditis. Hepatomegaly, ascites, and peripheral edema occur in more advanced cases.

Noninvasive Evaluation

The *chest film* often displays pulmonary congestion, reflecting the elevated ventricular diastolic pressure. Cardiomegaly is either mild or absent, and pleural effusions are seen in advanced disease. Atrial enlargement is common when AV regurgitation has developed. The **ECG** is seldom normal but frequently demonstrates only nonspecific repolarization changes. The findings of low-voltage, left axis deviation, and pseudomyocardial infarction should suggest an infiltrative process such as amyloidosis.[21]

Infiltrative diseases may be entirely confined to the heart or may be part of a more generalized systemic process. Complete blood count, erythrocyte sedimentation rate, serum protein electrophoresis, and renal and hepatic function studies should be undertaken. Additional blood studies (such as iron, iron binding, and ferritin) should be individualized.

Echocardiography confirms normal left and right ventricular size and systolic function and is useful for excluding hypertrophic cardiomyopathy or unsuspected valvular heart disease. Left ventricular wall mass is increased in patients with infiltrative diseases but may be normal in those with primary restrictive disease. The classic Doppler echocardiographic finding is rapid ventricular inflow and early cessation of flow in diastole. These filling characteristics result in a tall E-wave and a blunted A-wave (reflecting atrial inflow). However, the E:A ratio is load-dependent and cannot reliably define the extent or severity of diastolic dysfunction.[22] Echocardiographic findings are also often useful for differentiating restrictive cardiomyopathy from constrictive pericarditis. In patients with constriction, there are greater respiratory-dependent variations in left ventricular isovolumetric relaxation time and peak mitral valve velocity during early diastole. Echocardiography is not sufficiently accurate to quantify the degree of pericardial thickening or unequivocally establish a diagnosis of pericardial constriction.

Magnetic resonance imaging and computed tomography are quite useful for differentiating constrictive disease from restrictive cardiomyopathy. Both imaging techniques can accurately quantify the degree of pericardial thickening.

Invasive Evaluation

The characteristic hemodynamic feature of restrictive cardiomyopathy is a deep and rapid early decline in ventricular pressure at the onset of diastole followed by a rapid rise to a plateau phase in early diastole (Fig. 31–11). This dip and plateau in pressures has been termed the "square root" sign and is evident in both the atrial and the ventricular pressure tracings. The right atrial pressure is elevated and a prominent Y descent is noted. The X descent may also be rapid, and the combination may result in a characteristic M-waveform in the right atrial pressure tracing. Although both right- and left-sided filling pressures are elevated, patients with restrictive cardiomyopathy typically have left ventricular filling pressures that exceed right ventricular filling pressures by more than 5 mm Hg. This difference may be further accentuated by exercise.

Right ventricular endomyocardial biopsy is often useful in differentiating primary restrictive disease from an infiltrative process or constrictive pericarditis. Because of sampling error, a normal biopsy does not completely exclude the possibility of restrictive disease.

Differential Diagnosis

Restrictive cardiomyopathies must always be differentiated from constrictive pericarditis, a distinction that is not always easily made on the basis of clinical or hemodynamic findings (Table 31–10). In general, constrictive pericardial disease involves both ventricles equally and

Figure 31–11

Right ventricular (RV) and left ventricular (LV) pressure tracings in a patient with idiopathic restrictive cardiomyopathy. A dip-and-plateau pattern is seen in both ventricles, and diastolic filling pressures are elevated. The plateaus occur at different pressures, approximately 16 mm Hg for the RV tracing compared with 20 mm Hg for the LV tracing. The diagnosis of restrictive disease was confirmed by thoracotomy. ECG, electrocardiogram. (Redrawn from Benofti, J.R., Grossman, W., and Cohn, P.F.: The clinical profile of restrictive cardiomyopathy. Circulation 61:1206, 1980.)

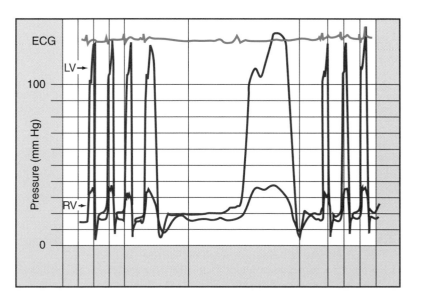

Table 31–10 Differentiation of Restrictive Cardiomyopathy from Constrictive Pericardial Disease

Feature	Restrictive Cardiomyopathy	Constrictive Pericarditis
Physical Examination		
Pulses paradoxus	Uncommon	Uncommon
Palpable apical impulse	May be present	Absent
S₃ gallop	May be present	Absent
AV regurgitation murmur	Common	Rare
Pericardial knock	Absent	May be present
Electrocardiogram		
Low voltage	Uncommon (exception: amyloidosis)	Commonly present
Chest Film		
Cardiomegaly	Mild LV prominence	Absent
Pericardial calcification	Absent	Seen in 30%–50%
Hemodynamics		
"Square root" sign	Frequently evident	Almost always
LV diastolic pressure exceeds RV diastolic pressure by 15 mm Hg during exercise, volume loading	Very common	Rare
Kussmaul's sign	Uncommon	Common (>80%)
MRI		
Pericardial thickening	Absent	Virtually always evident

Abbreviations: S₃, third heart sound: AV, atrioventricular; LV, left ventricular; RV, right ventricular; MRI, magnetic resonance imaging.

produces a plateau of filling pressures. Thus, in constrictive pericarditis, the left ventricular end-diastolic, left atrial, pulmonary capillary wedge, right ventricular end-diastolic, and right atrial pressures are within 5 mm of one another and have similar configurations. Conversely, restrictive cardiomyopathies tend to cause greater impairment of left than right ventricular diastolic filling. Thus, left-sided filling pressures almost always exceed those on the right side by more than 5 mm Hg; in questionable cases, provocative testing with a fluid load may be helpful to see if the right- and left-sided pressures diverge, a finding in restrictive cardiomyopathy. Further, the pulmonary artery systolic pressure is often above 50 mm Hg— a pressure level that is distinctly uncommon in constrictive disease. Patterns of diastolic filling, as determined by Doppler echocardiography or radionuclide ventriculography, may also help distinguish the two entities (see earlier). Magnetic resonance imaging is usually an essential study to differentiate the two conditions. In some cases, endomyocardial biopsy or, very rarely, surgical thoracotomy may be necessary to differentiate surgically correctable constrictive pericarditis from restrictive cardiomyopathy.

Prognosis and Treatment

The prognosis in restrictive cardiomyopathy is one of symptomatic progression; fewer than 10% of patients survive more than 10 years after the onset of symptoms.

Conventional treatment is directed toward relief of congestive symptoms. Diuretics are employed to reduce peripheral edema and ascites and to decrease exertional dyspnea. Although angiotensin-converting enzyme inhibitors and calcium channel blockers are often prescribed in an effort to improve diastolic filling, these agents must be used cautiously because of their peripheral vasodilating properties. No medical treatment has been shown to prolong survival. Corticosteroids and cytolytic agents may play a role in the treatment of specific causes of restrictive cardiomyopathy (see later).

Specific Causes of Restrictive Cardiomyopathy

Primary Restrictive Cardiomyopathy

Patients are considered to have a *primary* restrictive cardiomyopathy if they have a history of heart failure, normal left ventricular end-diastolic volume, elevation in ventricular filling pressures at catheterization, and the absence of an explainable cause for diastolic dysfunction, such as an infiltrative process, coronary artery disease, coronary vasculitis, or hypertrophic cardiomyopathy. Endomyocardial biopsy typically shows varying degrees of myocyte hypertrophy and interstitial fibrosis and differentiates this disorder from hypertrophic disease. Restrictive hemodynamics and complete heart block may be present in this disorder, despite the absence of significant fibrosis on biopsy. Complete heart block, skeletal myopathy, and a dominant pattern of inheritance have been described in a rare familial form. Mean survival has been reported to be approximately 9 years after symptom onset and 5 years after the development of heart failure.

Hypereosinophilic Syndrome

Endomyocardial fibrosis is a common form of restrictive disease in equatorial Africa but is rarely encountered in nontropical countries. Marked hypereosinophilia (>1500 eosinophils/mm³) of any cause can result in endomyocardial disease. The clinical diagnosis of idiopathic hypereosinophilic syndrome (so-called Loffler's endocarditis) is characterized by unexplained peripheral eosinophilia of greater than 6 months' duration and associated evidence of end-organ involvement. The heart is involved in more than 75% of patients. The central nervous system, kidneys, lungs, gastrointestinal tract, and skin are other common sites. Cardiac involvement is usually biventricular; endocardial fibrosis and thrombus formation are the characteristic pathologic lesions. Clinical features include weight loss, persistent fever, cough, skin rash, and heart failure. Although asymptomatic involvement may be present early in the disease, more than 50% of patients have symptoms of overt heart failure. AV valvular regurgitation is common owing to the extensive fibrosis. Likewise, large mural thrombi are often evident on echocardiography, and systemic embolization is a frequent complication. The echocardiogram commonly demonstrates localized thickening of the posterobasal left ventricular free wall with marked limitation of motion of the posterior mitral leaflet. The left ventricular apex may be obliterated by thrombus, and varying degrees of mitral and tricuspid regurgitation are present on Doppler echocardiography.

Therapy with corticosteroids and hydroxyurea may substantially improve survival. Medical therapy employing diuretics, afterload-reducing agents, and warfarin anticoagulation can often control symptoms. Surgical treatment offers symptomatic improvement once the fibrotic stage of the disease has developed.

Cardiac Amyloidosis

Amyloidosis is a systemic disease caused by extracellular deposition of insoluble amyloid protein fibrils within tissues.[21] Amyloid may be deposited in almost any organ, but clinically significant disease does not result unless there has been extensive infiltration. Primary amyloidosis is caused by the production of an amyloid protein composed of portions of immunoglobulin light chain (so-called AL amyloid) by a monoclonal population of plasma cells, often as a consequence of multiple myeloma. Secondary amyloidosis is caused by the production of a nonimmunoglobulin protein (termed AA) and is found in a variety of chronic inflammatory diseases. Six different forms of familial amyloidosis are now recognized and result from abnormal production of prealbumin protein. Finally, senile amyloidosis is due to production of yet another prealbumin protein. It is becoming increasingly common as the average age of the population increases. Although clinically significant cardiac involvement is present in up to 50% of patients with primary amyloidosis, the heart is involved in fewer than 10% of cases of secondary amyloidosis. Likewise, familial amyloidosis is only occasionally associated with overt cardiac

dysfunction and, then, only late in the course of the disease. Cardiac amyloidosis is more common in men than in women, and it is rarely seen before the age of 30 years, even in the familial forms.

Pathologically, the walls of both ventricles are firm, rubbery, and noncompliant. Amyloid is visible between myocardial fibers. The intramural coronary arteries and veins frequently also contain amyloid deposits.

The most common presentation of cardiac amyloid is that of right-sided heart failure due to restrictive physiology. Paroxysmal dyspnea and orthopnea are usually absent early in the disease. Although systolic function is typically normal at presentation, progressive deposition of amyloid frequently results in systolic dysfunction. The course of this disease is marked by the relentless progression of heart failure. Orthostatic hypotension consequent to autonomic nervous system involvement is a well-recognized occurrence.

The *ECG* is frequently abnormal. The most characteristic feature is diffusely diminished QRS voltage, which is evident in approximately 50% of all patients. Left axis deviation, atrial fibrillation, pseudo–myocardial infarction patterns, and ventricular arrhythmias are frequently evident with more severe infiltration.

Echocardiography is extremely sensitive for detecting clinically significant cardiac amyloid. Typical findings include increased ventricular wall thickness, small size of the left ventricular cavity, and atrial dilatation. The appearance of thickened ventricular walls and a granular, sparkling texture are highly suggestive of amyloidosis (Fig. 31–12). The sparkling pattern results from amorphous amyloid deposition that replaces collagen fibers within the myocardium. Echocardiographic findings also predict prognosis, with the poorest survival rates noted for patients with the greatest ventricular wall thickness.[22]

An abdominal fat pad aspirate is the single most useful

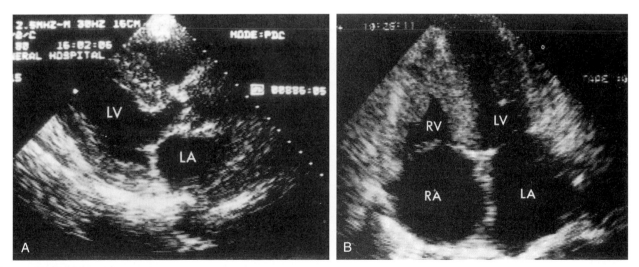

Figure 31–12

A, Parasternal long-axis echocardiographic image shows a "sparkling" granular myocardial texture in the interventricular septum in a patient with biopsy-proved amyloidosis. LV, left ventricle; LA, left atrium. *B,* An apical four-chamber echocardiographic image demonstrates biventricular hypertrophy in a patient with biopsy-proved amyloidosis. RV, right ventricle; RA, right atrium. (*A* and *B,* From Levine, R.A.: Echocardiographic assessment of the cardiomyopathies. *In* Weyman, A.E. [ed.]: Principles and Practice of Echocardiography. 2nd ed. Philadelphia, Lea & Febiger, 1994, p. 810.)

diagnostic technique, since it combines ease of performance, sensitivity, and specificity. Endomyocardial biopsy is useful for establishing the diagnosis of cardiac amyloidosis if the abdominal fat pad aspirate does not prove to be diagnostic.

The *treatment* of cardiac amyloidosis is generally palliative and ineffective. Diuretics should be judiciously used to control symptoms of venous congestion. Digitalis and calcium channel blockers are relatively contraindicated owing to their selective binding to amyloid fibers. Insertion of a permanent pacemaker is useful in patients with symptomatic conduction system disease or marked bradycardia. Several disease-specific treatment regimens have been studied, including prednisone, melphalan, and colchicine.[23] Although colchicine may be partially effective in familial amyloidosis, the results with other agents have been disappointing. Heart transplantation is contraindicated for primary amyloidosis owing to the early recurrence of amyloid deposits within the allograft.

Hemochromatosis

Hemochromatosis is characterized by excessive deposition of iron in a variety of tissues, including heart, liver, testes, and pancreas.[24] Cardiac involvement leads to a mixed dilated/restrictive cardiomyopathy with both systolic and diastolic dysfunction evident. The severity of myocardial dysfunction is directly proportional to the quantity of iron deposited within the myocardium.

Hemochromatosis may occur as a familial or idiopathic disorder, in association with a defect of hemoglobin synthesis, in chronic liver disease, or owing to excessive iron supplementation. Cardiac involvement is the presenting manifestation in up to 15% of patients and may include either arrhythmias or heart failure. Whereas repolarization abnormalities and supraventricular arrhythmias are common, AV conduction defects and ventricular tachyarrhythmias are rarely noted. Echocardiographic abnormalities typically include increased ventricular wall thickness, enlarged cardiac chambers, and systolic dysfunction. Cardiac involvement is usually evident from clinical, echocardiographic, and laboratory features. However, endomyocardial biopsy may occasionally be necessary to confirm the diagnosis.

Treatment should consist of repeated phlebotomy, which is most effective if instituted before irreversible end-organ damage has developed. Chelation therapy using desferrioxamine is most beneficial if begun early in the disease process, but this can provide clinical benefit even if symptomatic cardiomyopathy has developed. Combined heart-liver transplantation should be considered for selected patients with progressive heart failure who have not yet developed serious compromise in other end organs.

Cardiac Sarcoidosis

Sarcoidosis is a multisystem granulomatous disease that frequently involves the myocardium. Granulomatous involvement may involve any region of the heart, but the left ventricular free wall and interventricular septum are the most common sites. Although clinical involvement is

evident in only 5% of patients, cardiac involvement is present at autopsy in 20% to 30% of cases. Cardiac infiltration by granulomas is associated with progressive fibrosis and leads to increased left ventricular stiffness. Impaired systolic contractile function may also occur as the disease progresses. Endomyocardial biopsy is positive in approximately 50% of patients, but a negative biopsy does not exclude the diagnosis owing to the patchy nature of the disease. Myocardial sarcoidosis typically affects young or middle-aged adults of either gender and is usually associated with generalized sarcoidosis. The clinical spectrum includes ventricular arrhythmias, conduction system abnormalities, heart failure, and sudden cardiac death. Syncope is a common manifestation and requires prompt evaluation. ECG abnormalities may include repolarization abnormalities, varying degrees of AV block, and QS waves mimicking myocardial infarction. Myocardial imaging with thallium-201 or gallium-67 frequently demonstrates abnormal segmental uptake indicative of myocardial involvement.

The clinical course of the disease is highly variable, with a minority of patients having extensive myocardial involvement but few symptoms and others having rapid progression to death or transplantation. The most common cause of death is sudden cardiac death owing to ventricular tachyarrhythmias or high-grade AV block consequent to direct involvement of the conduction system.

Treatment of cardiac sarcoidosis remains unsatisfactory. Permanent pacing is useful when high-grade AV block is present. Antiarrhythmic treatment or cardioverter-defibrillator implantation is frequently required for patients with a recurrent ventricular tachyarrhythmia. Case reports have suggested that corticosteroids may halt disease progression or improve function, but controlled trials are lacking. Cardiac transplantation remains an option for individuals with progressive symptoms. Disease may recur in the cardiac allograft but is usually responsive to enhanced immunosuppression.

Chagas' Cardiomyopathy

Chagas' disease is characterized by severe myocarditis with trypanosomes demonstrated within cardiac myocytes. Following a latency period that averages 20 years after the initial and usually unrecognized infection, approximately 30% of infected individuals develop cardiac involvement. This is pathologically characterized by chronic myocarditis, focal and diffuse myocyte loss, extensive fibrosis, and areas of thinning of the ventricular free wall. The process is most commonly evident in the conduction system and at the left ventricular apex. Involvement of the conduction system almost always accompanies cardiac involvement, producing right bundle branch block or left anterior hemiblock, or both, in up to 80% of patients.[25] Myocardial involvement frequently leads to the formation of a narrow-necked apical left ventricular aneurysm. Localized areas of left ventricular akinesis or dyskinesis are also commonly seen and may mimic coronary artery disease. In the early phases of disease, a restrictive picture may predominate with diastolic dysfunction owing to the extent of myocardial replacement with fibrous tissue.

Treatment consists of the management of congestive

heart failure and the insertion of a pacemaker for advanced AV block. Public health measures including insecticides to eliminate the vector are important preventive measures.

Referral to Cardiologists

Unlike the dilated and hypertrophic forms, restrictive cardiomyopathy is rare and most patients should be referred to a cardiologist for consultation. The goals of such referral are (1) to differentiate primary restrictive disease from infiltrative causes, (2) to differentiate restrictive cardiomyopathy from constrictive pericarditis, (3) to develop the most appropriate treatment strategy, and (4) to evaluate patients for disease-specific treatment protocols or transplantation.

References

1. Richardson, P., McKenna, W., Bristow, M., et al.: Report of the 1995 World Health Organization International Society and Federation of Cardiology Task Force on the definition and classification of cardiomyopathies. Circulation 93:841–842, 1996.
2. DeSanctis, R.W., and Dec, G.W.: The cardiomyopathies. *In* Rubenstein, E., and Federman, D. (eds.): Scientific American Medicine. New York, Scientific American Medicine, 1995, pp. 1–27.
3. Durand, J.B., O'Connell, J.B., and Costanzo-Nordin, M.R.: Specific heart muscle disease. Curr. Opin. Cardiol. 7:445–456, 1992.
4. Kasper, E.K., Agema, W.R.P., Hutchins, G.M., et al.: The cause of dilated cardiomyopathy: A clinicopathologic review of 673 consecutive patients. J. Am. Coll. Cardiol. 23:586–590, 1994.
5. Stevenson, L.W., and Perloff, J.A.: The dilated cardiomyopathies. Cardiol. Clin. 6:187–231, 1988.
6. Dec, G.W., and Fuster, V.: Idiopathic dilated cardiomyopathy. N. Engl. J. Med. 331:1564–1575, 1994.
7. American College of Cardiology/American Heart Association Task Force Report: Guidelines for the evaluation and management of heart failure. J. Am. Coll. Cardiol. 26:1376–1398, 1995.
8. Baker, D.W., Jones, R., Hodges, J., et al.: Management of heart failure. III. The role of revascularization in the treatment of patients with moderately severe left ventricular systolic dysfunction. JAMA 272:1528–1534, 1994.
9. Maron, B.J.: Hypertrophic cardiomyopathy. Curr. Probl. Cardiol. 18:639–704, 1993.
10. Wigle, E.D., Rakowski, H., Kimball, B.P., and Williams, W.G.: Hypertrophic cardiomyopathy. Clinical spectrum and treatment. Circulation 92:1680–1692, 1995.
11. Marian, A.J., and Roberts, R.: Recent advances in the molecular genetics of hypertrophic cardiomyopathy. Circulation 92:1336–1347, 1995.
12. Rosenzweig, A., Watkins, H., Hwang, D.S., et al.: Preclinical diagnosis of familial hypertrophic cardiomyopathy by genetic analysis of blood lymphocytes. N. Engl. J. Med. 325:1753–1760, 1991.
13. Spirito, P., Seidman, C.E., McKenna, W.J., and Maron, B.J.: The managment of hypertrophic cardiomyopathy. N. Engl. J. Med. 336:775–785, 1997.
14. Maron, B.J., Thompson, P.D., Puffer, J.C., et al.: Cardiovascular preparticipation screening of competitive athletes. A statement for health professionals from the Sudden Death Committee (Clinical Cardiology) and Congenital Cardiac Defects Committee (Cardiovascular Disease in the Young), American Heart Association. Circulation 94:850–856, 1996.
15. Maron, B.J., Isner, J.M., and McKenna, W.J.: 26th Bethesda Conference: Recommendations for determining eligibility for competition in athletes with cardiovascular abnormalities. Task Force 3: Hypertrophic cardiomyopathy, myocarditis and other myopericardial diseases and mitral valve prolapse. J. Am. Coll. Cardiol. 24:880–885, 1994.
16. Cannon, R.O., Tripodi, D., Dilsizian, V., et al.: Results of permanent dual-chamber pacing in symptomatic nonobstructive hypertrophic cardiomyopathy. Am. J. Cardiol. 73:571–576, 1994.
17. Cohn, L.H., Trehan, H., and Collins, J.J.: Long-term follow-up of patients underoing myotomy/myectomy for obstructive hypertrophic cardiomyopathy. Am. J. Cardiol. 70:657–660, 1992.
18. Kushwaha, S., Fallon, J.T., and Fuster, V.: Restrictive cardiomyopathy. N. Engl. J. Med. 336:267–276, 1997.
19. Shabetai, R.: Pathophysiology and differential diagnosis of restrictive cardiomyopathy. Cardiovasc. Clin. 19:123–132, 1988.
20. Wynne, J., Braunwald, E.: The cardiomyopathies and myocarditides. *In* Fauci, A.S., Braunwald, E., Isselbacher, K.J., et al. (eds.): Harrison's Principles of Internal Medicine. 14th ed. New York, McGraw-Hill, 1998, pp. 1328–1334.
21. Kyle, R.A., and Gertz, M.A.: Primary systemic amyloidosis. Clinical and laboratory features in 474 cases. Semin. Hematol. 32:45–59, 1995.
22. Klein, A.L., Hatle, L.K., Taliercio, C.P., et al.: Prognostic significance of Doppler measures of diastolic function in cardiac amyloidosis. A Doppler echocardiographic study. Circulation 83:808–816, 1991.
23. Merlini, G.: Treatment of primary amyloidosis. Semin. Hematol. 132:60–79, 1995.
24. Adams, P.C., Kertesz, A.E., and Valberg, L.S.: Clinical presentation of hemochromatosis: A changing scene. Am. J. Cardiol. 90:445–449, 1991.
25. Hagar, J.M., and Rahimtoola, S.H.: Chagas' heart disease in the United States. N. Engl. J. Med. 325:763–768, 1991.

Index

Note: Page numbers in italics refer to illustrations; page numbers followed by t refer to tables